Practical Interventional Cardiology
Third Edition

Edited by
Ever D. Grech

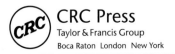

CRC Press
Taylor & Francis Group
Boca Raton London New York

CRC Press is an imprint of the
Taylor & Francis Group, an **informa** business

CRC Press
Taylor & Francis Group
6000 Broken Sound Parkway NW, Suite 300
Boca Raton, FL 33487-2742

© 2018 by Taylor & Francis Group, LLC

CRC Press is an imprint of Taylor & Francis Group, an Informa business

Printed and bound in India by Replika Press Pvt. Ltd.

No claim to original U.S. Government works

Printed on acid-free paper

International Standard Book Number-13: 978-1-4987-3509-4 (Pack- Hardbook and eBook)

Library of Congress Cataloging-in-Publication Data

Names: Grech, Ever D., editor.
Title: Practical interventional cardiology / [edited by] Dr Ever D. Grech.
Description: Third edition. | Boca Raton, FL : CRC Press, [2018] | Includes bibliographical references and index.
Identifiers: LCCN 2016052975| ISBN 9781498735094 (pack (hardbook and ebook) : alk. paper) | ISBN 9781498735100 (ebook) | ISBN 9781498735117 (ebook)
Subjects: | MESH: Coronary Artery Disease--surgery | Heart Diseases--surgery | Endovascular Procedures--methods
Classification: LCC RD598.35.C67 | NLM WG 300 | DDC 617.4/12--dc23
LC record available at https://lccn.loc.gov/2016052975

Visit the Taylor & Francis Web site at
http://www.taylorandfrancis.com

and the CRC Press Web site at
http://www.crcpress.com

Practical Interventional Cardiology

Dedication

For Lisa, Alexander, Frances and Mary

Contents

Foreword

In the spring of 1983, I attended Andreas Gruentzig's percutaneous transluminal coronary angioplasty (PTCA) teaching demonstration course in Emory University in Atlanta, Georgia. I was impressed and excited not only by Gruentzig's enthusiastic approach but also by that of many of the other participants who included Richard Myler, Simon Stertzer, Spencer King III, and the young fellow Bernie Meier. The live cases were of course thrilling, sometimes dramatic and always instructive due to the lively discussion about strategy, technique, the current balloon dilatation catheters, guiding catheters, guidewires, and accessories, their shortcomings and limitations and the rapid developments in the equipment aimed at improving success rates and reducing complications. Tips and tricks in achieving success and avoiding complications were priceless lessons learned. Schneider Medintag, USCI and Advanced Cardiovascular Systems were the major manufacturers of angioplasty equipment at that time and they and other companies blossomed as a result of working closely alongside these pioneers in interventional cardiology in their catheter laboratories. It would be this collaboration between interventional cardiologists and industry that would drive forwards the development of coronary intervention at an exponential pace. At about this time "over-the-wire" (OTW) balloon dilatation catheters were developed with the intention of making PTCA applicable to more than just proximal coronary artery lesions. Soon, however, the cumbersome nature of handling a 300 cm guidewire would lead to the introduction of a rapid exchange or Monorail balloon catheter by Bonzel in 1986 and this would eventually become the standard delivery system for coronary balloons and stents worldwide.

Over the next 10 years, my personal experience progressed rapidly from simple PTCA with Gruentzig's fixed wire balloon catheter to multilesion, multivessel and complex PTCA, coronary artery bypass grafts, chronic total occlusions, primary PTCA in acute myocardial infarction—initially with the OTW balloon dilatation catheter and then with the monorail device, directional coronary atherectomy, laser and rotational atherectomy, intracoronary stent implantation, and intracoronary ultrasound (IVUS) imaging. I learned much by meeting and watching great interventional cardiologists at work like Geoffrey Hartzler at the Mid-America Heart Institute, St. Luke's Hospital, Kansas City, Missouri, Bernie Meier in Bern, Switzerland,

John Simpson in Redwood City, California, and David Cumberland in Sheffield, but the seed of enthusiasm had germinated in Atlanta. The group photograph of all the participants at the meeting in 1983 hangs on my office wall in Liverpool and is a warm reminder not only of the friends and colleagues who were fortunate enough to be there too that year but also of the start of my passion for interventional cardiology. Perhaps you can recognize someone?

In just 40 years, the specialty of interventional cardiology has changed dramatically. Not only does it now include all aspects of coronary artery intervention but also fantastic imaging techniques such as IVUS, optical coherence tomography (OCT), and techniques for assessing coronary artery flow using pressure wire technology. A whole array of guidewires with carefully designed structures and behavioral characteristics and microcatheters have been introduced to help deal with the problem of chronically occluded arteries using new anterograde and retrograde approaches through the collateral bed. We have also reached a new era in coronary artery stenting with the availability of a wide range of stents with improved profile, flexibility, and deliverability with novel strut designs and drug delivery mechanisms and even a stent that is fully biodegradable once its scaffolding function and drug delivery tasks have been completed. Subspecialties of interventional cardiology have formed to deal with other cardiac pathologies and structural cardiac defects. For example, transcutaneous aortic valve implantation (TAVI) for the treatment of aortic valve stenosis is a good illustration of how the biomedical companies have rapidly developed the technology and reduced the size of the delivery systems to make the procedure more user-friendly, more successful, and less complicated with better outcomes for both patient and operator. Besides TAVI, percutaneous procedures to treat mitral stenosis, patent foramen ovale, atrial septal defect, and to occlude the left atrial appendage have all become standard procedures, less daunting for the experienced operator and highly successful for the patient. Femoral artery closure devices have been refined and adapted for use in both diagnostic and therapeutic interventional procedures. Alongside all this, radial artery catheterization for both diagnostic coronary angiography and for percutaneous coronary intervention (PCI) has become routine and now dominates as the favored route for PCI procedures in many catheter laboratories

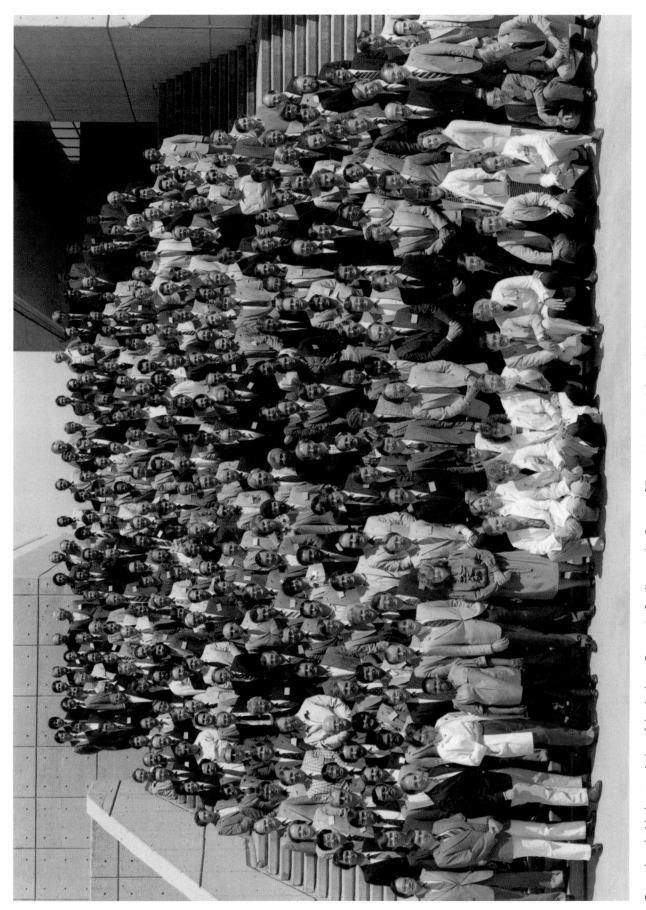

around the world. Radial artery closure devices have also been developed to make the procedures routine with few complications. In addition, there have been numerous concomitant developments in the pharmacology associated with intervention such as novel antiplatelet and antithrombotic therapy especially relevant for PCI in acute coronary syndromes and in particular acute myocardial infarction.

It goes without saying that to become skilled at interventional cardiology, trainees should spend time alongside senior colleagues who themselves are extremely experienced in the specialty, initially assisting and then becoming a supervised first operator before becoming an independent interventionist. There is no substitute for spending time in a busy catheter laboratory both watching and performing cases if one hopes to avoid learning from the same mistakes that the pioneers in interventional cardiology made during their early experiences. Attending and participating in courses in interventional cardiology, especially those presenting live case demonstrations are a fantastic medium for enhancing training and learning and many are still available and worth the time and expense for those dedicated to making a career in this exciting specialty. During my early years, balloon angioplasty courses in Emory University in Atlanta, San Francisco, Kansas City, Geneva, Toulouse, Paris, and London were always great fun and fantastic learning experiences where many friendships and working relationships were founded and developed. The courses were headed by the giants of coronary intervention who with the collaboration and financial help from the industry pushed forwards the evolution of the specialty. Transcatheter Cardiovascular Therapeutics has perhaps been one of the leading and most enjoyable of such international meetings over the last two decades. For many of us, our attendance at such venues was sponsored by industry and credit is due to them for our education and training. In return, representatives and product specialists from industry were regularly present with the interventionists in their laboratories during cases. Although this was often for their own education, it was also for providing advice on how to operate new devices and angioplasty equipment as well as collecting feedback on the performance of their latest device. Their input and advice frequently proved invaluable and they were considered part of the interventional team responsible for the success of procedures.

Besides live case demonstrations and national and international interventional cardiology meetings and symposia, journals of interventional cardiology and textbooks have remained an invaluable source of learning. Many of the textbooks on balloon angioplasty and interventional cardiology have been either written or edited by the great names in this specialty. In 1997, Ever Grech and myself assembled numerous talented contributors to our first edition of *Practical Interventional Cardiology* and were humbled by their knowledge, their generosity and their willingness to participate. Twenty years after Andreas Gruentzig's first PTCA, the book highlighted how rapidly the specialty had moved forwards. Five years later in 2002, the second edition had 36 chapters written by national and international colleagues updating the interventional fraternity on new procedures, new technologies, new pharmacology relevant to intervention, clinical trials in interventional cardiology, peripheral intervention, mitral balloon valvuloplasty, percutaneous intervention for structural cardiac defects and interventional electrophysiology as well as other relevant topics at that time.

Now we are treated to *Practical Interventional Cardiology*, 3rd edition, an enormous effort by my friend and colleague Ever Grech who has put together a fantastic textbook of interventional cardiology. It consists of 48 superb chapters on the many aspects of coronary artery intervention, interventional procedures for structural heart disease, invasive, and interventional electrophysiology, presentations on training programs and certification in Europe and the United States and the principles and practice of audit in interventional cardiology. The list of contributors is outstanding and again includes authors from major centers from around the globe—authors who are both experienced and respected by their peers in the interventional community. The book opens with a chapter on the Epidemiology and Pathophysiology of Coronary Artery Disease by Renu Virmani and colleagues and ends with a glimpse into the future of interventional cardiology by Steven L. Goldberg. The textbook is beautifully illustrated, contemporary, enjoyable, easy to read and well-referenced and should be recommended not only to those training in interventional cardiology, but to experienced interventionists, to catheter laboratory staff who share in interventional procedures, to those in industry who wish to familiarize themselves with the recent developments in intervention and to hospital and university libraries to make this knowledge available to everyone with an interest in this fascinating subject. It is evident from this book that progress in all aspects of interventional cardiology continues being driven by talented individuals worldwide. However, it is worth remembering how it all began, for truly this and subsequent generations of interventionists responsible for taking the specialty forwards into the future are ". . . standing on the shoulders of giants" (Isaac Newton, 1676).

David R. Ramsdale
Liverpool Heart and Chest Hospital
Liverpool, UK

Editor

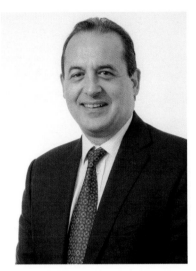

Dr. Ever D. Grech, MBBS (Lond), MD(Lond) FRCP, FACC is a consultant interventional cardiologist at South Yorkshire Cardiothoracic Centre, Northern General Hospital, Sheffield (Sheffield Teaching Hospitals NHS Foundation Trust), United Kingdom, and is an honorary senior clinical lecturer at the University of Sheffield. He graduated from St. Bartholomew's Hospital Medical College, University of London, and underwent postgraduate Cardiology training in the UK, as well as undertaking an Interventional Cardiology Fellowship at The London Health Sciences Centre, University of Western Ontario, Canada.

Dr. Grech has a wealth of experience in a wide range of cardiology interests. His specialist expertise is in the management of coronary heart disease and percutaneous coronary intervention (PCI), as well as aortic valve disease and transcatheter aortic valve implantation. He has also published a range of medical journals and textbooks, including two editions of the *ABC of Interventional Cardiology*. Dr. Grech is a Fellow of the Royal College of Physicians, a Fellow of the American College of Cardiology, a Member of the British Cardiovascular Society and the British Cardiovascular Intervention Society.

Contributors

Abdelkader Almalfi, MD, MRCP (UK), FACC
Texas Heart Institute
Houston, Texas

Abdallah Al-Mohammad, MD, FRCP, FESC, FACP
Northern General Hospital-Sheffield Teaching Hospitals
Sheffield, United Kingdom

Zulfiquar Adam, MB ChB, MRCP, MD
Northern General Hospital
Sheffield, United Kingdom

Javed Ahmed, MD, FRCP
Freeman Hospital
Newcastle upon Tyne, United Kingdom
and
Newcastle University
Newcastle upon Tyne, United Kingdom

Paolo Angelini, MD
Texas Heart Institute
Houston, Texas

Alejandro Aquino, MD
HonorHealth Heart Group
Scottsdale, Arizona

Ganesh Athappan

Tanvir Bajwa, MD
Aurora Cardiovascular Services
Aurora Sinai/Aurora St. Luke's Medical Centers
University of Wisconsin School of Medicine and Public
    Health
Milwaukee, Wisconsin

Stefan Bertog, MD
CardioVascular Center
Frankfurt, Germany

Gill Louise Buchanan, MBChB
Department of Cardiology
North Cumbria University Hospitals NHS Trust
Carlisle, United Kingdom

Michael W Cammarata, MD, MS
Department of Internal Medicine
Wake Forest Baptist Medical Center
Winston-Salem, North Carolina

Derek P Chew, MBBS, MPH
Southern Adelaide Local Health Network
Flinders University School of Medicine
Adelaide, South Australia

Tawfiq R Choudhury, MBBS, MD, MRCP, BSc
North Western Deanery
Manchester, United Kingdom

Antonio Colombo, MD
EMO-GVM Centro Cuore Columbus and San Raffaele
    Scientific Institute
Milan, Italy

George D Dangas, MD, PhD
Mount Sinai Medical Centre
New York City, New York

Jehangir Din, MBBS, MRCP, MD(Res)
Dorset Heart Centre
Royal Bournemouth Hospital
Bournemouth
Dorset, United Kingdom

Mohaned Egred, BSc (Hons) MB ChB MD FRCP FESC
Freeman Hospital and Newcastle University Institute of
Cellular Medicine
Newcastle upon Tyne, United Kingdom

Ted Feldman, MD, MSCAI, FACC, FESC
Evanston Hospital,
Evanston, Illinois

Stephen Fort, MD, MRCP, FRCPC
Kelowna General Hospital
British Colombia, Canada

Jennifer Franke, MD
CardioVascular Center
Frankfurt, Germany

Douglas G Fraser, MB, BChir, DM, FRCP, BA
University of Manchester and Manchester Royal Infirmary
Manchester, United Kingdom

Sameer Gafoor, MD
CardioVascular Center
Frankfurt, Germany

Amir Gahremanpour, MD, FACC
Texas Heart Institute
Houston, Texas

Amr S Gamal, MBBCh, MSc, MD
Freeman Hospital
Newcastle upon Tyne, United Kingdom
and
Cardiology Department
Zagazig University, Egypt

Pankaj Garg, MD (Hons), PhD, MRCP
Leeds Institute of Cardiovascular and Metabolic Medicine
    (LICAMM)
University of Leeds
Leeds, United Kingdom

Scot Garg, MB ChB, FRCP, PhD, FESC
Consultant Cardiologist
East Lancashire Hospitals NHS Trust
Blackburn, Lancashire, United Kingdom

Alessandra Giavarini, MD
NIHR Cardiovascular BRU Royal Brompton & Harefield
    NHS Foundation Trust
London, United Kingdom

Steven L Goldberg, MD, FACC, FSCAI
Tyler Heart Institute
Community Hospital of the Monterey Peninsula
Monterey, California

Lino Gonçalves, MD, MSc, PhD, FESC
University of Coimbra
Coimbra, Portugal

John P Greenwood, PhD, FRCP
Leeds Institute of Cardiovascular and Metabolic Medicine
    (LICAMM)
University of Leeds
Leeds, United Kingdom

Mayra Guerrero, MD, FACC, FSCAI
Evanston Hospital
Evanston, Illinois

Julian Gunn, MA, MB BChir, MD, MRCP
Department of Infection, Immunity and cardiovascular
    Disease
University of Sheffield
Sheffield, United Kingdom
and
Insigneo Institute for *in silico* Medicine
Sheffield, United Kingdom

Tarek Helmy, MD, FACC, FSCAI
St. Louis University School of Medicine
St. Louis, Missouri

Ziyad M Hijazi, MD, MPH, FACC, MSCAI, FAHA
Weill Cornell Medicine
Department of Pediatrics
Sidra Cardiac Program
Sidra Medical & Research Center
Doha, Qatar

David R Holmes, MD, FACC
Department of Cardiovascular Medicine
Mayo Clinic
Rochester, Minnesota

Marius Hornung, MD
CardioVascular Center
Frankfurt, Germany

Alfred Hurley, MD
Aurora Cardiovascular Services
Aurora Sinai/Aurora St. Luke's Medical Centers
University of Wisconsin School of Medicine and Public
    Health
Milwaukee, Wisconsin

Harriet Hurrell, MBBS, MRCP
Cardiology
Wexham Park Hospital
Wexham, Slough, Berkshire, United Kingdom

Kanji Inoue, MD
PTMC Institute
Kita-Ku, Kyoto, Japan
and
Kyoto University
Sakyo-Ku, Kyoto, Japan

Javaid Iqbal, MBBS, MRCP, PhD
South Yorkshire Cardiothoracic Centre
Sheffield Teaching Hospitals
NHS Foundation Trust, United Kingdom

Roy M John, MBBS, PhD
Department of Medicine, Brigham and Women's
    Hospital
Harvard Medical School
Boston, Massachusetts

Jonathan Kalman, MBBS, PhD, FRACP, FACC, FHRS
Royal Melbourne Hospital
Parkville, Victoria, Australia
and
University of Melbourne
Melbourne, Australia

Sanjog Kalra, MD, MSc, FRCPC
Einstein Health Network
Philadelphia, Pennsylvania

Se Hun Kang, MD
Department of Cardiology
CHA Bundang Medical Center, CHA University
Gyeonggi-do, Republic of Korea

Sunil Kapur, MD
Department of Medicine, Brigham and Women's Hospital
Harvard Medical School
Boston, Massachusetts

Dimitri Karmpaliotis, MD, PhD, FACC
Columbia University, New York

Gerry Kaye, MD, FRACP, FRCP(UK), FCSANZ, FHRS
Department of Cardiology
University of Queensland Medical School
Brisbane, Queensland, Australia
and
Princess Alexandra Hospital
Brisbane, Queensland, Australia

Jayant Khitha, MD
Aurora Cardiovascular Services
Aurora Sinai/Aurora St. Luke's Medical Centers
University of Wisconsin School of Medicine and Public
    Health
Milwaukee, Wisconsin

Lloyd W Klein, MD, FSCAI
Department of Medicine
Division of Cardiology
Advocate Illinois Masonic Medical Center & Rush Medical
    College
Chicago, Illinois

Frank D Kolodgie, PhD
CVPath Institute, Inc.
Gaithersburg, Maryland

John M Lasala, MD, PhD, FACC, MSCAI
Washington University School of Medicine-Barnes Jewish
    Hospital
St. Louis, Missouri

Justin Lee, MB, BCh, MD, FRCP, CCDS CEPS
Northern General Hospital
Honorary Senior Lecturer
University of Sheffield
Sheffield, United Kingdom

A Michael Lincoff, MD
Department of Cardiovascular Medicine
Cleveland Clinic Coordinating Center for Clinical Research
    (C5 Research)
Cleveland Clinic
Cleveland, Ohio

Mark S Link, MD
Tufts Medical Center
Cardiac Arrhythmia Center
Boston, Massachusetts

Kristel Longman, BSc, MBBS, MRCP
Dorset Heart Centre
Royal Bournemouth Hospital
Bournemouth
Dorset, United Kingdom

Giovannni Longo, MD
NIHR Cardiovascular BRU Royal Brompton & Harefield
    NHS Foundation Trust
London, United Kingdom

Amir Lotfi, MD, FSCAI
Department of Medicine
Division of Cardiology, Baystate Medical Center
Tufts University
Springfield, Massachusetts

Peter F Ludman MA, MD, FRCP
Queen Elizabeth Hospital
Birmingham University
Birmingham, United Kingdom

Christopher Madias, MD
Tufts Medical Center
Cardiac Arrhythmia Center
Boston, Massachusetts

Jaya Mallidi, MD, MHS
Department of Medicine
Division of Cardiology
Baystate Medical Center, Tufts University
Springfield, Massachusetts

Carlo Di Mario, MD, PhD
NIHR Cardiovascular BRU Royal Brompton & Harefield
    NHS Foundation Trust
NHLI Imperial College
London, United Kingdom

S Andrew McCullough, MD
Cardiology Division
Mount Sinai Medical Center, New York

Claire McCune, MB, BCh, BAO, MRCP
Craigavon Cardiac Centre,
Northern Ireland, United Kingdom

**Ian Menown, MB, BCh, BAO, MD, MRCP(UK),
    FRCP(Edin)**
Craigavon Cardiac Centre,
Northern Ireland, United Kingdom

Gary S Mintz, MD
Columbia University
New York City, New York

Javier Molina Martin de Nicolas, MD
Clinique Pasteur
Toulouse, France

Paul D Morris, BMedSci, MBChB, MRCP, PhD
University of Sheffield
Sheffield Teaching Hospitals NHS Foundation Trust
Sheffield, United Kingdom

Jeffrey W Moses, MD, FACC
Columbia University, Medical Centre
New York City, New York

Brian O'Murchu, MD
Temple University Hospital
Philadelphia, Pennsylvania

Peter O'Kane, BSc, MBBS, FRCP, MD(Res)
Dorset Heart Centre
Royal Bournemouth Hospital, Bournemouth
Dorset, United Kingdom

James Palmer, B.Med.Sci
University of Sheffield,
Sheffield, United Kingdom

Jayan Parameshwar, MD, FRCP
Advanced Heart Failure and Transplant Unit,
Papworth Hospital
Cambridge, United Kingdom

Seung-Jung Park, MD, PhD
Asan Medical Center, University of Ulsan
Seoul, South Korea

Stephen Pettit, PhD, MRCP
Advanced Heart Failure and Transplant Unit, Papworth
    Hospital
Cambridge, United Kingdom

Sven Plein, MD, PhD, FRCP
Leeds Institute of Cardiovascular and Metabolic Medicine
    (LICAMM)
University of Leeds
Leeds, United Kingdom

Sasan Raeissi, MD
Northwestern University Feinberg School of Medicine
Bluhm Cardiovascular Institute, Northwestern Memorial
Hospital
Chicago, Illinois

Varinder K Randhawa MD, PhD
London Health Sciences Centre
London, Ontario, Canada

Shabnam Rashid, BSc, MBChB
Leeds General Infirmary
Leeds, United Kingdom

David P Ripley, BSc (Hons), MBChB, MRCP (UK)
Leeds Institute of Cardiovascular and Metabolic Medicine
    (LICAMM)
University of Leeds
Leeds, United Kingdom

Rubén Rodríguez, MD
NIHR Cardiovascular BRU Royal Brompton & Harefield
    NHS Foundation Trust
London, United Kingdom

Dominic Rogers, MA, MD, FRCP
Northern General Hospital-Sheffield Teaching
Hospitals
Sheffield, United Kingdom

Fatemeh Sakhinia MB ChB, FRCR, EBIR
Sheffield Vascular Institute
Northern General Hospital, Sheffield
United Kingdom

Chris Sawh, MBBS, MRCP(UK), MRCP(London)
Northern General Hospital
Sheffield, United Kingdom

Patrick W Serruys, MD, PhD
International Centre for Circulatory Health Imperial
College
London, United Kingdom

Adeel Shahzad, MRCP
Trent Cardiac Centre
Nottingham, United Kingdom

Daniel M Shivapour, MD
Department of Cardiovascular Medicine
Cleveland Clinic
Cleveland, Ohio

Horst Sievert, MD
CardioVascular Center
Frankfurt, Germany

William H Spear, MD, FACC, FHRS
Consultants in Cardiology & Electrophysiology
Oak Lawn, Illinois

Goran Stankovic, MD
Department for diagnostic and catheterization
    laboratories
Clinical Center of Serbia
Medical School of Belgrade
Belgrade, Serbia

William G Stevenson, MD
Department of Medicine, Brigham and Women's Hospital
Harvard Medical School
Boston, Massachusetts

Ayyaz Sultan, MBBS, MRCP, FRCP, FACC
Royal Albert Edward Infirmary
Wigan, United Kingdom

Hussam S Suradi, MD, FACC, FSCAI
Rush Center for Congenital & Structural Heart Disease
Rush University Medical Center
Chicago, Illinois
and
St Mary Medical Center
Community HealthCare Network
Hobart, Indiana

Suneel Talwar, MBBS, MRCP, MD(Res)
Dorset Heart Centre
Royal Bournemouth Hospital
Bournemouth
Dorset, Massachusetts

Didier Tchétché, MD
Clinique Pasteur
Toulouse, France

Patrick Teefy, MD, FRCP
London Health Sciences Centre
Western University
London, Ontario, Canada

Steven M Thomas MRCP, FRCR, MSc EBIR
Sheffield Vascular Institute
Northern General Hospital
Sheffield, United Kingdom

Carlo E Uribe, MD, FSCAI
Texas Heart Institute
Houston, Texas

Isabelle Vandormael, MD
NIHR Cardiovascular BRU Royal Brompton & Harefield
    NHS Foundation Trust
London, Massachusetts

Sethumadhavan Vijayan, MBBS, MRCP
Department of Cardiology
Leeds General Infirmary
Leeds, United Kingdom

Renu Virmani, MD
CVPath Institute, Inc.
Gaithersburg, Maryland

Alain Vuylsteke, BSc, MA, MD, FRCA, FFICM
Cardiothoracic Intensive Care
Papworth Hospital
Cambridge, United Kingdom

Erik Wissner, MD, PHD, FACC, FHRS
Division of Cardiology
University of Illinois at Chicago
Chicago, Illinois

Kazuyuki Yahagi, MD
CVPath Institute, Inc.
Gaithersburg, Maryland

David X M Zhao, MD, PhD
Section on Cardiovascular Medicine
Department of Internal Medicine
Wake Forest Baptist Medical Center
Winston-Salem, North Carolina

Preface

2017 represents an important milestone in Interventional Cardiology as we celebrate both the 40th anniversary of the first percutaneous transluminal coronary angioplasty (PTCA) by Andreas Grüntzig in Zurich, Switzerland, and the 50th anniversary of the first coronary artery bypass surgery by Rene Favorolo in the USA. The first patient to undergo PTCA was 39-year-old Adolf Bachmann who is alive and well to this day. However, although clinically effective, acceptance of this new technique was by no means immediate. Skepticism and resistance was widespread for many years as PTCA faced a number of problems that required technical improvements and scientific validation.

As I browse through the second edition of *Practical Interventional Cardiology,* which was published 15 years ago, it is readily apparent that subsequent developments in Interventional Cardiology have been both astonishing and, in some instances, unexpected.

Astonishing, because the combination of new operator skills, superior equipment and new pharmacotherapy has led to a pronounced reduction in procedural risks, which has in turn propelled a truly exponential worldwide growth in percutaneous cardiovascular interventional procedures. The best illustration has to be the development of the intra-coronary stent. Since its tentative debut as a rigid, awkward and very expensive item, it has largely overcome its flaws (and rivals) to become the sleek, safe and highly effective device that has taken centre stage and is undeniably one of the linchpins of interventional cardiology. It is easy to forget that coronary intervention before the advent of the stent primarily consisted of balloon angioplasty. This was much riskier and unpredictable than today's procedures, which nearly always incorporate a stent (referred to as PCI), with surgical standby an absolute necessity, for good reason. Furthermore, the management of acute coronary syndromes (especially ST-segment elevation myocardial infarction) was regarded by many as 'tiger country,' where only pharmacotherapy was deemed to be safe despite the lack of efficacy and associated high mortality. Thankfully, those days are gone, and I do sometimes find myself feeling satisfied to have taken part in such an incredible transition in such a short space of time.

Unexpected, because no one foresaw the emergence of some of the new therapeutic interventions. The prime contender has to be the introduction and rapid growth in structural heart intervention, in particular percutaneous aortic valve implantation (TAVI). As initial concerns, such as access-site complications, para-valvular leaks and valve durability continue to be addressed, it is clear that this procedure has much further to go. It is also interesting to observe the variation in approaches currently being used to overcome the complex and difficult problems associated with percutaneous mitral valve intervention.

By highlighting these areas, I am aware that I have omitted many other important aspects and developments. Clearly, a lack of space will not allow me to expand here. However, I have ensured that these are given their rightful importance in this new and comprehensively updated edition. I am sure you will enjoy reading the chapters written by world leaders in their specialised fields.

Although it has been an onerous task to collate this third edition within tight time schedules so that it reflects current knowledge and practice in a rapidly changing field, it has been an immensely rewarding experience. I am very grateful to all the contributors of this book and have been humbled by their knowledge, their generosity and their willingness to participate. I am also thankful to our colleagues in industry for their assistance in providing technical details and data. I deeply appreciate the personal efforts, technical expertise and invaluable assistance of all at Taylor and Francis Group. In particular, I would like to mention Lance Wobus, Jessica Vega, Judith Simon (USA), Gabriel Schenk, Alice Oven, Drew Gwilliams and Ben O'Hara (UK) at Taylor & Francis Group, as well as Ramya Gangadharan (India) at diacriTech.

Ever D. Grech

South Yorkshire Cardiothoracic Centre,
Sheffield, United Kingdom

PART 1

Coronary artery disease

Epidemiology and pathophysiology of coronary artery disease

KAZUYUKI YAHAGI, FRANK D KOLODGIE, RENU VIRMANI

1.1 Epidemiology of coronary artery disease

Coronary artery disease (CAD) represents a global leading cause of death especially for middle- and high-income countries. In 2012, all-cause deaths were estimated as 56 million worldwide with 17.5 million deaths (31%) attributed to cardiovascular disease (CVD).[1] Ischemic heart disease represented 7.4 million (13%) of people, whilst 6.7 million (12%) died from stroke. In high-income countries, 70% of deaths occurred in ages greater than 70 years old mainly from chronic CVD, cancer, dementia, chronic obstructive lung disease and diabetes. On the contrary, the percentage of cardiovascular deaths in low-income countries is relatively low in comparison to infectious disease, lower respiratory infections, HIV/AIDS, diarrhoea, malaria and tuberculosis, which collectively account for almost one-third of all deaths.[1]

Despite the increase in the survival rates of CAD patients over the past few decades, the number of individuals with CVD is estimated to exceed more than 23.6 million by 2030.[2] Currently one in three adults in the United States (approximately 71.3 million) has some form of CVD, including more than 17 million with CAD and 10 million with angina pectoris.[3,4]

Age is the most powerful risk factor for CVD. Heart disease and stroke are the first and fourth leading causes of death in the United States and together, accounted for 29.4% of deaths in 2010.[5] After 40 years, the life-time risk of coronary heart disease is 49% in men and 32% in women, according to the findings of the Framingham Heart study.[6] Although the incidence of CAD in the United States is on the decline, observational studies have not yet shown a reduction in myocardial infarction (MI).[7,8] The National Registry of Myocardial Infarction with clinical data on 1.9 million acute myocardial infarction (AMI) patients from 2157 US hospitals between 1990 and 2006 has shown that the proportion of non-ST elevation MI (NSTEMI) increased from 14% to 59% ($p < .0001$), whereas the reported ST elevation MI (STEMI) cases decreased.[9] Hospital mortality rates, however, significantly fell amongst all patients (10.4%–6.3%), STEMI (11.5%–8.0%) and NSTEMI (7.1%–5.2%) from 1994 to 2006 (all $p < .0001$).

1.2 Native coronary atherosclerosis

The initial concept of atherosclerosis progression and plaque phenotypic change was established by Dr. Velican in the early 1980s who focused on morphological descriptions of fatty streak lesions to advanced fibroatheromatous plaques complicated by haemorrhage, calcification, ulceration and thrombosis.[10,11] Similarly, Dr. Michael Davies, a pathologist devoted to the study of plaque rupture and its associated features, described in detail the characteristics of plaque disruption and the role of inflammation in lesion instability.[12,13] The work of various pioneers in the field of atherosclerosis lacked uniform terminology and classification relative to how lesions progress and become the focal point of acute coronary syndromes. This gap was eventually addressed by the American Heart Association consensus group led by Dr. Stary[14,15] in the 1990s where lesions were classified into six different numerical categories relative to severity. One of the main weaknesses of the American Heart Association (AHA) classification was that the atherosclerotic plaque procession is complicated and not easily categorised by numerical groups. Moreover, the reference to a numeric nomenclature was found incomplete by our laboratory considering that under the AHA classification, all luminal thrombi were thought to exclusively arise from plaque rupture, excluding other causative entities like plaque erosion and nodular calcification.[16] Also, the AHA scheme failed to describe an important precursor lesion to rupture, the thin-cap fibroatheroma (TCFA) or 'vulnerable plaque'. These limitations prompted us to develop a modified version of the AHA classification initially published in 2000 and recently modified in 2015[16,17] (Figures 1.1 and 1.2, and Table 1.1).

Numeric AHA lesion types I–IV were essentially replaced by descriptive terminology to include adaptive intimal thickening, intimal xanthoma, pathologic intimal thickening (PIT) and fibroatheroma (FA) with recognised progressive lesion morphology of early and late FAs. AHA lesion types V and VI were abandoned since they failed to account for distinct morphologies of plaque rupture, erosion and calcified nodule that give rise to luminal thrombosis or support the profile of controlled lesions in stable angina patients. The AHA terminology also does not adequately address the concept of silent thrombi and vascular healing, which also includes silent or symptomatic chronic total occlusions (CTO) despite their presence in over 30% of sudden coronary deaths (SCDs), where the first manifestation of symptoms may indeed be sudden death itself.

Descriptive terms that are associated with lesion stability such as fibrous or fibrocalcific, and nodular calcification in the absence of thrombosis – that are observed more commonly in patients presenting with stable angina, and with or without long-standing diabetes mellitus and end-stage renal disease – were recently introduced by our laboratory (Figures 1.1 and 1.2, and Table 1.1).[17] Our updated SCD registry of subjects whose first manifestation was CAD showed an absence of acute thrombus or organising thrombi in over 30% of SCD cases with healed MI note in half these cases, whilst in the other half there is only severe coronary narrowing involving one or more coronary arteries (Table 1.2).[18]

1.3 Non-atherosclerotic intimal lesions

1.3.1 Intimal thickening and fatty streaks

For 35% of neonates, the intima/media ratio is 0.1 at birth, and thereafter it continuously increases by up to 0.3 in 2 years.[19] Intimal thickening in the absence of atherosclerosis is considered the earliest vascular change consisting primarily

of smooth muscle cells (SMCs) and extracellular matrix. Although intimal thickening is more frequently recognised in atherosclerosis-prone arteries, coronary, carotid, abdominal and descending aorta, and iliac artery,[20] it is regarded as a flow-related adaptive change as the proliferative activity is very low and supported by an anti-apoptotic phenotype.[21, 22]

On the contrary, the first of the inflammatory lesion is termed 'fatty streak' or intimal xanthomatous plaque, which is primarily composed of superficial collections of surface foam cells derived from circulating monocytes and from the uptake of lipids by SMCs. In humans, intimal xanthomas are capable of regression especially in the thoracic aorta and right coronary artery in young individuals aged 15–30 years as initially described in early studies[23, 24] and more recently in the 'Pathologic Determinants of Atherosclerosis in Youth' study.[25] Although the precise mechanisms involved in the initiation and regression of the intimal xanthoma are unknown, the early progressive lesions are thought to arise from SMC death in areas of 'lipid pools' classified as PIT. Therefore, a better understanding of this process may help unlock the point-of-no-return in the process of atherosclerotic change.

1.4 Progressive atherosclerotic lesions

1.4.1 Pathologic intimal thickening

PIT is considered the earliest of progressive change and is primarily composed of well-developed SMCs near the lumen embedded in hyaluronan, proteoglycans and type III collagen matrix (Figure 1.3).[26] The lesions are located in proximity to the media, characterised by areas devoid of SMCs but rich in hyaluronan and proteoglycans versican, biglycan and decorin admixed with neutral lipids and free cholesterol (Figure 1.4).[26] Apoptotic SMCs within the lipid pool are recognised by a thickened basement membrane on periodic acid Schiff (PAS) staining[27] and are thought to support continued intimal growth. The relationship of lipid pool formation to the deposition of select proteoglycans and attraction of lipids with lack of SMC, however, still remains unclear. There is cause to believe, however, substitutions in the glycosaminoglycans chain on proteoglycans are the initial proatherogenic steps that promote the binding of atherogenic lipoproteins.[28, 29]

Another important lesion hallmark of PITs is the adluminal accumulation of macrophages, and although not observed in all cases, this finding particularly near branch points may be associated with a more advanced stage of the disease.[28] The lipid pools may also exhibit free cholesterol, represented by varying degrees of fine crystalline structures, but never in excess. The absence of macrophages with the lipid pools suggests that the free cholesterol in PIT is of non-inflammatory origin. Moreover, the lipid pools show evidence of microcalcification (~0.5 μm, but typically <15 μm) admixed with SMC remnants, as well as with calcium hydroxyapatite crystals, are best appreciated by transmission electron microscopy and cannot be seen by other imaging modalities such as multi-slice computed tomography (MSCT), intravascular

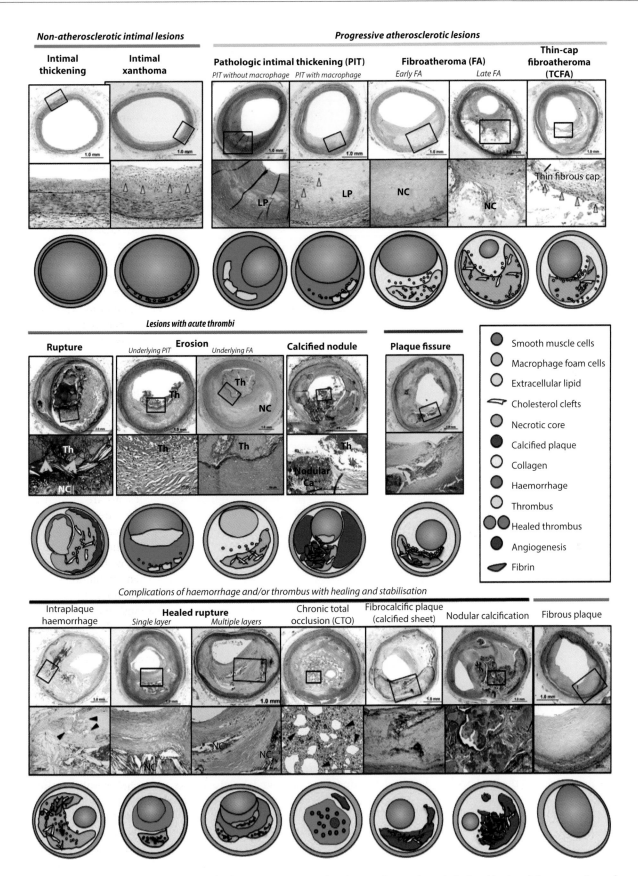

Figure 1.1 Human coronary lesions' morphologies categorised as 'non-atherosclerotic intimal lesions', 'progressive atherosclerotic lesions', 'lesions with acute thrombi' and other lesion morphologies/features. Ca2+, calcium; LP, lipid pool; NC, necrotic core; Th, thrombus. Yellow arrowheads = macrophages; yellow arrows = fibrous cap; black arrowheads = neoangiogenesis. (Reproduced from Yahagi K et al., *Nat. Rev. Cardiol.*, 13, 79–98, 2015. With permission.)

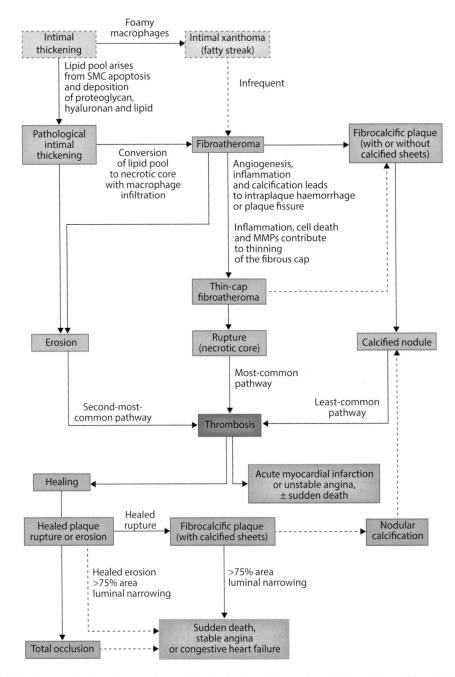

Figure 1.2 Simplified scheme for classifying atherosclerotic lesions. (Reproduced from Yahagi K et al., *Nat. Rev. Cardiol.*, 13, 79–98, 2015. With permission.)

ultrasound (IVUS) or optical coherence tomography (OCT).[30] Whether microcalcifications play a significant role in the evolution or progression of the lipid pool is yet to be determined.

1.4.2 Fibroatheroma

Distinguished from the lipid pool lesions of PIT, FAs consist of an acellular necrotic core containing cellular debris and notable depletion in extracellular matrix, best appreciated by picrosirius red staining. The necrotic core is encapsulated by a thick fibrous cap consisting of SMCs within a proteoglycan–collagen matrix,[31] which is considered a critical component of lesion stability, whilst on the contrary, fibrous cap thinning invariably occurs prior to plaque rupture.

In our laboratory, FAs are subclassified into those with 'early' and 'late' necrosis as this distinction may further enable us to better understand how necrotic cores develop. Early necrosis is identified by macrophage infiltration into lipid pools coinciding with a substantial increase in free cholesterol and diminution of extracellular matrix. Similar to PITs, lesions with early necrotic cores characteristically maintain expression of hyaluronan, versican, and biglycan and type III collagen, which are typically absent in more advanced plaques with late necrosis, presumably by matrix

Table 1.1 Updated classification of atherosclerotic lesions based on morphology

Types of lesions	Subtypes of lesions	Morphological description
Non-atherosclerotic intimal lesions	Intimal thickening	Natural accumulation of smooth muscle cells (SMCs) in the absence of lipid, macrophage foam cells and thrombosis.
	Intimal xanthoma	Superficial accumulation of foam cells without a necrotic core, fibrous cap or thrombosis.
Progressive atherosclerotic lesions	Pathological intimal thickening	Plaque rich in SMCs, with hyaluronan and proteoglycan matrix and focal accumulation of extracellular lipid. Absence of thrombosis.
	Fibroatheroma (FA)	During early necrosis: focal macrophage infiltration into areas of lipid pools with an overlying fibrous cap. During late necrosis: loss of matrix and extensive cellular debris with an overlying fibrous cap. With or without calcification. Absence of thrombosis.
	Intraplaque haemorrhage or plaque fissure	Large necrotic core (size >10% of plaque area) with haemorrhage, and plaque area shows presence of angiogenesis. Necrotic core communicates with the lumen through a fissure. Minimal tear without obvious thrombus.
	Thin-cap FA (TCFA)	A thin, fibrous cap (<65 μm) infiltrated by macrophages and lymphocytes, with rare or no SMCs and relatively large underlying necrotic core (>10% of plaque area). Intraplaque haemorrhage and/or fibrin might be present. Absence of thrombosis.
Lesions with acute thrombi	Plaque rupture	TCFA with cap disruption. Thrombosis is present and might or might not be occlusive. The luminal thrombus communicates with the underlying necrotic core.
	Plaque erosion	Can occur on pathological intimal thickening or on a FA. Thrombosis is present and might or might not be occlusive. No communication of the thrombus with the necrotic core.
	Calcified nodule	Eruptive (shedding) of calcified nodule with an underlying fibrocalcific plaque with minimal or no necrosis. Thrombosis is usually not occlusive.
Healed lesions	Healed plaque rupture, erosion, or calcified nodule	Healed lesion composed of SMCs, proteoglycans, and collagen type III with or without underlying disrupted fibrous cap, necrotic core, or nodular calcification. Lesions can contain large areas of calcification with few inflammatory cells and have a small or no necrotic core. The fibrotic or fibrocalcific collagen-rich plaque is associated with significant luminal stenosis. Absence of thrombosis.

Source: Reproduced from Yahagi K et al., *Nat. Rev. Cardiol.*, 13:79–98, 2015. With permission.

Table 1.2 Distribution of culprit plaques by sex and age in sudden coronary death (n = 442)

	Acute thrombi (n = 236)			No acute thrombi (stable severe CAD) (n = 206)		
	Rupture	Erosion	Calcified nodule	Organised thrombi (CTO)	No thrombi	Total
Men						
<50 years	82 (48%)	34 (20%)	3 (2%)	16 (9%)	36 (21%)	171
≥50 years	59 (31%)	14 (7%)	6 (3%)	46 (24%)	63 (34%)	188
Total (men)	141 (39%)	48 (13%)	9 (3%)	62 (17%)	99 (28%)	359
Women						
<50 years	3 (6%)	16 (36%)	0 (0%)	4 (9%)	21 (48%)	44
≥50 years	10 (26%)	6 (15%)	3 (8%)	8 (21%)	12 (31%)	39
Total (women)	13 (16%)	22 (27%)	3 (4%)	12 (14%)	33 (40%)	83
Total	154 (35%)	70 (16%)	12 (3%)	74 (17%)	132 (30%)	442

Source: Reproduced from Yahagi K et al., *Atherosclerosis*, 239, 260–267, 2015. With permission.
Organised thrombi with healed myocardial infarction (MI) = 62/74 (84%). No thrombi (stable plaque) with healed MI = 1/132 (54%). CAD, coronary artery disease; CTO, chronic total occlusion.

	Movat		Macrophages	T-lymphoytes
PIT w/o mac				
PIT with mac				
EFA				
LFA				

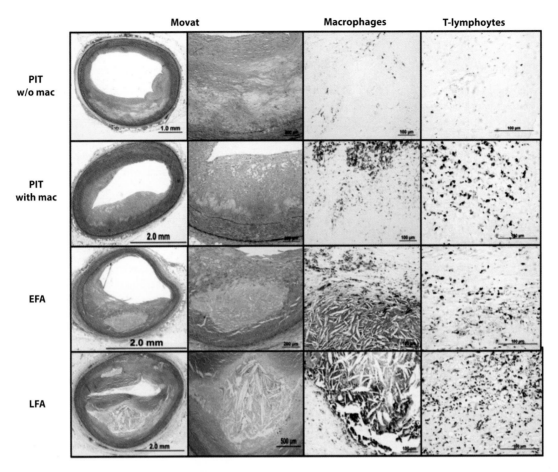

Figure 1.3 Representative histologic sections showing pathologic intimal thickening (PIT) without macrophage (mac) infiltration, PIT with macrophages, early and late fibroatheroma (EFA and LFA, respectively). The left two columns represent low- and high-power images of sections stained with Movat Pentachrome, and the right three columns show high-power images of immunohistochemical stains for macrophages (CD68), T lymphocytes (CD45RO) and vasa vasorum (CD31/CD34). (Reproduced from Otsuka F et al., *Atherosclerosis*, 241, 772–782, 2015. With permission.)

proteases produced by macrophage (Figure 1.4).[26] Notably, the majority of macrophages within the areas of necrotic core display features of apoptotic cell death. Free cholesterol is visualised as empty clefts by routine histopathologic sectioning and this is another discriminating feature of the late necrotic core.[32, 33] The death of macrophages has been attributed to defective phagocytic clearance 'efferocytosis' of apoptotic cells and is thought to contribute further to the expansion of the necrotic core.[33,34]

1.4.3 Thin-cap FA

Morphologically, fibrous cap thinning is the main recognised feature of lesion instability. The TCFA, traditionally designated as vulnerable plaque, essentially resembles plaque rupture, although there is an absence of luminal thrombosis and an intact, but thin fibrous cap.[31,35] The necrotic core is generally smaller with fewer numbers of infiltrating macrophages and overall less calcification compared with plaque rupture. The fibrous cap is predominantly composed of collagen type I and contains varying degrees of macrophages and fewer lymphocytes with a paucity or absence of SMCs. Fibrous cap thickness is the main attribute of plaque vulnerability and thin caps are defined pathologically as ≤ 65 μm since the thinnest portion of remnant ruptured caps is 23 ± 19 μm, whilst 95% of the TCFA caps measure <64 μm.[36] On the contrary, a single clinical OCT study of ruptured plaques report cap thicknesses of 49 ± 19 μm,[37] which may be more true in-life considering that formaldehyde fixation and dehydration can lead to 20%–25% shrinkage of the tissues.

1.5 Coronary thrombosis

1.5.1 Plaque rupture

Oftentimes plaque rupture is fatal and is characterised by a relatively large necrotic core with an overlying focally discontinuous thin fibrous cap and superimposed thrombus. The luminal thrombus near the rupture site is platelet rich (white thrombus), whereas the propagated thrombus at the proximal and distal ends is typically composed of layered fibrin admixed with erythrocytes (red thrombus). Notably, the luminal thrombus resultant from plaque rupture is not always occlusive.

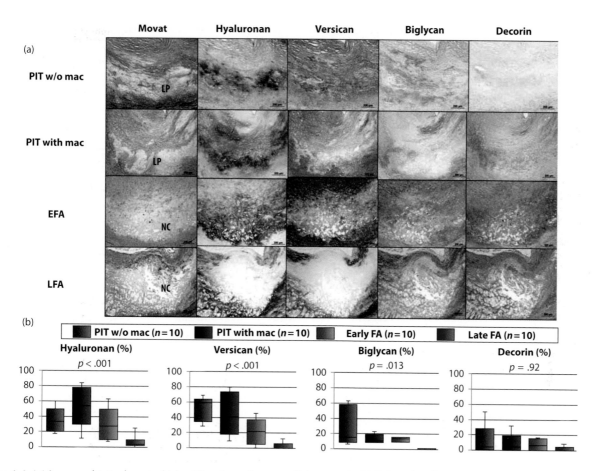

Figure 1.4 **(a)** Immunohistochemical identification of extracellular matrix (ECM) molecules hyaluronan and proteoglycan (versican, biglycan and decorin) in progressive human coronary plaques. Movat Pentachrome staining shows lipid pool (LP) with or without macrophage infiltration in pathologic intimal thickening (PIT) and necrotic core (NC) formation in early (EFA) and late fibroatheromas (LFA). There is intense immunstaining of hyaluronan in LPs of PIT, whereas early NCs show partial loss of staining and late NC exhibits almost complete absence of hyaluronan. A gradual decrease in versican was also noted from PIT without macrophages in LFA, where the staining was nearly absent in the late NC. Immunohistochemical reaction to biglycan and decorin were relatively weak; however, the expression of biglycan in LFA was significantly less as compared with PIT and EFA. **(b)** Quantitative assessment of hyaluronan and proteoglycan (versican, biglycan and decorin) showed a significant decrease in hyaluronan, versican and biglycan from PIT to EFA and LFA. (Reproduced from Otsuka F et al., *Atherosclerosis*, 241, 772–782, 2015. With permission.)

Plaque rupture presumably occurs at its weakest point, often near shoulder regions; however, we have observed an equivalent number of disrupted fibrous caps at their midpoint particularly when rupture occurs during exertion, whilst those dying at rest tend to occur at shoulder regions.[38] Thus, different pathophysiologic and biomechanical processes may be involved in the actual rupture event. Fibrous cap thinning has been linked to infiltrating macrophages together with their release matrix metalloproteinase (MMP),[39] which further weakens the cap along with high shear stress.[40] Other underlying factors include microcalcification and iron accumulation within the fibrous cap[41] and macrophage cell death.[42] Once the fibrous cap is breeched, the necrotic core contents are exposed to the circulating blood initiating a coagulation cascade principally involving platelets in response to the exposed lipids and tissue factor and other pro-coagulants present in the necrotic core.

1.5.2 Plaque erosion

Plaque rupture of an atherosclerotic plaque had been uniformly accepted as the primary causative event in SCDs.[43] This widely held paradigm was predicated on morphologic data from autopsy as well as angiographic imaging studies in which the presence of surface irregularities was interpreted as plaque rupture.[12,44] Meanwhile, in the middle of the 1990s data were presented that indicated the occurrence of plaque erosion is another mechanism of acute coronary thrombi in the absence of plaque rupture. In a series of 20 patients who died with acute MI, van der Wal et al. found plaque ruptures in 60% of lesions with thrombi, whilst the remaining 40% showed 'superficial erosion'.[45]

Our experience is similar where plaque erosion is considered an important substrate for coronary thrombosis in patients dying from sudden death or from AMI, with an increased frequency noted in women.[16,17,46,47] In contrast to ruptures, the thrombus in erosions is confined to the luminal surface without evidence of fissures or communication with an underlying necrotic core. The term 'erosion' is used as it applies to the general lack of surface endothelium.

Unlike prominent fibrous cap inflammation described in ruptures, eroded surfaces contain fewer macrophages (rupture 100% vs. erosion 50%, $p < .0001$) and T lymphocytes (rupture 75% vs. erosion 32%, $p < .004$).[46,48] Cell activation, indicated by human leukocyte antigen - antigen D related (HLA-DR) staining, was identified in macrophages and T cells in 25 (89%) plaque ruptures and in 8 (36%) plaque erosions ($p = .0002$). Besides, eroded plaques tend to be eccentric lesions with the base of the lesion being rich in SMCs and proteoglycans with a relatively intact media. Intriguingly, the density of myeloperoxidase (MPO) positive cell within the thrombus was significantly higher in erosion than in ruptures (erosion: 1632 ± 709 cells/mm^2, rupture: 759 ± 410 cells/mm^2, $p = .0015$), whilst subadjacent plaque surfaces failed to show significant difference between lesion types (erosion: 438 ± 280 cells/mm^2, rupture: 540 ± 468 cells/mm^2, $p = .98$). Differences in the cellular composition of luminal thrombi between rupture and erosion may influence vascular healing, as women with erosion more frequently showed a greater prevalence of organising thrombi compared with those with rupture.[49]

1.5.3 Calcified nodule

The calcified nodule is considered the least frequent lesion capable of inducing luminal thrombosis. Heavily calcified plates with fragmented calcified debris (nodules) embedding in areas of fibrous tissue or fibrin with an absence or

small necrotic core characterise these plaques. In this case, the fibrous-rich surface is breeched by fragments of calcified plates, where nodules protrude into the lumen accompanied by an overlying thrombus. Fibrin is often present between nodules along with osteoblasts and osteoclasts, and inflammatory cells consistent with bony spicules.[16] Calcified nodules are particularly more common in older males and tend to occur in the right or left anterior descending coronary artery, although more frequently observed in carotid arteries.

1.6 Episodic rupture and healing lesions

1.6.1 Healed plaque rupture

Plaque progression beyond 40%–50% luminal narrowing is thought to occur secondary to repeat thrombosis with subsequent vascular healing (Figure 1.5). Healed plaque ruptures (HPR) as shown by Davies et al. were detected microscopically as breaks in the fibrous cap, with an overlying repair reaction consisting of SMCs, proteoglycans and/or a collagen depending on the phase of healing.[50] Early healed repair sites are rich in proteoglycans along with collagen type III, which is eventually replaced by collagen type I.

The frequency of HPRs increase coincides with lumen narrowing[50] such that for plaques with 0%–20% diameter stenosis, the incidence of HPRs was 8%; for plaques with 21%–50% stenosis, the incidence of HPRs was 19%; and for lesions with >50% narrowing, the incidence of HPRs was 73%. In our experience, 61% of autopsied hearts from SCD victims show HPRs with the highest incidence observed in stable plaques (80% HPRs), followed by acute

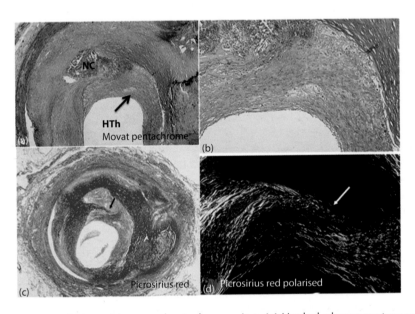

Figure 1.5 Healed plaque rupture lesion with severe luminal narrowing. **(a)** Healed-plaque rupture exhibiting a lipid-rich haemorrhagic necrotic core with cholesterol clefts, showing a collagenous proteoglycan-rich neointima overlying on old disrupted fibrous cap (HTh, healed thrombus, arrow, Movat Pentachrome). **(b)** High-power view of the healed fibrous cap. **(c)** Serial sections stained by picrosirius red showing an area of dark-red collagen (type I) surrounding a lipid-rich haemorrhagic core. **(d)** Image of the same section in 'C' under polarised light clearly delineates newer bluish–greenish collagen (type III) covering lighter reddish–yellowish fibrous cap disruption (type I collagen). (Reproduced from Burke A et al., *Circulation*, 103, 934–940, 2001. With permission.)

plaque rupture (75% HPRs) and then by plaque erosion (9% HPRs).[51] Multiple healed ruptures with layering were more common in segments with acute and healed ruptures, and the per cent luminal narrowing was dependent of the number of healed ruptured sites and was significantly greater for acute ruptures relative to healed ones (79% ± 15% vs. 66% ± 14%, p = .0001). Although the prevalence of silent ruptures in the clinical setting remains unknown, a recent large computed tomography (CT)–angiography study in 3158 patients showed that HPR was an independent predictor of acute coronary syndrome (ACS), although no differences were observed in a number of patients with or without HPR.[52]

1.6.2 Chronic total occlusion

CTO resulting from an occlusive luminal thrombus is a common finding, observed in 17% of SCDs at autopsy.[17] Clinically, CTO is defined as a high-grade native coronary stenosis with thrombolysis in myocardial infarction (TIMI) grade 0–1 flow typically of at least 3-month's duration with a prevalence of 15%–20% in individuals who undergo diagnostic cardiac catheterisation.[53] We recently reported that CTOs of long duration (LD)-CTO (matrix consisting of collagen) demonstrated severe negative remodelling, whereas CTOs of short duration (SD)-CTO (matrix consisting predominantly of proteoglycan with fibrin) demonstrated organising occlusive thrombi with larger underlying necrotic cores that are markedly less negatively remodelled.[54] These morphologic differences along with abrupt and tapering patterns present in proximal and distal lumens, respectively, likely affect successful recanalisation with percutaneous procedures which could be antegrade or retrograde. Further, CTOs in patients with coronary artery bypass grafts exhibit the most calcification and are more difficult to open percutaneously.[54]

1.6.3 Calcified plaque

Calcification of atherosclerotic coronary plaques significantly varies amongst lesions with no direct correlation with the disease severity or lesion vulnerability. Together there are multiple factors which affect calcification such as age/gender,[55] renal failure, vitamin D levels and other aspects of bone metabolism,[56] diabetes[57] and genetic control.[58]

Pathologic calcification in atherosclerosis is initiated by cell death both of SMC and macrophages. Apoptotic SMCs are considered to be a source of plaque calcification by active or passive processes involving mineralisation of cell organelles or through the release of matrix vesicles, a process similar to those observed in bone formation. Histologically, early calcifications are observed as collections of fine granular purple material of >0.5 µm in size[59] Macrophage cell death is considered yet another source of early calcium deposition, recognised as small blocky calcifications (typically <15 µm), which are morphologically distinct from SMCs. Microcalcifications derived from the apoptotic SMC and macrophages generally are observed in lipid pools and early infiltration of macrophages within the forming necrotic core. However, speckles

or fragments of calcification appear on the abluminal aspect of the necrotic core near the internal elastic lamina, in FAs, TCFAs and ruptured plaques. The precise mechanism(s) underlying the extension of calcifications, however, are less clear and may involve coalescence and other plaque components such as lipids, collagen and proteoglycans, eventually evolving into calcified plates/sheets. In heavily calcified burned-out lesions, there are little, if any, macrophage or other inflammatory cell, and the centre of the necrotic core may calcify or remain uncalcified.[30] Calcified plates may fracture, which results in the formation of nodular calcification that is accompanied by fibrin deposition.[30]

1.7 Pathology of neoatherosclerosis

In-stent atherosclerosis called 'neoatherosclerosis' has been reported as untoward complication of coronary stent implants, which leads to late drug-eluting stents (DES)/bare-metal stent (BMS) failure from restenosis or stent thrombosis due to plaque rupture (Figure 1.6).[60,61] Neoatherosclerosis is histologically identified by lipid-laden foamy macrophages with or without complications of a necrotic core and/or calcification within the nascent intima.[60] In all cases, necrotic cores of neoatherosclerosis do not communicate with the underlying native plaques. Clusters of macrophage-derived foam cells within the peri-strut regions or near the luminal surface constitute the most frequent and earliest lesion of neoatherosclerosis. Resident macrophages are often observed on the luminal aspect of the stent, which undergo apoptotic cell death giving rise to necrotic cores and more advanced fibroatheromatous plaques. Intraplaque haemorrhage derived from the lumen or, to a lesser extent, 'leaky' adventitial vasa vasorum near struts with or without fibrin deposits may also exist. Similar to native coronary atherosclerosis, it is also conceivable that infiltration of foamy macrophages within the neointima results in the thinning of fibrous cap, forming a TCFA, or the necrotic core may be formed close to the lumen giving rise to a TCFA with complications of in-stent plaque rupture.

Similar to native disease calcification is another feature of neoatherosclerosis generally involving stents with long-term implant duration. The morphologic character of calcification varies widely from microcalcification to calcified sheet. Calcification in neoatherosclerosis attributed to DES may also be associated with persistent fibrin deposition around stent struts, which is more commonly observed in paclitaxel-eluting stents (PES) but to a lesser extent in sirolimus-eluting stents (SES).

1.8 Prevalence of neoatherosclerosis

The overall prevalence of neoatherosclerosis, as shown by our laboratory, is significantly greater in first-generation DES compared with BMS (31% vs. 16%, p < .001).[60] Furthermore, the median stent duration is significantly less for DES compared with BMS (420 days vs. 2160 days, p < .001).[60] The earliest atherosclerotic change is characterised by macrophage

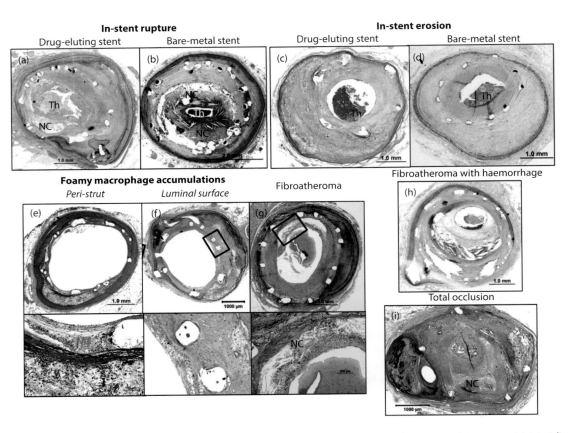

Figure 1.6 Causes of late and very late stent thrombosis attributed to neoatherosclerosis and 'restenosis' (a)–(d) and progression of neoatherosclerosis (e)–(i). Histological and schematic images are shown. Very late stent thrombosis (VLST) from in-stent plaque rupture with underlying neoatherosclerosis associated with (a) PES and (b) BMS. (c) VLST from in-stent erosion with underlying neoatherosclerosis associated with an SES. (d) Late stent thrombosis from in-stent erosion in the presence of restenosis associated with a BMS. Foamy macrophage accumulation (e) around struts in a cobalt-chromium everolimus-eluting stent, and (f) on the luminal surface within PES. (g) Fibroatheroma (FA) with necrotic core within neointima of PES. (h) LFA with intraplaque haemorrhage within BMS. (i) Chronic total occlusion in a case of restenosis in an SES with underlying neoatherosclerosis. BMS, bare-metal stent; Mφ, macrophage; NC, necrotic core; PES, paclitaxel-eluting stent; SES, sirolimus-eluting stent; Th, thrombus; LFA, late fibroatheroma. (Reproduced from Yahagi K et al., *Nat. Rev. Cardiol.*, 13, 79–98, 2015. With permission.)

foam cells, which have been observed as early as 70 days for PES and 120 days for SES, and much later, 900 days for BMS. Necrotic cores were observed with equal frequency in PES and SES within 1 year (PES = 270 days; SES = 360 days), whilst the earliest duration when necrotic core formation in BMS was significantly longer (900 days). Moreover, the unstable feature of neoatherosclerosis (TCFA and in-stent plaque rupture) was identified within 2 years following first-generation DES and 5 years following BMS implantation.[60] Finally, multiple logistic regression analysis showed that younger patients, long implant duration, SES and PES usage, and presence of unstable plaque underlying the stent were identified as independent factors for the development of neoatherosclerosis.[60]

The earliest finding of neoatherosclerosis in second-generation cobalt-chromium everolimus-eluting stent (CoCr-EES) was detected in 270-day implants, which was longer than first-generation SES (120 days) and PES (70 days).[62] The incidence of neoatherosclerosis, however, in CoCr-EES (29%) did not differ significantly from SES (35%)

and PES (19%).[62] A comparison of neoatherosclerotic lesion characteristic amongst stent cohorts failed to show any differences, although the dominant morphology for CoCr-EES and PES was foamy macrophage clusters (CoCr-EES = 67%; PES = 87%), which was less frequently observed for SES (32%).[62] Notably, unstable features of neoatherosclerosis recognised as TCFA or plaque rupture were not observed for CoCr-EES.

In clinical practice, late stent failure including stent thrombosis and late in-stent restenosis has emerged as major issues following both BMS and DES implantation.[63–66] Recently, we have investigated the association between neoatherosclerosis and late stent failure from our autopsy stent registry including 614 stented lesions in native coronary arteries (Figure 1.7).[61] The overall frequency of all cause very late stent thrombosis (VLST) (>1 year) was 3% in BMS, 19% in first-generation DES and 0% for second-generation DES. In-stent plaque rupture accounts for 83% of VLST in BMS and 15% of VLST in first-generation DES. Interestingly, beyond 3 years following

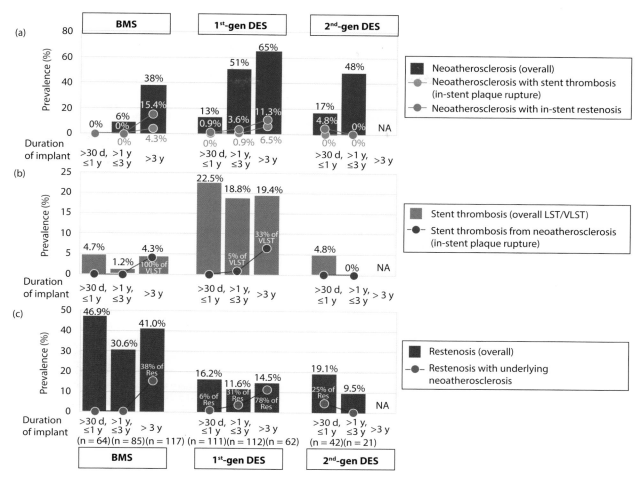

Figure 1.7 **(a)** Prevalence of neoatherosclerosis in BMS, first- and second-generation DES stratified by duration of implant (bar graphs) along with the prevalence of restenosis (green line) and thrombosis (orange line) in the lesions with neo-atherosclerosis and late stent failure. **(b)** Prevalence of overall stent thrombosis, in association with neoatherosclerosis (in-stent plaque rupture). **(c)** Prevalence of in-stent restenosis and its association with underlying neoatherosclerosis. BMS, bare-metal stent; LST/VLST, late and very late stent thrombosis; Res, restenosis. (Reproduced from Otsuka F et al., *Eur. Heart J.*, 36, 2147–2159, 2015. With permission.)

stent implantation, all VLST in BMS and 33% of VLST in first-generation DES were attributed to in-stent plaque rupture (Figure 1.7). In-stent restenosis with underlying neo-atherosclerosis was most frequent in BMS (6.8%) followed by first-generation DES (4.2%), and the least frequent in second-generation DES (3.2%), whilst the duration of the implant was longer in BMS compared with first- and second-generation DES. In BMS, restenosis with underlying neoatherosclerosis was exclusively observed beyond 3 years with a prevalence of 15.4% (Figure 1.7).

1.9 Conclusions

Luminal thrombosis and SCD are predominately due to plaque rupture, followed by erosion and least frequently in calcified nodules. The TCFA likely represents an appropriate target for the diagnosis and treatment of patients at risk for the future coronary events.

Late de novo neoatherosclerosis is a recently recognised substrate occurring from an accelerated disease process, which is now a recognised contributing factor of late in-stent restenosis or thrombosis attributed to percutaneous coronary intervention (PCI) and stenting. It is important to emphasise that the timing with respect to the onset of neoatherosclerosis is within months to a few years where plaque rupture with clinical events occur more rapidly than for native coronary disease, which generally progresses over decades before presentation with symptoms.

Finally, understanding and treating this worldwide epidemic of coronary disease are highly challenging, where it is imperative to have a comprehensive understanding of coronary plaque pathology, particularly in the setting of interventional treatment and management. Therefore, we hope that the pathophysiological features of atherosclerosis as described in this chapter will aid both physicians involved in the daily clinical practice as well as those involved in basic research and scientists developing new treatment modalities.

References

1. WHO Mortality Database, May 2014 update. World Health Organization, Department of Health Statistics and Information Systems, Geneva, Switzerland. World Health Organization, 2014. http://www.who.int/healthinfo/statistics/mortality_rawdata/en/index.html.

2. Laslett LJ et al. The worldwide environment of cardiovascular disease: Prevalence, diagnosis, therapy, and policy issues: A report from the American College of Cardiology. *J Am Coll Cardiol* 2012; 60 (25 Suppl): S1–49.

3. Fihn SD et al. ACCF/AHA/ACP/AATS/PCNA/SCAI/STS guideline for the diagnosis and management of patients with stable ischemic heart disease: A report of the American College of Cardiology Foundation/American Heart Association task force on practice guidelines, and the American College of Physicians, American Association for Thoracic Surgery, Preventive Cardiovascular Nurses Association, Society for Cardiovascular Angiography and Interventions, and Society of Thoracic Surgeons. *Circulation* 2012; 126(25): e354–e471.

4. Lloyd-Jones D et al. Heart disease and stroke statistics—2010 update: A report from the American Heart Association. *Circulation* 2010; 121(7): e46–e215.

5. Heron M. Deaths: Leading causes for 2010. National vital statistics reports: From the Centers for Disease Control and Prevention, National Center for Health Statistics. *Natl Vital Stat Sys* 2013; 62(6): 1–96.

6. Lloyd-Jones DM et al. Lifetime risk of developing coronary heart disease. *Lancet* 1999; 353(9147): 89–92.

7. Furman MI et al. Twenty-two year (1975 to 1997) trends in the incidence, in-hospital and long-term case fatality rates from initial Q-wave and non-Q-wave myocardial infarction: A multi-hospital, community-wide perspective. *J Am Coll Cardiol* 2001; 37(6): 1571–1580.

8. Roger VL et al. Trends in incidence, severity, and outcome of hospitalized myocardial infarction. *Circulation* 2010; 121(7): 863–869.

9. Rogers WJ et al. Trends in presenting characteristics and hospital mortality among patients with ST elevation and non-ST elevation myocardial infarction in the National Registry of Myocardial Infarction from 1990 to 2006. *Am Heart J* 2008; 156(6): 1026–1034.

10. Velican C and Velican D. Discrepancies between data on atherosclerotic involvement of human coronary arteries furnished by gross inspection and by light microscopy. *Atherosclerosis* 1982; 43(1): 39–49.

11. Velican D and Velican C. Atherosclerotic involvement of the coronary arteries of adolescents and young adults. *Atherosclerosis* 1980; 36(4): 449–460.

12. Davies MJ, and Thomas A. Thrombosis and acute coronary-artery lesions in sudden cardiac ischemic death. *N Engl J Med* 1984; 310(18): 1137–1140.

13. Davies MJ. Stability and instability: Two faces of coronary atherosclerosis. The Paul Dudley White Lecture 1995. *Circulation* 1996; 94(8): 2013–2020.

14. Stary HC et al. A definition of the intima of human arteries and of its atherosclerosis-prone regions. A report from the Committee on Vascular Lesions of the Council on Arteriosclerosis, American Heart Association. *Arterioscler Thromb* 1992; 12(1): 120–134.

15. Stary HC et al. A definition of advanced types of atherosclerotic lesions and a histological classification of atherosclerosis. A report from the Committee on Vascular Lesions of the Council on Arteriosclerosis, American Heart Association. *Arterioscler Thrombo Vasc Biol* 1995; 15(9): 1512–1531.

16. Virmani R et al. Lessons from sudden coronary death: A comprehensive morphological classification scheme for atherosclerotic lesions. *Arterioscler Thromb Vasc Biol* 2000; 20(5): 1262–1275.

17. Yahagi K et al. Pathophysiology of native coronary, vein graft, and in-stent atherosclerosis. *Nat Rev Cardiol.* 2016; 13(2): 79–98.

18. Yahagi K et al. Sex differences in coronary artery disease: Pathological observations. *Atherosclerosis* 2015; 239(1): 260–267.

19. Ikari Y et al. Neonatal intima formation in the human coronary artery. *Arterioscler Thromb Vasc Biol.* 1999; 19(9): 2036–2040.

20. Nakashima Y et al. Distributions of diffuse intimal thickening in human arteries: Preferential expression in atherosclerosis-prone arteries from an early age. *Virchows Arch* 2002; 441(3): 279–288.

21. Orekhov AN et al. Cell proliferation in normal and atherosclerotic human aorta: Proliferative splash in lipid-rich lesions. *Atherosclerosis* 1998; 139(1): 41–48.

22. Imanishi T et al. Expression of cellular FLICE-inhibitory protein in human coronary arteries and in a rat vascular injury model. *Am J Pathol* 2000; 156(1): 125–137.

23. Velican C. Relationship between regional aortic susceptibility to atherosclerosis and macromolecular structural stability. *J Atheroscler Res* 1969; 9(2): 193–201.

24. Velican C. A dissecting view on the role of the fatty streak in the pathogenesis of human atherosclerosis: Culprit or bystander? *Med Interne* 1981; 19(4): 321–337.

25. McGill HC Jr et al. Effects of coronary heart disease risk factors on atherosclerosis of selected regions of the aorta and right coronary artery. PDAY Research Group. Pathobiological Determinants of Atherosclerosis in Youth. *Arterioscler Thromb Vasc Biol* 2000; 20(3): 836–845.

26. Otsuka F et al. Natural progression of atherosclerosis from pathologic intimal thickening to late fibroatheroma in human coronary arteries: A pathology study. *Atherosclerosis* 2015; 241(2): 772–782.

27. Kockx MM et al. Luminal foam cell accumulation is associated with smooth muscle cell death in the intimal thickening of human saphenous vein grafts. *Circulation* 1996; 94(6): 1255–1262.

28. Nakashima Y et al. Early human atherosclerosis: Accumulation of lipid and proteoglycans in intimal thickenings followed by macrophage infiltration. *Arterioscler Thromb Vasc Biol* 2007; 27(5): 1159–1165.

29. Nakashima Y et al. Early atherosclerosis in humans: Role of diffuse intimal thickening and extracellular matrix proteoglycans. *Cardiovasc Res* 2008; 79(1): 14–23.

30. Otsuka F et al. Has our understanding of calcification in human coronary atherosclerosis progressed? *Arterioscler Thromb Vasc Biol* 2014; 34(4): 724–736.

31. Virmani R et al. Lessons from sudden coronary death: A comprehensive morphological classification scheme for atherosclerotic lesions. *Arterioscler Thromb Vasc Biol* 2000;20(5): 1262–1275.

32. Bao L et al. Sitosterol-containing lipoproteins trigger free sterol-induced caspase-independent death in ACAT-competent macrophages. *J Biol Chem* 2006; 281(44): 33635–33649.

33. Tabas I. Cholesterol and phospholipid metabolism in macrophages. *Biochim Biophys Acta* 2000; 1529(1–3): 164–174.

34. Tabas I et al. Evidence that the initial up-regulation of phosphatidylcholine biosynthesis in free cholesterol-loaded macrophages is an adaptive response that prevents cholesterol-induced cellular necrosis. Proposed role of an eventual failure of this response in foam cell necrosis in advanced atherosclerosis. *J Biol Chem* 1996; 271(37): 22773–22781.

35. Kolodgie FD et al. Pathologic assessment of the vulnerable human coronary plaque. *Heart* 2004; 90(12): 1385–1391.

36. Burke AP et al. Coronary risk factors and plaque morphology in men with coronary disease who died suddenly. *N Engl J Med* 1997; 336(18): 1276–1282.

37. Kubo T et al. Assessment of culprit lesion morphology in acute myocardial infarction: Ability of optical coherence tomography compared with intravascular ultrasound and coronary angioscopy. *J Am Coll Cardiol* 2007;50(10): 933–939.

38. Burke AP et al. Plaque rupture and sudden death related to exertion in men with coronary artery disease. *JAMA* 1999; 281(10): 921–926.

39. Sukhova GK et al. Evidence for increased collagenolysis by interstitial collagenases-1 and -3 in vulnerable human atheromatous plaques. *Circulation* 1999; 99(19): 2503–2509.

40. Gijsen FJ et al. Strain distribution over plaques in human coronary arteries relates to shear stress. *Am J Physiol Heart Circ Physiol* 2008; 295(4): H1608–H1614.

41. Vengrenyuk Y et al. A hypothesis for vulnerable plaque rupture due to stress-induced debonding around cellular microcalcifications in thin fibrous caps. *Proc Natl Acad Sci USA* 2006; 103(40): 14678–14683.

42. Kolodgie FD et al. Localization of apoptotic macrophages at the site of plaque rupture in sudden coronary death. *Am J Pathol* 2000; 157(4): 1259–1268.

43. Falk E et al. Coronary plaque disruption. *Circulation* 1995; 92(3): 657–671.

44. Ambrose JA et al. Angiographic morphology and the pathogenesis of unstable angina pectoris. *J Am Coll Cardiol* 1985; 5(3): 609–616.

45. van der Wal AC et al. Site of intimal rupture or erosion of thrombosed coronary atherosclerotic plaques is characterized by an inflammatory process irrespective of the dominant plaque morphology. *Circulation* 1994; 89(1): 36–44.

46. Farb A et al. Coronary plaque erosion without rupture into a lipid core. A frequent cause of coronary thrombosis in sudden coronary death. *Circulation* 1996; 93(7): 1354–1363.

47. Kramer MC et al. Histopathological features of aspirated thrombi after primary percutaneous coronary intervention in patients with ST-elevation myocardial infarction. *PloS One* 2009; 4(6): e5817.

48. Kolodgie FD et al. Differential accumulation of proteoglycans and hyaluronan in culprit lesions: Insights into plaque erosion. *Arterioscler Thromb Vasc Biol* 2002; 22(10): 1642–1648.

49. Kramer MC et al. Relationship of thrombus healing to underlying plaque morphology in sudden coronary death. *J Am Coll Cardiol* 2010; 55(2): 122–132.

50. Mann J, and Davies MJ. Mechanisms of progression in native coronary artery disease: Role of healed plaque disruption. *Heart* 1999; 82(3): 265–268.

51. Burke AP et al. Healed plaque ruptures and sudden coronary death: Evidence that subclinical rupture has a role in plaque progression. *Circulation* 2001; 103(7): 934–940.

52. Motoyama S et al. Plaque characterization by coronary computed tomography angiography and the likelihood of acute coronary events in mid-term follow-up. *J Am Coll Cardiol* 2015; 66(4): 337–346.

53. Kahn JK. Angiographic suitability for catheter revascularization of total coronary occlusions in patients from a community hospital setting. *Am Heart J* 1993; 126(3 Pt 1): 561–564.

54. Sakakura K et al. Comparison of pathology of chronic total occlusion with and without coronary artery bypass graft. *Eur Heart J* 2014; 35(25): 1683–1693.

55. Burke AP et al. Effect of menopause on plaque morphologic characteristics in coronary atherosclerosis. *Am Heart J*.2001; 141(2 Suppl): S58–S62.

56. Watson KE et al. Active serum vitamin D levels are inversely correlated with coronary calcification. *Circulation* 1997; 96(6): 1755–1760.

57. Burke AP et al. Coronary calcification: Insights from sudden coronary death victims. *Z Kardiol* 2000; 89(2 Suppl): 49–53.

58. Keso T et al. Polymorphisms within the tumor necrosis factor locus and prevalence of coronary artery disease in middle-aged men. *Atherosclerosis* 2001; 154(3): 691–697.

59. Proudfoot D, and Shanahan CM. Biology of calcification in vascular cells: Intima versus media. *Herz* 2001; 26(4): 245–251.

60. Nakazawa G et al. The pathology of neoatherosclerosis in human coronary implants bare-metal and drug-eluting stents. *J Am Coll Cardiol* 2011; 57(11): 1314–1322.

61. Otsuka F et al. Neoatherosclerosis: Overview of histopathologic findings and implications for intravascular imaging assessment. *Eur Heart J* 2015; 36(32): 2147–2159.

62. Otsuka F et al. Pathology of second-generation everolimus-eluting stents versus first-generation sirolimus- and Paclitaxel-eluting stents in humans. *Circulation* 2014; 129(2): 211–223.

63. Yamaji K et al. Very long-term (15 to 20 years) clinical and angiographic outcome after coronary bare metal stent implantation. *Circ Cardiovasc Interv* 2010; 3(5): 468–475.

64. Doyle B et al. Outcomes of stent thrombosis and restenosis during extended follow-up of patients treated with bare-metal coronary stents. *Circulation* 2007; 116(21): 2391–2398.

65. Wenaweser P et al. Incidence and correlates of drug-eluting stent thrombosis in routine clinical practice. 4-Year results from a large 2-institutional cohort study. *J Am Coll Cardiol* 2008; 52(14): 1134–1140.

66. Natsuaki M et al. Late adverse events after implantation of sirolimus-eluting stent and bare-metal stent: Long-term (5–7 years) follow-up of the Coronary Revascularization Demonstrating Outcome study-Kyoto registry Cohort-2. *Circ Cardiovasc Interv* 2014; 7(2): 168–179.

Radiation protection, image archiving and communication systems

FATEMEH SAKHINIA, STEVEN M THOMAS

Radiation protection

2.1 Introduction

Diagnostic and interventional fluoroscopic procedures are certainly on the rise and the reliance on imaging is increasing amongst clinicians and other medical professionals. However, with growing number of procedures, the amount of radiation that staff and patients are exposed to also increases and this is a growing concern.

Medical staff are known to receive the highest occupational radiation doses, and the important group amongst these are interventional cardiologists and radiologists who perform procedures frequently.[1] Therefore, protection from the stochastic and deterministic effects of radiation is paramount.

Although now there is no hard evidence so that the staff currently performing x-ray–guided therapeutic procedures are more prone to developing cancers than the ordinary population, individual cases of radiation-induced osteonecrosis, cataracts, brain tumours and aplastic anaemia are well recorded.

European and national guidelines require medical staff working within an interventional cardiology or radiology environment to have specific training in radiation protection. Undertaking such training is now a legal requirement in Europe for these staff.[2] This training focuses on various measures for radiation protection as well as behavioural components, and we will expand on these in this chapter.

2.2 Radiation units

To quantify the amount of radiation received by patients, physical quantities such as Kerma and absorbed dose as well as their International System of Units (SI) unit, the Grey (Gy), is used. The Gy is defined as the energy deposited per unit mass of the material, measured in joules per kilogram. The rate of absorbed dose is measured in Greys per second.

Alpha, gamma and x-rays are forms of ionising radiation, which cause different rates of energy deposition within the cell, and the Sievert (Sv) is the unit of dose equivalent, which takes this into account. For medical radiation protection purposes, units of radiation are usually very small and measured in mGy, mSV, μGy or μSv.

2.3 Risk estimates

The level of radiation required to produce acute effects is largely related to the dose. Ionising radiation has two main biological effects, which include stochastic and deterministic effects. Stochastic effects are statistical in nature, arising by chance. These include cancer and genetic abnormalities.

The characteristic feature of deterministic or non-stochastic effects is having a threshold dose below which the effect will not occur. Above this threshold dose, the likelihood of the effect occurring increases significantly. Deterministic effects have an immediate and very predictable alteration to the tissue.

Table 2.1 Threshold doses for deterministic effects

Effect	Threshold dose (Gy)
Skin erythema	2–5
Irreversible skin damage	20–40
Hair loss	2–5
Sterility	2–3
Cataracts (lens of eye)	5
Lethality (whole body)	3–5
Foetal abnormality	0.1–0.5

Source: Williams JR and Allisy-Roberts P, *Farr's Physics for Medical Imaging*, Saunders, Philadelphia, pp. 23–47, 2007.

These include radiation cataracts and skin changes such as erythema, ulcers, telangiectasia and dermal atrophy. Severe injuries can involve the subcutaneous fat as well as muscles (Table 2.1).[3]

2.4 Fundamentals of radiation protection

Radiation exposure is currently a major concern in interventional cardiology. The variety and complexity of cases are rapidly increasing, leading to longer fluoroscopy times and thus more radiation dose to patient and staff.

Radiation protection is aimed at preventing occurrence of deterministic as well as risks of stochastic effects, mainly cancer. Therefore, dose limits are set in the interventional cardiology laboratory and other departments who use ionising radiation. Regulatory bodies require the workers to aim at keeping their occupational exposure doses lower than the set limits, and also to implement the principles of optimised protection.[4]

Radiation protection rules proposed by the International Commission on Radiological Protection (ICRP), published in 1991, were the basis of the European Directives, which in turn inform the current legislation in the United Kingdom.[3]

ICRP introduced three main radiation protection principles, which include justification, optimisation and occupational dose limits.

1. Justification
   The use of ionising radiation should demonstrate a clear benefit outweighing the risks to those who are liable to be exposed. Therefore, a clinician requesting or directing an examination requiring x-rays must carefully consider the need for it in terms of the relative risks and benefits.
   The operator should be absolutely certain that any examination requiring radiation exposure, such as angiography, is necessary and consider the likelihood of the examination influencing patient management and clinical outcome.[3] Alternatives such as magnetic resonance imaging or ultrasound/echocardiography should be considered if that is practical and likely provide the necessary clinical information.
2. Optimisation (ALARA/ALARP principle)
   ICRP has stated that the principle of optimisation is that in using ionising radiation, the dose should be as low

Table 2.2 Dose limits for occupational exposure

Dose quantity	Occupational dose limit
Effective dose	20 mSv per year averaged over five consecutive years (100 mSv in 5 years), and 50 mSv in any single year
Equivalent dose in: lens of the eye	20 mSv in a year, averaged over defined periods of five years, with no single year exceeding 50 mSv
Skin	500 mSv in a year
Extremities (hands and feet)	500 mSv in a year

Source: Adapted from ICRP, Duran A et al., *Catheter Cardiovasc Interv.*, 81, 562–567, 2013.

as reasonably achievable (ALARA). The UK legislation terminology is as low as reasonably practicable (ALARP).

The design of equipment and x-ray output control during fluoroscopy should be maintained and dose efficient. Technique selection to produce diagnostic images at the lowest possible dose is essential. Operator technique to minimise screening times and restrict views should be advocated. There should be a system for quality assurance to ensure optimum equipment performance.
3. Dose limitation
   Dose limits apply to those who are employed to work with radiation and the general public who are likely to have exposure as a result of work activity. Operators should be fully aware of dose limits and should therefore limit diagnostic and therapeutic examinations accordingly. Strict dose limits apply to staff. It is important to note that dose limits do not apply to patients and the control of patient dose is exclusively based on the justification and optimisation principles. There is, however, a requirement to record sufficient information so that an estimate of dose to the patient can subsequently be made if necessary. This can then be checked against the reference dose levels on the upper quartile of national patient surveys (Table 2.2).[4]

European directives determine UK legislation on health and safety and regulations of ionising radiation are based on recommendations of ICRP. Current regulations governing staff and public safety are the Ionising Radiations Regulations 1999 (IRR99), which apply to all work places. The IRR99 is not directed at patient safety from radiation, other than for the equipment for medical exposures.[3]

Ionising Radiation Medical Exposure Regulations 2000 (IRMER) are a separate European directive concerned with patient protection in the UK law. IRMER emphasises the responsibilities of the employer and the requirements for justification and optimisation of individual exposures. In addition to the employer, IRMER identified three key persons who have a role in respect of diagnostic x-ray examinations: the referrer initiating a request, the practitioner considering whether an examination is justifiable in terms of its risks and benefits and the operator who carries out the practical side of exposure after authorisation.[3]

Interventional cardiologists are amongst the health care professionals who are generally entitled to act as IRMER practitioners.

2.5 Staff protection

In order to decrease the absorbed dose to the patient and staff the radiation protection principles of time, distance and shielding have to be followed.

Dose is directly related to time, so half the time leads to half the dose. Only essential staff should be in the cardiac catheter angiography room or suite where they will be exposed to radiation during angiography procedures (Figures 2.1 and 2.2).

2.5.1 Dosimetry

Using dosimeters in cardiac laboratories is paramount to establishing the occupational doses received by interventional cardiologists and other staff, and this then means that it is possible to assess whether adequate radiation protection is taking place or improvements need to be made.

It is recommended that interventional cardiologists be monitored on a monthly basis to facilitate the prompt identification of high doses and implement necessary changes.[4]

It is recommended that interventional cardiology departments advocate a policy for their personnel to wear two dosimeters, one under the lead apron and one at a collar level outside the lead apron. The dosimeter worn under the apron is proposed to give a good estimate of the effective dose and the one worn outside the protective garments can provide a good estimate of the dose delivered to the unprotected skin and eye lens.[4]

Further dosimeters can be used on forehead or hands in the form of ring dosimeters to assess eye lens or hand tissues.

Baumann et al. recently published a study looking at how real-time quantitative display of radiation exposure during angiographic procedures can significantly decrease staff radiation dose.[5] The importance of this topic was also discussed in 2010 at the board of Cardiovascular and Interventional Radiological Society of Europe, which recently created and implemented guidelines alongside the American Society of Interventional Radiology, under the title *Occupational Radiation Protection for Interventionalists*.[6]

A busy interventional cardiologist who takes all the necessary personal protection precautions is unlikely to have an annual effective dose more than 10 mSv, and is more likely to be in the range of 1–4 mSv.[4]

It is usually deemed appropriate to investigate a radiation dose of 2 mSv or above per month in order to not only protect the individual but also optimise the safety of other staff and patients. ICRP recently lowered their dose limit for the lens of the eye, which has already triggered investigations in many interventional cardiology facilities and led to practice modifications.

2.5.2 Protective tools

The most effective way of staff protection from radiation is to exclude them from the angiography room. These rooms are designed in such a way that the radiation doses received outside of the room are equal to or generally very much lower than the public dose limit.[3]

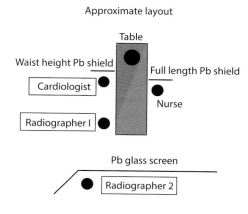

Approximate layout

Cardiologist	Position	Av dose (μSv)
	Forehead	13.6
	Left hand	19.3
Nurse	Right shoulder	18

	Angiography	PTCA
	(μSv per procedure)	
Cardiologist	11	25
Nurse	4.1	9.5
Radiographer 1	1	3.9
Radiographer 2	0	0

Figure 2.1 Average radiation dose received by a laboratory team during coronary angiography and PTCA.

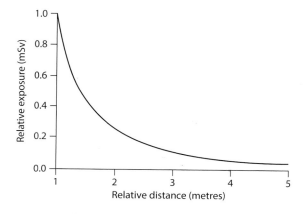

Figure 2.2 Reduction of radiation intensity according to the inverse square law.

Even with protective lead shielding placed close to the primary beam, the dose to the operator is not inconsiderable and varies at different body sites. The aim of lead aprons is to protect sensitive parts of the body, the bone marrow being the most sensitive.

The dose received by the operators is generally not from the direct beam but scattered radiation from the patient. The attenuation or loss of intensity of the x-ray beam as it passes through matter is exponential (Figure 2.3). Therefore small amounts of shielding of appropriate density can greatly reduce the intensity of the x-ray beam. 0.5 mm of lead, which is the standard thickness of lead in an apron, can reduce the intensity of the beam by 90%.

Various types of shielding in the angiography room can result in substantial dose reduction for the practitioner. These include table-suspended lead skirts, ceiling-suspended screens, lead gowns, leaded eyeglasses, mobile shields and disposable patient drapes.[4]

Interventional cardiology procedures in paediatrics may be carried out using biplanar systems and the operator is often standing closer to the patient than in adults, which can undoubtedly increase the scatter dose, however, lower dose rates and smaller beams are required in imaging smaller patients, which may compensate for these other factors.

Arterial access choice and patient arm position are also important factors in predicting the amount of scatter dose from the patient. Radial artery access has been demonstrated to reduce patient dose.[7]

Personal protective devices include lead aprons, thyroid shields, eyeglasses and lead-coated gloves. The main protection tool worn by interventional cardiologists is the wrap-around aprons with thyroid shields. They should be sized to fit the individual properly to allow comfort and aid in being able to wear them throughout the working day and especially during long complex procedures.

Lead eyeglasses should have protective side shields as well to provide more protection. They can be used as an alternative to ceiling-suspended shields.

The operator should always keep their hands out of the primary beam.

Key points for safe practice in interventional cardiology catheter labs include minimising fluoroscopy time and number of acquired images. Use of available patient dose reduction techniques, collimation, protective shielding and appropriate imaging equipment with sound quality assurance program is paramount. Appropriate radiation protection training, emphasis on wearing personal dosimeters at all times and knowing the dose limits and your individual doses are also crucial.

2.6 Patient protection

Cardiac patients are increasingly exposed to cumulative diagnostic and therapeutic procedures using ionising radiation, such as coronary angiography, percutaneous coronary intervention (PCI) and nuclear cardiology (Table 2.3).

Modern digital imaging can cause higher doses than cine imaging. However, the other advantages of digital imaging outweigh this potential disadvantage. Digital screening provides a relatively small dose compared with digital acquisition. It is therefore wise to acquire images only when it is necessary to obtain a record or when post-acquisition viewing of the recorded image will reduce the fluoroscopy time. The size of the field of view is also very important; increasing the field size from 14-inch to 16-inch more than trebles the entrance dose.

2.7 Digital cardiac angiography

Quantitative coronary angiography (QCA) has progressed a lot over the last few decades. From the early 1980s, images used to be acquired using very expensive cinefilm projectors onto 35-mm cinefilms, with optimal zooming for analysis. Modern digital imaging allows the drastic reduction of frame rates without compromising the image quality, and with an advantage of achieving high resolutions up to 512 or 1024 pixels.

The main difference between cinefilm and modern digital acquisition was that coronary arteries were displayed as bright arteries on a darker background, resulting in a 'pincushion' distortion caused by the concave input screen of the image intensifier.[8]

In digital imaging, arteries are visualised as dark structures on a bright background, with no geometric distortion from the modern flat panel x-ray detectors. There have been numerous studies comparing the previous cinefilms to the current digital imaging, and they have validated that there are no significant differences in accuracy and precision between the two techniques and in fact the high contrast

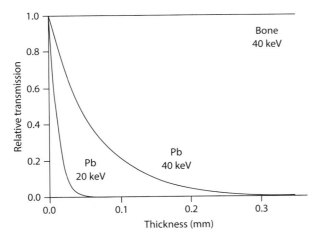

Figure 2.3 Absorption/transmission of x-rays by different thicknesses of lead and bone at different energies (keV, kilo electron volts).

Table 2.3 Average effective dose

Coronary angiography	5–10 mSV
Percutaneous coronary intervention	7–20 mSV
Nuclear cardiology	6–15 mSV

resolution of digital imaging compensates for the high spatial resolution of the 35-mm cinefilm.[8]

Digital imaging has also allowed for a reduction in radiation dose and contrast usage, compared with the cinefilm angiography. This is because digital imaging provides high detection efficiency, requires fewer retakes with less scope for poor technique and less need for repeat examinations as image will not be lost or unavailable.

2.8 Conclusion

Interventional cardiology demands an increasing awareness of the principles of time, distance and shielding as well as clinical judgement. Staff exposures can be reduced by the proper configuration of radiographic equipment and the use of shielding. Real-time dose exposure monitoring may also allow behavioural changes and reduced exposure.

One of the major advancements for the future may involve complete elimination of ionising radiation from the catheter lab and the need for wearing lead aprons, by replacement of the angiography system with magnetic resonance imaging (MRI) image guidance.[9]

Image archiving and communication systems

Prior to the advent of digital imaging, cinefilm was widely used in hospital cardiac labs. A typical cardiac angiographic study consisted of 2000–3000 images in 512-matrix format. Given the available film standards and quality in the early 1980s, cinefilm provided excellent quality for reviewing cardiac angiographic images. The 1990s also brought an introduction of digital images into the fairly buoyant digital market. Despite several manufactures launching digital solutions as early as 1986, cinefilm remained popular well into the late 1990s in many countries, despite its inherent susceptibility to damage and fogging, providing a truly universal standard for imaging, which could be accessed and viewed on any non-vender-specific projection system.

It was, however, difficult to copy and store. A patient's study became a precious source of images, with a danger of being lost or destroyed.

Hospitals that chose a digital solution early, found digital data storage volumes astronomically high and struggled to justify the cost of approximately 500–700 megabytes for one angiographic study.

Huge advances in digital technology in the mid-1990s with the digital revolution saw the costs of memory and storage spiral downward as manufacturers embraced this technology. The restrictions mentioned above placed by cinefilm, caused cardiologists to clamour for alternatives. Many expressed a strong opinion on trying to keep the native resolution of the acquired image in a digital format rather than converting to a cine film, or a video tape recorder (VTR) format. So after a short romance with other formats such as super VHS, they started exploring solutions with their colleagues in radiology.

2.9 DICOM

The collaboration between the American College of Radiologists (ACR) and the National Electrical Manufactures Associations (NEMA) in the United States resulted in development of an imaging standard called Digital Imaging and Communications in Medicine (DICOM),[10] which facilitated a communication standards between different imaging equipment and manufacturers allowing them to integrate but at the same time allowing them the freedom of end user experience.

2.10 CD medical

DICOM standards allowed the development of CD ROM/ MEDICAL as the standardised medium for image exchange.

> **Advantages of CD ROM over film**
> - Compact and requires a smaller space for storage
> - Rapid access
> - Encryption
> - No deterioration
> - Does not need processing
> - Low cost

2.11 Picture archiving and communication systems

Despite the convenience and the elegance of a CD, the obvious benefits of accessing the images by multiple cardiovascular departments at the same time and not having to physically carry CD ROMs from hospital to hospital, or room to room led to the adoption of Picture Archiving and Communication Systems (PACS).

Picture Archiving and Communication Systems were given the acronym PACS in the early 1980s and although the idea was aired in meetings as early as the 1970s, the idea came into its current form in 1984 in the United States. The bare essentials of PACS involve the ability to integrate different modalities like, digital plain film, digital subtraction angiography (DSA), computed tomography (CT) and MRI together into a common accessible standard. This allowed the clinical teams to be able to access the medical imaging information rapidly anywhere where there was a workstation to facilitate collaboration and coordinate patient care. The key components include

> - Image acquisition
> - Image display
> - Image transportation/Network
> - Image archiving
> - Image management

PACS along with the integrated local hospital systems aims to provide a single point of access from workstations for a seamless workflow and access from thin clients (smaller computers utilising servers for their main computing power) for review. It is only limited by the size of the network.

Accessing and storing such vast amounts of data can become a cumbersome and expensive process. Many systems rely on magnetic disks, optical disks and magnetic tapes. These disks are held in server stations in arrays called storage area networks (SAN), linked with either fibre optical or network cable. Often the storage is built at two levels, a short-term rapid access point, where the images for reporting are stored and can be accessed immediately with almost a zero lag time and a longer archive storage utilising slower but less expensive discs such as the Worm Drives, which are permanent storage solutions.

These storage devices must conform to national guidelines for life span; typically 5–7 years.

When accessing the PACS images the most recent images are imported to the workstations' random access memory (RAM), while the older and larger image files are stored in a local server ready for rapid access. Despite vast advances in RAM and the advent of double data rate DDR4 RAM, older networks are still limited by bandwidth and the lack of the latest cable (CAT6 and Optical).

Back up of such data also needs to be robust and often many myriads of back up configurations can be used from simple redundant arrays of independent disks (RAID), to more elaborate systems, which are beyond the scope of discussion.

2.12 Digital coronary angiography

Modern fluoroscopic images are acquired by allowing x-rays to impinge on a caesium iodide input screen coupled to an image intensifier. This amplifies the light produced on the input screen by accelerating photoelectrons through a potential difference of 20–30 kV. As the input screen is generally 35 cm and the output screen 2.5 cm, there is considerable increase in signal but also loss of spatial resolution. It is the gain of a bright image that makes it possible to study moving structures like the heart. A television (TV) camera picks up the images produced and the consequent video signal passed through an analogue-digital converter (ADC). The image matrix produced can vary in size, but $1024 \times 1024 \times 8$ is usually adequate. A frame rate required to monitor the passage of contrast media through the coronary arteries varies but is around 30 frames per second. Such units, producing vast amounts of data, present special problems for PACS. Ten seconds' worth of real-time cardiac imaging at 30 frames per second generates 300 megabytes of image data. To put this in context, this much data is equivalent to 12 abdominal CT scans.

CD-Recordable is a good solution to this problem. It is a spin-off of both the DICOM standard and the establishment of the CD-Recordable as a standard exchange medium.

CD technology is already a consumer standard in CD digital audio, CD interactive (CDI) and CD ROM.

2.13 Advancements in cardiac imaging

Three-dimensional (3D) imaging is one of the major advancements in cardiovascular imaging, which allows on-table imaging similar to a CT-like 3D image, allowing for better navigation and planning of vessels and other structures. Some catheter labs also allow the fusion or overlay of these 3D rotational CT or MR angiographic images on the live 2D fluoroscopic images for better accuracy. One of the examples is the use of this technology in trans-catheter valve replacement (TAVR) procedures for precise device placement.

Next steps in imaging will be the introduction of free-floating holographic 3D imaging in cardiac catheter labs, allowing interventionalists to interact with the images and even slice them into various planes and cross sections for better planning and navigation at the tableside.[9]

Information technology will also entail exciting advancements beyond standard reporting and PACS. 3D printing will allow 3D images to be printed into a resin-based 3D model for better visualisation of anatomy, and aiding production of custom-made implantable devices, such as heart valves.

2.14 Conclusion

Over the recent years, PACS has increased the efficiency of cardiology as a whole with numerous benefits including better patient care. Its value lies in convenience, reliability, speed of image retrieval and display and the flexibility of image data use.

Telecardiology is now widely used, where patient images are easily accessible across different regions and hospitals as well as community centres and primary care. This has allowed networking and collaborative approach to patient management across different cardiac centres, ultimately providing optimal patient care to a wider community, with the help of experts in non-local centres.

References

1. Roberto Sanchez et al. Staff radiation doses in a real-time display inside the angiography room. *Cardiovas Interv Radiol* 2010; 33: 1210–1214.
2. The Ionising Radiation (Protection of Persons Undergoing Medical Examinations or Treatments) Regulations SI778/1988. Her Majesty's Stationary Office, London.
3. Williams JR and Allisy-Roberts P. *Farr's Physics for Medical Imaging*. Philadelphia, PA: Saunders, 2007, pp. 23–47.
4. Duran A et al. A summary of recommendations for occupational radiation protection in interventional cardiology. *Catheter Cardiovasc Interv* 2013; 81: 562–567.
5. Baumann F et al. The effect of realtime monitoring on dose exposure to staff within an interventional radiology setting. *Cardiovas Interv Radiol* 2015; 38: 1105–1111.

6. Miller DL et al. Occupational radiation protection in interventional radiology: A joint guideline of the Cardiovascular and Interventional Radiology Society of Europe and the Society of Interventional Radiology. *J Vasc Interv Radiol* 2010; 21: 607–615.

7. Sun Z et al. Radiation-induced noncancer risks in interventional cardiology: Optimisation of procedures and staff and patient dose reduction. *Biomed Res Int* 2013; 2013: 976962.

8. Reiber JH. Introduction to QCA, IVUS and OCT in interventional cardiology. *Int J Cardiovasc Imaging*, 2011; 27: 153–154.

9. Fornell D. The cath lab of the future. *Diagnostic and Interventional Cardiology.* 2014.

10. National Electrical Manufacturers Association. *Digital Imaging and Communications in Medicine (DICOM).* NEMA Standards Publications P53. Washington DC: NEMA, 1994.

3

Non-invasive cardiac imaging for the interventionist

PANKAJ GARG, DAVID P RIPLEY, JOHN P GREENWOOD, SVEN PLEIN

3.1 Introduction

Cardiovascular imaging plays an important role in the assessment of patients with coronary artery disease (CAD). Non-invasive anatomical or functional imaging can provide information on coronary artery anatomy and course, left ventricular (LV) size and function, myocardial ischaemia and viability. These parameters can help the interventional cardiologist choose the best treatment strategy for a given patient and also provides pivotal prognostic information. The main non-invasive cardiac imaging modalities which guide intervention in the assessment of CAD are echocardiography (ECHO), computed tomography coronary angiography (CTCA), radionuclide myocardial perfusion scintigraphy (MPS), cardiovascular magnetic resonance (CMR) imaging and positron emission tomography (PET).

3.2 Stable chest pain assessment

Stable CAD is a leading cause of death and disability worldwide with substantial associated cost. In the United States alone 15.4 million people have CAD costing the US economy $109 billion/year[1]; in the United Kingdom there are an estimated 2.0 million people with angina costing the National Health Service £7.0 billion/year.[2] The use of non-invasive anatomical and functional imaging as part of the

management of patients with CAD is defined in national and international practice guidelines.[3,4] Many of these guidelines recommend assessment of pre-test likelihood of significant CAD in patients presenting with stable chest pain of suspected cardiac origin (Table 3.1). The 2013 European Society of Cardiology (ESC) guidelines on the management of stable CAD recommend non-invasive imaging for those with a pre-test likelihood of CAD of between 15% and 85%.[4] Guidelines also recommend a baseline resting echocardiogram for all patients with suspected CAD to rule out alternative causes of angina, to identify regional wall motion abnormality (RWMA), for measurement of LV ejection fraction (EF) for risk stratification and evaluation of diastolic function. The available non-invasive imaging tests have varying levels of evidence and different clinical roles.

3.2.1 Anatomical imaging

3.2.1.1 Computed tomography coronary artery calcium score

Computed tomography (CT) has high accuracy for the detection of the presence, extent and location of coronary artery calcification (CAC). CAC scoring may be used as a screening test to rule out of significant CAD with a calcium score of zero having a negative predictive value of 93% in a meta-analysis of

Table 3.1 Comparison of pre-test likelihood risk prediction models by sex and gender

Age	Type of chest pain	Diamond Forrester		Genders et al.		Duke (Prior et al.)[a]	
		Male	Female	Male	Female	Male	Female
35	Typical	70	26	59	28	30–88	10–78
	Atypical	22	4	29	10	8–59	2–39
	Non-anginal	5	1	18	5	3–35	1–19
45	Typical	87	55	69	37	51–92	20–79
	Atypical	46	13	38	14	21–70	5–43
	Non-anginal	14	3	25	8	9–47	2–22
55	Typical	92	79	77	47	80–95	38–82
	Atypical	59	32	49	20	45–79	10–47
	Non-anginal	21	8	33	12	23–59	4–25
65	Typical	94	90	84	58	93–97	56–84
	Atypical	67	54	59	28	71–86	20–51
	Non-anginal	28	2	44	17	49–69	9–29
75	Typical	–	–	89	68	–	–
	Atypical	–	–	69	37	–	–
	Non-anginal	–	–	54	24	–	–
80+	Typical	–	–	93	76	–	–
	Atypical	–	–	78	47	–	–
	Non-anginal	–	–	65	32	–	–

For the Duke score the mid-point for each decade is displayed.
[a] Prior et al. data are a range of pre-test probability depending on the presence or absence of hyperlipidaemia, smoking, diabetes mellitus, ST/T changes, Q waves and documented previous myocardial infarction.

18 studies.[2] The CAC score as a screening test offers substantial cost saving and lower false-positive results over the use of exercise tolerance testing (ETT).[5] However, recent data suggests that 12% of patients with significant CAD (mainly in the form of soft plaque) will be missed by CAC assessment only.[6]

3.2.1.2 CT coronary angiography

Current generation multidetector CT (MDCT) scanners acquiring 64 slices and above can reliably image the major coronary arteries with a spatial resolution of 0.3–0.5 mm, which is only slightly lower than that of invasive coronary angiography (ICA). Radiation exposure through CTCA has continued to fall, driven by prospective gating acquisition technology and other technological advances, and with modern CT scanners, routine CTCA can be performed with a dose of 2 mSv or less. CTCA has been endorsed as an appropriate investigation by the American College of Cardiology Foundation (ACCF) Appropriate Use Criteria for the investigation of patients with chest pain.[7] The particular strength of CTCA lies in its ability to rule out CAD with a negative predictive value of up to 99%. However, the positive predictive value of CTCA is lower and ranges from 64% to 100%, in part because of false-positive results due to 'blooming' artefact associated with coronary calcification and intracoronary stents (Figure 3.1). However, technological progress, for example dual energy imaging, reduces this limitation and improves imaging of calcified lesions and stents. A CTCA negative for coronary atheroma is associated with a good prognosis with annual mortality

of 0.65% as opposed to 1.99% in those with non-obstructive atheroma.[8]

In the planning of interventional procedures CTCA can be used to identify the ostium and anatomical course of vessels that cannot be selectively cannulated on ICA, imaging of aortic bypass grafts from unanticipated locations, demonstration of flush occlusions of aortic grafts and the presence, course and anatomy of anomalous coronary arteries. In addition, the role of CTCA role in guiding coronary intervention in chronic total occlusion (CTO) is expanding. Unlike ICA, which is limited by its two-dimensional projection and luminal contrast enhancement, CTCA can identify the length, trajectory and tortuosity of the occluded segment and the severity and distribution of calcification, all of which are important predictors of procedural success.[9,10] Other methods are under development that may further enhance the role of CTCA in guiding interventional procedures. Real-time hybrid CTCA and ICA image registration[11] may be used for selecting the best working angulations for reducing foreshortening and vessel overlapping, determining stent size and location and providing a reference vessel path and structure in CTO. Mathematical modelling of contrast flow within the coronary artery allows the functional assessment of stenosis comparable to invasive fractional flow reserve (FFR). The clinical utility of this CT-FFR measurement is currently subject to large scale randomised research.

The role of CTCA following re-vascularisation is less clear. In terms of diagnosing flow limiting disease post-CABG, the ACCF Appropriate Use Criteria classify the

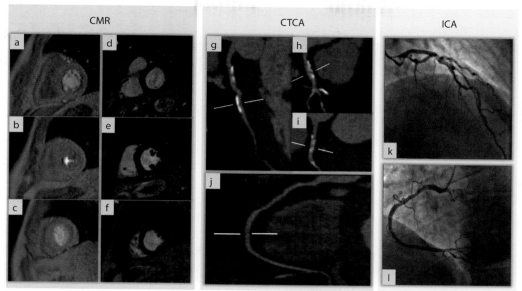

Figure 3.1 Multimodality imaging in a 53-year-old patient who presented with stable chest pain. Panels (a, c) demonstrate normal first-pass stress perfusion on cardiac magnetic resonance imaging. Panels (d, f) demonstrate no evidence of scar on late gadolinium enhancement (LGE) CMR Panels (g–i) are multiplane reconstructed images of the left coronary system on cardiac computed tomography (CT) angiography. Panel g demonstrates the course of left main stem and left anterior descending artery. There is evidence of coronary calcification of the left main stem (LMS) and the left anterior descending (LAD) artery. A closer look at the LMS (h, i) reveals a heterogeneous plaque comprising of soft plaque (dark area) and calcium deposits (hard plaque). Panel j demonstrates minor soft plaque in the proximal segments of the right coronary artery. Panels (k, l) demonstrate invasive coronary angiography (ICA) in the same patient. Even though computed tomography coronary angiography (CTCA) had raised concerns of >50% stenosis in the LMS, ICA and stress perfusion CMR confirmed that the lesion was non-significant.

routine use of CTCA as an inappropriate/uncertain indication or a Class IIb indication, Level of Evidence: C.[12,13] For the assessment of in-stent restenosis after percutaneous coronary intervention the sensitivity of CTCA remains less accurate than ICA due to blooming artefact from the metallic stent struts, although this is less of a problem with latest generation scanners, which have demonstrated better accuracy for the evaluation of coronary stents.[14]

3.2.2 Functional imaging

3.2.2.1 Stress ECHO

Stress ECHO with a physical (treadmill or bicycle), pharmacological (predominantly dobutamine, Table 3.2) or electrical stress (via pacing) allows the assessment of myocardial ischaemia, function and viability. Stress ECHO is the most widely disseminated and inexpensive technique for the assessment of CAD.

The ACCF Appropriate Use Criteria recommend stress ECHO for the investigation of ischaemia in the symptomatic patient with a low pre-test likelihood of CAD and uninterpretable electrocardiogram (ECG) or for patients who are unable to exercise and with intermediate and high pre-test likelihood of CAD irrespective of ECG and exercise status. Stress ECHO is also recommended in asymptomatic patients with new onset LV dysfunction, history of sustained ventricular tachycardia (VT), frequent premature ventricular contractions

(PVCs), exercise-induced VT or non-sustained VT, syncope with intermediate or high CAD risk or troponin elevation without symptoms or additional evidence of acute coronary syndrome (ACS).[15] The 2013 ESC guidelines for the management of stable CAD give a Class I recommendation for non-invasive stress testing of patients with a pre-test probability of 15%–85% and recognise stress ECHO as an imaging option.

Exercise stress ECHO is preferred when feasible due to the additional physiological data that can be acquired during the test, such as exercise time and workload. Pharmacological stress is recommended when there are resting wall motion abnormalities, for concurrent viability and ischaemia assessment, and when exercise is not possible.[16] Trans-pulmonary contrast ultrasound agents must be used when two or more myocardial segments are not seen. This improves visualisation of the endocardial surface and improves diagnostic accuracy[17] (Figure 3.2). A normal stress ECHO is associated with a statistically lower likelihood of hard cardiac events compared with an abnormal stress echo ($p = .001$).[18] A normal stress ECHO implies an excellent prognosis yielding an annual risk of 0.54%.[19]

3.2.2.2 Myocardial perfusion scintigraphy

Radionuclide MPS enables evaluation of cardiac perfusion and function in patients with suspected CAD. MPS has been endorsed in the ACCF Appropriate Use Criteria for investigating patients with stable chest pain as an appropriate test

Table 3.2 Comparison of common pharmacologic agents used for stress testing

	Dobutamine	Adenosine	Regadenoson	Dipyridamole
Compound	Synthetic catecholamine	Endogenous vasodilator of purine derivative	Purine derivative	Pyrimidine derivative
Mechanism of action	Alpha-1, beta-1, and beta-2 stimulation increases myocardial O2 demand and secondary vasodilatation	Stimulation of adenosine receptor A2A causing coronary vasodilation	Stimulates A2A adenosine receptor causes coronary vasodilation	Blocks reuptake of endogenous adenosine causing coronary vasodilation
Onset of action	1–2 minutes	Immediate onset	1–4 minutes	7–15 minutes
Half-life	2 minutes	<15 seconds	30 minutes	30–45 minutes
Dose	5–40 µg/kg per minute, depending upon heart rate response	140–210 mcg/kg per minute for 4–6 minutes	Regadenoson 0.4 mg/5 mL	40 mcg/kg per minute for 4 minutes (maximum 0.56 mg/kg)
Haemodynamic effects	Target heart rate 85% of maximum predicted heart rate	Slight increase in heart rate and slight decrease in blood pressure (BP) (adenosine more than dipyridamole)	Slight increase in heart rate and slight decrease in BP	Slight increase in heart rate and slight decrease in BP
Side effects	Most common palpitations, hot flush and chest pain, most serious non-sustained ventricular tachycardia, non-fatal myocardial infarction	Chest pain and tightness but resolve rapidly; transient atrio-ventricular block	Dyspnoea, headache, and flushing	Most common chest pain

where the pre-test likelihood is intermediate to high.[20] In the low pre-test likelihood group, it is still appropriate to use MPS to rule out myocardial ischaemia, if the ECG is uninterpretable. Similarly, the current ESC guidelines endorse MPS for patients with intermediate pre-test likelihood for CAD.

MPS requires the administration of a radioactive perfusion tracer (also called a radiopharmaceutical or radio-isotope), which is usually administered intravenously, and a gamma camera system, utilising single-photon emission computed tomography (SPECT), for the detection of the gamma photons. MPS images are usually acquired at rest and at stress, most commonly using pharmacological stress with the vasodilators adenosine, dipyridamole or regadenoson (Table 3.2). Mainly, 2-day rest-first MPS protocols are used but increasingly 1-day stress-only imaging is being performed. The benefit of the rest-stress MPS protocol is that it also provides information on the presence or absence of myocardial infarction and viability (Figure 3.3).

MPS is a diagnostic tool for the detection of myocardial ischaemia. It is a well-validated, accurate and non-invasive technique with a sensitivity as high as 90% for the detection of angiographically defined coronary disease.[21] Data

derived from large population studies demonstrate the prognostic value of MPS. In a pooled analysis of 20,963 patients from 16 published studies in the literature with a follow-up of slightly more than 2 years, the hard event rate, that is cardiac death and non-fatal myocardial infarction (MI), was only 0.7% per year.[22]

3.2.2.3 Cardiovascular magnetic resonance

CMR is an expanding imaging modality for the functional and anatomical assessment of a wide range of cardiovascular disease. CMR is safe, does not use ionising radiation, provides prognostic information, changes clinical outcomes and guides management (Table 3.3).[23,24]

CMR is increasingly included in both national and international clinical guidelines for the investigation of patients presenting with stable chest pain.[3,4,25] The ESC guidelines on the management of stable CAD give a Class I recommendation for non-invasive stress testing for those patients with a pre-test probability of 15%–85%, with stress perfusion CMR being one of the recommended imaging options.[4]

A stress CMR study takes around 30–60 minutes and typically includes cine images in multiple planes for

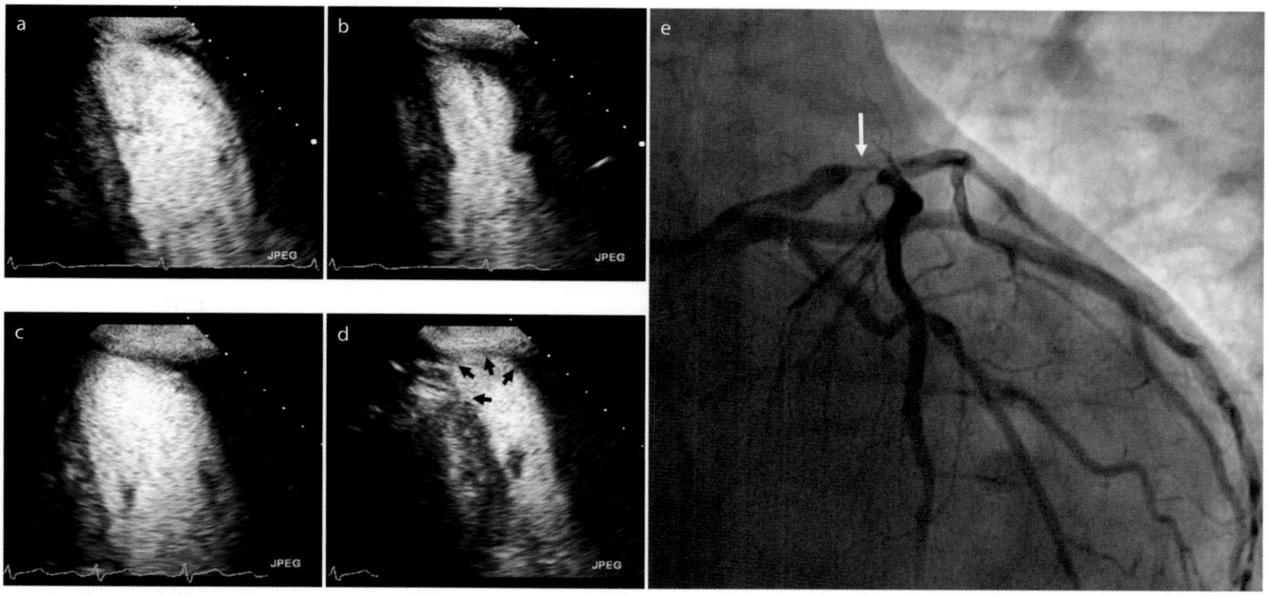

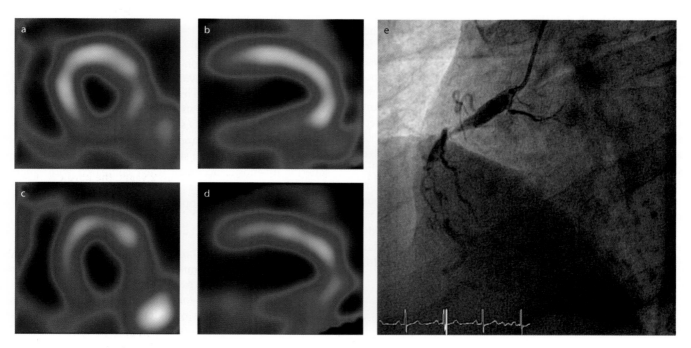

Figure 3.2 Contrast enhanced stress echocardiography (stress ECHO) in a 47-year-old male patient who presented to the local chest pain clinic with stable symptoms. Panels (a, b) demonstrate resting end-diastolic **(a)** and end-systolic **(b)** frames of the two chamber view on contrast enhanced stress-ECHO. Panels **(c, d)** demonstrate end-diastolic (c) and end-systolic (d) frames of the two chamber view at peak stress. In the peak stress end-systolic frame (d), apical dyskinesia (black arrows) is seen with hypercontractility of all other segments. Panel **(e)** demonstrates severe stenosis of the left anterior descending artery (white arrow) at subsequent elective diagnostic ICA.

Figure 3.3 Single photon emission computed tomography myocardial perfusion scintigraphy (MPS) in a 60-year-old male patient who presented with mild shortness of breath and typical cardiac chest pain. Panels **(a)** (short-axis) and **(b)** (long-axis) are rest MPS images demonstrating reduced perfusion to the basal and mid inferior wall. This is suggestive of sub-endocardial scar. Panels **(c)** (short-axis) and **(d)** (long-axis) are stress MPS images demonstrating reduced perfusion in the infarct and peri-infarct zone which is involving five to six segments (>10% myocardial ischaemic burden). This scan suggested that the patient had an inferior infarct and some preserved viable myocardium and significant ischaemia in the right coronary artery territory. Panel **(e)** demonstrates chronic total occlusion of the proximal right coronary artery at subsequent elective diagnostic ICA.

Table 3.3 Comparison of all the imaging modalities in patients presenting with stable and acute onset chest pain of uncertain origin

	TTE/SE	CTCA	MPS/PET	CMR
Bedside	+++	−	−	−
Low cost	+++	+	+	−
Ionising radiation exposure	−	++	++	−
Feasibility of use in cath lab	+++	−	−	−
Availability in non-tertiary centre	+++	++	++	+
Coronary anatomy/plaque tissue characterisation	−	+++	−	+
Regional wall motion	++	+	++	+++
Scar	+	−	++	+++
Viability	+	−	++	+++
Myocardial oedema	−	−	−	+++
Differential diagnosis	+	+++	−	−
• Pulmonary embolus	−	−	−	+++
• Myocarditis	+	+	−	++
• Pericarditis	−	+++	−	++
• Chest infection (consolidation)	−	+++	−	+++

Abbreviations: CMR, cardiovascular magnetic resonance imaging; CTCA, computed tomography coronary angiography; MPS, myocardial perfusion scanning; PET, positron emission tomography; SE, stress echocardiography; TTE, transthoracic echocardiography.

assessment of LV volumes and global and regional function, stress and rest perfusion for the detection of myocardial ischaemia and late gadolinium enhancement (LGE) for the delineation of scar (Figure 3.4). The combination of these above techniques in a single multiparametric examination allows the quantification of ischaemic burden and assessment of myocardial viability, which can be used to risk-stratify patients and guide re-vascularisation. The use of CMR as a first-line diagnostic tool in patients presenting with chest pain has been subject to clinical trials showing high diagnostic accuracy for the detection of significant CAD.[26,27] One recent meta-analysis demonstrated a pooled sensitivity of 89% (95% confidence interval [CI]: 88%–91%) and specificity of 76% (95%CI: 73%–78%).[28] Non-invasive coronary angiography by CMR is not recommended for the detection of coronary artery stenosis, but like CTCA, it can identify the presence and anatomical course of anomalous coronary arteries.[29]

As for other functional tests, a normal stress CMR study is associated with a very low major adverse cardiovascular event rate and an excellent 1-year prognosis in patients with suspected CAD.[30]

3.2.2.4 Positron emission tomography

Cardiac PET is a nuclear medicine technique using intravenous injection of a radiotracer for the evaluation of perfusion and viability. PET can be used to quantify both perfusion and metabolism as well as determine myocardial viability. PET requires the use of cyclotron-produced positron-emitting isotopes (e.g. [82]rubidium, ^{13}N-ammonia). Although there is less evidence than for MPS, meta-analyses have suggested that PET has higher sensitivity for the detection of CAD than MPS, including in women and obese patients,[31,32] likely

due to its higher spatial resolution. The ESC guidelines for the management of stable chest pain include PET as an non-invasive stress imaging option.[4] PET is the gold standard test for the non-invasive quantification of myocardial blood flow, allowing the detection of microvascular disease.

3.2.2.5 Hybrid imaging

Hybrid applications of non-invasive imaging are becoming available that typically involve anatomical imaging (CTCA) combined with functional imaging for ischaemia (PET, MPS) (Figure 3.5). This combination offers a promising algorithm for the evaluation of CAD since it allows anatomical detection of coronary stenosis and assessment of a lesion's haemodynamic significance in a single study and it seems to offer superior diagnostic accuracy when compared with single modality imaging.[33] Other combinations including PET and CMR are also being developed.

3.2.2.6 Which test for which indication?

For the detection of CAD in patients with stable symptoms, guidelines generally recommend the use of CTCA for lower risk patients in view of its excellent negative predictive value. In intermediate risk patients and in those where ICA has shown coronary stenosis of indeterminate functional significance, the value of stress ECHO, MPS, CMR and PET is generally considered to be similar and the choice of one of these methods is often determined by local availability and expertise. CTCA with CT-FFR may play a future role in this patient group. In patients with a history of myocardial infarction, scar imaging with LGE CMR appears to provide the best assessment of residual myocardial viability to guide re-vascularisation, although no large-scale clinical trials have yet demonstrated its clinical value.

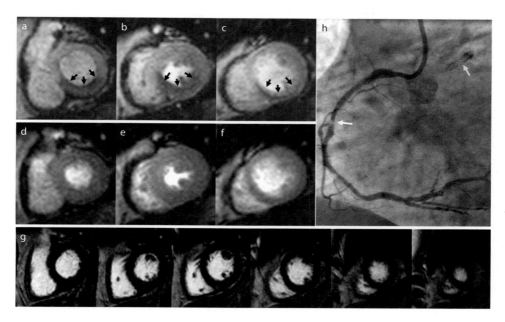

Figure 3.4 First-pass stress perfusion cardiac magnetic resonance (CMR) imaging in a 57-year-old female patient. The patient had a history of coronary artery disease with percutaneous intervention to the left anterior descending artery 2 years ago and represented with stable chest pain symptoms. Panels **(a–c)** demonstrate three-slice stress perfusion images from base to apex. A perfusion defect is seen in the inferior wall in all three slices (black arrows), involving at least six segments (36% myocardial ischaemic burden). Panels **(d–f)** demonstrate three-slice rest perfusion images from base to apex showing no perfusion defects. Panel **(g)** shows LGE images of the complete ventricle with normal signal distribution in all segments suggesting that this patient has not had previous myocardial infarction. Panel **(h)** demonstrates severe stenosis of the mid-right coronary artery (white arrow) at subsequent elective diagnostic ICA. The previous stent in the left anterior descending artery can be noted in this view (yellow arrow).

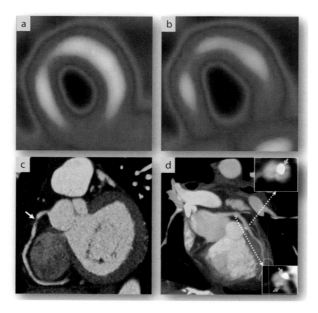

Figure 3.5 Single photon emission computed tomography (CT) imaging (functional imaging) and echocardiogram (ECG)-gated cardiac CT (anatomical imaging) in a 75-year-old female patient who presented with cardiac sounding chest pain. Panel **(a)** (rest myocardial perfusion scintigraphy [MPS] images) demonstrates reduced perfusion to the inferior wall suggesting sub-endocardial scar in the segment. Panel **(b)** (stress MPS images) demonstrates marked perfusion defect at stress, suggestive of significant ischaemia in the inferior segments. CT coronary angiography demonstrates soft-plaque in the proximal right coronary artery **(c)**, which is greater than 75% of the lumen diameter, suggesting a significant coronary lesion. The left coronary arteries did not have any significant coronary stenosis **(d)**, however, coronary calcification (orange arrows in both sub-panels) was identified at the level of proximal and mid left anterior descending artery. A minor soft plaque was seen in the proximal segment (red arrows in inferior sub-panel).

3.3 Acute chest pain assessment

Acute chest pain remains one of the main symptoms of presentation and admission to hospital. It contributes approximately 20%–40% of all medical admissions. Even though contemporary biomarkers of myocardial injury are very sensitive in detecting ACS, their specificity tends to be low.

Cardiac imaging can contribute to the diagnosis of ACS, in particular when combined with the clinical history, ECG findings and cardiac biomarkers. When cardiac imaging is used appropriately in this setting, it can reduce the number of missed ACS, filter out those who were wrongly diagnosed as ACS and guide the management of those with confirmed ACS.

In patients with confirmed ACS, cardiac imaging can be used to confirm the presence of ischaemia in the culprit vessel territory and detect ischaemia in non-culprit coronary territories. In addition, non-invasive imaging provides information on the extent of infarction and presence of residual viable myocardium to guide re-vascularisation decisions. Furthermore, functional non-invasive imaging can complement diagnostic ICA to determine the functional significance of any observed coronary lesions and the extent of ischaemia to inform the choice of the re-vascularisation strategy.

The available non-invasive imaging tests have different strengths and limitations in the setting of acute chest pain presentations and thus differ in their clinical use.

3.3.1 Echocardiography

Bedsides transthoracic ECHO has been endorsed by both European and American guidelines as the first-line imaging modality with Class 1, level C evidence for the diagnosis of RWMA in patients with acute chest pain where the initial ECG and troponin results are equivocal.[34,35] Using ECHO in this context can speed up diagnostic time and facilitate rapid reperfusion therapy if warranted.[36] In patients with acute chest pain, a bedside echo provides structural information of any acute mechanical complication secondary to ACS, for example, papillary muscle rupture, ventricular septal defect and mitral regurgitation. If the echo windows are not adequate for interpretation, use of contrast can improve the detection of RWMA and can allow detection of perfusion defects. Contrast ECHO can also provide incremental mid-term (30 days) and long-term (2 years) prognostic information over a modified thrombolysis in myocardial infarction (mTIMI) score[37] in patients with suspected ACS (Table 3.4).

3.3.2 Stress ECHO

Similar to resting echo, stress ECHO has also been endorsed by guidelines in patients with suspected ACS with Class I, level A evidence.[15,34] Its role is mainly in patients with no resting chest pain, normal ECG, negative troponins and a low-risk score. Several studies have demonstrated high sensitivity (85%) and specificity (95%) for stress ECHO to diagnose ACS.[38] A negative stress ECHO also provides reassuring prognostic information in such patient populations. A prospective, double-blind, multicentre stress ECHO study of 377 low-risk patients presenting to the emergency department with acute chest pain demonstrated a 6-month risk of composite cardiac events of 4% in patients with a negative stress ECHO and 30.8% in patients with a positive stress ECHO ($p < .0001$).[39]

3.3.3 Cardiac computed tomography

CTCA has been endorsed by the 'Appropriate Use Criteria for Cardiac Computed Tomography' and by the ESC guidelines as an appropriate test in the context of acute chest pain

Table 3.4 Pitfalls of imaging modalities in patients presenting with acute onset chest pain

Imaging modality	Pitfalls
TTE	• Poor endocardial definition reduces diagnostic yield • Quantification not as reliable as other techniques • Reliability is questionable when symptoms subside
CTCA	• Coronary calcium interferes with interpretation • Functionally non-significant lesions (moderate stenosis) can lead to increased invasive angiograms • Patients with fast heart rates, atrial fibrillation and abnormal renal function may not be eligible • Entails radiation exposure and iodinated contrast (nephrotoxic)
Rest MPS	• Patients with fast heart rates, atrial fibrillation and abnormal renal function may not be eligible • Entails radiation exposure • Soft-tissue (breast) attenuation artefacts reduce the diagnostic accuracy of the test
CMR	• Approximately 5% patients suffer from claustrophobia in CMR • Patients with fast heart rates, high burden of ventricular ectopics are challenging to acquire good images • Ferro-magnetic implants may not be eligible for CMR • Patients with severe renal impairment are contraindicated to have gadolinium-based contrast

CMR, cardiovascular magnetic resonance imaging; CTCA, computed tomography coronary angiography; MPS, myocardial perfusion scanning; TTE, transthoracic echocardiography.

patients with non-diagnostic ECGs, normal/equivocal bio-markers in the low/intermediate pre-test probability group with class IIa, level B evidence.[7,34] CTCA is an alternative to ICA to exclude ACS and other causes of chest pain (pulmonary embolus, consolidation, aortic dissection, etc.). A recent meta-analysis of CTCA in this setting demonstrated high sensitivity (93%) and specificity (90%) to predict major cardiovascular events (MACE) at 30 days.[40] There is some evidence to suggest that incorporation of CTCA in the emergency department to assess suspected ACS patients may lead to an increase in requests for invasive diagnostic angiography.[41] Long-term outcome studies have shown excellent prognosis if the initial CTCA was negative.[42]

3.3.4 Myocardial perfusion scintigraphy

MPS has been endorsed both by the American 'Appropriate Use Criteria for Cardiac Radionuclide' and the ESC guidelines as an appropriate test for patients with suspected ACS where ECG and biomarkers fail to confirm the diagnosis.[34,43] In a pooled analysis of several studies with greater than 2000 patients, rest MPS has demonstrated similar high sensitivity (90%) and specificity (80%) to diagnose ACS in these chest pain patients.[44] A negative rest MPS has also been shown

to provide modest short-term prognosis (3% MACE with negative MPS versus 10%–30% MACE with positive MPS) and long-term prognosis (0% MI/death versus 11% MI/8% cardiac death; $p < .001$).[45,46] Even though rest MPS is a reasonable rule out test, its sensitivity in patients who no longer have chest pain is much lower and also rest MPS cannot differentiate acute ischaemia from an old infarct unless a follow-up scan in a pain free state is performed.

Initial stress MPS in low-risk patients is safe and has similar performance to rest MPS alone.[47] After the initial chest pain has settled, a stress–rest MPS protocol to detect inducible hypoperfusion is more accurate and has greater prognostic value than rest MPS alone.[48]

3.3.5 Cardiovascular magnetic resonance

Stress CMR has been endorsed both by the American and the ESC guidelines with Class I, level A evidence for its role in the assessment of acute chest pain patients when initial ECG and cardiac biomarkers are non-diagnostic.[13,34] Compared with the other imaging modalities, multiparametric CMR can provide the most comprehensive information on ischaemia, myocardial oedema, scar and regional wall dysfunction (Figure 3.6). In the context of raised

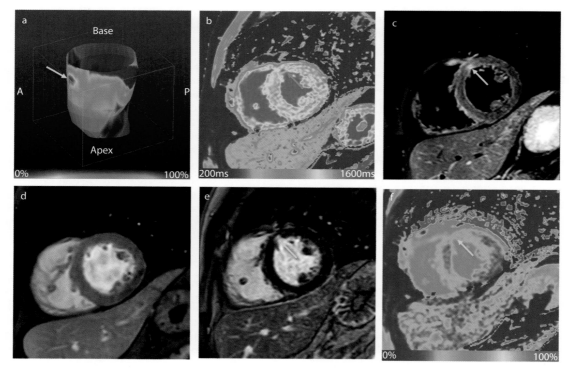

Figure 3.6 Multi-parametric cardiac magnetic resonance (CMR) imaging in a patient with suspected acute coronary syndrome (ACS). (a) Three-dimensional wall motion colour-map demonstrating an area of hypokinesia and akinesia (yellow arrow). (b) Short-axis native T1-map demonstrating elevated T1 in the anterior wall (green arrow), suggestive of tissue oedema. (c) T2-weighted imaging demonstrating myocardial oedema in the same segment (yellow arrow). (d) Early gadolinium enhancement imaging demonstrating absence of microvascular obstruction. (e) LGE imaging showing a small subendocardial scar in the anterior wall (yellow arrow). (f) Extracellular volume (ECV) calculated from the pre-/post-contrast T1-maps demonstrates a small area of ECV expansion (myocardial oedema/infarction) in the same segments (yellow arrow). (Adapted from Garg et al., Nat Card Rews, 2016.)[49]

biomarkers, CMR can help differentiate myocardial infarction and other causes of acutely raised cardiac biomarkers like acute myocarditis. Several small-scale studies have demonstrated feasibility and safety of CMR in acute chest pain patients and have shown high diagnostic accuracy for the detection of ACS (sensitivity 96%–84% and specificity of 85%–83% for CAD).[50] The addition of T2-weighted imaging for assessment of myocardial oedema can further increase the detection of acute myocardial infarction.[51] Similar to other imaging modalities, patients with negative stress CMR have excellent short-/long-term prognosis.[52]

3.3.6 Which test for which indication?

In the initial assessment of patients with acute chest pain, who do not have an indication for urgent invasive angiography, bedside ECHO and CT can aid the diagnosis of ACS and the differential diagnosis of other conditions. In patients with a diagnosis of ACS, all functional imaging tests (stress ECHO, CMR or MPS) can complement invasive assessment in the catheter laboratory by providing information on the presence and extent of inducible ischaemia. For assessment of scar extent, CMR appears to be the most appropriate test. CMR is also the most useful test for the differential diagnosis of patients with ACS presentation and angiographically normal coronary arteries, as myocarditis, cardiomyopathy (including Tako-tsubo cardiomyopathy), and focal infarction following spontaneous reperfusion can be reliably identified and differentiated.

References

1. Heidenreich PA et al. Forecasting the future of cardiovascular disease in the United States: A policy statement from the American Heart Association. *Circulation* 2011; 123: 933–44.
2. Liu JLY, et al. The economic burden of coronary heart disease in the UK. *Heart* 2002 Dec; 88(6):597–603.
3. Fihn SD et al. 2012 ACCF/AHA/ACP/AATS/PCNA/SCAI/STS guideline for the diagnosis and management of patients with stable ischemic heart disease: A report of the American College of Cardiology Foundation/American Heart Association task force on practice guidelines, and the. *Circulation* 2012; 126: e354–471.
4. Montalescot G et al. 2013 ESC guidelines on the management of stable coronary artery disease: The Task Force on the management of stable coronary artery disease of the European Society of Cardiology. *Eur Heart J* 2013; 34: 2949–3003.
5. Raggi P et al. Evaluation of chest pain in patients with low to intermediate pretest probability of coronary artery disease by electron beam computed tomography. *Am J Cardiol* 2000; 85: 283–886.
6. Gottlieb I et al. The absence of coronary calcification does not exclude obstructive coronary artery disease or the need for revascularization in patients referred for conventional coronary angiography. *J Am Coll Cardiol.* 2010 Feb 16;55(7):627–634.
7. Taylor AJ et al. ACCF/SCCT/ACR/AHA/ASE/ASNC/NASCI/SCAI/SCMR 2010 appropriate use criteria for cardiac computed tomography. A report of the American College of Cardiology Foundation Appropriate Use Criteria Task Force, the Society of Cardiovascular Computed Tomography, the American College of Radiology, the American Heart Association, the American Society of Echocardiography, the American Society of Nuclear Cardiology, the North American Society for Cardiovascular Imaging, the Society for Cardiovascular Angiography and Interventions, and the Society for Cardiovascular Magnetic Resonance. *J Am Coll Cardiol* 2010; 56: 1864–94.
8. Chow BJW et al. Incremental prognostic value of cardiac computed tomography in coronary artery disease using confirm coronary computed tomography angiography evaluation for clinical outcomes: An international multi-center registry. *Circ Cardiovasc Imaging* 2011; 4: 463–72.
9. García-García HM et al. Computed tomography in total coronary occlusions (CTTO registry): Radiation exposure and predictors of successful percutaneous intervention. *EuroIntervention* 2009; 4: 607–16.
10. Cho JR et al. Quantification of regional calcium burden in chronic total occlusion by 64-slice multi-detector computed tomography and procedural outcomes of percutaneous coronary intervention. *Int J Cardiol* 2010; 145: 9–14.
11. Roguin A et al. Novel method for real-time hybrid cardiac CT and coronary angiography image registration: Visualising beyond luminology, proof-of-concept. *EuroIntervention* 2009; 4: 648–53.
12. Budoff MJ et al. Assessment of coronary artery disease by cardiac computed tomography: A scientific statement from the American Heart Association Committee on Cardiovascular Imaging and Intervention, Council on Cardiovascular Radiology and Intervention, and Committee on C. *Circulation* 2006; 114: 1761–91.
13. Hendel RC et al. ACCF/ACR/SCCT/SCMR/ASNC/NASCI/SCAI/SIR 2006 appropriateness criteria for cardiac computed tomography and cardiac magnetic resonance imaging: A report of the American College of Cardiology Foundation Quality Strategic Directions Committee Appropriateness C. *J Am Coll Cardiol* 2006; 48: 1475–97.
14. Yang WJ et al. High-definition computed tomography for coronary artery stents imaging compared with standard-definition 64-row multidectector computed tomography: An initial in vivo study. *J Comput Assist Tomogr* 2012; 36: 295–300.
15. Douglas PS et al. ACCF/ASE/AHA/ASNC/HFSA/HRS/SCAI/SCCM/SCCT/SCMR 2011 Appropriate use criteria for echocardiography. A report of the American College of Cardiology Foundation Appropriate Use Criteria Task Force, American Society of Echocardiography, American Heart Association, American Society of Nuclear Cardiology, Heart Failure Society of America, Heart Rhythm Society, Society for Cardiovascular Angiography and Interventions, Society of Critical Care Medicine, Society of Cardiovascular Computed Tomography, and Society for Cardiovascular Magnetic Resonance Endorsed by the American College of Chest Physicians. *J Am Coll Cardiol* 2011; 57: 1126–66.
16. Marwick TH. Stress echocardiography. *Heart* 2003; 89: 113–8.

17. Plana JC et al. A randomized cross-over study for evaluation of the effect of image optimization with contrast on the diagnostic accuracy of dobutamine echocardiography in coronary artery disease The OPTIMIZE Trial. *JACC Cardiovasc Imaging* 2008; 1: 145–52.

18. Marcovitz PA et al. Value of dobutamine stress echocardiography in determining the prognosis of patients with known or suspected coronary artery disease. *Am J Cardiol* 1996; 78: 404–8.

19. Metz LD et al. The prognostic value of normal exercise myocardial perfusion imaging and exercise echocardiography: A meta-analysis. *J Am Coll Cardiol* 2007; 49: 227–37.

20. Wolk MJ et al. ACCF/AHA/ASE/ASNC/HFSA/HRS/SCAI/ SCCT/SCMR/STS 2013 multimodality appropriate use criteria for the detection and risk assessment of stable ischemic heart disease. *J Am Coll Cardiol* 2014; 63: 380–406.

21. de Jong MC et al. Diagnostic performance of stress myocardial perfusion imaging for coronary artery disease: A systematic review and meta-analysis. *Eur Radiol* 2012; 22: 1881–95.

22. Klocke FJ et al. ACC/AHA/ASNC guidelines for the clinical use of cardiac radionuclide imaging– executive summary: A report of the American College of Cardiology/American Heart Association Task Force on Practice Guidelines (ACC/ AHA/ASNC) Committee to Revise the 1995 Guidelines. *J Am Coll Cardiol* 2003; 42: 1318–33.

23. Bruder O et al. European Cardiovascular Magnetic Resonance (EuroCMR) registry – Multi national results from 57 centers in 15 countries. *J Cardiovasc Magn Reson* 2013; 15: 9.

24. Flett AS et al. The prognostic implications of cardiovascular magnetic resonance. *Circ Cardiovasc Imaging* 2009; 2: 243–50.

25. McMurray JJ et al. ESC Guidelines for the diagnosis and treatment of acute and chronic heart failure 2012: The Task Force for the Diagnosis and Treatment of Acute and Chronic Heart Failure 2012 of the European Society of Cardiology. Developed in collaboration with the Heart. *Eur Heart J* 2012; 33: 1787–847.

26. Greenwood JP et al. Cardiovascular magnetic resonance and single-photon emission computed tomography for diagnosis of coronary heart disease (CE-MARC): A prospective trial. *Lancet (London, England)* 2012; 379: 453–60.

27. Schwitter J et al. MR-IMPACT II: Magnetic Resonance Imaging for Myocardial Perfusion Assessment in Coronary artery disease Trial: Perfusion-cardiac magnetic resonance vs. single-photon emission computed tomography for the detection of coronary artery disease: A comparative. *Eur Heart J* 2013; 34: 775–81.

28. Jaarsma C et al. Diagnostic performance of noninvasive myocardial perfusion imaging using single-photon emission computed tomography, cardiac magnetic resonance, and positron emission tomography imaging for the detection of obstructive coronary artery disease: A meta-anal. *J Am Coll Cardiol* 2012; 59: 1719–28.

29. Ripley DP et al. The distribution and prognosis of anomalous coronary arteries identified by cardiovascular magnetic resonance: 15-year experience from two tertiary centres. *J Cardiovasc Magn Reson* 2014; 16: 34.

30. Greenwood JP et al. Prognostic value of cardiovascular magnetic resonance and single-photon emission computed tomography in suspected coronary heart disease: Long-term follow-up of a prospective, diagnostic accuracy cohort study. *Ann Intern Med* 2016 Jul 5;165(1):1.

31. Sampson UK et al. Diagnostic accuracy of rubidium-82 myocardial perfusion imaging with hybrid positron emission tomography/computed tomography in the detection of coronary artery disease. *J Am Coll Cardiol* 2007; 49: 1052–8.

32. Nandalur KR et al. Diagnostic performance of positron emission tomography in the detection of coronary artery disease: A meta-analysis. *Acad Radiol* 2008; 15: 444–51.

33. Slomka PJ et al. Quantitative analysis of myocardial perfusion SPECT anatomically guided by coregistered 64-slice coronary CT angiography. *J Nucl Med* 2009; 50: 1621–30.

34. Hamm CW et al. ESC Guidelines for the management of acute coronary syndromes in patients presenting without persistent ST-segment elevation: The Task Force for the management of acute coronary syndromes (ACS) in patients presenting without persistent ST-segment elevation. *Eur Heart J* 2011; 32: 2999–3054.

35. Steg PG et al. ESC Guidelines for the management of acute myocardial infarction in patients presenting with ST-segment elevation. *Eur Heart J* 2012; 33: 2569–619.

36. Mohler ER et al. Clinical utility of troponin T levels and echocardiography in the emergency department. *Am Heart J* 1998; 135: 253–60.

37. Tong KL et al. Myocardial contrast echocardiography versus Thrombolysis In Myocardial Infarction score in patients presenting to the emergency department with chest pain and a nondiagnostic electrocardiogram. *J Am Coll Cardiol* 2005; 46: 920–7.

38. Conti A et al. Assessment of patients with low-risk chest pain in the emergency department: Head-to-head comparison of exercise stress echocardiography and exercise myocardial SPECT. *Am Heart J* 2005; 149: 894–901.

39. Bholasingh R et al. Prognostic value of predischarge dobutamine stress echocardiography in chest pain patients with a negative cardiac troponin T. *J Am Coll Cardiol* 2003; 41: 596–602.

40. Takakuwa KM et al. A meta-analysis of 64-section coronary CT angiography findings for predicting 30-day major adverse cardiac events in patients presenting with symptoms suggestive of acute coronary syndrome. *Acad Radiol* 2011; 18: 1522–8.

41. Hulten E et al. Outcomes after coronary computed tomography angiography in the emergency department: A systematic review and meta-analysis of randomized, controlled trials. *J Am Coll Cardiol* 2013; 61: 880–92.

42. Nasis A et al. Long-term outcome after CT angiography in patients with possible acute coronary syndrome. *Radiology* 2014; 272: 674–82.

43. Hendel RC et al. ACCF/ASNC/ACR/AHA/ASE/SCCT/ SCMR/SNM 2009 Appropriate Use Criteria for Cardiac Radionuclide Imaging: A Report of the American College of Cardiology Foundation Appropriate Use Criteria Task Force, the American Society of Nuclear Cardiology, the American Col. *J Am Coll Cardiol* 2009; 53: 2201–29.

44. Sechtem U et al. Non-invasive imaging in acute chest pain syndromes. *Eur Heart J Cardiovasc Imaging* 2012; 13: 69–78.

45. Heller GV et al. Clinical value of acute rest technetium-99m tetrofosmin tomographic myocardial perfusion imaging in

patients with acute chest pain and nondiagnostic electro-cardiograms. *J Am Coll Cardiol* 1998; 31: 1011–7.

46. Tatum JL et al. Comprehensive strategy for the evaluation and triage of the chest pain patient. *Ann Emerg Med* 1997; 29: 116–25.

47. Duvall WL et al. Stress-only Tc-99m myocardial perfusion imaging in an emergency department chest pain unit. *J Emerg Med* 2012; 42: 642–50.

48. Fesmire FM et al. The Erlanger chest pain evaluation protocol: A one-year experience with serial 12-lead ECG monitoring, two-hour delta serum marker measurements, and selective nuclear stress testing to identify and exclude acute coronary syndromes. *Ann Emerg Med* 2002; 40: 584–94.

49. Garg P et al. Noninvasive cardiac imaging in suspected acute coronary syndrome. *Nat Rev Cardiol* 2016 May;13(5):266–275.

50. Plein S et al. Assessment of non-ST-segment elevation acute coronary syndromes with cardiac magnetic resonance imaging. *J Am Coll Cardiol* 2004; 44: 2173–81.

51. Cury RC et al. Cardiac magnetic resonance with T2-weighted imaging improves detection of patients with acute coronary syndrome in the emergency department. *Circulation* 2008; 118: 837–44.

52. Miller CD et al. Stress CMR imaging observation unit in the emergency department reduces 1-year medical care costs in patients with acute chest pain: A randomized study for comparison with inpatient care. *JACC Cardiovasc Imaging* 2011; 4: 862–70.

Coronary intravascular ultrasound (IVUS)

AMR S GAMAL, JAVED AHMED, GARY S MINTZ

Coronary angiography has been the gold standard for assessment of coronary anatomy since first performed by Mason Sones in 1958.[1] However, the coronary angiogram has many limitations; it gives us information about the patency of the arterial lumen (lumenography) but no information about the vessel wall. In addition, it depends on the visual estimation of the severity of lesion which could be misleading as we compare the diseased part of the vessel to a nearby presumed normal reference segment which is not always the case. This is clearly evident when we examine patients who have minimal coronary artery disease (CAD) on invasive coronary angiography despite the presence of extensive disease on coronary computed tomography (CT) angiography. Furthermore, assessment of lesion severity has shown to be unreliable with significant inter-observer and intra-observer variability.[2]

In 1972, Bom et al. developed the first ultrasound imaging catheter for use in humans.[3] This was used within the cardiac chambers to obtain internal dimensions and to assess heart valves. Work on coronary intravascular ultrasound (IVUS) started in 1982 and by 1988 the first coronary images were recorded.[4]

The use of IVUS allows excellent visualisation not only of the vessel lumen but also of the surrounding vessel wall providing a detailed assessment of the extent of CAD for proper decision-making.[5-7] This is dependent on a physical property of sound waves which penetrate well through the vessel wall. Additionally, the extent of disease and the reference vessel size could be easily measured which is very important for guidance of stent placement and procedural success. Furthermore, IVUS can differentiate plaque components by their acoustic characteristics.[8]

IVUS has been used for many years in clinical situations such as ambiguous lesion, assessment of left main stenosis and evaluation of restenosis and stent thrombosis (ST). Additionally, it has been the cornerstone for research trials evaluating the response of the vascular bed after percutaneous transluminal coronary angioplasty (PTCA) or implantation of bare-metal stents (BMS), drug-eluting stents (DES) and more recently bioresorbable vascular scaffolds (BVS).

Moreover, IVUS has been used to monitor progression or regression of the burden of atherosclerotic plaque in various trials and for surveillance for development and progression of transplant vasculopathy in cardiac transplant patients. Without IVUS, such information would be only available through autopsy studies.

By knowing the composition of the plaque, IVUS can help with strategic planning; for example by guiding the use of specialised interventional techniques, such as the use of rotational atherectomy in heavily calcified lesions or directional atherectomy in bifurcation lesions or lesions with a large plaque burden. It has also been important in chronic total occlusions (CTO) intervention by guiding wire position into the true distal lumen.

4.1 Principle of IVUS examination

IVUS is based upon the same principles used for ultrasound elsewhere in the body. It utilises a monorail catheter with an ultrasound transducer at its tip to generate a two-dimensional cross-sectional image of the coronary artery similar to a histologic cross section. Due to their different acoustic properties, the intima, media and adventitia are readily differentiated.

For the purpose of guiding percutaneous coronary intervention (PCI) procedures, we select the worst lesion site (minimal luminal diameter [MLD]) and compare it to a relatively normal, adjacent reference site.

Basically IVUS has three major components: a catheter incorporating a miniaturised ultrasound transducer, a pullback device and a console containing the electronics necessary to reconstruct the image.[5-8]

4.1.1 IVUS catheters

Depending on the manufacturer, current IVUS catheters in use range from 20 to 60 MHz for coronary imaging and 10 to 20 MHz for peripheral imaging. With increasing frequency, radial resolution is improved which comes at the expense of tissue penetration.

Currently, two types of IVUS catheter designs are available for use: solid state and rotational. The catheter is usually centred in the lumen of the vessel. Depending on the type of the IVUS catheter used, its diameter ranges from 0.87 to 1.17 mm, which could be used as a reference for sizing of balloons and stents (Table 4.1). Short monorail catheters are accompanied by a guidewire artefact that is not seen with the long-monorail solid-state catheter.

4.1.1.1 Solid-state (phased electronic array) IVUS

The IVUS catheter has multiple transducer elements that are mounted in an annular way at the tip of the imaging catheter. Those elements are activated sequentially in a rotational fashion in order to generate an ultrasound beam. The resulting ultrasound information is then transferred to a computer system which in turn generates a cross-sectional, real-time image. The only commercially available solid-state catheter currently available (Volcano Corporation) has 64 separate transducer elements and uses a 20 MHz scanning frequency. These catheters are 3.5 French in size at the transducer and are compatible with a 5-French guiding catheter over a 0.014" (inch) guidewire. Larger devices are also available for use over both 0.018- and 0.035" wires and are designed for use in the peripheral vessels and aorta. Electronic systems can also provide simultaneous coloration of blood flow. In addition to the conventional grey-scale IVUS images, the Volcano solid-state catheters perform radiofrequency IVUS, also known as virtual histology or VH-IVUS.

4.1.1.2 Rotational (mechanical) IVUS

The IVUS catheter has a single transducer element located at its tip that is rotated by an external motor drive attached

Table 4.1 Comparison of different coronary IVUS catheters

	Boston Scientific		Volcano			ACIST
	OptiCross™	Atlantis™	Eagle eye™ Gold	Eagle eye™ Platinum	Revolution™	Kodama™ HD IVUS
Transducer design	Rotational	Rotational	Phased array	Phased array	Rotational	Rotational
Transducer frequency	40 MHz	40 MHz	20 MHz	20 MHz	45 MHz	40–60 MHz
Transducer profile	2.6 Fr/0.87 mm	3.2 Fr/1.07 mm	3.5 Fr/1.17 mm	3.5 Fr/1.17 mm	3.2 Fr/1.07 mm	3.2 Fr/1.07 mm
Transducer max OD + GW	0.054"/1.37 mm (0.040" + 0.014")	0.061"/1.55 mm (0.047" + 0.014")	0.056"/1.42 mm (0.042" + 0.014")	0.056"/1.42 mm (0.042" + 0.014")	0.060"/1.52 mm (0.046" + 0.014")	0.061"/1.55 mm (0.047" + 0.014")
Guide catheter compatibility	5 Fr/1.67 mm	6 Fr/2.0 mm	5 Fr/1.67 mm	5 Fr/1.67 mm	6 Fr/2.0 mm	6 Fr/2.0 mm
Tip to transducer distance	20 mm	20 mm	≤10.5 mm	≤10 mm	30 mm	20 mm

OD, outer diameter; GW, guidewire; IVUS, intravascular ultrasound to the proximal end of the catheter at 1800 rpm (30 revolutions per second).

As the transducer rotates, ultrasound information is generated, and after it is reflected from tissue, collected to generate a circumferential cross-sectional image. As the rotating transducer sits inside the catheter, there is a very short rapid exchange portion at the tip of the catheters for use with a 0.014" guidewire. Currently, there are four commercially available rotational coronary imaging catheters (Boston Scientific, Volcano, Infraredx and ACIST). The OptisCross Boston Scientific coronary catheter is 2.6 French in size, is compatible through a 5-French catheter, and uses a 40-MHz scanning frequency. The Volcano rotational catheter has a 3.2-French crossing profile and is compatible through a 6-French sheath and uses a scanning frequency of 45 MHz. The Infraredx device has a 3.2-French crossing profile is compatible through a 6-French sheath and uses a 40-MHz scanning frequency; the Infraredx catheter also provides the ability to perform near-infrared spectroscopy (NIRS) in addition to IVUS. The ACIST device incorporates the first high-definition transducer that images at 60 MHz. It has 3.2-French crossing profile and is compatible through a 6-French guiding catheter (Table 4.1).

4.1.2 Pullback device

The transducer pullback can be done either manually or using a motorised pullback device which withdraws the catheter at a constant speed (between 0.25 and 1 mm/s; most frequently, 0.5 mm/s), although ACIST allows pullback at 20 mm/s.[6,7]

Assessment of lesion length by IVUS is only possible using motorised transducer pullback. Other advantages of motorised pullback are (1) controlled catheter withdrawal so no segment of the vessel is skipped or imaged too quickly by withdrawing the catheter too rapidly, (2) the ability to concentrate on images without having to pay attention to catheter manipulation, (3) volumetric measurements, (4) consistent and systematic IVUS image acquisition among different operators and (5) uniform and reproducible image acquisition for multicentre and serial studies. Disadvantages of motorised pullback are (1) even at very slow pullback speeds, it is possible to skip over very focal lesions, (2) not enough attention may be paid to important regions of interest and (3) it is not possible to have the transducer 'sit' at one specific site in the vessel. Manual transducer pullback should be at a slow rate similar to motorised pullback. Advantages of manual catheter pullback are that it is possible to concentrate on specific regions of interest by having the transducer 'sit' at a specific site in the vessel. Disadvantages of manual catheter pullback include (1) it is easy to skip over significant pathology by pulling the transducer back too quickly or unevenly, (2) length and volume measurements cannot be performed and (3) antegrade and retrograde manual catheter movement can be confusing when the study is reviewed at a later date.

4.1.3 Imaging console

The imaging console includes the hardware and software which are used to convert the IVUS signal into the image as well as the monitor and recording devices.

4.2 IVUS examination technique

Prior to imaging, intravenous heparin with a target activated coagulation time (ACT) > 200–250 s. Heparin should be routinely given to prevent thrombus formation over the IVUS catheter. Most interventionalists use a 6- or 7-French guiding catheter. An 0.014-in angioplasty guidewire is passed distal to the lesion of interest. A stable guiding catheter position with good support is highly recommended since current ultrasound catheters have less trackability and a larger profile than those of modern balloon angioplasty catheters. Intracoronary nitroglycerin (100–200 µg) is routinely used immediately prior to each imaging run both to prevent the occasional case of coronary spasm, a complication seen in 2% of patients[6] and to achieve maximal epicardial coronary vasodilatation. The IVUS catheter is then advanced over the guidewire with the imaging transducer beyond the area of interest.

In manual pullback, the operator will do a controlled slow withdrawal of the transducer across the area of interest. With motorised pullback, an external 'sled' is attached to the proximal portion of the catheter which when activated will provide a steady withdrawal of the catheter at a predetermined speed. Using a pullback speed of 0.5 mm/s and a frame rate of 30 images/s, 60 images will be produced from a pullback through a 1-mm segment. Faster pullbacks are associated with fewer frames per 1-mm segment. With solid-state catheters, the entire catheter is slowly pulled back while with rotational catheters the internal imaging catheter is slowly withdrawn leaving the outer catheter in place beyond the lesion.

4.3 Image interpretation

When you look at the IVUS image, you have to recognise the four essential different components: the catheter, the lumen, the vessel wall and the adjacent structures.

1. **The lumen:** The flowing blood exhibits a characteristic echogenic pattern of described as a swirling or speckling pattern. This blood 'speckle' helps in image interpretation to separate the lumen from the vessel wall. In addition, it is useful to make out whether a dissection plane is connected to the lumen.

2. **The vessel wall:** Ultrasound is reflected at tissue interfaces when the change in acoustic impedance becomes abrupt. In the coronary arterial wall, two interfaces can be recognised: one at the border between blood and the leading edge of the intima (i.e. the luminal border) and the other at the interface between the media and adventitia referred to as the external elastic membrane

(EEM), representing the outer border of the artery. The trailing edge of the intima is indistinct, merging into the media. The outer border of the adventitia is poorly defined and cannot be reliably differentiated from the surrounding tissues. In young subjects, the normal value for intimal thickness is 0.15 ± 0.07 mm. Most investigators use 0.25–0.50 mm as the upper limit of normal (Figure 4.1).[9,10]

3. **The adjacent structures:** The adjacent structures, such as arterial side-branches, cardiac veins and the pericardium, can be differentiated depending on the size of the artery and the depth of penetration and the zoom factor or scale.[11] Compared with optical coherence tomography (OCT), IVUS can image the perivascular structures owing to its higher penetration which of course decreases with higher frequency systems.

The arterial side-branches appear first at the periphery of the image and then join the imaged vessel on subsequent images during the pullback. On the other hand, the course of a cardiac vein is either parallel to or crossing the imaged coronary artery and unlike side-branches never joins the artery. Therefore, looking through the images back and forth help to differentiate veins from side-branches. The adjacent structures serve as landmarks to match images from serial examinations.

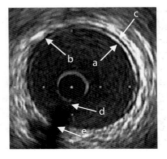

Figure 4.1 An example of a normal coronary artery with intima (**a**), media (**b**) and adventita (**c**). Note the thickness of the normal media. The maximum intimal/medial thickness (measured from the leading edge of the intima to the leading edge of the adventitia) is 0.15 mm. Also note the minimal guidewire artefact (**d**) with shadowing (**e**). (Courtesy of Gary Mintz.)

4. **IVUS image artefacts:** There are some artefacts which could affect the quality and sometimes the interpretation of the generated IVUS image:[12]

a. *Guidewire artefact:* All IVUS catheters are monorail designs. Because the rotating transduce design has a short monorail distal to the transduce, an artefact generated by the wire lying to one side of the catheter is common. (This is not seen with solid state catheters.) The wire looks bright and is followed by a narrow angle beam of acoustic shadowing similar to calcium. Saying that, however, pulling the guidewire out during imaging run is not recommended so that the access to the vessel maintained secure (Figure 4.2).

b. *Non-uniform rotational distortion (NURD):* This type of artefact occurs only in rotating IVUS systems and is related to mechanical bending of the driving cable that rotates the catheter. This leads to oscillations of rotational transducer speed from cycle to cycle which is seen as a visible distortion of the image.[12] This could occur for a number of reasons like having acute bends in the artery, kinking of the imaging sheath, tortuous guide catheter shape or very small guiding-catheter lumen. The most frequent and easily correctable cause is excessive tightening of the haemostatic valve. In extreme cases, fracture of the driving cable could occur (Figure 4.3).

c. *Ring down artefacts:* They are seen as bright halos of variable thickness surrounding the catheter.[12] They are caused by acoustic oscillations in the transducer, which result in high-amplitude ultrasound signals that obscure the area immediately adjacent to the catheter. Ring-down artefacts create a zone of uncertainty adjacent to the transducer surface. This artefact is present in all types of IVUS catheters; however, it is more common in solid-state systems that attempt to minimise such artefacts by performing a 'ringdown' once the catheter is placed into the vessel. This acts like a mask or digital subtraction over this area in the centre of the image.[6]

d. *Reverberation artefact:* These artefacts are caused by secondary, false echoes of the same structure. They lie along the axial path of the ultrasound beam as it penetrates tissue. This gives the false impression of a second interface at multiples of the

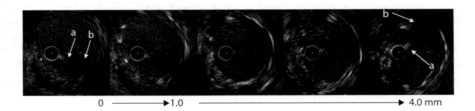

0 ————►1.0 ————————————————————► 4.0 mm

Figure 4.2 Two guidewire artefacts (**a**) with shadowing (**b**). Note that the guidewire appearance and location change during pullback. Guidewire artefacts are seen only with short-monorail intravascular ultrasound (IVUS) catheters unless there is a second guidewire in the lumen. (Courtesy of Gary Mintz.)

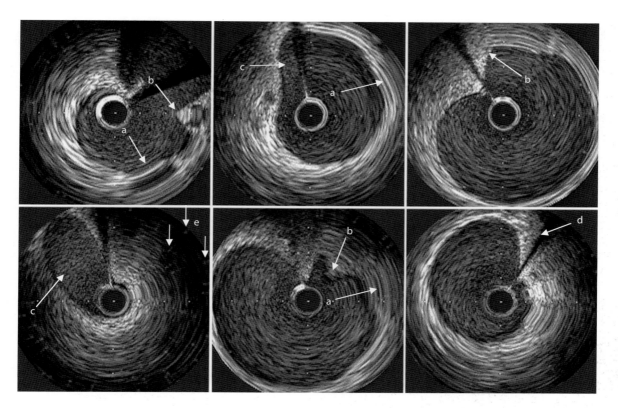

Figure 4.3 Six panels illustrate different appearances of non-uniform rotational distortion (NURD). NURD occurs only with mechanical systems. Part of the image is expanded in its circumferential sweep and part is compressed. The image can appear smeared **(a)**, lumpy **(b)** or very elliptical **(c)**. Note how the guidewire artefact is also compressed **(d)**. In addition, note the radiofrequency noise – the bursts of white dots – indicated by the white arrows **(e)**. (Courtesy of Gary Mintz.)

distance from the transducer to the first structure. Reverberations are more common from strong echo reflectors such as calcium, stent metal, guiding catheters and guidewires (Figure 4.4).

e. ***Motion artefact:*** This type of artefact may happen in both mechanical and electronic catheters which can move as much as 5 mm longitudinally between diastole and systole.[13] This could hinder accurate assessment of the length of the lesion.

f. ***Coronary pulsations:*** Similar to the motion artefact which occur in the longitudinal access, characteristic changes in the diameter of the coronary arteries also occur during the cardiac cycle. In normal coronary arteries although the maximal vessel size happens during systole, maximal flow is found in diastole because at that time the resistance to flow in the intra-myocardial capillaries reaches its minimum.[14,15] A reversal of this phenomenon is seen in presence of muscle bridge where the minimum diameter is reached during systole because of contraction of the muscle surrounding the vessel.

g. ***Obliquity, eccentricity and problems of vessel curvature:*** Current IVUS imaging systems assume that the vessel is circular, the catheter is central in the artery and that the transducer is parallel to the long axis of it.[6] However, in clinical practice, this is not always the case. In fact, both transducer obliquity and vessel curvature can lead to elliptical image distortion. Transducer obliquity is to be considered in large vessels where it can lead to overestimation of dimensions and a distortion of image quality.[16] This reduction in quality of image mainly happens because the amplitude of the echo reflected from an interface is dependent on the angle at which the beam strikes the interface. Accordingly, the signals are strongest when the catheter is coaxial in the vessel because the beam strikes the target at a 90° angle.[6]

h. ***Slow flow (blood speckle):*** With increasing transducer frequency or when the blood velocity is decreased, blood speckle is more prominent that it may obscure the blood–tissue interface particularly with echolucent plaque, thrombus or neointima. This becomes more problematic when the catheter is across a tight stenosis because of stagnation or rouleaux formation. Flushing of the vessel with saline or contrast medium during IVUS imaging can help to identify lumen from vessel wall.[6] Conversely, blood speckle is rarely seen with the 20-MHz solid-state device (Figure 4.5a and b).

i. ***Side lobes:*** These are extraneous beams of ultrasound that are generated from the edges of the

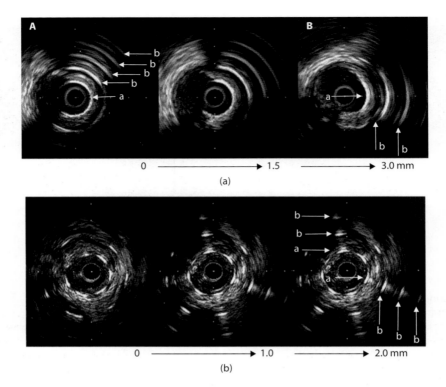

Figure 4.4 Reverberations are false, repetitive echoes of the same structure that give the impression of second, third, etc., interfaces at fixed multiple distances from the transducer. In both examples, true structures are indicated by the arrows a; and the false structures (reverberations) are indicated by the arrows b. The reverberations follow the same contours as the true structures. The top example shows reverberations from calcium. In this example, the 'true' calcium is closer to the transducer in panel **(a)** compared with panel **(b)**; this leads to more reverberations that are closer together in panel (a) compared with panel (b). (Note that these strong, multiple reverberations are seen mostly after rotational atherectomy.) The bottom example shows reverberations from stent struts. Reverberations are analogous to looking in one mirror with another mirror behind you. (Courtesy of Gary Mintz.)

individual transducer elements (Figure 4.6). They follow the circumferential sweep of the beam. Side lobes are more problematic when imaging stents or other strong reflecting structures (e.g. calcium). They are also partly caused by high gain settings. Side lobes may obscure the true lumen and stent borders.

j. *Air bubbles artefact:* Small trapped air bubbles can degrade image quality. They can cause either a weak image or a variety of artefacts. This problem occurs only with mechanical systems. Recent improvements in transducer housing design have made it more difficult to trap air bubbles (Figure 4.7a and b).

5. **Atheroma morphology:** The ultrasound morphologic appearance of plaques has been compared with histology in freshly explanted arteries.[17,18] This provided the basis for ultrasound classification of in vivo atherosclerotic plaque morphology. However, ultrasound cannot detect and quantify specific histologic contents.[6]

a. *Echolucent ('soft') plaques:* The low echogenicity is attributed to high lipid content in a mostly cellular lesion.[19-25] However, a necrotic zone within the plaque, an intramural haemorrhage, or a thrombus could produce a similar appearance on IVUS. The term 'soft' refers to the acoustic signal that arises from low echogenicity not to the structural or mechanical characteristics of the plaque,[6] so some do not use this term to avoid confusion (Figure 4.8).

b. *Echodense ('fibrous') plaques:* These represent the majority of atherosclerotic lesions. Their echogenicity is intermediate between echolucent and highly echogenic calcific plaques.[19-25] However, with increasing fibrous tissue content, the echogenicity of the tissue is increased; and very dense fibrous plaques may produce so much attenuation and acoustic shadowing that they may be misclassified as calcified (Figure 4.9).

c. *Calcific plaques:* These will be discussed in detail in Section 4.3.

d. *Mixed plaques:* Plaques more often contain tissues with different acoustical subtypes like fibrofatty or fibrocalcific.[6] Such mixed plaques could be seen in the same cross section or in adjacent cross sections (Figure 4.10).

e. *Thrombus:* A thrombus is usually seen as an intraluminal mass, often with a layered, lobulated, or pedunculated appearance.[26,27] It is

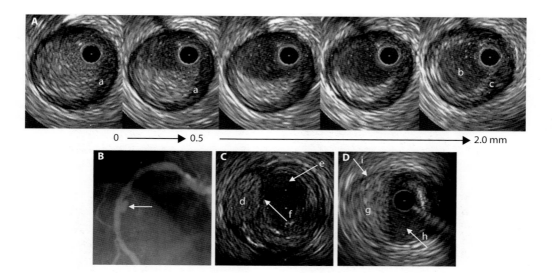

Figure 4.5 (I) Ultrasound is reflected from aggregated blood cells. This is called blood speckle, and it limits the ability to differentiate lumen from tissue (particularly hypoechoic structures such as soft plaque, neointima and thrombus). The intensity of blood speckle increases exponentially as transducer frequency increases and as blood flow velocity decreases. Stasis leading to rouleaux formation and exaggerated blood speckle is most evident when the catheter is across a tight stenosis or when blood is trapped in a false lumen or cavitated structure. Panel A shows intraluminal blood stasis (**a**) where the intima is totally obscured. Moving the transducer re-establishes flow and 'unmasks' the true lumen (b) and plaque (**c**). Compare the static blood speckle (a) with that of moving blood (**b**). A second example of blood stasis causing intense blood speckle is shown in the complex/ruptured plaque in panel B (white arrow) and panel C. Note that the evacuated plaque cavity (**d**) is filled with blood that is more echodense compared with the flowing blood (**e**) in the lumen. Presumably the intravascular ultrasound (IVUS) catheter 'sealed' the ruptured plaque cavity causing the trapped blood to aggregate and become intensely reflective. Note the thin flap of tissue (**f**) separating the cavity from the true lumen. A third example of blood stasis causing intense blood speckle is shown in panel D. Post-intervention, blood accumulated with the blind pouch of a medial dissection, aggregated, and became intensely echo-reflective (**g**) compared with flowing blood in the lumen (**h**). The trapped blood eliminated the echolucent appearance of the media, obscuring the media–adventia border (**i**). This phenomenon has been called an intramural hematoma. (Courtesy of Gary Mintz.)

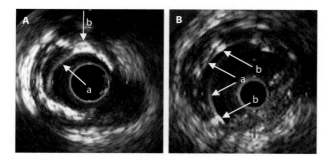

Figure 4.6 Side lobes (a) are intense reflections from the edges of strong echo-reflectors – i.e. from calcium (b in panel a) or stent metal (c in panel b). Side lobes follow the circumferential sweep of the intravascular ultrasound (IVUS) image, whether that sweep is created mechanically or electronically. In particular, it is important not to confuse side lobes with the flap of a dissection (panel a); this confusion is more of an issue in non-stented arteries. (Courtesy of Gary Mintz.)

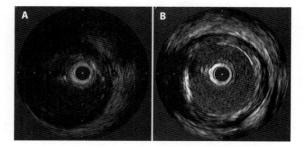

Figure 4.7 An air bubble is the most common cause of a weak image when using a mechanical scanner, and the most common manifestation of an air bubble is a weak image (panel A). Flushing the catheter will expel the bubble and improve the image (panel B). If the catheter contains a large amount of air, it is probably safer to remove and re-prep the catheter to avoid air embolisation. (Courtesy of Gary Mintz.)

usually echolucent or shows a variable grey-scale with speckling. Blood flow in micro-channels may also be apparent within some thrombi. Stagnant blood flow with a greyish-white accumulation of specular echoes within the vascular lumen can resemble a thrombus. This could be differentiated with injection of contrast or saline which disperses the stagnant flow and

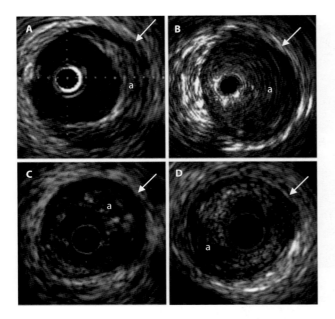

Figure 4.8 Soft plaque **(a)** – also called hypoechoic plaque – as imaged by four different intravascular ultrasound (IVUS) machines. Soft plaque is a misnomer since it is not soft to the touch. Rather, it is 'visually' soft. It is also called hypoechoic plaque, in that it is less echo-reflective when compared with the adventitia (white arrows). A = CVIS (now SciMed/Boston Scientific), B = InterTherapy, C = Hewlett-Packard and D = Endosonics (now Volcano). (Courtesy of Gary Mintz.)

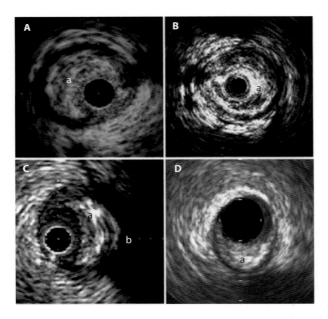

Figure 4.9 Fibrotic (hyperechoic, non-calcific) plaque as imaged by four different intravascular ultrasound (IVUS) machines. In each of these examples, there is evidence of hyperechoic plaque **(a)** – plaque that is as bright or brighter than the adventitia. There is no shadowing in panels A, B, and D. In panel C, the shadowing **(b)** is either from deep calcium or from attenuation. A = Hewlett-Packard, B = InterTherapy, C = CVIS (now SciMed/Boston Scientific) and D = Endosonics (now Volcano). (Courtesy of Gary Mintz.)

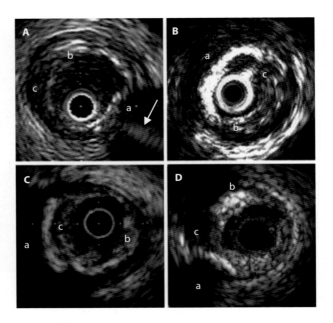

Figure 4.10 Mixed plaque as imaged by four different intravascular ultrasound (IVUS) machines. Each panel contains calcium **(a)**, fibrotic plaque **(b)**, and soft plaque **(c)** without any one dominant plaque type. A = CVIS (now SciMed/Boston Scientific), B = InterTherapy, C = Hewlett-Packard and D = Endosonics (now Volcano). Note that the reverberations from the guidewire in panel (a) (white arrow) continue even into the area shadowed by the calcium. (Courtesy of Gary Mintz.)

clears the lumen. However, IVUS diagnosis of thrombus is usually presumptive as no one feature is pathognomonic (Figure 4.11a and b).[6]

f. **Stent*struts*:** The metallic prosthesis of endovascular stents are strongly echo-reflective. They create a third IVUS boundary between the lumen and the EEM. On tracing the stent, it is important not to mistake guidewire for a sent strut because both are strong echo-reflectors. The appearance of different stent designs and the ease or difficulty in measuring stent cross-sectional area (CSA) can be seen in Figure 4.12. In general, most tubular-slotted or multicellular stents have a similar appearance. However, measurement of stent CSA is more reliable with tubular-slotted or multicellular stents (or coil stents that have a similar appearance) compared with the clam-shell stent design. It is important to note that the thickness of the endothelial layer covering a stent is below the resolution of IVUS; so, re-endothelialisation in the absence of intimal hyperplasia(IH) accumulation appears as a stent without overlying tissue. High-gain settings should be avoided when imaging the struts to avoid creating the side lobes (Figure 4.6).

6. ***Intimal hyperplasia (IH):*** The intimal hyperplasia of early-mid in-stent restenosis often appears as tissue with

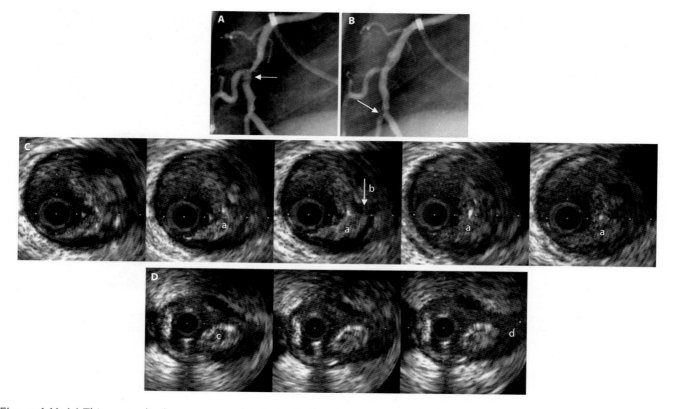

Figure 4.11 **(a)** This example shows an unstable lesion before intervention (white arrow in panel A) and after balloon angioplasty (panel B); note the new, post-balloon angioplasty filling defect at the origin of the acute marginal branch in panel B (white arrow). Pre-intervention IVUS (panel C) shows many features of a thrombus: a lobulated, pedunculated mass (a); a distinct interface with the underlying vessel wall (b); and in real-time, blood speckle within the lesion. Post-balloon angioplasty IVUS (panel d) shows the thrombus (c) that has embolised into the acute marginal branch. (Courtesy of Gary Mintz.)

very low echogenicity, sometimes less echogenic than the blood speckle in the lumen. The intimal hyperplasia of late in-stent restenosis often appears more echogenic (Figure 4.13a and b).[6]

4.4 Role of IVUS in the presence of calcium

Ultrasound has a much higher sensitivity than fluoroscopy in the detection of coronary calcification.[28,29] Calcific plaques appear as bright echoes that hinder the penetration of ultrasound beam beyond. This lack of penetration, referred to as 'acoustic shadowing', makes it impossible to detect the whole thickness of calcium by IVUS because only the leading edge is visualised. Calcium can also produce reverberations – oscillation of the ultrasound beam between the transducer and the leading edge of calcium with each oscillation producing a secondary, pseudo-interface behind the actual leading edge of the calcium. Shadowing is more sensitive while reverberations are more specific.

The relationship between presence of calcium and stability of plaques is unclear. Whereas large calcification is frequently associated with lesion stability, micro-calcifications are usually found in lipid-rich necrotic core characteristic of unstable plaques.[30,31]

The distribution of calcium could be either superficial where the leading edge of the acoustic shadowing appears within the most shallow 50% of the plaque plus media thickness or deep where the leading edge of the acoustic shadowing appears within the deepest 50% of the plaque plus media thickness.

An electronic protractor can be used to measure the arc of calcium in degrees. Semi-quantitative grading is more commonly used where the number of quadrants subtended by calcium is counted and is given a number from 0 (no calcium) to 4 (circumferential calcium). The length of the calcific plaques can be additionally measured longitudinally by using motorised not manual transducer pullback (Figure 4.14a through c).[6]

A comprehensive IVUS report should not only comment on the presence of calcium but also include additional data about the distribution (qualitative) and the arc of calcium (quantitative) for proper interventional planning.[6]

4.5 Practical integration and basic measurements

Accurate procedural information is critical, especially when reviewing cases after completion. It is helpful if online

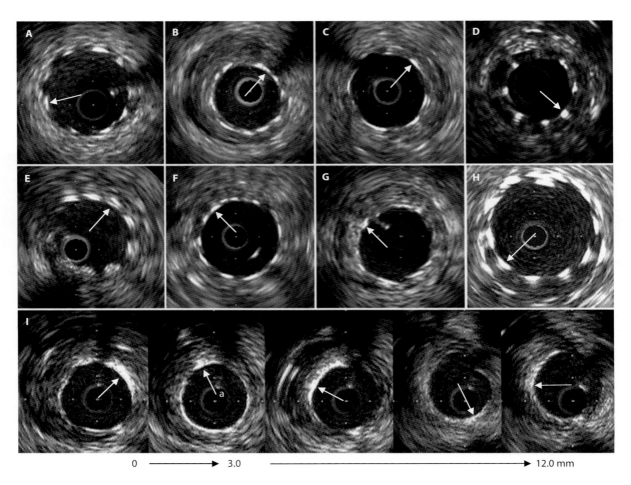

Figure 4.12 This example illustrates nine different types of stents; the white arrow shows the stent metal in each image slice. Most tubular-slotted or multicellular stents have a similar appearance: A =NIR, B = MultiLink, C = AVE GFX, D = Duet, E = Paragon and F = Palmaz–Schatz. Some coiled stents – such as the CrossFlex (G) or the Wiktor stent – have an appearance that is like a tubular-slotted/multicellular stent. The mesh Wallstent (H) also has a similar appearance, but it has more stent metal. The design of the Gianturco–Roubin-II stent (I) results in an IVUS appearance that varies almost mm by mm over the length of the stent. With the exception of one cross section (a), a complete stent circumference is usually not seen. Consequently, it is difficult to identify and measure the minimum stent cross-sectional area (CSA). (Courtesy of Gary Mintz.)

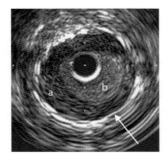

Figure 4.13 (a) Intimal hyperplasia (a) can be less echodense than blood speckle (b). Stent CSA measured 12.9 mm², lumen CSA measured 4.8 mm², and intimal hyperplasia CSA measured 8.1 mm². The stent is indicated by the white arrow. (Courtesy of Gary Mintz.)

procedural information is annotated onto the ultrasound system's video screen: (1) the timing of IVUS imaging (e.g. pre-intervention), (2) the procedure being performed and (3) the target lesion location. All IVUS instruments have internal clocks, and the time is automatically recorded onto the image if the clock is properly set. It is ideal to note the 'time' that corresponds to the centre of the lesion. In the absence of systematic pre-intervention imaging, recording the 'time' corresponding to the lesion may be the only way to identify the target lesion on subsequent review. Digital acquisition and limited storage are provided; however, it is important to avoid overwriting studies on the console before archiving them permanently.

Imaging should always include careful uninterrupted imaging of (1) at least 10 mm of distal reference, (2) the lesion or stented site (s) and (3) the entire proximal reference back to the aorta at least once during the procedure. This is equally important in assessing a previously treated lesion site. When using IVUS, we strongly recommend that the entire artery be imaged back to the aorto-ostial junction at least once during the procedure since it will provide additional information about the proximal vessel (e.g. the left main coronary

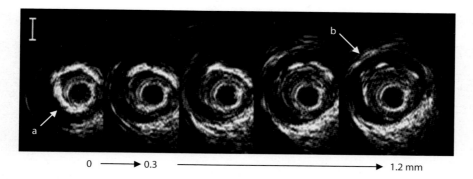

Figure 4.14 Calcium **(a)** shadows the deeper arterial structures, including the external elastic membrane (EEM) **(b)**. Moving the transducer proximally or, as in this example, distally – even just a small amount – can unmask the EEM. (Courtesy of Gary Mintz.)

artery [LMCA]) when the primary concern is the left anterior descending (LAD) but will not add to the cost of the procedure. Measurements should be made offline after the imaging run is complete, not when the catheter is in the vessel; this saves procedure time and minimises patient ischaemia.

4.5.1 Lumen measurements

Lumen measurements depend on using the interface between the lumen and the intimal leading edge. The intima could be easily detected in normal subjects because it has different acoustic properties compared with both the media and the lumen. The leading edge of this echogenic layer represents the boundary of the lumen. However, in young normal people (e.g. post-transplantation), the vessel wall will appear having only a single-layer; and it will be difficult to make out the intima as a separate layer from the media. The most inner part of this intima–media layer could still be differentiated from the lumen and be used as a marker for luminal border.

After defining the lumen border, the following lumen measurements are obtained. Measurements should be performed relative to the centre of the lumen, rather than relative to the centre of the IVUS catheter:

Lumen CSA: The area bounded by the luminal border.
Minimum lumen diameter: The shortest diameter through the centre point of the lumen.
Maximum lumen diameter: The longest diameter through the centre point of the lumen.
Lumen area stenosis: Reference lumen CSA minus minimum lumen CSA/reference lumen CSA. The reference segment used should be specified (proximal, distal, largest or average).[6]

4.5.2 EEM measurements

The EEM is identified as a discrete interface at the border between the media and the adventitia. It is better to use the term *EEM CSA* instead of alternative descriptions like 'vessel area' or 'total vessel area'. EEM circumference and area cannot be measured accurately at sites where large side-branches originate or in presence of extensive calcification because of acoustic shadowing. If acoustic shadowing involves a relatively small arc (90°), planimetry of the circumference can be performed by extrapolation from the closest identifiable EEM borders, although measurement accuracy and reproducibility will be reduced. If the calcification arc is more than 90°, EEM measurements should not be reported. The EEM could also be obscured by some stent designs. Disease-free coronary arteries are circular. With the development of atherosclerosis, the arteries may remodel into a non-circular configuration.[6]

4.5.3 Atheroma measurement

Because media thickness cannot be measured accurately (the leading edge of the media is not a well-defined acoustic structure), IVUS cannot determine the true atheroma area. As a result, IVUS studies in non-stented arteries use the EEM and lumen CSA measurements to calculate a surrogate for true atheroma area, the plaque plus media (P&M) area. (in stented arteries the stent forms a third measurable structure). In practice, the inclusion of the media into the atheroma area does represent a major limitation of IVUS because the media constitutes only a very small fraction of the atheroma CSA. Complete quantification of a non-stented lesion is possible by tracing the EEM and lumen areas of the proximal reference, lesion and distal reference and calculating the following measurements (Figure 4.15):[6]

Plaque plus media (or atheroma) CSA: The EEM CSA minus the lumen CSA.
Maximum plaque plus media (or atheroma) thickness: The largest distance from the intimal leading edge to the EEM along any line passing through the centre of the lumen.
Minimum plaque plus media (or atheroma) thickness: The shortest distance from intimal leading edge to the EEM along any line passing through the luminal centre of mass.
Plaque plus media (or atheroma) eccentricity: Maximum plaque plus media thickness divided by the minimum plaque plus media thickness.

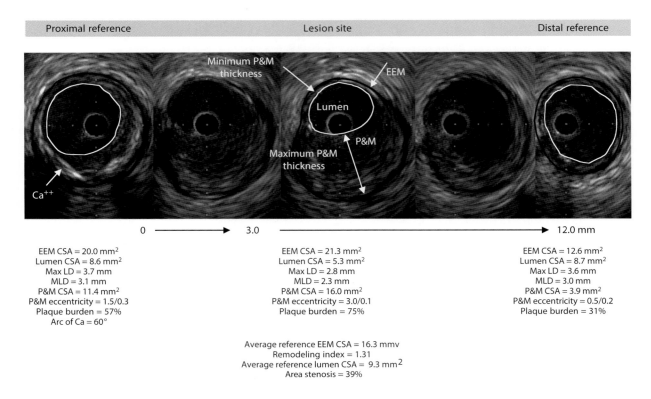

| Proximal reference | Lesion site | Distal reference |

EEM CSA = 20.0 mm²
Lumen CSA = 8.6 mm²
Max LD = 3.7 mm
MLD = 3.1 mm
P&M CSA = 11.4 mm²
P&M eccentricity = 1.5/0.3
Plaque burden = 57%
Arc of Ca = 60°

EEM CSA = 21.3 mm²
Lumen CSA = 5.3 mm²
Max LD = 2.8 mm
MLD = 2.3 mm
P&M CSA = 16.0 mm²
P&M eccentricity = 3.0/0.1
Plaque burden = 75%

EEM CSA = 12.6 mm²
Lumen CSA = 8.7 mm²
Max LD = 3.6 mm
MLD = 3.0 mm
P&M CSA = 3.9 mm²
P&M eccentricity = 0.5/0.2
Plaque burden = 31%

Average reference EEM CSA = 16.3 mmv
Remodeling index = 1.31
Average reference lumen CSA = 9.3 mm²
Area stenosis = 39%

Figure 4.15 A complete set of intravascular ultrasound (IVUS) measurements in a non-stented artery is shown. The black line highlights each external elastic membrane, and the white line indicates each image slice's lumen. Max LD, maximum lumen diameter; MLD, minimum lumen diameter. The P&M CSA has also been called the atheroma CSA; and the plaque burden has also been called the atheroma burden. (Courtesy of Gary Mintz.)

Plaque (or atheroma) burden: Plaque plus media CSA divided by the EEM CSA.

4.5.4 Lesion length measurement

Assessment of lesion length by IVUS is only possible using motorised transducer pullback (number of seconds × pullback speed).

4.5.5 Stent measurements

Complete quantification of a stented lesion is possible by tracing the EEM and lumen areas of the proximal and distal reference and the EEM, lumen, and stent areas of the stented lesion and calculating the following measurements:

Stent CSA: The area bounded by the stent border.
Minimum stent diameter: The shortest diameter through the centre of mass of the stent.
Maximum stent diameter: The longest diameter through the centre of mass of the stent.
Stent symmetry: Maximum stent diameter divided by minimum stent diameter.
Stent expansion: The minimum stent CSA compared with the predefined reference area, which can be the proximal, distal, largest, or average reference area.

Similarly, the length of the stent can be only measured in motorised pullback systems.

4.6 Guiding stent implantation

In day-to-day terms, the following is an algorithm for IVUS-guided stent implantation:

- Perform pre-intervention IVUS to measure reference vessel size and measure lesion length.
- Select stent size using maximum reference lumen diameter whether proximal or distal to the lesion (or for experienced users, midwall measurements).
- Select stent length based on distance between proximal and distal references.
- Determine the maximum achievable stent dimension assuming a 0% residual stenosis.
- Implant a stent according to conventional techniques.
- Repeat IVUS to assess MSA. If the MSA is adequate, stop. If the MSA is inadequate, perform additional higher-pressure inflations and, if necessary, use a larger balloon. If there is malapposition, select a balloon sized to the distance between the non-apposed intima and inflate at low pressures. Check to make sure that there are no complications.

These steps are, conceptually, little different from angiography-guided stent implantation.

4.6.1 Stent sizing

Reference segments by IVUS are rarely normal (see above); rather, they are the most 'normal-looking' cross sections proximal and distal to the minimal lumen area (MLA) but (in general) within the same coronary segment, i.e. the cross sections with the largest lumens and the least amount of plaque. IVUS reference lumen dimension measurements typically indicates that a larger device can be used without having to resort to midwall or media-to-media stent sizing as advocated by some authorities. IVUS 'true vessel', 'media-to-media' or midwall dimensions reflect the amount of angiographically silent disease and the extent of positive remodelling, not just vessel size; this measurement will be even larger than reference lumen dimensions. Sizing to the IVUS reference lumen dimension is safe and effective, especially if followed by IVUS-guided fine-tuning of the final minimum stent area (MSA). Sizing to IVUS midwall or media-to-media dimensions is more aggressive and requires more experience and caution.

Angiography measures lesion length from shoulder-to-shoulder in the least foreshortened projection. sHowever, it is not always possible to eliminate foreshortening, vessel tortuosity or bend points. IVUS measures lesion length by tracking the transducer through the coronary artery during motorised pullback regardless of bend points, tortuosity or foreshortening. IVUS reference segment identification and stent length selection ensure that secondary plaques proximal and distal to the stenosis will be covered by the stent.

4.7 Clinical applications of IVUS

4.7.1 Assessment of intermediate non-left main coronary artery (non-LMCA) stenosis

The two-dimensional representation of coronary anatomy provided by angiography is limited in distinguishing intermediate lesions that require stenting from those that simply need appropriate medical therapy. This is particularly obvious in diseased reference vessel, foreshortening, tortuous vessels, calcification, lesion eccentric lesions and poor contrast opacification. A challenging question for interventional cardiologist has been always to treat or to leave moderately severe lesions which are 40%–70% severe. Such lesions are clinically important because it has been proposed that acute myocardial infarctions originate from those lesions.

Fractional flow reserve (FFR) is the gold standard for diagnosing flow limiting intermediate coronary stenosis. Research has been done to investigate the use of IVUS for this purpose mainly by trying to set a definite MLA cut-off point below which a diagnosis of physiologic significance is made. However, the use of anatomical tool to detect a functional relevance is a matter of debate. First, there is huge discrepancy in the size of coronary arteries so saying that one cut-off cannot fit all vessel sizes. Cut-offs have ranged from 2.0. to 4.0 mm^2 with 3.0 mm^2 being the most common in western patients and 2.4 mm^2 being the most common in eastern Asian patients. In addition, there are many factors other than MLA that could still influence the significance of a coronary lesion like lesion length and amount of myocardium supplied. Finally, the negative predictive value is consistently higher than the positive predictive value indicating that while it might be possible to use IVUS to decide not to treat an intermediate lesion in certain clinical situations (an MLA >3.0 mm^2 is rarely ischaemia producing), the converse is not acceptable; and IVUS alone should not be used to justify stent implantation especially in borderline situations. Table 4.2 shows some studies evaluating IVUS in non-LMCA stenosis.

4.7.2 Assessment of intermediate LMCA stenosis

Decisions for revascularisation have been made based on visual estimation of severity of lesion on angiography. However, angiographic evaluation of the left main is poor with the greatest inter- and intra-observer variability of all coronary segments. This is related to significant foreshortening, ostial angulation and streaming of contrast medium from the catheter tip. In addition, LMCA disease is usually diffuse that may even extend into proximal left anterior descending (LAD) and left circumflex (LCX) with no healthy reference segment. The following studies have highlighted the inaccuracy of angiography in LMCA stenosis assessment.

- Hermiller et al.[56] in 1993, showed that LMCA disease can be unrecognised and appear normal on the coronary angiogram.
- Coronary Artery Surgery Study (CASS),[57] where 870 angiograms were analysed by two readers for evaluating the reproducibility of interpretation of angiograms found that LMCA analysis was the least reproducible.
- Lindstaedt et al.[58] in 2007 reported an assessment of 51 patients in whom unanimous correct assessment of LMCA severity by four experienced interventional cardiologists was only 29%. Correct lesion classification was achieved in less than 50% by each. This means that in more than 50% of cases, visual estimation of LMCA disease was incorrect.
- Hamilos et al.[59] in 2009 showed that two reviewers either (1) disagreed whether the LM was significant (26%) or (2) agreed but were wrong in their assessment when compared with FFR (23%).
- Chakrabarti et al.[60] in 2014 reported that in 11.2% (17 of 152) of patients with 'core laboratory' LMCA disease assessment were considered to be normal by clinical site analysis in the NCDR, whereas 56.7% (177 of 312) of patients that were listed as having LMCA disease by clinical site analysis in the NCDR had no LMCA lesion by core laboratory analysis.
- Toth et al.[61] in 2014 compared FFR and QCA %DS in 2986 patients (4086 LMCA and non-LMCA lesions). The greatest variation in the accuracy of the 50% DS cut-off was seen in the 152 LMCA lesions (area under the curve, AUC = 0.55).

Table 4.2 Intravascular ultrasound (IVUS) studies evaluating use of minimal lumen area (MLA) and other parameters for predicting ischaemia in non–left main coronary artery (LMCA) lesions

Reference	Versus	No. of lesions	% abn	Inclusion criteria	Mean MLA (mm²)	MLA cut-off (mm²)	Other independent IVUS anatomic determinants	PPV	NPV
Abizaid et al.[32]	CFR<2.0	112	40%		4.4	4.0			
Nishioka et al.[33]	SPECT	70	65%		4.3	4.0			
Takagi et al.[34]	FFR<0.75	51	49%		3.9	3.0			
Briguori et al.[35]	FFR<0.75	53	23%	40%–70% DS	3.9	4.0	Lesion length	46%	96%
Takayama and McB[36]	FFR	14	50%	>2.5 mm vessels	3.5		MLA divided by lesion length		
Lee et al.[37]	FFR<0.75	94	40%	30%–75% DS<3 mm vessels	2.3	2.0	Lesion length Plaque burden		
Kang et al.[38]	FFR<0.8	236	21%	30%–75% DS	2.6	2.4	LAD Plaque burden	37%	96%
Ahn et al.[39]	SPECT	170	26%		2.1	2.1	Plaque burden	39%	91%
Ben-Dor et al.[40]	FFR<0.75	92	19%	40%–70% DS >2.5 mm vessels	3.6	2.8	Lesion length		
	FFR<0.8					3.2			
Koo et al.[41]	FFR<0.8	267	33%	30%–70% DS Proximal or Mid	3.0	3.0	Proximal or mid LAD	47%	
Ben-Dor et al.[42]	FFR<0.8	205	26%	40%–70% DS >2.5 mm vessels		3.1			
Kang et al.[43]	FFR<0.8	784	29%	30%–90% DS		2.4	LAD Lesion length Plaque rupture	48%	90%
Koh et al.[44]	FFR<0.8	38	37%	40%–70% DS Ostial MV		3.5	Plaque burden	69%	87%
		55	27%	40%–70% DS Ostial SB				<50%	
Kwan et al.[45]	FFR<0.8	169	59%	40%–99% DS LAD	3.0	3.0	Plaque burden	84%	82%

(Continued)

Table 4.2 (continued) Intravascular ultrasound (IVUS) studies evaluating use of minimal lumen area (MLA) and other parameters for predicting ischaemia in non–left main coronary artery (LMCA) lesions

Reference	Versus	No. of lesions	% abn	Inclusion criteria	Mean MLA (mm²)	MLA cut-off (mm²)	Other independent IVUS anatomic determinants	PPV	NPV
Gonzalo et al.[46] 2012	FFR<0.8	51	46%	40%–70% DS 0% DS	2.6	2.4		67%	65%
Waksman et al.[47]	FFR<0.8	334	25%	40%–80% DS >2.5 mm vessels	5.6	3.1	LAD Plaque burden	40%	83%
Kang et al.[48]	FFR<0.8	493 males 207 females	43% males 27% females	>30% DSLAD	2.6 2.5	2.5 2.5		63% male 42% female	81% male 93% female
Lopez-Palop et al.[49]	FFR<0.8	61	49%	40%–70% DS ≥20 mm length	2.7	3.1	Lesion length	67%	93%
Cui et al.[50]	FFR<0.8	206	26%	40%–70% DS >2.5 mm vessels	3.9	3.2	Plaque burden	53%	85%
Yang et al.[51]	FFR<0.8	206	44%	40%–70% DS Prox/mid LAD >3.0 mm vessel	3.1	3.2 (Prox) 2.5 (Mid)	Lesion length		
Naganuma et al.[52]	FFR<0.8	169	30%	40%–70% DS	3.0	2.7	Plaque burden	59%	90%
Voros et al.[53]	FFR<0.75	323	27%	40%–99% DS	3.7	2.7		39%	93%
Han et al.[54]	FFR<0.8	169	39%		3.1	2.8		49%	73%
Cho et al.[55]	FFR <0.8	945	40%	30%–70% DS	3.1	3.0	Plaque burden	50%	72%

CFR, coronary flow rate; FFR, fractional flow rate; DS, disease; IVUS, intravascular ultrasound; MLA, minimal lumen area; MV, main vessel; NPV, negative predictive value; PPV, positive predictive value; SB, side branch; SPECT, single-photon emission computed tomography.

Therefore, when making management decisions regarding the LMCA, angiography is often not adequate. Studies have shown that untreated obstructive (>50%) LMCA disease is associated with poor outcome.[62] However, non-obstructive LMCA disease is associated with normal survival; and bypass surgery for non-haemodynamically significant stenosis could result in early graft closure.[63] Therefore, finding another diagnostic modality for intermediate LMCA lesions has become imperative. However, most patients with LMCA disease have associated disease in the LAD and/or LCX that might impact the accuracy of FFR measurements. Compared with FFR, IVUS has an additional advantage to accurately assess the anatomy of the LMCA, the reference size of the vessel and involvement of LAD and LCX ostia if stent implantation is required. IVUS can also detect the presence and extent of calcification, which is useful in proper lesion preparation before stent insertion, debulking of calcium with rotational atherectomy, or vessel dilatation with the help of non-compliant balloons.

On one hand, there is better correlation between IVUS and FFR in assessing LMCA than in assessing non-LMCA lesions due to limited variability in each of left main stem (LMS) length (short), LMS size (large) and amount of supplied myocardium. However, like FFR, IVUS assessment of LMCA has practical limitations especially for distal LMS lesions, where it is necessary to image from both the LAD and LCX as it is not possible to assess the LCX from an LAD-to-left main stem (LMS) pullback, and it is not possible to assess the LAD from an LCX-to-LMS pullback.

Most studies have found MLA and MLD to be the two most independent IVUS parameters for predicting ischaemia having single-photon emission computed tomography (SPECT) and FFR as the reference. Table 4.3 shows IVUS studies evaluating the use of MLA and MLD for predicting ischaemia in intermediate LMCA lesions. However, an MLA of <6 mm^2 and a MLD < 2.8 mm are the most accepted cut-offs for a significant LMCA stenosis in Western patients. Although heavily debated, these standards for IVUS evaluation of physiologically significant LMCA stenosis are recognised in the 2011 American College of Cardiology/American Heart Association (ACC/AHA) guidelines.[64] According to the LITRO Study Group (Spanish Working Group on Interventional Cardiology) trial,[65] IVUS can be safely used to defer a LMCA lesion with MLA > 6.0 mm^2. In LMCA lesions with an MLA 5.0–6.0 mm^2, there is a grey zone among different studies where we do recommend doing FFR to assess functional significance.

4.7.3 In-stent restenosis and thrombosis

Compared with BMS, DES has significantly reduced the rates of in-stent restenosis (ISR) by decreasing neointimal hyperplasia. However, the rate of stent thrombosis (ST) is slightly higher with DES. Because some mechanical factors like stent underexpansion and malappositon have proved to be related to ISR in BMS, a lot of studies in the DES era have addressed the additional advantage of using IVUS for stent optimization.

4.8 Better outcomes with IVUS guidance

Two meta-analyses of seven randomised IVUS versus angiographic-guided BMS implantation trials showed that IVUS guidance reduced restenosis, repeat revascularisation, and major adverse cardiac events (MACE) but not death or MI; and ST was not reported.

Five meta-analyses of the published IVUS versus angiographic-guided DES studies (the most recent including 29,068 patients from 17 registries and three randomised trials) – as well as propensity score matching sub-studies and sub-analyses of high-risk lesions and unstable patient subsets – showed that IVUS guidance reduced overall MACE including early and late ST and myocardial infarction (MI) and mortality during follow-up of at least 1 year. These meta-analyses did not include eight additional publications (four randomised and four registry studies); seven of eight reported better outcomes with IVUS guidance, and four of the seven were randomised studies. (It should be noted that the eighth study also showed no outcomes benefit to intracoronary physiology.)

The angiography versus IVUS optimisation (AVIO) trial was the first major randomised trial comparing IVUS-guided versus angiographic-guided DES implantation.[72] Post-procedure MLD and use of larger post-dilation balloons were significantly higher in the IVUS group. Although the study was not powered for clinical endpoints, there was no difference in myocardial infarction, target lesions/vessel revascularisation (TLR/TVR) or cardiac death at 30 days or 24 months.

The outcomes of IVUS guidance versus angiographic guidance of DES were again addressed in The Assessment of Dual Antiplatelet Therapy With Drug-Eluting Stents (ADAPT-DES) study that mainly assessed the relationship between platelet reactivity and other clinical and procedural variables with subsequent ST.[73] During the procedure, IVUS guidance changed the strategy in 74% of patients. At 1 year follow-up, there was a significant difference in the rate of definite/probable ST being lower in the IVUS-guided group compared with the angiography-guided one. Despite the longer vessel segment covered by longer stents, there was a significant reduction in peri-procedural myocardial infarction, target vessel myocardial infarction combined endpoint of MACE (cardiac death, ST or myocardial infarction) and ischaemic-driven TLR/TVR in the IVUS-guided group.

Table 4.3 IVUS studies evaluating use of MLA and MLD for predicting ischaemia in intermediate LMCA lesions

Reference	Versus	N lesions	Mean MLA	MLA cut-off	Other independent IVUS parameters	Comments
Abiziad et al.[66]	12 months follow-up study	122			MLD <3	No specific cut-off suggested MLD was the most important predictor of cardiac events
Lindstaedt et al.[67]	FFR<0.75 99Tc-Mibi-Spect	44				44 months follow-up for MACE
Jasti et al.[68]	FFR<0.75	55	7.65	5.9	MLD<2.8 (the most sensitive and specific)	11 months follow-up for ischaemia
Fassa et al.[69]	Getting lower range of normal (normal mean –2 SD)	121 (reference MLA was then applied on 214 patients with inter-mediate LM disease for outcome)		7.5		Data from patients with normal or near normal LMS40 months follow-up for MACE
de la Torre Hernandez et al.[65]	Revalidation of pre-defined MLA cut-off	354		6.0		24 months follow-up for MACE
Kang et al.[70]	FFR<0.8 FFR<0.75	55	4.9	4.8 4.1	Plaque rupture	No follow-up
Park et al.[71]	FFR<0.8	112	4.8	4.5	Plaque rupture	No follow-up

VUS, intravascular ultrasound; MLA, minimal lumen area; MLD, minimal luminal diameter; LMCA, left main coronary artery.

Two other randomised trials deserve particular mention. In one trial of percutaneous CTO revascularisation, 402 patients were randomised to IVUS versus angiographic guidance after guidewire crossing; according to the intention-to-treat analysis, IVUS guidance was associated with a lower MACE of 2.6% versus 7.1% (p=0.035) along with a reduction in death/MI and repeat revascularisation. (The per-protocol differences in MACE – comparing PCI procedures that were actually guided by IVUS versus those that were guided by angiography alone – were even greater: 2.2% versus 8.4%, p=0.005.) In the IVUS-XLP trial 1400 patients with long lesions were randomised to IVUS versus angiographic guidance; all patients were treated with the same metallic DES; IVUS guidance was associated with a lower MACE rate of 2.9% versus 5.8% (intention-to-treat, p=0.007); and as previously noted in the subgroup of IVUS-guided patients with a post-intervention MLA greater than the distal reference lumen area, the MACE rate was only 1.5%. The most likely explanation was studies showing that angiographic guidance achieved, on average, only 75% of the predicted minimum stent diameter and 67% of the predicted MSA. IVUS guidance minimised contrast use (median of 20.0 mL) even when compared with a contrast conservation, angiography-guided stent implantation strategy (median of 64.5 mL, p < 0.0001); this can be particularly important in patients with renal insufficiency. As a result, meta-analysis of the eight randomised IVUS-guided versus angiography-guided DES implantation studies showed that IVUS guidance was associated with a reduction in the risk of MACE by 41%, mortality by 54%, ST by 51% and ischaemia-driven target lesion revascularisation by 40%.

For unprotected LMCA intervention, there is a lack of randomised trials and most data are derived from registries,[74–76] so it is a Class IIb recommendation (expert opinion) to use IVUS for guiding LMCA interventions in the ACC/AHA guidelines 2011.[64] The Revascularization Unprotected Left Main Coronary Artery Stenosis: Comparison of Percutaneous Coronary Angioplasty Versus Surgical Revascularization (MAIN-COMPARE) registry[75] has shown that the risk of 3-year MACE and mortality was significantly lower in patients undergoing IVUS guided DES implantation. However, IVUS did not reduce the 3 years risk of MACE or mortality after BMS.

Recently, similar results to the MAIN-COMPARE registry were obtained from a pooled analysis of four registries of LMCA intervention. IVUS guidance leads to the use of larger balloons and stents and significant reduction in overall mortality, combined endpoint of death, MI and TLR and ST.[77]

These benefits of IVUS-guided DES implantation are directly related to reduction in under-expansion of stents, as a result of use of larger balloons and stents, and more recognition of mechanical problems and geographical miss (edge dissections, plaque burden at the stent edge >50%, etc.).

4.9 IVUS optimum stent implantation criteria

4.9.1 Stent expansion

Stent expansion is the most important criterion of optimal stent implantation. Additional high-pressure balloon inflations may be necessary to correct stent under-expansion.

The multicenter ultrasound stenting in coronaries (MUSIC) criteria which were met in 80% of patients in the MUSIC study[78] included (1) complete apposition of the entire stent against the vessel wall: (a) MLA ≥90% of the average reference lumen area or ≥100 % of lumen area of the reference segment with the lowest lumen area, (b) MLA >9.0 mm^2 or (c) MLA ≥80% of the average reference lumen area or ≥90% of lumen area of the reference segment with the lowest lumen area. (2) Symmetric stent expansion. However, these criteria could not be replicated in subsequent studies with only 48% of patients in the AVID study[79] and 56% in the OPTICUS study[80] fulfilling those criteria.

The RESIST study[81] used stent CSA≥80% of the mean proximal and distal reference vessel CSA as the IVUS criterion for optimal stent expansion, which was achieved in only 77% of patients with adequate angiographic results. On the other hand, in the TULIP trial,[82] optimal stent implantation by IVUS necessitated complete stent apposition plus MLD ≥80% of the mean of proximal and distal reference diameters and MLA ≥ distal reference lumen area. This was fulfilled in 89% of patients.

The Angiography Versus IVUS Optimization (AVIO) trial[72] proposed new IVUS criteria for optimal stent deployment where the diameter of the post-dilatation balloon is chosen on the basis of the average media-to-media diameters of the vessel at different points of the stented area. Optimal stent expansion was defined as 70% ± 10% of the cross-sectional area of the inflated post-dilatation balloon. This was achieved, however, in only 48% of patients. Tables 4.4 and 4.5 show IVUS criteria for ISR and thrombosis, respectively, in different studies.

Table 4.4 Studies evaluating ISR by IVUS

Study	No. of patients	IVUS parameters of ISR	Comments
Kasaoka et al.[90]	1173 patients with 1633 stented lesions divided into 891 patients (1224 lesions) without restenosis and 282 patients (409 lesions) with restenosis	The most important predictor of restenosis was stent CSA and total stent length.	
Fuji et al.[91]	48 previous ISR lesions (11 recurrent ISR)	Stent under-expansion is the cause of failure after sirolimus-eluting stent (SES) implantation treatment of ISR. Geographical miss was found in 3/11 lesions. MSA was <5 mm^2 in 9/11 lesions.	
Sonoda et al.[92]	122 cases (72 SES and 50 BMS)	MSA was correlated to stent patency at follow up. SES had less biologic variability, more predictable long-term stent patency with post-procedure MSA and lower optimal MSA threshold (5.0 mm^2 compared with 6.5 mm^2 with BMS).	8 months follow-up

(Continued)

Table 4.4 (continued) Studies evaluating ISR by IVUS

Study	No. of patients	IVUS parameters of ISR	Comments
Sakurai et al.[93]	317 edges of 167 stents which had 18 edge stenosis on follow-up	A large percentage of plaque area in the reference segment and a larger edge stent area/reference minimum lumen area were related to edge stenosis on follow-up.	Study of interaction of sirolimus drug-eluting stents and vessel margin on 8 months follow-up
Hong et al.[94]	543 (449 patients)	Final minimum stent area<5.5 mm^2 and stent length>40 mm were the only independent predictors of angiographic restenosis.	Involved 6 months angiographic follow-up
Costa et al.[95]	1557 patients treated with SESs were assessed for occurrence of geographic miss (GM) (longitudinal (LGM; injured or diseased segment not covered by SES) or axial GM (balloon-artery size ratio <0.9 or >1.3)	GM occurred was the most independent factor associated with increased risk of TVR and myocardial infarction at 1 year (more with longitudinal GM).	
Liu et al.[96]	20 definite stent thrombosis patients were compared with 50 risk-factor-balanced ISR patients and 50 risk-factor-balanced 'no-event' patients with no thrombosis or ISR	Under-expansion is a risk factor for both stents thrombosis and restenosis (more significant in the thrombosis group). Under-expansion leading to thrombosis is usually more severe, diffuse and proximal in location.	
Doi et al.[97]	1580 patients (PES 1098, BMS 482)	Post-intervention MSA was the best predictor of future ISR in both the PES and BMS(cut-offs of stent patency at 9 months were 5.7 mm^2 for PES and 6.4 mm^2 for BMS).	9 months follow-up
Kang et al.[98]	394	IH was the general mechanism of ISR irrespective of the presence of under-expansion. However, under-expansion associated with longer stent length is still an important preventable mechanism of ISR by providing more room for intimal hyperplasia.	
Choi et al.[99]	355 lesions (45 ISR)	A smaller minimum stent area was the independent predictor of ISR after primary PCI for STEMI. Additional factors are diabetes, BMS use and longer stent length.	13 months follow-up from the HORIZONS-AMI Trial IVUS sub-study
Kang et al.[100]	175 patients with ISR of a single coronary artery (angiographic stenosis >50%), had a comparison of quantitative coronary angiography and IVUS with SPECT	The independent determinants for a positive SPECT were, in-segment IVUS-MLA<1.9 mm^2, stent under-expansion (MLA <5 mm^2), proximal location of the IVUS-MLA. Other factors are diabetes, in-segment angiographic diameter stenosis >69.5%	

(Continued)

Table 4.4 (continued) Studies evaluating ISR by IVUS

Study	No. of patients	IVUS parameters of ISR	Comments
Song et al.[101]	990 lesions (541 SES, 220 ZES and 229 EES)	Smaller post-procedural MSA predicted angiographic restenosis of the first and second generation DES with nearly similar cut-off values (5.5, 5.4 and 5.3 mm^2 for SES, EES and ZES, respectively).	9-months follow-up
Kang et al.[102]	126	Post-PCI MLD ≤ 2.4 mm and SER≤70%.	Done in CTO patients

IVUS, intravascular ultrasound; ISR, in-stent restenosis; BMS, bare-metal stents; CSA; CTO, chronic total occlusions; DES, drug-eluting stent; EES, everolimus-eluting stents; HORIZONS-AMI, Harmonizing Outcomes with Revascularization and Stents in Acute Myocardial Infarction; IH, intimal hyperplasia; MSA, minimum stent area; PCI, percutaneous intervention; SER; STEMI, ST segment elevation myocardial infarction; SPECT, ZES, zotarolimus-eluting stents.

Table 4.5 Studies evaluating stent thrombosis (ST) by IVUS

	No. of patients	IVUS parameters of ST	Comments
Cheneau et al.[103]	7484 without acute MI who were treated with PCI and underwent IVUS imaging during the intervention. 27 of them had angiographically documented sub-acute closure <1 week after PCI.	Sub-acute ST is related to inadequate post-procedure lumen dimensions (stent under-expansion), alone or in combination with other procedure related abnormal lesion morphologies (dissection, thrombus or tissue prolapse).	
Alfonso et al.[104]	50 consecutive patients with ST were enrolled. Thirty-eight of them were excluded for different reasons. In the remaining 12 patients, the thrombosed stent was studied by IVUS before intervention.	Severe stent under-expansion was present in most patients. Stent-related dissections, stent malapposition and significant inflow/outflow disease were also common.	
Fujii et al.[105]	15 patients with ST after SES implantation were compared with 45 matched control patients who had no evidence of stentthrombosis.	The independent predictors of ST were stent under-expansion (80% of ST group had an MSA <5 mm^2 and a significant residual reference segment stenosis. Stent malapposition was not significantly different between the two groups.	A retrospective study
Okabe et al.[106]	44 (14 lesions with ST and 30 control lesions).	A smaller minimum stent area and residual disease at the stent edges.	
Liu et al.[96]	20 definite ST patients were compared with 50 risk-factor-balanced ISR patients and 50 risk-factor-balanced 'no-event' patients with no thrombosis or ISR.	Under-expansion is a risk factor for both stents thrombosis and restenosis (more significant in the thrombosis group). Under-expansion leading to thrombosis is usually more severe, diffuse and proximal in location.	
Choi et al.[107]	12 patients with definite/probable early ST were compared with 389 patients without early ST.	Smaller stent lumen area <5 mm^2 and inflow/outflow disease (residual stenosis or dissection within 10 mm from stent edge) but not acute malapposition were associated with early ST after intervention in acute MI.	Substudy of HORIZON AMI study Done on acute MI patients

HORIZONS-AMI, Harmonizing Outcomes with Revascularization and Stents in Acute Myocardial Infarction; ISR, in-stent restenosis; IVUS, intravascular ultrasound; MI, myocardial infarction; PCI, percutaneous coronary intervention.

Finally and most recently, the IVUS-XLP study[83] showed that the simple criterion of a MSA greater than the distal reference lumen was associated with a 1-year MACE rate of only 1.5%. This seems to be a most reasonable and achievable endpoint to define optimal stent expansion.

4.9.2 Geographical miss and stent edge dissection

The second most important determinant of optimal stent implantation is the absence of geographical miss – defined as a stent edge plaque burden <50% and no significant stent edge dissection. Addition stents may be necessary to correct geographical miss. Geographical miss (GM) is simply defined as a stent missing a plaque after a PCI. This occurs as a result of incorrect stent edge landing zones and is essentially a marker of failed PCI, although the patient does not have an immediate event. It may be more problematic with DES compared with BMS. In the STLLR trial, which addressed the issue of GM, the incidence was surprisingly very high around 65%.[84] GM is associated with stent edge stenosis.

IVUS is commonly used to detect and direct the treatment of dissections (Figure 4.16) and other complications after intervention.[85–89]. *Dissection is classified on IVUS into five degrees of severity:*

Intimal: Limited to the intima or atheroma, and not extending to the media.
Medial: Extending into the media.

Adventitial: Extending through the external elastic membrane (EEM), consistent with perforation.
Intramural hematoma: An accumulation of blood within the medial space, displacing the internal elastic membrane inward and EEM outward. Entry and/or exit points may or may not be observed.
Intra-stent: Separation of neointimal hyperplasia from stent struts, usually seen after treatment of ISR.

The severity of a dissection can be quantified according to

1. Depth (into plaque – useful only in describing intimal dissections that do not reach the media)
2. Circumferential extent (in degrees of arc) using a protractor centred on the lumen
3. Length using motorised transducer pullback
4. Size of residual lumen which is arguably the most important parameter

Additional details of a dissection may include the presence of a false lumen, the identification of mobile flap(s), the presence of calcium at the dissection border and dissections in close proximity to stent edges (Figure 4.16).[6]

4.9.3 Malpposition

A final word about acute stent malapposition. Expansion refers to stent dimensions; apposition refers to the contact between the stent struts and the vessel wall. Under-expansion and malapposition can occur together or

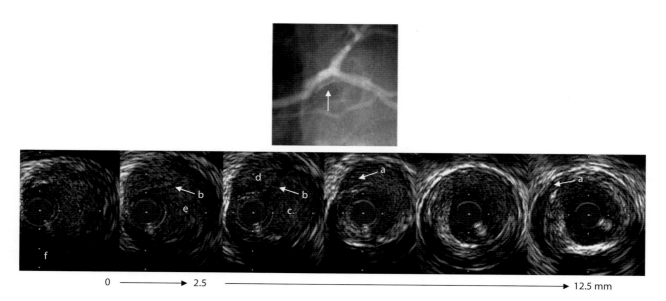

0 ———→ 2.5 —————————————————————————→ 12.5 mm

Figure 4.16 This dissection (white arrow in the angiogram) occurred during guiding catheter engagement. Intravascular ultrasound (IVUS) imaging showed a dissection plane (intimal flap) that distally was at the junction of plaque and normal vessel wall (a), while proximally was a thin membrane (b), separating true lumen (c) from false lumen (d). The true minimum lumen CSA (e) measured 8.1 mm². The thin proximal intimal flap looked echolucent compared with the blood speckle in the true and false lumina because of the reduced echogenicity of the intimal flap and because its thickness was near or below the resolution of the transducer. Notice that the pullback continued until the aorta (f) was seen. (Courtesy of Gary Mintz.)

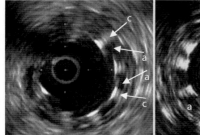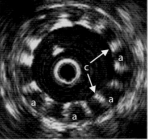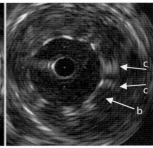

Figure 4.17 Three examples of acute stent malapposition are shown. Notice the space between the stent strut and the intima (a), the blood speckle behind the stent struts (b) and the multiple reflections from the malapposed stent struts that produce a characteristic rectangular appearance (c). (Courtesy of Gary Mintz.)

separately but apposition is different from expansion; and the two terms should not be used interchangeably. Despite widespread misconceptions, there are little data suggesting that isolated acute incomplete stent apposition is associated with adverse long-term outcomes – as long as the stent is well-expanded (Figure 4.17).

References

1. Sones FM. Cine coronary angiography. *Mod Concepts Cardiovasc Dis* 1962; 31: 735–38.
2. Topol EJ, and Nissen SE. Our preoccupation with coronary luminology. The dissociation between clinical and angiographic findings in ischemic heart disease. *Circulation* 1995; 92(8): 2333–42.
3. Bom N et al. An ultrasonic intracardiac scanner. *Ultrasonics* 1972; 10(2): 72–76.
4. Marco J et al. Intracoronary ultrasound imaging: Initial clinical trials (abstract). *Circulation* 1989; 80:II–374.
5. Nissen SE, and Yock P. Intravascular ultrasound: Novel pathophysiological insights and current clinical applications. *Circulation* 2001; 103: 604–16.
6. Mintz GS et al. American College of Cardiology Clinical Expert Consensus Document on Standards for Acquisition, Measurement and Reporting of Intravascular Ultrasound Studies (IVUS). A report of the American College of Cardiology Task Force on Clinical Expert Consensus Documents. *J Am Coll Cardiol* 2001; 37: 1478–92.
7. Di Mario C et al. Clinical application and image interpretation in intracoronary ultrasound. Study Group on Intracoronary Imaging of the Working Group of Coronary Circulation and of the Subgroup on Intravascular Ultrasound of the Working Group of Echocardiography of the European Society of Cardiology. *Eur Heart J* 1998; 19: 207–29.
8. Yamagishi M et al. Morphology of vulnerable coronary plaque: Insights from follow-up of patients examined by intravascular ultrasound before an acute coronary syndrome. *J Am Coll Cardiol* Jan 2000; 35: 106–11.
9. St Goar FG et al. Intravascular ultrasound imaging of angiographically normal coronary arteries: An in vivo comparison with quantitative angiography. *J Am Coll Cardiol* 1991; 18: 952–58.
10. Fitzgerald PJ et al. Intravascular ultrasound imaging of coronary arteries. Is three layers the norm? *Circulation* 1992; 86: 154–58.
11. Fitzgerald PJ et al. Orientation of intracoronary ultrasonography: Looking beyond the artery. *J Am Soc Echocardiogr* 1998; 11: 13–19.
12. ten Hoff H et al. Imaging artifacts in mechanically driven ultrasound catheters. *Int J Card Imaging* 1989; 4: 195–99.
13. Batkoff BW, and Linker DT. Safety of intracoronary ultrasound: Data from a Multicenter European Registry. *Cathet Cardiovasc Diagn* 1996; 38: 238–41.
14. Ge J et al. Intravascular ultrasound imaging of angiographically normal coronary arteries: A prospective study in vivo. *Br Heart J* 1994; 71: 572–78.
15. Tsutsui H et al. Influence of coronary pulsation on volumetric intravascular ultrasound measurements performed without ECG-gating. Validation in vessel segments with minimal disease. *Int J Cardiovasc Imaging* 2003; 19: 51–57.
16. Di Mario C et al. The angle of incidence of the ultrasonic beam: A critical factor for the image quality in intravascular ultrasonography. *Am Heart J* 1993; 125: 442–48.
17. Palmer ND et al. In vitro analysis of coronary atheromatous lesions by intravascular ultrasound; reproducibility and histological correlation of lesion morphology. *Eur Heart J* 1999; 20: 1701–06.
18. Peters RJ et al. Histopathologic validation of intracoronary ultrasound imaging. *J Am Soc Echocardiogr* 1994; 7: 230–41.
19. Nishimura RA et al. Intravascular ultrasound imaging: In vitro validation and pathologic correlation. *J Am Coll Cardiol* 1990; 16: 145–54.
20. Metz JA et al. Intravascular ultrasound: Basic interpretation. *Cardiol Clin* 1997; 15: 1–15.
21. Lockwood GR et al. In vitro high resolution intravascular imaging in muscular and elastic arteries. *J Am Coll Cardiol* 1992; 20: 153–60.
22. Gussenhoven EJ et al. Arterial wall characteristics determined by intravascular ultrasound imaging: An in vitro study. *J Am Coll Cardiol* 1989; 14: 947–52.
23. Potkin BN et al. Coronary artery imaging with intravascular high-frequency ultrasound. *Circulation* 1990; 81: 1575–85.
24. Hodgson JM et al. Intracoronary ultrasound imaging: Correlation of plaque morphology with angiography, clinical syndrome and procedural results in patients undergoing coronary angioplasty. *J Am Coll Cardiol* 1993; 21: 35–44.
25. Rasheed Q et al. Intracoronary ultrasound-defined plaque composition: Computer-aided plaque characterization and correlation with histologic samples obtained during directional coronary atherectomy. *Am Heart J* 1995; 129: 631–37.

26. Siegel RJ et al. Histopathologic validation of angioscopy and intravascular ultrasound. *Circulation* 1991; 84: 109–17.

27. Kearney P et al. Differences in the morphology of unstable and stable coronary lesions and their impact on the mechanisms of angioplasty. An in vivo study with intravascular ultrasound. *Eur Heart J* 1996; 17: 721–30.

28. Mintz GS et al. Target lesion calcification in coronary artery disease: An intravascular ultrasound study. *J Am Coll Cardiol* 1992; 20: 1149–55.

29. Tuzcu EM et al. The dilemma of diagnosing coronary calcification: Angiography versus intravascular ultrasound. *J Am Coll Cardiol* 1996; 27: 832–38.

30. Schmermund A, and Erbel R. Unstable coronary plaque and its relation to coronary calcium. *Circulation* 2001; 104: 1682–87.

31. Schoenhagen P, and Tuzcu EM. Coronary artery calcification and end stage renal disease. Vascular biology and clinical implications. *Cleve Clin J Med* 2002; 69 (Suppl 3): S12–S20.

32. Abizaid A et al. Clinical, intravascular ultrasound, and quantitative angiographic determinants of the coronary flow reserve before and after percutaneous transluminal coronary angioplasty. *Am J Cardiol* 1998; 82(4): 423–28.

33. Nishioka T et al. Clinical validation of intravascular ultrasound imaging for assessment of coronary stenosis severity: Comparison with stress myocardial perfusion imaging. *J Am Coll Cardiol* 1999; 33(7): 1870–78.

34. Takagi A et al. Clinical potential of intravascular ultrasound for physiological assessment of coronary stenosis: Relationship between quantitative ultrasound tomography and pressure-derived fractional flow reserve. *Circulation* 1999; 100(3): 250–55.

35. Briguori C et al. Intravascular ultrasound criteria for the assessment of the functional signifi cance of intermediate coronary artery stenoses and comparison with fractional flow reserve. *Am J Cardiol* 2001; 87(2): 136–41.

36. Takayama T, and Hodgson JM. Prediction of the physiologic severity of coronary lesions using 3D IVUS: Validation by direct coronary pressure measurements. *Catheter Cardiovas Interv* 2001; 53(1): 48–55.

37. Lee CH et al. New set of intravascular ultrasound-derived anatomic criteria for defining functionally significant stenoses in small coronary arteries (results from intravascular ultrasound diagnostic evaluation of atherosclerosis in Singapore [IDEAS] study). *Am J Cardiol* 2010; 105(10): 1378–84.

38. Kang SJ et al. Validation of intravascular ultrasound-derived parameters with fractional flow reserve for assessment of coronary stenosis severity. *Circ Cardiovasc Interv* 2011; 4(1): 65–71.

39. Ahn JM et al. Validation of minimal luminal area measured by intravascular ultrasound for assessment of functionally significant coronary stenosis comparison with myocardial perfusion imaging. *JACC Cardiovasc Interv* 2011; 4(6): 665–71.

40. Ben-Dor I et al. Correlation between fractional flow reserve and intravascular ultrasound lumen area in intermediate coronary artery stenosis. *EuroIntervention* 2011; 7: 225–33.

41. Bon-Kwon Koo et al. Optimal intravascular ultrasound criteria and their accuracy for defining the functional significance of intermediate coronary stenoses of different locations. *J Am Coll Cardiol Intv* 2011; 4(7): 803–11.

42. Ben-Dor I et al. Intravascular ultrasound lumen area parameters for assessment of physiological ischemia by fractional flow reserve in intermediate coronary artery stenosis. *Cardiovasc Revasc Med* 2012; 13(3): 177–82.

43. Soo-Jin Kang et al. Usefulness of minimal luminal coronary area determined by intravascular ultrasound to predict functional significance in stable and unstable angina pectoris. *Am J Cardiol* 2012; 109(7): 947–53.

44. Jin-Sin Koh et al. Relationship between fractional flow reserve and angiographic and intravascular ultrasound parameters in ostial lesions. Major epicardial vessel versus side branch ostial lesions. *J Am Coll Cardiol Intv* 2012; 5(4): 409–15.

45. Kwan TW et al. Optimized quantitative angiographic and intravascular ultrasound parameters predicting the functional significance of single de novo lesions in the left anterior descending artery. *Chin Med J* 2012; 125(23): 4249–53.

46. Gonzalo N et al. Morphometric assessment of coronary stenosis relevance with optical coherence tomography: A comparison with fractional flow reserve and intravascular ultrasound. *J Am Coll Cardiol* 2012; 59(12): 1080–89.

47. Waksman R et al. Intravascular ultrasound versus optical coherence tomography guidance. *J Am Coll Cardiol* 2013; 62(17): 532–40.

48. Kang SJ et al. Sex differences in the visual-functional mismatch between coronary angiography or intravascular ultrasound versus fractional flow reserve. *JACC Cardiovasc Interv* 2013; 6: 562–68.

49. Lopez-Palop R et al. Correlation between intracoronary ultrasound and fractional flow reserve in long coronary lesions. A three-dimensional intracoronary ultrasound study. *Rev Esp Cardiol (Engl Ed)* 2013; 66: 707–14.

50. Cui M et al. Usefulness of lumen area parameters determined by intravascular ultrasound to predict functional significance of intermediate coronary artery stenosis. *Chin Med J (Engl)* 2013; 126: 1606–11.

51. Yang HM et al. Relationship between intravascular ultrasound parameters and fractional flow reserve in intermediate coronary artery stenosis of left anterior descending artery: Intravascular ultrasound volumetric analysis. *Catheter Cardiovasc Interv* 2014; 83: 386–94.

52. Naganuma T et al. The role of intravascular ultrasound and quantitative angiography in the functional assessment of intermediate coronary lesions: Correlation with fractional flow reserve. *Cardiovasc Revasc Med* 2014; 15: 3–7.

53. Voros S et al. Prospective, head-to-head comparison of quantitative coronary angiography, quantitative computed tomography angiography, and intravascular ultrasound for the prediction of hemodynamic significance in intermediate and severe lesions, using fractional flow reserve as reference standard (from the ATLANTA I and II Study). *Am J Cardiol* 2014; 113: 23–29.

54. Han JK et al. Optimal intravascular ultrasound criteria for defining the functional significance of intermediate coronary stenosis: An international multicenter study. *Cardiology* 2014; 127: 256–62.

55. Cho YK et al. Usefulness of combined intravascular ultrasound parameters to predict functional significance of coronary artery stenosis and determinants of mismatch. *EuroIntervention* 2015; 11(2): 163–70.

56. Hermiller JB et al. Unrecognized left main coronary artery disease in patients undergoing interventional procedures. *Am J Cardiol* 1993; 71(2): 173–76.

57. Fisher LD et al. Reproducibility of coronary arteriographic reading in the coronary artery surgery study (CASS). *Cathet Cardiovasc Diagn* 1982; 8(6): 565–75.

58. Lindstaedt M et al. How good are experienced interventional cardiologists at predicting the functional significance of intermediate or equivocal left main coronary artery stenoses? *Int J Cardiol* 2007; 120(2): 254–61.

59. Hamilos M et al. Long-term clinical outcome after fractional flow reserve-guided treatment in patients with angiographically equivocal left main coronary artery stenosis. *Circulation* 2009; 120: 1505–12.

60. Chakrabarti AK et al. Angiographic validation of the American College of Cardiology Foundation – the Society of Thoracic Surgeons Collaboration on the Comparative Effectiveness of Revascularization Strategies study. *Circ Cardiovasc Interv* 2014; 7: 11–18.

61. Toth G et al. Evolving concepts of angiogram: Fractional flow reserve discordances in 4,000 coronary stenoses. *Eur Heart J* 2014; 35: 2381–88.

62. Conley MJ et al. The prognostic spectrum of left main stenosis. *Circulation* 1978; 57(5): 947–52.

63. Cameron A et al. Left main coronary artery stenosis: Angiographic determination. *Circulation* 1983; 68(3): 484–89.

64. Levine GN et al. 2011 ACCF/AHA/SCAI guideline for percutaneous coronary intervention. A report of the American college of cardiology Foundation/American heart association task force on practice guidelines and the society for cardiovascular angiography and interventions. *J Am Coll Cardiol* 2011; 58(24): e44–e122.

65. de la Torre Hernandez JM et al. Prospective application of pre-defined intravascular ultrasound criteria for assessment of intermediate left main coronary artery lesions results from the multicenter LITRO study. *J Am Coll Cardiol* 2011; 58(4): 351–58.

66. Abizaid AS et al. One-year follow-up after intravascular ultrasound assessment of moderate left main coronary artery disease in patients with ambiguous angiograms. *J Am Coll Cardiol* 1999; 34: 707–15.

67. Lindstaedt M et al. Invasive assessment of the borderline left main coronary artery stenosis—comparison with 99Tc-MIBI SPET (abstr). *Eur Heart J* 2004; 25 Suppl: 429.

68. Jasti V et al. Correlations between fractional flow reserve and intravascular ultrasound in patients with an ambiguous left main coronary artery stenosis. *Circulation* 2004; 110(18): 2831–36.

69. Fassa AA et al. Intravascular ultrasound-guided treatment for angiographically indeterminate left main coronary artery disease: A long-term follow-up study. *J Am Coll Cardiol* 2005; 45(2): 204–11.

70. Kang SJ et al. Intravascular ultrasound-derived predictors for fractional flow reserve in intermediate left main disease. *JACC Cardiovasc Interv* 2011; 4(11): 1168–74.

71. Park SJ et al. Intravascular ultrasound-derived minimal lumen area criteria for functionally significant left main coronary artery stenosis. *JACC Cardiovasc Interv* 2014; 7(8): 868.

72. Chieffo A et al. A prospective, randomized trial of intravascular-ultrasound guided compared with angiography guided stent implantation in complex coronary lesions: The AVIO trial. *Am Heart J* 2013; 165(1): 65–72.

73. Witzenbichler B et al. Relationship between intravascular ultrasound guidance and clinical outcomes after drug-eluting stents: The assessment of dual antiplatelet therapy with drug-eluting stents (ADAPT-DES) study. *Circulation* 2014; 129(4): 463–70.

74. Agostoni P et al. Comparison of early outcome of percutaneous coronary intervention for unprotected left main coronary artery disease in the drug-eluting stent era with versus without intravascular ultrasonic guidance. *Am J Cardiol* 2005; 95(5): 644–47.

75. Park SJ et al. Impact of intravascular ultrasound guidance on long-term mortality in stenting for unprotected left main coronary artery stenosis. *Circ Cardiovasc Interv* 2009; 2(3): 167–77.

76. Puri R et al. Optimizing outcomes during left main percutaneous coronary intervention with intravascular ultrasound and fractional flow reserve: The current state of evidence. *JACC Cardiovasc Interv* 2012; 5(7): 697–07.

77. de la Torre Hernandez JM et al. Clinical impact of intravascular ultrasound guidance in drug-eluting stent implantation for unprotected left main coronary disease: Pooled analysis at the patient-level of 4 registries. *JACC Cardiovasc Interv* 2014; 7(3): 244–54.

78. de Jaegere P et al. Intravascular ultrasound-guided optimized stent deployment. Immediate and 6 months clinical and angiographic results from the multicenter ultrasound stenting in coronaries study (MUSIC study). *Eur Heart J* 1998; 19(8): 1214–23.

79. Russo RJ et al. A randomized controlled trial of angiography versus intravascular ultrasound-directed bare-metal coronary stent placement (the AVID trial). *Circ Cardiovasc Interv* 2009; 2(2): 113–23.

80. Mudra H et al. Randomized comparison of coronary stent implantation under ultrasound or angiographic guidance to reduce stent restenosis (OPTICUS study). *Circulation* 2001; 104(12): 1343–49.

81. Schiele F et al. Impact of intravascular ultrasound guidance in stent deployment on 6-month restenosis rate: A multicenter, randomized study comparing two strategies – With and without intravascular ultrasound guidance. RESIST study group. REStenosis after ivus guided STenting. *J Am Coll Cardiol* 1998; 32(2): 320–28.

82. Oemrawsingh PV et al. Thrombocyte activity evaluation and effects of ultrasound guidance in long intracoronary stent placement. Intravascular ultrasound guidance improves angiographic and clinical outcome of stent implantation for long coronary artery stenoses: Final results of a randomized comparison with angiographic guidance (TULIP study). *Circulation* 2003; 107(1): 62–67.

83. Sung-Jin Hong et al. Effect of intravascular ultrasound–guided vs angiography-guided everolimus-eluting stent implantation. The IVUS-XPL Randomized Clinical Trial. *JAMA* 2015; 314 (20): 2155–63.

84. Costa MA et al. Impact of stent deployment procedural factors on long-term effectiveness and safety of sirolimus-eluting stents (Final Results of the Multicenter Prospective STLLR Trial. *Am J Cardiol* 2008; 101(12): 1704–11

85. Losordo DW et al. How does angioplasty work? Serial analysis of human iliac arteries using intravascular ultrasound. *Circulation* 1992; 86: 1845–58.

86. Potkin BN et al. Arterial responses to balloon coronary angioplasty: An intravascular ultrasound study. *J Am Coll Cardiol* 1992; 20: 942–51.

87. Braden GA et al. Qualitative and quantitative contrasts in the mechanisms of lumen enlargement by coronary balloon angioplasty and directional coronary atherectomy. *J Am Coll Cardiol* 1994; 23: 40–48.

88. van der Lugt A et al. Comparison of intravascular ultrasonic findings after coronary balloon angioplasty evaluated in vitro with histology. *Am J Cardiol* 1995; 76: 661–66.

89. Honye J et al. Morphological effects of coronary balloon angioplasty in vivo assessed by intravascular ultrasound imaging. *Circulation* 1992; 85: 1012–25.

90. Kasaoka S et al. Angiographic and intravascular ultrasound predictors of in-stent restenosis. *J Am Coll Cardiol* 1998; 32(6): 1630–35.

91. Fujii K et al. Contribution of stent underexpansion to recurrence after sirolimus-eluting stent implantation for in-stent restenosis. *Circulation* 2004; 109(9): 1085–88.

92. Sonoda S et al. Impact of final stent dimensions on long-term results following sirolimus eluting stent implantation: Serial intravascular ultrasound analysis from the SIRIUS trial. *J Am Coll Cardiol* 2004; 43: 1959–63.

93. Sakurai R et al. Predictors of edge stenosis following sirolimus-eluting stent deployment (a quantitative intravascular ultrasound analysis from the SIRIUS trial). *Am J Cardiol* 2005; 96(9): 1251–53.

94. Hong MK et al. Intravascular ultrasound predictors of angiographic restenosis after sirolimus-eluting stent implantation. *Eur Heart J* 2006; 27: 1305–10.

95. Costa MA et al. Impact of stent deployment procedural factors on long-term effectiveness and safety of sirolimus-eluting stents (final results of the multicenter prospective STLLR trial). *Am J Cardiol* 2008; 101(12): 1704–11.

96. Liu X et al. Intravascular ultrasound assessment of the incidence and predictors of edge dissections after drug eluting stent implantation. *JACC Cardiovasc Interv* 2009; 2: 997–1004.

97. Doi H et al. Impact of post-intervention minimal stent area on 9-month follow-up patency of paclitaxel-eluting stents. An integrated intravascular ultrasound analysis from the TAXUS IV, V, and VI and TAXUS ATLAS Workhorse, Long Lesion, and Direct Stent Trials. *JACC Cariovasc Interv* 2009; 2(12): 1269–75.

98. Kang SJ et al. Mechanisms of in-stent restenosis after drug-eluting stent implantation: Intravascular ultrasound analysis. *Circ Cardiovasc Interv* 2011; 4(1): 9–14.

99. Choi SY et al. Usefulness of minimum stent cross sectional area as a predictor of angiographic restenosis after primary percutaneous coronary intervention in acute myocardial infarction (from the HORIZONS-AMI Trial IVUS substudy). *Am J Cardiol* 2012; 109(4): 455–60.

100. Kang SJ et al. Predictors for functionally significant. In-stent restenosis. An integrated analysis using coronary angiography, IVUS, and myocardial perfusion imaging. *JACC Cardiovasc Imaging* 2013; 6(11): 1183–90.

101. Song HG et al. Intravascular ultrasound assessment of optimal stent area to prevent in-stent restenosis after zotarolimus-, everolimus-, and sirolimus-eluting stent implantation. *Catheter Cardiovasc Interv* 2014; 83(6): 873–78.

102. Kang J et al. Intravascular ultrasound and angiographic predictors of in-stent restenosis of chronic total occlusion lesions. *PLoS ONE* 10(10): 1–15.

103. Cheneau E et al. Predictors of subacute stent thrombosis: Results of a systematic intravascular ultrasound study. *Circulation* 2003; 108(1): 43–47.

104. Alfonso F et al. Findings of intravascular ultrasound during acute stent thrombosis. *Heart* 2004; 90: 1455–59.

105. Fuji K et al. Stent under expansion and residual reference segment stenos are related to stent thrombosis after sirolimus-eluting stent implantation: An intravascular ultrasound study. *JACC* 2005; 45: 995–98.

106. Okabe T et al. Intravascular ultrasound parameters associated with stent thrombosis after drug-eluting stent deployment. *Am J Cardiol* 2007; 100(4): 615–20.

107. Choi SY et al. Intravascular ultrasound findings of early stent thrombosis after primary percutaneous intervention in acute myocardial infarction: A Harmonizing Outcomes with Revascularization and Stents in Acute Myocardial Infarction (HORIZONS-AMI) substudy. *Circ Cardiovasc Interv* 2011; 4(3): 239–47.

New intravascular imaging techniques (optical coherence tomography"OCT" and optical frequency domain imaging"OFDI")

AMR S GAMAL, JAVED AHMED

5.1 Introduction

Optical coherence tomography (OCT) is an evolving intra-coronary imaging modality that performs high-resolution cross-sectional images of biological structures, including coronary arteries. It acts like an optical biopsy yielding real time and in situ visualisation of vascular microstructure and pathology without the need for an excisional biopsy.[1] This technology was originally developed for retinal imaging but shortly the indications have expanded to visualise the coronary arteries.

5.2 Principle

OCT is a catheter-based invasive imaging system that uses light instead of ultrasound. OCT catheter utilises a single optical fibre that both emits light and records the reflection from the coronary wall structures whilst simultaneously rotating and being pulled back along the artery. By measuring the echo time delay and the signal intensity after its reflection or back-scattering, a scan of the segment of interest is performed.[2] It uses light in the infrared spectrum with central wavelength ranging from 1250 to 1350 nm.[3]

The very short wave length of light leads to extremely high speed of light compared with ultrasound, which represents the fundamental difference between optical and ultrasound-based imaging. In tissues, the speed of light is nearly 3×10^8 m/s compared with 1500 m/s for ultrasound. The ideal resolution for intravascular ultrasound (IVUS), 100 µm, requires a time delay of 100 nanoseconds to detect sound echoes. This time delay, also called time resolution, is within the range of electronic detection of IVUS machines. On the other hand, the detection of light echoes requires much higher time resolution. A time resolution of ~30 femtoseconds (3×10^{15} seconds) is required for measurement of distances with a 10 µm resolution, the typical resolution for OCT imaging. Accordingly, direct measurement of time delays between optical echoes by usual electronic means is extremely difficult and measurement methods such as interferometry are required for OCT imaging. Interferometry depends on coherence, a physical property of light waves that makes them capable of generating interference when combined.[4]

The light emitted from a low coherence source like infrared diode or a femtosecond laser passes through an interferometer, which splits the light beam into halves. The first half goes to the patient (sample arm), whilst the other one travels a predefined distance that ends in a mirror (reference arm). After leaving the tissue, signals coming from the two arms are combined by a detector. Interference occurs when the distances travelled by both arms are roughly equivalent creating a pattern of high and low intensities that are analysed by the OCT system to determine the amount of backscatter in relation to the delay time and accordingly the depth of tissue.

5.3 Characteristics of OCT image

OCT is characterised by very high image resolution. The axial resolution of OCT is 10–20 μm, whilst it is typically only 100–200 μm with IVUS. This superior resolution of OCT helps as an essential tool in assessment of the intimal layer of the coronary vessel. However, this high resolution occurs at the expense of low tissue penetration. The current maximum tissue penetration with OCT is approximately 1.5–3 mm compared with 10 mm for IVUS. This limits the assessment of some vessel structures like external elastic lamina particularly in the presence of highly attenuating tissues like lipid plaques or dense blood in the lumen. Accordingly plaque volume is better measured with IVUS, which has higher tissue penetration and less attenuation.

5.4 Types of OCT systems

There are two main types of OCT systems:

1. **Time domain OCT (TD-OCT):** Commercially available as M2 and M3 OCT systems (Light Lab Imaging, Westford, MA, USA).
2. **Newly developed frequency domain or Fourier domain OCT (FD-OCT):**
   Currently available FD-OCT systems are
   a. The C7-XR/ILUMIEN™ system from St. Jude ILUMIEN™ Medical/Light Lab Imaging, Westford, MA, USA) (Figure 5.1).
   b. The OFDI system from Terumo Corporation (Tokyo, Japan) (Figure 5.1).
   c. The LVOCT™ system from Volcano Corporation.

In TD-OCT systems, an over-the-wire low-pressure occlusion balloon catheter with distal flush ports (Helios, Goodman, Nagoya, Japan) is used to infuse saline or Ringer's Lactate at approximately 0.5 mL/s to displace blood during imaging acquisition. Optimal imaging was limited by prolonged occlusion times.[5] In this OCT system, the position of the mirror at the end of the reference arm is varied by few millimetres to produce known echo delays. This mechanical scanning of the reference mirror limits the maximum

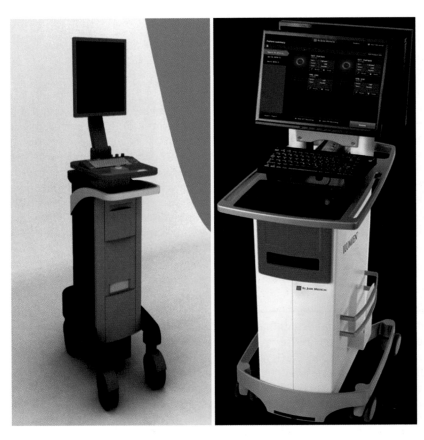

Figure 5.1 OFDI Terumo (left panel) and OCT ILUMIEN (right panel). (Courtesy of Terumo Corporation and St. Jude Medical, respectively.)

acquisition rate. Accordingly, the pullback speed is limited as well to get an acceptable lateral and longitudinal resolution; forty to fifty seconds are required for an entire OCT pullback.

On the other hand, in FD-OCT systems, the reference arm mirror is fixed but the wavelength of the light source is swept. In these systems, frequency encoding is employed to resolve the depth of scattering structures. This makes these systems significantly faster by simultaneously detecting light reflections from all echo delays. A 4- to 6-cm-length epicardial coronary vessel could be scanned in 3–5 seconds using a single, high-rate (4 cc/s) bolus injection of contrast that replaces occlusion balloon and produces a blood-free environment. These systems can acquire 100 frames/s, reaching pullback speeds up to 20 mm/s with no need for balloon occlusion.[5]

5.5 Colour mapping

The intensity of OCT signal is mapped into a colour scale that is displayed on a monitor. The main colours used are grey scale (low intensity is black, high intensity is white) inverted grey scale, sepia scale, ranging from black (low OCT signal) through brown, gold, yellow and white (high OCT signal) and less commonly colour mappings (e.g. rainbow-like).

5.6 OCT imaging acquisition technique

In the old Lightlab TD-OCT, an over-the-wire balloon catheter (Helios) is first passed distally to the segment of interest over an angioplasty guidewire (0.014-in.). This balloon has a maximum external diameter of 1.5 mm, which makes it compatible with large 6-F guiding catheters. The guidewire is then exchanged for the OCT ImageWire, then the occlusion balloon is pulled back and repositioned in a healthy proximal segment. The balloon is highly compliant and is inflated at minimal pressure, usually between 0.4 and 0.7 atm with a dedicated inflator. This helps clearing of blood from the imaging field. A contrast injector pump is set at an infusion rate of 0.5–1.0 cc/s until blood is totally cleared. The solution is injected through the end-hole distal port of the occlusion balloon catheter and should start several seconds before balloon occlusion. The pullback speed can be adjusted from 0.5 to 3.0 mm/s.[6]

In the newer generation FD-OCT systems, after the removal of the catheter from the packaging (Dragonfly catheter [DUO C7 and OPTIS], St. Jude Medical, Westford, MA, USA), a 3 cc syringe is used to flush the side arm of the catheter with non-diluted contrast. The catheter is then connected to the console and then advanced over the wire to be parked distally in the coronary vessel beyond the segment of interest. Again, at least a 6Fr-guiding catheter is required for the FD-OCT imaging. Coaxial alignment of the guiding catheter is important and should be confirmed by injection of a small contrast flush through the guide catheter prior to imaging.[6]

Manual contrast injection through the guide catheter using the manifold syringe initiates the automated OCT pullback. In addition, contrast injection in those systems is also needed for clearance of blood as balloon occlusion is not used. The average rate of contrast injection should be 4 cc/s to assure complete blood clearance. For non-occlusion techniques, iodinated contrast media is preferred over saline or Ringer's lactate because the former high viscosity solutions are much better in completely removing blood. The pullback speeds for FD-OCT systems typically ranges from 10 to 40 mm/s. Imaging of 4–6 cm of coronary artery segments can be achieved with 10–15 mL of contrast per pullback.[6]

5.7 Image interpretation

5.7.1 OCT artefacts

Some OCT artefacts are similar to those seen with IVUS, and others are unique to OCT. Knowledge of these artefacts is important to guide proper image interpretation.[6,7]

1. **Residual blood (blood swirling):** The high scattering of red blood cells (RBCs) causes significant light attenuation and may preclude imaging of the underlying vessel wall depending on the density of the blood. Care must be taken not to mistake this artefact for thrombus or some other specific intravascular finding. However, the presence of diluted blood does not appear to affect area measurements as long as the lumen surface is still clearly defined (Figure 5.2).
2. **Nonuniform rotational distortion (NURD):** This type of artefact occurs less frequently in OCT compared with IVUS imaging probably related to the smaller profile and simplified rotational mechanics of OCT wires. It appears as smearing of the OCT signal in the lateral or circumferential direction. It is the result of variation in the rotational speed of the spinning optical fibre caused by either by vessel tortuosity, passage across a tight lesion, a crimped imaging sheath or its constriction by a tight haemostatic valve (Figure 5.3).
3. **Motion or sew-up artefact** is the result of rapid movement of the artery, wire or catheter leading to single-point misalignment of the intimal border (Figure 5.4).
4. **Saturation artefact** occurs when light is reflected off a highly reflective surface (metal, wire or stent strut) leading to production of signals with amplitudes that exceed the normal dynamic range of the detector. This appears as streaking scan lines of different intensity along the axial direction of the reflector (Figure 5.5).
5. **Fold-over artefact** is more specific to the new generation FD-OCT and occurs when the vessel is larger than the ranging depth leading to the appearance of folding over of a portion of the vessel in the periphery of the image. This is particularly seen in large vessels and side branches (Figure 5.6).
6. **Bubble artefact** occurs when small gas bubbles or other impurities are present in the silicon lubricant used to reduce friction between the sheath and the revolving optic fibre in TD-OCT and occasionally the FD-OCT systems. They can attenuate the signal along a region of

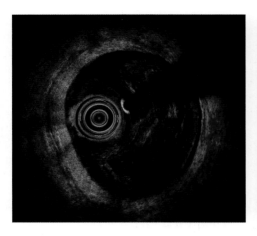
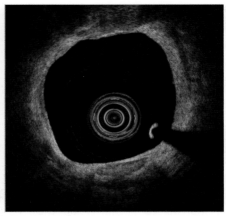

Figure 5.2 Blood swirling (left panel) compared with clear vessel lumen (right panel). (Courtesy of St. Jude Medical.)

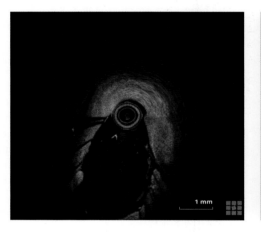
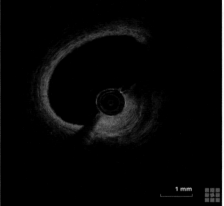

Figure 5.3 OCT NURD artefact: seen from 12 to 3 o'clock in left panel (note the metallic stent artefacts in the rest of the image) and from 3 to 6 o'clock in right panel. (Courtesy of Amr Gamal.)

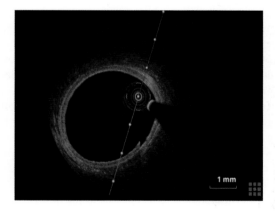

Figure 5.4 Sew-up artefact at 5 o'clock. (Courtesy of St. Jude Medical.)

the vessel wall leading to difficult interpretation of tissue characterisation and plaque morphology. Sometimes gas bubbles lead to shadowing of the underlying vessel wall similar to guidewire artefact. However, the gas bubbles are contained within the catheter sheath whilst the guidewire is out of the catheter sheath into the lumen.

7. **Artefacts related to eccentric wire position:**
   Eccentricity of the image wire in the vessel lumen can lead to longer distance the light travels to reach the opposite wall and consequently decreasing the lateral resolution. This artefact has been also named the 'merry-go-round' effect.

8. **Multiple reflections artefacts** occur when the light is reflected against specular surfaces many times at a reflection distance equal to the phase of light creating phantom structures. These reflections appear as circular lines around the catheter when light bounces the inner facets of the catheter or as multiple strut reflections in the vessel when light bounces the original struts.

9. **Tangential signal drop out:** It occurs when the catheter is near or touching vessel wall leading to parallel direction of the optical beam in relation to the vessel surface. As a result, the optical beam is attenuated as it passes through the superficial part of the vessel wall resulting in signal poor appearance of the underlying vessel wall. This could be misinterpreted as lipid pools or necrotic core (Figure 5.7).

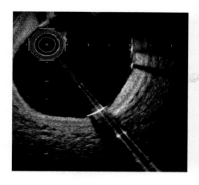
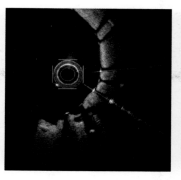
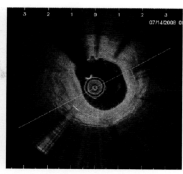

Figure 5.5 OCT saturation artifact appearing as laser beam crossing stent struts (Courtesy of Terumo corporation and St. Jude medical respectively.)

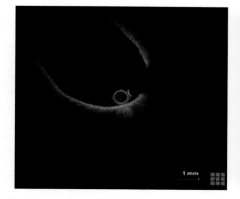
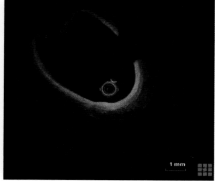

Figure 5.6 Fold over artifact from 9 to 12 o'clock. Note the large size of the vessel (Courtesy of Amr Gamal.)

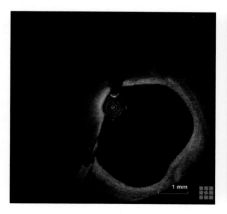
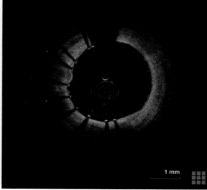

Figure 5.7 **Left panel**: Tangential tissue dropout (from 7 to 1 O'Clock). Note the catheter touching the vessel wall at 11 O'Clock and the wire artifact at 12 O'Clock, **right panel**: Blooming artifact (around the struts from 5 to 7 o'clock) appear as circumferential glare. (Courtesy of Amr Gamal.)

10. **Blooming:** Highly reflecting structures like stent struts create the appearance of a glare that is smeared along the stent surface and falsely enlarges the dimensions of struts. This blooming artefact may affect the quantification of strut coverage and should be considered when assessing the apposition of struts (Figure 5.7).
11. **Metallic struts and guidewires:** Light cannot penetrate metals so it creates a shadow on the sides of guidewires, metallic stent struts and radiopaque markers of bioabsorbable vascular scaffolds (BVS) (Figures 5.7 and 5.8). This back shadowing is different from blooming artefact, which is more of a circumferential glare. The size of the shadow depends on the location of the metallic structure to the imaging catheter and the vessel wall being larger if the metallic structure is closer to the imaging catheter and/or farther from the vessel wall. The direction of the shadow is away from the OCT catheter and it hinders visualisation of the underlying vessel wall structures. For example, in metallic stents, the endoluminal part of the strut rather than the entire strut thickness is visualised, which should also be considered when assessing the stent struts apposition to the vessel

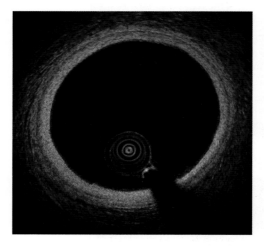

Figure 5.8 Wire shadowing artefact (at 1 o'clock). (Courtesy of Amr Gamal.)

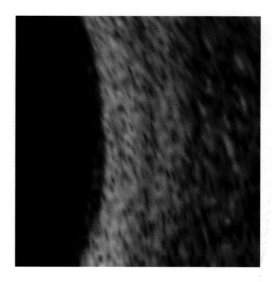

Figure 5.9 **Upper panel** shows normal vessel wall, lumen and imaging catheter with wire artifact at 5 O'Clock. **Lower panel** shows magnified vessel wall with 3-layered structure: intima, media, and adventitia (courtesy of St. Jude medical).

wall. The same applies to guidewire which appears crescent shaped as the back side of the wire is not visualised. On the other hand, in optically translucent stents like BVS, the entire strut thickness could be visualised. A similar phenomenon occurs on the abluminal side of opaque objects as blood, thrombus and macrophages where the drop in signal intensity leads to creation of a shadow behind those structures.

12. **Speckle** is a grainy noise within the OCT image and is technically caused by the way of OCT image formation. It is seen everywhere in the image particularly in signal poor areas and its size becomes bigger as we go away from the imaging catheter.

13. **Scattering and focus artefacts:** Scattering of light away from the imaging focus decreases OCT signal intensity and accordingly lateral resolution. Accordingly, structures like stent struts which are far from the focus or are imaged though blood or thick neointimal tissue may appear dimmer and larger than they are.

14. **Elongation of the imaging wire at the start of pullback:** It is typically seen with TD-OCT system where at the beginning of pullback, the optic fibres in those systems elongate. This is related to the fact that the optical fibres in TD-OCT are not contained in the catheter sheath. This appears as fluctuation in the size of the wire in a cross-sectional view which affects the accuracy of measurement.

5.7.2 Criteria used for describing lesions on OCT

The following criteria are commonly used in OCT to identify lesion morphology:

1. **Backscatter (signal intensity):** Backscattering is a term used to describe signal intensity. Lesion with high backscattering will appear bright (signal rich) and vice versa.
2. **Attenuation:** Attenuation is used to describe penetration beyond the lumen. In a lesion with low attenuation, the lumen and underlying vessel wall can be evaluated whilst with high attenuation lesions, this will be difficult.
3. **Borders** (sharply or poorly delineated).
4. **Consistency** (homogenous or heterogeneous).

5.7.3 Normal vessel wall on OCT

OCT is capable of defining the tri-laminar structure (intima, media and adventitia) of the vessel with an accuracy comparable to histology. In OCT, the innermost layer is the intima which appears as high backscattering signal rich layer. It is usually seen in young individuals. Next to the intima is the media which is a homogeneous low backscattering signal poor layer. The outermost layer is the adventitia, which is a high backscattering and heterogeneous layer. The internal and external elastic membranes (also called internal and external elastic laminae; IEM or IEL and EEM or ELL respectively) appear as high backscattering thin lines separating the intima from the media and the media from the adventitia, respectively.[8] The thickness of IEL and EEL is around 20 μm (Figure 5.9).

5.7.4 Lesion morphology on OCT

1. **Non-atherosclerotic intimal thickening:** It exhibits homogeneous signal rich, low attenuating appearance with an intimal thickness between 300 and 600 μm. The media is visualised in ≥ 3 quadrants (Figure 5.10).
2. **Pathological intimal thickening (PIT) or fibrous plaques:** It exhibits homogeneous signal rich, low attenuating appearance with an intimal thickness more than 600 μm (Figure 5.11).[7]
3. **Fibrocalcific plaque:** It exhibits signal poor, high attenuating heterogenous appearance with sharply demarcated borders (leading, trailing and/or lateral edges). It shows evidence of both fibrous tissue and calcium. Microcalcifications are not well defined (Figures 5.12 and 5.13).[7]
4. **Fibroatheroma (fatty plaques):** This plaque shows evidence of both lipid (necrotic core) and fibrous tissue (fibrous cap) (Figures 5.14 through 5.17 and 5.19).
   a. **Necrotic core:** It exhibits signal poor, high attenuating homogeneous appearance with poorly delineated borders. It may also show features of macrophages, cholesterol crystals or microcalcifications. The necrotic core is covered by a fibrous cap.[7]
   b. **Fibrous cap:** It appears as a homogenous signal rich layer with low attenuation.[7]
   c. **Thin-cap fibroatheroma (TCFA):** A fibroatheroma where the minimum fibrous cap thickness is less than a predetermined threshold (65 μm). Additionally, the arc subtended by the necrotic core should be greater than 90° (one quadrant)[7] (Figure 5.15).
   d. **Thick-cap fibroatheroma:** A fibroatheroma where the minimum fibrous cap thickness is greater than 65 μm (Figure 5.16).
5. **Mixed plaque:** It shows a mixture of evidence of either calcium, lipid or fibrous tissue.[7]
6. **Macrophages:** They appear as signal-rich, distinct or confluent punctate accumulations with high attenuation of the underlying tissue giving it the false appearance of underlying lipid pool or necrotic core. Accordingly, a relatively normal artery can falsely appear as a TCFA. However, the overall image should be thoroughly assessed as macrophages are only considered in the context of fibroatheroma as no validation studies have been performed on normal vessel wall or intimal hyperplasia.

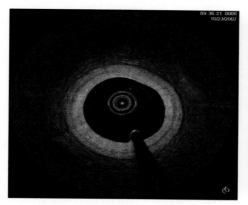 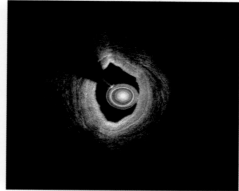

Figure 5.10 Mild (nonatherosclerotic) intimal thickening on both OCT ILUMIEN (left panel) and OFDI (right panel). (Courtesy of St. Jude Medical and Terumo Corporation, respectively.)

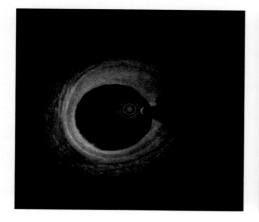 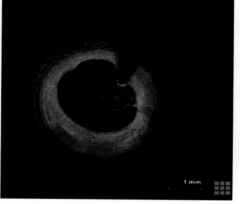

Figure 5.11 Shows pathological intimal thickening on OFDI (left panel) and ILUMIEN St. Jude OCT (right panel) (Courtesy of Terumo corporation and Amr Gamal respectively.)

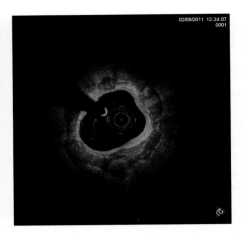

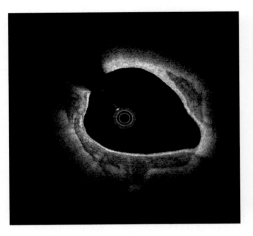

Figure 5.12 **Left panel** shows calcified plaque extending from 9 to 12 O'Clock, **right panel** shows nearly complete arc of Calcium napkin ring) (Courtesy of St. Jude Medical.)

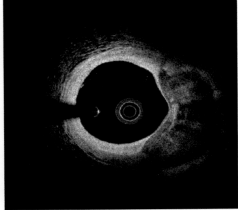

Figure 5.13 Shows calcified plaque extending from 1 to 3 and from 4 to 10 o'clock (left panel) and from 2 to 6 o'clock (right panel) (Courtesy of Terumo corporation.)

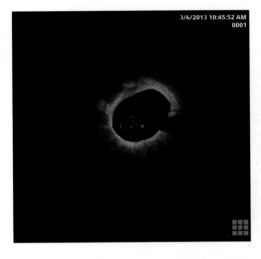

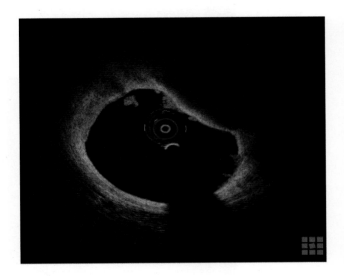

Figure 5.14 Thin-cap fibroatheroma (TCFA) with necrotic core and overlying fibrous cap from 3 to 11. Note the macrophages accumulation from 10 to 12 o'clock. (Courtesy of St. Jude Medical.)

Figure 5.15 Thin-cap fibroatheroma (TCFA) with an underlying lipid pool from 12 to 4 o'clock. (Courtesy of Amr Gamal.)

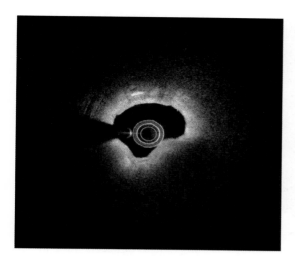

Figure 5.16 Thick-cap fibroatheroma on OFDI shows a large necrotic core from 3 to 8 o'clock covered by a thick fibrous cap. Note cholesterol crystals at 12 o'clock. (Courtesy of Amr Gamal)

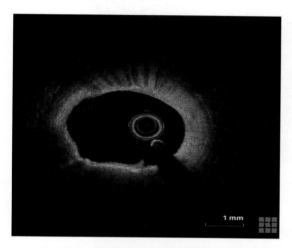

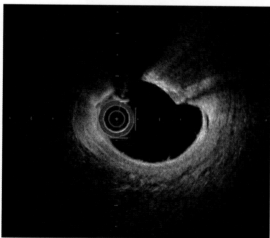

Figure 5.17 Macrophage appears as highly backscattering accumulations within the artery wall with backshadowing. Macrophages could be either scattered as in upper panel (from 10 to 1 o'clock) or confluent as in lower panel (from 1 to 3 o'clock). (Courtesy of Amr Gamal and Javed Ahmed.)

In fibrotheroma, macrophages are seen at the boundary between the bottom of the cap and the top of a necrotic core (the most characteristic feature differentiating it from thin fibrous cap). Another differentiating point is that macrophages-induced attenuation appears as interrupted usually multiple linear shadowings (not confluent as with TCFA). Shadowing is not caused by macrophages themselves but rather by their content of large pools of lipid (fat- laden macrophages or foam cells) that cause significant light attenuation. Macrophage accumulations should be differentiated from microcalcifications, cholesterol crystals, IEM or EEM (Figure 5.17).[7]

7. **Microvessels:** They appear as round or oval structures with black (signal poor) content appearing as sharply delineated voids. With atherosclerotic disease progression and intimal thickening exceeding 500 μm, hypoxia occurs, which stimulates the growth of microvessels from the adventitia (also called vasa plaquorum). If these vascular channels exceed a diameter of 200 μm on OCT, a differential diagnosis of side branches should be considered. Inspection of multiple adjacent frames will help to diagnose microvessel, which typically grows from the periadventitial vessels towards the media and intima not traversing the luminal border, unlike the side branch which typically connects with the lumen at some point (Figure 5.18).[7]

8. **Cholesterol crystals:** They appear as thin, linear regions (needle shaped crystals) of high intensity, usually associated and located deeper within a lipid plaque. However, there is no definite histopathological validation for this feature (Figure 5.19).[7,9]

9. **Thrombus:** It appears as a mass either attached to vessel wall, stent struts or the catheter itself or floating within the lumen. Two types are recognised:[7]
   a. **Red (RBC-rich) thrombus:** Characterised by highly backscatter and a high attenuation (resembles blood) (Figure 5.20).
   b. **White (platelet-rich) thrombus:** Characterised by less backscattering (more translucent), homogeneous and low attenuation (Figure 5.21).

10. **Dissections:** They appear as disruptions in the luminal vessel contour that could be intimal, medial, adventitial, intramural hematoma or intrastent (will be discussed later).[7]

11. **Aneurysm:** It appears as a cavity-like structure which may be true or false depending on the disruption of EEM creating a true and false lumen.

12. **Metallic stent struts:** They are clearly observed on OCT images as small bright line segments. Because of the fact that light does not pass through metals, it is strongly reflected on the endoluminal surface of stent struts creating a hyperintense signal, usually named as 'blooming' with a shadow seen behind the blooming.[10] With healing and growth of the neointima over the stent, the intensity of the blooming decreases. As the abluminal surface of the strut is not seen, assessment of strut apposition does need subtraction of the strut thickness (Figure 5.22).

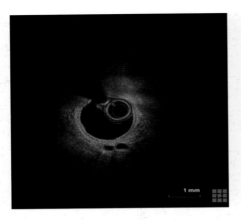
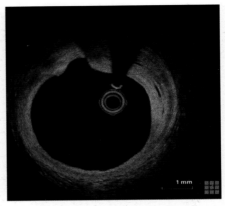

Figure 5.18 Intimal vessels, appear as well-delineated low backscattering voids within the intima from 12 to 3 o'clock in the right panel and 5 to 6 o'clock in the left panel. Note the fibroatheromatous plaque in the left panel and the fibrous one in the right panel. (Courtesy of Amr Gamal.)

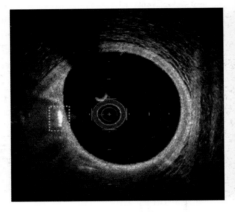
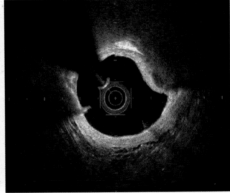

Figure 5.19 **Cholesterol crystals** appear as linear high backscattering areas within the plaque at 9 o'clock (left panel), and from 12 to 1 o'clock (right panel) (Courtesy of Terumo corporation and Amr Gamal respectively.)

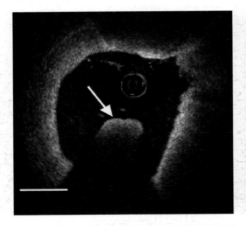
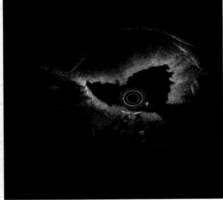

Figure 5.20 **Left panel:** Red thrombus at 6 o'clock (white arrow), **right panel:** red thrombus from 9 to 2 o'clock. In both it appears as a protruding mass into the lumen with high backscattering and attenuation (Courtesy of St. Jude Medical and Terumo corporation respectively.)

13. **Bioabsorbable stents (bioresorbable vascular scaffolds, BVS):** They are clearly seen on OCT as box-shaped structures with dark content as the light is diffusely reflected from the strut borders.[10] They reflect and scatter OCT light more weakly than metallic stents. As the abluminal surface of the strut is clearly seen, assessment of strut apposition does not need subtraction of the strut thickness (Figure 5.23).

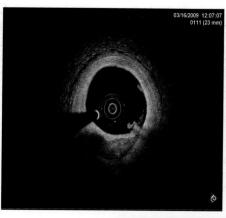
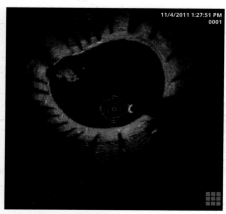

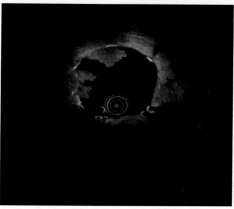

Figure 5.21 White thrombus appears as homogeneous backscattering mass with low attenuation attached to the surface of coronary artery(note the underlying calcific plaque in left upper panel) or stent struts (note the underlying stent struts in right upper panel and lower panel) (Courtesy of St.Jude Medical and Terumo corporation respectively.)

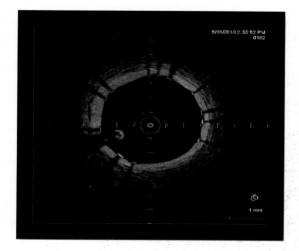

Figure 5.22 Metallic stent struts with bright inner surface and shadowing behind. (Courtesy of St. Jude Medical.)

Figure 5.23 Bioabsorbable vascular scaffolds (BVS) struts (translucent) seen in the upper part of the image and metallic struts in the lower part (dark). (Courtesy of St. Jude Medical.)

5.8 Clinical applications of OCT

5.8.1 Diagnostic assessment of coronary atherosclerosis

Using tissue histology as the reference, a number of validation studies[8,11–14] have helped the international OCT community to define the lesions' morphology on OCT. In this chapter, we use the modified American Heart Association (AHA) classification by Virmani et al.[15] Based on this classification, the following morphological lesions of pre-atherosclerosis/atherosclerosis can be seen on OCT:

a. **Non-atherosclerotic intimal changes** such as intimal thickening and fatty streaks (intracellular lipid) may gradually occur in the normal vessel with advancing age. Physiologically, it is considered as an adaptive response to mechanical stress caused by variation in flow, wall tension and shear stress. Pathologically, intimal thickening is caused by accumulation of smooth muscle cells with absence of lipid or macrophage foam cells. The normal intimal thickness is less than 300 μm on OCT. In non-atherosclerotic intimal thickening, the thickness of the intima is above the normal range (300 μm) but still below that for atherosclerotic lesion (600 μm). It displays homogeneous signal rich, low attenuating appearance. The media is visible in three or more quadrants. Fatty streaks cannot be distinguished from intimal thickening on OCT.

b. **PIT or fibrous plaques:** Pathologically, it represents accumulation of smooth muscle cells within a matrix rich in proteoglycans. It may contain extracellular lipids with no necrotic core and it has an intact extracellular matrix, which differentiates it from fatty plaques. However, the distinction between intracellular and extracellular lipids is not possible on OCT and hence an arbitrary cut-off point of 600 μm is used to differentiate normal intimal thickening from a pathological one. Similar to normal intimal thickening, PIT (fibrous plaques) appears as a homogenous signal rich low attenuating layer. It should be noted that these plaques may contain some calcium or lipid but they are limited to less than one quadrant. Due to the low attenuation properties of the fibrous plaque, it is often still possible to visualise the underlying media. Sometimes, very thick fibrous intima may cause strong light attenuation resembling fatty plaques.

c. **Fibroatheromas (fatty or lipid plaques):** With the progression of atherosclerosis, the disintegration of the extracellular matrix by collagenases leads to the formation of necrotic core, which is the distinguishing feature of fibroatheroma. Although necrotic core is considered as an advancing stage of lipid pool after destruction of extracellular matrix, both of them display homogeneous signal poor high attenuating areas. Whilst it is proposed that the light attenuation caused by necrotic core is greater than that caused by lipid pools, this differentiation cannot be made by OCT and so they are denoted together. Because PIT contains extracellular lipid pool, which has nearly the same OCT appearance of necrotic core, a plaque is called PIT when lipid pool/necrotic core is less than one quadrant and a fibroatheroma when the lipid pool/necrotic core is one or more quadrant. This lipid pool/necrotic core is covered by fibrous cap, which appears as a homogenous

signal rich layer. This cap could be thin (TCFA) or thick (thick cap fibroatheroma). This differentiation is important in assessing the risk of plaque rupture and subsequent thrombosis (plaque vulnerability). A fibrous cap thickness of 65 μm is used as a cut-off point to differentiate between the two subtypes. Due to the high attenuation of fatty plaques, visualising the underlying media is not possible.

d. **Fibrocalcific plaque:** From previous histology studies, it is known that coronary calcification correlates with plaque burden.[16] On OCT, calcific plaques appear as low-scattering, signal-poor areas with low attenuation. Although signal-poor appearance is also characteristic of lipid pool/necrotic core, two main criteria differentiate calcified plaques from fatty ones; first, the borders of calcified plaques are well delineated whilst those of fatty plaques are indistinct. Second, the calcified plaques are characterised by low attenuation and accordingly it is feasible to delineate the underlying vessel wall, whilst fatty plaques display high attenuating appearance.

5.8.2 Assessment of plaque vulnerability

A vulnerable plaque is a term that refers to a thrombosis prone plaque leading to acute coronary syndrome (ACS) or sudden cardiac death. Here we are going to discuss in detail rupture prone plaques as an example of vulnerable plaques. The precursors of plaque erosion and calcium nodules, as other substrates of ACS, are not well defined. From the current understanding of plaque biology, we can find that around 80% of plaque rupture occurs in an inflamed TCFA.[17] TCFA are characterised by three essential components: a thin fibrous cap, a lipid core and inflammatory cell cap infiltration.

a. **Thin fibrous cap:** A fibrous cap thickness of 65 μm has been traditionally used as the cut-off point for TCFA and accordingly higher risk of plaque rupture. However, it has been demonstrated by OCT that the patterns of fibrous cap thickness and plaque rupture vary significantly. For example, in 93% of cases of acute myocardial infarction with exertional symptoms, the fibrous cap thickness is 90 μm whilst in 57% of cases of acute myocardial infarction having symptoms at rest the thickness of the fibrous cap is 50 μm.[18]

b. **Lipid core:** As the light does not penetrate deeply into the necrotic core, and is absorbed by the lipid tissue, it is difficult to quantify the extent of lipid core or to evaluate remodelling.[8] It is agreed that lipid accumulation in two or more quadrants is required to complete the definition of TCFA.

c. **Inflammation:** The thin fibrous cap of fibroatheroma is infiltrated by macrophages. These inflammatory cells can occur isolated and spread or more often clustered together appearing as dots or band, respectively. Due to their large size and high lipid content, they yield strong optical signals. Clusters of macrophages can appear as bright spots along the fibrous cap casting a very dark shadow.[19]

Collections of macrophages have strong attenuating properties, which lead to casting of a laterally sharply demarcated shadow. This is a typical characteristic which can help to differentiate a band of macrophages overlying a fibroatheroma from a true TCFA.

Another characteristic of advanced plaque which is closely related to inflammation is the development of microvessels. With gradually increasing plaque volume, these nurturing vessels are seen growing from the adventitia into the inner layers of the vessel wall and the plaque. Because they are naturally communicating with both the periadventitial vasculature and the lumen of the coronary artery, their blood content is flushed during an OCT pullback. Depending on whether they are cut in a cross-sectional or longitudinal fashion, the appearance of these micro-vessels could be either round or oval respectively with luminal content similar to the blood vessel lumen. These vascular channels are usually relatively small in size. Inspection of adjacent frames is essential to differentiate larger channels from small side branches, which appear coming in from the vascular lumen whilst micro-vessels typically never transverse the intima.

5.8.3 Acute coronary syndrome

Three main types of vulnerable plaques have been described on OCT; TCFA with plaque rupture, plaque erosion and calcium nodules. They are the physiologic substrates of ACS in 2/3, 1/3 and 1/20 of cases, respectively.[15] In addition, intraluminal thrombi are often observed in the context of ACS. These thrombi could be either red or white thrombi (described earlier). These thrombi are either attached to the surface of the plaque or floating within the lumen. Jia et al. have proposed new criteria for the culprit lesion classification in patients with ACS that covered the gap of lacking OCT-based diagnostic criteria for OCT erosion and OCT calcified nodule (OCT-CN).[20]

a. **Plaque rupture:** A ruptured plaque is a plaque with a structural defect or discontinuity in the fibrous cap that covers the lipid-rich necrotic core of the plaque, thereby exposing the thrombogenic core of the plaque to the circulating blood.[17] Unlike pathology, the presence of overlying thrombus is not required for OCT diagnosis. Actually, patients with these plaques may have already received antithrombotics or thrombolytics before imaging. This the most common cause of ACS accounting for 44% of cases according to a more recent study (Figure 5.24).[20]

b. **Plaque erosion:** Plaque erosion is defined as the loss and/or dysfunction of endothelial cells lining

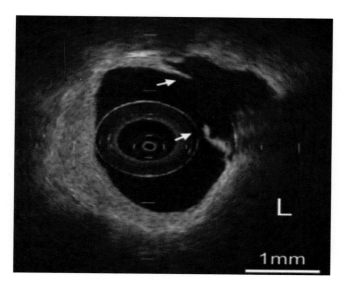

Figure 5.24 Plaque rupture from 12 to 2 o'clock. (Courtesy of St. Jude Medical.)

the plaque with no structural gap of plaque architecture using pathological criteria.[21] This leads to thrombosis through exposure of proteoglycans and smooth muscle cells to the flowing blood. Although the absence of endothelial cells is an essential pathological criterion for plaque erosion, it cannot be detected on OCT despite its high resolution. Accordingly, OCT definition of plaque erosion is mainly a diagnosis of exclusion requiring the absence of a fibrous cap rupture. It has to remembered that the presence of thrombus hinders the assessment of the underlying the culprit lesion which may further complicate OCT diagnosis of plaque erosion. Jia et al.[20] have proposed the use of definite OCT erosion and probable OCT erosion to aid in the diagnosis of plaque erosion:

i.   Definite OCT erosion refers to the presence of attached thrombus overlying an intact and visualised plaque.

ii. Probable OCT erosion refers to either (a) irregularity of luminal surface at the culprit lesion without overlying thrombus or (b) presence of thrombus attenuating the underlying plaque without superficial lipid, or calcification immediately proximal or distal to the site of thrombus.

In comparison to plaque rupture, the underlying plaque exhibits features of early lesions mainly PIT or fibrous plaque or less frequently fibroatheromas with thick fibrous cap and less necrotic core, less calcification and less plaque burden.[15,20–22] Unlike plaque rupture, the thrombus burden in plaque erosion is usually not massive with larger lumen and preserved vascular structure. This has led to the hypothesis that patients with erosion may be stabilised more effectively by antithrombotic treatment and that stents implantation may not be needed if the lumen is not significantly compromised after thrombectomy. Thirty-one per cent of cases of ACS are caused by plaque erosion (Figure 5.25).[20]

c. **Calcified nodule (CN) or disruptive calcified plaque:** CN refers to disruptive nodular calcification protruding into the lumen with overlying thrombus. From this definition, we can understand that fibrous cap disruption is essential for its diagnosis. The underlying calcified plaque shows evidence of protruding calcification, superficial calcium and the presence of substantive calcium proximal and/ or distal to the lesion. A CN should not be confused with nodular calcification within a thin fibrous cap, which does not induce thrombosis. Calcified nodules are the least common cause of acute coronary syndrome accounting for 8% of cases.[20] Calcified nodules are usually the culprit for ACS in heavily calcified tortuous arteries, older patients and men. Mid RCA and LAD are predominantly involved as a result of maximum torsion stress (Figure 5.26).

5.8.4 OCT guided coronary intervention

a. **Use of OCT prior to intervention for decision making (to treat or not to treat).**

The use of OCT for guiding decision making will differ depending on the clinical situation.

In **stable angina,** the information needed for deciding intervention is more quantitative (reduction in flow caused by plaque volume) rather than qualitative (plaque morphology). Of course, the morphology of plaque is still needed for strategic planning of how to properly treat a particular lesion.

In such clinical scenario, it is important to identify the physiological significance of coronary stenosis particularly for intermediate stenosis (40%–70% visual stenosis severity). Being an anatomical tool, intravascular OCT, similar to IVUS, is unable to accurately predict physiology when compared with today's gold standard, fractional flow reserve (FFR).[23] This is attributed to the large variation of vessel sizes, recruitment of micro-vessels, vessels supplying infarcted myocardium or vessels supplying more than one coronary territory (collaterals). All those factors preclude single cross-section lumen analysis to accurately assess the haemodynamic significance of a lesion. Compared with IVUS, intravascular OCT-derived minimal lumen area (MLA) has a tendency to be smaller.[24] Many studies are trying to define the 'OCT-equivalent' of the IVUS data.

The first study done by Stefano et al. was to evaluate the use of OCT for the assessment of intermediate coronary artery stenosis. In this study, no significant correlation could be observed between physiologic assessment by FFR and morphologic quantitative parameters by OCT.[23]

In a study done by Gonzalo et al.,[9] it was found that OCT has a moderate diagnostic efficiency in identifying the functional significance of coronary stenosis. In all vessel sizes, OCT was also found to have slightly higher diagnostic efficiency than IVUS. However, OCT was significantly better than IVUS in vessels <3 mm in diameter. There has been a concern about the applicability of previously reported IVUS cutoff points in small vessels.[25] In addition, it was interestingly found that the optimal diagnostic cutoff values for use of OCT and IVUS in functional stenosis assessment

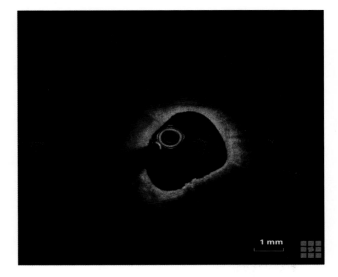

Figure 5.25 Plaque erosion: an irregular luminal surface with an overlying little white thrombus at 5 o'clock. There is no evidence of rupture. (Courtesy of Amr Gamal and Javed Ahmed)

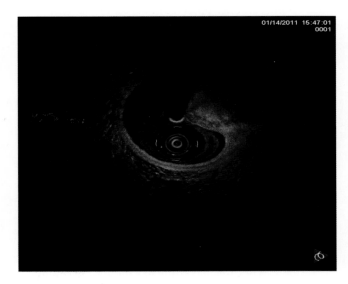

Figure 5.26 Disruptive calcified plaque from 12 to 3 o'clock. (Courtesy of St. Jude Medical.)

are much lower than the customarily applied 4 mm² IVUS-derived cutoff value.[26] MLA was found in this study to be the best OCT parameter to predict functional significance. An OCT-derived MLA cutoff point of 1.95 mm² showed a moderate diagnostic efficiency with a considerable sensitivity of 82% but a low specificity of 63%. This means that in cases where OCT-derived MLA is less than 1.95 mm², a more specific test for evaluating functional significance is needed to avoid unnecessary interventions.

It could be speculated that the higher diagnostic efficacy of OCT over IVUS and the better delineation of the lumen-vessel boundary obtained with OCT facilitate automatic tracing and measurement of the lumen area with an excellent reproducibility.[27]

Another small study was performed by Shiono et al.[28] on 62 lesions for defining the OCT criteria for predicting physiologically significant intermediate coronary lesions. OCT-derived MLA <1.91 mm², MLD <1.35 mm and percent lumen area stenosis (AS) >70.0% were the best cutoff values to correlate with an FFR <0.75.

In the ongoing FFR or OCT guidance to revascularise intermediate coronary stenosis using angioplasty (FORZA) trial, the OCT criteria used for defining functional significance and accordingly warranting intervention are the following: percentage of AS is ≥75% or 50%–75% with a minimal lumen area <2.5 mm² or if a major plaque ulceration is detected. This trial is performed on a larger number of patients and is expected to provide a useful guidance for the management of patients with intermediate coronary artery disease using the OCT criteria.[29]

In conclusion, from the few studies performed so far to assess the OCT use for predicting functional significance, it could be inferred that OCT is slightly more efficient than IVUS in the assessment of functional stenosis severity, particularly in vessels <3 mm (where the IVUS catheter could be occlusive) and in irregular calcified plaque (where the resolution of OCT for defining the intimal luminal border is much higher). In addition, it is noted that those studies mainly focused on the assessment on intermediate non–left main stem (LMS) stenosis.

Unlike IVUS, we do not have definitive studies using an OCT-determined MLA of the left main coronary artery to determine functional significance. However, with increasing use of this technology in the catheterisation lab and with limited variability of size of LMS compared with non-LMS arteries, we could infer that the currently accepted IVUS value of 6.0 mm² would be lower with OCT and accordingly, if an OCT-derived MLA of the left main is 6.0 mm² or more, percutaneous coronary intervention (PCI) could safely be deferred at this time. If LMS size is in the grey zone between 4.8 and 6.0 mm², OCT could be done particularly with concomitant LMS and proximal left anterior descending (LAD) disease and unequivocal pullback.[30] However, it should be emphasised that due to technical issues regarding the inability to clear blood for optimal image quality particularly for ostial or large LMS, IVUS has been so far the gold standard imaging modality for LMS assessment.[31]

In acute coronary syndrome (discussed earlier):

b. **OCT for detailed vessel assessment at the time of PCI (how to optimise what you treat):**

Assessment of lumen geometry remains the cornerstone of intravascular imaging criteria to evaluate disease severity and guide interventional procedures. Determination of appropriate vessel diameter is one of the most important decisions prior to PCI for selection of appropriate stent and balloon size. OCT utilises the size of the catheter as a reference (around 3.06 mm) to infer the size of the vessel. Nowadays, the integrated consoles 'auto-calibrate' with four markers that have to be correctly aligned to the outermost border of the catheter to get proper vessel sizing. Accurate markers positioning is crucial as it has been found that 1% change in magnitude can result in up to a 14% error in area measurements.[32]

OCT provides an accurate measurement of reference lumen diameters, especially the proximal reference, and the MLA at the level of the plaque. Other relevant interventional parameters like percentage lumen obstruction and percent neointimal hyperplasia (NIH) could be also accurately assessed on OCT. In addition, OCT can define the culprit lesion, its length and the presence of other vulnerable plaques at risk of rupture. Other morphological features in the culprit lesion could also be assessed like the presence and extent of calcification, plaque ulceration or rupture with intraluminal thrombus or if there is intimal dissection close to the plaque. Besides, in bifurcational lesions, it gives valuable information regarding the status of the side branch which help in deciding the best strategy for an individual patient.

c. **OCT for coronary evaluation after PCI with metallic stents (assessing result and looking for possible complications):**

OCT is also important to assess the result of PCI and its possible complications.

i. **Stent expansion:**

OCT provides important information about the luminal diameter and area of the stented coronary segment that correlates with the risk of restenosis.

ii. **Stent strut apposition:**

This refers to the relationship between individual stent struts and vessel wall.

Malapposition (also called incomplete stent apposition) is separation of at least one stent strut from the underlying vessel wall in the absence of a side branch.[7]

It is important to differentiate between:

1. Malapposition occurring immediately after stent implantation (acute malapposition), typically related to the implantation technique.
2. Malapposition occurring on follow up (late malapposition). The latter is further subdivided into persistent (starts at the time of PCI and then persists) or late acquired (not seen at the time of PCI but develops on follow up). Serial OCT imaging at baseline and on follow up is required to distinguish between the two types.

Stent malapposition should not be confused with stent underexpansion which mainly refers to the stent area on its own or in relation to a reference. It should be noted that whilst there has been a consistent association between stent underexpansion and acute or subacute stent thrombosis in IVUS studies, the same association was not present in isolated acute stent malapposition.[33] By affecting endothelialisation and coverage of stent struts, acute stent malapposition mainly impacts long-term outcome including late stent thrombosis.[34]

However, some IVUS studies have shown that malapposition may occur in 10%–20% of drug-eluting-stents (DES) without any clinical implications, which again doubts the clinical importance of stent malapposition.[35] With the widespread use of OCT, we may be able to find mechanisms explaining why some

malapposed stent struts are at risk of late stent thrombosis.

Interestingly, despite the proven efficacy of DES over bare-metal stent (BMS), it has been found that late stent malapposition is more common with DES.[36] One of the proposed mechanisms is vessel remodelling caused by chronic inflammatory reaction to the drug polymer.[37] Another mechanism could be the dissolution of thrombus trapped between the stent and the vessel wall.

Stent strut apposition in diseased vessels with irregular luminal contour is classified into (1) embedded, where the endoluminal strut order is either completely buried or just touching the luminal vessel contour or (2) protruding, where the endoluminal strut order is above the luminal vessel contour with a strut lumen distance not exceeding the actual strut thickness (to be differentiated from malapposition).

By definition, malapposition is present when the strut is not in contact with the vessel wall. Because the light cannot penetrate the metallic struts, only the endoluminal surface of the struts is seen on OCT.

To overcome this, malapposition is calculated by subtracting the actual stent thickness from the distance from the midpoint of strut reflection to the vessel wall. The actual strut thickness is the sum of stent strut thickness, polymer thickness, and the axial resolution of OCT (varying from 10 to 20 mm) (Figures 5.27 through 5.32).

iii. **Plaque protrusion (also called intrastent prolapse or tissue prolapse):**
Tissue prolapse is defined as the convex-shaped projection of tissue through recently implanted stent struts into the lumen without disruption

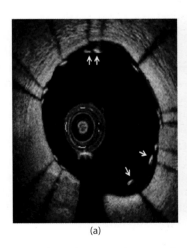
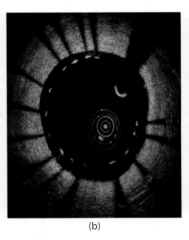
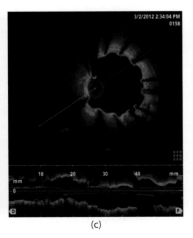

(a)　　　　　　　　　　(b)　　　　　　　　　　(c)

Figure 5.27 Panel **(a)** shows malapposed struts at 12 and 5 o'clock, panel **(b)** shows circumferential newly implanted strut malapposition, panel **(c)** shows late stent malapposition on follow-up. (Courtesy of St. Jude Medical.)

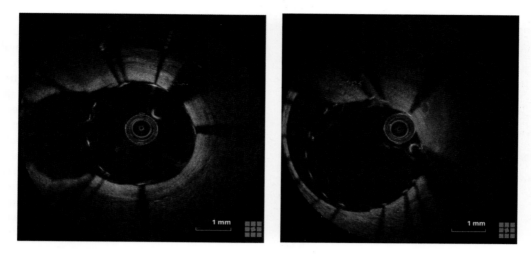

Figure 5.28 **Left panel** shows side branch strut from 7 to 11 o'clock, **right panel** shows malapposed struts from 6 to 11, protruding struts from 3 to 6 and embedded struts from 12 to 3 o'clock. (Courtesy of Amr Gamal.)

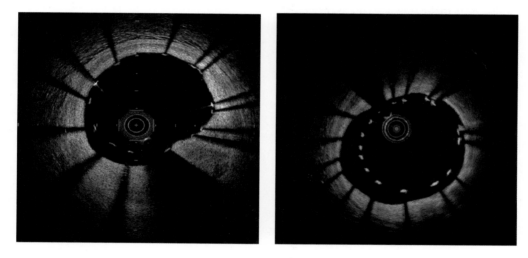

Figure 5.29 **Left panel:** shows well apposed metallic stent struts from 10 to 6 o'clock and malapposed struts in the rest of the image, **right panel:** shows circumferentially malapposed metallic stent struts (Courtesy of Terumo corporation.)

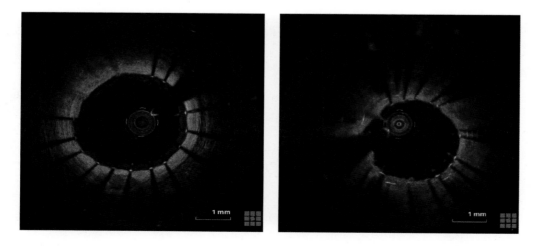

Figure 5.30 Newly implanted well apposed metallic stent struts which are protruding in left panel and embedded in right panel. (Courtesy of Amr Gamal.)

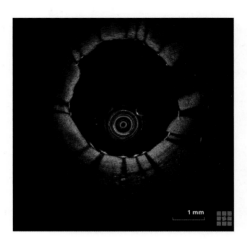

Figure 5.31 Another example of well apposed metallic DES strut. Note the protruding struts from 5 to 9 and embedded struts from 10 to 4 o'clock. (Courtesy of Amr Gamal.)

of the luminal surface continuity.[7,37] The extent of protrusion could be quantified using either prolapse area or prolapse length (prolapse depth, defined as the distance from the arc connecting two adjacent struts to the point of maximum protrusion). Tissue prolapse could be also characterised based on the protruding tissue composition (i.e. fibrous, calcific or lipid plaques). In a study evaluating post-PCI lesions with both IVUS and OCT, tissue prolapse was identified in 95% with OCT versus 18% with IVUS.[38] The relationship between OCT detected prolapse and tissue composition, stent type or clinical setting is unclear. Nevertheless, it is seen more frequently in lipid-rich plaques and in acute coronary syndromes.[7,37] Current studies have suggested that tissue prolapse is not associated with clinical events in short or mid-term (Figure 5.33).[37,39]

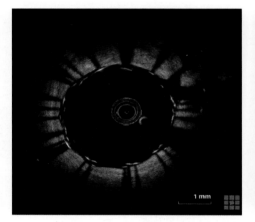
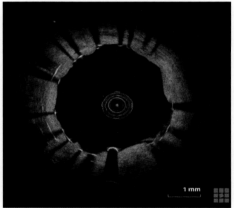

Figure 5.32 **Left panel:** shows 2 layers of newly implanted metallic stent struts (overlapping) (Note the bright reflection of all stent struts), **right panel:** shows a layer of newly implanted metallic DES on top of underlying layer of previously implanted metallic DES (Note the difference in brightness of reflection between the new stent and the old stent struts) (Courtesy of Amr Gamal.)

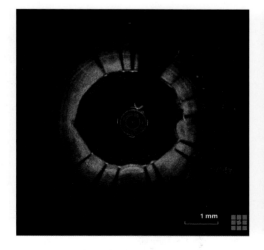
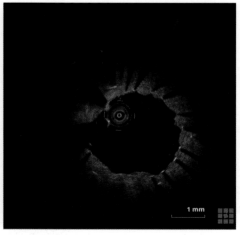

Figure 5.33 Two different cases with tissue prolapse between metallic stent struts. (Courtesy of Amr Gamal.)

iv. **Edge dissection:**
Implantation of coronary stents can cause an iatrogenic injury to the vessel wall leading sometimes to dissection at the transition between the rigid stent and the adjacent vessel wall. The incidence of dissection following stent implantation ranges from 1.7% to 6.4% on angiography[40] to 7.8% to 19.3% on IVUS.[41] The much higher resolution of OCT compared with both angiography and IVUS has resulted in more frequent recognition of dissections after PCI.[42] Angiographic and IVUS detected dissections have been associated with early stent thrombosis and adverse cardiac events.[43]

Stent edge dissections are defined as disruptions in the luminal vessel contour proximal or distal to the stent.[42] OCT detected coronary dissections are classified according to one of the following parameters: depth, length, area and opening distance.

Depth is defined as the distance from the luminal surface to the junction point with the vessel wall at the base of the flap. **Length** is the distance from the tip of flap to the junction point of the flap with the vessel wall. **Area** is identified with planimetry of a region outlined by lumen contours incorporating and interpolating the flap.

Opening distance is the distance from the tip of the flap to the lumen contour along a line projected through the gravitational centre of the lumen.[44] Additional descriptors of the severity of a dissection include (1) presence of flaps, cavities or double lumen dissections,[42] (2) circumferential extent (in degrees of arc) using a protractor, (3) dissection length using motorised transducer pullback and (4) size of residual lumen (cross-sectional area [CSA]).

Dissections can also be classified into five main categories:[7]

a. **Intimal:** Limited to the intima or atheroma and not extending to the media. Small intimal dissections are also called intimal disruptions with unknown significance.
b. **Medial:** Extending into the media.
c. **Adventitial:** Extending through the EEM into the adventitia.
d. **Intramural haematoma:** An accumulation of [blood or] flushing media within the medial space, splitting it and displacing the IEM inwards and EEM outwards. Entry and/or exit points may or may not be observed.
e. **Intrastent:** Separation of intima or neointimal hyperplasia from stent struts.

In a study, it was observed that distal edge dissections were more frequent than proximal ones. The main independent predictors of stent edge dissection are the presence of atherosclerotic plaque at stent edges, angle of calcification in fibrocalcific plaques (cutoff is 72°), minimum fibrous cap thickness in lipid-rich plaques (cutoff is 80 μm), presence of TCFAs, stent and lumen eccentricity, stent-to-lumen diameter and area ratios. Only 22.6% of OCT detected dissections were treated. It has been proposed that OCT detected angiographically silent dissections, non-flow limiting dissections, dissections with longitudinal length <1.75 mm, with <2 concomitant flaps, flap depth <0.52 mm, flap opening <0.33 mm and not extending deeper than the media layer are not associated with increased adverse outcome and can be left untreated (Figures 5.34 and 5.35).[44]

v. **Assessment of vascular healing (strut coverage, restenosis and neoatherosclerosis):**
After inflating a balloon or implanting a stent, vascular healing starts leading to the formation of neointima covered by endothelium. This layer of tissue covering the luminal stent surface is needed for preventing the contact between stent and blood components and accordingly stent thrombosis. On the other extreme is the in-stent restenosis that is due to excess neointimal tissue formation sometimes leading to obstruction of a previously implanted stent.

Due to the high resolution of OCT, it is able to visualise tissue coverage of struts and assess response to stent implantation.[45] Being very thin, the neointimal covering is usually below the resolution threshold of IVUS. Struts are termed covered when tissue is identified over the entire circumference of the struts and uncovered when tissue is absent.[7] Stent struts uncovering represents delayed healing process and could be related to the underlying plaque composition (i.e. necrotic core of TCFA has been associated with poor healing[46]), stent struts malapposition[47] or other not fully established factors.

OCT is able to not only detect in-stent restenosis, but also describe the restenotic tissue in detail that helps in better understanding of mechanisms of stent failure. Implantation-related factors like smaller post-PCI MLA and greater residual stenosis are associated with decreased long-term patency of DES and could be easily identified on OCT. In addition, three-dimensional (3D) OCT has a niche in the diagnosis of stent fracture which could be missed on angiography.[48] The appearance of restenotic tissue on OCT could be further differentiated into layered, homogeneous or heterogeneous neointima.[49]

Restenosis has been thought to be due to exclusively dense fibrotic tissue growth and

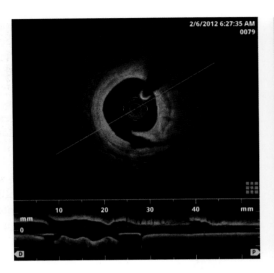
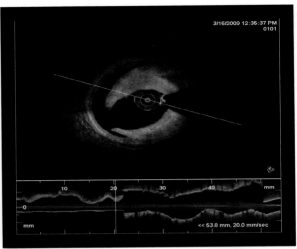

Figure 5.34 Coronary dissection: **Left panel** shows small coronary dissection extending into the media, **right panel** shows larger coronary dissection. (Courtesy of St. Jude Medical.)

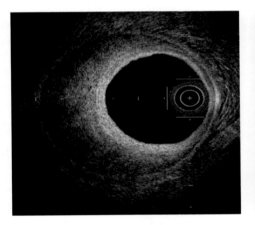
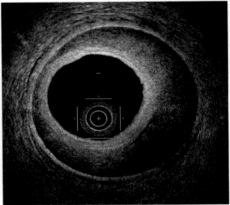

Figure 5.35 Shows intramural haematoma having the typical crescent like appearance within the media (Courtesy of Terumo Corporation.)

the end spectrum of in-stent tissue healing. However, with the use of OCT, we have realised that restenosis is not only fibrous tissue thickening (signal rich area with low attenuation), but with time, there could be also evidence of atherosclerotic disease within the neointima between the previously implanted stent and the lumen. This atherosclerosis, also called neoatherosclerosis, could be in the form of lipid plaque (signal poor region and invisible struts), thin capped fibroatheromas, ruptured caps with overlying platelet rich thrombus within stents or even calcification.[50] Consequently, late stent thrombosis cannot be exclusively attributed to exposed stent struts without endothelialisation, but also due to vulnerable plaques within the restenotic fibrous tissue. In a study done by Taniwaki et al., neoatherosclerosis was evident in 15% of lesions 5 years after DES implantation.

Neoatherosclerosis was more common in lesions treated with paclitaxel than sirolimus DES, and fibroatheromas were more common than fibrocalcific lesions. Macrophage accumulations were frequent but microvessels and surface erosions were rare and no plaque ruptures were seen (Figures 5.36 through 5.39).[50]

vi. **In-stent thrombosis:**
Stent thrombosis (ST) is a rare but potentially life-threatening complication of stent implantation. Thrombus formation inside a stent can result in partial or complete occlusion of the lumen which could be complicated by myocardial infarction (in 70% of cases) and death (in 40% of cases).[51]

ST could be classified according to the time of occurrence in relation to stent implantation into early (<1 month), late (1 month to 1 year) and very late (>1 year).[52]

Whilst early ST is mainly caused by inadequate inhibition of platelet aggregation

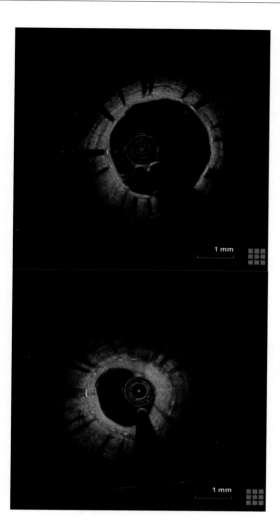

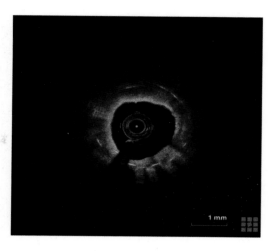

Figure 5.37 In-stent restenosis with low backscattering neointima (necrotic core) covered with a thin fibrous cap (TCFA). (Courtesy of Amr Gamal).

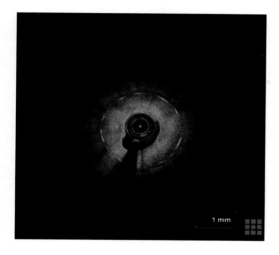

Figure 5.36 **Top panel** shows covered metallic stent struts with a thin layer of neointima, **Bottom panel** shows in-stent restenosis with high backscattering neointima (composed of fibrous tissue) (note the difference in stent struts reflection between the two frames, which represents the temporal difference since the time of stent implantation). (Courtesy of Amr Gamal.)

Figure 5.38 Severe in-stent restenosis with high backscattering neointima (composed of fibrous tissue). (Courtesy of Amr Gamal.)

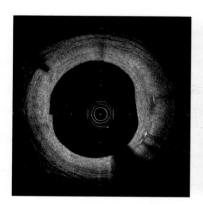
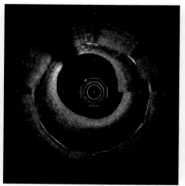
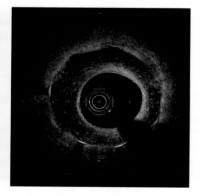

Figure 5.39: Shows 3 different types of restenotic tissue (neointima) on OCT which could be either layered, homogeneous or heterogeneous (from left to right) (Courtesy of Terumo Corporation.)

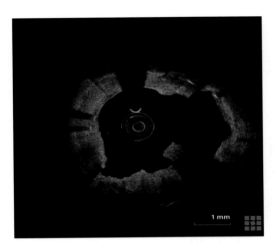

Figure 5.40 Red thrombus overlying low backscattering neointima (late stent thrombosis). (Courtesy of Amr Gamal and Javed Ahmed.)

in addition to procedural factors like edge dissection or stent underexpansion, late and very late ST are caused by delayed healing and unendothelialised struts, positive remodelling or neoatherosclerosis inside the previously implanted stent with subsequent plaque rupture.[53,54] The high-resolution power of OCT compared to IVUS allows the detection of even small thrombi (13% versus 0% identified with OCT and IVUS, respectively).[38] As mentioned before, OCT detected thrombi could be either red (RBCs rich) or white (platelet rich). OCT allows not only the accurate differentiation between the two types of stent thrombosis but also gives an insight into its underlying mechanism. However, OCT assessment of stent thrombosis has a limited evaluation of stent struts behind a red thrombus due to high attenuation of light so data like strut apposition or coverage are difficult to be assessed. In addition, the low penetration power of OCT makes the assessment of EEM and accordingly positive remodelling and late stent malapposition as a cause of late ST extremely difficult. These two scenarios are better assessed by IVUS (Figure 5.40).

5.8.5 OCT in assessment of Bioresorbable Vascular Scaffolds (BVS)

Unlike metallic stents, the BVS are quite rigid and less elastic and accordingly the stent scaffolds could be easily deformed by excessive expansion. This means that careful sizing of the scaffolds to the coronary artery dimensions is crucial. Another major difference is that the stent polymers are not visible under X-ray. The Absorb BVS (Abbott Vascular, Santa Clara, CA, USA) have two radio-opaque markers on both ends of the scaffold but the stent polymer backbone is not seen after deployment.[55,56] The high resolution of OCT, compared with IVUS, offers detailed assessment of the vascular scaffolds by providing the following data.

   i. **Guiding decision making:**

Similar to metallic stents, OCT can guide decision making and optimise treatment strategy. Prior to stenting, appropriate sizing of the scaffolds relative to the size of the vessel is essential to avoid overexpansion of the scaffolds. Being rigid, these stents have limitation in their expansion ability, for example; Absorb BVS allows only for a maximum over- expansion of 0.5 mm above the nominal scaffold diameter otherwise, scaffold fracture usually follows. This means that although proper stent sizing is important with all stents it is more crucial with BVS because in other types of stents we can still do postdilatation with high pressure balloon inflations and their size will increase depending on the compliance chart of the stent used. In addition, OCT gives detailed information about the morphology of the plaque which is essential for deciding the appropriate strategy of lesion preparation (e.g. balloon dilatation or rotablation depending on the burden of calcification). Again, although lesion preparation is important with virtually all types of stents it is more crucial with BVS owing to their high crossing profile due to much thicker stent struts (114–228 μm in the currently available BVS).[57] OCT is also essential to assess the junction between two adjacent BVS which are preferable to be just abutting or minimally overlapping to avoid the drawback of having two layers of thick struts particularly in small vessels (Figure 5.41).

  ii. **Prediction of strut fracture:**

By applying strain to the strut polymer, the stressed struts appear elongated than the adjacent struts and have two white high signal intensity nuclei inside the dark box. Those nuclei, also called scattering centres (SC) do not typically reach the axial or the transverse axis of the strut edges and so appear as dot inside a box. This is different to the OCT appearance of confluent or bifurcating struts which also have high-intense signal in the core of the strut. However, this signal reaches the axial edges of the strut (Figures 5.42 and 5.43).

 iii. **Assessment of stent expansion, apposition and presence of edge dissection:**

OCT accurately assesses both strut expansion relative to the distal and proximal reference segments and to side branches and strut apposition against the vessel wall. These data are very important as inadequate strut expansion

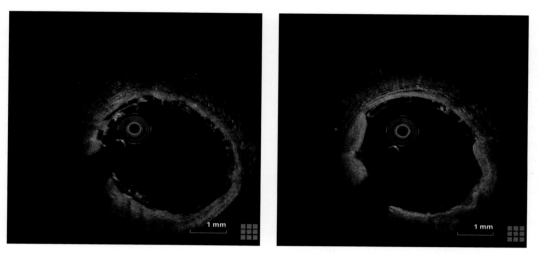

Figure 5.41 **Left panel** shows overlapping two bioabsorbable vascular scaffolds (BVS) struts, **right panel** shows well-apposed BVS struts with evidence of plaque prolapse (note the box shaped thicker struts and the clearly visible abluminal surface). (Courtesy of Amr Gamal and Mohaned Egred.)

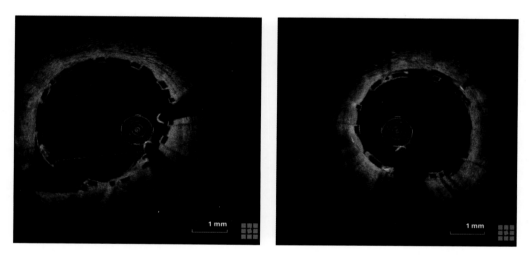

Figure 5.42 Box-shaped bioabsorbable vascular scaffolds (BVS) struts with bifurcating or confluent strut at 8 o'clock (left panel) and at 7 and at 11 o'clock in right panel. (Courtesy of Amr Gamal and Mohaned Egred.)

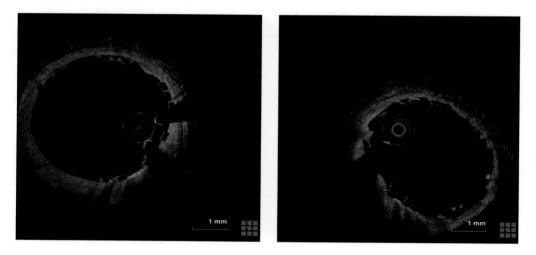

Figure 5.43 Well-apposed bioabsorbable vascular scaffolds (BVS) struts with stressed struts at 12 and 6 o'clock (left panel) and from 4 to 6 o'clock (right panel). (Courtesy of Amr Gamal and Mohaned Egred.)

or apposition is associated with non-laminar blood flow that could initiate platelet activation, thrombosis or restenosis.[58] At baseline, strut apposition could be classified into (1) protruding struts: less than one half of the strut thickness is impacted in the vessel wall, (2) embedded struts: more than a half of the strut thickness is impacted in the vessel wall, (3) incomplete strut apposition (ISA): there is a separation of the backside of the struts from the vessel wall, (4) side branch strut: The strut is located opposite a side branch with no contact with the vessel wall (Figures 5.44 through 5.46).[59] In addition, OCT helps to detect BVS edge dissection and evaluate its severity in the same way as mentioned earlier with metallic stent edge dissection (Figure 5.47).

iv. **Assessment of strut coverage:**
Similar to the metallic stents, late and very late scaffold thrombosis is caused by either absence of neointimal covering or its exaggerated presence with subsequent development of neotheroscelrosis inside the scaffold.[60] OCT is very sensitive in the detection of very thin neointimal layer overlying the stents. In case of excess neointimal covering, OCT allows both reliable quantification and characterisation of the neointimal tissue.[60] On follow-up, strut coverage is classified into (1) apposed and covered strut: the four corners of the strut polymers have lost the right angle with signs of tissue coverage and (2) apposed and uncovered strut: the right angle shape of one of the two endoluminal strut corners is preserved with no signs of tissue coverage (Figures 5.48 through 5.51).[59]

v. **Assessment of strut degradation:**
The pattern of degradation of the scaffold struts and the changes in their appearance over

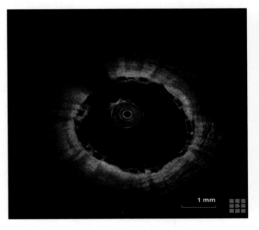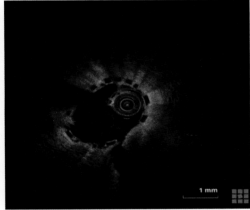

Figure 5.44 Well-apposed bioabsorbable vascular scaffolds struts which could be protruding (left panel) or embedded (right panel from 7 to 5 o'clock). (Courtesy of Amr Gamal and Mohaned Egred.)

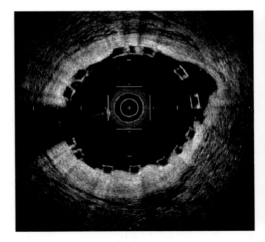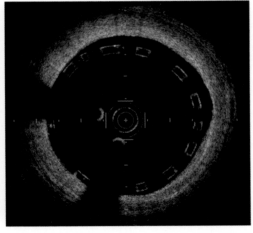

Figure 5.45 **Left panel:** shows well apposed (protruding) BVS struts (note side branch struts from 2 to 3 o'clock), **right panel:** shows malapposed BVS struts from 11 to 6 o'clock (Courtesy of Terumo corporation.)

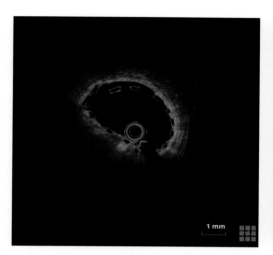
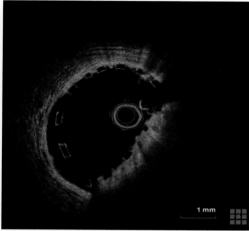

Figure 5.46 **Left panel** shows malapposed bioabsorbable vascular scaffolds (BVS) struts from 9 to 1, protruding struts from 1 to 5 and embedded struts from 5 to 9 o'clock, **right panel** shows malapposed BVS struts from 6 to 11. (Courtesy of Amr Gamal and Mohaned Egred.)

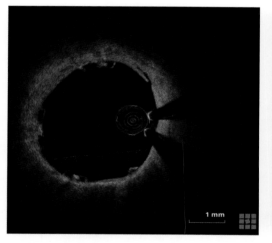
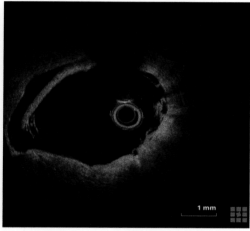

Figure 5.47 **Left panel** shows small bioabsorbable vascular scaffolds (BVS) edge dissection confined to the intima (note the two wires artefacts at 3 o'clock), **right panel** shows larger BVS edge dissection extending into the media. (Courtesy of Amr Gamal.)

time are best detected on OCT.[61] In a preclinical study comparing OCT findings with the corresponding histology in coronary arteries of healthy swine after BVS implantation, the box-shaped appearance of the scaffold struts is still detectable on OCT at 2 years. However, on histology, it was found that the polymeric material is no longer present and that this persistent box-shaped structures represent struts replaced by proteoglycans. At the 4-year follow-up, both OCT and histology confirmed the absence and complete degradation of the struts.[62] Similar results were obtained in human-based study where the scaffold struts have disappeared on 5 years follow-up.[63] The struts have become integrated between

the overlying neointima and the underlying plaque creating a homogenous signal-rich, low-attenuating layer that is needed to separate the lumen from the thrombogenic plaque components after resorption of the scaffolds polymers. The minimum thickness of this layer was found to be 150 μm and its homogenous low attenuation properties point towards the absence of high-risk wall components such as necrotic core and macrophages.[64] This means that this layer could protect against very late scaffold thrombosis.[65] Ormiston et al.[61] have proposed definitions for resorbable struts of one type of scaffolds (preserved box, open box, dissolved bright box and dissolved black box).

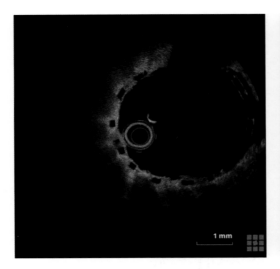
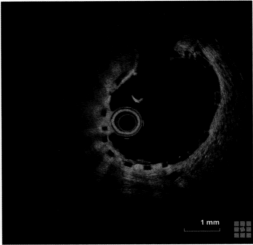

Figure 5.48 **Left panel** shows uncovered malapposed bioabsorbable vascular scaffolds (BVS) struts from 1 to 3, uncovered protruding struts from 4 to 6, covered embedded struts from 6 to 12 o'clock, **right panel** shows uncovered protruding BVS struts from 12 to 5 and covered embedded struts from 6 to 11 o'clock. (Courtesy of Amr Gamal and Mohaned Egred.)

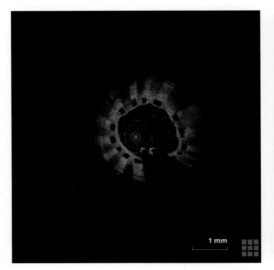
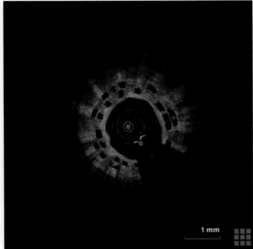

Figure 5.49 **Left panel**: covered embedded bioabsorbable vascular scaffolds (BVS) struts with thin high backscattering neointima (fibrous tissue), **right panel**: mild in-stent restenosis (ISR) of high backscattering neointima (fibrous tissue) overlying two layers of overlapping BVS struts. (Courtesy of Amr Gamal and Mohaned Egred.)

5.9 3 Dimensional OCT

The unique ability of OCT to reconstruct 3D image has allowed better visualisation of the stents particularly in complex lesions.[66] In bifurcational lesions, we could confirm re-crossing of side branch wire through the most distal cell.

5.10 Limitations of OCT

1. Limited penetration: As mentioned earlier, OCT is unreliable in the assessment of plaque volume or deeper part of diseased vessel wall. Although an excellent agreement has been reported between OCT and IVUS in measurement of lumen area and diameter in non-diseased vessels, smaller lumen and stent areas have been consistently observed with OCT in diseased vessels. Accordingly, when OCT for PCI guidance, it is important to depend on lumen criteria rather than media-to-media values, as used in IVUS studies.

2. Poor interpretation of tissue covered by thrombus. Thrombi, especially red thrombi, casts a shadow over the underlying vessel wall, making assessment of underlying plaque or healing of the stent struts (both are commonly associated with stent thrombosis) unreliable.

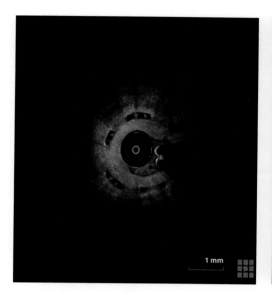

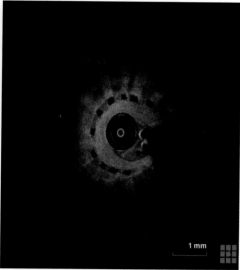

Figure 5.50 Severe ISR of high backscattering neointima (fibrous tissue) inside previously implanted bioabsorbable vascular scaffolds (BVS) (note the stressed struts appearance in left panel). (Courtesy of Amr Gamal and Mohaned Egred.)

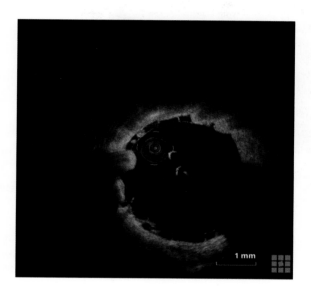

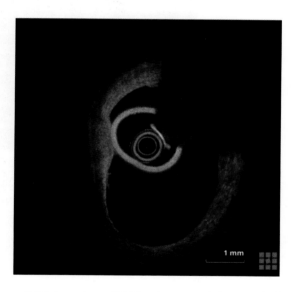

Figure 5.51 Red thrombus at 9 o'clock overlying uncovered protruding bioabsorbable vascular scaffolds (BVS) struts. (Courtesy of Amr Gamal and Mohaned Egred.)

Figure 5.52 Imaging of LMS using a guideliner with disengaged guiding catheter. Note the yellow ring of guideliner around the imaging catheter with guidewire artefact at 1 o'clock. (Courtesy of Amr Gamal and Mohaned Egred.)

3. Difficult assessment of large vessels including ostial LMS: As mentioned earlier in this chapter, it is difficult to clear blood to obtain a good-quality image particularly for ostial or large LMS. However, there are some case reports about ameliorating blood removal for OCT of ostial LMS through the 'backflow method' using a guide extension catheter (mother and child catheter or guideliner). This is first entails installing the guideliner alone in LMS with disengagement of the guiding catheter to avoid pressure wedge. This is followed by pullback of OCT through the guide extension catheter. This technique makes use of both the coaxial alignment and the translucency of the plastic component of the guideliner to infrared light, which allows the assessment of the surrounding vessel wall without backshadowing (Figures 5.52 and 5.53).

4. The need for use of less contrast in patients with heart failure or renal impairments: This could be partially ameliorated by use of guide extension catheter to decrease the contrast used to the minimum possible.

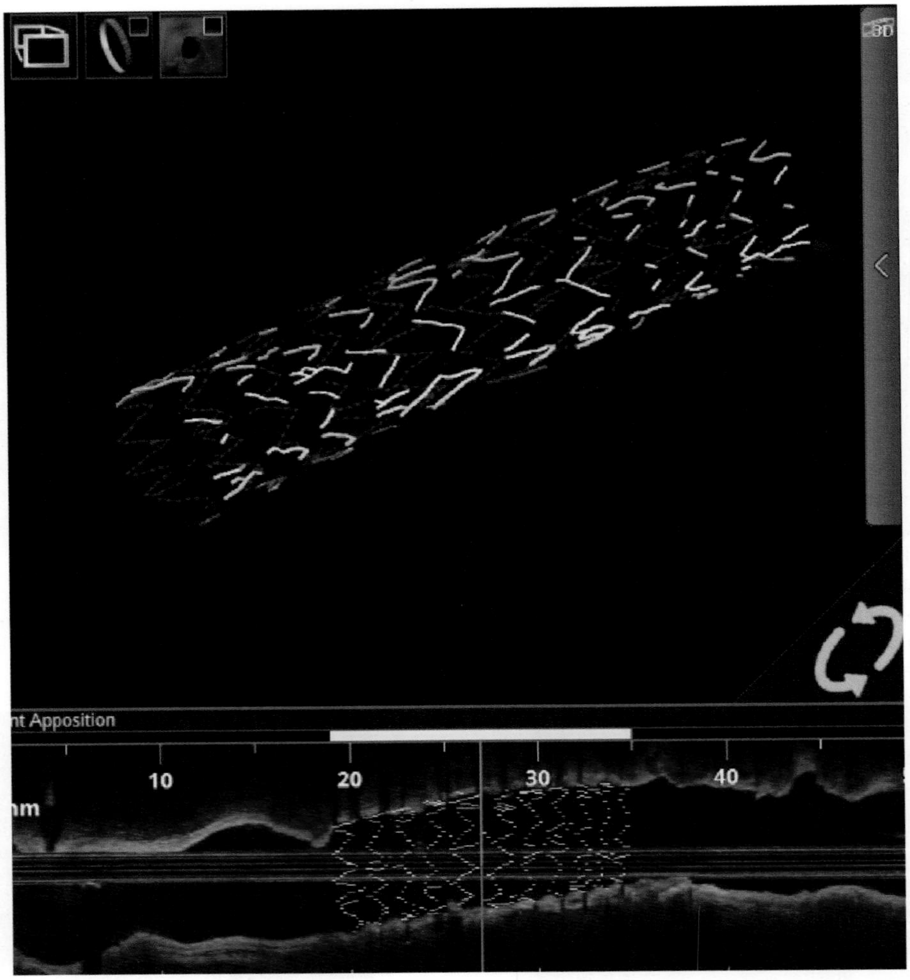

Figure 5.53 **Upper panel** shows 3 Dimensional strut mapping of a DES after taking out the vessel wall and it confirmed well expansion of the stent struts, **Lower panel:** shows longitudinal OCT reconstruction of the same stent inside the vessel wall and confirmed well apposition of the stent to the vessel wall (Courtesy of Amr Gamal and Javed Ahmed.)

References

1. Fujimoto JG et al. Biomedical imaging and optical biopsy using optical coherence tomography. *Nat Med* 1995; 1: 970–2.
2. Huang D et al. Optical coherence tomography. *Science* 1991; 254: 1178–81.
3. Prati F et al. Expert review on methodology, terminology, and clinical applications of optical coherence tomography: Physical principles, methodology of immune acquisition, and clinical application for assessment of coronary arteries and atherosclerosis. *Eur Heart J* 2010; Feb 31(4): 401–15.
4. Schmitt JM. Optical coherence tomography (OCT): A review. *IEEE J Sel Top Quant Electr* 1999; 5(4): 1205–15.
5. Barlis P, and Schmitt JM. Current and future developments in intracoronary optical coherence tomography imaging. *EuroIntervention* 2009; 4: 529–34.
6. Hiram G, et al. Intracoronary optical coherence tomography: A comprehensive review clinical and research application. *JACC Interv* 2009; 2: 1035–46.
7. Tearney G et al. Consensus standard for acquisition, measurement, and reporting of intravascular optical coherence tomography studies. A report from the international working group for intravascular optical coherence tomography standardization and validation. *J Am Coll Cardiol* 2012; 59: 1058–72.
8. Yabushita H et al. Characterization of human atherosclerosis by optical coherence tomography. *Circulation* 2002; 106: 1640–45.
9. Gonzalo N et al. Morphometric assessment of coronary stenosis relevance with optical coherence tomography: A comparison with fractional flow reserve and intravascular ultrasound. *J Am Coll Cardiol* 2012; 59: 1080–9.
10. Mehanna EA et al. Assessment of coronary stent by optical coherence tomography, methodology and definitions. *Int J Cardiovasc Imaging* 2011; 27(2): 259–69.
11. Kawasaki M et al. Diagnostic accuracy of optical coherence tomography and integrated backscatter intravascular ultrasound images for tissue characterization of human coronary plaques. *J Am Coll Cardiol* 2006; 48(1):81–88
12. Manfrini O et al. Sources of error and interpretation of plaque morphology by optical coherence tomography. *Am J Cardiol* 2006; 98(2): 156–9.

13. Rieber J et al. Diagnostic accuracy of optical coherence tomography and intravascular ultrasound for the detection and characterization of atherosclerotic plaque composition in ex-vivo coronary specimens: A comparison with histology. *Coron Artery Dis* 2006; 17(5): 425–30.

14. Goderie T P M et al. Combined optical coherence tomography and intravascular ultrasound radio frequency data analysis for plaque characterization. Classification accuracy of human coronary plaques in vitro. *Int J Cardiovasc Imaging* 2010; 26(8): 843–50.

15. Virmani R et al. Lessons from sudden coronary death: A comprehensive morphological classification scheme for atherosclerotic lesions. *Arterioscler Thromb Vasc Biol* 2000; 20(5): 1262–75.

16. Sangiorgi G et al. Arterial calcification and not lumen stenosis is highly correlated with atherosclerotic plaque burden in humans: A histologic study of coronary artery segments using nondecalcifying methodology. *J Am Coll Cardiol* 1998; 31(1): 126–33.

17. Schaar JA et al. Terminology for high-risk and vulnerable coronary artery plaques. Report of a meeting on the vulnerable plaque, June 17 and 18, 2003, Santorini, Greece. *Eur Heart J* 2004; 25: 1077–82.

18. Tanaka A et al. Distribution and frequency of thin-capped fibroatheromas and ruptured plaques in the entire culprit coronary artery in patients with acute coronary syndrome as determined by optical coherence tomography. *Am J Cardiol* 2008; 102: 975–9.

19. MacNeill BD et al. Focal and multi-focal plaque macrophage distributions in patients with acute and stable presentations of coronary artery disease. *J Am Coll Cardiol* 2004; 44: 972–9.

20. Jia H et al. *In vivo* diagnosis of plaque erosion and calcified nodule in patients with acute coronary syndrome by intravascular optical coherence tomography. *J Am Coll Cardiol* 2013; 62(19): 1748–58.

21. Farb A et al. Coronary plaque erosion without rupture into a lipid core. A frequent cause of coronary thrombosis in sudden coronary death. *Circulation* 1996; 93(7): 1354–63.

22. Kramer MC et al. Relationship of thrombus healing to underlying plaque morphology in sudden coronary death. *J Am Coll Cardiol.* 2010; 55(2): 122–32.

23. Stefano GT et al. Utilization of frequency domain optical coherence tomography and fractional flow reserve to assess intermediate coronary artery stenoses: Conciliating anatomic and physiologic information. *Int J Cardiovasc Imaging* 2011; 27: 299–308.

24. Bezerra HG et al. Optical coherence tomography versus intravascular ultrasound to evaluate coronary artery disease and percutaneous coronary intervention. *JACC Cardiovasc Interv* 2013; 6: 228–36.

25. Costa MA et al. Anatomical and physiologic assessments in patients with small coronary artery disease: Final results of the Physiologic and Anatomical Evaluation Prior to and After Stent Implantation in Small Coronary Vessels (PHANTOM) trial. *Am Heart J* 2007; 153: 296e1–7.

26. Magni V et al. Evaluation of intermediate coronary stenosis with intravascular ultrasound and fractional flow reserve: Its use and abuse. *Catheter Cardiovasc Interv* 2009; 73: 441–8.

27. Gonzalo N et al. Reproducibility of quantitative optical coherence tomography for stent analysis. *EuroIntervention* 2009; 5: 224–32.

28. Shiono Y et al. Optical coherence tomography-derived anatomical criteria for functionally significant coronary stenosis assessed by fractional flow reserve. *Circ J* 2012; 76(9): 2218–25.

29. Burzotta F et al. Fractional flow reserve or optical coherence tomography guidance to revascularize intermediate coronary stenosis using angioplasty (FORZA) trial: Study protocol for a randomized controlled trial. *Trials* 2014; 15: 140.

30. Kang SJ et al. Intravascular ultrasound-derived predictors for fractional flow reserve in intermediate left main disease. *JACC Cardiovasc Interv* 2011; 4: 1168–74.

31. Fujino Y et al. Frequency-domain optical coherence tomography assessment of unprotected left main coronary artery disease-a comparison with intravascular ultrasound. *Catheter Cardiovasc Interv* 2013; 82: E173–83.

32. Bezerra HG et al. Intracoronary optical coherence tomography: A comprehensive review. *JACC Cardiovasc Interv* 2009; 2: 1035–46.

33. Teruo O et al. Intravascular ultrasound parameters associated with stent thrombosis after drug-eluting stent deployment. *Am J Cardiol* 2007; 100(4): 615–20.

34. Gutiérrez-Chico JL et al. Delayed coverage in malapposed and side-branch struts with respect to well-apposed struts in drug-eluting stents: In vivo assessment with optical coherence tomography. *Circulation* 2011; 124(5): 612–23.

35. Cook S et al. Impact of incomplete stent apposition on long-term clinical outcome after drug-eluting stent implantation. *Eur Heart J* 2012; 33(11): 1334–43.

36. Hassan AK et al. Late stent malapposition risk is higher after drug-eluting stent compared with bare-metal stent implantation and associates with late stent thrombosis. *Eur Heart J* 2010; 31(10): 1172–80.

37. Gonzalo N et al. Optical coherence tomography assessment of the acute effects of stent implantation on the vessel wall: A systematic quantitative approach. *Heart* 2009; 95(23): 1913–9.

38. Kubo T et al. OCT compared with IVUS in a coronary lesion assessment: The OPUSCLASS study. *JACC Cardiovasc Imaging* 2013; 6(10): 1095–104.

39. Kume T et al. Natural history of stent edge dissection, tissue protrusion and incomplete stent apposition detectable only on optical coherence tomography after stent implantation – Preliminary observation. *Circ J* 2012; 76(3): 698–703.

40. Giuseppe GL et al. On behalf of the RECIPE (Real-world Eluting-stent. Incidence, predictors, and outcomes of coronary dissections left untreated after drug-eluting stent implantation. *Eur Heart J* 2006; 27: 540–46.

41. Liu X et al. Intravascular ultrasound assessment of the incidence and predictors of edge dissections after drug-eluting stent implantation. *JACC Cardiovasc Interv* 2009; 2(10): 997–1004.

42. Gonzalo N et al. Relation between plaque type and dissections at the edges after stent implantation: An optical coherence tomography study. *Int J Cardiol* 2011; 150(2): 151–5.

43. Alfonso F et al. Findings of intravascular ultrasound during acute stent thrombosis. *Heart* 2004; 90(12): 1455–9.

44. Chamie D et al. Incidence, predictors, morphological characteristics, and clinical outcomes of stent edge dissections detected by optical coherence tomography. *JACC Cardiovasc Interv* 2013; 6(8): 800–13.

45. Suzuki Y et al. In vivo comparison between optical coherence tomography and intravascular ultrasound for detecting small degrees of in-stent neointima after stent implantation. *JACC Cardiovasc Interv* 2008; 1(2): 168–73.

46. Finn AV et al. Does underlying plaque morphology play a role in vessel healing after drug-eluting stent implantation? *JACC Cardiovasc Imaging* 2008; 1(4): 485–88.

47. Joner M et al. Pathology of drug-eluting stents in humans: Delayed healing and late thrombotic risk. *J Am Coll Cardiol* 2006; 48(1): 193–202.

48. Okamura T, and Matsuzaki M. Sirolimus-eluting stent fracture detection by three-dimensional optical coherence tomography. *Catheter Cardiovasc Interv* 2012; 79: 628–32.

49. Gonzalo N et al. Optical coherence tomography patterns of stent restenosis. *Am Heart J* 2009; 158(2): 284–93.

50. Taniwaki M et al. Frequency and type of neoatherosclerosis five years after drug-eluting stent implantation: An optical coherence tomography study. *J Am Coll Cardiol* 2012; 60.

51. Wenaweser P et al. Incidence and correlates of drug-eluting stent thrombosis in routine clinical practice. 4-year results from a large 2-institutional cohort study. *J Am Coll Cardiol* 2008; 52(14): 1134–40.

52. Cutlip DE et al. Academic Research Consortium. Clinical end points in coronary stent trials: A case for standardized definitions. *Circulation* 2007; 115(17): 2344–51.

53. Windecker S, and Meier B. Late coronary stent thrombosis. *Circulation* 2007; 116: 1952–65.

54. Takano M et al. Two cases of coronary stent thrombosis very late after bare-metal stenting. *JACC Cardiovasc Interv* 2009; 2: 1286–87.

55. Tamai H et al. Initial and 6-month results of biodegradable poly-l-lactic acid coronary stents in humans. *Circulation* 2000; 102(4): 399–404.

56. Ormiston JA et al. A bioabsorbable everolimus-eluting coronary stent system for patients with single de-novo coronary artery lesions(ABSORB): A prospective open-label trial. *Lancet* 2008; 371(9616): 899–907.

57. Gutierrez-Chico JL et al. Quantitative multi-modality imaging analysis of a fully bioresorbable stent: A head-to-head comparison between QCA, IVUS and OCT. *Int J Cardiovasc Imaging* 2012; 28(3): 467–78.

58. Foin N et al. Incomplete stent apposition causes high shear flow disturbances and delay in neointimal coverage as a function of strut to wall detachment distance: Implications for the management of incomplete stent apposition. *Circ Cardiovasc Interv* 2014; 7(2): 180–9.

59. Gomez-Lara J et al. Serial analysis of the malapposed and uncovered struts of the new generation of everolimus-eluting bioresorbable scaffold with optical coherence tomography. *JACC Cardiovasc Interv* 2011; 4(9): 992–1001.

60. Gomez-Lara J et al. Head-to-head comparison of the neointimal response between metallic and bioresorbable everolimus-eluting scaffolds using optical coherence tomography. *JACC Cardiovasc Interv* 2011; 4(12): 1271–80.

61. Ormiston JA et al. A bioabsorbable everolimus-eluting coronary stent system for patients with single de-novo coronary artery lesions(ABSORB): A prospective open-label trial. *Lancet* 2008; 371(9616): 899–907.

62. Onuma Y et al. Intracoronary optical coherence tomography and histology at 1 month and 2, 3, and 4 years after implantation of everolimus-eluting bioresorbable vascular scaffolds in a porcine coronary artery model: An attempt to decipher the human optical coherence tomography images in the ABSORB trial. *Circulation*. 2010; 122(22): 2288–300.

63. Karanasos A et al. OCT assessment of the long-term vascular healing response 5 years after everolimus-eluting bioresorbable vascular scaffold. *J Am Coll Cardiol* 2014; 64(22): 2343–56.

64. Ughi GJ et al. Automated tissue characterization of in vivo atherosclerotic plaques by intravascular optical coherence tomography images. *Biomed Opt Express* 2013; 4: 1014–30.

65. Virmani R et al. Pathology of the vulnerable plaque. *J Am Coll Cardiol* 2006; 47(Suppl): C13–8.

66. Farooq V et al. Three-dimensional optical frequency domain imaging in conventional percutaneous coronary intervention: The potential for clinical application. *Eur Heart J* 2013; 34(12): 875–85.

6

Fractional flow reserve: Invasive and non-invasive assessment to guide percutaneous coronary interventions

JAYA MALLIDI, AMIR LOTFI, LLOYD W KLEIN

6.1 Introduction

Fractional flow reserve (FFR) is considered the gold standard for invasively assessing the physiologic significance of coronary artery stenosis. This technique has become an integral adjunct to coronary angiography for identifying ischaemic lesions and an invaluable tool in guiding clinical decision making regarding revascularisation. Measuring FFR optimises the benefit of percutaneous coronary interventions (PCI) and distinguishes stenoses responsible for ischaemia from functionally insignificant ones. FFR improves clinical outcomes and saves resources compared

with PCI guided by angiography alone. Its use should be expanded for the following reasons:

1. Coronary angiography is limited in its ability to demonstrate the clinical significance of intermediate coronary lesions (40%–70%). Numerous confounding factors exist which limit the accuracy of the angiogram. These factors include eccentricity, calcification, contrast streaming, branch overlap and vessel foreshortening – all of which cause significant interobserver variability.[1] This ambiguity can be easily overcome by FFR assessment.

2. In patients with single-vessel coronary artery disease (CAD), non-invasive stress test correlates well with angiography. However, in patients with multi-vessel disease, non-invasive stress testing is less reliable to identify ischaemia producing lesions.[2] Hence, FFR is invaluable in identifying ischaemic lesions in multi-vessel disease.

3. Several randomised clinical trials validated favourable long clinical outcomes with FFR-guided revascularisation in patients with stable single or multi-vessel stable CAD.[3-5]

Despite convincing evidence supporting FFR-guided revascularisation, physiological lesion assessment is underutilised in real-world practice. In an analysis from the National Cardiovascular Data Registry, only 6.1% of the 61,874 attempted coronary interventions of intermediate lesions used FFR.[6] Park et al.[7] coined the term 'functional angioplasty' for the strategy that incorporates FFR into revascularisation decisions. This chapter aims to review the concepts of FFR and the literature supporting deferral of revascularisation based on it. Further, the limitations and pitfalls of FFR and use of non-invasive FFR to guide revascularisation are also discussed.

6.2 Definition and concept of FFR

Pijl et al.[8] first introduced the term 'FFR' in 1993. FFR is defined as the ratio of myocardial blood flow in a coronary artery in the presence of epicardial stenosis and myocardial blood flow in the same artery in the hypothetical absence of stenosis under conditions of maximal hyperaemia. Routinely, FFR of a coronary lesion is measured as the ratio of mean distal coronary pressure measured beyond the lesion (P_d) to the mean aortic pressure (P_a) during maximal hyperaemia (Figure 6.1).[8,9] The pressure distal to the lesion is measured using a high-fidelity pressure sensor mounted 3 cm from the tip of a 0.014-inch guidewire. An example of FFR-guided

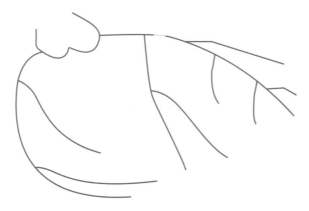

Figure 6.1 Principles in measuring fractional flow reserve (FFR). P_d, pressure distal to the lesion; P_a, proximal aortic pressure; P_v, coronary venous pressure. (Reprinted from *Textbook of Interventional Cardiology*, Seventh Edition, edited by Eric J. Topol and Paul S. Teresstein, Intracoronary pressure and flow measurements, Kern, M.J. et al., 85–107, Copyright (2016), with permission from **Elsevier**.)

clinical decision making in a patient with intermediate coronary artery stenosis based on angiogram is illustrated in Figure 6.2.

The central concept to measurement of FFR is the assumption that coronary blood flow is proportional to pressure when myocardial resistance is minimal and constant. Under resting conditions, the myocardial resistance is constantly changing based on myocardial oxygen demand, blood pressure, contrast injection and coronary vasomotion. Hence, FFR is measured only after achieving maximal hyperaemia, where the microvascular resistance is minimal and constant, using pharmacologic agents such as intravenous adenosine, contrast, intracoronary adenosine, nitroprusside and papaverine. A condition for accurate FFR measurements is that microvascular resistance is reduced maximally and remains stable during the measurement. In a normal vessel without stenosis, the distal coronary pressure is equal to the aortic pressure. In the presence of epicardial stenosis, the resistance to flow causes turbulence and loss of energy resulting is a drop of pressure distal to the coronary stenosis.[10] Pijl et al.[8] validated the concept of FFR by proving the proportional nature of pressure and coronary flow under maximal hyperaemia in instrumented dogs and subsequently in humans.[11]

A simplified derivation of FFR is presented in Figure 6.1. The pressure drop across the stenosis is directly related to the flow rate in an exponential manner. A vasodilating drug is administered to abolish vasomotor tone and, thus, to minimise microvascular resistance. Under this condition, blood flow across the stenosis is assumed to be maximal producing the maximal achievable pressure gradient. By measuring the ratio of the coronary pressure distal to the stenosis to aortic pressure, the percentage of normal coronary flow, or the fraction of normal flow (hence FFR), is calculated. FFR has a normal value of 1.0. FFR for a stenotic vessel is expressed as a decimal or fraction of this value. A fundamental assumption of FFR is that, at maximal vasodilation, the relationship between coronary perfusion pressure and flow is proportional and linear, that is, that a stenosis affects distal coronary pressure to the same degree as it affects flow.[12] Another important assumption is that coronary venous pressure (P_v) is considered to be negligible compared with aortic or distal coronary pressure.[12] Hence, FFR is an extremely useful invasive index as it is reproducible, not affected by haemodynamic changes, accounts for collateral flow, independent of microvasculature vessels.[13]

6.3 Can revascularisation be deferred based on FFR in stable CAD?

Several randomised trials proved favourable for long-term clinical outcomes with deferral of revascularisation based on FFR in patients with stable CAD.[14-16] Whilst the American College of Cardiology/American Heart Association (ACC/AHA) guidelines for PCIs[17] and the current consensus guidelines endorsed by Society of Cardiovascular Angiography

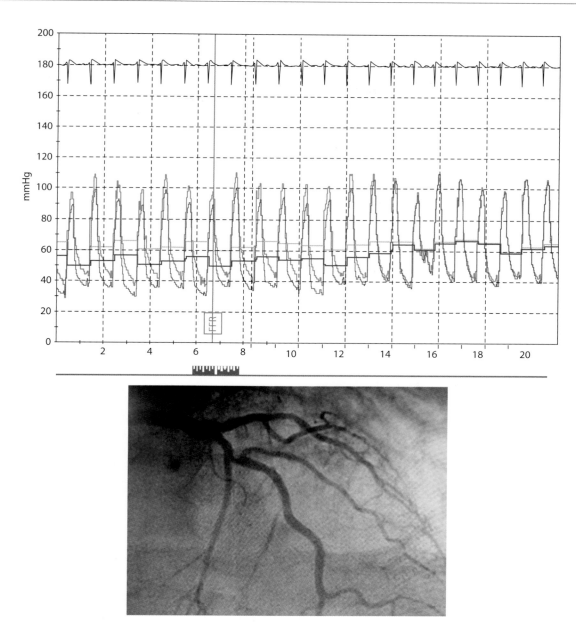

Figure 6.2 Angiographic image of an intermediate stenosis of left anterior descending coronary artery and associated fractional flow reserve (FFR) measurement of 0.83 in a 78-year-old gentleman with chest pain. Since the measured FFR value was consistent with a nonhaemodynamically significant lesion, revascularisation was not performed and patient was treated with medical therapy.

and Intervention (SCAI)[18] support the use FFR in intermediate coronary lesions to guide revascularisation decisions in patients with stable CAD as a Class II a recommendation, the latest guidelines by the European Society of Cardiology/European Society of Cardiothoracic Surgery (ESC/ESCS)[19] support it as a Class I a recommendation, especially when evidence of ischaemia is not available based on any other prior tests.

Pijls et al.[20] performed the first study that validated the use of FFR in intermediate single-vessel CAD amongst 45 patients by comparing it to the results of non-invasive stress tests. In this study, all patients with moderate coronary stenosis and chest pain underwent bicycle exercise testing, thallium scintigraphy, stress echocardiography with dobutamine and quantitative coronary angiogram with FFR. In 21 patients with an FFR less than 0.75, reversible ischaemia was demonstrated on at least one non-invasive stress test. In 21 of the 24 patients with an FFR of 0.75 or higher, there was no ischaemia detected on any of the non-invasive tests. No revascularisation was required in any of these patients during the following 14 months. FFR has a sensitivity of 88% and a specificity of 100% for identifying ischaemic lesions. This study established the FFR cutoff value of 0.75 for identifying ischaemia producing lesions.

The following are the three landmark randomised trials, which strongly support deferral of revascularisation based on FFR in patients with stable CAD.

6.3.1 Deferral versus performance of PCI of functionally nonsignificant coronary stenosis (DEFER)[3,14]

DEFER is the first randomised trial that further supported deferral of revascularisation based on FFR in single-vessel CAD. In this study, 325 patients with intermediate single-vessel CAD were randomised to deferral of revascularisation or performance of PCI if the FFR was greater than 0.75. All patients with FFR < 0.75 were revascularised. At 24 months, the event-free survival rates (death, myocardial infarction, repeat revascularisation) were similar between the deferral and the performance groups (89% versus 83%, p = .27).[14] Even after 15 years of follow-up, the rate of death was not different between the deferral and the performance groups (33.0% versus 31.1%, p = .79) with the rate of myocardial infarction being significantly lower in the deferral group (2.2% versus 10%, p = .03, Figure 6.3).[3]

6.3.2 FFR-guided PCI versus angiography for guiding PCI in multi-vessel disease

In FFR-guided PCI versus angiography for guiding PCI in multi-vessel disease (FAME 1),[4,15] a total of 1005 patients with multi-vessel disease (defined as coronary artery stenosis of at least 50% of vessel diameter in at least two major epicardial vessels) with stable (67%) and unstable (33%) angina were enrolled. Prior to randomisation, all lesions that require PCI were identified angiographically. Patients were then randomised to two groups – angiography-guided PCI or FFR-guided PCI. In the FFR-guided PCI group, only lesions with FFR < 0.80 were revascularised. The number of angiographically significant lesions per patient was not different between the two groups (2.7 versus 2.8, p = .34). The following are the important findings from this study (Figure 6.4):

- At 1 year, the primary composite endpoint (death, nonfatal myocardial infarction and repeat revascularisation) was significantly lower in the FFR-guided PCI group compared with the angiography group (13.2% versus 18.3%, p = .02).[15] At 5-year follow-up, there was no significant difference in the rates of major

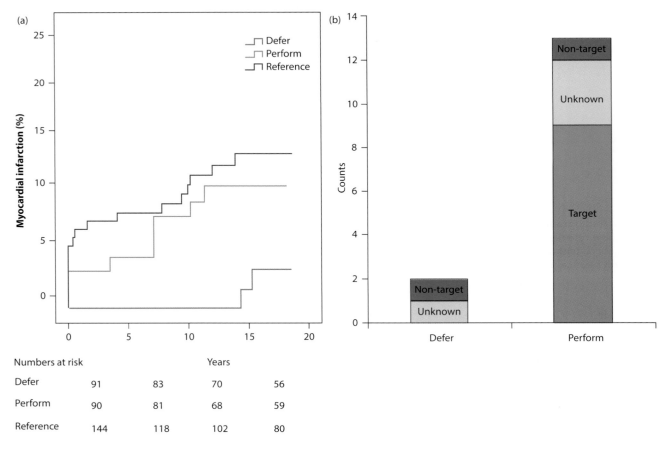

Numbers at risk

				Years
Defer	91	83	70	56
Perform	90	81	68	59
Reference	144	118	102	80

Figure 6.3 Fifteen-year results from deferral versus performance of PCI of functionally nonsignificant (DEFER). **(a)** Kaplan Meier estimates of myocardial infarction and **(b)** relation of myocardial infarction with study vessel territory. (Reprinted from Zimmermann, F.M. et al., *Eur Heart J.*, 36, 45, 2015. With permission.)

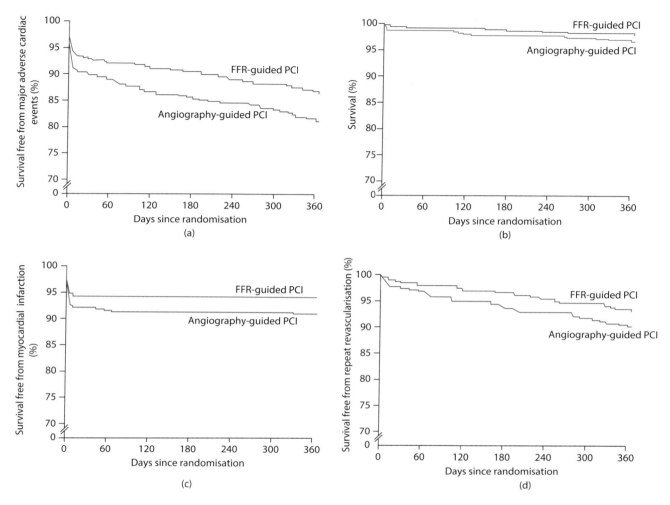

Figure 6.4 **(a–d)** The FFR-guided PCI versus angiography for guiding PCI in multi-vessel disease (FAME 1) study results. Kaplan Meier survival curves at 2 years according to study group. FFR, fractional flow reserve; PCI, percutaneous coronary intervention. (Reprinted from Tonino, P.A. et al., *N Engl J Med.*, 360, 3, 2009.)

cardiovascular events in both groups (28% FFR group versus 31% angiography group, $p = .31$).[4]
- There was no difference in the percentage of patients who remained angina free at 1 year (81% FFR group versus 78% angiography group, $p = .20$).[15]
- The number of stents used per patients was significantly lower in the FFR-guided PCI group ($1.9 + 1.3$ versus $2.7 + 1.2$, $p < .001$).[15]

6.3.3 FFR-guided PCI versus medical therapy in stable CAD

In FFR-guided PCI versus medical therapy in stable CAD (FAME 2),[5,16] 1220 patients with stable CAD, with at least one angiographically significant stenosis (>50%), were recruited. Patients who had at least one functionally significant stenosis (FFR ≤ 0.80) were randomised to FFR-guided PCI plus optimal medical therapy or optimal medical therapy alone

(888 patients). Patients without a single functionally significant stenosis (FFR > 0.80) were enrolled in a separate registry (332 patients). The following are the most important findings of the study (Figure 6.5):

- At 1 year, the primary endpoint (composite of death, nonfatal myocardial infarction and hospitalisation requiring) was significantly lower in the FFR-guided PCI plus medical therapy compared with medical therapy alone (4.3% versus 12.7%, $p < .001$).[16] The study recruitment was in fact halted at 1220 patients instead of the planned 1632 patients because of this significant difference in primary endpoint. The difference in primary endpoint was predominantly driven by urgent revascularisation (1.6% in FFR-guided PCI group versus 11.1% in medical therapy group, $p < .001$). There was no significant difference in the rate of myocardial infarction or death between the groups.[16]

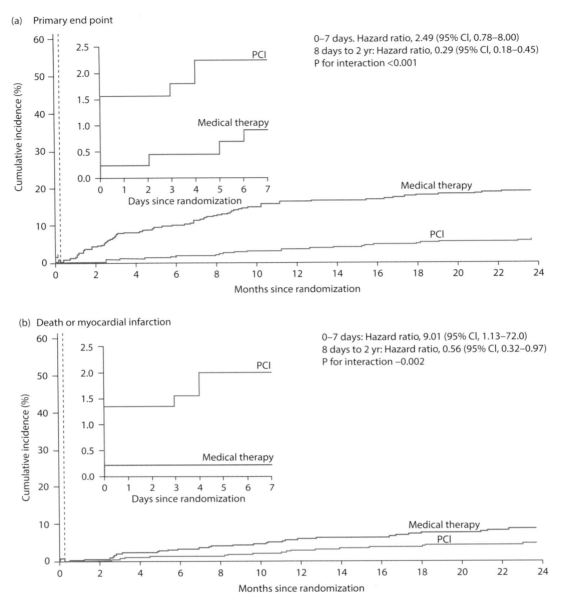

Figure 6.5 The FFR-guided PCI versus medical therapy in stable CAD (FAME 2) study results. Kaplan Meier curves for land mark analysis. **(a)** Cumulative incidence of primary endpoint (a composite of death from any cause, nonfatal myocardial infarction or any revascularisation). **(b)** Cumulative incidence of death or myocardial infarction in first 7 days and in 24 months. (Reprinted from De Bruyne, B. et al., *N Engl J Med.*, 371, 13, 2014. With permission.)

- Even at the 2-year follow-up, similar results were reported – primary endpoint was significantly lower in the FFR-guided PCI group (8.1% versus 19.5%, p < .001), without any difference in rates of death or myocardial infarction.[5]
- In a further analysis of the data from FAME 2, the rate of death or myocardial infarction from 8 days to 2 years (excluding the periprocedural events) was noted to be lower in the FFR-guided PCI group (4.6% versus 8.0%, p = .04).[5]
- Favourable outcomes were noted in patients enrolled in the registry without evidence of ischaemia (with FFR > 0.80), with the lowest rate of primary endpoint of 3.0% at 1 year and 9.0% at 2 years.[5,16]

In a recent meta-analysis of study and patient level data, Johnson et al.[21] demonstrated a graded relationship of the FFR numerical value to clinical outcomes as modulated by medical therapy versus revascularisation. The identification of ischaemia by FFR is not dichotomous based on the value of 0.75 or 0.80.[21] Instead, ischaemia exists as a graded continuum based on the numerical value of FFR.[21] Hence, the benefit of revascularisation compared with medical therapy in improving clinical outcomes increases with decreasing FFR value (Figure 6.6).[21] FFR-guided clinical decision making not only resulted in half as many revascularisations as those in angiography-based strategy, but also with 20% fewer adverse events and 10% better relief of angina.[21] Also,

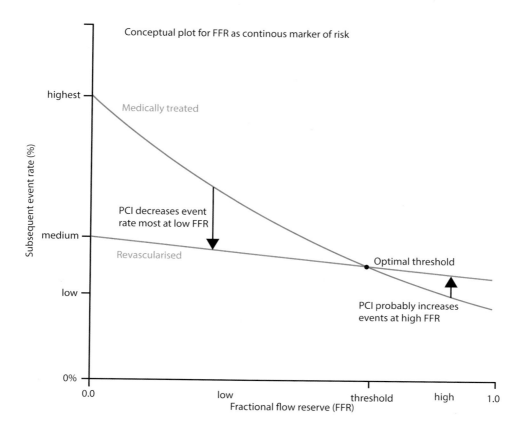

Figure 6.6 Conceptual relationship between fractional flow reserve (FFR) and outcomes. FFR is related to subsequent outcomes in a graded fashion. Lesions with low FFR values are associated with increased risk of subsequent major cardiovascular events and hence have the greatest benefit from revascularisation whilst revascularisation can be deferred in lesions with normal or high FFR values. (Reprinted from Johnson, N.P. et al., *J Am Coll Cardiol.*, 64, 16, 2014. With permission.)

FFR measured immediately after PCI has a prognostic value in determining the subsequent clinical events.[22]

In summary, in patients with stable CAD, FFR-guided revascularisation strategy compared with angiography-guided strategy decreases unnecessary revascularisation procedures and has favourable long-term clinical outcomes.

6.4 Can revascularisation be deferred based on FFR in specific lesion subsets?

Accurate measurement of FFR is technically challenging in certain clinical situations such as tandem or bifurcations lesions, left main stenosis or in acute coronary syndromes (ACS) due of unique haemodynamic changes that occur in each of these situations. In all the large-scale randomised trials supporting FFR-guided revascularisation, patients with these clinical scenarios were not included. Hence, the existing literature supporting FFR-guided revascularisation in each of these situations is limited and not as robust as in patients with stable CAD.

6.4.1 Tandem lesions

In tandem or serial lesions (defined as two lesions separated by a angiographically normal segment in between), each

lesion limits the maximal hyperaemic flow through the other lesion.[23] This interaction limits the use of the simple formula of Pd/Pa across each lesion for measuring FFR. Therefore, Pd/Pa measured across a distal lesion in the presence of a proximal lesion that is different from the calculated FFR for the same distal lesion after the treatment of proximal lesion and vice versa.

De Bruyne et al.[23] developed complex formulae to predict FFR across each lesion as if the other lesion was not present. However, these formulae involve the measurement of coronary wedge pressure (Pw) and cannot be used easily in everyday clinical setting. A more practical approach to measuring FFR in tandem lesions involves the repetitive pressure pullback technique described as follows (Figure 6.7):[24]

- The FFR pressure wire is positioned beyond the most distal lesion. If the measured FFR with this wire position (across all lesions) is greater than 0.80, no revascularisation is recommended. If the FFR ≤ 0.80, the pressure pullback technique should be performed.
- During maximal hyperaemia, the pressure wire is pulled back from beyond the distal lesion across the proximal lesion. The lesion across which there is maximum pressure gradient is first revascularised. It is

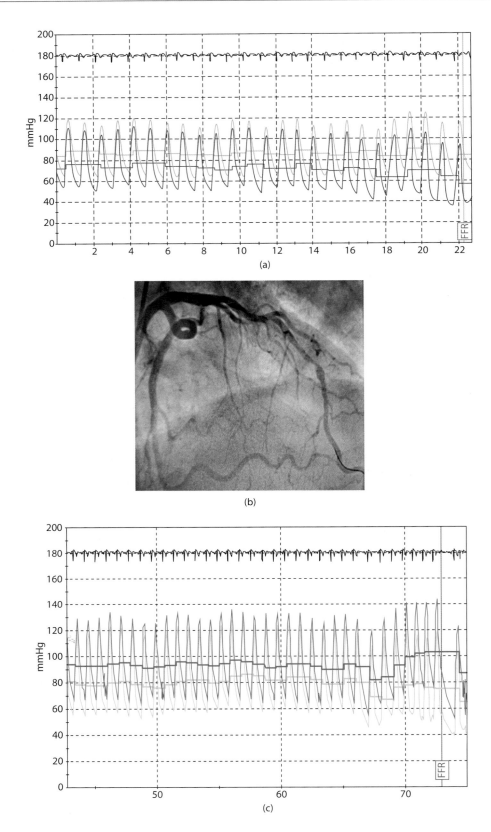

Figure 6.7 Use of fractional flow reserve (FFR) in tandem lesions. **(a)** Angiographic image of tandem lesions (lesion A and B) in left anterior coronary artery in a 64-year-old gentleman with exertional angina. **(b)** FFR of 0.67 measured across both the lesions. A pullback technique showed that the maximum gradient was across the proximal lesion A. **(c)** Angiographic image after stenting proximal lesion. FFR of 0.73 suggestive of haemodynamic significance, across the distal lesion B, after stenting the proximal lesion. Subsequently the distal lesion was also stented.

important to not measure separate FFR lesion values. The pressure gradient across each lesion should be used to determine which one should be treated first.

- After stenting the lesion with the maximum pressure gradient, FFR is measured across the remaining lesion using the standard technique. The second stenosis is also treated if the FFR is significant.

In a prospective cohort study involving 131 patients from two large Korean centres, Kim et al.[25] demonstrated the safety of FFR-guided revascularisation using the pullback pressure technique in tandem lesions. In this study, revascularisation was deferred in 61% of the lesions based on FFR. During a mean follow-up of 501 + 311 days, there were no clinical events related to deferred lesions. Hence, in patients with tandem lesions, repetitive pullback technique is a practical, safe and effective approach of measuring FFR to determine which lesion has a greater pressure drop and requires stenting first.

6.4.2 Bifurcation or ostial lesions

Angiographic assessment of an ostial lesion of a side branch prior to intervention or that produced by 'jailing' of the side branch after stenting is extremely difficult because of complex angulation, vessel overlap, foreshortening, stent struts across the branch and the eccentricity of the plaque.[26] Also, interventions involving bifurcation lesions are complex and associated with poor clinical outcomes compared with non-bifurcation lesions.[27] Provisional stenting of the side branch is the recommended strategy rather than routine complex intervention involving the stenting of main and side branch vessels.[27] Given the difficulty in accurate anatomic evaluation and poor clinical outcomes associated with complex bifurcation inventions, it is of paramount importance to determine the functional significance of side branch before embarking on performing a high-risk complex intervention (Figure 6.8).

There are no large-scale randomised trials supporting the deferral of revascularisation based on FFR in bifurcation lesions. Koo et al.[28] performed a prospective cohort study in patients with jailed side branches. Side branch FFR was measured in 91 patients. Intervention was performed only if the FFR <0.75. Only 27% of all the side branch lesions were noted to be functionally significant. In rest of the patients, side branch intervention was deferred based on the FFR results. When compared to the conventional group (patients with bifurcation lesions treated without FFR guidance) of 110 patients, there was no difference in the 9-month cardiac event rates (4.6% FFR group versus 3.7 conventional group, $p = .7$). Off note, the number of complex side branch interventions was significantly lower in the FFR-guided group (30% versus 45%, $p = .03$).

The following are a few practical tips when measuring FFR of the jailed side branches:[24]

- The FFR pressure wire should be advanced carefully through the main vessel stent struts, ensuring not to damage the pressure sensor by jailing the wire against the stent struts.
- A workhorse wire can be used to engage the side branch and then exchanged for a FFR wire through an exchange microcatheter. This is probably easier than trying to wire a side branch with FFR wire, which has reduced torquability compared to a workhorse wire.
- When interpreting the FFR of the ostial side branch, lesions in the distal part of the side branch vessel as well as in the proximal part of the main vessel should be taken into consideration.

In summary, angiographic evaluation of bifurcation lesions is often not accurate. Though, measuring FFR in side

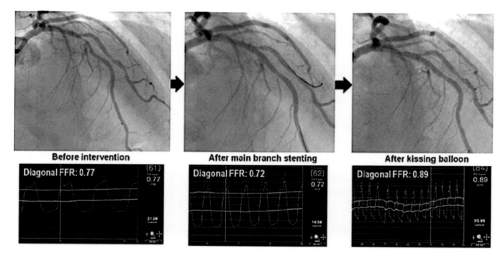

Figure 6.8 Use of fractional flow reserve (FFR) for provisional stenting strategy for a side branch. After main branch stenting, the side branch ostial lesion became functionally significant. After kissing balloon inflation, FFR increased to 0.89 despite angiographically significant residual disease. (Reprinted from Koo, B.K, and De Bruyne, B., *EuroIntervention*, 6, 2010. With permission.)

branches may be technically more challenging than in main vessels, deferral of revascularisation based on FFR is safe and reduces unnecessary high complex interventions associated with poor clinical outcomes.

6.4.3 Left main coronary artery disease

Assessment of intermediate left main coronary artery (LMCA) stenosis based on angiography alone is challenging given its short segment, reverse tapering at the ostium, contrast streaming, overlapping branches and lack of distinct reference segment.[29] Hence, significant interobserver variability is noted in evaluation of equivocal or intermediate LMCA stenosis and the functional significance of such a lesion should not be based on angiographic assessment alone.[30]

Despite the enhanced ambiguity in assessment of LMCA lesions by angiography compared to other lesions, to date there are no large-scale randomised trials comparing FFR-guided strategy to angiography alone guided strategy in guiding revascularisation decisions of intermediate unprotected LMCA stenosis. A recently published meta-analysis of six prospective cohort studies involving a total of 525 patients evaluated the use of FFR for clinical decision making in ambiguous LMCA stenosis.[31] Patients were divided into two groups – medical therapy or deferred group and revascularisation group – based on measured FFR of LMCA stenosis. There was no significant difference in the rate of all-cause mortality or nonfatal myocardial infarctions between the two groups, though the rate of subsequent revascularisations was higher in the deferred group (Figure 6.9).[31] A FFR cut-off value of 0.75–0.80 is recommended by the current consensus guidelines to guide revascularisation decisions in patients with ambiguous LMCA stenosis.[17]

The following are important technical issues that should be taken into account when measuring FFR of LMCA stenosis:

- Overestimation of FFR is theoretically possible if the LMCA disease is associated with significant downstream disease in either the left anterior descending

(LAD) or in the left circumflex artery (LCx). However, unless there is severe proximal stenosis of the LAD or the LCx, FFR of LMCA can be measured by placing the pressure wire in the non-diseased vessel. The minimal impact of downstream disease on FFR measurement of LMCA was demonstrated by Fearon et al.[32] in 25 patients by creating intermediate LMCA stenosis and LAD or LCx stenosis with a deflated balloon catheter after PCI of the LAD/LCx or both. Since downstream disease usually overestimates FFR, a numerical value of less than 0.75 will accurately identify LMCA stenosis that requires revascularisation.

- Though intracoronary ultrasound (IVUS) provides anatomical data, its use is recommended when the FFR value of LMCA stenosis is between 0.80 and 0.85. In a study by Jasti et al.,[33] an IVUS minimal luminal area of 5.9 mm^2 and a minimal lumen diameter of 2.8 mm were associated with physiologically significant LMCA stenosis.

- When measuring FFR of LMCA, care should be taken to always disengage the guide from the LMCA ostium to prevent dampening of the pressure waveforms.

In summary, clinical significance of intermediate LMCA stenosis is difficult to assess based on angiography alone. Though measuring FFR of LMCA stenosis is technically challenging, limited evidence from prospective cohort studies supports favourable long-term clinical outcomes if revascularisation of LMCA stenosis is deferred based on FFR.

6.4.4 Acute coronary syndromes

Measurement of FFR is based on the assumption of minimal and constant myocardial resistance during period of maximal hyperaemia. In ACS, several factors such as acute rise in filling pressures, downstream embolisation into the microvasculature, extent and duration of ischaemia and acute wall stress result in dynamic changes in microvascular resistance and dysfunction.[34] Hence, at least

Study name	Odds ratio	Lower limit	Upper limit	z-Value	p-Value	Odds ratio and 95% CI
Bech	1.316	0.332	5.207	0.391	0.696	
Jimenez–Navarro	0.625	0.087	4.491	−0.467	0.640	
Legutko	0.889	0.112	7.061	−0.111	0.911	
Lindstaedt	0.952	0.269	3.367	−0.076	0.940	
Courtis	3.394	1.072	10.741	2.079	0.038	
Hamilos	1.415	0.658	3.043	0.889	0.374	
	1.434	0.875	2.349	1.431	0.152	

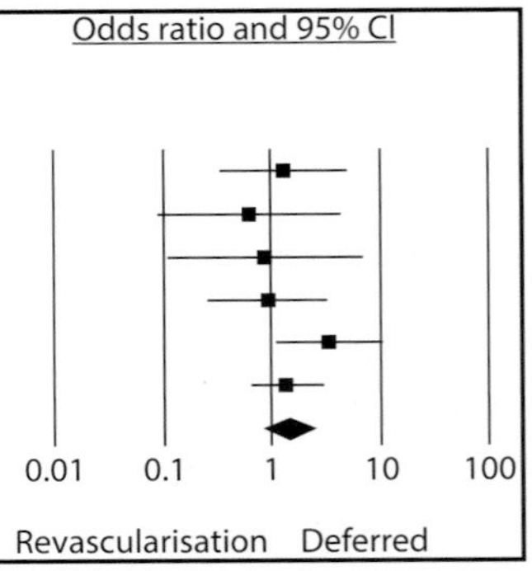

0.01 0.1 1 10 100

Revascularisation   Deferred

Figure 6.9 Results from meta-analysis of six prospective control trials to define long-term outcomes of patients in whom ambiguous left main revascularisation were deferred based on fractional flow reserve (FFR). There was no statistically significant difference in primary endpoint (composite of all-cause mortality, nonfatal myocardial infarction and revascularisation) between revascularised and deferred groups based on an FFR (odds ratio [OR]: 1.43, 95% confidence interval [CI]: 0.88–2.35, p = .15). (Reprinted from Mallidi, J. et al., *Catheter Cardiovasc Interv*, 2015. With permission.)

theoretically, maximal hyperaemia is difficult to achieve and FFR is often overestimated especially in the culprit vessel in ACS. However, recent studies have validated the use of FFR in nonculprit vessels in ST segment elevation myocardial infarction (STEMI)[35,36] and in all vessels in non-ST segment myocardial infarction,[37] where the dynamic nature of microvascular resistance is not as profound as in the culprit vessel in STEMI.

1. STEMI – Can FFR be used to guide revascularisation in nonculprit vessel?

   The appropriate management of nonculprit vessel with significant stenosis in terms of the need and timing of revascularisation in patients presenting with STEMI is unknown. Whilst the current guidelines recommend treatment of only the culprit vessel at the time of primary PCI,[38] the results from recently published randomised trials were controversial and did not convincingly support any particular strategy.[36,39]

   Ntalians et al.[35] showed that FFR measured in the nonculprit vessel during the acute phase did not change at follow-up after 35 days. So FFR measured in the acute phase in the nonculprit vessel in STEMI in patients with multi-vessel disease may be useful in risk stratification and reducing additional non-invasive testing. DANAMI – 3 – PRIMULTI[36] is an open-label, randomised trial involving 627 patients with STEMI and multi-vessel disease, conducted at two centres in Denmark. After PCI of the culprit vessel, patients were randomised into two groups – no further invasive treatment or FFR-guided complete revascularisation 2 days later prior to discharge. The primary endpoint was a composite of all-cause mortality, nonfatal reinfarction and ischaemia-driven revascularisation. At 1 year, the rate of primary events was significantly lower in FFR-guided complete revascularisation patients (13% versus 22%, p = .004). However, this difference was predominantly driven by repeat revascularisation rates and there was no significant difference in all-cause mortality or nonfatal myocardial infarction between the two groups. Future randomised trials are warranted to clarify whether FFR-guided complete revascularisation should be performed at index admission or later and if this would affect long-term clinical outcomes.

2. Non-ST segment myocardial infarction – Can FFR be used to guide revascularisation?

   The literature supporting the use of FFR to guide revascularisation in patients with non-ST segment elevation myocardial infarction (NSTEMI) is limited. In the FAME 1 study,[14] 328 patients out of 1005 patients enrolled with multi-vessel disease had unstable angina or NSTEMI. In a subgroup analysis of these patients, Sels et al.[40] showed that there is no difference in benefit from FFR-guided PCI for patients with NSTEMI and stable angina. The absolute risk reduction in major cardiovascular events was similar in patients with NSTEMI and stable angina (5.1% versus 3.7%, p = .92).

The number of stents used in the FFR-guided PCI group was significantly lower than in angiography-guided group (1.9 ± 1.5 versus 2.9 ± 1.1, p < .01).

FFR versus angiography in guiding management to optimise outcomes in NSTEMI (FAMOUS NSTEMI)[37] is the only multicentre, randomised trial conducted specifically amongst NSTEMI patient to evaluate the outcomes of FFR-guided revascularisation. In this study, 350 NSTEMI patients with more than 30% stenosis in at least one vessel were randomised to FFR-guided revascularisation strategy or angiography-guided standard care. FFR was disclosed to the operator in the FFR-guided group and it was measured, but not disclosed in the other group. Change in the treatment plan based on FFR was observed in 21.6% of patients. The number of patients who underwent revascularisation at index hospitalisation was significantly lower in the FFR-guided group (77.3% versus 86.8%, p = .02). There was no difference between the two groups in major cardiovascular events. Though limited, based on these studies, deferral of revascularisation based on FFR patients with NSTEMI, is safe and helps in reducing unnecessary interventions.

6.5 What are the pitfalls of invasive FFR measurements?

Since revascularisation decisions and subsequent long-term clinical outcomes are based on FFR, interventional cardiologists should pay close attention whilst measuring it to avoid the following common pitfalls, which can result in erroneous measurements.

1. Equipment-related factors such as improper zeroing, loose connections, malfunctioning pressure transducers, miscalibration of the haemodynamic recorder and leaving the introducer needle in the Tuohy–Borst connector are often the most common factors that result in over or underestimation of FFR.[41] Pressure wire drift can also result in erroneous measurements. When there is a gradient across the lesion, but the pressure tracings are identical in shape, pressure drift should be suspected. This can be confirmed by pulling the pressure sensor to guide tip and noting if there is there is any difference in the guide catheter and pressure wire measurements. If there is a difference, normalisation should be performed and FFR should be repeated again.[41,42]

2. Procedure-related factors such as inadequate hyperaemia (due to inadequate dosing, lack of guide catheter engagement or use of side hole catheter when administering intracoronary adenosine, or giving adenosine through an extremely small peripheral vein), guide catheter damping, incorrect placement of the pressure sensor can result in false negative results.[41]

3. Physiological factors such as coronary vasospasm, guidewire whipping phenomenon due to placement of

the sensor in small distal braches can cause erroneous results. Nitroglycerine should always be administered before measuring FFR to avoid coronary vasospasm.[42]

4. FFR measurement is technically more challenging in special clinical situations such as tandem and bifurcation lesions, left main disease and ACS as described earlier.

5. Haemodynamic factors that increase extravascular compressive forces, such as tachycardia (reduced diastolic duration) and an increased left ventricular end diastolic pressure (LVEDP), can increase hyperaemic microvascular resistance and raise FFR. Pv is not negligible in this situation.

6. FFR is sensitive to the size of the perfusion territory, since this factor can influence the coronary flow rate and thus the pressure drop across the stenosis.[11]

7. The minimal lumen diameter and lesion length also influence FFR. These factors are not considered in the angiographic interpretation of stenosis severity, but are influential in their haemodynamic significance.

8. Microvascular dysfunction can impair drug-induced coronary vasodilation, resulting in a blunted flow response and an elevated FFR.[11]

6.6 Can non-invasive FFR be used to guide revascularisation?

Coronary computed tomography angiography (CCTA) is a non-invasive, purely anatomic imaging modality, used commonly to rule out obstructive CAD. With CCTA, often the degree of stenosis is overestimated, prompting increased downstream testing and referral for invasive coronary angiography.[43] Though other non-invasive stress tests such as stress echocardiography and myocardial perfusion scintigraphy provide information regarding ischaemia burden, these tests have poor discrimination in identifying specific lesions causing ischaemia, especially in patients with multivessel disease.[2] Hence, there is a need for accurate non-invasive functional testing to identify if a specific coronary lesion produces ischaemia or not.

Recently, with advances in computational fluid dynamics, coronary flow and pressure can be derived from the traditional CCTA images, without modifying any protocols and without administration of additional medications. Measurement of FFR from CCTA images (FFR_{CTA}) requires the application of mathematical models of coronary physiology and the laws of physics governing fluid dynamics to the anatomic model of coronary arteries derived from CCTA. A simulation model is used to derive FFR to determine the decrease in coronary microvasculature as if adenosine was administered. These scientific principles used to calculate FFR from CCTA images have been well described by Taylor et al.[44]

The following are important studies that support the use of this novel modality, FFR_{CTA} in detecting ischaemia producing lesions and guiding revascularisation.

6.6.1 Diagnosis of ischaemia causing coronary stenosis by non-invasive FFR computed from coronary computed tomographic angiogram (DISCOVER FLOW)

This is a multicentre, prospective study[45] involving 103 stable patients with suspected or known CAD who underwent CCTA, FFR_{CTA}, invasive coronary angiography and invasive FFR. FFR_{CTA} was found to have a per-vessel accuracy, sensitivity, specificity, positive predictive value and negative predictive value of 84.3%, 87.9%, 82.2%, 73.9% and 92.2%, respectively, in comparison to 58.5%, 91.4%, 39.6%, 46.5% and 88.9%, respectively, for CCTA. Hence, FFR_{CTA} augments the diagnostic accuracy of CCTA for detection and exclusion of ischaemia causing coronary lesions.

6.6.2 Determination of FFR by anatomic computed tomography angiography

Similar to the DISCOVER FLOW trial, Determination of FFR by anatomic computed tomographic angiography (DeFACTO)[46] is a multicentre, prospective cohort study involving 252 patients with suspected or known CAD. Even in this study, FFR_{CTA} was noted to have improved discrimination for identifying ischaemic lesions compared with CCTA alone (AUC of 0.81 for FFR_{CTA} compared with appropriate use criteria (AUC) of 0.68 for CCTA alone, $p < .001$), though the pre-specified primary outcome of this study (to achieve the per patient diagnostic accuracy such that the lower boundary of one-sided 95% confidence interval estimate exceeded 70%) was not achieved. The diagnostic accuracy, sensitivity, specificity, positive predictive value and negative predictive value of FFR_{CTA} plus CCTA on a per patient basis were noted to be 73%, 90%, 54%, 67% and 84%, respectively.

6.6.3 Analysis of coronary blood flow using CT angiography: Next steps

Analysis of coronary blood flow using CT angiography: next steps (NXT)[47] is also a prospective multicentre trial involving 254 patients with suspected CAD. In all patients, CCTA/ FFR_{CTA} was performed before invasive coronary angiography. In contrast to the previous studies, in this study the latest generation software and computational algorithms were used to measure FFR_{CTA}. There was a very good correlation between FFR_{CT} and invasive FFR ($r = 0.82$, $p < .001$). The per-patient specificity for identifying myocardial ischaemia was remarkably higher for FFR_{CTA}, compared with CCTA alone (79% versus 34%).

A recent meta-analysis of all retrospective and prospective studies comparing the diagnostic performance of CCTA and FFR_{CTA} showed that FFR_{CTA} significantly increases the specificity of identifying functionally significant stenosis as identified by invasive FFR on a per patient level (43% versus 72%, $p = .004$).[48]

6.6.4 Clinical outcomes of FFR by computed tomographic angiography-guided diagnostic strategies versus usual care in patients with suspected CAD: The prospective longitudinal trial of FFR$_{CTA}$: Outcomes and resource (PLATFORM)

This is the first study designed to evaluate the clinical outcomes of measuring FFR$_{CT}$.[49] In this prospective cohort study utilising a comparative effectiveness observational design, 584 patients with new onset chest pain without known CAD, but with intermediate likelihood of obstructive CAD with planned non-emergent, non-invasive or invasive cardiovascular testing to evaluate for suspected CAD were enrolled. Patients were enrolled into tow cohorts – usual planned care or CCTA/FFR$_{CTA}$. On invasive angiography, no obstructive CAD was found in 12% of patients in the CCTA/FFR$_{CTA}$ group, compared with 73% in the usual care arm ($p < .0001$). In both the groups, the clinical event rates (death, myocardial infarction and unplanned revascularisation) were extremely low. These results suggest that CCTA/FFR$_{CT}$ may be a feasible alternative to invasive angiography in stable patients presenting with new onset chest pain with intermediate risk of CAD. Figure 6.10[50] shows an example where FFR$_{CTA}$ was used in conjunction with CTA and invasive angiography.

In summary, FFR$_{CTA}$ is emerging as a powerful non-invasive tool for assessment of flow limiting coronary artery lesions. Computational flow dynamic models can be used to not only measure FFR across a lesion, but also predict the FFR after virtual stenting without any modifications to the CCTA acquisition protocols or administration of additional medications. All the prospective cohort studies have established its high diagnostic value and correlation with invasive FFR. In contrast to regular CCTA alone, use of FFR$_{CTA}$ may help in reducing the referrals to invasive angiogram. However, the definitive benefit in terms of cost effectiveness and long-term clinical outcomes of incorporating FFR$_{CT}$ in routine clinical practice to guide revascularisation decisions needs to be established by future trials.

6.7 Conclusion

FFR is the gold standard for assessing the physiological significance of intermediate lesions based on coronary angiography. It ought to be the single measure of PCI appropriateness when there is any uncertainty as to the significance of a stenosis. Instead of relying solely on angiographic criteria of severity when there is no stress test present, or when the stress test/anatomic results are discordant, FFR should be the final authority. 'Functional angioplasty' (performing PCI on lesions responsible for ischaemia and treating medically those that are not), as opposed to complete anatomic revascularisation (performing PCI on all lesions that appear angiographically significant), is the preferred decision-making process.

Deferral of revascularisation based on FFR for patients with single and multi-vessel stable CAD is cost effective and associated with good long-term clinical

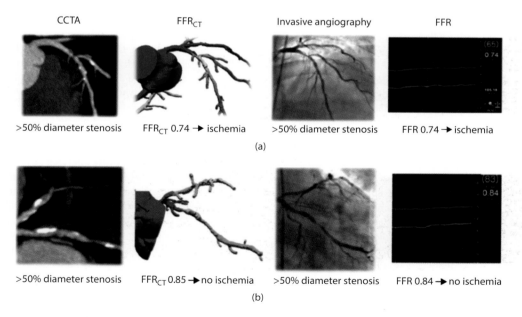

CCTA	FFR$_{CT}$	Invasive angiography	FFR
>50% diameter stenosis	FFR$_{CT}$ 0.74 → ischemia	>50% diameter stenosis	FFR 0.74 → ischemia

(a)

>50% diameter stenosis	FFR$_{CT}$ 0.85 → no ischemia	>50% diameter stenosis	FFR 0.84 → no ischemia

(b)

Figure 6.10 Non-invasive detection of lesion specific ischaemia by FFR$_{CTA}$. **(a)** Example of epicardial lesion deemed significant on computed coronary angiography (CCTA) and invasive angiography, noted to be haemodynamically significant by FFR$_{CTA}$ and invasive FFR. **(b)** FFR$_{CTA}$ reduces the total number of false positive CCTA findings. An example of calcified plaque that appears obstructive based on CCTA and invasive angiography is shown to be haemodynamically not significant by both FFR$_{CTA}$ and invasive FFR. (Reprinted from Danad, I. et al., *Interv Cardiol Clin.*, 4, 4, 2015. With permission.)

outcomes. Though measuring FFR is technically challenging, FFR-guided revascularisation strategy can be safely extended to other clinical scenarios outside of focal lesions in stable CAD such as tandem, bifurcation lesions, left main stenosis and to ACS Non-invasive physiological assessment using FFR_{CTA} is an emerging tool with high diagnostic accuracy and potential to reduce unnecessary invasive angiograms and percutaneous interventions.

References

1. Zir LM et al. Interobserver variability in coronary angiography. *Circulation* 1976; 53(4): 627–32.
2. Ragosta M et al. Comparison between angiography and fractional flow reserve versus single-photon emission computed tomographic myocardial perfusion imaging for determining lesion significance in patients with multivessel coronary disease. *Am J Cardiol* 2007; 99(7): 896–902.
3. Zimmermann FM et al. Deferral vs. performance of percutaneous coronary intervention of functionally non-significant coronary stenosis: 15-year follow-up of the DEFER trial. *Eur Heart J* 2015; 36(45): 3182–88.
4. van Nunen LX et al. Fractional flow reserve versus angiography for guidance of PCI in patients with multivessel coronary artery disease (FAME): 5-year follow-up of a randomised controlled trial. *Lancet* 2015; 386(10006): 1853–60.
5. De Bruyne B et al. Fractional flow reserve–guided PCI for stable coronary artery disease. *N Engl J Med* 2014; 371(13): 1208–17.
6. Dattilo PB et al. Contemporary patterns of fractional flow reserve and intravascular ultrasound use among patients undergoing percutaneous coronary intervention in the United States: Insights from the national cardiovascular data registry. *J Am Coll Cardiol* 2012; 60(22): 2337–39.
7. Park SJ et al. Paradigm shift to functional angioplasty new insights for fractional flow reserve- and intravascular ultrasound-guided percutaneous coronary intervention. *Circulation* 2011; 124(8): 951–57.
8. Pijls NH et al. Experimental basis of determining maximum coronary, myocardial, and collateral blood flow by pressure measurements for assessing functional stenosis severity before and after percutaneous transluminal coronary angioplasty. *Circulation* 1993; 87(4): 1354–67.
9. Kern MJ et al. Intracoronary pressure and flow measurements. In: Eric J. Topol and Paul S. Terestein (editors), *Textbook of interventional Cardiology*, 7th Edition. Philadelphia, PA: Elsevier, 2016, pp. 85–107.
10. Duncker DJ, and Bache RJ. Regulation of coronary vasomotor tone under normal conditions and during acute myocardial hypoperfusion. *Pharmacol Ther* 2000; 86(1): 87–110.
11. De Bruyne B et al. Coronary flow reserve calculated from pressure measurements in humans. Validation with positron emission tomography. *Circulation* 1994; 89(3): 1013–22.
12. Crystal GJ, and Klein LW. Fractional flow reserve: Physiological basis, advantages and limitations, and potential gender differences. *Curr Cardiol Rev* 2014; 11(3): 209–19.
13. De Bruyne B et al. Simultaneous coronary pressure and flow velocity measurements in humans feasibility, reproducibility, and hemodynamic dependence of coronary flow velocity reserve, hyperemic flow versus pressure slope index, and fractional flow reserve. *Circulation* 1996; 94(8): 1842–49.
14. Bech GJW et al. Fractional flow reserve to determine the appropriateness of angioplasty in moderate coronary stenosis a randomized trial. *Circulation* 2001; 103(24): 2928–34.
15. Tonino PA et al. Fractional flow reserve versus angiography for guiding percutaneous coronary intervention. *N Engl J Med* 2009; 360(3): 213–24.
16. De Bruyne B et al. Fractional flow reserve–guided PCI versus medical therapy in stable coronary disease. *N Engl J Med* 2012; 367(11): 991–1001.
17. Levine GN et al. 2011 ACCF/AHA/SCAI guideline for percutaneous coronary intervention: A report of the American College of Cardiology Foundation/American Heart Association Task Force on Practice Guidelines and the Society for Cardiovascular Angiography and Interventions. *J Am Coll Cardiol* 2011; 58(24): e44–e122.
18. Lotfi A et al. Expert consensus statement on the use of fractional flow reserve, intravascular ultrasound, and optical coherence tomography. *Catheter Cardiovasc Interv* 2014; 83(4): 509–18.
19. Windecker S Kolh, P et al. 2014 ESC/EACTS Guidelines on myocardial revascularization. *Eur Heart J* 2014, p.ehu278.
20. Pijls NH et al. Measurement of fractional flow reserve to assess the functional severity of coronary-artery stenoses. *N Engl J Med* 1996; 334(26): 1703–08.
21. Johnson NP et al. Prognostic value of fractional flow reserve: Linking physiologic severity to clinical outcomes. *J Am Coll Cardiol* 2014; 64(16): 1641–54.
22. Samady H et al. Baseline fractional flow reserve and stent diameter predict optimal post-stent fractional flow reserve and major adverse cardiac events after bare-metal stent deployment. *JACC: Cardiovasc Intervent* 2009; 2(4): 357–63.
23. De Bruyne B et al. Pressure-derived fractional flow reserve to assess serial epicardial stenoses theoretical basis and animal validation. *Circulation* 2000; 101(15): 1840–47.
24. Mallidi J, and Lotfi A. Fractional flow reserve for the evaluation of tandem and bifurcation lesions, left main, and acute coronary syndromes. *Intervent Cardiol Clin* 2015; 4(4): 471–80.
25. Kim HL et al. Clinical and physiological outcomes of fractional flow reserve-guided percutaneous coronary intervention in patients with serial stenoses within one coronary artery. *JACC: Cardiovasc Intervent* 2012; 5(10): 1013–18.
26. Koo BK, and De Bruyne B. FFR in bifurcation stenting: What have we learned? *EuroIntervent: J EuroPCR Collaboration with the Working Group on Intervent Cardiol Eur Soc Cardiol* 2010; 6: J94–98.
27. Gao XF et al. Stenting strategy for coronary artery bifurcation with drug-eluting stents: A meta-analysis of nine randomised trials and systematic review. *EuroIntervent: J EuroPCR in Collaboration with the Working Group on Intervent Cardiol Eur Soc Cardiol* 2014; 10(5): 561–69.
28. Koo BK et al. Physiological evaluation of the provisional side-branch intervention strategy for bifurcation lesions using fractional flow reserve. *Eur Heart J* 2008; 29(6): 726–732.
29. Puri R et al. Optimizing outcomes during left main percutaneous coronary intervention with intravascular ultrasound

and fractional flow reserve: The current state of evidence. *JACC: Cardiovasc Intervent* 2012; 5(7): 697–707.

30. Lindstaedt M et al. How good are experienced interventional cardiologists at predicting the functional significance of intermediate or equivocal left main coronary artery stenoses? *Int J Cardiol* 2007; 120(2): 254–61.

31. Mallidi J et al. Long-term outcomes following fractional flow reserve-guided treatment of angiographically ambiguous left main coronary artery disease: A meta-analysis of prospective cohort studies. *Catheter Cardiovasc Interv* 2015.

32. Fearon WF et al. The impact of downstream coronary stenosis on fractional flow reserve assessment of intermediate left main coronary artery disease: Human validation. *JACC: Cardiovasc Intervent* 2015; 8(3): 398–403.

33. Jasti V et al. Correlations between fractional flow reserve and intravascular ultrasound in patients with an ambiguous left main coronary artery stenosis. *Circulation* 2004; 110(18): 2831–36.

34. Tamita K et al. Effects of microvascular dysfunction on myocardial fractional flow reserve after percutaneous coronary intervention in patients with acute myocardial infarction. *Catheter Cardiovasc Interv* 2002; 57(4): 452–59.

35. Ntalianis A et al. Fractional flow reserve for the assessment of nonculprit coronary artery stenoses in patients with acute myocardial infarction. *JACC: Cardiovasc Intervent* 2010; 3(12): 1274–81.

36. Engstrøm T et al. Complete revascularisation versus treatment of the culprit lesion only in patients with ST-segment elevation myocardial infarction and multivessel disease (DANAMI-3—PRIMULTI): An open-label, randomised controlled trial. *Lancet* 2015; 386(9994): 665–71.

37. Layland J et al. Fractional flow reserve vs. angiography in guiding management to optimize outcomes in non-ST-segment elevation myocardial infarction: The British Heart Foundation FAMOUS–NSTEMI randomized trial. *Eur Heart J* 2015; 36(2): 100–11.

38. O'Gara PT et al. 2013 ACCF/AHA guideline for the management of ST-elevation myocardial infarction: A report of the American College of Cardiology Foundation/American Heart Association Task Force on Practice Guidelines. *J Am Coll Cardiol* 2013; 61(4): e78–e140.

39. Gershlick AH et al. Randomized trial of complete versus lesion-only revascularization in patients undergoing primary percutaneous coronary intervention for STEMI and multivessel disease: The CvLPRIT trial. *J Am Coll Cardiol* 2015; 65(10): 963–72.

40. Sels JWE et al. Fractional flow reserve in unstable Angina and non–ST-segment elevation myocardial infarction: Experience from the FAME (Fractional flow reserve versus Angiography for Multivessel Evaluation) study. *JACC: Cardiovasc Intervent* 2011; 4(11): 1183–89.

41. Seto AH et al. Limitations and pitfalls of fractional flow reserve measurements and adenosine-induced hyperemia. *Interv Cardiol Clin* 2015; 4(4): 419–34.

42. Fearon WF. Fractional flow reserve-guided percutaneous coronary intervention. In: Mathew J. Price (editors), *Coronary Stenting. A Companion to Topol's Textbook of Interventional Cardiology*. Chapter 11. Philadelphia, PA: Elsevier Saunders, 2014, pp. 126–32.

43. Shreibati JB et al. Association of coronary CT angiography or stress testing with subsequent utilization and spending among Medicare beneficiaries. *Jama* 2011; 306(19): 2128–36.

44. Taylor CA et al. Computational fluid dynamics applied to cardiac computed tomography for noninvasive quantification of fractional flow reserve: Scientific basis. *J Am Coll Cardiol* 2013; 61(22): 2233–41.

45. Koo BK et al. Diagnosis of ischemia-causing coronary stenoses by noninvasive fractional flow reserve computed from coronary computed tomographic angiograms: Results from the prospective multicenter DISCOVER-FLOW (Diagnosis of ischemia-causing stenoses obtained via noninvasive fractional flow reserve) study. *J Am Coll Cardiol* 2011; 58(19): 1989–97.

46. Min JK et al. Diagnostic accuracy of fractional flow reserve from anatomic CT angiography. *Jama* 2012; 308(12): 1237–45.

47. Nørgaard BL et al. Diagnostic performance of noninvasive fractional flow reserve derived from coronary computed tomography angiography in suspected coronary artery disease: The NXT trial (Analysis of coronary blood flow using CT angiography: Next steps). *J Am Coll Cardiol* 2014; 63(12): 1145–55.

48. Gonzalez JA et al. Meta-analysis of diagnostic performance of coronary computed tomography angiography, computed tomography perfusion, and computed tomography-fractional flow reserve in functional myocardial ischemia assessment versus invasive fractional flow reserve. *Am J Cardiol* 2015; 116(9): 1469–78.

49. Douglas PS et al. Clinical outcomes of fractional flow reserve by computed tomographic angiography-guided diagnostic strategies vs. usual care in patients with suspected coronary artery disease: The prospective longitudinal trial of FFRCT: Outcome and resource impacts study. *Eur Heart J* 2015: p. 444.

50. Danad I et al. Noninvasive fractional flow reserve derived from coronary computed tomography angiography for the diagnosis of lesion-specific Ischemia. *Intervent Cardiol Clin* 2015; 4(4): 481–89.

New concepts in coronary physiological assessment

PAUL D MORRIS, JULIAN GUNN

7.1 Introduction

The emergence of sensor-tipped angioplasty guidewires has enabled invasive coronary angiography to move beyond simple *anatomical* lumenographic assessment into the realms of *physiological* assessment. When it comes to coronary revascularisation, prognostic benefit is limited to those with demonstrable ischaemia.[1] Accordingly, revascularisation should be targeted at is chaemia-causing, that is, physiologically significant, lesions. Traditional visual and quantitative coronary angiographic assessment methods are unreliable in identifying physiological lesion significance,[2,3] whereas adjunctive fractional flow reserve (FFR) has been shown to be associated with a number benefits including improved patient and economic outcomes.[4,5] Whilst FFR has become accepted as the 'gold-standard' method for determining coronary lesion significance, it has its limitations, and a number of other indices are now available to aid decision-making. This chapter explores the basic principles which underpin physiological coronary assessment and reviews alternative indices which can be used to complement FFR, in order to build up a more comprehensive understanding of the underlying pathophysiology which can be used to improve management decisions.

7.2 The coronary compartments

The coronary circulation comprises three compartments. The first is the large epicardial coronary artery compartment (>500 μm), easily visualised on the coronary angiogram. In the undiseased state, these conduction vessels offer little resistance to flow and there is therefore little pressure gradient along their course. The second is the pre-arteriolar compartment (150–500 μm), and the third is the arteriolar/capillary compartment (<150 μm), collectively known as the coronary microvasculature (CMV) (Figure 7.1). The CMV offers more than 90% of the resistance to blood flow and this is the site of coronary blood flow regulation. Regulation of CMV tone and therefore coronary microvasculature resistance (CMVR) govern coronary blood flow. CMVR is widely heterogeneous in health and disease, even under maximal flow (hyperaemic) conditions.[6–8]

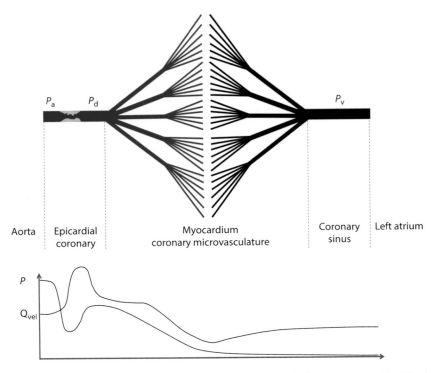

Figure 7.1 The coronary circulation with epicardial stenosis is demonstrated diagrammatically. The bottom graph demonstrates how the pressure (P) and flow velocity (Q_{vel}) vary along the length of the circulation. P_a, proximal (aortic) pressure; P_d, distal pressure; P_v, venous pressure. (Courtesy of Morris PD.)

7.3 Coronary vascular haemodynamics

Pressure drives flow through the cardiovascular system according to the hydraulic equivalent of Ohm's law (Equation 7.1):

$$\Delta P = Q \cdot R \qquad (7.1)$$

where ΔP = pressure gradient, Q = mass flow rate and R = resistance (comprising both epicardial and CMVR). Across the entire coronary system ΔP, therefore, represents the aortic pressure (P_a) minus the right atrial venous pressure (P_v). Although P_v does, therefore, influence blood flow (Q), it is generally accepted as negligible and is disregarded.

In contrast to other human circulations, coronary blood flow is reduced during systole, when driving pressure (P_a) is highest, and is augmented during diastole when driving pressure falls. This occurs because CMVR is elevated during systole due to myocardial contraction. This effect is reversed during diastole, when coronary blood flow predominates. Whilst this has clinical relevance in many pathological conditions (e.g. aortic valve disease, hypertrophic cardiomyopathy), most physiological indices incorporate flow and pressure values, time-averaged over at least one cardiac cycle.

Both the epicardial and CMV components of the circulation offer resistance to coronary blood flow, and the sum of these two resistances determines total coronary flow at a given pressure gradient. In the undiseased state, epicardial arteries offer minimal resistance to flow. This is not the case

in the CMV, in which coronary blood flow remains constant despite variation in blood pressure (*myogenic* control, in which vessel tone is proportional to driving pressure), and responds to metabolic demands (*metabolic* control, in which vessel tone is inversely proportional to metabolic activity).

In the presence of a coronary stenosis, epicardial resistance becomes significant, causing a trans-lesional pressure drop with a corresponding reduction in distal myocardial (and CMV) perfusion pressure (P_d) (Figure 7.1). Initially, autoregulatory mechanisms compensate by reactive CMV vasodilatation which ensures that adequate coronary blood flow is maintained. As stenosis severity increases beyond approximately 50% diameter loss, autoregulatory mechanisms are sufficient to maintain flow under resting conditions, but not under exercise conditions when ischaemia occurs, corresponding to the exertional symptoms of stable angina. Autoregulation continues to compensate for epicardial luminal narrowing, until the point when CMV dilatation is maximal and flow reserve is exhausted. At this point, even a slight increase in either stenosis severity or myocardial metabolic demand can no longer be compensated for, and pain occurs during minimal exertion or at rest. According to the original work by Gould et al. in the 1970s, this corresponds to a lumen diameter loss of approximately 85%.[9,10]

Under hyperaemic flow conditions, CMVR is minimised, autoregulatory responses are abolished and flow becomes dependent upon pressure. The relationship between flow and pressure under maximal hyperaemia is relevant to understanding the rationale behind indices of coronary physiology. The magnitude of the coronary arterial pressure gradient has been incorporated into a number of clinical indices of coronary physiology as a marker of lesion significance. Trans-stenotic flow dynamics are demonstrated in Figure 7.2. There are two primary contributors to the pressure drop. The first, and most significant in the presence of a stenosis, is captured by Bernoulli's law, which states that kinetic (blood flow velocity) and potential (blood pressure) energy are interchangeable (Equation 7.2). According to Bernoulli, any increase in flow velocity (which must occur when vessel diameter reduces) occurs simultaneously with a decrease in pressure and vice versa. Thus, Bernoulli pressure losses occur secondary to convective acceleration of blood flow through narrowed segments. They increase linearly with blood density (ρ) but *quadratically* with flow velocity (V):

$$\Delta P = \frac{1}{2}\rho(V_2^2 - V_1^2) \qquad (7.2)$$

As flow decelerates distal to the lesion, kinetic energy is lost and, according to Bernoulli, pressure recovers. In reality, even if the reference vessel diameter is restored, full pressure recovery does not occur in the post-stenotic region due to flow separation, vortex and eddy current formation. These effects are not captured by Bernoulli.

The second source of pressure loss is explained by Poiseuille's law (Equation 7.3). Poiseuille pressure losses result from viscous friction between adjacent lamina of flowing blood. Poiseuille pressure (P) losses increase *linearly* with flow and are dependent upon blood viscosity (μ), vessel length (L) and, critically, the fourth power of the radius (R):

$$\Delta P = \frac{8\mu QL}{\pi R^4} \qquad (7.3)$$

Relative to the Bernoulli pressure loss, this is likely to be significant only in the context of less severe stenoses or in the absence of any appreciable stenosis.

So the total pressure loss down the artery (ΔP) is equal to the sum of the Bernoulli and Poiseuille pressure losses (Equation 7.4):

$$\Delta P = K_1 Q + K_2 Q^2 \qquad (7.4)$$

where K_1 and K_2 are case-specific coefficients of the luminal anatomy and the rheological properties of blood. The first term accounts for Poiseuille losses and the second, Bernoulli losses. Because of the squared velocity term, in the presence of a stenosis, the Bernoulli term dominates. In the absence of stenosis, the equation approximates the Poiseuille term alone and the ΔP–Q plot becomes mostly linear. The terms of this equation uniquely characterise the relationship between flow and pressure (ΔP–Q relationship) on an artery-by-artery basis. Figure 7.3 represents the ΔP–Q relationship in three severities of stenosis.

Whilst these basic haemodynamic laws remain central to understanding coronary physiology, they are a simplification based upon idealised circumstances which fail to fully capture the complex haemodynamic effects of vessel tortuosity or the effects of dynamic (pulsating) vascular flow. Furthermore, they do not represent the influence of the CMVR. This is one reason why predicting the physiological significance of a lesion using measures derived from anatomical assessment, such as quantitative coronary angiography (QCA), intravascular ultrasound (IVUS) and optical coherence tomography (OCT), has failed to provide satisfactory results.[11,12]

The ΔP–Q relationship in a case of epicardial coronary stenosis is demonstrated in Figure 7.4.[13] The blue line represents the baseline flow condition (Q_b) which, due to autoregulation, is relatively flat within the physiological pressure range. Outside of the physiological range, compensatory mechanisms become exhausted and flow becomes dependent upon pressure. The dotted red line represents hyperaemic flow conditions in the presence of a stenosis. The dotted grey line represents the same artery without

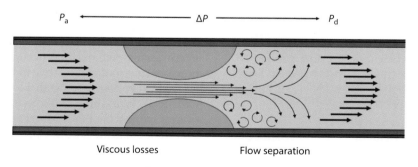

P_a ⟵ ΔP ⟶ P_d

Viscous losses   Flow separation

Convective acceleration   Pressure recovery

Figure 7.2 Trans-stenotic flow dynamics. Initially laminar flow with parabolic velocity profile (left) accelerates across a stenosis (middle). The vena contracta is demonstrated diagrammatically just beyond the neck of the stenosis. Flow separation, vortices and eddy currents occur in the post-stenotic region resulting in energy losses and incomplete pressure recovery. Thus the Bernoulli equation alone fails to accurately predict the trans-lesional pressure gradient. Note that P_d is also influenced by the distal coronary microvasculature resistance (CMVR) which is not represented in this diagram. (Courtesy of Morris PD.)

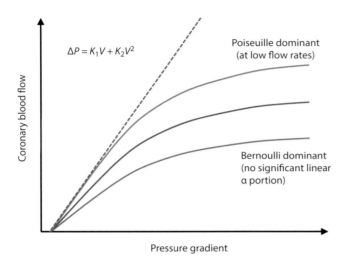

$$\Delta P = K_1 V + K_2 V^2$$

Poiseuille dominant
(at low flow rates)

Bernoulli dominant
(no significant linear
a portion)

Coronary blood flow

Pressure gradient

Figure 7.3 Pressure and flow relationship in the presence of stenosis. In this idealised diagram, the green, blue and red lines represent mild, moderate and severe stenoses. The dotted grey line represents a hypothetical normal artery without stenosis. The equation describes the P–Q plot. Each unique geometry is characterised by different K_1 and K_2 coefficients. Without a stenosis, the equation simplifies to the linear Poiseuille term which explains the interrupted grey line. (Courtesy of Morris PD.)

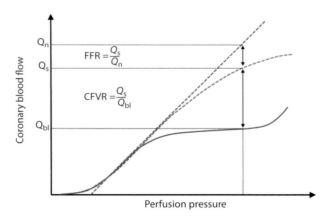

Q_n

$FFR = \dfrac{Q_s}{Q_n}$

Q_s

$CFVR = \dfrac{Q_s}{Q_{bl}}$

Q_{bl}

Coronary blood flow

Perfusion pressure

Figure 7.4 Pressure (P) and flow (Q) relationships in coronary flow velocity reserve (CFVR) and fractional flow reserve (FFR). Q_s, trans-stenotic flow; Q_n, flow through a hypothetically normal artery; Q_{bl}, flow at baseline. See text for explanation immediately above. (Adapted from van de Hoef et al., *Nat Rev Cardiol*, 10, 8, 2013.)

stenosis. In this hypothetical situation the P–Q relationship straightens because Bernoulli forces are eradicated (no stenosis) and linear Poiseuille forces dominate. In the presence of a stenosis, hyperaemic flow is restricted (relative to the hypothetical normal artery) and the line curves towards the pressure axis due to (nonlinear) Bernoulli forces (dotted red line). As the severity of the stenosis increases, hyperaemic flow (Q_s) becomes more limited relative to flow in the hypothetical normal artery (Q_n). This decreases the value of both

coronary flow reserve (CFR) (Q_s/Q_b) and FFR (Q_s/Q_n). Note that in the context of FFR, distal and proximal pressures are used as surrogates for flow. It should also be noted that the x axis intercept is not at zero but at a value just above venous pressure, termed pressure at zero-flow (P_{zf}). The coronary wedge pressure (P_w) is slightly greater and incorporates the influence of collateral flow.[13]

7.4 Why look beyond FFR?

Using FFR to guide coronary revascularisation in the cardiac catheter laboratory is associated with a number of advantageous clinical and economic outcomes.[3,4,14–18] Moreover, relative to other indices of coronary physiology, FFR is relatively simple to measure and is largely reproducible.[19] Therefore, FFR has become the 'gold-standard' investigation for diagnosing lesion significance. FFR estimates the percentage coronary flow restriction caused by proximal coronary disease, relative to an identical but hypothetically nonstenosed artery. A particular strength of FFR is that it automatically incorporates the influence of the distal CMVR vessels and that of any collateral flow. However, no single index of coronary physiology is perfect. It is important for operators to understand the potential limitations when interpreting FFR.

7.5 Flow rather than pressure

Although FFR is an index of *flow* reserve, flow is not incorporated into its calculation. Instead, the ratio of distal to proximal pressure (P_d/P_a) is used as a surrogate. This is acceptable, providing a number of assumptions hold true, but some are controversial.[13] FFR assumes that pharmacologically induced minimal CMVR is stable and constant pre- and post–percutaneous coronary intervention (PCI), implying that changes in perfusion pressure (e.g. P_d and P_a) do not affect the CMVR. This may not be a valid assumption because distal vascular tone is affected by the perfusion pressure in the process of autoregulation, even under hyperaemic conditions. There is a positive correlation between lesion severity and CMVR, which normalises when the lesion is treated with PCI,[20] and restoration of P_d by PCI induces a reduction in CMVR below the level of corresponding reference vessels, suggesting that long-term microvascular remodelling occurs by exposure to a low-pressure environment.[21] This indicates that more severe lesions will be associated with a lower P_d and thus a higher CMVR. In turn, this would result in an increased P_d, thus overestimating the FFR. Consequently, physiologically significant lesions might be inappropriately left untreated.

7.6 Is a single FFR threshold valid?

The original Deferral versus Performance of PCI of Functionally Nonsignificant Coronary Stenosis (DEFER) trial applied a 0.75 threshold, whereas the later Fractional Flow Reserve Versus Angiography for Multivessel Evaluation (FAME) trials used 0.80.[14,22] Both values are associated with positive trial outcomes data and, whilst a binary approach (single threshold point) is highly convenient and broadly works as a population average for decision-making (do or do not revascularise), does a patient truly benefit from full revascularisation if their FFR is 0.79 but not at all if it is 0.81? Perhaps a more continuous approach might be better. Recent work suggests that there is a 'dose–response' gradient for FFR < 0.75, through the 'grey zone' of 0.75–0.80, to FFR > 0.80 (ref). The issues of reproducibility and accuracy are also relevant. Analysis of the DEFER trial data revealed that, for borderline FFR values falling between 0.77 and 0.83, repeatability was just below 80%.[23] In clinical practice, this means that there is a 20% chance that a lesion will be reclassified (as significant or nonsignificant) if FFR is repeated 10 minutes later. The closer the initial value is to the 0.80 threshold, the higher the chance of reclassification on repeat measurement. There are also issues of 'drift' when the pressure wire has been in place for some time and that the guide catheter is not 'plugged' in the coronary ostium.[24] FFR must not be measured too soon after hyperaemia induction otherwise lesion significance may be overestimated. The measurement must be taken during the stable period which occurs at between 60 and 90 seconds in most people.[25] Furthermore, can a single scheme adequately represent all patients? Does an octogenarian, with multiple comorbidities, taking a multitude of cardiovascular drugs, require the same flow reserve as a 50-year-old marathon runner? It is unlikely that the former will spend much (if any) time in a maximally hyperaemic (and therefore potentially ischaemic) state. We require a more sophisticated approach, and this can be informed by deeper understanding of coronary physiology. FFR is, after all, simply another test with which to help clinical decision-making and cannot be the sole arbiter.

7.7 Is hyperaemia 'standard'?

FFR is based upon the assumption that maximal, stable hyperaemia (i.e. minimised CMVR) can be consistently attained with a standard dose and regimen of adenosine. However, variability of dose, dosing strategy and response to treatment may be relevant.[8,26,27] Adenosine is one of the many influences regulating CMVR, and the CMVR response to a hyperaemic stimulus demonstrates interindividual[6,8] and intra-individual variability between adjacent myocardial territories.[8] Furthermore, compared with the standard regime, incrementally larger doses of adenosine can induce progressively lower FFR values.[26,27] The currently applied ischaemic thresholds were determined by the standard protocol without validation using higher doses. Although FFR is influenced by the CMV, it cannot provide information regarding the state of the CMV. In theory, this means that lesion significance may be masked by occult coronary microvascular disease (CMVD). The independence of FFR from other dynamic physiological factors such as arterial and venous pressure has similarly been challenged.[28] Some of these limitations can be overcome by combining pressure measurements with those of coronary flow.

7.8 Measuring coronary blood flow

Coronary blood flow can be measured with either Doppler or thermistor-equipped 0.014-inch angioplasty guidewires.

The Doppler wire (FloWire®, Philips Volcano, Zaventem, Belgium) can be used to measure flow velocity at any point along the artery. Usually, the tip of the wire will be positioned in the proximal arterial segment with the tip, ideally, oriented co-axially. The console (ComboMap®, Philips Volcano) software displays a Doppler velocity signal as a function of time and calculates a number of velocity-based parameters including average peak velocity (APV). The range-gate (sampling volume) is a 2 mm deep dome positioned at 5–7 mm from the wire tip across a 30° arc. By incorporating the whole vessel diameter within the range-gate, the flow can be calculated (Equation 7.5):

$$Q(cm^3/s) = 0.5 \cdot APV \cdot (D^2\pi)/4 \qquad (7.5)$$

A combined pressure- and Doppler-sensitive wire (ComboWire®, Philips Volcano) is also produced, which can be useful for determining hyperaemic stenosis resistance (HSR, see below).

A thermistor-equipped angioplasty wire may also be used to estimate flow using the thermodilution method. One manufacturer produces a pressure wire, which also incorporates proximal and distal thermistors (PressureWire™, St Jude Medical, Minnesota). With the distal thermistor positioned >5 cm from the guiding catheter tip, 3 mL of room-temperature saline is injected via the guide catheter. The drop in temperature is recorded by both thermistors and the mean transit time (T_{mn}) is calculated (s) from the thermodilution curve. The average of three recordings is used. Mass flow rate can be calculated if the vessel volume can be estimated from the diameter (Equation 7.6):

$$Q = \frac{vol}{T_{mn}} \qquad (7.6)$$

7.9 Challenges in measuring flow

Both techniques are technically challenging. Flow measurement is largely restricted to research and is performed in a small minority of cases. Doppler signal artefact is commonly encountered with inadequate signal acquisition in up to 15% of cases.[29] Even an adequate Doppler signal may not reflect true flow because the wire measures flow *velocity*, and the wire may not be orientated to detect peak velocity which generally occurs in the centre of the vessel. Secondary flow patterns, disturbed or rapidly fluctuating flow, or a large velocity gradient in the sample volume further impact accuracy. These effects occur commonly near bifurcations, the stenosis itself and downstream of catheters. High amplitude, low-frequency wall artefact is often problematic when the sample volume is close to the vessel wall.[30] In other words, flow measurement is highly directional, whereas pressure is nondirectional; so the orientation of a flow wire is critical, whereas that of a pressure wire is immaterial. Measurement of pressure (and hence FFR) is, therefore, much easier and more reliable than measurement of flow using current technology.[29,31,32]

7.10 Coronary flow reserve

Measurement of coronary blood flow is incorporated into a number of coronary physiological indices, including indices of stenosis resistance, CMVR and CFR. CFR is defined as the ratio of coronary blood flows under hyperaemic and baseline conditions and is therefore the increase in flow from baseline to maximal hyperaemia. CFR reflects vasodilatory reserve, which progressively declines as epicardial disease increases. Just like FFR (pressure ratio), CFR (a ratio of two flows) is dimensionless, without units. CFR can be calculated with either the Doppler (Equation 7.7) or thermodilution (Equation 7.8) methods. In each case, flow is measured at baseline ($_{BL}$) and then under hyperaemic ($_{hyp}$) conditions:

$$CFR_{Doppler} = \frac{APV_{hyp}}{APV_{BL}} \qquad (7.7)$$

$$CFR_{therm} = \frac{T_{mn-BL}}{T_{mn-hyp}} \qquad (7.8)$$

Doppler is more commonly used to calculate the CFR, whereupon it is often known as coronary flow velocity reserve (CFVR). A normal CFR is a reflection of a healthy epicardial *and* microvascular circulation, whereas an abnormal CFR (<2.0) could be due to resistance in either the epicardial or CMV compartments, without being able to distinguish which. CFR is also vulnerable to alterations in the prevailing haemodynamic conditions under both baseline and hyperaemic flow[33]; it is reduced, for example, by tachycardia due to an increase in basal flow and a decrease in hyperaemic flow.[34] The challenges in measurement of flow, discussed above, further limit the utility of CFR.

The effect of pathological CMV physiology can be minimised by relating CFR in the index artery to that in an undiseased artery under identical conditions. This is known as relative CFR (rCFR). A normal rCFR is considered to be >0.80, and abnormal <0.65. However, a normal rCFR of c1.0 only indicates CFR equivalence, not normality. Since rCFR requires interrogation of a normal reference vessel, it is unsuitable in three-vessel disease.

7.11 Combining pressure and flow measurements

There are limitations associated with assessing pressure (FFR) and flow (CFR) *independently*. FFR and CFR are both influenced by CMV disease (in opposite directions), yet neither index generates any information about the state of the CMV nor can they differentiate epicardial from CMV disease. The implications of independent pressure or flow results are outlined in Table 7.1. Many of these problems can be circumvented by the concurrent measurement of pressure *and* flow. Furthermore, this approach yields additional value by enabling the calculation of resistance (R). According to the hydraulic equivalent of Ohm's law (Equation 7.9):

$$\Delta P = Q \cdot R \quad \rightarrow \quad R = \frac{\Delta P}{Q} \qquad (7.9)$$

Since flow through the system is constant at each level, if P_a and P_d are known (from pressure-wire assessment), flow is measured, and coronary venous pressure is assumed negligible, both epicardial and CMVRs can be calculated (Equations 7.10 and 7.11):

$$R_{sten} = \frac{P_a - P_d}{Q} \qquad (7.10)$$

and

$$R_{CMV} = \frac{P_d - P_v}{Q} \qquad (7.11)$$

Thus, combined *P–Q* assessment allows a more complete understanding of the entire coronary circulation. The physiological state of the CMV and its relative influence on FFR can be inferred and small vessel (CMV) disease can be discriminated from epicardial disease. Figure 7.5 demonstrates

Table 7.1 Implication of normal and abnormal flow and pressure indices

Test	Result	Implication
CFR	Normal (≥2.0)	Healthy epicardial *and* microvascular compartments (but influenced also by variability in baseline measurement)
	Abnormal (<2.0)	Unhealthy microvascular *or* significant epicardial stenosis
FFR	Normal (>0.80)	No significant benefit from revascularisation of epicardial disease
	Abnormal (≤0.80)	Likely significant benefit from revascularisation of epicardial disease

CFR, coronary flow reserve; FFR, fractional reserve flow.

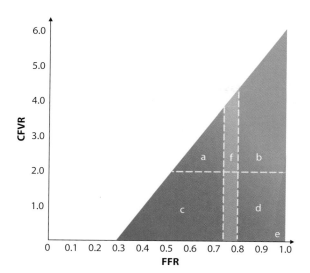

Figure 7.5 Pressure and flow measurement during invasive coronary angiography. Zone (a) indicates epicardial disease with healthy coronary microvasculature (CMV). Zone (b) indicates healthy epicardial and CMV physiology. Zone (c) indicates concordance between fractional flow reserve (FFR) and coronary flow velocity reserve (CFVR) results. Zone (d) indicates normal FFR with reduced flow reserve associated with predominately microvascular disease. Zone (e) indicates those patients with microvascular angina with pure CMV involvement. Only with combined physiological assessment can these individual zones be distinguished. Zone (f) indicates the grey zone in FFR threshold between 0.75 and 0.80. (Adapted from van de Hoef et al., *Circ Cardiovasc Interv*, 7, 3, 2014; Johnson, N.P. et al., *JACC Cardiovasc Imaging*, 5, 2, 2012.)[35,36]

schematically the pathological spectrum of epicardial and CMV physiology relative to the commonly used indices of intra-coronary pressure (FFR) and flow (CFVR).[35,36] Figures 7.6 and 7.7 demonstrate two cases where pressure and flow results are discordant. These relationships can be used practically to calculate indices of stenosis and myocardial resistance which are useful during patient assessment in the catheter laboratory, particularly in the context of discordant pressure and flow results.

7.12 Indices of stenosis resistance

7.12.1 Hyperaemic stenosis resistance

HSR incorporates both pressure and flow. It is the ratio of the mean trans-lesional pressure gradient ($\overline{\Delta P}$) and APV ideally measured by a combined flow- and pressure-sensitive angioplasty wire (ComboWire®, Philips Volcano), positioned distal to the target coronary lesion. It is calculated as the ratio of trans-lesional pressure gradient (ΔP) and APV (Equation 7.12):

$$HSR = \frac{\overline{\Delta P}}{APV} \qquad (7.12)$$

In the absence of disease, and therefore pressure gradient, HSR is equal to zero. HSR provides a more refined physiological assessment which quantifies the degree of coronary resistance attributable exclusively to the stenosis.[37] An HSR of >0.80 mmHg/cm/s is the threshold for ischaemia.[38] HSR is independent of variations in the haemodynamic conditions and is highly reproducible.[31,38]

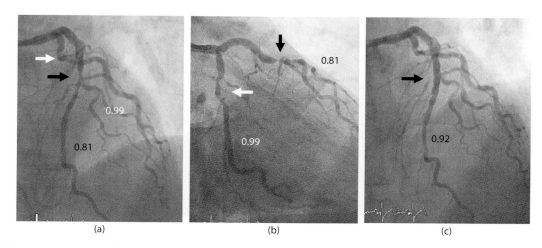

Figure 7.6 Discordant pressure-flow results and the influence of coronary microvasculature (CMV) disease. A 69-year-old male presented with chronic stable angina. Coronary angiography demonstrated lesions in the left anterior descending (LAD, black arrows) and circumflex (white arrows) arteries. The fractional flow reserve (FFR) and coronary flow reserve (CFR) in the circumflex were normal at 0.99 and 2.2, respectively. Surprisingly, the FFR in the LAD fell (just) in the normal range at 0.81 (see plates [a] and [b]) but the CFR was abnormal at 1.7. The hyperaemic microvascular resistance (HMR) was high in the LAD which explains why the FFR results did not match what might be expected from visual angiographic analysis. The LAD lesion underwent PCI. Post-PCI, the FFR improved to 0.92.

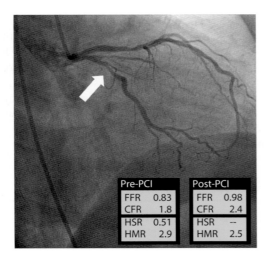

Figure 7.7 Discordant physiological results. A 55-year-old woman presented with exertional chest pain. Coronary angiography revealed a moderate stenosis in the left circumflex artery (arrow). The physiological results are shown. The fractional flow reserve (FFR) was normal at 0.83 but the coronary flow reserve (CFR) was reduced at 1.80. This suggests a significant influence from coronary microvascular disease. Combined assessment (pressure and flow) allowed the hyperaemic stenosis and myocardial resistance indices to be calculated. The hyperaemic stenosis resistance (HSR) and hyperaemic myocardial resistance (HMR) were 0.51 (normal) and 2.9 (elevated) respectively. Given the clear history of chest pain, the operator stented the circumflex lesion. Post-PCI, the FFR had improved to 0.98 and the CFR to 2.4

An advantage over FFR is that the calculation of HSR is robust despite naturally occurring variations in maximal hyperaemia because of the inclusion of the $\Delta P/Q$ ratio.[38] In a three-way comparison HSR was superior to both FFR and CFR in identifying physiological lesion significance. Its performance was particularly impressive in cases demonstrating physiologically discordant results between FFR and CFVR.[38] In a study of 181 intermediate coronary lesions, discordance between FFR and CFR was observed in 28%.[6] Patients with a normal FFR (<0.75) but abnormal CFVR (<2.0) had a significantly increased CMVR, masking the apparent significance of an epicardial lesion. Thus, HSR enabled the relative influence of epicardial and CMV disease to be distinguished.

The same group performed a similar study of 186 intermediate lesions and followed patients for 12 months. The highest rate of major adverse cardiovascular events (MACE) was observed in those with concordant abnormal values, an intermediate rate in those with discordant results and the lowest rate in those with concordant normal values (33.3% vs. 19.7% vs. 5.4%, $p = .008$). HSR was a better predictor of MACE than both FFR and CFVR.[39] In a study of 157 intermediate lesions followed up over ten years, 37 % demonstrated discordance between FFR and CFR. Those with a normal FFR but abnormal CFVR had a significantly increased MACE rate.

Conversely, those with normal CFVR but abnormal FFR had an outcome equivalent to those with concordant normal tests.

Baseline stenosis resistance (BSR) is the ratio of the pressure gradient across the stenosis to the basal APV measured under baseline (B) flow conditions, averaged over a cardiac cycle[32] (Equation 7.13):

$$BSR = \frac{P_d^B - P_a^B}{APV^B} \qquad (7.13)$$

The ischaemic threshold is quoted as 0.66 mmHg/cm/s. The advantage of this index is that it combines pressure and flow and does not require induction of hyperaemia, which itself has associated problems, summarised above. In a comparison with HSR, FFR and CFR at detecting ischaemia, as defined by single-photon emission computed tomography (SPECT), BSR was comparable to FFR and CFR. However, HSR was superior to BSR and CFR.[32] In a similar comparison, combining myocardial perfusion scintigraphy (MPS) and HSR as the reference standard, baseline stenosis resistance (BSR), instantaneous wavefree ratio (iFR) (see below) and FFR all demonstrated similar diagnostic accuracy.[40]

7.12.2 Indices of coronary microvascular resistance

The same pressure and flow measurements allow estimation of CMVR by calculating either velocity-based hyperaemic microvascular resistance (HMR) or thermodilution-based index of microvascular resistance (IMR). This can be performed assuming a zero coronary venous pressure (P_v) or correcting with measured right atrial pressure during right heart catheterisation (rarely performed). These indices provide objective data regarding the state of the CMV and help to identify and diagnose CMVD. This is particularly important in the context of an abnormal CFR but normal FFR. Often this is attributed to CMVD but may also occur secondary to diffuse epicardial disease or abnormal baseline conditions. Both methods provide an objective measure of CMVR which augments the diagnostic and prognostic assessment.

7.12.3 Hyperaemic microvascular resistance

For HMR a combination wire is required. It is the ratio of P_d and flow[6] (Equation 7.14). P_d is used as a surrogate of the pressure gradient (assuming a venous pressure of zero) and APV is used as a surrogate of flow:

$$HMR = \frac{P_d - P_v}{APV} = \frac{P_d}{APV} \qquad (7.14)$$

The units are mmHg·s/cm. No definite threshold value has yet been defined, although a value of 1.9 is associated with a healthy CMV and 2.4 is associated with abnormal CFR.[6,39] In the absence of epicardial disease, P_a can be substituted for P_d. HMR helps to explain discordance in FFR and CFVR[6] and adds value to the quantification of FFR by improving the diagnostic accuracy after adjustment for the IMR.[41] In the context of acute myocardial infarction (MI), HMR correlates with infarct size and predicts the presence of regional wall motion abnormalities.[42]

7.12.4 Index of microvascular resistance

IMR is a measure of the minimal CMVR. It is measured under hyperaemic flow conditions and is calculated from the mean transit time (T_{mn}) via the thermodilution method (Equation 7.15)[43]:

$$IMR = (P_d - P_v) \cdot T_{mn} = P_d \cdot T_{mn} \qquad (7.15)$$

Normal IMR is <25 mmHg/s.[44] Due to the potential confounding influence of collateral vessels and elevated venous pressure, coronary wedge pressure (e.g., measured distal to an inflated balloon during PCI) and left atrial pressure should be included in the calculation.[45] However, this is rarely done in practice.[46] IMR is highly reproducible, less variable than CFR and, in the context of AMI, predicts negative outcomes.[47,48] IMR has also been shown to be useful in identifying CMVD in patients with chest pain and normal coronary arteries.

7.13 Instantaneous wavefree ratio

Whereas FFR represents the trans-lesional pressure ratio during hyperaemia averaged over the entre cardiac cycle, iFR measures the pressure ratio from mid to end diastole under resting conditions. iFR makes use of the wave-free, high-flow, diastolic period when CMVR is at its lowest basal level. During this phase, the ratio of P_d to P_a demonstrates high agreeability with FFR.[49] iFR is measured using a pressure-sensitive wire in the same way as FFR but without the induction of hyperaemia. Software within the external module uses specialised algorithms to identify the diastolic wave-free period and calculate the P_d/P_a ratio within this zone. An iFR ≤0.90 has a diagnostic accuracy of 80% to predict FFR ≤ 0.80. The central concept of iFR is the notion that resting (diastolic) CMVR is equivalent to the mean hyperaemic resistance.[50,51] Although iFR requires the passage of a pressure wire, it does not require induction of hyperaemia, which is its key advantage.[52]

iFR has a high diagnostic accuracy for the diagnosis of ischaemia causing lesions as defined by an FFR of <0.80 (area under receiver operating characteristic [ROC] curve = 0.93), iFR correlating closely with FFR ($r = 0.9$) in a preliminary study of 118 cases.[49] In contrast to FFR, iFR is resistant

to spontaneous beat-to-beat variability. A hybrid iFR–FFR approach is proposed as an adenosine-saving strategy, in which an iFR < 0.86 indicates intervention and an iFR > 0.93 deferral, intermediate results requiring adenosine administration and FFR measurement. This approach generated good results in the hybrid iFR study[53] but less accurate evaluations are reported by other groups.[50,51] The lack of a true gold-standard method for identifying ischaemia causing lesions has left room for debate as to the relative value of iFR compared with FFR,[54] with some data suggesting that iFR use may even be superior to FFR.[55] Data from two large outcome trials which together will study iFR and FFR in over 4500 patients are awaited (NCT02053038, NCT02166736).

7.14 Challenges in accepting physiological assessment

Unlike previous tests, which were validated against established, but inaccurate, non-invasive tests, FFR has been shown to improve clinical outcomes in large trials. Future innovations will need to demonstrate similar clinical benefit. Despite the well-documented benefits of using even simple indices such as FFR, adoption rates are low. Even in the United Kingdom and United States where the use of FFR is amongst the highest, FFR is used in only about 6% of PCI cases[56] and almost no purely diagnostic angiographic studies. Physiological assessment adds complexity, expense, invasiveness and time to the procedure. It requires a PCI operator and an angioplasty capable catheterisation laboratory. Many cardiologists and surgeons rely on familiarity and confidence in their own visual assessment. A major challenge, therefore, is to change attitudes, and increase adoption of these techniques, something which requires the demonstration of clinical benefit from clinical trials.

7.15 Where next?

If FFR represents the first major step towards the use of adjunctive physiological assessment in the catheter laboratory to guide management, perhaps the next steps will be towards combined pressure and flow assessment because of the additional clinical and prognostic information generated.[35] The measurement of coronary flow is rare in routine interventional practice and is mostly restricted to research centres. Measuring coronary blood flow velocity with Doppler tipped coronary wires is technically challenging for many operators, whereas pressure measurement acquisition is much simpler. A major challenge will be to develop user-friendly and reliable methods for measuring coronary flow. It may be that information from perfusion magnetic resonance (MR) or even computed tomography (CT) can be used objectively to compliment invasive measurements.

Both HSR and BSR require further clinical validation before they are adopted into routine clinical practice.

7.16 Computing FFR

An alternative to acquiring physiological measurements invasively is to use computational fluid dynamics (CFD) processing to compute coronary physiology. Several groups have applied CFD analysis to estimate 'virtual FFR' (vFFR) from images of the coronary arteries, obtained by CT or by invasive angiography. Although this presents fresh challenges, promising early results have been demonstrated.[57] An example is demonstrated in Figure 7.8. When this approach reaches maturity, indices of coronary physiology, such as FFR, could be made available to closer to 100% of those who undergo PCI. This may be of particular importance for patients who are being assessed for bypass surgery and who do not currently have the opportunity for invasive pressure or flow wire assessment.

7.17 Is there a 'best test' to diagnose myocardial ischaemia?

How do the indices of ischaemia discussed here compare with non-invasive tests? Non-invasive tests such as SPECT, stress echocardiography and CMRI provide information about the location and extent of myocardial ischaemia and detect ischaemia caused by either epicardial or CMV disease but, with the possible exception of CT perfusion, they cannot distinguish between these two aetiologies. Table 7.2 summarises the European guidelines regarding investigations

used in coronary artery disease (CAD)/ischaemic heart disease (IHD).[58] Anatomical tests provide detailed information specific to the artery or even an individual lesion but ignore the functional consequences of disease and do not detect CMV disease at all. Catheter laboratory-based functional tests have the advantage of providing combined anatomic and functional data at an artery-, or even lesion-specific level. Importantly, indices such as FFR reveal the potential value of revascularisation, a key factor in clinical decision-making. However, they cannot estimate the myocardial ischaemic burden. Because these tests are deployed in the catheter laboratory during invasive angiography, they can also be used to directly guide decisions about the mode and strategy of treatment. The literature is confusing because of wide variability in terms of which investigation is used as the 'gold' standard, the criteria used to define significant CAD and whether the reported accuracy is defined on a per-patient or per-vessel basis.

The value of an individual test is determined by a wide range of individual, patient-specific factors (e.g. clinical stability, age, frailty, gender, comorbidities, mobility, heart rate, arrhythmia, body mass index) which must be weighed against heterogeneous investigation-specific factors (such as radiation exposure, invasiveness, habitus, sensitivity and specificity) and other considerations such as the strength of supporting evidence, available resources, cost and local expertise. Although guideline documents are helpful, these case-specific factors are often underrepresented. Table 7.3 summarises some of the key considerations of the major investigations used in the diagnosis and assessment of stable CAD. Table 7.4 and Figure 7.9 summarise some of the major physiological indices.

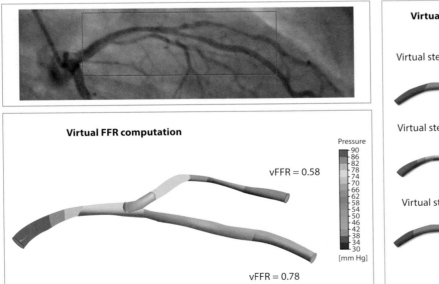
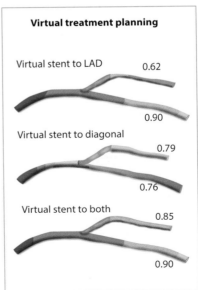

Figure 7.8 Virtual coronary physiology. Computer modelling has been used to calculate the pressure gradient along diseased LAD and diagonal coronary arteries. Modelling has also allowed the physiological impact of a variety of stenting strategies to be assessed (right). This information is potentially useful when planning PCI strategy.

Table 7.2 Recommendations and level of supporting evidence for investigations indicated in the investigation of CAD/IHD

Test	Asymptomatic		Symptomatic					
			Pretest probability of CAD[a]					
			Low (<15%)		Intermediate (15%–85%)		High (>85%)	
	Class	Level	Class	Level	Class	Level	Class	Level
ICA	III	A	III	A	IIb	A	I	A
CTCA	III	B	III	C	IIa	A	III	B
Stress echo	III	A	III	A	I	A	III	A
MPS SPECT	III	A	III	A	I	A	III	A
MPS PET	III	B	III	C	I	A	III	B
Stress MRI	III	B	III	C	I	A	III	B

Source: Windecker, S. et al., *Eur Heart J.*, 35, 37, 2014.
ICA, invasive coronary angiography; CTCA, coronary computed tomography; echo, echocardiography; SPECT, single photon emission computed tomography; PET, photon emission tomography; MPS, myocardial perfusion scintigraphy ; MRI, magnetic resonance imaging; CAD, coronary artery disease.
[a] See Figure 1.2.1.

Table 7.3 Practical and methodological considerations (pros and cons) of the major investigations used in IHD

Investigation	Radiation exposure	Coronary anatomical data	Myocardial functional data (detects ischaemia)	Capable of directly guiding PCI	Invasive	Applicable to a largely unselected patient cohort	Discriminates epi- from endocardial disease
Invasive anatomical tests							
ICA	Yes	Yes	No	Yes	Yes	Yes	No
CTCA	Yes	Yes	No	No	No	No	No
Non-invasive functional tests							
Exercise ECG	No	No	Yes	No	No	No	No
Stress echo	No	No	Yes	No	No	Yes	No
MPS (SPECT)	Yes	No	Yes	No	No	Yes	No
MPS (PET)	Yes	No	Yes	No	No	Yes	No
Perfusion MRI	No	No	Yes	No	No	Yes[a]	No
CT perfusion	Yes	Yes[b]	Yes	No	No	No	Yes[b]
ICA-based functional tests							
FFR	Yes	Yes	Yes	Yes	Yes	Yes	No
CFVR	Yes	Yes	Yes	Yes	Yes	Yes	No
HSR (also allows HMR)	Yes	Yes	Yes	Yes	Yes	Yes	Yes

Red and green shading indicates positive and negative attributes. ICA, invasive coronary angiography; CTCA, coronary computed tomography; echo, echocardiography; SPECT, single photon emission computed tomography; PET, photon emission tomography; MPS, myocardial perfusion scintigraphy; MRI, magnetic resonance imaging; ECG, electrocardiography; CT, computed tomography; FFR, fractional flow reserve; CFVR, coronary flow velocity reserve; HSR, hyperaemic stenosis resistance.
[a] Standard MRI exclusions (claustrophobia and ferromagnetic prostheses).
[b] Potentially, if performed as hybrid procedure with CTCA protocol.

Table 7.4 Summary of the major intracoronary physiological indices

Index	Definition	Hyperaemia induction	Threshold for abnormality	Procedural requirements	Information generated	Limitations
FFR	$= P_d / P_a$	Y	≤ 0.80	Pressure wire assessment. Induction of hyperaemia.	Percentage flow limitation caused by proximal stenosis/es and therefore value of putative revascularisation.	No information about the CMV. Use of pressure as a surrogate of flow relies on a number of assumptions.
CFR therm'	$= T_{mn}^{BL} / T_{mn}^{hyp}$	Y	< 2.0	Average of three recordings.	Degree of flow limitation secondary to disease of either epicardial or CMV vessels.	Variability in baseline physiology / haemodynamics can also reduce CFR. Average of three recordings for BL and hyperaemic measurements.
CFVR Doppler	$= Q_{vel}^{hyp} / Q_{vel}^{BL}$	Y	< 2.0	Doppler flow velocity wire assessment in index vessel.	Degree of flow limitation secondary to disease of either epicardial or CMV vessels.	Variability in baseline physiology / haemodynamics can also reduce CFR.
rCFR	$= CFVR^{sten} / CFVR^{norm}$	Y	< 0.65	Doppler flow velocity wire assessment in index and normal reference vessel.	Degree of flow limitation relative to a 'normal' reference vessel. Less susceptible to variability in baseline physiology than CFVR.	Also requires measurement in a normal reference artery. Unsuitable in three-vessel disease. Can be 'normal' even if flow is globally reduced by CV dysfunction.
IMR	$= P_d \cdot T_{mn}$	Y	< 25 mmHg $\cdot$s^{-1}	Pressure wire and thermodilution assessment.	Index of myocardial resistance.	Few centres have experience with thermodilution method.
HMR	$= P_d / Q_{vel}$	Y	Not fully established but upper limit of normal considered 1.85–2.05 mmHg cm $\cdot$s^{-1}.	Combined pressure and flow assessment distal to epicardial lesion/s.	Coronary microvascular resistance.	Normal values and role in management decisions not yet established.
HSR	$= P_d - P_a / Q_{vel}$	Y	>0.80 mmHg cm^{-1} $\cdot$s	Combined pressure and flow assessment distal to epicardial lesion/s.	Trans-lesional epicardial resistance. Independent of baseline haemodynamic conditions.	Measuring Doppler flow velocity distal to a lesion can be challenging.

(Continued)

Table 7.4 (continued) Summary of the major intracoronary physiological indices

Index	Definition	Hyperaemia induction	Threshold for abnormality	Procedural requirements	Information generated	Limitations
BSR	$= P_d - P_a / Q_{vel}$	N	Not fully established but >0.66 mmHg cm^{-1} ·s considered abnormal	Combined pressure and flow assessment distal to epicardial lesion/s.	Trans-lesional epicardial resistance measured at baseline.	Not as effective as HSR at identifying ischaemia-causing lesions.
iFR	$= P_d / P_a$ during diastolic, wave-free period	N	>0.93 normal; <0.86 abnormal, 0.86–0.93 undergo FFR	Pressure wire assessment.	No induction of hyperaemia needed.	Whether iFR represents equivalence to FFR is controversial. Long-term outcome data awaited.

P = pressure. Pressure is used as mean. CMV, coronary microvascular vessels; FR, instantaneous wavefree ratio; HSR, hyperaemic stenosis resistance; BSR, baseline stenosis resistance; HMR, hyperaemic microvascular resistance; IMR, index of microvascular resistance; CFVR, coronary flow velocity reserve; rCFR, relative CFR; CFR, coronary flow reserve; FFR, fractional flow reserve; BL, baseline; CV, cardiovascular.

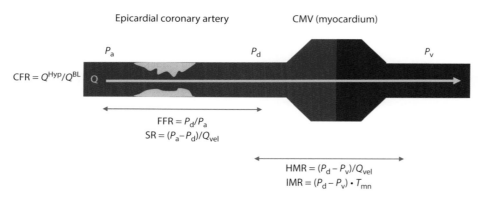

Figure 7.9 A summary of some of the major coronary physiological indices. When calculating indices of stenosis resistance, P_v is often disregarded and P_d is used. CMV, coronary microvascular vessels; CFR, coronary flow reserve; Q, flow; Hyp, hyperaemia; BL, baseline; P_a, proximal pressure; P_d, distal pressure; P_v, venous pressure; FFR, fractional flow reserve; SR, stenosis resistance; vel, velocity; HMR, hyperaemic stenosis resistance; IMR, index of stenosis resistance; T_{mn}, mean transit time. (Courtesy of Morris PD.)

7.18 Summary

Compared with visual angiographic assessment, physiological lesion assessment is superior in terms of identifying ischaemia-causing lesions, and optimising treatment decisions. A number of techniques are now available to the interventionist. A good understanding of the underlying principles of coronary physiology can aid interpretation of images and decision-making. The ease, simplicity and reproducibility of measuring FFR has meant that cardiologists currently rely almost exclusively on this test. However, no index of coronary physiology is perfect and other indices can be used to build up a more comprehensive picture of the underlying coronary pathophysiology. Future developments may involve combined assessment of pressure and flow because this 'unlocks' valuable information regarding the state of the CMV. However, this will require advances in how coronary flow is assessed, which may involve adopting new technology such as computational techniques based upon coronary imaging.

References

1. Shaw LJ et al. Optimal medical therapy with or without percutaneous coronary intervention to reduce ischemic burden: Results from the Clinical Outcomes Utilizing Revascularization and Aggressive Drug Evaluation (COURAGE) trial nuclear substudy. *Circulation* 2008; 117(10): 1283–91.
2. Topol EJ, and Nissen SE. Our preoccupation with coronary luminology. The dissociation between clinical and

angiographic findings in ischemic heart disease. *Circulation* 1995; 92(8): 2333–42.

3. Tonino PA et al. Angiographic versus functional severity of coronary artery stenoses in the FAME study fractional flow reserve versus angiography in multivessel evaluation. *J Am Coll Cardiol* 2010; 55: 2816–21.

4. Zhang D et al. Fractional flow reserve versus angiography for guiding percutaneous coronary intervention: A meta-analysis. *Heart* 2015; 101(6): 455–62.

5. Fearon WF et al. Economic evaluation of fractional flow reserve-guided percutaneous coronary intervention in patients with multivessel disease. *Circulation* 2010; 122(24): 2545–50.

6. Meuwissen M et al. Role of variability in microvascular resistance on fractional flow reserve and coronary blood flow velocity reserve in intermediate coronary lesions. *Circulation* 2001; 103(2): 184–87.

7. Austin RE, Jr. et al. Profound spatial heterogeneity of coronary reserve. Discordance between patterns of resting and maximal myocardial blood flow. *Circ Res* 1990; 67(2): 319–31.

8. Chareonthaitawee P et al. Heterogeneity of resting and hyperemic myocardial blood flow in healthy humans. *Cardiovasc Res* 2001; 50(1): 151–61.

9. Gould KL et al. Physiologic basis for assessing critical coronary stenosis. Instantaneous flow response and regional distribution during coronary hyperemia as measures of coronary flow reserve. *Am J Cardiol* 1974; 33(1): 87–94.

10. Gould KL et al. Compensatory changes of the distal coronary vascular bed during progressive coronary constriction. *Circulation* 1975; 51(6): 1085–94.

11. Ben-Dor I et al. Intravascular ultrasound lumen area parameters for assessment of physiological ischemia by fractional flow reserve in intermediate coronary artery stenosis. *Cardiovasc Revasc Med* 2012; 13(3): 177–82.

12. Gonzalo N et al. Morphometric assessment of coronary stenosis relevance with optical coherence tomography: A comparison with fractional flow reserve and intravascular ultrasound. *J Am Coll Cardiol* 2012; 59(12): 1080–89.

13. van de Hoef TP et al. Fractional flow reserve as a surrogate for inducible myocardial ischaemia. *Nat Rev Cardiol* 2013; 10(8): 439–52.

14. Bech GJ et al. Fractional flow reserve to determine the appropriateness of angioplasty in moderate coronary stenosis: A randomized trial. *Circulation* 2001; 103(24): 2928–34.

15. Tonino PA et al. Fractional flow reserve versus angiography for guiding percutaneous coronary intervention. *N Engl J Med* 2009; 360(3): 213–24.

16. De Bruyne B et al. Fractional flow reserve-guided PCI versus medical therapy in stable coronary disease. *N Engl J Med* 2012; 367(11): 991–1001.

17. Li J et al. Long-term outcomes of fractional flow reserve-guided vs. angiography-guided percutaneous coronary intervention in contemporary practice. *Eur Heart J* 2013; 34(18): 1375–83.

18. Frohlich GM et al. Long-term survival in patients undergoing percutaneous interventions with or without intracoronary pressure wire guidance or intracoronary ultrasonographic imaging: A large cohort study. *JAMA Intern Med* 2014; 174(8): 1360–66.

19. Johnson NP et al. Repeatability of fractional flow reserve despite variations in systemic and coronary hemodynamics. *JACC Cardiovasc Interv* 2015; 8(8): 1018–27.

20. Chamuleau SA et al. Association between coronary lesion severity and distal microvascular resistance in patients with coronary artery disease. *Am J Physiol Heart Circ Physiol* 2003; 285(5): H2194–200.

21. Verhoeff BJ et al. Influence of percutaneous coronary intervention on coronary microvascular resistance index. *Circulation* 2005; 111(1): 76–82.

22. Pijls NH et al. Fractional flow reserve versus angiography for guiding percutaneous coronary intervention in patients with multivessel coronary artery disease: 2-year follow-up of the FAME (Fractional Flow Reserve Versus Angiography for Multivessel Evaluation) study. *J Am Coll Cardiol* 2010; 56(3): 177–84.

23. Petraco R et al. Fractional flow reserve-guided revascularization: Practical implications of a diagnostic gray zone and measurement variability on clinical decisions. *JACC Cardiovasc Interv* 2013; 6(3): 222–25.

24. Pijls NH et al. Practice and potential pitfalls of coronary pressure measurement. *Catheter Cardiovasc Interv* 2000; 49(1): 1–16.

25. Tarkin JM et al. Hemodynamic response to intravenous adenosine and its effect on fractional flow reserve assessment: Results of the Adenosine for the Functional Evaluation of Coronary Stenosis Severity (AFFECTS) study. *Circ Cardiovasc Interv* 2013; 6(6): 654–61.

26. De Luca G et al. Effects of increasing doses of intracoronary adenosine on the assessment of fractional flow reserve. *JACC Cardiovasc Interv* 2011; 4(10): 1079–84.

27. Rioufol G et al. 150 microgram intracoronary adenosine bolus for accurate fractional flow reserve assessment of angiographically intermediate coronary stenosis. *EuroIntervention: Journal of EuroPCR in Collaboration with the Working Group on Interventional Cardiology of the European Society of Cardiology* 2005; 1(2): 204–07.

28. Siebes M et al. Influence of hemodynamic conditions on fractional flow reserve: Parametric analysis of underlying model. *Am J Physiol Heart Circ Physiol* 2002; 283(4): H1462–70.

29. Kern MJ. Coronary physiology revisited: Practical insights from the cardiac catheterization laboratory. *Circulation* 2000; 101(11): 1344–51.

30. Hartley CJ. Review of intracoronary Doppler catheters. *Int J Cardiac Imaging* 1989; 4(2–4): 159–68.

31. Siebes M et al. Single-wire pressure and flow velocity measurement to quantify coronary stenosis hemodynamics and effects of percutaneous interventions. *Circulation* 2004; 109(6): 756–62.

32. van de Hoef TP et al. Diagnostic accuracy of combined intracoronary pressure and flow velocity information during baseline conditions: Adenosine-free assessment of functional coronary lesion severity. *Circ Cardiovasc Interv* 2012; 5(4): 508–14.

33. Hoffman JI. Problems of coronary flow reserve. *Ann Biomed Eng* 2000; 28(8): 884–96.

34. McGinn AL et al. Interstudy variability of coronary flow reserve. Influence of heart rate, arterial pressure, and ventricular preload. *Circulation* 1990; 81(4): 1319–30.

35. van de Hoef TP et al. Physiological basis and long-term clinical outcome of discordance between fractional flow reserve and coronary flow velocity reserve in coronary stenoses of intermediate severity. *Circ Cardiovasc Interv* 2014; 7(3): 301–11.

36. Johnson NP et al. Is discordance of coronary flow reserve and fractional flow reserve due to methodology or clinically relevant coronary pathophysiology? *JACC Cardiovasc Imaging* 2012; 5(2): 193–202.

37. Kern MJ et al. Physiological assessment of coronary artery disease in the cardiac catheterization laboratory: A scientific statement from the American heart association committee on diagnostic and interventional cardiac catheterization, council on clinical cardiology. *Circulation* 2006; 114(12): 1321–41.

38. Meuwissen M et al. Hyperemic stenosis resistance index for evaluation of functional coronary lesion severity. *Circulation* 2002; 106(4): 441–46.

39. Meuwissen M et al. The prognostic value of combined intracoronary pressure and blood flow velocity measurements after deferral of percutaneous coronary intervention. *Catheter Cardiovasc Interv* 2008; 71(3): 291–97.

40. van de Hoef TP et al. Head-to-head comparison of basal stenosis resistance index, instantaneous wave-free ratio, and fractional flow reserve: Diagnostic accuracy for stenosis-specific myocardial ischaemia. *EuroIntervention:* 2015 Dec;11(8):914–925. doi: 10.4244/EIJY14M08_17.

41. van de Hoef TP et al. Impact of hyperaemic microvascular resistance on fractional flow reserve measurements in patients with stable coronary artery disease: Insights from combined stenosis and microvascular resistance assessment. *Heart* 2014; 100(12): 951–59.

42. Teunissen PF et al. Doppler-derived intracoronary physiology indices predict the occurrence of microvascular injury and microvascular perfusion deficits after angiographically successful primary percutaneous coronary intervention. *Circ Cardiovasc Interv* 2015; 8(3): e001786.

43. Fearon WF et al. Novel index for invasively assessing the coronary microcirculation. *Circulation* 2003; 107(25): 3129–32.

44. Kobayashi Y, and Fearon WF. Invasive coronary microcirculation assessment--current status of index of microcirculatory resistance. *Circulation Journal: Official Journal of the Japanese Circulation Society* 2014; 78(5): 1021–28.

45. Aarnoudse W et al. Myocardial resistance assessed by guidewire-based pressure-temperature measurement: In vitro validation. *Catheter Cardiovasc Interv* 2004; 62(1): 56–63.

46. Yong AS et al. Calculation of the index of microcirculatory resistance without coronary wedge pressure measurement in the presence of epicardial stenosis. *JACC Cardiovasc Interv* 2013; 6(1): 53–58.

47. Ng MK et al. Invasive assessment of the coronary microcirculation: Superior reproducibility and less hemodynamic dependence of index of microcirculatory resistance compared with coronary flow reserve. *Circulation* 2006; 113(17): 2054–61.

48. Fearon WF et al. Prognostic value of the index of microcirculatory resistance measured after primary percutaneous coronary intervention. *Circulation* 2013; 127(24): 2436–41.

49. Sen S et al. Development and validation of a new adenosine-independent index of stenosis severity from coronary wave-intensity analysis: Results of the ADVISE (ADenosine Vasodilator Independent Stenosis Evaluation) study. *J Am Coll Cardiol* 2012; 59(15): 1392–402.

50. Johnson NP et al. Does the instantaneous wave-free ratio approximate the fractional flow reserve? *J Am Coll Cardiol* 2013; 61(13): 1428–35.

51. Berry C et al. VERIFY (VERification of Instantaneous Wave-Free Ratio and Fractional Flow Reserve for the Assessment of Coronary Artery Stenosis Severity in EverydaY Practice): A multicenter study in consecutive patients. *J Am Coll Cardiol* 2013; 61(13): 1421–27.

52. Petraco R et al. Classification performance of instantaneous wave-free ratio (iFR) and fractional flow reserve in a clinical population of intermediate coronary stenoses: Results of the ADVISE registry. *EuroIntervention:* 2013 May 20;9(1):91–101. doi: 10.4244/EIJV9I1A14.

53. Petraco R et al. Hybrid iFR-FFR decision-making strategy: Implications for enhancing universal adoption of physiology-guided coronary revascularisation. *EuroIntervention: Journal of EuroPCR in Collaboration with the Working Group on Interventional Cardiology of the European Society of Cardiology* 2013; 8(10): 1157–65.

54. Jeremias A et al. Multicenter core laboratory comparison of the instantaneous wave-free ratio and resting Pd/Pa with fractional flow reserve: The RESOLVE study. *J Am Coll Cardiol* 2014; 63(13): 1253–61.

55. Sen S et al. Diagnostic classification of the instantaneous wave-free ratio is equivalent to fractional flow reserve and is not improved with adenosine administration. Results of CLARIFY (Classification Accuracy of Pressure-Only Ratios Against Indices Using Flow Study). *J Am Coll Cardiol* 2013; 61(13): 1409–1420.

56. Ludman PF. BCIS audit returns adult interventional procedures January 2013 to December 2013. *Br Cardiovasc Intervent Soc* 2014.

57. Morris PD et al. "Virtual" (computed) fractional flow reserve: Current challenges and limitations. *JACC Cardiovasc Interv* 2015; 8(8): 1009–17.

58. Windecker S et al. 2014 ESC/EACTS guidelines on myocardial revascularization: The task force on myocardial revascularization of the European Society of Cardiology (ESC) and the European Association for Cardio-Thoracic Surgery (EACTS) developed with the special contribution of the European Association of Percutaneous Cardiovascular Interventions (EAPCI). *Eur Heart J* 2014; 35(37): 2541–619.

Overview of randomised trials of percutaneous coronary intervention: Comparison with medical and surgical therapy

JAVAID IQBAL, AYYAZ SULTAN, PATRICK W SERRUYS

Coronary artery disease remains among the top most causes of morbidity and mortality globally. There have been substantial improvements in medical therapy to prevent and treat coronary artery disease. However, patients with prognostically significant disease or anginal symptoms despite optimal medical therapy (OMT) require coronary revascularisation with either coronary artery bypass grafting (CABG) or percutaneous coronary intervention (PCI). CABG was the main revascularisation modality during the second half of 20th century; however, PCI has now become the preferred mode of revascularisation in patients with one- or two-vessel disease. Nevertheless, the optimal therapy in patients with multi-vessel disease and/or unprotected left main stem (LMS) disease has remained debatable and is the subject of many clinical trials in recent years. This chapter discusses the current status and the evidence-based use of PCI in the treatment of patients with coronary artery disease.

8.1 Introduction

Treatment of coronary artery disease, both medically and invasively, has seen marked improvements in the last few decades. Development of surgical revascularisation techniques in the latter half of the 20th century revolutionised the treatment of coronary artery disease.[1] Vasilii Kolesov performed anastomosis between the left internal mammary artery (LIMA) and left circumflex artery in a man in 1962.

Rene Favaloro used saphenous vein graft (SVG) as bypass conduit in 1967. Reed was the first surgeon to perform the operation using cardiopulmonary bypass. CABG has shown superiority over medical therapy for prognosis and symptomatic relief; however, there are operative risks that may make it less attractive option in certain groups of patients.

Andreas Gruentzig performed the first balloon angioplasty in 1977.[2] Although it was a huge advancement in the treatment of coronary artery disease, outcomes were compromised by acute vessel closure due to dissection or elastic recoil, late vascular remodelling and neointimal proliferation.[3] Coronary stents were, therefore, developed to address these issues.[4] The Belgium Netherlands Stent Arterial Revascularisation Therapies Study (BENESTENT) and the North American Stent Restenosis Study (STRESS) demonstrated superiority of the stents over balloon angioplasty.[5,6] However, there was a significant risk of in-stent restenosis over medium and long-term follow-up of these bare metal stents (BMS).[7] Drug eluting stents (DES) were therefore developed and have shown reduction in restenosis and target vessel revascularisation (TVR) compared with BMS.[8,9] The concerns about stent thrombosis (ST) with the first generation DES[10,11] led to the development of novel polymers, anti-platelet agents and the newer generation of DES.[12,13] Cobalt–chromium and platinum–chromium have superseded steel as the material of choice for stents and biocompatible and biodegradable polymers have largely replaced the permanent synthetic polymers.[14] These stent platforms are being combined with newer anti-proliferative drugs including everolimus, zotarolimus and biolimus. The 'newer generation' DES have shown superiority over the 'original' DES, in terms of preventing complications or the need for repeat revascularisation.[15–18] This chapter discusses the current status and the evidence-based use of PCI in the treatment of patients with coronary artery disease, with a particular emphasis on comparison with other treatment modalities.

8.2 Revascularisation versus medical therapy

Whilst studies for the treatment of coronary artery disease have usually compared two treatment options, MASS (Medicine, Angioplasty or Surgery Study) and MASS-II trials are unique for comparing the three treatment modalities. MASS was a modest size ($n = 214$), single-centre study of patients with stable angina, normal ventricular function and a proximal stenosis of the left anterior descending artery who were randomly assigned to undergo CABG ($n = 70$), balloon angioplasty ($n = 72$) or medical therapy alone ($n = 72$). The predefined primary study endpoint was the combined incidence of cardiac death, myocardial infarction or refractory angina requiring revascularisation. At an average follow-up period of 3 years, a primary endpoint had occurred in only two patients (3%) assigned to bypass surgery compared with 17 assigned to angioplasty (24%) and 12 assigned to medical therapy (17%) ($p = .0002$, angioplasty vs. bypass surgery; $p = .006$, bypass surgery vs. medical treatment; $p = .28$, angioplasty vs. medical treatment). There was no difference in mortality or infarction rates among the groups. However, no patient allocated to bypass surgery needed revascularisation, compared with eight and seven patients assigned, respectively, to coronary angioplasty and medical treatment ($p = .019$).[19]

MASS-II ($n = 611$) was the next step to compare CABG ($n = 203$), PCI with BMS ($n = 205$) or OMT ($n = 203$) group. The 1-year mortality rates were similar in the three groups (CABG 4.0% vs. PCI 4.5% vs. OMT 1.5%, $p = .23$). The 1-year survival rates without Q-wave MI were 98% for CABG, 92% for PCI, and 97% for OMT ($p = .01$). After 1-year follow-up, 1.97% of OMT patients and 8.78% of PCI patients underwent additional interventions, compared with only 0.5% of CABG patients ($p = .08$). Although underpowered for outcomes, MASS-II has shown no difference in survival between OMT and revascularisation (OMT 69%, CABG 74.9%, PCI 75.1%, $p = .089$) at 10-year follow-up.[20] However, for the primary composite endpoint of mortality, Q-wave MI and repeat revascularisation, CABG was superior to other therapies (CABG 33% vs. PCI 42.4% vs. OMT 59.1%, $p = .01$). Compared with PCI and OMT, repeat revascularisation was five times lower among patients with CABG; however, in this trial PCI was performed using BMS. There has been no randomised trial comparing OMT, CABG and PCI with DES in a head-to-head fashion.

8.2.1 CABG versus medical therapy

The superiority of CABG over medical therapy has been demonstrated in multiple studies (e.g. the European Coronary Surgery Study, the Veteran's Administration Coronary Artery Bypass Surgery Cooperative Study Group and the Coronary Artery Surgery Study) and meta-analyses, confirming a survival advantage conferred by CABG in patients with unprotected LMS or three-vessel disease, particularly in those with severe symptoms, early positive exercise tests and impaired left ventricular (LV) function.[21,22] However, it should be noted that only patients at high (4.8%) or moderate (2.5%) annual mortality risk gained a clinically and statistically significant improvement in survival. Among patients without involvement of the proximal left anterior descending (LAD) disease, mortality lowered with surgical therapy for patients with three-vessel disease. In patients who would not get survival benefit with CABG, surgery can still be considered to improve functional capacity and quality of life (if not accomplished with OMT). However, no overall impact of CABG surgery on subsequent infarction has been demonstrated. This is due to an excess of infarction in the perioperative period among those assigned to surgery, even though the subsequent risk is lower during extended follow-up.

8.2.2 PCI versus medical therapy

Multiple studies have also compared outcomes of PCI and medical therapy. The initial studies (e.g. ACME [Angioplasty Compared to Medicine], RITA-2 [Randomised Intervention Treatment of Angina], AVERT [Atorvastatin versus Revascularization Treatment], TIME [Trial of Invasive versus Medical Therapy in Elderly], MASS [Medicine, Angioplasty or Surgery Study]) comparing balloon angioplasty or PCI with BMS against medical therapy have limited relevance to current practice as both medical therapy (lipid lowering, anti-platelet, secondary prevention drugs) and PCI techniques/technology have significantly improved in recent years.

Clinical Outcomes Utilizing Revascularization and Aggressive Drug Evaluation (COURAGE) trial ($n = 2287$) compared OMT alone versus PCI plus OMT for treating patients with significant one-, two- and three-vessel disease without LMS involvement and found no significant difference in the composite endpoint of death or non-fatal myocardial infarction (MI) at a median follow-up of 4.6 years (hazard ratio [HR] for the PCI group 1.05, 95% confidence interval [CI] 0.87–1.27, $p = .62$) (Figure 8.1).[23] Both groups were also equal in terms of freedom from angina at 5 years. During 6 years follow-up, 21% patients in the PCI group had additional revascularisation, as compared with 33% of those in the OMT group (HR 0.60, 95% CI 0.51–0.71, $p < .001$).[23] However, it should be noted that in nuclear sub-study of

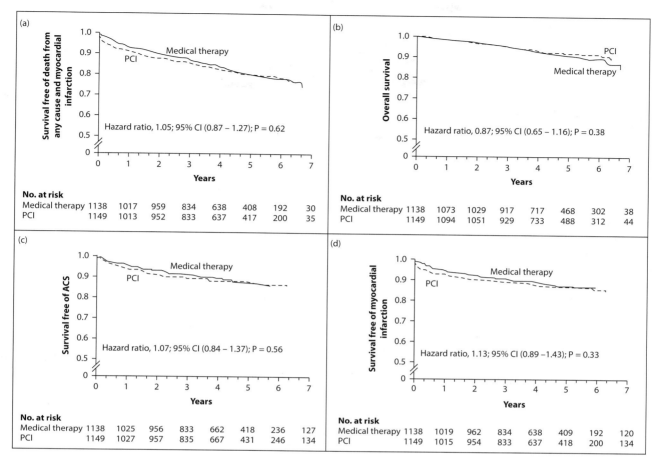

Figure 8.1 Comparison of optimal medical therapy versus percutaneous coronary intervention in the COURAGE trial. Kaplan–Meier curves showing that patients treated with optimal medical therapy (OMT) and percutaneous coronary intervention (PCI) had similar outcomes for the primary composite endpoint of all-cause death and non-fatal myocardial infarction **(panel a)**, all-cause death **(panel b)**, hospitalisation for acute coronary syndromes **(panel c)** and acute myocardial infarction **(panel d)** over 4.6 years follow-up.

COURAGE trial, reduction in ischaemic myocardium was greater with PCI group (2.7% vs. 1.6%, $p < .0001$).[24]

There are multiple meta-analyses comparing OMT with PCI and most reported no mortality benefit, increased non-fatal periprocedural MI and reduced need for urgent revascularisation with PCI compared with OMT.[25,26] However, it has also been shown recently that in patients with stable CAD and functionally significant stenosis, PCI guided by fractional flow reserve (FFR) along with the best available medical therapy, as compared with OMT alone, decreased the need for urgent revascularisation; but in patients without ischaemia, the outcome was favourable with OMT alone.[27]

We can conclude that OMT should be considered as a first-line therapy in patients with one- or two-vessel disease not involving LMS or proximal LAD. While PCI will reduce the stenosis of haemodynamically significant lesions causing angina, it may not prevent future MI, which is often due to the rupture of mild lesions. It is therefore imperative to acknowledge the importance and complimentary value of OMT for patients with CAD undergoing coronary revascularisation.[28]

8.3 PCI versus CABG surgery

8.3.1 Single-vessel disease

Both PCI and CABG are highly effective in providing symptom relief for patients with severe single vessel coronary artery disease. Neither procedure is associated with an unequivocal reduction in mortality. PCI can provide good outcomes in such patients and may be the preferred revascularisation strategy.[29] PCI can also provide long-term improvement in quality of life similar to CABG in this group of patients.[30]

Among patients with single-vessel disease, treatment of isolated LAD coronary artery disease has remained debatable due to the prognostic significance of lesions at this location. Historically, proximal LAD disease has been treated with CABG, as data from multiple trials and two meta-analyses reported a two- to fourfold increase in recurrence of angina and TVR in PCI group. However, there was no significant difference in mortality, MI or stroke.[31,32] Patients undergoing CABG had longer hospital stay, required more blood transfusions and were more likely to have post-procedural arrhythmias.[32] Recent advances in PCI technology (especially use of DES) have made data from old trials somewhat redundant. A small randomised controlled trial (RCT) comparing sirolimus DES against minimally invasive direct coronary artery bypass (MIDCAB) showed that PCI is non-inferior to MIDCAB at 12-month follow-up with respect to MACE and relief in symptoms.[33] Another study compared 1-year outcomes among all patients in New York who underwent CABG surgery or PCI with DES for isolated proximal LAD disease between 2008 and 2010.[34] CABG and DES groups did not significantly differ for mortality or mortality, MI and/or stroke, but repeat revascularisation rates were lower for CABG (7.09% vs. 12.98%, $p = .0007$). After further adjustment with Cox proportional hazards models, there were still no significant differences in 3-year mortality rates (HR 1.14, 95% CI 0.70–1.85) or mortality, MI and/or stroke rates (HR 1.15, 95% CI 0.76–1.73); however, repeat revascularisation rate remained significantly lower for CABG patients (HR 0.54, 95% CI 0.36–0.81). Based on these data, it can be concluded that PCI is a reasonable choice for the treatment of isolated proximal LAD disease.[35]

8.3.2 Multi-vessel disease

There is a large spectrum of heterogeneity in what is classified as 'multi-vessel disease'. A patient with discrete lesions of the right coronary and circumflex arteries who has a normal left ventricle or a patient with diffuse three-vessel disease and a poor ejection fraction can be rightly classified under the term 'multi-vessel disease', yet the prognoses, risks and potential benefits of revascularisation vary considerably. Synergy between percutaneous coronary intervention with Taxus and cardiac surgery (SYNTAX) score has emerged as a good marker of extent and complexity of coronary disease and is recommended to be used in clinical practice.[35] CABG has been the standard of care for stable patients with multi-vessel CAD, over many decades. While recent advances in PCI have made it technically possible to intervene in complex lesions, technical feasibility is not, by itself, a definite indication to intervene.

While there have been numerous randomised trials of PCI versus CABG in multi-vessel disease, most trials (with the exception of the MASS-II and SYNTAX trials) only enrolled around 5%–10% of the total potentially eligible population, raising questions about applicability of results to daily practice.[36] Furthermore, the initial trials (e.g. RITA, EAST [emory angioplasty versus surgery], GABI [German angioplasty vs bypass investigation], CABRI [coronary angioplasty versus bypass revascularisation investigation], ERACI [Argentine randomized study: coronary angioplasty vs. coronary bypass surgery in multivessel disease], ARTS [arterial revascularization therapies], SoS [stent or surgery]) showing superiority of CABG over balloon angioplasty or PCI with BMS for patients with multi-vessel disease have limited applicability in contemporary practice.[37] A large meta-analysis of 23 RCTs comparing PCI with plain old balloon angioplasty (POBA) or bare-metal stent (BMS) ($n = 5019$) versus CABG ($n = 4944$) reported that there was no mortality difference between PCI and CABG but a significantly higher rate of stroke in CABG (1.2% vs. 0.06%, $p = .002$) and TVR in PCI (46% vs. 9.8%, $p < .001$).[38] Hlatky et al. performed a collaborative analysis comparing POBA and BMS with CABG and reported no difference in mortality (PCI 15% vs. CABG 16%, $p = .12$) at a median of follow-up of 5.9 years.[39] Another meta-analysis of the four RCTs comparing BMS versus CABG in multi-vessel disease showed a similar rate of the composite of death, stroke or MI and a significantly higher rate of TVR in PCI treated patients at 5-year follow-up.[40]

With the advent of DES, indirect comparison against CABG was attempted by the addition of DES arms to the original BMS-CABG trials, as in ARTS-II and ERACI-III. ARTS-II study showed higher rates of repeat revascularisation in PCI arm (20.8% vs. 9.0%, $p < .001$) but no difference in survival between PCI with DES and CABG (DES 94.5% vs. CABG 92.6%) at 5-year follow-up.[41] ERACI-III also reported similar events rate in CABG (5.7%) and PCI with DES (9.8%) groups at 3-year follow-up.[42] Comparison between CABG and PCI with DES in various registries has produced mixed results: Asan Medical registry showed no difference in mortality at 5-year follow-up[43]; New York registry reported similar unadjusted survival (PCI 93.7% vs. CABG 93.4%), but different risk-adjusted survival (PCI 94.0% vs. CABG 92.7%, $p = .03$) at 18 months[44]; and ACCF and STS Database Collaboration on the Comparative Effectiveness of Revascularization Strategies (ASCERT) reported no mortality difference at 1 year (PCI 6.55% vs. CABG 6.24%, HR 0.95; 95% CI 0.90–1.0) but lower mortality with CABG at 4 years (PCI 20.8% vs. CABG 16.4%, HR 0.79; 95% CI 0.76–0.82).[45]

SYNTAX is the largest clinical trial of patients with multi-vessel randomised to revascularisation with PCI or CABG and followed-up for 5 years. In 1800 randomised patients, 12.4% of CABG and 17.8% of PCI patients reached the primary composite endpoint ($p = .002$) of death (3.5% vs. 4.4%; $p = .37$), MI (3.3% vs. 4.8%; $p = .11$), stroke (2.2% vs. 0.6%; $p = .003$) or repeat revascularisation (5.9% vs. 13.5%; $p < .001$) at 1 year.[46] At 5 years, the composite endpoint was significantly more in PCI arm (PCI 37.3% vs. CABG 26.9%, $p < .001$), all cause death (PCI 13.9% vs. CABG 11.4%, $p = .10$), MI (PCI 9.7% vs. CABG 3.8%, $p < .001$), stroke (PCI 2.4% vs. CABG 3.7%, $p = .09$) and repeat revascularisation (PCI 25.9% vs. CABG 13.7%, $p < .001$). The sub-group analyses (whilst acknowledging limitations of this approach) of the trial have shown that in the tercile of patients with the lowest SYNTAX scores (0–22) there was no significant difference in mortality (PCI 8.9% vs. CABG 10.1%, $p = .64$), MI (PCI 7.8% vs. CABG 4.2%, $p = .11$), stroke (PCI 1.8% vs. CABG 4.0%, $p = .11$), TVR (PCI 23.0% vs. CABG 16.9%, $p = .056$) and major adverse cardiovascular and cerebrovascular events (MACCE) (PCI 32.1% vs. CABG 28.6%, $p = .43$) between the two groups. However, CABG outperformed PCI in middle (23–32 score) tercile (PCI 36.0% vs. CABG

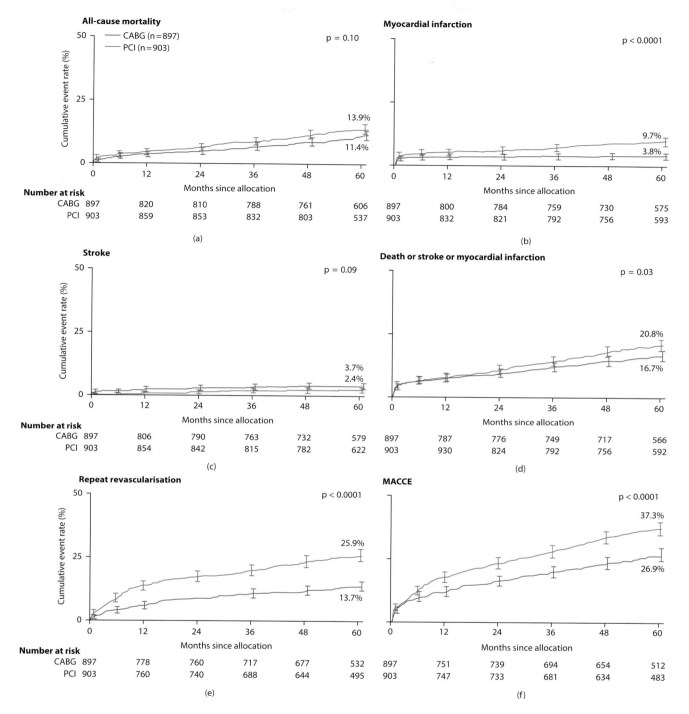

Figure 8.2 **(a–f)** Comparison of percutaneous coronary intervention versus coronary artery bypass grafting in the synergy between percutaneous coronary intervention with TAXUS and cardiac surgery (SYNTAX) trial at 5-year follow-up.

25.8%, p = .008) and high (≥33 score) tercile (PCI 44.0% vs. CABG 26.8%, p < .001) for MACCE at 5 years.[47] In the highest tercile (>33 score), PCI patients had higher all cause death (HR 1.84, 95% CI 1.19–2.83, p = .005) and cardiac death (HR 2.99, 95% CI 1.62–5.53, p = .0002) (Figure 8.2). These outcomes are also consistent with several other studies and registry data.[44,45] SYNTAX trial, however, used first generation DES, which have now been superseded by newer generation DES and it is postulated that comparison may be different between CABG and newer generation DES.

Randomised Comparison of Coronary Artery Bypass Surgery and Everolimus-Eluting Stent Implantation in the Treatment of Patients with Multivessel Coronary Artery Disease (BEST) is a recently reported prospective, randomised and non-inferiority trial, comparing PCI with everolimus-eluting stents versus CABG. After the enrolment of 880 patients (PCI = 438; CABG = 442), the study was terminated early owing to slow enrolment. At 2 years, the primary endpoint had occurred in 11.0% of the patients in the PCI group and in 7.9% of those in the CABG group (p = .32 for non-inferiority). At longer-term follow-up (median, 4.6 years), the primary endpoint had occurred in 15.3% of the patients in the PCI group and in 10.6% of those in the CABG group (HR 1.47, 95% CI 1.01–2.13, p = .04). No significant differences were seen between the two groups in the occurrence of a composite safety endpoint of death, myocardial infarction or stroke. However, the rates of repeat revascularisation and MI were significantly higher after PCI than after CABG.[48] A recent observational study of 34,819 eligible patients elected propensity-based 9223 patients who received PCI with everolimus-eluting stents and 9223 who underwent CABG. At a mean follow-up of 2.9 years, PCI with everolimus-eluting stents, as compared with CABG, was associated with a similar risk of death (3.1% vs. 2.9% per year; HR 1.04, 95% CI 0.93–1.17, p = .50), higher risks of myocardial infarction (1.9% vs. 1.1% per year; HR 1.51, 95% CI 1.29–1.77, p < .001), repeat revascularisation (7.2% vs. 3.1% per year; HR 2.35, 95% CI 2.14–2.58, p < .001) and a lower risk of stroke (0.7% vs. 1.0% per year; HR 0.62, 95% CI 0.50–0.76, p < .001). The higher risk of MI with PCI than with CABG was not significant among patients with complete revascularisation but was significant among those with incomplete revascularisation (p = .02 for interaction).[49]

Taking together the currently available evidence, we would recommend following the strategy supported by SYNTAX data, that is to prefer CABG in patients with SYNTAX scores >22, whereas PCI as well as CABG can be considered for those with SYNTAX score 22 or less. However, it is imperative to highlight that many other factors, including patient preference, comorbidities, local expertise and resources and expected completeness of revascularisation, etc., will also play a role in decision making.

8.3.3 Unprotected LMS disease

Cohen and Gorlin published a case series of CABG in unprotected LMS in 1975 showing a long-term mortality benefit.[50] Subsequently, several registries and RCTs confirmed the survival benefit of CABG over medical treatment in moderate to high-risk groups.[21,51] PCI has remained a class III indication (i.e. the procedure is generally not effective and may even be harmful) for this indication in international guidelines,[52,53] largely due to historical data comparing POBA or BMS with CABG.

Several RCTs have compared PCI with DES against CABG for the treatment of LMS stenosis (Table 8.1). The Study of Unprotected Left Main Stenting Versus Bypass Surgery (LEMANS) trial was the first randomised trial of PCI (n = 52) versus CABG (n = 53). The primary outcome of MACE at 1 year was similar in the two groups, despite higher perioperative complications in CABG group and higher TVR in PCI group.[54] This trial has now 10-year

follow-up data available showing that mortality (21.6% vs. 30.2%, p = .41), MI (8.7% vs. 10.4%; p = .62), stroke (4.3% vs. 6.3%, p = .68) and repeat revascularisation rates (26.1% vs. 31.3%; p = .64) were similar between PCI and CABG.[55] However, the results of this trial may not be applicable to contemporary practice as only 72% of the CABG group received a LIMA graft and only 35% of PCI group received DES. Another prospective, multi-centre RCT (n = 101) attempted to address these limitations by assigning 201 patients with unprotected LMS disease to undergo PCI with sirolimus-eluting stenting (n = 100) or CABG using predominantly arterial grafts. The combined rates for death or MI were comparable (CABG 7.9% vs. PCI, 5.0%; non-inferiority p < .001). Freedom from angina was similar in both groups, whereas repeat vascularisation was higher in PCI arm and perioperative complications including stroke were higher in CABG arm.[56] In Premier of Randomised Comparison of Bypass Surgery versus Angioplasty Using Sirolimus-Eluting Stent in Patients with Left Main Coronary Artery Disease (PRECOMBAT) trial, 600 patients with unprotected LMS stenosis were randomised to undergo CABG (n = 300 patients) or PCI with sirolimus-eluting stents (n = 300). At 2-year follow-up, PCI was non-inferior to CABG for MACCE (12.2% vs. 8.1%, HR with PCI 1.50, 95% CI 0.90–2.52, p = .12). However, ischaemia- driven TVR was higher in PCI group (9.0% vs. 4.2%; HR 2.18, 95% CI 1.10–4.32, p = .02).[57] At 5 years, MACCE outcomes were still comparable in PCI or CABG-treated patients (17.5% vs. 14.3%, p = .26). The two groups did not differ significantly in terms of death from any cause, myocardial infarction or stroke as well as their composite (8.4% vs. 9.6%, p = .66). Ischaemia-driven target vessel revascularisation remained more frequent in the PCI group than in the CABG group (11.4% and 5.5%, p = .012).[58] In the LMS subgroup of the SYNTAX trial, there was no difference in MACCE between the treatment groups (CABG 31% vs. PCI 37%, p = .12) at 5 years.[47] Analysing MACCE on the basis of SYNTAX score terciles indicated that both PCI and CABG may provide optimal revascularisation in lower (CABG 32% vs. PCI 30%, p = .74) and middle (CABG 32% vs. PCI 33%, p = .88) terciles, but for high score tercile CABG is clearly superior (CABG 30% vs. PCI 47%, p = .003).[47] Two recent large clinical trials, NOBLE (Coronary Artery Bypass Grafting Vs Drug Eluting Stent Percutaneous Coronary Angioplasty in the Treatment of Unprotected Left Main Stenosis) and EXCEL (Evaluation of Xience Versus Coronary Artery Bypass Surgery for Effectiveness of Left Main Revascularisation), have compared PCI with newer generation DES versus CABG.[59,60] In NOBLE (n = 1201), there was no difference in mortality (12% vs. 9%, P = 0.77) and stroke (5% vs. 2%, P = 0.073) but higher rates of non-procedural MI (7% vs. 2%, P = 0.004) and revascularisation (16% vs. 10%, P = 0.032) in PCI group.[59] In EXCEL (n = 1905), there was no difference in mortality (PCI: 8.2% vs. CABG: 5.9%, P = 0.11), cardiac death (PCI: 4.4% vs CABG: 3.7%, P = 0.48), stroke and MI at 3-years; however, ischemia-driven revascularisation was higher in PCI arm (12.6% vs. 7.5%, P < 0.001).[60]

Table 8.1 Clinical trials comparing PCI with DES and CABG for left main stem disease

Trial	n	Mean Syntax score	Follow-up	Mortality	MI	Stroke	Repeat Revas	MACE/MACCE
				PCI vs. CABG outcomes (%)				
LEMANS	105	25	1 year	1.9 vs. 7.5, p = 0.37	2 vs. 6, p = ns	0 vs. 4, p = NS	30 vs. 10, p = 0.01	28.8 vs. 24.5, p = 0.29
Boudriot et al.	201	24	1 year	2.0 vs. 5.0, p = ns	3.0 vs. 3.0, p = ns	-	14 vs. 6, pn = 0.35	19.0 vs. 13.9, p = 0.13
PRECOMBAT	600	25	5 years	5.7 vs. 7.9, p = 0.32	2 vs. 1.7, p = .76	0.7 vs. 0.7, p = .99	11.4 vs. 5.5, p = 0.012	16.8 vs. 13.7, p = 0.24
SYNTAX Left Main	701	30	5 years	12.8 vs. 14.6, p = 0.53	8.2 vs. 4.8, p = 0.10	1.5 vs. 5.3, p = .03	26.7 vs. 15.5, p < 0.01	36.9 vs. 31, p = 0.12
NOBLE	1201	22	5 year	12.0 vs. 9.0, p = 0.77	7.0 vs. 2.0, p = 0.004	5.0 vs. 2.0, p = 0.07	16 vs. 10, p = 0.03	29 vs. 19, p = 0.007
EXCEL	1905	21	3 year	8.2 vs. 5.9, p = 0.11	8.0 vs. 8.3, p = 0.64	2.3 vs. 2.9, p = 0.37	12.9 vs. 7.6, P < 0.001	14.7 vs. 15.4, p = 0.98

PCI = Percutaneous coronary intervention, CABG = Coronary artery bypass graft, MI = Myocardial infarction, MACE = Major adverse cardiac events, MACCE = Major adverse cardiac and cerebrovascular events, ns = non-significant

A meta-analysis of four trials (LEMANS, PRECOMBAT, Boudriot et al. and SYNTAX LMS) including 1611 patients has shown that PCI, as compared with CABG, was associated with a significant reduction in risk of stroke, an increased risk of repeat revascularisation, a similar risk of mortality or MI, resulting in a higher risk of MACE but a similar risk of MACCE.[61] Similarly a recent meta-analysis of five trials (excluding LEMANS) has shown similar results.[62] The trails included in this meta-analysis had differences in inclusion/exclusion criteria, complexity of coronary disease (LMS bifurcation disease, Syntax score, etc.), technical aspect of the procedure (type of stent, use of intravascular ultrasound, use of arterial grafts), definition of clinical endpoints, and duration of follow-up. Despite these differences, it is reassuring to see that both PCI and CABG provided effective treatment of unprotected LMS disease with no difference in survival. There are trends towards less stroke in PCI treated patients and less MI in CABG treated patients. The main advantage seen with CABG was reduction in repeat revascularisation. This difference persisted even with the use of DES. However, one may argue that without impact on survival, need for revascularisation is not a hard endpoint and many patients would accept it to avoid the need for CABG. Nevertheless, it is also important to consider that patients with LMS may have varying degree of anatomical complexities leading to different outcomes. PCI of non-distal LMS has favourable clinical and angiographic outcomes, whereas PCI of complex LMS bifurcation or trifurcation may be associated with poorer outcomes.[63-66] There are reports suggesting that simple bifurcation lesions treatable with a one-stent approach may have better results compared with 'complex' bifurcation lesions treated with a two-stent approach. There are limited data on long-term outcomes for patients with LMS bifurcation disease treated with CABG or PCI with DES. However, a study compared the long-term treatment effects of PCI with DES (n = 556) and CABG (n = 309) in LMS bifurcation disease. After adjusting for covariates, the cumulative rates of death (HR 0.95, 95% CI 0.62–1.45) or composite of death, MI and stroke (HR 0.97, 95% CI 0.64–1.48) were not significantly different between the two groups over a 5-year follow-up period. However, repeat revascularisation remained higher in the PCI group (HR 4.42, 95% CI 2.39–8.18). The long-term outcomes were comparable between simple stenting and complex stenting groups except for TVR (HR 1.94, 95% CI 1.22–3.10).[67]

Based on these recent data, PCI may be considered for patients with coronary anatomy that is associated with a low risk of procedural complication and/or clinical conditions that predict an increased risk of adverse surgical outcomes. We recommend that patients with LMS disease and SYNTAX scores between 0 and 32 can be treated with PCI using DES when technically feasible, whereas in patients with SYNTAX scores ≥ 33, CABG surgery should remain the standard treatment. We also believe that future iterations of guidelines should also update PCI for LMS to a class I (level of evidence A), for patients with Syntax score ≤ 32.

8.4 PCI versus CABG for patients with diabetes mellitus

Diabetes is a risk factor for both revascularisation strategies.[68] Although some studies have reported no difference between PCI and CABG outcomes in patients with diabetes, data from dedicated trials reported clear advantage of CABG over PCI, as discussed below.

In the CARDia (Coronary Artery Revascularisation in Diabetes) trial comparing PCI and CABG in diabetic patients with multi-vessel disease, repeat revascularisation was more frequently in the PCI group (9.9% vs. 2.0%, $p < .001$), even in DES PCI group (7.3% vs. 2.0%, $p < .013$); however, there was no significant difference in 1-year mortality (PCI 3.2% vs. CABG 3.3%, $p = .83$) or the 1-year MACCE (PCI 10.2% vs. CABG 11.8%).[69] Bypass angioplasty revascularization investigation 2 diabetes (BARI 2D) trial randomised 2368 patients with both type 2 diabetes and coronary artery disease to undergo either prompt revascularisation with intensive medical therapy or intensive medical therapy alone. At 5 years, survival rate was same for patients with type 2 diabetes and stable ischaemic heart disease irrespective of the treatment with OMT only and CABG surgery or PCI with OMT (88.3% vs. 87.7%; $p = .89$). OMT is therefore an acceptable first-line strategy for diabetic patients with less severe coronary disease. BARI 2D, however, supported the CABG as the preferred revascularisation method for diabetic patients with stable multi-vessel disease.[70] A subgroup analysis of 452 diabetic patients in the SYNTAX trial demonstrated a higher rate of MACCE for diabetic patients treated with PCI, but did not find any mortality difference.[68] At 5-year follow-up, PCI was associated with significantly higher rates for MACCE (PCI 46.5% vs. CABG 29.0%, $p < .001$) and repeat revascularisation (PCI 35.3% vs. CABG 14.6%, $p < .001$). There was no statistical difference in all-cause death (PCI 19.5% vs. CABG 12.9%, $p = .065$), stroke (PCI 3.0% vs. CABG 4.7%, $p = .34$) or MI (PCI 9.0% vs. CABG 5.4%, $p = .20$).[71] Future Revascularisation Evaluation in Patients With Diabetes Mellitus: Optimal Management of Multivessel Disease (FREEDOM) is the largest ($n = 1900$) contemporary trial in patients with diabetes and multi-vessel coronary disease randomised to either PCI with first generation DES (51% PES, 43% SES) or CABG. All patients were prescribed currently recommended medical therapies for the control of diabetes, hypertension and dyslipidaemia, and were followed-up for a median of 3.8 years. The mean age was 63.1 ± 9.1 years, 29% were women, median diabetes duration of 10.2 ± 8.9 years, 32% on insulin therapy and 83% had three-vessel disease. The primary endpoint (composite of death from any cause, non-fatal MI or stroke) occurred more frequently in the PCI group (26.6% vs. 18.7%, $p = .005$)[72] (Figure 8.3). The benefit of CABG was driven by differences in both death from any cause (10.9% vs. 16.3%, $p = .049$) and rates of MI (6.0% vs. 13.9%, $p < .001$).[72] However, the incidence of stroke was higher in the CABG group (PCI 2.4% vs. CABG 5.2%, $p = .03$).[72] Based on these data, CABG should be the revascularisation option of choice for patients with

Primary outcome

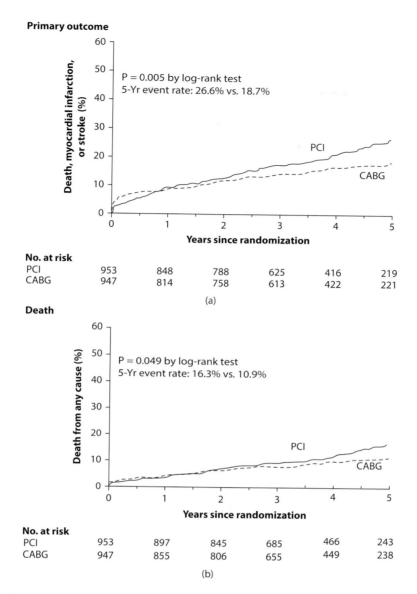

P = 0.005 by log-rank test
5-Yr event rate: 26.6% vs. 18.7%

No. at risk

PCI	953	848	788	625	416	219
CABG	947	814	758	613	422	221

(a)

Death

P = 0.049 by log-rank test
5-Yr event rate: 16.3% vs. 10.9%

No. at risk

PCI	953	897	845	685	466	243
CABG	947	855	806	655	449	238

(b)

Figure 8.3 Comparison of percutaneous coronary intervention versus coronary artery bypass grafting for diabetic patients in the FREEDOM trial. Kaplan–Meier curves showing that diabetic patients treated with coronary artery bypass grafting (CABG) had lower rates of the composite primary outcome of death, myocardial infarction or stroke **(panel a)** and death from any cause **(panel b)**, compared with diabetic patient treated with percutaneous coronary intervention (PCI).

multi-vessel disease and diabetes mellitus. However, in diabetic patients with relatively less complex disease (e.g. lower SYNTAX score), both PCI and CABG can be considered.

8.5 Summary and recommendations

OMT can be the initial strategy for majority of patients with mild symptoms and non-prognostic coronary disease. Single-vessel disease can usually be treated with PCI. Multi-vessel disease can also be treated with PCI if patient is not diabetic and disease is not extensive (SYNTAX score> 22), in which case CABG should be the first choice. It must be remembered that the three modes of therapy are not utilised in a mutually exclusive fashion, but in fact are complementary. In clinical practice, both PCI and

CABG surgery may be used in the same patient at different times, while OMT and aggressive risk factor reduction must be used in all patients with significant coronary artery disease. The selection of revascularisation strategy for patients with complex coronary disease remains challenging and it is strongly recommended to adopt a multidisciplinary heart-team approach for decision making after careful consideration of relevant data.[73] It is best to avoid *ad hoc* PCI in stable patients with complex coronary disease and these cases should be discussed in heart team before a deferred revascularisation (PCI or CABG) procedure. There are various tools available to help heart team in selecting optimal strategy. EuroSCORE and the SYNTAX score have been shown to predict adverse outcomes in studies with both PCI and CABG arms.[47,74] The recently proposed SYNTAX score II, combining anatomical and clinical factors, may provide an evidence-based approach for decision-making process.[75] It is important to acknowledge that all risk models have their limitations; informed patient consent and clinical judgement of heart team remain vital.

References

1. Head SJ et al. Coronary artery bypass grafting: Part 1—The evolution over the first 50 years. *Eur Heart J* 2013; 34: 2862–2872.
2. Gruntzig A. Transluminal dilatation of coronary-artery stenosis. *Lancet* 1978; 1: 263.
3. Bauters C et al. Mechanisms and prevention of restenosis: From experimental models to clinical practice. *Cardiovasc Res* 1996; 31: 835–846.
4. Sigwart U et al. Intravascular stents to prevent occlusion and restenosis after transluminal angioplasty. *N Engl J Med* 1987; 316: 701–706.
5. Serruys PW et al. A comparison of balloon-expandable-stent implantation with balloon angioplasty in patients with coronary artery disease. Benestent study group. *N Engl J Med* 1994; 331: 489–495.
6. Fischman DL et al. A randomized comparison of coronary-stent placement and balloon angioplasty in the treatment of coronary artery disease. Stent restenosis study investigators. *N Engl J Med* 1994; 331: 496–501.
7. Chen MS et al. Bare metal stent restenosis is not a benign clinical entity. *Am Heart J* 2006; 151: 1260–1264.
8. Morice MC et al. A randomized comparison of a sirolimus-eluting stent with a standard stent for coronary revascularization. *N Engl J Med* 2002; 346: 1773–1780.
9. Stone GW et al. A polymer-based, paclitaxel-eluting stent in patients with coronary artery disease. *N Engl J Med* 2004; 350: 221–231.
10. McFadden EP et al. Late thrombosis in drug-eluting coronary stents after discontinuation of antiplatelet therapy. *Lancet* 2004; 364: 1519–1521.
11. Daemen J et al. Early and late coronary stent thrombosis of sirolimus-eluting and paclitaxel-eluting stents in routine clinical practice: Data from a large two-institutional cohort study. *Lancet* 2007; 369: 667–678.
12. Kedhi E et al. Stent thrombosis: Insights on outcomes, predictors and impact of dual antiplatelet therapy interruption from the SPIRIT II, SPIRIT III, SPIRIT IV and COMPARE trials. *EuroIntervention* 2012; 8: 599–606.
13. Stefanini GG et al. Biodegradable polymer drug-eluting stents reduce the risk of stent thrombosis at 4 years in patients undergoing percutaneous coronary intervention: A pooled analysis of individual patient data from the ISAR-TEST 3, ISAR-TEST 4, and LEADERS randomized trials. *Eur Heart J* 2012; 33: 1214–1222.
14. Iqbal J et al. Coronary stents: Historical development, current status and future directions. *Br Med Bull* 2013; 106: 193–211.
15. Stone GW et al. Comparison of an everolimus-eluting stent and a paclitaxel-eluting stent in patients with coronary artery disease: A randomized trial. *JAMA* 2008; 299: 1903–1913.
16. Palmerini T et al. Stent thrombosis with drug-eluting and bare-metal stents: Evidence from a comprehensive network meta-analysis. *Lancet* 2012; 379: 1393–1402.
17. Serruys PW et al. Comparison of zotarolimus-eluting and everolimus-eluting coronary stents. *N Engl J Med* 2010; 363: 136–146.
18. Serruys PW et al. From metallic cages to transient bioresorbable scaffolds: Change in paradigm of coronary revascularization in the upcoming decade? *Eur Heart J* 2012; 33: 16–25b.
19. Hueb WA et al. The Medicine, Angioplasty or Surgery Study (MASS): A prospective, randomized trial of medical therapy, balloon angioplasty or bypass surgery for single proximal left anterior descending artery stenoses. *J Am Coll Cardiol* 1995; 26: 1600–1605.
20. Hueb W et al. Ten-year follow-up survival of the Medicine, Angioplasty, or Surgery Study (MASS II): A randomized controlled clinical trial of 3 therapeutic strategies for multivessel coronary artery disease. *Circulation* 2010; 122: 949–957.
21. Yusuf S et al. Effect of coronary artery bypass graft surgery on survival: Overview of 10-year results from randomised trials by the coronary artery bypass graft surgery trialists collaboration. *Lancet* 1994; 344: 563–570.
22. Jeremias A et al. The impact of revascularization on mortality in patients with nonacute coronary artery disease. *Am J Med* 2009; 122: 152–161.
23. Boden WE et al. Optimal medical therapy with or without PCI for stable coronary disease. *N Engl J Med* 2007; 356: 1503–1516.
24. Shaw LJ et al. Optimal medical therapy with or without percutaneous coronary intervention to reduce ischemic burden: Results from the Clinical Outcomes Utilizing Revascularization and Aggressive Drug Evaluation (COURAGE) trial nuclear substudy. *Circulation* 2008; 117: 1283–1291.
25. Trikalinos TA et al. Percutaneous coronary interventions for non-acute coronary artery disease: A quantitative 20-year synopsis and a network meta-analysis. *Lancet* 2009; 373: 911–918.
26. Stergiopoulos K, and Brown DL. Initial coronary stent implantation with medical therapy vs medical therapy alone for stable coronary artery disease: Meta-analysis of randomized controlled trials. *Arch Intern Med* 2012; 172: 312–319.
27. De Bruyne B et al. Fractional flow reserve-guided PCI versus medical therapy in stable coronary disease. *N Engl J Med* 2012; 367: 991–1001.
28. Iqbal J et al. Optimal medical therapy improves clinical outcomes in patients undergoing revascularization with percutaneous coronary intervention or coronary artery bypass grafting: Insights from the synergy between percutaneous coronary intervention with TAXUS and cardiac surgery (SYNTAX) trial at the 5-year follow-up. *Circulation* 2015; 131: 1269–1277.
29. Wijns W et al. Guidelines on myocardial revascularization. *Eur Heart J* 2010; 31: 2501–2555.
30. Brorsson B et al. Quality of life of chronic stable angina patients 4 years after coronary angioplasty or coronary artery bypass surgery. *J Intern Med* 2001; 249: 47–57.
31. Aziz O et al. Meta-analysis of minimally invasive internal thoracic artery bypass versus percutaneous

revascularisation for isolated lesions of the left anterior descending artery. *BMJ* 2007; 334: 617.

32. Kapoor JR et al. Isolated disease of the proximal left anterior descending artery comparing the effectiveness of percutaneous coronary interventions and coronary artery bypass surgery. *JACC Cardiovasc Interv* 2008; 1: 483–491.

33. Thiele H et al. Randomized comparison of minimally invasive direct coronary artery bypass surgery versus sirolimus-eluting stenting in isolated proximal left anterior descending coronary artery stenosis. *J Am Coll Cardiol* 2009; 53: 2324–2331.

34. Hannan EL et al. Coronary artery bypass graft surgery versus drug-eluting stents for patients with isolated proximal left anterior descending disease. *J Am Coll Cardiol* 2014; 64: 2717–2726.

35. Windecker S et al. 2014 ESC/EACTS Guidelines on myocardial revascularization: The task force on myocardial revascularization of the European Society of Cardiology (ESC) and the European Association for Cardio-Thoracic Surgery (EACTS) developed with the special contribution of the European Association of Percutaneous Cardiovascular Interventions (EAPCI). *Eur Heart J* 2014; 35: 2541–2619.

36. Taggart DP, and Thomas B. Ferguson lecture. Coronary artery bypass grafting is still the best treatment for multivessel and left main disease, but patients need to know. *Ann Thorac Surg* 2006; 82: 1966–1975.

37. Hoffman SN et al. A meta-analysis of randomized controlled trials comparing coronary artery bypass graft with percutaneous transluminal coronary angioplasty: One- to eight-year outcomes. *J Am Coll Cardiol* 2003; 41: 1293–1304.

38. Bravata DM et al. Systematic review: The comparative effectiveness of percutaneous coronary interventions and coronary artery bypass graft surgery. *Ann Intern Med* 2007; 147: 703–716.

39. Hlatky MA et al. Coronary artery bypass surgery compared with percutaneous coronary interventions for multivessel disease: A collaborative analysis of individual patient data from ten randomised trials. *Lancet* 2009; 373: 1190–1197.

40. Daemen J et al. Long-term safety and efficacy of percutaneous coronary intervention with stenting and coronary artery bypass surgery for multivessel coronary artery disease: A meta-analysis with 5-year patient-level data from the ARTS, ERACI-II, MASS-II, and SoS trials. *Circulation* 2008; 118: 1146–1154.

41. Serruys PW et al. 5-year clinical outcomes of the ARTS II (Arterial Revascularization Therapies Study II) of the sirolimus-eluting stent in the treatment of patients with multivessel de novo coronary artery lesions. *J Am Coll Cardiol* 2010; 55: 1093–1101.

42. Rodriguez AE et al. Late loss of early benefit from drug-eluting stents when compared with bare-metal stents and coronary artery bypass surgery: 3 years follow-up of the ERACI III registry. *Eur Heart J* 2007; 28: 2118–2125.

43. Park DW et al. Long-term comparison of drug-eluting stents and coronary artery bypass grafting for multivessel coronary revascularization: 5-year outcomes from the Asan medical center-multivessel revascularization registry. *J Am Coll Cardiol* 2011; 57: 128–137.

44. Hannan EL et al. Drug-eluting stents vs. coronary-artery bypass grafting in multivessel coronary disease. *N Engl J Med* 2008; 358: 331–341.

45. Weintraub WS et al. Comparative effectiveness of revascularization strategies. *N Engl J Med* 2012; 366: 1467–1476.

46. Serruys PW et al. Percutaneous coronary intervention versus coronary-artery bypass grafting for severe coronary artery disease. *N Engl J Med* 2009; 360: 961–972.

47. Mohr FW et al. Coronary artery bypass graft surgery versus percutaneous coronary intervention in patients with three-vessel disease and left main coronary disease: 5-year follow-up of the randomised, clinical SYNTAX trial. *Lancet* 2013; 381: 629–638.

48. Park SJ et al. Trial of everolimus-eluting stents or bypass surgery for coronary disease. *N Engl J Med* 2015; 372: 1204–1212.

49. Bangalore S et al. Everolimus-eluting stents or bypass surgery for multivessel coronary disease. *N Engl J Med* 2015; 372: 1213–1222.

50. Cohen MV, and Gorlin R. Main left coronary artery disease. Clinical experience from 1964-1974. *Circulation* 1975; 52: 275–285.

51. Caracciolo EA et al. Comparison of surgical and medical group survival in patients with left main equivalent coronary artery disease. Long-term CASS experience. *Circulation* 1995; 91: 2335–2344.

52. Silber S et al. Guidelines for percutaneous coronary interventions. The task force for percutaneous coronary interventions of the European society of cardiology. *Eur Heart J* 2005; 26: 804–847.

53. Smith SC, Jr et al. ACC/AHA/SCAI 2005 guideline update for percutaneous coronary intervention summary article: A report of the American College of Cardiology/American Heart Association Task Force on Practice Guidelines (ACC/AHA/SCAI writing committee to update the 2001 guidelines for percutaneous coronary intervention). *Circulation* 2006; 113: 156–175.

54. Buszman PE et al. Acute and late outcomes of unprotected left main stenting in comparison with surgical revascularization. *J Am Coll Cardiol* 2008; 51: 538–545.

55. Buszman PE et al. Left main stenting in comparison with surgical revascularization: 10-year outcomes of the (left main coronary artery stenting) LE MANS trial. *JACC Cardiovasc Interv.* 2016; 9: 318–327.

56. Boudriot E et al. Randomized comparison of percutaneous coronary intervention with sirolimus-eluting stents versus coronary artery bypass grafting in unprotected left main stem stenosis. *J Am Coll Cardiol* 2011; 57: 538–545.

57. Park SJ et al. Randomized trial of stents versus bypass surgery for left main coronary artery disease. *N Engl J Med* 2011; 364: 1718–1727.

58. Ahn JM et al. Randomized trial of stents versus bypass surgery for left main coronary artery disease: 5-year outcomes of the PRECOMBAT study. *J Am Coll Cardiol* 2015; 65: 2198–2206.

59. Makikallio T et al. Percutaneous coronary angioplasty versus coronary artery bypass grafting in treatment of unprotected left main stenosis (NOBLE): A prospective, randomised, open-label, non-inferiority trial. *Lancet* 2016; 388: 2743–2752.

60. Stone GW et al. Everolimus-Eluting Stents or Bypass Surgery for Left Main Coronary Artery Disease. *N Engl J Med* 2016; 375: 2223–2235.

61. Ferrante G et al. Percutaneous coronary intervention versus bypass surgery for left main coronary artery

disease: A meta-analysis of randomised trials. *EuroIntervention* 2011; 7: 738–746, 731.

62. Nerlekar N et al. Percutaneous coronary intervention using drug-eluting stents versus coronary artery bypass grafting for unprotected left main coronary artery stenosis: A meta-analysis of randomized trials. *Circ Cardiovasc Interv* 2016; 9.

63. Valgimigli M et al. Short- and long-term clinical outcome after drug-eluting stent implantation for the percutaneous treatment of left main coronary artery disease: Insights from the Rapamycin-Eluting and Taxus Stent Evaluated At Rotterdam Cardiology Hospital registries (RESEARCH and T-SEARCH). *Circulation* 2005; 111: 1383–1389.

64. Chieffo A et al. Favorable long-term outcome after drug-eluting stent implantation in nonbifurcation lesions that involve unprotected left main coronary artery: A multi-center registry. *Circulation* 2007; 116: 158–162.

65. Palmerini T et al. Ostial and midshaft lesions vs. bifurcation lesions in 1111 patients with unprotected left main coronary artery stenosis treated with drug-eluting stents: Results of the survey from the italian society of invasive cardiology. *Eur Heart J* 2009; 30: 2087–2094.

66. Valgimigli M et al. Distal left main coronary disease is a major predictor of outcome in patients undergoing percutaneous intervention in the drug-eluting stent era: An integrated clinical and angiographic analysis based on the Rapamycin-Eluting Stent Evaluated At Rotterdam Cardiology Hospital (RESEARCH) and Taxus-Stent Evaluated At Rotterdam Cardiology Hospital (T-SEARCH) registries. *J Am Coll Cardiol* 2006; 47: 1530–1537.

67. Chang K et al. Long-term outcomes of percutaneous coronary intervention versus coronary artery bypass grafting for unprotected left main coronary bifurcation disease in the drug-eluting stent era. *Heart* 2012; 98: 799–805.

68. Banning AP et al. Diabetic and nondiabetic patients with left main and/or 3-vessel coronary artery disease: Comparison of outcomes with cardiac surgery and paclitaxel-eluting stents. *J Am Coll Cardiol* 2010; 55: 1067–1075.

69. Kapur A et al. Randomized comparison of percutaneous coronary intervention with coronary artery bypass grafting in diabetic patients. 1-year results of the CARDia (coronary artery revascularization in diabetes) trial. *J Am Coll Cardiol* 2010; 55: 432–440.

70. Bari 2D Study Group et al. A randomized trial of therapies for type 2 diabetes and coronary artery disease. *N Engl J Med* 2009; 360: 2503–2515.

71. Kappetein AP et al. Treatment of complex coronary artery disease in patients with diabetes: 5-year results comparing outcomes of bypass surgery and percutaneous coronary intervention in the SYNTAX trial. *Eur J Cardiothorac Surg* 2013.

72. Farkouh ME et al. Strategies for multivessel revascularization in patients with diabetes. *N Engl J Med* 2012.

73. Head SJ et al. The rationale for heart team decision-making for patients with stable complex coronary artery disease. *Eur Heart J* 2013.

74. Rodes-Cabau J et al. Nonrandomized comparison of coronary artery bypass surgery and percutaneous coronary intervention for the treatment of unprotected left main coronary artery disease in octogenarians. *Circulation* 2008; 118: 2374–2381.

75. Farooq V et al. Anatomical and clinical characteristics to guide decision making between coronary artery bypass surgery and percutaneous coronary intervention for individual patients: Development and validation of SYNTAX score II. *Lancet* 2013; 381: 639–650.

Adjunctive pharmacotherapy and coronary intervention

DANIEL M SHIVAPOUR, DEREK P CHEW, A MICHAEL LINCOFF

9.1 Introduction

It is essential for interventionists performing percutaneous coronary interventions (PCI) to have a thorough understanding of periprocedural anti-thrombotic therapies, which mitigate thrombotic as well as bleeding risks related to the procedure. During PCI, patients are at risk for thrombus formation both as a result of the mechanical disruption of coronary plaque and vascular endothelium by the procedure itself, as well as propagation and embolisation of ruptured plaque and thrombosis from the underlying pathology when PCI is performed in the setting of acute coronary syndromes (ACS). The resulting activation of platelets and the coagulation cascade produce a platelet–fibrin clot that can lead to partial or complete obstruction of the vessel; thus, important complications of PCI include intra-procedural and post-procedural thrombotic events, which can lead to death, myocardial infarction (MI), recurrent ischaemia and need for urgent repeat re-vascularisation. Recognition and understanding of these risks have led to adjunctive pharmacologic management with anti-platelet and anticoagulant medications before, during and after PCI. This has become a highly evidence-based discipline guided by decades of rigorous investigation and has resulted in improved survival and reduced morbidity and forms a cornerstone in the pharmacologic management of coronary artery disease (CAD). Whilst several other categories of medications, such as beta blockers, angiotensin converting enzyme (ACE)-inhibitors and 3-hydroxy-3-methylglutaryl (HMG) coenzyme A reductase inhibitors ('statins') also have a robust evidence-supported roles in the long-term treatment of CAD, anti-thrombotic agents are the only acute therapies which have been convincingly shown to reduce ischaemic events associated with PCI. This chapter reviews the science supporting the adjunctive pharmacologic therapy during and after PCI and provides an overview of each of the categories of agents used.

9.2 Anti-platelet therapy

9.2.1 Platelet activation

Anti-platelet agents are amongst the most important adjunctive medications given in the setting of PCI, and a thorough understanding of platelet activation and interaction with vascular endothelium is needed to understand the mechanism of action of these agents. During ACS, when an atherosclerotic plaque erodes or ruptures within a coronary artery, the lipid-rich necrotic core and sub-endothelial matrix are exposed to circulating pro-thrombotic factors. Von Willebrand Factor (vWF) plays a key role in the initiation of thrombosis, as it binds to the sub-endothelial matrix and subsequently attracts platelets through a combination of shear stress forces and binding at the glycoprotein (GP)

Ib receptor. The binding of vWF to the GP Ib receptor is an important step in the platelet activation pathway via the $P2Y_{12}$ adenosine diphosphate (ADP) receptor. As the initial ruptured plaque defect in the coronary endothelium is covered by activated platelets, this promotes further platelet recruitment and activation to the site of injury in a paracrine fashion. This complex process is mediated through platelet-derived factors including ADP and thromboxane A2 (TXA-2). The activation of platelets produces a conformational change in the glycoprotein IIb/IIIa receptors, which are essential to the formation of thrombus through facilitation of platelet cross-linking with fibrinogen.

In addition to the mechanisms described above, procedural aspects inherent to PCI such as catheter and wire manipulation may also cause vascular endothelial injury and platelet activation, resulting in a prothrombotic state even outside of the ACS context described above. Indwelling interventional equipment can be intrinsically thrombogenic, either transiently (as is the case for removable equipment, such as coronary wires and balloons) or permanently (as is the case for stents). Similarly, angioplasty and stent deployment also cause platelet activation and endothelial disruption, further promoting thrombosis. Therefore, in order to rapidly and effectively interrupt both the underlying pathophysiologic (e.g. ACS) as well as PCI procedural aspects contributing to platelet activation, a combination of multiple anti-platelet agents is employed to target different steps in the process.

9.2.2 Aspirin

Aspirin (acetylsalicylic acid or ASA) is a cornerstone of effective anti-platelet therapy. The enzyme cyclo-oxygenase-1 (COX-1) is responsible for the conversion of arachidonic acid into TXA-2 within platelets, a potent platelet aggregator and endothelial vasoconstrictor, which subsequently facilitates the further activation of other platelets. Aspirin exerts its anti-platelet effects by irreversibly inhibiting the COX-1 enzyme, effectively blocking the synthesis of TXA-2. Since platelets do not synthesise new enzymes, the functional defect induced by aspirin therapy persists for the life of the platelet.

The evidence for aspirin comes from several clinical trials and subsequent meta-analyses showing that it lowers ischaemic morbidity and mortality rates by as much as 50% in ACS.[1] Whilst these early trials were completed prior to the advent of PCI, they clearly and consistently demonstrated aspirin is beneficial in patients with established cardiovascular disease. The only randomised trial comparing aspirin versus placebo in the setting of PCI was designed to evaluate the prevention of early restenosis after percutaneous transluminal coronary angioplasty (PTCA). Whilst periprocedural treatment with a combination of aspirin and dipyridamole did not reduce the 6-month rate of restenosis after successful PTCA, it markedly reduced the incidence of MI during or soon after PTCA. Subsequent trials examined aspirin versus aspirin plus dipyridamole and found no added benefit from the addition of dipyridamole, indicating

the periprocedural ischaemic benefits were conferred by the effects of aspirin.

Initial therapy prior to elective PCI in patients not already on aspirin therapy, and for any patients with suspected or confirmed ACS, should include a 325 mg dose of non-enteric-coated chewable ASA to allow for rapid absorption, followed by indefinite low-dose maintenance therapy (81 mg daily) for those patients with confirmed ACS or in whom PCI is performed. Recent evidence from the CURRENT-OASIS 7 trial, which included a large subgroup of 17,263 patients undergoing PCI, has shown there is no benefit to a higher 325 mg daily maintenance dose, and it is associated with higher rates of bleeding complications.[2]

9.2.3 $P2Y_{12}$ receptor blockade

The addition of a second oral anti-platelet agent to aspirin ('dual anti-platelet therapy' or DAPT) marked a significant advance in contemporary pharmacotherapy for PCI. Historically, early anti-thrombotic therapy following coronary stent placement included aspirin, dipyridamole, heparin and warfarin, and resulted in very high rates of bleeding complications as well as persistently high rates of stent thrombosis. In the late 1990s, several landmark trials convincingly demonstrated that combined anti-platelet therapy (aspirin and thienopyridine), as compared with conventional anticoagulant therapy, after PCI reduced the incidence of both thrombotic and bleeding complications.

Several medications are available to inhibit platelet activity at the level of the $P2Y_{12}$ ADP receptor that provides an additive anti-platelet effect to the TXA-2 inhibition by aspirin. There are three oral thienopyridines (clopidogrel, prasugrel and ticlopidine) approved by the United States Food and Drug Administration (FDA) which irreversibly inhibit ADP-mediated platelet activation and aggregation by binding to the platelet $P2Y_{12}$ receptor. Non-thienopyridine agents include ticagrelor and cangrelor, which do not require metabolic activation and lead to a reversible $P2Y_{12}$ receptor inhibition, in contrast to thienopyridines. Ticlopidine was the first approved agent and was used in many of the early historical trials; however, due to its delayed onset of action and unfavourable haematologic adverse events it is no longer used in contemporary treatment. Clopidogrel, considered a 'second-generation' agent, along with the 'third-generation' prasugrel and ticagrelor, is currently used as oral agents. Cangrelor was recently approved and is an intravenous medication which combines desirable properties of both a rapid onset of action with a short duration of effect. After a review of the individual agents, this section will also examine the evidence for pre-treatment with and duration of DAPT therapy in the setting of PCI.

9.2.4 Clopidogrel

Clopidogrel is an irreversible, 'second generation' $P2Y_{12}$ receptor antagonist. As a pro-drug, it requires conversion into its active metabolite by the hepatic cytochrome P450

2C19 isoenzyme. It has a variable time to peak effect of approximately 2–4 hours depending on the loading dose chosen. The foundation for its use in PCI in a non-ST-elevation myocardial infarction and unstable angina (NSTE ACS) patient population was established by the sub-group analysis of the Clopidogrel to Prevent Recurrent Events (CURE) Trial, which demonstrated a 28% relative reduction (9.6% vs. 13.2%, $p < .001$) of composite endpoints including cardiovascular death, non-fatal MI and stroke, at the expense of more major bleeding (3.7% vs. 2.7%, $p = .001$).[3] The subsequent Clopidogrel and Metoprolol in Myocardial Infarction (COMMIT) Trial also demonstrated a highly significant 9% proportional reduction in death, re-infarction or stroke (9.2% vs. 10.1%; $p = .002$) when clopidogrel was added to standard aspirin therapy in a predominantly ST-elevation MI (STEMI) patient population (93% STEMI, 7% NSTE ACS).[4]

Dual anti-platelet therapy with aspirin and a P2Y$_{12}$ inhibitor should be initiated as soon as possible after presentation for all patients with ACS. As clopidogrel may particularly increase bleeding in patients who undergo coronary artery bypass surgery (CABG), guidelines recommend stopping clopidogrel at least 5 days prior to CABG. Concerns regarding CABG-related bleeding have led some clinicians to delay clopidogrel administration until a patient's coronary anatomy is angiographically defined. Unless there is a very high suspicion that the patient will require urgent surgery, we advocate for the early administration of clopidogrel so as to not withhold its anti-ischaemic benefits from the vast majority of patients who will not require urgent surgical re-vascularisation.

The required activation of the pro-drug clopidogrel by the hepatic cytochrome P450 2C19 (CYP2C19) system creates important therapeutic considerations. Genetic polymorphisms of CYP2C19 and some medications, such as omeprazole, have been associated with pharmacokinetic/pharmacodynamic (PK/PD) effects on clopidogrel activation. Observational studies have suggested an association with worse outcomes in patients with slow conversion; however, randomised studies using genetic polymorphisms and platelet function testing to guide more aggressive anti-platelet therapy have thus far failed to show a clinical benefit of treatment modifications based upon such testing. As such, we do not recommend regular use of functional or genetic testing in routine clinical practice. There has only been one randomised controlled trial testing co-administration of clopidogrel and omeprazole, and it did not show an effect of omeprazole on cardiovascular outcomes.[5]

9.2.5 Prasugrel

Prasugrel is a 'third generation' thienopyridine that irreversibly inhibits the P2Y$_{12}$ receptor. Whilst it is also a pro-drug requiring hepatic metabolism to its active metabolite, this conversion requires fewer enzymatic steps and thus occurs with a more rapid and less variable pharmacodynamic profile than with clopidogrel. Its metabolism is not dependent

on the CYP2C19 isoenzyme, and proton pump inhibitors are not known to have any clinically significant PK/PD interaction with prasugrel. No inactive metabolite is formed by this process (by comparison, 85% of clopidogrel is converted to inactive metabolite), resulting in not only more rapid but also more intense peak inhibition from prasugrel compared with clopidogrel. The foundation for prasugrel's use was established by the TRITON-TIMI 38 Trial, which demonstrated a lower rate of composite endpoints, including cardiovascular death, nonfatal MI and nonfatal stroke (9.9% vs. 12.1%, $p < .001$), as well as a lower risk of in-stent thrombosis in patients with acute coronary syndromes (MI or unstable angina) who underwent PCI (1.1% vs. 2.4%, $p < .001$).[6] However, these ischaemic benefits were again at the expense of a higher rate of non-CABG major bleeding including fatal bleeding (2.4% vs. 1.8%, $p = .03$). An important sub-group of patients who had a net negative outcome was those with a prior history of stroke or transient ischaemia attack (TIA), and prasugrel use in such patients is not recommended. Additional populations in which special caution is advised include patients over 75 years of age and patients weighing <60 kg as increased bleeding complications were noted in these groups. In an important distinction from the CURE trial, NSTE ACS patients in TRITON-TIMI 38 only received the prasugrel loading dose after their coronary anatomy was angiographically defined and percutaneous re-vascularisation planned, and in most cases prasugrel should be held for 7 days prior to CABG due to the higher bleeding risk.

9.2.6 Ticagrelor

Ticagrelor is a 'third generation' reversible P2Y$_{12}$ antagonist that is an active drug and does not require hepatic conversion to an active metabolite (unlike the thienopyridines). It exhibits the most rapid onset, greatest inhibition and least individual variability of the oral P2Y$_{12}$ agents. The foundation of its use was established by the PLATO trial in which ticagrelor demonstrated a lower rate of composite cardiovascular events (death, MI and stroke; 9.8% vs. 11.7%, $p < .001$) with fewer cases of in-stent thrombosis and without a significantly increased risk of major bleeding compared with clopidogrel.[7] There was, however, a higher incidence of non-CABG major bleeding including intra-cranial haemorrhage in the ticagrelor group (4.5% vs. 3.8%, $p = .03$). It is important to recognise several key differences from the PLATO trial design and results when compared with the TRITON-TIMI 38 trial, which established prasugrel use. First, in PLATO ticagrelor was administered 'upstream' at the time of randomisation and prior to coronary angiography, which more closely fits contemporary patterns of ACS management. In addition, there was a significant benefit from ticagrelor not only amongst those patients who subsequently received re-vascularisation with PCI, but also in those who were managed medically ('conservative management') as well.

The anti-platelet effects of ticagrelor attenuate more quickly than the thienopyridines because of its reversible pharmacokinetics. However, because platelet function is recovering a higher level of inhibition, studies have found comparable residual platelet inhibition at 72 hours following the last dose of either clopidogrel or ticagrelor.[8] Whilst labelling still recommends holding ticagrelor for 5 days prior to CABG, experienced surgical centres can often operate earlier with acceptable bleeding outcomes.

In addition to its anti-platelet effects at the $P2Y_{12}$ receptor outlined above, recent studies have suggested possible 'pleiotropic' effects of ticagrelor due to its biological effects on adenosine.[9] Patients with ACS were found to have significantly higher adenosine plasma concentrations 6 hours after ticagrelor loading compared with clopidogrel loading, and ticagrelor-treated patients (but not clopidogrel-treated patients) demonstrate reduced in vitro uptake of exogenous adenosine by erythrocytes. Whilst these early findings are still only hypothesis generating, a number of reported clinical effects of ticagrelor (e.g. improved endothelial function) could be compatible with an adenosine-mediated effect and this warrants further dedicated investigation.

Also in contrast to the other $P2Y_{12}$ agents discussed above, the use of ticagrelor is explicitly contraindicated in patients with severe hepatic dysfunction and another agent should be considered. Similar to clopidogrel and prasugrel, the use of ticagrelor in moderate liver dysfunction has not been well studied. Ticagrelor may infrequently interact with other agents affecting CYP3A4 metabolism. Specifically, concomitant use of ticagrelor should be avoided with strong CYP3A4 inducers (e.g. rifampin, carbamazepine, dexamethasone, phenobarbital, and phenytoin) or strong CYP3A4 inhibitors (e.g. ketoconazole, ritonavir, nefazodone).

9.2.7 Cangrelor

Cangrelor is an intravenous (non-thienopyridine) adenosine triphosphate analogue, which reversibly inhibits the $P2Y_{12}$ ADP receptor. It was approved for use by the FDA in June 2015 as an adjunct to PCI in patients who have not been treated with a $P2Y_{12}$ agent and who are not being given a glycoprotein IIb/IIIa receptor inhibitor (GPI). Major advantages of cangrelor when compared with other anti-platelet agents are its rapid onset of action and rapid return of platelet function after its discontinuation. Two trials (CHAMPION PLATFORM and CHAMPION PCI) evaluated its use in patients with ACS or stable angina requiring PCI and both failed to show clinical superiority compared with clopidogrel alone for a composite endpoint of death, MI or ischaemia-driven re-vascularisation.[10,11] A third trial (CHAMPION PHOENIX) studied patients undergoing urgent or elective PCI and found a composite primary efficacy endpoint (death, MI, ischaemia-driven re-vascularisation or stent thrombosis) occurred less often in the cangrelor group, without significant difference in the rate of severe or life-threatening bleeding at 48 hours.[12] The most notable difference in design of the CHAMPION PHOENIX trial compared with the earlier cangrelor trials was that it used a more sophisticated and detailed definition

for PCI-related MI. In a pooled analysis of patient-level data from the three CHAMPION trials (comprised of 12% STEMI, 57% NSTE ACS, 31% stable disease), cangrelor lowered the rate of the primary composite efficacy end point of death, MI, ischaemia-driven re-vascularisation or stent thrombosis at 48 hours compared with control (clopidogrel or placebo) (3.8% vs. 4.7%; odds ratio [OR] 0.81; 95% confidence interval [CI] 0.71–0.91).[13] Mild, but not major, bleeding was increased with cangrelor (16.8% vs. 13.0%).

9.3 Pre-treatment with dual anti-platelet therapy

The optimal timing and dose of $P2Y_{12}$ blockade for PCI have been the subject of considerable investigation. Multiple studies have compared 'pre-treatment' or 'upstream' treatment with DAPT at various intervals prior to PCI versus administration at the time of PCI. Optimal clopidogrel dosing was examined in a pre-specified subgroup analyses from the CURRENT-OASIS 7 trial, which showed that a 600 mg loading dose demonstrated a nominally significant reduction ($p = .03$ for interaction) for the primary outcome of death, MI or stroke, as well as stent thrombosis, within 30 days compared with the 300 mg loading dose for the 17,263 patients who underwent PCI, whereas no benefit of the higher dose was observed in the 7823 patients who did not undergo PCI.[2]

With respect to the timing of clopidogrel pre-treatment before PCI, a 2012 meta-analysis of patients who actually received PCI, which included the CREDO, PCI-CURE and PCI-CLARITY trials and overall combined 37,814 patients showed that clopidogrel pre-treatment was not associated with a reduction of death (absolute risk 1.54% vs. 1.97%; OR 0.80; 95% CI 0.57–1.11; $p = .17$) but was associated with a lower risk of major cardiac events (9.83% vs. 12.35%; OR 0.77; 95% CI 0.66–0.89; $p < .001$) including MI.[14]

As noted earlier, prasugrel was not initially evaluated for upstream use as the TRITON-TIMI 38 trial administered the prasugrel loading dose after coronary anatomy was angiographically defined for patients with NSTE ACS. The subsequent ACCOAST trial (A comparison of prasugrel at the time of percutaneous coronary intervention or as pre-treatment at the time of diagnosis in patients with non-ST-segment elevation myocardial infarction.) in 4033 patients with non-ST elevation ACS did not demonstrate a benefit of pre-treatment with prasugrel for reduction of the rate of major ischaemic events within 30 days, although the time difference between prasugrel administration in the two arms of that trial was only 4.4 hours. Major bleeding was increased in patients who received pre-treatment, primarily amongst those who did not undergo PCI but had nevertheless received the pre-treatment bolus of prasugrel.[15]

Ticagrelor pre-treatment was further studied in the ATLANTIC trial in 1862 patients with suspected STEMI randomised to (in-ambulance) pre-treatment versus dosing in the catheterisation laboratory at the time of PCI. The rate of the primary composite endpoint of death, MI, stroke, urgent coronary re-vascularisation or stent thrombosis was not significantly different between the study groups. However, definite stent thrombosis was significantly reduced in the ticagrelor pre-treatment group at 24 hours, with preservation of the effect at 30 days.[16] This was almost certainly a real effect, as subsequent analyses demonstrated a significant difference in platelet inhibition between the two treatment arms, which persisted until 6 hours post-PCI and lends support for treating as early as possible with ticagrelor in the setting of STEMI. A possible explanation for the difference in findings observed between the clopidogrel pre-treatment trials and the more contemporary trials with prasugrel and ticagrelor is that the clopidogrel trials reflected a larger difference in timing between the two treatment arms with a drug that has a long time to effect; whereas, the prasugrel and ticagrelor pre-treatment trials were more likely negative due to the relatively short differences in timing between the treatment arms with drugs that have considerably faster times to effect than clopidogrel.

Patients presenting with STEMI are an important and unique patient population to consider when applying the pre-treatment data described earlier. Multiple trials have demonstrated that contemporary $P2Y_{12}$ blockers, including both ticagrelor and prasugrel, exhibit an initial delay in the onset of their anti-platelet action in the setting of STEMI compared with baseline pharmacokinetic (PK)/pharmacodynamics (PD) studies obtained in healthy volunteers. Whilst the exact mechanism for this is not known, it is hypothesised that this could be attributed to impaired absorption of the drugs in the setting of STEMI and/or simply reflects the extremely pro-thrombotic milieu present. Concurrent use of analgesic medications (e.g. morphine) in STEMI patients could further contribute by slowing gastric absorption of oral agents. These findings may provide an expanded role for bridging with the rapidly acting intravenous agent cangrelor in STEMI populations, given that its unique PK/PD features make it well suited to cover the initial anti-platelet action gap from prasugrel or ticagrelor in STEMI.

9.4 Duration of dual anti-platelet therapy

The optimal duration of DAPT after PCI is not known and likely depends on integrating multiple patient-specific ischaemic and bleeding risks. The DAPT trial is the largest of the randomised trials that have compared longer with shorter duration DAPT after PCI. It randomly assigned 9961 patients who had been successfully treated with 12 months of aspirin and either clopidogrel or prasugrel to continue receiving the same $P2Y_{12}$ receptor blocker or placebo for an additional 18 months (on the background of all patients continuing low-dose maintenance aspirin). The rates for both co-primary endpoints of stent thrombosis and a composite of all-cause mortality, MI or stroke were significantly lower with prolonged DAPT (0.4% vs. 1.4; HR 0.29, 95% CI 0.17–0.48 for stent thrombosis, and 4.3% vs. 5.9%; HR 0.71, 95% CI 0.59–0.85 for the composite endpoint). The reduction in events with prolonged DAPT was mostly attributable to a lower rate of MI (2.1% vs. 4.1%; HR 0.47, $p < .001$); however, moderate and

severe bleeding rates were significantly increased in patients treated with prolonged DAPT (2.5% vs. 1.6%, $p = .001$).[17]

Of note, the rate of all-cause mortality was slightly higher in the prolonged DAPT group (2.0% vs. 1.5%; HR 1.36, 95% CI 1.00–1.85); however, this was driven by increased non-cardiac deaths (1.0% vs. 0.5, $p = .002$), with no differences in cardiovascular deaths. Additional pre-specified sub-analyses suggested a greater benefit of prolonged DAPT in patients who received PCI for ACS (p-interaction = .03). Furthermore, the rate of MI not related to the stented site was also lower in patients treated with prolonged DAPT (1.8% vs. 2.9%; HR 0.59; $p < .001$), accounting for 55% of the total reduction in MI seen with prolonged DAPT. This suggests there may be a possible benefit from DAPT attributable to the prevention of adverse events from plaque rupture at sites remote from the stented index lesion.

Of note, other smaller randomised trials, including PRODIGY, DES-LATE and ARCTIC-Interruption, did not show a decrease in ischaemic events with prolonged DAPT.[18–20] These and other trials have been studied together in several meta-analyses including up to 10 randomised control trials and representing over 30,000 patients, which have found a significantly lower rate of MI and stent thrombosis with prolonged DAPT at the expense of significantly higher rates of bleeding. The small increase in overall mortality with prolonged DAPT beyond 12 months, as seen in the DAPT trial, was also noted in all but two of the subsequent meta-analyses. The largest meta-analysis on the topic was presented at the European Society of Cardiology in August 2015 and examined patients presenting with or having a history of MI, finding significantly lower rates of a composite endpoint (cardiovascular death, MI or stroke) in patients receiving prolonged DAPT.[21] Cardiovascular death was significantly reduced without an increase noted in non-cardiovascular death or all-cause mortality in the prolonged DAPT group, highlighting the importance of extended anti-platelet therapy in patients with prior MI. Intracranial haemorrhage and fatal bleeding events were rare and not significantly different between the groups; however, similar to prior analyses major bleeding was significantly increased in the prolonged DAPT group.

In a meta-analysis, which included only studies comparing shorter duration (3–6 months) to 12 months of therapy (including the SECURITY, ITALIC, ISAR-SAFE, OPTIMISE, EXCELLENT, RESET and PRODIGY trials), there was no significant difference in the risk of all-cause death (HR 0.89, 95% CI 0.66–1.20) for 6 months of DAPT compared with 12 months or longer.[22] However, each trial was noted to have one or more significant limitations, such as small sample size or enrolment of lower-risk patients, and there was significant heterogeneity amongst the included trials.

In summary, the optimal duration of DAPT must be tailored to the individual patient taking into account specific bleeding and ischaemic risks, as well as cost. Our practice is to continue DAPT for at least 12 months following drug-eluting stent placement, and in patients who have tolerated this, continue either their current agent for up to 30 months, or for patients taking a third-generation $P2Y_{12}$ consider switching to clopidogrel for months 13–30 based on individualised bleeding risk.

9.5 Glycoprotein IIb/IIIa receptor inhibitors

Glycoprotein IIb/IIIa receptor inhibitors (GPI) are intravenous medications that inhibit platelet aggregation and thrombus formation by preventing the binding of fibrinogen or circulating vWF on the platelet surface. The three agents currently approved by the US FDA are abciximab, eptifibatide and tirofiban. Abciximab is a Fab fragment of a humanised murine antibody that exhibits a very strong affinity for the glycoprotein receptor. Whilst it has a short plasma half-life (approximately 30 minutes), abciximab's strong binding results in platelet inhibition, which continues for hours to days after the infusion is stopped. Eptifibatide, a small-molecule cyclic heptapeptide and tirofiban, a synthetic non-peptide antagonist, both reversibly inhibit the IIb/IIIa receptors on the platelet surface with a shorter duration of action (half-life approximately 2 hours with platelet activity normalising approximately 4 hours after discontinuation).

At proper doses, all three GPI agents are very potent inhibitors of platelet aggregation; however, their clinical use has been diminishing as much of their supporting evidence came prior to the contemporary era of routine oral DAPT. Several, large randomised control trials have investigated GPI use in multiple contexts, including ACS and elective PCI. When reviewing this literature, it is important to carefully understand the indications and the patient populations studied in each of these trials, as these factors influence the noted differences in results and the relative benefits and risks may vary significantly based on the context in which the medication is being given. Table 9.1 presents a brief summary of select, landmark GPI trials in the setting of PCI. Multiple trials examining abciximab and eptifibatide with aspirin and heparin in high-risk and NSTE ACS patients undergoing PCI found 30%–50% reductions in short-term ischaemic endpoints at the expense of increased bleeding. Whilst bleeding complications were reduced by adjustments in weight-based dosing of GPI's and concurrent lowering of heparin dosing, minor bleeding and the risk of thrombocytopenia remained elevated. More recent trials reflecting routine use of clopidogrel early in the course of treatment or bivalirudin in PCI did not demonstrate an incremental benefit for ischaemic outcomes with the routine addition of GPI. Therefore, current guidelines for management of patients with ACS call for dual, not triple anti-platelet therapy (ASA and usually oral $P2Y_{12}$ antagonists rather than GPI), with the addition of GPI reserved for selected patients who remain unstable, have a large thrombus burden on angiography, or have very high-risk clinical features.

9.5.1 Anticoagulants

An understanding of the coagulation cascade, along with its interactions with platelets and vascular endothelium, is essential in order to limit the thrombotic and bleeding risks inherent to PCI procedures. Anticoagulant agents specifically target the soluble coagulation cascade consisting of proteins required to form fibrin clots. The effects of thrombin on the activation of platelets, conversion of fibrinogen to fibrin and activation of factor XIII all contribute to fibrin cross-linking and clot stabilisation. Anticoagulants, such as unfractionated heparin, low molecular weight heparins (LMWH), direct thrombin inhibitors, and fondaparinux have a fundamental role in the periprocedural management of patients undergoing PCI.

9.5.2 Unfractionated heparin

Unfractionated heparin (UFH) is a glycosaminoglycan of varying molecular weights that accelerates the action of anti-thrombin (formerly known as anti-thrombin III), the enzyme that inactivates thrombin and factor Xa, thereby preventing conversion of fibrinogen to fibrin. Initial dosing is weight-based, and at traditional dosing of 50–70 units/kg commonly used in PCI it has a dose-dependent half-life of 30–60 minutes. A distinct advantage of UFH is that its anticoagulant effect can be followed (and subsequent dosing titrated to achieve) by routine activated partial thromboplastin times (aPTT) or point-of-care activated clotting times (ACT) in the catheterisation laboratory, with common ACT targets ranging from 250 to 300 seconds for UFH monotherapy or 200 to 250 seconds when used with concurrent GPI (or if being conservative in the setting of increased bleeding risk or other patient-specific factors). Of note, this ideal ACT range has not been re-examined in the era of routine $P2Y_{12}$ receptor blocker use. Additional advantages include its widespread availability, low cost, rapid clearance after the infusion is discontinued, and the ability to reverse its anticoagulant effects with protamine in urgent situations. Potential disadvantages include the higher incidence of heparin-induced thrombocytopenia (HIT) with UFH compared with other heparin preparations, platelet activation, inability to inhibit clot-bound thrombin due to steric hindrance, circulating inhibitors and inconsistent PK/PD due to non-specific binding to multiple other proteins.

Unfractionated heparin can be thought of as a 'legacy drug' – whilst its use in PCI and ACS has been widespread for over 20 years, its supporting evidence base does not meet the standard of nearly every other drug discussed in this chapter. There is no randomised control trial establishing its use in PCI; rather, there are only smaller trials examining the relationships between ACT and efficacy and bleeding. Similarly, there are no randomised placebo-controlled trials establishing UFH use in STEMI. The majority of its evidence and foundation for its use in ACS was highlighted by a meta-analysis of six relatively small randomised controlled trials in NSTE ACS patients that demonstrated a 33% reduction in death or MI amongst unstable angina patients treated with aspirin plus UFH compared with those treated with aspirin alone.[23]

Table 9.1 Select major trials of GP IIb/IIIa inhibitors

Trial name, year	GPI studied	Number of patients	Trial design	Results	Comments
EPIC, 1994	Abciximab	2099	Prospective, double blind, high-risk patients (ACS or 'high-risk anatomy') on ASA and heparin randomised to abciximab vs. placebo.	At 30 days, there was a 30% reduction in the primary composite endpoint.	These benefits were subsequently present out to 6 months and 3 years.
EPILOG, 1997	Abciximab	2792	Prospective, double blind trial in patients undergoing elective or urgent PCI randomised to abciximab with standard-dose, weight-adjusted heparin; low-dose, weight-adjusted heparin; or placebo with standard-dose, weight-adjusted heparin.	At 30 days, the composite event rate was 11.7% in the placebo group, 5.2% in the abciximab/ low-dose heparin group, and 5.4% in the abciximab/ standard-dose heparin group.	These benefits were achieved without a significant increase in major bleeding and were subsequently demonstrated to remain favourable at one year follow-up.
EPISTENT, 1998	Abciximab	2399	Prospective, randomised assignment to stent plus placebo; stent plus abciximab; or balloon angioplasty plus abciximab.	At both 30 days and 6 months, the primary endpoint was lowest in the stent plus abciximab group.	The benefits were present regardless of whether the stent was elective or urgent.
PURSUIT, 1998	Eptifibatide	10,948	Prospective, double-blind, random assignment to eptifibatide vs. placebo for up to 72 hours.	At 30 days, the eptifibatide group had lower rates of the primary composite endpoint (14.2% vs. 15.7%).	The benefit was apparent by 96 hours and persisted through 30 days.
PRISM-PLUS, 1998	Tirofiban	1915	Prospective, double-blind, ACS patients randomised to IV heparin, tirofiban, or IV heparin plus tirofiban prior to PCI.	At 7 days, the composite endpoint was lowest in the patients who received IV heparin plus tirofiban.	At 30 days, the benefit of the IV heparin plus tirofiban combination remained and there was no significant increase in major bleeding.

Abbreviations: ACS, acute coronary syndrome; ASA, aspirin; IV, intravenous; PCI, percutaneous intervention.

9.5.3 Enoxaparin

LMWH are a group of agents derived from UFH that act via anti-thrombin and preferentially inhibit Factor Xa more than thrombin. Three LMWH agents have been approved by the FDA for clinical use: enoxaparin, dalteparin and tinzaparin. Enoxaparin is the most rigorously studied of all the LMWH in the setting of ACS and is the agent typically used in the United States. Enoxaparin exhibits much less binding to plasma proteins and endothelial cells than UFH, giving it a more consistent and predictable anticoagulant effect. When given intravenously, enoxaparin has a time to peak effect of 5–10 minutes, compared with 3–5 hours when administered subcutaneously. Enoxaparin's 5- to 7-hour half-life is dose independent; however, dose adjustment is required in patients with renal insufficiency.

The majority of trials using LMWH in PCI have been in the setting ACS; the evidence base supporting its use during routine elective PCI is much weaker. Multiple early trials demonstrated a reduction in death and MI amongst conservatively managed NSTE ACS patients (not undergoing routine re-vascularisation) treated with enoxaparin compared with UFH; however, in patients undergoing early invasive management LMWH was non-inferior to UFH for ischaemic endpoints but was associated with increased bleeding.[24–27] Select findings from the major clinical trials which provide the foundational evidence supporting LMWH use in PCI are summarised in Table 9.2. Similar to the preceding discussion reviewing the GPI historical trials, it is important to carefully examine the indications, patient populations and co-interventions in each of these trials as they significantly contribute to the noted differences in results and influence the relative benefits and risks of a given treatment strategy in a particular patient. For example, only one of the landmark NSTE ACS trials (SYNERGY) utilised contemporary dual anti-platelet therapy (aspirin plus oral $P2Y_{12}$ or GPI).

A recent high-quality meta-analysis examined multiple clinical trials to compare the relative safety and efficacy of enoxaparin to UFH in PCI.[34] Notably, it included over 30,000 patients and captured a full spectrum of PCI populations (from stable angina patients undergoing elective PCI to primary PCI in STEMI). Enoxaparin was associated with significant reductions in death (relative risk [RR] 0.66; 95% CI 0.57–0.76; $p < .001$), composite endpoint of death and MI (RR 0.68; 95% CI 0.57–0.81; $p < .001$) and major bleeding (RR 0.80; 95% CI 0.60–0.85; $p < .001$). In sub-group analyses, enoxaparin's mortality benefit was primarily driven by patients with STEMI, although non-statistically significant trends towards lower mortality were also seen in both elective PCI and NSTE ACS patient populations. All PCI groups, however, consistently demonstrated statistically significant reductions in bleeding with enoxaparin compared with UFH. Notable limitations of this meta-analysis include that it was not performed with individual patients' data, approximately one-third of the patients included came from studies that were not randomised, and $P2Y_{12}$ usage patterns, such as pre-treatment, are not well detailed. However, we still believe its conclusions are robust and valid.

In contemporary practice with routine dual-anti-platelet therapy and the increasing utilisation of radial artery access for PCI, LMWH use in the United States is still primarily focused on NSTE ACS patients selected for conservative management. Large-scale trials incorporating current management techniques would likely be required to definitively establish the role for LMWH as first-line therapy in primary invasive management. Unlike UFH, enoxaparin is not reversible with protamine, and its anti-coagulant effect is not able to be monitored in the catheterisation laboratory with routine labs (aPTT or ACT). Special dosing consideration is required when using LMWH in very obese patients, the elderly, or those with significant renal insufficiency; whilst we prefer UFH in these patients, if LMWH is used anti-Xa levels should be followed carefully. HIT occurs at lower rates with LMWH than with UFH; however, platelet counts should be still be monitored routinely after treatment.

9.5.4 Bivalirudin

Bivalirudin is a synthetic 20-amino acid direct thrombin inhibitor that exerts anti-thrombotic effects by reversibly binding to both clot-bound and circulating free thrombin. It has a half-life of 25 minutes and a response that is linearly proportional to its dosing, with coagulation parameters returning to baseline approximately 1–2 hours after its discontinuation in patients with normal renal function. Bivalirudin has several intrinsic advantages over UFH and LMWH in the setting of PCI: it does not require a cofactor (such as anti-thrombin), it has no known natural inhibitors (such as platelet factor 4), it has a more predictable bio-availability and does not directly activate platelets. Unlike UFH, bivalirudin does not require periprocedural monitoring with ACT levels after it is administered. Special dosing of bivalirudin infusions is required in patients with renal insufficiency based on the severity of renal impairment, and its use should be avoided in patients with end-stage renal disease. Special caution should also be exercised with its use in patients at extremes of weight and the elderly.

Bivalirudin has been the focus of multiple randomised clinical trials over a 20-year period, comparing it with various anticoagulation regimens (most notably against UFH and against UFH + GPI) in nearly all PCI settings (elective PCI, NSTE ACS and STEMI). Select findings from the major clinical trials which provide the foundational evidence supporting bivalirudin use in PCI are summarised in Table 9.3. In early trials, bivalirudin alone was consistently found to reduce the incidence of major bleeding by approximately 40% compared with UFH + GPI, without a significant increase in composite ischaemic events. Although a higher incidence of acute stent thrombosis was observed in patients with STEMI, that may (e.g. EUROMAX trial) or may not (e.g. MATRIX trial) be able to be reduced by prolonging the bivalirudin infusion after PCI, long-term mortality was similar with or reduced by bivalirudin compared with heparin + GPI. For several years bivalirudin monotherapy had largely replaced the use of UFH + routine GPI in patients undergoing PCI. However, several concurrent advances in contemporary PCI such as radial artery access, newer thinner stent designs with second-generation anti-proliferative drugs, and improved third-generation $P2Y_{12}$ anti-platelet agents have led to the re-evaluation of bivalirudin against UFH-only regimens. In several of these recent trials (including NAPLES-III, MATRIX and HEAT-PPCI), bivalirudin was not found to significantly reduce bleeding, and in one trial in a contemporary STEMI population (HEAT-PPCI) UFH alone reduced composite

Table 9.2 Select major trials of LMWH by indication

Trial name, year	LMWH studied	Number of patients	Trial design	Results	Comments
Conservatively managed NSTE ACS (non-invasive)					
ESSENCE, 1997[24]	Enoxaparin	3,171	Unstable angina or acute NSTEMI patients treated with ASA received enoxaparin vs. UFH therapy for a minimum of 48 hours to a maximum of 8 days.	**Composite:** At 30 days, enoxaparin had a lower rate of composite endpoint events (death, MI, or recurrent angina) (19.8% vs. 23.3% for UFH, p = .016). **Major Bleeding:** There was no difference between the groups in the 30-day incidence of major bleeding complications (6.5% vs. 7.0%). **Repeat Re-vascularisation:** The need for repeat re-vascularisation procedures at 30 days was significantly less in the patients assigned to enoxaparin (27.1% vs. 32.2%, p = .001).	Revascularisation was not intended in this trial. These benefits were maintained at 12 months for both the composite endpoint (32% vs. 36% for UFH, p = .022) and the need for repeat re-vascularisation (36 vs. 41%, p = .002).
TIMI-11B, 1999[25]	Enoxaparin	3,910	Unstable angina or acute NSTEMI patients treated with ASA received enoxaparin vs. UFH therapy for a minimum of 3 days. This trial also included an outpatient phase (to day 43).	**Composite:** At 8 days, enoxaparin had a lower rate of composite endpoint events (death, MI, or urgent revascularisation) (12.4% vs. 14.5% for UFH, p = .048). **Major Bleeding:** There was no difference between the groups in the pre-discharge incidence of major bleeding complications (1.5% vs. 1.0%).	Revascularisation was not intended in this trial. The benefit of enoxaparin was limited to patients with elevated troponin.
Elective PCI					
REDUCE, 1996[28]	Reviparin	612	Single-lesion CAD patients treated with PTCA randomised to fixed-dose LMWH vs. UFH. Patients also received low-dose SQ reviparin or placebo injections for 28 following PCI.	**Composite:** There was no difference between the groups for the composite endpoint of death, MI, need for re-intervention or bypass surgery at 30 days (33.3% vs. 32%; p = .707). **Major Bleeding:** There was no difference between the groups in major bleeding complications observed within the 35 days following PTCA.	There were no differences between the groups in the incidence of angiographic restenosis over 30 weeks; however, a secondary endpoint for the requirement of bailout intervention was reduced in the reviparin group (2.0% vs. 6.9%; p = .003).

(Continued)

Table 9.2 (Continued) Select major trials of LMWH by indication

Trial name, year	LMWH studied	Number of patients	Trial design	Results	Comments
STEEPLE, 2006[29]	Enoxaparin	3,528	Either 0.5 or 0.75 mg/kg enoxaparin vs. UFH (targeted to ACT and stratified by provisional GPI use).	**Composite:** The 0.5 mg/kg enoxaparin dose reduced composite bleeding events by 31% at 48 hours (5.9% vs. 8.5%; $p = .01$), whilst the 0.75 mg/kg dose was no different than UFH. Also, target anticoagulation levels were achieved in significantly more patients in both enoxaparin groups (0.5 mg/kg dose, 79%; 0.75 mg/kg dose, 92%) than patients who received UFH (20%, $p < .001$).	There was no difference in ischaemic outcomes; however, the trial was not powered to provide a definitive comparison of efficacy in the prevention of ischaemic events.
Early-invasive management of NSTE ACS					
A–Z Trial, 2004[30]	Enoxaparin	3,987	Unstable angina or acute NSTEMI randomised to receive either enoxaparin or UFH in combination with ASA and tirofiban.	**Composite:** At 7 days, there was no significant difference in the incidence of composite endpoint events (death, MI, or refractory ischaemia) (8.4% vs. 9.4% for UFH, $p = .048$). **Major Bleeding:** The incidence of major bleeding complications was higher with enoxaparin (0.9% vs. 0.4%, $p = .05$).	74% of patients met NSTEMI criteria, and an early invasive strategy was pursued in 55% of study patients. In a pre-specified subgroup analysis, there was no difference in outcome for the patients treated with an early invasive strategy, whereas there was a significant reduction in the primary endpoint for patients treated with a conservative (non-invasive) strategy.
SYNERGY, 2004[31]	Enoxaparin	10,027	Unstable angina or acute NSTEMI patients planned for an early invasive strategy randomised to receive either enoxaparin or UFH in combination with ASA plus either P2Y$_{12}$ or GPI.	**Composite:** At 30 days, there was no significant difference in the incidence of composite endpoint events (death or nonfatal MI) (14.0% vs. 14.5% for UFH). **Major Bleeding:** The incidence of in-hospital major bleeding complications was higher with enoxaparin (9.1% vs. 7.6%, $p = .008$).	There remained no difference in composite endpoint rates at 6 and 12 months. In NSTE ACS patients with high bleeding risk who are treated with contemporary dual anti-platelet therapy and undergoing an early invasive strategy, UFH may be preferable to enoxaparin due to the increased bleeding risk highlighted by this trial.

(Continued)

Table 9.2 (*Continued*) Select major trials of LMWH by indication

Trial name, year	LMWH studied	Number of patients	Trial design	Results	Comments
STEMI					
ATOLL, 2011[32]	Enoxaparin	910	STEMI patients randomised 1:1 to either 0.5 mg/kg enoxaparin vs. UFH administered pre-hospital (in ambulance).	**Composite:** There was no significant difference in the incidence of composite endpoint (death, complication of MI, procedure failure, or major bleeding) events at 30 days (28% vs. 34%, $p = .06$).	The main secondary endpoint (composite of death, recurrent ACS, or urgent re-vascularisation) was significantly reduced in the enoxaparin treatment arm (7% vs. 11%; $p = .015$).
FINESSE, 2010[33]	Enoxaparin	2,452	STEMI patients randomised to either enoxaparin vs. UFH in primary PCI or facilitated PCI with GPI + half-dose reteplase.	**Composite:** There was significantly less death, MI, urgent re-vascularisation, or refractory ischaemia at 30 days in the enoxaparin treatment arm (5.3% vs. 8%; $p = .0005$) as well as all-cause mortality through 90 days (3.8% vs. 5.6%; $p = .046$).	Non-intracranial major/minor bleeding was not significantly different between the groups, and 33% of patients in the trial were treated with facilitated PCI.

Abbreviations: LMWH, low molecular weight heparins; NSTE ACS, non-ST-elevation acute coronary syndrome; NSTEMI, non-ST-elevation myocardial infarction; UFH, unfractionated heparin; MI, myocardial infarction; ASA, aspirin; GPI, glycoprotein IIb/IIIa receptor inhibitors; CAD, Coronary artery disease; PCI, percutaneous coronary intervention; ACT, activated clotting time; PTCA, percutaneous transluminal coronary angioplasty; SQ, subcutaneous.

Table 9.3 Select major trials of bivalirudin by indication

Trial name, year	Number of patients	Trial design	Results	Comments
Elective PCI				
REPLACE 2, 2003[35]	6,010	Patients undergoing elective PCI (or urgent PCI without MI) randomised to UFH + GPI vs. bivalirudin with provisional GPI.	**Composite**: No difference in the primary composite endpoint (death, MI, urgent repeat re-vascularisation, or in-hospital major bleeding) at 30 days. **Major bleeding**: Bivalirudin significantly reduced in-hospital major bleeding rates (2.4% vs. 4.1%; $p < .001$).	All patients received aspirin and 85% received $P2Y_{12}$. Provisional GPI used in 7.2% of patients in the bivalirudin group.
NAPLES III, 2015[36]	837	Consecutive biomarker negative patients at increased bleeding risk undergoing elective PCI were randomised to UFH vs. bivalirudin alone.	**Composite**: No difference in the primary composite endpoint of in-hospital major bleeding.	Small, single-centre study of patients undergoing elective PCI with 100% femoral access used.
Early-invasive Management of NSTE ACS				
Bivalirudin Angioplasty Study, 1995[37,38]	4,098	Patients with unstable angina or post-infarct angina undergoing PTCA randomised to high-dose UFH alone or bivalirudin.	**Composite**: No significant difference in the composite primary endpoint (in-hospital death, MI, abrupt vessel closure, or rapid clinical deterioration of cardiac origin). However, a subsequently published re-analysis of the trial dataset reported bivalirudin significantly reduced composite primary endpoint events at 7 days ($p = .039$) and 90 days ($p = .012$), with a trend towards reduced events at 180 days. **Major bleeding**: Patients treated with bivalirudin had lower incidence of bleeding (3.8% vs. 9.8%; $p < .001$).	No coronary stenting performed in this trial, limiting its generalisability to contemporary practice. No routine GPI use in this trial.
ACUITY, 2006[39]	13,819	Patients with NSTE ACS randomised to bivalirudin alone vs. bivalirudin + GPI vs. heparin (UFH or LMWH) + GPI.	**Composite**: No differences in the primary composite endpoint (death, MI, unplanned re-vascularisation) at 30 days. **Major bleeding**: Bivalirudin alone reduced major bleeding compared with heparin + GPI or bivalirudin + GPI (3.1% vs. 5.7% vs. 5.3%, respectively; $p < .001$).	The sub-study of 7789 patients that underwent PCI similarly found no differences in the primary ischaemic endpoint, with again less bleeding in the bivalirudin alone treatment arm (driven predominantly by fewer access site and retroperitoneal haemorrhages).

(Continued)

Table 9.3 (Continued) Select major trials of bivalirudin by indication

Trial name, year	Number of patients	Trial design	Results	Comments
ISAR-REACT 3, 2008[40]	4,570	Patients with stable or unstable angina undergoing PCI treated with 600 mg clopidogrel randomised to bivalirudin vs. very high-dose UFH monotherapy.	**Composite**: No significant difference in the composite primary endpoint (death, MI, urgent target vessel re-vascularisation). **Major bleeding**: Bivalirudin reduced major bleeding complications (3.1% vs. 4.6%; $p = .008$) compared with very high-dose UFH.	The UFH dose used in this trial (140 unit/kg) was much higher than is used in contemporary interventional practice (50–70 unit/kg). No routine GPI use in this trial.
ISAR-REACT 4, 2011[41]	1,721	Patients with NSTE ACS randomised to bivalirudin alone vs. UFH + GPI.	**Composite**: No significant difference in the composite primary endpoint (death, MI, urgent target vessel re-vascularisation). **Major bleeding**: Bivalirudin reduced major bleeding complications (2.6% vs. 4.6%; $p = .02$) compared with UFH + GPI.	
MATRIX, 2015[42]	7,213	Patients with NSTE ACS randomised to bivalirudin vs. UFH. Patients in the bivalirudin group were subsequently randomly assigned to receive or not to receive a post-PCI bivalirudin infusion.	**Composite**: No significant difference in the composite primary endpoint (death, MI, or stroke). Post-PCI continuation of bivalirudin infusion did not significantly decrease the rate of urgent target-vessel re-vascularisation, definite stent thrombosis, or net adverse clinical events compared with bivalirudin infusion during the PCI procedure only. **Major bleeding**: No significant difference in the rates of reduced major bleeding complications.	
STEMI				
HORIZONS-AMI, 2008[43]	3,602	Patients with STEMI randomised to UFH + GPI vs. bivalirudin during PCI (with provisional GPI allowed if clinically needed).	**Composite**: No significant difference in the composite primary endpoint (death, MI, urgent target vessel re-vascularisation, or stroke) at 30 days. **Major bleeding**: Bivalirudin alone reduced major bleeding complications (4.9% vs. 8.3%; $p < .001$) compared with UFH + GPI.	Provisional GPI used in 7.2% of patients in the bivalirudin group with large thrombus burden. Bivalirudin reduced cardiovascular death (1.8% vs. 2.9%; $p = .03$) and all-cause mortality (2.1% vs. 3.1%; $p = .047$) at 30 days; however, bivalirudin was associated with an increased risk of acute stent thrombosis within 24 hours of PCI (1.3% vs. 0.4%; $p < .001$).

(Continued)

Table 9.3 (*Continued*) Select major trials of bivalirudin by indication

Trial name, year	Number of patients	Trial design	Results	Comments
EUROMAX, 2013[44]	2,218	Patients with STEMI randomised to UFH + provisional GPI vs. bivalirudin during PCI and continued for at least four hours post-procedure (with provisional GPI allowed if clinically needed).	**Composite:** No significant difference in the composite primary endpoint (death, MI, urgent target vessel re-vascularisation, or stroke) at 30 days. **Major bleeding:** Bivalirudin alone reduced major bleeding complications (2.6% vs. 6.0%; $p < .001$) compared with UFH + GPI.	Reflective of contemporary PCI practice, with all patients receiving DAPT (including 40% with third generation agents prasugrel or ticagrelor) and over 45% of patients with radial artery access. Bivalirudin was again associated with an increased risk of acute stent thrombosis (1.6% vs. 0.5%; $p = .02$) despite prolonged infusion after PCI. There was also a trend towards higher rates of re-infarction at 30 days, although the study was not adequately powered to assess this.
HEAT-PPCI, 2014[45]	1,829	Patients with STEMI randomised to UFH vs. bivalirudin during PCI (with provisional GPI allowed in both arms if clinically needed).	**Composite:** UFH demonstrated significantly lower rates of the composite primary endpoint (death, MI, urgent target vessel re-vascularisation, or stroke) at 28 days (5.7% vs. 8.7%; $p = .01$) compared with bivalirudin. **Major bleeding:** No significant difference in the rates of major bleeding complications.	Reflective of contemporary PCI practice, with over 90% of patients receiving DAPT including third generation agents prasugrel or ticagrelor and over 75% of patients with radial artery access. Rates of "bailout" GPI use were not significantly different between the groups (13% in the bivalirudin group; 15% in the UFH group). Again noted was a greater risk of re-infarction with bivalirudin, driven by increased acute stent thrombosis (3.4% vs. 0.9%; $p = .001$).
BRIGHT, 2015[46]	2,194	Patients with STEMI randomised to UFH vs. UFH + GPI vs. bivalirudin with a post-PCI infusion.	**Composite:** Bivalirudin reduced the rates of the primary composite endpoint (all-cause death, MI, ischaemia-driven target vessel re-vascularisation, stroke, or bleeding) at 30 days vs. UFH and UFH + GPI (8.8% vs. 13.2% vs. 17.0%, respectively; $p < .001$). **Major bleeding:** Bivalirudin reduced major bleeding compared with UFH alone or UFH + GPI (4.1% vs. 7.5% vs. 12.3%, respectively; $p < .001$).	No differences in stent thrombosis were noted within 24 hours, at 30 days, or at 1 year.

Abbreviations: UFH, unfractionated heparin; ASA, aspirin; NSTE ACS, non-ST-elevation acute coronary syndrome; MI, myocardial infarction; GPI, glycoprotein IIb/IIIa receptor inhibitors; PCI, percutaneous coronary intervention; PTCA, percutaneous transluminal coronary angioplasty; LMWH, low molecular weight heparins; DAPT, dual anti-platelet therapy.

ischaemic events compared with bivalirudin. Another such trial (BRIGHT), again in a contemporary STEMI population, however, found ischaemic events and major bleeding reduced by bivalirudin compared with UFH.

A recent high-quality meta-analysis examined 16 bivalirudin trials in nearly 34,000 patients to compare the relative safety and efficacy of bivalirudin with UFH in PCI, stratified according to the use of GPI.[47] In their analyses, ischaemic complications were slightly more frequent amongst patients receiving bivalirudin-based regimens compared with UFH-based regimens (risk ratio 1.09, 95% confidence interval 1.01–1.17), regardless of the clinical indication for PCI or the GPI strategy used. The impact of bivalirudin on bleeding, however, was significantly impacted by the GPI strategy used. There was no significant difference found in bleeding in comparisons of bivalirudin monotherapy versus UFH monotherapy; it is noteworthy that the one large trial comparing bivalirudin to UFH monotherapy that observed increased bleeding with UFH monotherapy used much higher doses (140 unit/kg) of UFH than are conventionally used in contemporary PCI. Therefore, in the contemporary PCI era where GPI are not routinely used, the role of bivalirudin over standard dose (70 unit/kg) UFH monotherapy with third-generation DAPT is less clear.

9.5.5 Fondaparinux

Fondaparinux is a synthetic analogue of the heparin pentasaccharide that causes an anti-thrombin-mediated, selective inhibition of Factor Xa; its effect is exclusively on factor Xa with no action on thrombin. It can be administered subcutaneously with a time to peak effect of 2.5 hours and a half-life of approximately 20 hours in patients with normal renal function, which allows for predictable anticoagulant effects with once daily dosing. The foundation for its use comes from two large randomised clinical trials for the treatment of ACS, which included patients treated with PCI. The OASIS-5 trial, in which approximately 40% of patients underwent PCI, found NSTE ACS patients treated with fondaparinux had non-inferior rates of the composite endpoint (death, MI or refractory ischaemia) at 9 and 30 days; however, the fondaparinux treatment group had significantly lower rates of major bleeding (2.4% vs. 5.1%, $p < .00001$) when compared with enoxaparin, with or without adjunctive GPI. At 6 months fondaparinux produced a significant reduction in all major endpoints; however, in the subset of patients who underwent PCI there was no difference in the primary endpoint at any time point.[48]

In the subsequent OASIS-6 trial, which examined fondaparinux versus UFH in a higher-risk STEMI population, results were largely similar. Adjunctive GPI administration was again allowed, with adjustment of fondaparinux and UFH dosing in these patients. Overall, the fondaparinux treatment arm had significantly lower rates of the primary composite endpoint (9.7% vs. 11.2%; 95% CI 0.77–0.96; $p = .008$) at 9 days, with benefits persisting out to 6 months.[49] Like OASIS-5, however, in the 29%

of patients who underwent primary PCI fondaparinux was not superior to UFH. Of particular importance, in both trials, fondaparinux was associated with increased catheter-related thrombus formation ($p < .001$) as well as higher overall rates of coronary complications (e.g. abrupt vessel closure, no reflow, perforation; $p = .04$) during PCI.

These findings led to the FUTURA (Fondaparinux with UnfracTionated heparin dUring Revascularization in Acute coronary syndromes)/OASIS-8 trial which evaluated the addition of low-dose versus standard dose UFH to fondaparinux during PCI. In the NSTE ACS population studied, there was no difference in the primary composite endpoint (major bleeding, minor bleeding or access site complications) or pre-specified secondary endpoints (composite bleeding at 48 hours, death, MI, or target vessel revascularisation within 30 days) between the low-dose and standard dose groups. Catheter thrombosis incidence was lower than in the prior OASIS trials, however, there was no significant difference between the low- versus standard-UFH dosing populations.[50]

Therefore, in contemporary practice the use of fondaparinux is typically reserved for patients with a high risk of bleeding selected for a conservative management strategy, as it has not been shown to have added benefit over UFH or LMWH in patients undergoing PCI. Because of the unique concerns with catheter thrombosis and fondaparinux, it is not recommended for use as the sole anticoagulant agent during PCI and it is important that patients treated with fondaparinux who go on to have PCI performed do so with the addition of other anti-thrombotic therapy, such as UFH or bivalirudin.

9.6 Concluding remarks

The adjunctive pharmacotherapy is used in coronary intervention a highly evidence-based discipline that is guided by decades of rigorous investigation. Whilst considerable attention has been given to the technological advances in PCI itself, the majority of benefit with regard to improving survival, reducing morbidity and modifying the progression of CAD can be attributed to the significant advances in the concurrent medical therapies used. This chapter has provided a broad overview of each of the categories of anti-thrombotic agents used in the periprocedural period with PCI. A fundamental goal of therapy is to achieve a robust anti-thrombotic effect using a combination of anti-platelet and anti-thrombotic medications whilst at the same time limiting the associated risks of bleeding. To achieve this goal through the choice of a 'patient-tailored' anti-thrombotic regimen, the interventionist needs to combine a careful assessment of thrombotic and bleeding risks with the knowledge of the anti-thrombotic pharmacology. Aspirin remains a cornerstone of therapy, and should be given in combination with a second anti-platelet agent (most commonly $P2Y_{12}$ antagonists rather than GPI), with the addition of GPI reserved for selected circumstances. Whilst there are multiple anti-coagulants with significant supporting evidence, unfractionated heparin has remained a durable choice and has many properties which make its use favourable (e.g. widespread availability, low cost, short duration, easy point-of-care monitoring and rapid reversal with protamine). Several new anti-thrombotic agents are currently under investigation, and the 'holy grail' for new anti-thrombotic therapies remains to achieve a predictable, uniform response that offers improved efficacy without unacceptably increasing haemorrhagic complications. Together with optimisation of modifiable cardiovascular risk factors such as hypertension, dyslipidaemia, smoking status and diabetes mellitus, the importance of a comprehensive evidence-based pharmacologic approach for the management of patients before, during and after PCI for any indication cannot be overemphasised.

References

1. Antithrombotic Trialists C. Collaborative meta-analysis of randomised trials of antiplatelet therapy for prevention of death, myocardial infarction, and stroke in high risk patients. *BMJ* 2002; 324(7329): 71–86.
2. Investigators C-O et al. Dose comparisons of clopidogrel and aspirin in acute coronary syndromes. *N Engl J Med* 2010; 363(10): 930–42.
3. Fox KA et al. Benefits and risks of the combination of clopidogrel and aspirin in patients undergoing surgical revascularization for non-ST-elevation acute coronary syndrome: The Clopidogrel in Unstable angina to prevent Recurrent ischemic Events (CURE) Trial. *Circulation* 2004; 110(10): 1202–8.
4. Chen ZM et al. Addition of clopidogrel to aspirin in 45,852 patients with acute myocardial infarction: Randomised placebo-controlled trial. *Lancet* 2005; 366(9497): 1607–21.
5. Bhatt DL et al. Clopidogrel with or without omeprazole in coronary artery disease. *N Engl J Med* 2010; 363(20): 1909–17.
6. Wiviott SD et al. Prasugrel versus clopidogrel in patients with acute coronary syndromes. *N Engl J Med* 2007; 357(20): 2001–15.
7. Wallentin L et al. Ticagrelor versus clopidogrel in patients with acute coronary syndromes. *N Engl J Med* 2009; 361(11): 1045–57.
8. Gurbel PA et al. Randomized double-blind assessment of the ONSET and OFFSET of the antiplatelet effects of ticagrelor versus clopidogrel in patients with stable coronary artery disease: The ONSET/OFFSET study. *Circulation* 2009; 120(25): 2577–85.
9. Cattaneo M et al. Adenosine-mediated effects of ticagrelor: Evidence and potential clinical relevance. *J Am Coll Cardiol* 2014; 63(23): 2503–9.
10. Bhatt DL et al. Intravenous platelet blockade with cangrelor during PCI. *N Engl J Med* 2009; 361(24): 2330–41.
11. Harrington RA et al. Platelet inhibition with cangrelor in patients undergoing PCI. *N Engl J Med* 2009; 361(24): 2318–29.
12. Bhatt DL et al. Effect of platelet inhibition with cangrelor during PCI on ischemic events. *N Engl J Med* 2013; 368(14): 1303–13.
13. Steg PG et al. Effect of cangrelor on periprocedural outcomes in percutaneous coronary interventions: A pooled analysis of patient-level data. *Lancet* 2013; 382(9909): 1981–92.
14. Bellemain-Appaix A et al. Association of clopidogrel pretreatment with mortality, cardiovascular events, and major bleeding among patients undergoing percutaneous coronary intervention: A systematic review and meta-analysis. *JAMA* 2012; 308(23): 2507–16.
15. Montalescot G et al. Pretreatment with prasugrel in non-ST-segment elevation acute coronary syndromes. *N Engl J Med* 2013; 369(11): 999–1010.
16. Montalescot G et al. Prehospital ticagrelor in ST-segment elevation myocardial infarction. *N Engl J Med* 2014; 371(11): 1016–27.
17. Mauri L et al. Twelve or 30 months of dual antiplatelet therapy after drug-eluting stents. *N Engl J Med* 2014; 371(23): 2155–66.
18. Lee CW et al. Optimal duration of dual antiplatelet therapy after drug-eluting stent implantation: A randomized, controlled trial. *Circulation* 2014; 129(3): 304–12.
19. Collet JP et al. Dual-antiplatelet treatment beyond 1 year after drug-eluting stent implantation (ARCTIC-Interruption): A randomised trial. *Lancet* 2014; 384(9954): 1577–85.
20. Campo G et al. Short- versus long-term duration of dual antiplatelet therapy in patients treated for in-stent restenosis: A PRODIGY trial substudy (Prolonging dual antiplatelet treatment after grading stent-induced intimal hyperplasia). *J Am Coll Cardiol* 2014; 63(6): 506–12.
21. Udell JA et al. Long-term dual antiplatelet therapy for secondary prevention of cardiovascular events in the subgroup of patients with previous myocardial infarction: A collaborative meta-analysis of randomized trials. *Eur Heart J* 2016; 37(4): 390–9.
22. Palmerini T et al. Short- versus long-term dual antiplatelet therapy after drug-eluting stent implantation: An individual patient data pairwise and network meta-analysis. *J Am Coll Cardiol* 2015; 65(11): 1092–102.
23. Oler A et al. Adding heparin to aspirin reduces the incidence of myocardial infarction and death in patients with unstable angina. A meta-analysis. *JAMA* 1996; 276(10): 811–5.
24. Cohen M et al. A comparison of low-molecular-weight heparin with unfractionated heparin for unstable coronary artery disease. Efficacy and safety of subcutaneous enoxaparin in non-Q-wave coronary events study group. *N Engl J Med* 1997; 337(7): 447–52.
25. Antman EM et al. Enoxaparin prevents death and cardiac ischemic events in unstable angina/non-Q-wave myocardial infarction. Results of the thrombolysis in myocardial infarction (TIMI) 11B trial. *Circulation* 1999; 100(15): 1593–601.
26. Ferguson JJ et al. Enoxaparin vs unfractionated heparin in high-risk patients with non-ST-segment elevation acute coronary syndromes managed with an intended early invasive strategy: Primary results of the SYNERGY randomized trial. *JAMA* 2004; 292(1): 45–54.
27. de Lemos JA et al. Enoxaparin versus unfractionated heparin in patients treated with tirofiban, aspirin and an early conservative initial management strategy: Results from the A phase of the A-to-Z trial. *Eur Heart J* 2004; 25(19): 1688–94.

28. Karsch KR et al. Low molecular weight heparin (reviparin) in percutaneous transluminal coronary angioplasty. Results of a randomized, double-blind, unfractionated heparin and placebo-controlled, multicenter trial (REDUCE trial). Reduction of restenosis after PTCA, early administration of reviparin in a double-blind unfractionated heparin and placebo-controlled evaluation. *J Am Coll Cardiol* 1996; 28(6): 1437–43.

29. Montalescot G et al. Enoxaparin versus unfractionated heparin in elective percutaneous coronary intervention. *N Engl J Med* 2006; 355(10): 1006–17.

30. Blazing MA et al. Safety and efficacy of enoxaparin vs unfractionated heparin in patients with non-ST-segment elevation acute coronary syndromes who receive tirofiban and aspirin: A randomized controlled trial. *JAMA* 2004; 292(1): 55–64.

31. Mahaffey KW et al. High-risk patients with acute coronary syndromes treated with low-molecular-weight or unfractionated heparin: Outcomes at 6 months and 1 year in the SYNERGY trial. *JAMA* 2005; 294(20): 2594–600.

32. Montalescot G et al. Intravenous enoxaparin or unfractionated heparin in primary percutaneous coronary intervention for ST-elevation myocardial infarction: The international randomised open-label ATOLL trial. *Lancet* 2011; 378(9792): 693–703.

33. Montalescot G et al. Enoxaparin in primary and facilitated percutaneous coronary intervention A formal prospective nonrandomized substudy of the FINESSE trial (Facilitated INtervention with Enhanced Reperfusion Speed to Stop Events). *JACC Cardiovasc Interv* 2010; 3(2): 203–12.

34. Silvain J et al. Efficacy and safety of enoxaparin versus unfractionated heparin during percutaneous coronary intervention: Systematic review and meta-analysis. *BMJ* 2012; 344: e553.

35. Lincoff AM et al. Bivalirudin and provisional glycoprotein IIb/IIIa blockade compared with heparin and planned glycoprotein IIb/IIIa blockade during percutaneous coronary intervention: REPLACE-2 randomized trial. *JAMA* 2003; 289(7): 853–63.

36. Briguori C et al. Novel approaches for preventing or limiting events (Naples) III trial: Randomized comparison of bivalirudin versus unfractionated heparin in patients at increased risk of bleeding undergoing transfemoral elective coronary stenting. *JACC Cardiovasc Interv* 2015; 8(3): 414–23.

37. Bittl JA et al. Treatment with bivalirudin (Hirulog) as compared with heparin during coronary angioplasty for unstable or postinfarction angina. Hirulog angioplasty study investigators. *N Engl J Med* 1995; 333(12): 764–9.

38. Bittl JA et al. Bivalirudin versus heparin during coronary angioplasty for unstable or postinfarction angina: Final report reanalysis of the bivalirudin angioplasty study. *Am Heart J* 2001; 142(6): 952–9.

39. Stone GW et al. Bivalirudin in patients wi th acute coronary syndromes undergoing percutaneous coronary intervention: A subgroup analysis from the Acute Catheterization and Urgent Intervention Triage strategy (ACUITY) trial. *Lancet* 2007; 369(9565): 907–19.

40. Kastrati A et al. Bivalirudin versus unfractionated heparin during percutaneous coronary intervention. *N Engl J Med* 2008; 359(7): 688–96.

41. Kastrati A et al. Abciximab and heparin versus bivalirudin for non-ST-elevation myocardial infarction. *N Engl J Med* 2011; 365(21): 1980–9.

42. Valgimigli M et al. Bivalirudin or unfractionated heparin in acute coronary syndromes. *N Engl J Med* 2015; 373(11): 997–1009.

43. Stone GW et al. Bivalirudin during primary PCI in acute myocardial infarction. *N Engl J Med* 2008; 358(21): 2218–30.

44. Steg PG et al. Bivalirudin started during emergency transport for primary PCI. *N Engl J Med* 2013; 369(23): 2207–17.

45. Shahzad A et al. Unfractionated heparin versus bivalirudin in primary percutaneous coronary intervention (HEAT-PPCI): An open-label, single centre, randomised controlled trial. *Lancet* 2014; 384(9957): 1849–58.

46. Han Y et al. Bivalirudin vs heparin with or without tirofiban during primary percutaneous coronary intervention in acute myocardial infarction: The BRIGHT randomized clinical trial. *JAMA* 2015; 313(13): 1336–46.

47. Cavender MA, and Sabatine MS. Bivalirudin versus heparin in patients planned for percutaneous coronary intervention: A meta-analysis of randomised controlled trials. *Lancet* 2014; 384(9943): 599–606.

48. Fifth Organization to Assess Strategies in Acute Ischemic Syndromes I et al. Comparison of fondaparinux and enoxaparin in acute coronary syndromes. *N Engl J Med* 2006; 354(14): 1464–76.

49. Yusuf S et al. Effects of fondaparinux on mortality and reinfarction in patients with acute ST-segment elevation myocardial infarction: The OASIS-6 randomized trial. *JAMA* 2006; 295(13): 1519–30.

50. Steg PG et al. Low-dose vs standard-dose unfractionated heparin for percutaneous coronary intervention in acute coronary syndromes treated with fondaparinux: The FUTURA/OASIS-8 randomized trial. *JAMA* 2010; 304(12): 1339–49.

Percutaneous transluminal coronary intervention: History, techniques, indications and complications

GANESH ATHAPPAN, BRIAN O'MURCHU

10.1 History

It has been almost 40 years since Andreas Gruentzig performed the first human percutaneous transluminal coronary angioplasty (PTCA), marking a major milestone in the treatment of cardiovascular disease.[1] As that day dawned, in September 1977, Greuntzig stood on broad shoulders. The pioneering work of Forssmann in 1929 had ushered in the era of percutaneous cardiac catheterisation, when he had courageously inserted a catheter into his own right atrium via the left basilic vein in seeking 'a safer approach for intracardiac drug injection'.[2] Cardiac catheters were first used for diagnostic purposes in 1941 by Cournand[3,4] and Richards[5] and were later developed for selective coronary angiography by Sones[6,7] and Judkins.[8] In 1964, catheters were used by Dotter for mechanical 'dilation' of stenosis in peripheral arteries (hence the term 'dottering').[9–13] Whilst a combination of complications and scepticism ensured that the diamond would remain rough, other workers, notably Zeitler and Schoop in Europe, continued to probe the possibilities contained within the therapeutic envelope.[14–16]

By the mid-1970s, Gruentzig, a pupil of Zeitler, developed a prototype catheter with a dual lumen, which allowed inflation of a distal tip balloon, made of low-compliance polyvinyl chloride (PVC).[17] Encouraging preliminary results in peripheral arteries spurred Gruentzig to miniaturise this balloon catheter for use in coronary arteries.[18,19] In 1976, coronary angioplasty was successfully performed in canine and post-mortem human coronary arteries.[18] In May 1977,

the first human coronary angioplasties were performed.[20] During elective multi-vessel coronary artery bypass grafting (CABG), Gruentzig and Myler with Hanna and Turina in San Francisco and Zurich advanced a balloon catheter retrogradely through the coronary arteriotomy (which would be used for graft insertion) into a proximal stenosis and performed an inflation/deflation cycle.[21,22] Post-operative angiography showed reduction in the angioplasty-treated stenosis. In September of 1977, Gruentzig, working in Zurich, performed the first PTCA, soon followed by reports from Gruentzig and his colleagues.[1,23,24]

In 1986, Sigwart et al. was first to report the implantation of a metallic stent in a living human coronary artery.[25] Schatz and co-workers subsequently developed the first balloon expandable stent.[26] Coronary stents were initially limited to use in abrupt or threatened closure occurring during PTCA.[27] In the ensuing years, numerous randomised and non-randomised trials established the effectiveness of coronary stenting in a wide array of acute and chronic ischemic coronary syndromes.[28,29] This experience fuelled exponential growth such that by 1999, stents were used in nearly 85% of percutaneous coronary intervention (PCI) procedures.[30] The post-millennial introduction of anti-restenotic drug elution from a stent platform had a hugely favourable impact on the problem of restenosis.[31,32] Recently, fully bioabsorbable stent platforms have reached clinical use.[33,34] Currently PCI is the most widely used re-vascularisation strategy worldwide. Niche devices directed at specific lesions (chronic total occlusions, calcified lesions, bifurcation lesions) fill out the interventional quiver and a variety of refinements and new interventional devices continue to emerge.

In this chapter we briefly discuss the growth and evolution of PCI technology along with its indications and complications.

10.2 Technique and technology

PCI is performed most commonly through either the femoral or the radial artery. The brachial cut down approach is rarely ever used in the current era. In the first era (1977–1980), coronary angioplasty equipment was cumbersome. Guiding catheters had high profiles, with poor memory and torque control. Dilatation catheters also had high profiles and low balloon burst points (5 atm). There were no guidewires. This primitive equipment resulted in a high percentage (25%–30%) of unsuccessful, though uncomplicated, procedures. Technical advances occurred rapidly in the early 1980s with the development of introducer sheaths[35,36] and bonded multilayered guiding catheters with an inner surface of Teflon (to decrease friction), a middle layer of woven mesh (for torque control) and an outer layer of polyurethane (to maintain form).[37] Various catheter configurations with softer tips are now widely available for vessels with atypical proximal segments.[37,38] In addition to standard Judkins and Amplatz configurations, many other shapes were developed and are now in routine usage. These newer iterations of guiding catheters have very thin walls (i.e. large lumens) and accommodate various devices (e.g. guideliner, simultaneous balloons and stents, rotational and orbital atherectomy burrs). Most importantly, typical guide catheter outer diameter has decreased to 6F. Even smaller guides are occasionally used, although perhaps at the price of less optimal imaging.

The prototype balloon angioplasty catheter, developed by Gruentzig in 1976, had a central lumen to allow perfusion and pressure transduction. In 1979, in an attempt to improve steerability, a short wire was fixed onto the distal tip. In 1982, Simpson[39,40] developed a moveable long guidewire, which could be advanced through the central lumen. This was a major breakthrough and allowed better directional control and access to distal arterial sites. Guidewire technology has since evolved rapidly to meet the demands of complex coronary interventions. Contemporary guidewire configurations vary in diameter from 0.009 to 0.018 in. and are predominantly composed of a combination of nitinol and stainless steel. These newer wires improved flexibility, torque transmission, trackability and support accounting for the success and growth in PCI.[41] Specialty wires used to treat chronic total occlusions have also been developed.

Balloon catheters have similarly undergone a rapid evolution to the current ultrasophisticated models. Fixed-wire systems are long obsolete.[42–45] Contemporary monorail or over-the-wire balloon catheters are of low profile, have greater trackability and lower cost than earlier versions. Polyethylene terephthalate (PET) has now been replaced by polyether-block-amide (Pebax) that has increased flexibility. Compliant and non-compliant balloons, scoring and cutting balloons have been added to our armamentarium.

The introduction of stents in 1986 revolutionised the field of PCI. The first stent to be implanted in a human coronary artery was the self-expanding stainless steel WALLSTENT® (Schneider AG), by Sigwart et al. in 1986.[25] This was soon superseded by balloon expandable technology with introduction of the Palmaz-Schatz® (Johnson & Johnson) stent in 1987.[46,47] The first FDA approved stent was the Cook Gianturco-Roubin stent, used for acute, or threatened, closure following coronary angioplasty.[27] Two landmark trials[28,29] published in 1993, the Belgium Netherlands Stent Arterial Revascularization Therapies Study (BENESTENT) and the North American Stent Restenosis Study (STRESS), established the role of coronary stents in reducing restenosis and led to a rapid growth of PCI technology. First generation drug-eluting stents[48] have been eclipsed by the second generation.[49,50] Recently, both partially and fully bioabsorbable stent scaffolds have entered clinical use.[33]

A discussion of developments in cardiac imaging is beyond the scope of this chapter. However, the importance of individualised radiographic projections cannot be overemphasised and reflects the demands of the interventional rather than the diagnostic cardiologist. Digital and high-resolution imaging allowing immediate playback and on-line quantitative analysis add to the improvement in success rates. In addition, fractional flow reserve (FFR), intravascular ultrasound (IVUS) and optical coherence tomography (OCT) with angiographic coregistration have enhanced the assessment of lesion morphology and composition. Robotic PCI is an intriguing technique that has begun to capture attention.[51]

10.3 Indications: Appropriate use

In the infancy of PTCA, criteria for patient selection were rigorous – refractory angina and single-vessel atherosclerotic coronary disease with normal or well-preserved left ventricular function in patients who were, otherwise, good candidates for CABG.[52] The ideal PTCA lesion was a proximal, discrete, concentric and non-calcified stenosis which did not involve major branches or angulations.[52] However, this initial application of PTCA to low-risk clinical situations steadily widened to include those with more complex clinical and morphologic characteristics.[53,54]

Currently, PCI is by far the most common means to achieve coronary re-vascularisation and is safely and successfully performed in acute coronary syndromes,[55] the very elderly,[56] in post-CABG patients and in those with severe left ventricular dysfunction. Similarly, the application of PCI has extended to patients with high-risk or complex coronary patho-anatomy, such as unprotected left main disease,[57] chronic total occlusions,[58] multi-vessel disease,[59,60] bifurcation lesions and calcified and un-dilatable lesions. Many of these patients would otherwise have required CABG in the early days of PCI.

With the twin goals of enhancing the clinical application of PCI and of deterring overuse, criteria for the appropriate use of PCI emerged in 2009[61] from a collaborative effort of the American College of Cardiology Foundation (ACCF), the American Heart Association (AHA), the Society for Cardiovascular Angiography and Interventions (SCAI), Society of Thoracic Surgeons (STS), the American Association for Thoracic Surgery (ATS) and the American Society of Nuclear Cardiology (ASNC). Based on the available scientific data and complemented by expert opinion, a panel of 17 experts developed appropriate use criteria (AUC) for PCI that applied to 180 potential clinical scenarios (expanded in 2012 to 198 scenario).[62] The concept of appropriateness as defined by RAND/UCLA methodology in the 1980s was used by the panellists to grade appropriateness. In addition to benefit/risk concerns, the cost and resource utilisation were also factored in developing the AUC. A procedure was deemed 'appropriate' if, by a sufficiently wide margin, the health benefit was likely to exceed the health risk and 'inappropriate' if the health risk was likely to exceed the health benefit. A middle ground in which the appropriateness of PCI was 'uncertain' was also identified, indicating a knowledge gap. More recently, alternative terminology has been suggested, replacing 'uncertain' with 'may be appropriate' and 'inappropriate' with 'rarely appropriate'.[63] It was hoped and anticipated that implementation of AUC would act as a powerful stimulus to optimise the quality and cost/benefit of PCI and to deter inappropriate procedures. Such has been the case, since the introduction of AUC for PCI both the volume of non-acute PCI and the rate of inappropriate use have fallen.[64]

Based on firm data demonstrating a 2% absolute mortality benefit of PCI over thrombolytic therapy, primary PCI is appropriate in ST elevation Myocardial infarction (STEMI) if performed within 12 hours of symptom onset.[65,66] At facilities without onsite PCI capability (a majority of all hospitals), transfer for primary PCI (rather than thrombolytic therapy) is recommended if the delay to mechanical reperfusion is likely to be less than 60 minutes.[67,68] When the delay to catheterisation and PCI is likely to be more than 60 minutes, the optimal strategy appears to be the administration of thrombolytic therapy (absent a contraindication), transfer to a PCI-capable facility (if applicable) and early catheterisation (between 3 and 24 hours)[69] and PCI when amenable anatomy is encountered. Facilitated PCI (defined as thrombolytic or IIB/IIIA therapy followed by immediate transfer for immediate PCI) has an unfavourable risk/benefit ratio[70,71] and is discouraged. Urgent catheterisation (and PCI if anatomy is amenable) is also indicated for most patients with failed thrombolysis,[72] cardiogenic shock, electrical instability or persistent ischemic symptoms (irrespective of the time delay from MI onset). PCI in stable symptom-free patients presenting more than 12 hours from symptom onset is inappropriate.[73] PCI of a non-infarct related artery lesion is considered appropriate in the setting of cardiogenic shock or with recurrent myocardial ischemia and/or high-risk findings on non-invasive stress testing.

Recent randomised controlled data in the STEMI setting have generated considerable debate on the risk/benefit/appropriateness of PCI performed for amenable lesions in non-infarct related arteries.[74]

In other patient cohorts with acute coronary syndromes (UA/NSTEMI), PCI of the culprit artery improves composite clinical outcome (death and non-fatal MI) for patients with high-risk (TIMI risk score >4) and intermediate-risk features (e.g. TIMI score 3–4).[75] In UA/NSTEMI patients with low TIMI (≤2) or GRACE scores (≤108), PCI of the culprit artery is considered to be of uncertain benefit.[62] In patients with multi-vessel disease and high risk TIMI score re-vascularisation of multiple coronary arteries is considered appropriate when the culprit artery cannot be clearly determined.

In non-acute coronary syndromes the appropriateness of PCI is based on the interplay of clinical, non-invasive and angiographic factors.[62] First comes an assessment of the severity of angina (which can be absent; asymptomatic) based on Canadian Cardiovascular Society Class[76] (I, II, III or IV) and of the extent of anti-anginal therapy. The next factor to be considered is the extent of ischemia on non-invasive testing, a predictor of clinical outcome. Depending on the stress imaging technique that is used, high-risk findings are associated with a >3% per year cardiac mortality, intermediate risk with a 1%–3% per year cardiac mortality and low-risk findings with <1% per year cardiac mortality. Low-, intermediate- and high-risk findings of each non-invasive stress modality are outlined in Table 10.1. The severity of coronary artery disease (1-, 2- or 3-vessel disease, with or without proximal LAD or left main coronary disease) also factors into the appropriateness of PCI. Appropriate indications are shown in the tables from the ACC/AHA guidelines. In patients referred for coronary angiography without non-invasive testing, FFR should be used to guide re-vascularisation. In FAME I,[77] FFR-guided PCI reduced the occurrence of the composite end point of death, myocardial infarction and repeat re-vascularisation compared to angiographic guidance. In the more recent FAME II,[78] patients with an FFR of <0.80 were randomly assigned to PCI or to optimal medical therapy. Whilst patients randomised to PCI underwent urgent re-vascularisation less frequently than their medically treated counterparts, a benefit in terms of hard endpoints (death, non-fatal MI) was not observed. IVUS can also be used to identify lesions for which re-vascularisation may be appropriate. An IVUS minimal luminal area (MLA) of 6 mm^2 in the left main coronary artery and 4 mm^2 in other vessels have been validated as a guide to re-vascularisation.[79,80]

10.4 Complications

The widespread application of intra-coronary stents and use of dual anti-platelet therapy have contributed to an overall decrease in complications in the current era of PCI.[81,82] Complications can be categorised in a variety of ways. We propose this practical approach to categorise them as systemic complications (death,

Table 10.1 Low, Intermediate, and High Risk Findings of Various Non-Invasive Stress Modality

Stress test	Low risk	Intermediate risk	High risk
Exercise Stress Test	• DTS ≥ 5	• DTS score −10 to +4 • ≥1 mm ST depression at peak exercise	• DTS score of ≤ −11 • ≥2 mm ST segment depression at peak exercise, low work load or persisting in recovery • Exercise induced ST elevation, VT or Vfib
Exercise/Pharmacological Nuclear Stress MPI	• Normal Stress test • Ischemia involving <10% of LV myocardium • Summed stress score of <4 (normal) or 4–8 (mild) • Summed difference score <2 (normal) or 2–4 (mild)	• Ischemia involving 10%–20% of LV myocardium • Ischemia <10% of LV myocardium and LVEF <35 • Summed stress score 9–13 • Summed difference score 5–8	• Ischemia involving >20% of LV myocardium • Scar in >10% of LV myocardium • Resting LVEF <35%–40% • Moderate sized ischemia (10%–20% of LV myocardium) in diabetics • Stress-induced multiple perfusion defects of moderate size • Transient ischemic dilation or increased lung uptake with Thallium • Summed stress score >13 or Summed difference score >8
Stress Echocardiography	• Normal stress testing	• Small wall motion abnormality involving 1–2 segments or 1 coronary bed	• Stress-induced LV dysfunction (LV dilation or peak LVEF < 45% or drop in LVEF < 10%) • Wall motion abnormality in >2 segments or 2 coronary beds • WMA with low dose dobutamine or at low heart rate (<120 bpm)
Cardiac CT	• Agaston Calcium score <100 or no coronary stenosis	• Agaston Calcium score of 100–299 • 1 vessel CAD or ≥2 vessel moderate (50%–69% stenosis) CAD	• Agaston Calcium >400 • Multi-vessel CAD (≥70% stenosis) or Left main stenosis (>50%)

myocardial infarction, stroke, contrast-induced nephropathy or allergic reaction), vascular access site complications (bleeding, infection and vascular injury including occlusion, dissection, perforation, pseudoaneurysm, arteriovenous fistula) and local intra-coronary complications (coronary perforation, dissection, abrupt vessel closure, no reflow/slow flow, side branch closure, spasm, air embolism and thrombosis).

10.4.1 Systemic complications

In an analysis of the NCDR CathPCI database of patients undergoing PCI between 2004 and 2007, the overall in-hospital mortality rate was 1.27%, ranging from 0.65% in elective PCI to 4.81% in STEMI.[83] More recent data from the New York State PCI registry showed that the overall in-hospital/30-day death rate for the 47,045 PCIs included in the 2012 analysis was 1.0%.[84] In non-emergent PCI's, the death rate was 0.29%. Factors associated with an increased risk of PCI-related mortality include advanced age, female gender, comorbidities, multi-vessel CAD, high-risk lesions and the setting of PCI (e.g. STEMI, urgent or emergency procedure, cardiogenic shock). Several models have been developed to calculate mortality and risk during PCI, namely the British Columbia PCI risk score,[85] Mayo clinic risk score,[86] Massachusetts general PCI risk calculator, Cadillac risk score,[87] and more recently the SCAI PCI risk calculator.[88]

The incidence of periprocedural MI varies from 5% to 30%.[89] A clinically relevant MI has recently been defined as an increase in the level of CK-MB of at least 10 times the upper limit of normal (ULN) within 48 hours after a PCI when baseline levels are normal and as an increase in troponin I or T of at least 70 times the ULN in the absence of CK-MB.[90] However, if an ECG shows new pathologic Q-waves in at least two contiguous leads or a new persistent left bundle branch block, then the threshold is lowered to at least five times and at least 35 times the ULN for CK-MB and troponin, respectively. Older definitions of MI have included elevation of cTn values >3–5 times the ULN occurring within 48 hours of the procedure (in patients with normal baseline values).[91,92]

Contrast induced nephropathy (CIN) is acute kidney injury within 48 hours after contrast administration. Whilst several definitions of CIN exist, perhaps the most widely applied is an increase in serum creatinine concentration of >0.5 mg/dL (>44 μmol/L) or 25% above baseline.[93] Pre-existing renal dysfunction, diabetes mellitus, congestive heart failure, shock, STEMI, female sex, older age, hypotension and anaemia are important predictors of CIN after PCI. The reported incidence of CIN varies from 1% to 50%. In a recent analysis of the NCDR cath PCI registry, Tsai et al.[94] reported a 7% incidence of CIN and 0.3% incidence of dialysis after PCI. A simple rule of thumb to limit CIN is to use a maximum contrast volume of 3.7 times the estimated glomerular filtration rate (eGFR).[95]

Stroke is an infrequent but potentially devastating complication after PCI with a reported incidence of approximately 0.3%–0.4%.[96] Independent predictors of stroke include age, female sex, renal failure and prior history of stroke or transient ischemic attack (TIA).

10.4.2 Vascular complications

Vascular complications after PCI are an important cause of morbidity and mortality. Their reported incidence after femoral PCI is in the order of 5.4%–20%.[97] Radial access for PCI has consistently been shown to reduce vascular complications when compared to the femoral route. In the STEMI–RADIAL study[98] major bleeding and vascular complications were significantly lower in the radial compared to the femoral arm (1.4% vs. 7.2%). Similarly in an analysis of the NCDR REGISTRY Rao et al. reported a significantly lower risk of bleeding with the radial access (OR 0.42 95% CI 0.31–0.56).[99] Radial artery spasm is the most common vascular complication of radial PCI, is usually temporary and rarely requires more than vasodilator and analgesic therapy. Radial artery occlusion is reported to occur in 1%–10% of patients after radial PCI.[100] Most radial artery occlusion is clinically silent, due to dual (radial and ulnar) arterial supply to the hand. Its importance lies in the fact that radial occlusion may preclude subsequent ipsilateral radial access or harvesting of the radial artery as a conduit for CABG.

10.4.3 Local coronary complications

Complete penetration of the arterial wall by a tear or dissection leads to coronary perforation, which occurs at a rate of 0.2%–0.8%.[101] It occurs more frequently during complex PCI such as debulking, tortuosity, chronic total occlusion, calcified lesions and coronary graft interventions. Ellis et al.[102] classified coronary perforation as a continuum of increasing severity and clinical consequence: Type I, extraluminal crater without extravasation; Type II, epicardial fat or myocardial blush; Type III, extravasation through frank (>1 mm) perforation; and Type IV, cavity spilling into the left ventricle, right ventricle or coronary sinus. A type V distal perforation caused by guidewires was recently proposed by Muller et al.[103] Types I and II perforation is usually self-limited whilst Type III perforation is frequently associated with cardiac tamponade. Management of perforation begins with reversal of anticoagulation when possible and prolonged balloon inflation proximal to and at the site of perforation. Tamponade requires immediate pericardiocentesis and deployment of a covered stent to seal the perforation should be considered (Figure 10.1a through 10.1d). An optimal Heart Team approach should include an alert to cardiothoracic surgery, since surgery may be necessary. When small, perforations that flow into a cavity (Type IV) usually do not require any treatment. Type V perforations can be successfully treated with coils or gel foam if unresponsive to initial measures.

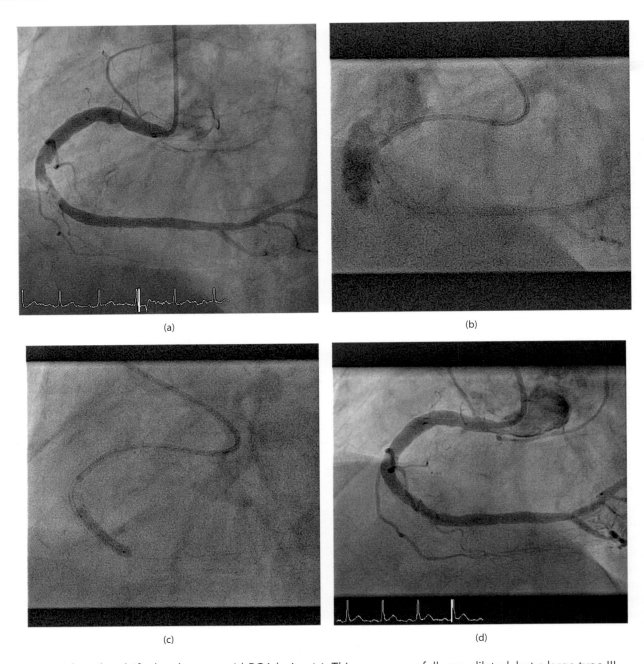

(a)

(b)

(c)

(d)

Figure 10.1 A heavily calcified and severe mid-RCA lesion (a). This was successfully pre-dilated, but a large type III perforation ensued after stent deployment (b) resulting in cardiac tamponade. Heparin reversal with protamine, intermittent balloon inflations to reduce coronary extravasation, emergency pericardiocentesis and deployment of a covered stent (c) resulted in successful sealing of the perforation and resolution of haemodynamic disturbance (d). (Courtesy of Dr. E.D. Grech South Yorkshire Cardiothoracic Centre, Sheffield, UK.)

Coronary dissection occurs when splitting of the arterial wall layers occurs. It is the most common angiographic complication during PCI. The NHLBI classifies coronary dissection into six grades (A–F) according to angiographic appearance.[104] In Type A dissection there is a minor radiolucency within the coronary lumen whilst, in Type B, a parallel track or double lumen separated by a radiolucent area is seen only during contrast injection. Both are considered relatively benign. Type C dissection is characterised by persistence of extraluminal dye following contrast injection. Type D refers to a spiral dissection. Type E is a dissection with new filling defects, Type F is dissection with impaired flow rate or total occlusion. Prolonged inflation (>30 minutes) of a perfusion balloon, intended to tack up the dissection flap, has been effectively replaced by stenting in the current era. During stenting of a dissection, further extension of dissection and either antegrade or retrograde propagation of intramural hematoma (Figure 10.2a through d) can increase risk and complexity of the salvage operation.

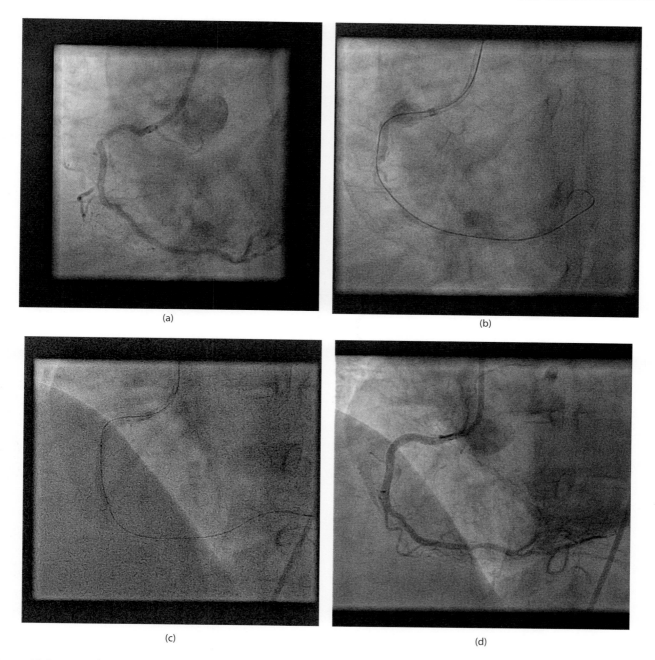

(a)

(b)

(c)

(d)

Figure 10.2 A significant discrete in-stent restenotic proximal RCA lesion (a), which was dilated with a 3.0 mm angioplasty balloon. This resulted in a proximal ballooning intra-coronary haematoma which extended distally causing an external compressive occlusion of the coronary artery just beyond the distal edge of the stent (b). Deployment of two drug-eluting stents in the proximal and mid-RCA (c) relieved the external haematoma compression and restored brisk antegrade flow (d). (Courtesy of Dr. E.D.Grech. South Yorkshire Cardiothoracic Centre, Sheffield, UK.)

Rarely, ostial coronary dissection can propagate into the aortic root and extend into the ascending aorta[105] (Figure 10.3a through d).

The incidence of abrupt closure/acute occlusion and subacute closure (<24 hours) has declined[106] from 3% in the PTCA era to 0.3% in the current era of intra-coronary stents and effective dual anti-platelet therapy. The mechanism of abrupt closure includes coronary dissection, thrombosis and vasospasm. Less frequently, air embolisation and vessel-to-vessel distal embolisation can occur. Patients will often become hemodynamically unstable and must first be resuscitated and stabilised, with intubation and mechanical ventilation and mechanical circulatory support if needed. Activated clotting time (ACT) should be therapeutic. Intra-coronary stenting has become the cornerstone of management of abrupt or threatened closure due to dissection; thrombectomy may occasionally be useful when thrombus formation is prominent.

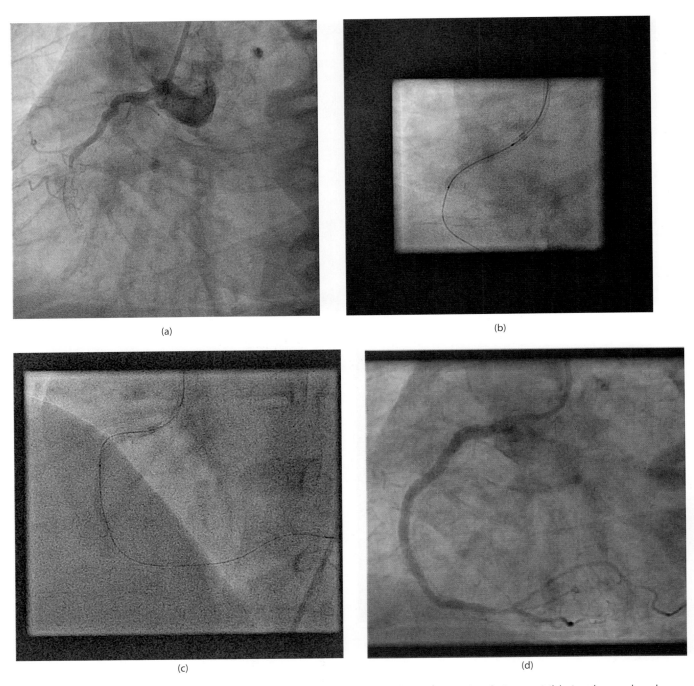

(a)

(b)

(c)

(d)

Figure 10.3 (a) A totally occluded proximal RCA which had been stented 5 years previously (stent visible just beyond occlusion). This was recanalised and dilated with an angioplasty balloon (b) resulting in coronary dissection which propagated proximally into the aortic root wall (c). Deployment of a drug-eluting stent successfully sealed the dissection with only minimal contrast entering the aortic dissection (d). Subsequent CT scan confirmed a small area of aortic dissection adjacent to the RCA ostium with no aortic valve involvement. (Courtesy of Dr. E.D. Grech. South Yorkshire Cardiothoracic Centre, Sheffield, UK.)

10.5 Summary and conclusions

Since the introduction of PTCA in September 1977, many millions of patients worldwide have benefitted from this remarkable technique. With the emergence of coronary stents, success rates have been exceptional (>95%) and restenosis is now uncommon when drug-eluting stents are used. Procedural failure and major complications will continue to be a concern. The 'last great frontier' for PCI has long been that of CTO. Several new devices, technologies and techniques have been developed and deployed to tackle these and other complex lesion subsets. The allure of a clinically superior and fully bioabsorbable stent platform may be just that allure. Future studies will determine if bioabsorbable stents represent the next revolution in interventional cardiology.

PCI has come a very long way on its 40-year odyssey and is now more effectively and more safely performed than at any time. Advances in technology notwithstanding, experience and wisdom are invaluable. I frequently think of two particular observations that were made to this author (B.O.M.) over two decades ago, observations that remain salient to this day. During an interview for interventional fellowship at Scripps, it was Richard Schatz who enunciated to me his 'Top Ten Steps to Successful Coronary Stenting'. They were #1 Guide. #2 Guide. #3 Guide. #4 Guide. #5 . . . ! And it was John Bresnahan at Mayo Clinic who said 'Once that balloon goes up, there's only so much you can control. The rest is between the balloon, the patient and her maker!' Planning, experience and integrity will always be the cornerstones of successful PCI.

References

1. Gruntzig A. Transluminal dilatation of coronary-artery stenosis. *Lancet* 1978; 1(8058): 263.
2. Forssmann W. Die sonderrung des rechten Hertzens. *Klin Wochenschr* 1929; 8: 2085–7.
3. Cournand AF. Catheterization of the right auricle in man. *Proc Soc Exp Biol Med* 1941; 46: 462–6.
4. Cournand AF et al. Measurement of cardiac output in man using the technique of catheterization of the right auricle. *J Clin Invest* 1945; 24: 106–16.
5. Richards DW. Cardiac output in the catheterization technique in various clinical conditions. *Fed Proc* 1945: 215–20.
6. Sones FM, Jr., and Shirey EK. Cine coronary arteriography. *Mod Concepts Cardiovasc Dis* 1962; 31: 735–8.
7. Proudfit WL et al. Selective cine coronary arteriography. Correlation with clinical findings in 1,000 patients. *Circulation* 1966; 33(6): 901–10.
8. Judkins MP. Selective coronary arteriography. I. A percutaneous transfemoral technic. *Radiology* 1967; 89(5): 815–24.
9. Dotter CT, and Judkins MP. Transluminal treatment of arteriosclerotic obstruction. Description of a new technic and a preliminary report of its application. *Circulation* 1964; 30: 654–70.
10. Dotter CT et al. Transluminal dilatation of atherosclerotic stenosis. *Surg Gynecol Obstet* 1968; 127(4): 794–804.
11. Dotter CT et al. Transluminal iliac artery dilatation. Nonsurgical catheter treatment of atheromatous narrowing. *JAMA* 1974; 230(1): 117–24.
12. Dotter CT. Transluminal angioplasty. *Am J Roentgenol* 1980; 135(5): 997–8.
13. Dotter CT. Transluminal angioplasty: A long view. *Radiology* 1980; 135(3): 561–64.
14. Zeitler E et al. The treatment of occlusive arterial disease by transluminal catheter angioplasty. *Radiology* 1971; 99(1): 19–26.
15. Zeitler E et al. Selective coronary arteriography. *Vasa* 1975; 4(2): 133–44.
16. Zeitler E. Percutaneous dilatation and recanalization of iliac and femoral arteries. *Cardiovasc Intervent Radiol* 1980; 3(4): 207–12.
17. Gruntzig A. Percutaneous recanalisation of chronic arterial occlusions (Dotter principle) with a new double lumen dilatation catheter (author's translation). *Rofo* 1976; 124(1): 80–6.
18. Gruntzig A. Percutaneous dilatation of experimental coronary artery stenosis – description of a new catheter system. *Klin Wochenschr* 1976; 54(11): 543–5.
19. Grüntzig A et al. Coronary transluminal angioplasty. *Circulation* 1976; 56: 84.
20. Turina M. Beginning of percutaneous coronary interventions: Zurich 1976–1977. *J Thorac Cardiovasc Surg* 2011; 141(6): 1342–3.
21. Gruentzig AR et al. Coronary percutaneous transluminal angioplasty: Preliminary results (abstr). *Circulation* 1978; 58 (Suppl II): II–56.
22. Gruentzig AR et al. Coronary transluminal angioplasty (abstr). *Circulation* 1977; 84 (Suppl III): III–55–III–56.
23. Gruntzig AR et al. Nonoperative dilatation of coronary-artery stenosis: Percutaneous transluminal coronary angioplasty. *N Engl J Med* 1979; 301(2): 61–8.
24. Stertzer SH MR et al. Transluminal coronary artery dilatation. *Pract Cardiol* 1979; 5: 25–30.
25. Sigwart U et al. Intravascular stents to prevent occlusion and restenosis after transluminal angioplasty. *N Engl J Med* 1987; 316(12): 701–6.
26. Schatz RA et al. Clinical experience with the Palmaz-Schatz coronary stent. *J Am Coll Cardiol* 1991; 17(6 Suppl B): 155B–159B.
27. Roubin GS et al. Intracoronary stenting for acute and threatened closure complicating percutaneous transluminal coronary angioplasty. *Circulation* 1992; 85(3): 916–27.
28. Serruys PW et al. A comparison of balloon-expandable-stent implantation with balloon angioplasty in patients with coronary artery disease. Benestent Study Group. *N Engl J Med* 1994; 331(8): 489–95.
29. Fischman DL et al. A randomized comparison of coronary-stent placement and balloon angioplasty in the treatment of coronary artery disease. Stent Restenosis Study Investigators. *N Engl J Med* 1994; 331(8): 496–501.
30. Holmes DR, Jr. et al. Results of Prevention of Restenosis with Tranilast and its Outcomes (PRESTO) trial. *Circulation* 2002; 106(10): 1243–50.
31. Kirtane AJ et al. Safety and efficacy of drug-eluting and bare metal stents: Comprehensive meta-analysis of randomized trials and observational studies. *Circulation* 2009; 119(25): 3198–206.
32. Marroquin OC et al. A comparison of bare-metal and drug-eluting stents for off-label indications. *N Engl J Med* 2008; 358(4): 342–52.
33. Ellis SG et al. Everolimus-eluting bioresorbable scaffolds for coronary artery disease. *N Engl J Med* 2015; 373(20): 1905–15.
34. Kimura T et al. A randomized trial evaluating everolimus-eluting absorb bioresorbable scaffolds vs. everolimus-eluting metallic stents in patients with coronary artery disease: ABSORB Japan. *Eur Heart J* 2015; 36(47): 3332–42.
35. Hillis LD. Percutaneous left heart catheterization and coronary arteriography using a femoral artery sheath. *Cathet Cardiovasc Diagn* 1979; 5(4): 393–9.
36. Grollman JH, Jr., and Hoffman RB. Does use of a vascular introducer sheath obviate need for catheter exchanges over a guidewire? *Cathet Cardiovasc Diagn* 1991; 23(1): 1–2.
37. Myler RK. *Transfemoral Approach to Percutaneous Angioplasty.* New York: Elsevier Biomedical, 1983.

38. Myler RK et al. Guiding catheter selection for right coronary artery angioplasty. *Cathet Cardiovasc Diagn* 1990; 19(1): 58–67.

39. Simpson JB et al. Update of clinical experience with a new catheter system for percutaneous transluminal coronary angioplasty. *Circulation* 1981; 64(Suppl IV): IV–252.

40. Simpson JB et al. A new catheter system for coronary angioplasty. *Am J Cardiol* 1982; 49(5): 1216–22.

41. Myler RK et al. A new flexible and deflectable tip guidewire for coronary angioplasty and other invasive and interventional procedures. *J Invasive Cardiol* 1992; 4(8): 393–7.

42. Finci L et al. Clinical experience with the Monorail balloon catheter for coronary angioplasty. *Cathet Cardiovasc Diagn* 1988; 14(3): 206–12.

43. Mooney MR et al. Monorail Piccolino catheter: A new rapid exchange/ultralow profile coronary angioplasty system. *Cathet Cardiovasc Diagn* 1990; 20(2): 114–9.

44. Myler RK et al. The balloon on a wire device: A new ultra-low-profile coronary angioplasty system/concept. *Cathet Cardiovasc Diagn* 1988; 14(2): 135–40.

45. Feldman RL et al. Randomized comparison of over-the-wire and fixed-wire balloon devices for coronary angioplasty. *J Invasive Cardiol* 1991; 3(3): 120–6.

46. Palmaz JC et al. Expandable intraluminal graft: A preliminary study. Work in progress. *Radiology* 1985; 156(1): 73–7.

47. Schatz RA et al. Clinical experience with the Palmaz-Schatz coronary stent. Initial results of a multicenter study *Circulation* 1991; 83(1): 148–61.

48. Morice MC et al. A randomized comparison of a sirolimus-eluting stent with a standard stent for coronary revascularization. *N Engl J Med* 2002; 346(23): 1773–80.

49. Alfonso F, and Fernandez C. Second-generation drug-eluting stents. Moving the field forward. *J Am Coll Cardiol* 2011; 58(1): 26–9.

50. Serruys PW et al. A randomised comparison of an everolimus-eluting coronary stent with a paclitaxel-eluting coronary stent: the SPIRIT II trial. *EuroIntervention* 2006; 2(3): 286–94.

51. Carrozza JP, Jr. Robotic-assisted percutaneous coronary intervention – filling an unmet need. *J Cardiovasc Transl Res* 2012; 5(1): 62–6.

52. Detre K et al. Percutaneous transluminal coronary angioplasty in 1985–1986 and 1977–1981. The National Heart, Lung, and Blood Institute Registry. *N Engl J Med* 1988; 318(5): 265–70.

53. Comparison of coronary bypass surgery with angioplasty in patients with multivessel disease. The Bypass Angioplasty Revascularization Investigation (BARI) Investigators. *N Engl J Med* 1996; 335(4): 217–25.

54. Rodriguez A et al. Argentine Randomized Study: Coronary Angioplasty with Stenting versus Coronary Bypass Surgery in patients with Multiple-Vessel Disease (ERACI II): 30-day and one-year follow-up results. ERACI II Investigators. *J Am Coll Cardiol* 2001; 37(1): 51–8.

55. Hochman JS et al. Early revascularization in acute myocardial infarction complicated by cardiogenic shock. SHOCK Investigators. Should We Emergently Revascularize Occluded Coronaries for Cardiogenic Shock. *N Engl J Med* 1999; 341(9): 625–34.

56. Fach A et al. Comparison of Outcomes of Patients With ST-Segment Elevation Myocardial Infarction Treated by Primary Percutaneous Coronary Intervention Analyzed by Age Groups (<75, 75 to 85, and >85 Years); (Results from the Bremen STEMI Registry). *Am J Cardiol* 2015; 116(12): 1802–9.

57. Morice MC et al. Five-year outcomes in patients with left main disease treated with either percutaneous coronary intervention or coronary artery bypass grafting in the synergy between percutaneous coronary intervention with taxus and cardiac surgery trial. *Circulation* 2014; 129(23): 2388–94.

58. Hoebers LP et al. Contemporary overview and clinical perspectives of chronic total occlusions. *Nat Rev Cardiol* 2014; 11(8): 458–69.

59. Garg S et al. Five-year outcomes of percutaneous coronary intervention compared to bypass surgery in patients with multivessel disease involving the proximal left anterior descending artery: An ARTS-II sub-study. *EuroIntervention* 2011; 6(9): 1060–7.

60. Rodriguez AE et al. Revascularization strategies of coronary multiple vessel disease in the Drug Eluting Stent Era: One year follow-up results of the ERACI III Trial. *EuroIntervention* 2006; 2(1): 53–60.

61. Patel MR et al. ACCF/SCAI/STS/AATS/AHA/ASNC 2009 Appropriateness Criteria for Coronary Revascularization: A report by the American College of Cardiology Foundation Appropriateness Criteria Task Force, Society for Cardiovascular Angiography and Interventions, Society of Thoracic Surgeons, American Association for Thoracic Surgery, American Heart Association, and the American Society of Nuclear Cardiology Endorsed by the American Society of Echocardiography, the Heart Failure Society of America, and the Society of Cardiovascular Computed Tomography. *J Am Coll Cardiol* 2009; 53(6): 530–53.

62. Patel MR et al. ACCF/SCAI/STS/AATS/AHA/ASNC/HFSA/SCCT 2012 appropriate use criteria for coronary revascularization focused update: A report of the American College of Cardiology Foundation Appropriate Use Criteria Task Force, Society for Cardiovascular Angiography and Interventions, Society of Thoracic Surgeons, American Association for Thoracic Surgery, American Heart Association, American Society of Nuclear Cardiology, and the Society of Cardiovascular Computed Tomography. *J Thorac Cardiovasc Surg* 2012; 143(4): 780–803.

63. Harrington RA. Appropriate use criteria for coronary revascularization and the learning health system: A good start. *JAMA* 2015; 314(19): 2029–31.

64. Desai NR et al. Appropriate use criteria for coronary revascularization and trends in utilization, patient selection, and appropriateness of percutaneous coronary intervention. *JAMA* 2015; 314(19): 2045–53.

65. Steg PG et al. ESC guidelines for the management of acute myocardial infarction in patients presenting with ST-segment elevation. *Eur Heart J* 2012; 33(20): 2569–619.

66. O'Gara PT et al. 2013 ACCF/AHA guideline for the management of ST-elevation myocardial infarction: A report of the American College of Cardiology Foundation/American Heart Association Task Force on Practice Guidelines. *Circulation* 2013; 127(4): e362–425.

67. Andersen HR et al. A comparison of coronary angioplasty with fibrinolytic therapy in acute myocardial infarction. *N Engl J Med* 2003; 349(8): 733–42.

68. Bonnefoy E et al. Comparison of primary angioplasty and pre-hospital fibrinolysis in acute myocardial infarction (CAPTIM) trial: A 5-year follow-up. *Eur Heart J* 2009; 30(13): 1598–606.

69. Cantor WJ et al. Routine early angioplasty after fibrinolysis for acute myocardial infarction. *N Engl J Med* 2009; 360(26): 2705–18.

70. Ellis SG et al. Facilitated percutaneous coronary intervention versus primary percutaneous coronary intervention: Design and rationale of the Facilitated Intervention with Enhanced Reperfusion Speed to Stop Events (FINESSE) trial. *A Heart J* 2004; 147(4): E16.

71. Assessment of the Safety and Efficacy of a New Treatment Strategy with Percutaneous Coronary Intervention (ASSENT-4 PCI) Investigators. Primary versus tenecteplase-facilitated percutaneous coronary intervention in patients with ST-segment elevation acute myocardial infarction (ASSENT-4 PCI): Randomised trial. *Lancet* 2006; 367(9510): 569–78.

72. Gershlick AH et al. Rescue angioplasty after failed thrombolytic therapy for acute myocardial infarction. *N Engl J Med* 2005; 353(26): 2758–68.

73. Malek LA et al. Late coronary intervention for totally occluded left anterior descending coronary arteries in stable patients after myocardial infarction: Results from the Occluded Artery Trial (OAT). *Am Heart J* 2009; 157(4): 724–732.

74. Wald DS et al. Randomized trial of preventive angioplasty in myocardial infarction. *N Engl J Med* 2013; 369(12): 1115–23.

75. Amsterdam EA et al. 2014 AHA/ACC Guideline for the Management of Patients with Non-ST-Elevation Acute Coronary Syndromes: A report of the American College of Cardiology/American Heart Association Task Force on Practice Guidelines. *J Am Coll Cardiol* 2014; 64(24): e139–228.

76. Campeau L. Letter: Grading of angina pectoris. *Circulation* 1976; 54(3): 522–3.

77. De Bruyne B et al. Fractional flow reserve-guided PCI versus medical therapy in stable coronary disease. *N Engl J Med* 2012; 367(11): 991–1001.

78. De Bruyne B et al. Fractional flow reserve-guided PCI for stable coronary artery disease. *N Engl J Med* 2014; 371(13): 1208–17.

79. Jasti V et al. Correlations between fractional flow reserve and intravascular ultrasound in patients with an ambiguous left main coronary artery stenosis. *Circulation* 2004; 110(18): 2831–6.

80. de la Torre Hernandez JM et al. Prospective application of pre-defined intravascular ultrasound criteria for assessment of intermediate left main coronary artery lesions: Results from the multicenter LITRO study. *J Am Coll Cardiol* 2011; 58(4): 351–8.

81. Seshadri N et al. Emergency coronary artery bypass surgery in the contemporary percutaneous coronary intervention era. *Circulation* 2002; 106(18): 2346–50.

82. Yang EH et al. Emergency coronary artery bypass surgery for percutaneous coronary interventions: Changes in the incidence, clinical characteristics, and indications from 1979 to 2003. *J Am Coll Cardiol* 2005; 46(11): 2004–9.

83. Peterson ED et al. Contemporary mortality risk prediction for percutaneous coronary intervention: Results from 588,398 procedures in the National Cardiovascular Data Registry. *J Am Coll Cardiol* 2010; 55(18): 1923–32.

84. https://www.health.ny.gov/statistics/diseases/.../docs/pci_2010-2012.pdf. health.ny.gov, 2015.

85. Hamburger JN et al. Percutaneous coronary intervention and 30-day mortality: The British Columbia PCI risk score. *Catheter Cardiovasc Interv* 2009; 74(3): 377–85.

86. Singh M et al. Bedside estimation of risk from percutaneous coronary intervention: The new Mayo Clinic risk scores. *Mayo Clin Proc* 2007; 82(6): 701–8.

87. Halkin A et al. Prediction of mortality after primary percutaneous coronary intervention for acute myocardial infarction: The CADILLAC risk score. *J Am Coll Cardiol* 2005; 45(9): 1397–405.

88. Brennan JM et al. Enhanced mortality risk prediction with a focus on high-risk percutaneous coronary intervention: Results from 1,208,137 procedures in the NCDR (National Cardiovascular Data Registry). *JACC Cardiovasc Interv* 2013; 6(8): 790–9.

89. Grines CL, and Dixon S. A nail in the coffin of troponin measurements after percutaneous coronary intervention. *J Am Coll Cardiol* 2011; 57(6): 662–3.

90. Moussa ID et al. Consideration of a new definition of clinically relevant myocardial infarction after coronary revascularization: An expert consensus document from the Society for Cardiovascular Angiography and Interventions (SCAI). *Catheter Cardiovasc Interv* 2014; 83(1): 27–36.

91. Thygesen K et al. Universal definition of myocardial infarction. *Circulation* 2007; 116(22): 2634–53.

92. Thygesen K et al. Third universal definition of myocardial infarction. *Glob Heart* 2012; 7(4): 275–95.

93. Tepel M et al. Contrast-induced nephropathy: A clinical and evidence-based approach. *Circulation* 2006; 113(14): 1799–806.

94. Tsai TT et al. Contemporary incidence, predictors, and outcomes of acute kidney injury in patients undergoing percutaneous coronary interventions: Insights from the NCDR Cath-PCI registry. *JACC Cardiovasc Interv* 2014; 7(1): 1–9.

95. Mehran R et al. A simple risk score for prediction of contrast-induced nephropathy after percutaneous coronary intervention: Development and initial validation. *J Am Coll Cardiol* 2004; 44(7): 1393–9.

96. Hamon M et al. Periprocedural stroke and cardiac catheterization. *Circulation* 2008; 118(6): 678–83.

97. Merriweather N, and Sulzbach-Hoke LM. Managing risk of complications at femoral vascular access sites in percutaneous coronary intervention. *Crit Care Nurse* 2012; 32(5): 16–29; quiz first page after 29.

98. Bernat I et al. ST-segment elevation myocardial infarction treated by radial or femoral approach in a multicenter randomized clinical trial: The STEMI-RADIAL trial. *J Am Coll Cardiol* 2014; 63(10): 964–72.

99. Rao SV et al. Trends in the prevalence and outcomes of radial and femoral approaches to percutaneous coronary intervention: A report from the National Cardiovascular Data Registry. *JACC Cardiovasc Interv* 2008; 1(4): 379–86.

100. Kotowycz MA, and Dzavik V. Radial artery patency after transradial catheterization. *Circ Cardiovasc Interv* 2012; 5(1): 127–33.

101. Chua SK LS, Shyu KG et al. Incidence, management, and Clinical Outcomes of Procedure- Related Coronary Artery Peforation: Analysis of 13,888 Coronary angioplasty procedures. *Acta Cardiol Sin* 2008; 24: 80–5.

102. Ellis SG et al. Increased coronary perforation in the new device era. Incidence, classification, management, and outcome. *Circulation* 1994; 90(6): 2725–30.
103. Muller O et al. Management of two major complications in the cardiac catheterisation laboratory: The no-reflow phenomenon and coronary perforations. *EuroIntervention* 2008; 4(2): 181–3.
104. Rogers JH, and Lasala JM. Coronary artery dissection and perforation complicating percutaneous coronary intervention. *J Invasive Cardiol* 2004; 16(9): 493–9.
105. Al Maluli H et al. Aortocoronary dissection: Long term follow up of a case managed with ostial stent. *Intervent Cardiol* 2015; 7(1): 13–7.
106. Almeda FQ et al. Frequency of abrupt vessel closure and side branch occlusion after percutaneous coronary intervention in a 6.5-year period (1994 to 2000) at a single medical center. *Am J Cardiol* 2002; 89(10): 1151–5.

Percutaneous coronary intervention of single- or multi-vessel disease

GILL LOUISE BUCHANAN

11.1 Introduction

Percutaneous coronary intervention (PCI) was first achieved by Andreas Gruntzig in 1977[1] and has subsequently become one of the most frequent therapeutic interventions performed within medicine.[2] In the early days of PCI, typically a single lesion would be addressed, in patients with preserved left ventricular function and minimal other co-morbidities. However, with significant recent advances in technology, including the new-generation drug-eluting stents (DES), adjunctive assessment tools (intravascular ultrasound, optical coherence tomography and fractional flow reserve [FFR]) and more potent anti-platelet agents, more complex multi-vessel disease (MVD) is frequently tackled by the interventional cardiologist. Hence, individual operators have gained increasing experience in dealing with such disease and outcomes have been favourable in the right patient setting.

It must be taken into account that not all single-vessel diseases are the same and can include a challenging chronic total occlusion (CTO) of the vessel or bifurcation disease with a heavy degree of calcification. A number of risk stratification tools have become available which help determine the appropriateness of PCI, irrespective of the number of vessels involved. It is imperative that in each individual case, baseline clinical and angiographic parameters are considered with appropriate discussion with the 'Heart Team' when necessary to choose the most effective revascularisation modality to provide favourable long-term outcomes for the patient. The aim of this discussion is to assess the role of PCI in the modern era for patients with single-vessel disease and MVD.

11.2 Decision-making and risk assessment

11.2.1 *The heart team*

When considering single-vessel coronary disease, it may be considered that such intervention is low risk for the individual, with generally short procedure times and excellent clinical outcomes. Hence, in general, single-vessel disease does not require a multi-disciplinary discussion. Figure 11.1 illustrates single-vessel disease appropriately treated with PCI. However, in specific contexts, such as proximal left anterior descending (LAD) artery disease or a CTO of this vessel unsuccessfully revascularised by PCI, a discussion is crucial (Figure 11.2). Furthermore, certain subgroups of patients, including those with diabetes mellitus (DM), do necessitate such consideration prior to intervention.

A recent addition to revascularisation guidelines has been the need for such a multi-disciplinary assessment by the 'Heart Team'. This group typically consists of interventional cardiologists, non-invasive cardiologists and cardiac surgeons, who provide a balanced deliberation as to the most effective method of revascularisation on an individual patient basis.[3] Factors taken into account include risk scores, the age and varying co-morbidities of the patient, in addition to patient preference and operator experience. Current European guidelines do state a Class I (Level of Evidence C) indication for patients to be discussed by the 'Heart Team' when decision-making is complex.[4]

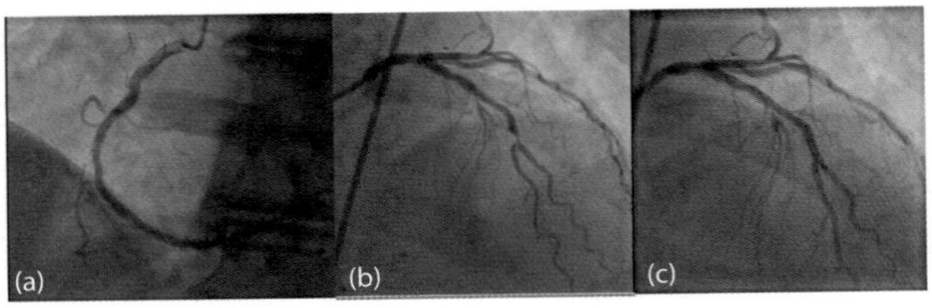

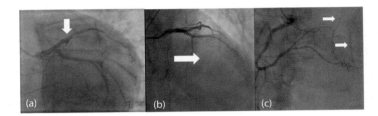

Figure 11.1 An illustration of single-vessel disease with a low SYNTAX score of 7, treated successfully with percutaneous coronary intervention. This 84-year-old male patient with a history of exertional chest discomfort was treated with implantation of a 3.0 × 14 mm drug-eluting dedicated bifurcation stent to the left anterior descending coronary artery. (a) Disease-free right coronary artery, (b) lesion prior to intervention and (c) excellent angiographic end result.

Figure 11.2 Angiographic images of an 82-year-old diabetic gentleman with single-vessel disease referred for coronary artery bypass grafting (SYNTAX score 24.5). (a and b) Chronic total occlusion of the left anterior descending coronary artery (arrowed) with unfavourable characteristics for percutaneous intervention. (c) Right coronary artery with evidence of collaterals (arrowed) to the left system.

11.2.2 Anatomical assessment and risk scores

To aid in the discussion with the Heart Team, a number of anatomically based scoring systems have been developed in order to allow a risk stratification for PCI. The most commonly used is the 'SYNergy between PCl with TAXus and cardiac surgery' (SYNTAX Score)[5] which enables assessment of the coronary lesions dependent on position within the coronary tree and extent of factors, such as presence of CTOs, bifurcation disease, aorto-ostial lesions and calcification, tortuosity, etc. The 5-year study data by risk tertiles (low risk: SYNTAX score <23; intermediate risk: 23–32; high-risk: >32) has shown no difference between PCI and coronary artery bypass grafting (CABG) in major adverse cardiovascular and cerebrovascular events (MACCE) in the low-risk tertile (PCI 32.1% vs. CABG 28.6%; $p = .43$). However, in both intermediate-risk (PCI 36.0% vs. CABG 25.8%; $p = .008$) and high-risk tertiles (PCI 44.0% vs. CABG 26.8%; $p < .0001$), the results suggested an advantage of CABG over PCI.

The drawback of the SYNTAX score is the lack of clinical variables and as such the SYNTAX Score II has recently been devised by adding baseline clinical features with strong associations with mortality at four years in the SYNTAX Study to those of the original anatomical SYNTAX Score (including age, creatinine clearance, left ventricular ejection fraction, peripheral vascular disease, female sex and chronic obstructive pulmonary disease).[6] A further concept recently described is that of the 'functional SYNTAX score'.[7] This has been demonstrated to be a better discriminator for adverse events in patients with MVD undergoing PCI, by incorporating only lesions which are ischaemic when evaluated by FFR. These newer risk scoring systems may better guide decision-making by the Heart Team for more complex patients.

11.3 Current guidelines for PCI

Both the current European Society of Cardiology (ESC) and the American College of Cardiology Foundation/American Heart Association/Society for Cardiovascular Angiography and Interventions (ACCF/AHA/SCAI) guidelines state a Class I (Level of Evidence A) indication for single-vessel PCI.[4,8] Indeed, PCI is also recommended as a Class I indication (Level of Evidence B) in MVD when the SYNTAX score is low (≤22).

Conversely, guidelines do not recommend PCI for MVD when the SYNTAX score is for intermediate risk (23–32) or high risk (>32), and in such patients, CABG should be the preferred treatment option in the absence of other significant co-morbidities that may render such an operation of prohibitive risk. Hence, it is important to assess each individual patient prior to determining whether PCI is a suitable revascularisation option.

11.4 What is the evidence for PCI?

11.4.1 Single vessel

The benefits of PCI over medical therapy have been demonstrated in a number of trials in those with single-vessel disease with regards to symptom control.[9–12] The 'Medicine, Angioplasty or Surgery' (MASS) study randomised 214 patients to CABG, PCI or optimal medical therapy (OMT) and demonstrated at 5 years that there was no difference in treatment option in the primary outcome of acute myocardial infarction (MI), death or refractory angina; however, PCI patients required more revascularisation procedures than CABG.[13] This study was performed before the development of contemporary coronary stents, and more recently the development of DES has led to significantly improved outcomes, with regards to rates of restenosis.[14,15]

11.4.2 Multi-vessel disease

Traditionally, the preferred option for the treatment of MVD has been CABG and in a large meta-analysis of major CABG studies, a definite benefit of surgery compared with medical therapy was shown.[16] More recently, CABG has been compared with PCI in this cohort of patients, with data suggesting no difference in mortality, but conversely a higher rate of revascularisation in those undergoing PCI.

The landmark clinical trial comparing PCI with DES versus CABG in MVD was the SYNTAX study. This large, international, prospective clinical trial randomised 1800 patients with MVD to either PCI with paclitaxel-eluting stents versus CABG. The primary study endpoint was non-inferiority of PCI in MACCE at one year, which was not met (PCI 17.8% vs. CABG 12.1%; $p = .002$), largely due to a significantly higher need for repeat revascularisation in those undergoing PCI (13.7% vs. 5.9%; $p < .001$). Of note, there was a higher rate of stroke in CABG patients (0.6% vs. 2.2%; $p = .003$). Importantly, there was no difference between revascularisation strategy in the occurrence of death, stroke or MI (PCI 7.6% vs. CABG 7.7%; $p = .98$).[17] At 5 years, there remained a difference in MACCE (PCI 37.3% vs. CABG 26.9%; $p < .0001$) as a consequence of the increased need for revascularisation with PCI (9.7% vs. 3.8%; $p < .0001$). Nonetheless, there were still no differences in all-cause mortality (PCI 11.4% vs. CABG 13.9%; $p = .10$) or indeed stroke (PCI 2.4% vs. CABG 3.7%; $p = .09$).[18] Figure 11.3 shows a patient with low SYNTAX score undergoing successful PCI for MVD, with conversely Figure 11.4 showing complex disease in a patient referred for CABG.

It must be taken into account that first generation DES were utilised in the SYNTAX study, which have now been demonstrated to be inferior to the new-generation DES, which require less repeat revascularisation.[19,20] The 'Clinical Evaluation of the Xience V Everolimus Eluting Coronary Stent System in the Treatment of Patients with de novo Native Coronary Artery Lesions' (SPIRIT) III and IV randomised trials demonstrated less target lesion revascularisation (3.7% vs. 7.4%; $p = .01$) with the everolimus-eluting

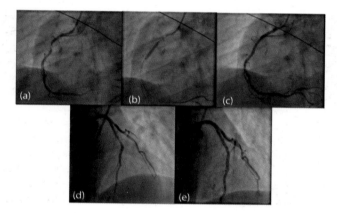

Figure 11.3 An illustration of the excellent angiographic results which can be achieved in the treatment of multi-vessel disease with percutaneous coronary intervention (PCI), utilising the new-generation drug-eluting stents. This 62-year-old female patient presented with a non-ST elevation myocardial infarction and underwent coronary angiography. The SYNTAX score was in the low tertile at 11. Focal lesion in the right coronary artery with pre (a), stent implantation (b) and post-PCI (c) images. Left anterior descending coronary artery pre-stenting (d) and post-stenting (e) were treated in a further procedure.

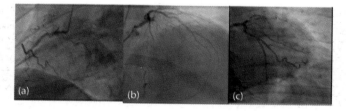

Figure 11.4 Angiographic images of a 71-year-old hypertensive male patient who presented with worsening anginal symptoms and significant coronary artery disease (SYNTAX score 44.5) referred for coronary artery bypass grafting. (a) The right coronary artery is chronically occluded. (b) A further chronic total occlusion of the left anterior descending coronary artery. (c) There is also the presence of a significant circumflex artery disease.

stents (EES) compared with the paclitaxel-eluting stents (as used in the SYNTAX study) in pooled data of 4689 patients undergoing MVD PCI.[21]

A more recent observational registry of 18,446 propensity matched patients with MVD compared PCI with EES versus CABG to a mean follow-up of 2.9 years. This demonstrated no difference in the primary end point of all-cause mortality (PCI 3.1% vs. CABG 2.9%; 95% CI 0.93–1.17; p = .50); however, again a higher rate of stroke was observed following CABG (PCI 0.7% vs. CABG 1.0%; p < .001). There remained a higher need for repeat revascularisation in those undergoing PCI (PCI 7.2% vs. CABG 3.1%; p < .001).[22]

A further study entitled 'Bypass Surgery Versus Everolimus Eluting Stent Implantation for Multi-Vessel Coronary Artery Disease' (BEST) on 880 patients with MVD randomised to PCI with EES versus CABG recently published results.[23] Of note, the study was terminated early due to slow enrolment, with only half the planned number of patients included, rendering the statistical power of the primary endpoint insufficient. Furthermore, the primary endpoint of death, MI and target vessel revascularisation (TVR) at one year did not reach non-inferiority (PCI 11.0% vs. CABG 7.9%; p = .32) and all other analyses are therefore only hypothesis generating.

11.4.3 Patients with diabetes mellitus

As mentioned earlier, a distinct subgroup of patients are those with DM, who often have more aggressive coronary disease, which is more likely to be MVD with diffuse involvement. Additionally, this high risk group of patients are more likely to develop in-stent restenosis following PCI and have lower longer term survival rates compared with CABG in disparity to patients without DM.[24,25]

The first study looking at this group was the 'Bypass Angioplasty Revascularization Investigation 2 Diabetes' (BARI-2D) trial, which specifically addressed revascularisation in DM and stable coronary artery disease. Overall, 2368 patients with DM and evidence of ischaemia were randomised to either OMT or revascularisation (PCI or CABG). At 5 years, in the PCI cohort there was no difference in freedom from MACCE compared with OMT (PCI 77.0% vs. OMT 78.9%; p = .15). However, in the CABG group (where patients had more widespread disease), the freedom from MACCE was significantly higher with revascularisation (CABG 77.6% vs. OMT 69.5%; p = .01).[26]

This led to a growing interest in research in this field and a number of trials were subsequently published. The 'Coronary Artery Revascularization in Diabetes' (CARDia) trial compared PCI versus CABG in 510 patients with DM. The primary composite endpoint of death, MI and stroke at one year did not show any difference between the two means of revascularisation (PCI 13.0% vs. CABG 10.5%; HR 1.25; 95% CI 0.75–2.09; p = .39); however, when repeat revascularisation was included in the endpoint, CABG had a greater benefit (19.3% vs. 11.3%; HR 1.77; 95% CI 1.11–2.82; p = .02).[27] It must be noted as a criticism of the study that

sirolimus-eluting stents (SES) were used in 69% of patients and bare-metal stents (BMS) in the other patients, which as discussed previously have been demonstrated to be inferior to contemporary DES.

A subgroup of patients with DM from the SYNTAX study also demonstrated higher rates of MACCE with PCI at 5 years (PCI 46.5% vs. CABG 29.0%; p < .001) again due to repeat revascularisation (PCI 35.3% vs. CABG 14.6%; p < .001). Encouragingly, there was no difference in the combined endpoint of death, stroke or MI (PCI 23.9% vs. 19.1%; p = .26).[28]

The 'Future Revascularization Evaluation in Patients with Diabetes Mellitus: Optimal management of Multi-Vessel Disease' (FREEDOM) study was the landmark trial in patients with DM and MVD, comparing PCI with DES to CABG. The primary composite outcome of all-cause mortality, non-fatal MI or non-fatal stroke at 5 years, showed CABG to be superior (PCI 26.6% vs. CABG 18.7%; p = .005) mainly due to mortality benefits (PCI 16.3% vs. CABG 10.9%; p = .049) and MI (PCI 13.9% vs. CABG 6.0%; p < .001). Of note, the greater benefit of CABG was present throughout all three SYNTAX tertiles.[29] To date, this is the only adequately powered randomised controlled trial comparing PCI with DES with CABG and has led to a recommendation of CABG over PCI in many diabetic patients. More work does need to be performed to assess the effect of treatment for DM on outcome, especially with regards to insulin.[30]

11.5 Complete versus incomplete revascularisation

A further question that can be deliberated by the Heart Team when deciding upon the approach to revascularisation is important to consider whether the aim is to provide complete revascularisation, functional revascularisation or purely for symptom control.

Complete revascularisation for the patient with MVD is most likely to be achieved with CABG; with a suggestion that complete revascularisation may have improved outcomes. Lower mortality (relative risk [RR] 0.82; 95% CI 0.68–0.99; p = .05) and non-fatal MI (RR 0.67; 95% CI 0.53–0.84; p < .01) has been demonstrated with complete revascularisation in a large meta-analysis of 37,116 patients with MVD who received either complete (n = 11,596) or incomplete (n = 25,520) revascularisation.[31] A subsequent meta-analysis of 89,883 patients showed similar results with lower long-term mortality (RR 0.71; 95% CI 0.65–0.77; p < .001). This study also reported more incomplete revascularisation following PCI compared with CABG (56.0% vs. 25.0%; p < .001).[32]

The functional significance of an anatomical lesion is also an important concept and the landmark 'Fractional Flow reserve versus Angiography for Multivessel Evaluation' (FAME) study was the first to assess this. Over 1000 patients with MVD (at least two vessels with >50% stenosis on angiography) were randomised to either angiographic-guided or FFR-guided procedures. In the FFR group, there was a significant reduction in MACCE (angiographic alone

22.8% vs. FFR 14.9%; p = .02) and notably one third of angiographically identified lesions were not functionally significant by FFR.[33] It is therefore possible that improved outcomes would be observed if complete revascularisation was done on a functional rather than anatomical basis. The FFR measurement combined with the SYNTAX score, the so-called 'functional SYNTAX score', has been piloted[7] and currently the FAME 3 study is recruiting 1500 patients to compare FFR-guided PCI versus CABG in patients with MVD with a primary endpoint of MACCE at 1 year.

A final theory is that of 'reasonable complete revascularisation',[34] which may be present with non-viable myocardium, jailed side branches or small vessels. The lesion can always be treated in the future if this becomes problematic, which is a feature exclusive to PCI. More work is needed in this area to determine the most effective approach to these complex patients, who may be anatomically challenging.

11.6 Summary

Since the introduction of PCI, rapid advances have led to changing indications from simple single-vessel disease to more complex anatomy and MVD. Encouragingly, with the exception of patients with DM, the majority of studies show no significant differences between PCI and CABG in death, stroke or MI. However, each individual patient is different and in the case of MVD should be considered with the multi-disciplinary 'Heart Team' to determine the best treatment option, taking into account both anatomical and clinical features.

Ongoing studies aim to assess more contemporary coronary stents in large multi-centre trials, which will assist in decision-making, particularly in those patients with MVD. The SYNTAX II study will include 450 all-comers with de novo three vessel diseases without left main stem involvement deemed suitable for PCI following screening with the SYNTAX II score and the 'Heart Team'. Following assessment with FFR and iFR, patients will undergo PCI with the SYNERGY™ stent (Boston Scientific, Natick, Massachusetts) with MACCE at 12 months compared with the historical SYNTAX cohort.

In conclusion, PCI is now commonly performed to revascularise patients with both single-vessel disease and MVD with excellent angiographic and clinical outcomes. The decision to perform PCI should not be based solely on the number of vessels involved but on the overall assessment of the individual patient. With growing data, this mode of revascularisation may well develop an increasing role in future clinical guidelines in the correct patient populations.

References

1. Gruntzig A. Transluminal dilatation of coronary-artery stenosis. *Lancet* 1978; 1: 263.
2. Stefanini GG, and Holmes DR, Jr. Drug-eluting coronary-artery stents. *N Engl J Med* 2013; 368: 254–65.
3. Head SJ et al. The rationale for Heart Team decision-making for patients with stable complex coronary artery disease. *Eur Heart J* 2013; 34(32): 2510–18.
4. Authors/Task Force m, Windecker S et al. 2014 ESC/EACTS Guidelines on myocardial revascularization: The Task Force on Myocardial Revascularization of the European Society of Cardiology (ESC) and the European Association for Cardio-Thoracic Surgery (EACTS). Developed with the special contribution of the European Association of Percutaneous Cardiovascular Interventions (EAPCI). *Eur Heart J* 2014; 35: 2541–619.
5. Sianos G et al. The SYNTAX Score: An angiographic tool grading the complexity of coronary artery disease. *EuroIntervention* 2005; 1: 219–27.
6. Farooq V et al. Anatomical and clinical characteristics to guide decision making between coronary artery bypass surgery and percutaneous coronary intervention for individual patients: Development and validation of SYNTAX score II. *Lancet* 2013; 381: 639–50.
7. Nam CW et al. Functional SYNTAX score for risk assessment in multivessel coronary artery disease. *J Am Coll Cardiol* 2011; 58: 1211–8.
8. Levine GN et al. 2011 ACCF/AHA/SCAI Guideline for Percutaneous Coronary Intervention. *J Am Coll Cardiol* 2011; 58(24): e44–122.
9. Parisi AF et al. A comparison of angioplasty with medical therapy in the treatment of single-vessel coronary artery disease. Veterans Affairs ACME Investigators. *N Engl J Med* 1992; 326: 10–6.
10. Alderman EL. Results from late-breaking clinical trials sessions at ACC '98. American College of Cardiology. *J Am Coll Cardiol* 1998; 32: 1–7.
11. Coronary angioplasty versus medical therapy for angina: The second Randomised Intervention Treatment of Angina (RITA-2) trial. RITA-2 trial participants. *Lancet* 1997; 350: 461–8.
12. Pitt B et al. Aggressive lipid-lowering therapy compared with angioplasty in stable coronary artery disease. Atorvastatin versus Revascularization Treatment Investigators. *N Engl J Med* 1999; 341: 70–6.
13. Hueb WA et al. Five-year follow-op of the medicine, angioplasty, or surgery study (MASS): A prospective, randomized trial of medical therapy, balloon angioplasty, or bypass surgery for single proximal left anterior descending coronary artery stenosis. *Circulation* 1999; 100: II107–13.
14. Morice MC et al. A randomized comparison of a sirolimus-eluting stent with a standard stent for coronary revascularization. *N Engl J Med* 2002; 346: 1773–80.
15. Colombo A et al. Randomized study to assess the effectiveness of slow- and moderate-release polymer-based paclitaxel-eluting stents for coronary artery lesions. *Circulation* 2003; 108: 788–94.
16. Yusuf S et al. Effect of coronary artery bypass graft surgery on survival: Overview of 10-year results from randomised trials by the Coronary Artery Bypass Graft Surgery Trialists Collaboration. *Lancet* 1994; 344: 563–70.
17. Serruys PW et al. Percutaneous coronary intervention versus coronary-artery bypass grafting for severe coronary artery disease. *N Engl J Med* 2009; 360: 961–72.
18. Mohr FW et al. Coronary artery bypass graft surgery versus percutaneous coronary intervention in patients with three-vessel disease and left main coronary disease: 5-year

follow-up of the randomised, clinical SYNTAX trial. *Lancet* 2013; 381: 629–38.

19. Stone GW. Everolimus-eluting versus paclitaxel-eluting stents in coronary artery disease. *N Engl J Med* 2010; 362: 1663–74.

20. Kedhi E et al. Second-generation everolimus-eluting and paclitaxel-eluting stents in real-life practice (COMPARE): A randomised trial. *Lancet* 2010; 375: 201–9.

21. Kereiakes DJ et al. Comparison of everolimus-eluting and paclitaxel-eluting coronary stents in patients undergoing multilesion and multivessel intervention: The SPIRIT III (A Clinical Evaluation of the Investigational Device XIENCE V Everolimus Eluting Coronary Stent System [EECSS] in the Treatment of Subjects With De Novo Native Coronary Artery Lesions) and SPIRIT IV (Clinical Evaluation of the XIENCE V Everolimus Eluting Coronary Stent System in the Treatment of Subjects with De Novo Native Coronary Artery Lesions) randomized trials. *JACC Cardiovasc Interv* 2010; 3: 1229–39.

22. Bangalore S et al. Everolimus-eluting stents or bypass surgery for multivessel coronary disease. *N Engl J Med* 2015; 372: 1213–22.

23. Park SJ et al. Trial of everolimus-eluting stents or bypass surgery for coronary disease. *N Engl J Med* 2015; 372: 1204–12.

24. Niles NW et al. Survival of patients with diabetes and multivessel coronary artery disease after surgical or percutaneous coronary revascularization: Results of a large regional prospective study. Northern New England Cardiovascular Disease Study Group. *J Am Coll Cardiol* 2001; 37: 1008–15.

25. Banning AP et al. Diabetic and nondiabetic patients with left main and/or 3-vessel coronary artery disease: Comparison of outcomes with cardiac surgery and paclitaxel-eluting stents. *J Am Coll Cardiol* 2010; 55: 1067–75.

26. Group BDS et al. A randomized trial of therapies for type 2 diabetes and coronary artery disease. *N Engl J Med* 2009; 360: 2503–15.

27. Kapur A et al. Randomized comparison of percutaneous coronary intervention with CABG in diabetic patients. 1-year results of the CARDia (Coronary Artery Revascularization in Diabetes) trial. *J Am Coll Cardiol* 2010; 55: 432–40.

28. Kappetein AP et al. Treatment of complex coronary artery disease in patients with diabetes: 5-year results comparing outcomes of bypass surgery and percutaneous coronary intervention in the SYNTAX trial. *Eur J Cardiothorac Surg* 2013; 43: 1006–13.

29. Farkouh ME et al. Strategies for multivessel revascularization in patients with diabetes. *N Engl J Med* 2012; 367: 2375–84.

30. Dangas GD et al. Long-term outcome of PCI versus CABG in insulin and non-insulin-treated diabetic patients: Results from the FREEDOM trial. *J Am Coll Cardiol* 2014; 64: 1189–97.

31. Aggarwal V et al. Clinical outcomes based on completeness of revascularisation in patients undergoing percutaneous coronary intervention: Meta-analysis of multivessel coronary artery disease studies. *EuroIntervention* 2012; 7: 1095–102.

32. Garcia S et al. Outcomes after complete versus incomplete revascularization of patients with multivessel coronary artery disease: A meta-analysis of 89,883 patients enrolled in randomized clinical trials and observational studies. *J Am Coll Cardiol* 2013; 62: 1421–31.

33. Tonino PA et al. Fractional flow reserve versus angiography for guiding percutaneous coronary intervention. *N Engl J Med* 2009; 360: 213–24.

34. Dauerman HL. Reasonable incomplete revascularization. *Circulation* 2011; 123: 2337–40.

Coronary stenting I: Intracoronary stents – Form and function

VARINDER K RANDHAWA, PATRICK TEEFY

12.1 Introduction

We practice interventional cardiology in an era when coronary stents are ubiquitous and utilised in well over 90% of cases. This was not always the case. Some interventional cardiologists recall a time when balloon angioplasty (occasionally supplemented by atherectomy debulking techniques) was the state-of-the-art modality for lesion dilatation and luminal optimisation. Despite limitations of arterial dissection, inherent risk of vessel closure and omnipresent restenosis, the foundation of interventional cardiology was built upon this practice introduced by Andreas Grüntzig along with Richard Myler (following the pioneering work of Charles Dotter) in 1977. Abrupt closure (vessel recoil, thrombosis, platelet aggregation and dissection) occurred in 4%–8% of patients, restenosis in 30%–50% and repeat revascularisation in 20%–30% of all patients.[1,2]

When coronary stents were introduced first by Sigwart and Puel in 1986 (self-expanding, elastic, macroporous tubular prosthesis woven from stainless steel; Wallstent, Medinvent, Lausanne, Switzerland) approximately a decade after the establishment of interventional programs, not all centres embraced the technology enthusiastically.[3] There was understandable uncertainty about implanting an irretrievable metallic object into a coronary artery with inherent risk of stent thrombosis (at a considerably higher incidence than current levels due to the use of oral anti-coagulation and lack of consistent post-deployment high-pressure balloon expansion). Moreover, they were comparatively expensive and somewhat cumbersome to utilise. The Palmaz-Schatz (Johnson & Johnson Interventional Systems, Warren, New Jersey) system consisted of a stent-mounted balloon covered by 5F protective sheath withdrawn to expose the stent once the lesion was crossed ideally requiring an 8F guiding catheter and adequate pre-dilatation.[4] Patients were not typically premedicated with blood thinners other than aspirin, necessitating dextran to be started in the cath lab in addition to heparin. Being available only in 15 mm length, they were not ideally suited for long or heavily calcified lesions. Hence, their initial role was predominately for bailout stabilisation of unstable dissections causing or threatening arterial closure from balloon angioplasty and/or atherectomy procedures often after prolonged use of perfusion balloon angioplasty.[3] Indeed, the Gianturco-Roubin stent (Cook Inc., Bloomington, Indiana), consisting of balloon-expandable coiled stainless steel wire wrapped in a clamshell-like configuration was approved by the U.S. Food and Drug Administration (FDA) for threatened closure associated with balloon angioplasty in 1993.

Two studies dramatically altered the utilisation of stents proving, through well-designed randomised controlled trials, that stents reduce the rate of restenosis. In the STRESS trial, Fischman et al. showed that the Palmaz-Schatz stent reduced the rate of restenosis from 42.1% (Percutaneous Transluminal Coronary Angioplasty [PTCA] group) to 31.6% (stent group), $p = .046$.[5] In the BENESTENT trial, Serruys et al. likewise demonstrated an absolute reduction in restenosis of 10% when utilising the Palmaz-Schatz stent, $p = .02$.[6] Stent thrombosis was to remain the Achilles' heel, necessitating prolonged hospital stays to initiate oral anticoagulation with its inherent haemorrhagic complications.

If the reduction in restenosis was the justification to utilise stents in a much broader array of cases, indeed as a preferred strategy, it was a paradigm shift in technique and pharmacologic protocol that dramatically reduced the rate of stent thrombosis, simplified the regime and expedited patient discharge. Initial studies by Colombo revealed that high-pressure balloon dilatation following stent deployment (guided by intravascular ultrasound) combined with dual anti-platelet therapy (aspirin plus the thienopyridine, ticlopidine) reduce stent thrombosis rates to <2%.[7–9]

Hence, these initial landmark studies, confirming a clinical utility for interventional treatment for coronary artery disease coupled with a reproducible, efficient and relatively low risk of major procedural and subsequent thrombotic complications, launched the modern stent era. The number and variety of stent designs increased thereafter, focused not only on the short localised lesions addressed in these initial studies but also long diffuse obstructive plaque, bifurcations, vein grafts and other complex anatomy.[10–12,13]

This chapter focuses on examples of currently available coronary stent technology with respect to their various forms, functions and clinical utility.

Stent is actually derived from a dental prosthesis designed by an English dentist Charles Stent in the nineteenth century. The first commercially available coronary stents consisted of unique designs. The Gianturco-Roubin stent consisted of a balloon-expandable coil stent, configured in such a way that the undulating loops of the single 316L stainless steel coil resembled a clamshell configuration. It was approved for acute or threatened closure within a coronary artery or vein graft. The Palmaz-Schatz stent composed of 316L stainless steel was a slotted tube design with two cylindrical 7-mm articulated segments connected by a 1-mm bridging strut mounted on a balloon catheter, providing longitudinal flexibility yet maintaining radial strength. The Wallstent (Medinvent-Schneider, Switzerland) was a cobalt alloy – platinum core with braided mesh design, self-expanding following retraction of the membrane sheath once advanced across the lesion. The size was selected to be slightly larger than the estimated reference vessel diameter to ensure radial strength and also prevent migration.[12]

With confirmation of efficacy in bailout for vessel closure (reducing recoil and dissection flap obstruction) as well as clinical impact on reducing restenosis, the number and variety of stents proliferated. Coil designs included the tantalum WIKTOR stent (Medtronic, Inc., Minneapolis, Minnesota) and unique modular designs such as the Bard XT (CR Bard, Murray Hill, New Jersey) consisted of zigzag modules welded to a flexible longitudinal spine.[14,15] Slotted tube designs included stainless steel BeStent 2 with two radio-opaque gold markers marking the proximal and distal ends of the stent (Medtronic, Inc.), the MultiLink (Advanced Cardiovascular Systems, Santa Clara, California), and the multicell NIR stent (Medinol, Tel Aviv, Israel, and later Boston Scientific) design.

Stent structure can be broken down into a number of fundamental characteristics critical in their function and performance.[16] Moreover, certain unique structural characteristics enable a particular stent to perform and be suitable for specific anatomic circumstances or lesion-specific situations. Hence, form and function are fundamentally intertwined. Rather than be an exhaustive list of every stent, the following is a more conceptual framework of the specific stent structural characteristics which are inherent or conducive to fulfilling/optimising this role. This chapter will discuss the interconnection between the various structural characteristics some of which are complementary, others competitive.

Table 12.1 Characteristics of the Ideal Coronary STENT

- Optimize lumen (desired lumen gain with reliable apposition and minimal strut thickness)
- Adequate tissue coverage and minimization of tissue prolapse
- Conformability to bends and tortuosity
- Strut design to allow sidebranch access/ intervention
- Minimal longitudinal deformation of vessel curvature
- Flexibility maintaining vasomotion/ prevent vessel kinking
- Biocompatibility to minimize thrombosis, inflammation, restenosis and neoatherosclerosis
- Inert and hypoallergenic
- Uniformity of drug delivery
- Robust randomized controlled clinical results with low MACE
- Deliverability (reliability and ease of delivery)
- Minimal impact (endothelial trauma) on proximal artery upon delivery
- Precision of implant upon deployment
- Optimal radial strength
- Lack of recoil in cross-sectional dimensions
- Lack of longitudinal foreshortening
- Fracture resistance
- Optimal radiopacity (frame visibility without obscuration of contrast-defined lumen)
- Range of sizes (length and diameters)
- Adequate range of final diameter within each designated stent size (post-deployment expansion without compromise of lesion coverage radially or longitudinally)
- Breadth of application (various lesion characteristics, saphenous vein grafts, bifurcations)
- Costs in line with global health care budgets

12.2 Basic stent characteristics

1. **Means of deployment**
   a. Balloon expandable
   b. Self-expanding
2. **Composition**
   a. Stainless steel (316L)
   b. Cobalt chromium
   c. Cobalt alloy (cobalt, nickel, chromium, molybdenum)
   d. Tantalum
   e. Nitinol

f. Platinum chromium (also contains iron, nickel, molybdenum)

g. Coating (inert and active components)

h. Biodegradable material

3. **Structural PATTERN – Architectural design**

a. **Mesh stents**

The original mesh stent (Wallstent) was composed of round wires of stainless steel woven together into a mesh-like sleeve. Since they were self-expanding a retractable sheath was necessary, with inherent limitations of deliverability due to the crossing profile of stent and sheath complex (Figure 12.1).

b. **Wire coil stent**

The coiled 'slinky' toy (Poof-Slinky, Inc, Canton, MI) is a great analogue to the coiled stent. The extreme flexibility of this instrument allows it to bend and flex down an incline or staircase yet maintain its form and structure. Such was the concept of the coiled wire stents. Undulations in the wire, mounted on a balloon catheter, provided great flexibility and hence deliverability during the initial years of stenting. There were, however, limitations in the performance of some of these stents. Adjacent loops or interdigitations could become displaced upon crossing the lesion or during balloon inflation, especially within a lesion of variable compliance, such that the expanded loops could be closely spaced in some regions and conversely relatively sparse in others potentially increasing the chance of tissue prolapse and/or incomplete lesion expansion. Hence, overall there was reduced and greater variability of radial strength of the stent scaffold (non-uniformity). Moreover, certain designs led to a rather unique structural problem in the event of stent dislodgment. Difficult vessel passage/lesion crossing could lead to longitudinal compression of the coil stent (concertina effect) or conversely, unravelling of the coil into a linear wire string upon withdrawal of a dislodged stent. A wire backbone on some of the stent designs (Gianturco-Roubin II stent) prevented these adversities but still had limitations of excessive tissue prolapse on the free edge of the loop. Newer designs have modified the coiled wire (helical design).

c. **Slotted tube**

Many of the initial stents in practice were essentially made from a cylindrical tube of metal from which the slots between the stent struts were either etched or laser cut. Radial strength was satisfactory but flexibility in early designs was suboptimal. The original Palmaz-Schatz stent, a 15-mm rigid slotted tube, was modified to the PS153 involving two 7-mm segments articulated with a 1-mm interconnecting bridge, allowing flexibility through

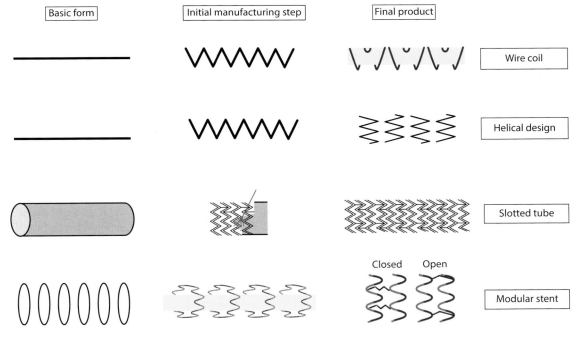

Figure 12.1 Basic stent designs. The various stent designs are illustrated. The **wire coil** consists of a single wire shaped in an undulating fashion into a tubular sleeve around the balloon catheter. The **helical design** is a modification of the wire coil, such that the single wire is arranged in a sinusoidal pattern circumferentially in a helical pattern on the balloon catheter, subsequently laser fused to adjacent loops at regular intervals. The **slotted tube** involves laser cutting of a cylindrical metal tube to form a lattice pattern. The **modular stent** consists of a series of rings (with crest and valley undulations, or peaks or crowns) fused with each other at various intervals. **Open** designs have larger gaps allowing more flexibility and side branch access, whereas the more regularly adjoined **closed** system is inherently less flexible, but provides better tissue coverage.

an articulation though potentially compromising lesion coverage and permitting tissue prolapse between the two segments (especially if the strut was positioned on the inner curvature of the tortuous segment).

d. **Modular design**

The modular design is a unique concept to maintain flexibility and preserve radial strength as well as lesion coverage. Figure 12.1 illustrates this concept. Individual rings have undulations (e.g. sinusoidal configuration, crowns or peaks) in circumferential arrangement, providing radial support, stacked serially in the longitudinal pattern (with the number of peaks adjusted in direct proportion to maximal vessel diameter – most available stents have two or three sizes, e.g. six and nine peaks per ring). Hence, this confers a high degree of flexibility. Each module ensures lesion coverage and the interdigitation of (laser-fused) struts, or connectors, provide architectural integrity and, as such, longitudinal strength. The periodicity of the interdigitating struts has an influence on flexibility. Closed-cell design signifies that the adjacent modular ring segments are fused/connected at every possible juxtaposed segment or crest. Closed-cell designs are less flexible but provide better tissue coverage (scaffolding). In the era of drug elution, the closed-cell designs may optimise uniformity of anti-proliferative/immunosuppressive drug delivery due to a higher metal-to-artery ratio and less variation in gap size within curved arterial segments leading to scaffolding uniformity. Open-cell designs, with a fraction of the number of connecting struts compared to close cell designs, permit greater flexibility/conformability with an acceptably small reduction of radial strength. There is, however, a potential for tissue prolapse due to the larger cell gaps. Open cells also enhance the ability to expand the cell space providing a larger diameter for access and stenting of side branches. The point of interconnection varies with the various open-cell design (e.g. peak-to-peak, peak-to-valley or mid strut).

e. **Helical designs**

Composed of single wire in a sinusoidal pattern arranged circumferentially in a helical pattern on the balloon catheter, this stent is subsequently laser fused at regular intervals. The design maintains flexibility and deliverability, yet preserves uniformity of radial strength and tissue coverage by reducing the loop deviation and displacement (e.g. Integrity, Medtronic, Inc.). Uniform cell size at flexion points is maintained. Longitudinal distortion is preserved by the helical design, and flexibility is insured with only two interconnections per revolution. Scaling is theoretically reduced due to uniformity of cell size at the flexion points. Hence, they may have particular advantage for tortuous and

calcified lesions. The helical arrangement of the continuous sinusoid pattern of a single wire coil is used for the RESOLUTE ONYX Stent (Medtronic, Inc.) This stent uses the unique CoreWire Technology having a denser core metal surrounded by a cobalt alloy outer layer ensuring radio-opacity and, due to thinner struts, improves deliverability without adversely affecting radial or longitudinal strength.

f. **Custom designs**

Hybrid designs include the closed-cell design at the edges and open-cell concept for the mid portion of the stent. This provides a mixture of stronger radial force at the ends, improved flexibility in the mid portion with enhanced side branch access in the segment if centred across the bifurcation.

Stents must be predictably deliverable despite the anatomic complexities of the coronary arteries (e.g. tortuosity, rigidity and calcification) necessitating a degree of flexibility, thin struts and reliable adherence to the balloon catheter. Once deployed, they must cover the lesion adequately to minimise tissue prolapse (including the greater and lesser curvatures of bends) maintaining radial strength to ensure adequate lumen expansion with minimal recoil and foreshortening. Adequate visualisation (radio-opacity) without obscuration is a desirable quality to allow fluoroscopic identification reducing geographic miss, facilitating precise post-deployment high-pressure balloon expansion as well as stent overlap but at the same time permitting enough luminal visualisation (i.e., presence of thrombus, tissue prolapse) and assessment of restenosis if patients return for angiography.

Hence, the additional features necessary in the engineering and stent design include:-

4. **Deliverability**

A stent is only useful if it can be deployed at the target lesion in the coronary artery. Modification of design over time has radically improved the ease of deliverability. The characteristics important in the ability of a standard stent to be delivered to a lesion are listed and discussed as follows.[17] Specialty stents, on the other hand, such as covered stents and those for bifurcations necessarily must sacrifice or compromise on some of these characteristics in order to fulfil their unique role. Factors such as in the balloon itself – its tapering and physical characteristics of the balloon catheter shaft – are also important aspects, though we will confide our discussion to the stents proper. Stent adherence to the balloon catheter was less secure and reliable in the past in comparison to current standards. Indeed the Palmaz-Schatz stent had a protective sheath, which was retracted once the pre-dilated lesion was crossed, minimising the risk of premature dislodgment prior to balloon expansion. As an alternative to this rather bulky profile and inherent limitations of delivery, interventional cardiologists would mount free stents on balloon catheters crimping the device by hand or utilising a standard crimping clamp before delivering the stent to the target lesion without a protective sheath. Some interventional cardiologists recall the not infrequent stent dislodgment and retracting expeditions of the undeployed stents from failed crossing attempts.

In terms of balloon-expandable stents, a major advancement came with the improved adherence of the stents to the wrapped/folded delivery balloon catheter. Protective outer delivery sheaths were no longer necessary, markedly improving the crossing profile. Improvements in the tapered leading edge of the balloon catheter, its profile and tracking capacity were other important factors enhancing deliverability. As a result, the balloon-expandable stents are the most frequently utilised delivery system for current interventional cardiology practice. Self-expanding stents by design necessitate a protective sheath retracted once the lesion is crossed, expanding and unfurling the stent as the sheath is withdrawn from distal to proximal. Newer designs have reduced the crossing profile and are accommodated into 6F guiding catheters.

A number of processes with quantifiable metrics are pertinent to stent deliverability. These include: (1) **pushability,** the ratio of distal force at the catheter tip as a specific proximal force is applied on the delivery system measured in newtons; (2) **trackability,** referring to the ability to advance stent/delivery system up to the lesion over the guidewire in a simulated anatomical setup (e.g. an angulated segment) and (3) **crossability,** relating to the ability of the distal portion of the stent system to pass through a luminal narrowing. Hence, the stent's profile is a very important aspect of crossability.

a. **Strut thickness and shape**
Strut architecture is complex and it is an intricate interplay amongst material composition, architectural pattern and thickness in order to maintain optimal deliverability, lesion coverage, fluoroscopic visibility and radial strength. Of the most frequently used stents in current practice, strut thickness varies roughly between 60 and 90 μm. These differences in strut thickness understandably can influence lesion crossing and performance particularly in tight and tortuous lesions. As such, many lesions are stented directly without pre-dilatation with confidence and dependability. Strut shape potentially may influence deliverability. Some stent struts are rounded in cross section (e.g. Integrity, ONYX, Medtronic, Inc.) whilst others have rounded rather than square corner edges, though overall influence in performance is probably minimal. Drug-coated stents necessitated an additional layer of polymer onto which the anti-proliferative/immunosuppressive agent is embedded adding additional thickness. The strut thickness of the bioabsorbable vascular scaffolding (Absorb, Abbott Vascular, Santa Clara, California) is considerably larger at 150 μm, a

compromise necessary to maintain architectural integrity and radial strength of the non-metallic poly-L-lactic acid composition. There seems to be a relationship between strut thickness and restenosis, with larger struts exacting more vascular injury and greater restenotic tendency.[18,19] Strut thickness also has an influence on stent thrombosis. Indeed, minimizing strut thickness and adequate expansion are critical in reducing thrombogenicity.[20]

b. **Flexibility**
The balloon-mounted, undeployed stent should have reasonable flexibility to allow passage through a tortuous and/or rigid arterial segment. The concept is understandable to anyone who has moved furniture. The upper mattress of the bed with its separate and flexible coils is relatively easy to move around corners or down an angulated staircase in comparison to the rigid frame of the box spring. Flexibility must be balanced with maintenance of radial strength and adequate lesion coverage.[21]

5. **Radial strength**
Radial strength is the quantitative measure of the resistance to extrinsic compression maintaining its scaffold structure. This resistance can be measured quantitatively and is important given the extrinsic forces of the moving vessel. Slotted tubes in general have greater radial strength than coil designs. Close cell designs also enhance radial strength but compromise conformability and side branch access compared with open-cell configurations.[22] Though stent thickness is proportionally related to radial strength, thicker struts incur greater vascular injury and potential for restenosis. Strut thickness has decreased over time (e.g. 152.6 μm Cypher, 88.6 μm XIENCE V).

Material composition is a critical feature in radial strength. Reduction of thickness of stainless steel reduces flexibility but compromises radial strength as well as visibility. Chromium–cobalt composition maintains radial strength with thinner struts (80 μm) with a slight improvement of visibility/radio-opacity. ORSIRO Stent (Biotrinik, Bulach, Switzerland) consists of ultrathin cobalt-chromium L605 struts (60 um), but covered with amorphous silicon carbide layer. With thinner struts, however, recoil is affected. Platinum chromium alloys permit thin strut architecture with preservation of radial strength/conformability and enhance radio-opacity.[23-26] Thinner struts also reduce vascular injury, reduce side branch occlusion and promote earlier and complete strut endothelial restoration. Maintaining radial strength is especially critical in aorto-ostial and calcific lesions. Hence, newer alloys optimise radial strength whilst reducing the unfavourable consequences of thick bulkier struts. Finally, the newer bioresorbable vascular scaffold systems are resorbed over time and hence the structure loses its radial strength but importantly only beyond the important first 6 months of vascular healing and remodelling.

6. **Recoil**

Recoil, the ability of the stent to maintain its immediate expanded diameter following balloon (or self-expansion) deployment is an important characteristic. There should be minimal recoil to prevent inadequate final stent diameter and malapposition and the inherent risk of stent thrombosis and restenosis. Balloon-expandable stents vary in the degree of recoil. The original self-expanding varieties were theoretically excellent in this regard but in calcified lesions had paradoxically more acute recoil compared to balloon-expandable stents.[27] The new STENTYS system (STENTYS, Paris, France) is nitinol-based and expands after deployment and hence can more aptly accommodate to the entire length of a tapered vessel or, in clot laden arteries at the site of plaque rupture following initial deployment, expanding and apposing the vessel wall as clot is eventually reabsorbed. Hence, minimising the recoil tendency is important in preventing malapposition and stent thrombosis.

As the largest coronary stents are expanded, there are differences in the maximal diameter achieved with a 6.0-mm high-pressure balloon dilatation – which may have relevance for left main or vein graft intervention. Inability to achieve the desired diameter, that is to say a significant degree of recoil, will result in stent malapposition. The minimal lumen internal diameter after inflation with a 6-mm non-compliant balloon at 14 atm varied depending on stent design (5.4 mm Integrity, 5.6 mm Xience Prime, 5.7 mm Promus Element and 5.9 mm Biomatrix). Deformation of the individual stent cell with over expansion of the stent can result in increased propensity of tissue prolapse and reduces the effective coverage by anti-proliferative/immunosuppressive agents. When approaching their stretching limit, stent struts become progressively straightened and may form a quasi-circular configuration. Cell opening diameters were largest with Biomatrix, intermediate with Integrity and smallest with the Element design in a study using *in vitro* micro-computed tomography (CT) analysis to assess the morphological stent changes after overexpansion of each stent design. Knowledge of these characteristics is important in choosing the appropriate stent for large vessels, especially the left main coronary artery.[28] Medtronic Inc. recently announced an expanded size matrix (4.5-5 mm) for the Resolute Onyx DES, of particular relevance to large vessels, especially the left main. The dense core metal is wrapped in a cobalt alloy outer layer for increased radio-opacity, has thinner struts to improve deliverability through challenging lesions while maintaining radial and longitudinal strength with its CoreWire Technology, and potentially preserves conformability in bifurcation lesions. Its utility in left main lesions allows interventional cardiology to better tackle unmet clinical needs in patients who are high-risk surgical candidates. The unexpanded stent profile still facilitates a transradial approach, for ease of operator use. Having a more sizeable DES that caters to the larger diameter of the left main artery prevents the need to post dilate and potentially overstretch smaller stents into this vessel, which impacts the ideal stent-to-artery ratio and drug concentration, and can disrupt the polymer coating and/or fracture the thin stent struts lending to higher rates of restenosis.

7. **Conformability**

Conformability, defined as the ability to maintain vessel tortuosity/vessel geometry following stent implantation. This property reduces potential for vascular injury that can occur with excessive vessel straightening and foreshortening. Once delivered to a lesion, it is desirable for the vessel to maintain an approximation of its original shape and motion through the cardiac cycle (see Figure 12.2).[29] Conformability can be quantified using the change in angulation and changes in curvature

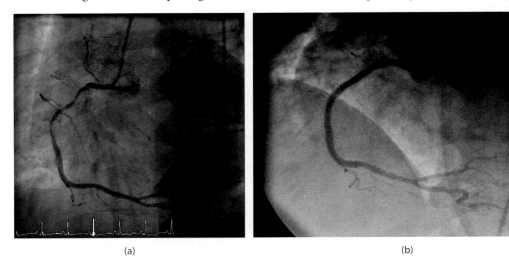

(a)   (b)

Figure 12.2 Conformability. **(a)** *De novo* lesion in proximal to mid–right coronary artery (RCA) with moderate tortuosity. **(b)** Following placement of an **open-celled single long modular** drug-eluting stent, a very conformable device, there is maintenance of the general curvature but loss of the more subtle bends in the vessel.

(1/radius of an approximated centreline of the involved segments). This is a complex relationship between stent and vessel architecture. Low conformability (excessive straightening of the curve segment can affect the adjacent non-stented segments occasionally leading to the juxta-stent kinking or pseudo-stenosis). On the other hand, excessive vasomotion of the stented segment can lead to stent fracture. The inner curvature of a tortuous segment has lower wall stress, which potentially could impart greater intimal hyperplasia within the implanted stent at that point. Hence, conformability has both positive and negative implications for the stented vessel.

Design characteristics and material clearly influence conformability of vascular stents. Open-cell designs impart greater flexibility and conformability, but sacrifice uniformity of scaffolding and, with less tissue coverage, may adversely affect distribution and effectiveness of anti-proliferative medication. Bioreabsorbable scaffold designs composed of poly-L-lactic acid have enhanced conformability compared with the MultiLink Vision stent.[30]

8. **Scaffolding**

Scaffolding refers to the ability of the stent to adequately cover the vessel wall and prevent plaque prolapse. Closed-cell (compared with open cell) designs have better scaffolding and radial force, which become more apparent on the greater curvature of a bend. The sacrifice is reduction in conformability and side branch access.

9. **Radio-opacity**

Visibility with fluoroscopic imaging is an important feature of coronary stents. Ensuring adequate lesion coverage and avoidance of geographic miss is paramount for stent deployment. In complex cases, necessitating precise placement proximal and distal to important side branches, ensuring adequate but not excessive stent overlap, in the absence of intravascular imaging modalities having confidence that full and uniform stent expansion is achieved are factors inherently linked to appropriate visualisation of the deployed stents. Post-deployment high-pressure balloon expansion depends on adequate stent edge visualisation. Imprecision can lead to under expansion of stent edges or, conversely, excessive balloon overhang with damage to the juxta-stent region. Stent visualisation can be particularly challenging in obese patients or densely calcified lesions. Excessive radio-opacity, on the other hand, obscures visualisation of the intra-stent region potentially affecting angiographic evaluation of restenosis. As radio-opacity was sacrificed for thinner stainless steel struts, gold markers were placed on the ends or used to coat stents. However, the coating leads to higher rates of restenosis. Platinum chromium is a superior balance of radio-opacity and the other important stent characteristics including maintenance of radial strength (e.g. PROMUS Premier stent). The ABSORB bioresorbable vascular scaffold system uses platinum makers at proximal and distal ends for fluoroscopic landmarking given the reduced radio-opacity of the structure per se.

10. **Side branch access**

There may be need to intervene upon side branches of significant size following main branch intervention as a prospective dedicated strategy or on a bail-out/provisional basis. Knowledge of the stent cell size dilatation capacity unique to that structure can be important in its selection for this very purpose. The diameter to which stent cells can be dilated varies with the type of stent as well as the angulation of the side branch from the main vessel. From a study evaluating stent cell dilatation capacity for the 3 mm stent size, even the stent with the lowest diameter side branch aperture, i.e., CYPHER (Cordis Corp., Miami Lakes, Florida) would still accommodate a 3 mm balloon or side branch stent. The ENDEAVOUR Stent (Medtronic, Inc., Minneapolis, Minnesota) had the largest diameter stent cell dilatation capacity at 6.3 mm with PROMUS (Boston Scientific, Maple Grove, Minnesota) and PROKINITIC (Biotrinik, Bulach, Switzerland) being intermediate.[31] If a cell is entered into a side branch for the purpose of balloon dilatation of an obstructing ostial plaque/dissection or a dedicated T-stent is intended, it is often preferable to enter the side branch distal to the most distal strut covering the ostium. This will allow some of the stent architecture to cover the proximal free wall of the side branch opposite the carina upon expansion. It should always be kept in mind that dilatation of the side branch ostium alone (through the stent cell) will deform the main stent just distal to the side branch. This can be rectified with the kissing balloon technique (followed by a proximal optimization dilatation).[32]

The following chart illustrates the relative degree of radio-opacity and advantages/disadvantages of these radiographic characteristics (Table 12.2):

Table 12.2 Advantages/disadvantages of coronary stent radio-opacity

Highly radio-opaque

Gives better impression of stent expansion

More accurate placement for overlapping serial stents

Stent-strut fracture is more evident

Obscures the in-stent visualization and assessment important to guide management for the possible restenosis (intravascular imaging may be required)

More radiolucent

Provides better visualization of in-stent material/debris (restenosis, thrombosis, tissue prolapse)

A challenge to ensure optimal stent overlap

Stent fracture is less evident

Extensive and dense calcification can obscure stent visualization

10. **Accuracy of placement**

Once the undeployed stent is positioned across the lesion, the operator requires confidence that it can be deployed precisely at this location to ensure the necessary coverage of the lesion and, in some cases, accurately avoid certain anatomical landmarks (e.g. side branches). One of the disadvantages of self-expanding stents is the skill needed to ensure accurate placement and expansion as the sheath is retracted (i.e., Newton's third law states that a slight forward advancement of the stent occurs as the sheath is withdrawn distally). The skilled operator can make the necessary adjustments to minimise this effect. Moreover, early recognition of geographic miss can be rectified by recapturing partially deployed stents in some of the models.

Current technology is predominantly balloon expandable. Independent of the stent itself is the issue of to-and-fro motion of the undeployed stent, which occasionally can lead to bobbing of the balloon stent catheter delivery system with the systolic/diastolic excursion of the heart. Ensuring adequate guiding catheter intubation, distal guidewire advancement and (very rarely) slowing of the heart rate with intravenous beta blocker can help overcome this phenomenon. The opaque markers on the balloon shaft referenced 0.4 mm beyond the proximal and distal stent edges facilitate precise placement and indeed markers have actually been manufactured on the stent edges themselves on some devices (the former BeStent and the current Absorb).

Newer radiographic capabilities such as *StentBoost* on Philips angiographic equipment enhances visualisation of the stent and especially helpful with subsequent precise high-pressure balloon inflation technique to ensure adequate edge expansion yet avoid trauma to adjacent non-stented segments as well as enable optimal visualisation for stent overlap.

One cannot overemphasise to the operator the importance of having the most optimal view of the diseased segment, to display it as longitudinal as possible, free of vessel overlap in order to ensure accurate device placement. Also important to consider is the potential for longitudinal shortening of stents upon expansion. The degree of shortening varies depending on material and stent design (up to 4% on average with some varieties, occasionally greater than 10%). Hence, a slightly longer stent to account for this issue may be necessary with certain designs.[33]

11. **Biocompatibility**

Stents and their coatings, including polymers and drug-eluting chemicals must be biocompatible to reduce the chance of hypersensitivity reactions and minimise thrombotic/restenotic tendencies from the material per se.

12.3 Drug-eluting stents

1. **Stents/scaffolds**

A number of fixed barriers on the stent surface were evaluated in the past (heparin, gold, silicon), but these coatings provided little benefit in reducing the restenotic process.[34] In order to reduce the frequency and prevent symptoms associated with restenosis, drug-eluting stents were eventually developed. The concept of drug-eluting stents (DES) involves the release of an anti-proliferative/immunosuppressive pharmacologic agent during the period of time when the vascular neointimal proliferative response is most active. A controlled and predictable release is the objective and achieved through either binding the chemical polymer coating to the stent strut surface or released through extrusion from ports on the abluminal surface.

Drug elution has certainly added a new dimension to coronary intravascular therapy.[35] Experience from the first-generation DES models has shown substantial clinical benefit in reducing restenosis balanced against small but definite rise in inflammatory response, late malapposition, impaired re-endothelialisation and late stent thrombosis. This knowledge is a testament to the rigid clinical plus angiographic/intravascular imaging surveillance of this cohort of patients. Research has focused on the stent platform (switch from the thick strut 316L stainless steel to thinner cobalt–chromium/platinum chromium platforms; bioreabsorbable scaffolds), the binding polymer, polymer-free abluminal reservoirs as well as the anti-proliferative/immunosuppressive agents themselves.

2. **Polymer coatings**

Polymers adhered to the stent surface bind and permit controlled release (elution) of the anti-proliferative/immunosuppressive medication. The polymers affixed to first-generation DES were permanent/durable consisting of SIBS (polystyrene-b-isobutylene-b-styrene) for TAXUS stent (Boston Scientific, Natick, Massachusetts) eluting 10% of paclitaxel over the first 10 days (the remainder fixed) and PEVA (polyethylene-co-vinyl acetate)/PBMA (polyhexyl methacrylate) for CYPHER stent (Cordis Corp, Miama, Florida) eluting 80% of the sirolimus during the first 30 days.

Polymer-induced chronic inflammation and impaired vascular healing potentially leading to late thrombosis was a concern with these first-generation devices. The risk of very late stent thrombosis was low (0.2%–0.6%/year) and was balanced by reduced repeat revascularisation and restenosis with its own inherent risk of myocardial infarction.[36]

Everolimus (XIENCE, Abbott Vascular and PROMUS, Boston Scientific) elution occurs (80%) over 30 days and zotarolimus (RESOLUTE, Medtronic, Inc.) elution occurs (80%) over the first 60 days, both from durable polymers, PMBA + PVDF – HFP (copolymer of vinylidene fluoride/hexafluoropropylene) and PMBA/polyhexyl methacrylate (PHMA)/olyvinylpyrrolidone (PVP)/polyvinyl acetate (PVA), respectively.

The novel EluNIR™ stent (EluNIR™, Medinol, Israel) elutes ridaforolimus from the 80 um-thin cobalt-chromium alloy (95%) over 180 days linked to a durable elastomer polymer coating, which further eliminates irregularities and prevents cracking or peeling on the stent surface through a smooth elastic surface that provides uniform drug elution to the vessel wall. Kandzari and colleagues, in reporting their BIONICS study, showed comparable target lesion failure of 5.4% at 12 months for EluNIR™ and Resolute Integrity stents (p=0.0013 for non-inferiority), and non significant stent thrombosis of 0.4% vs 0.8%, respectively. The NIREUS study also revealed non-inferiority of 6 month angiographic in-stent late loss, and non-significance of 12 month

Biodegradable polymers are available and early studies demonstrate safety and efficacy compared to durable-based polymer systems in treatment of simple de novo lesions, rather than of chronic total occlusions.[39] The biolimus BIOMATRIX drug-eluting stent (Biosensors International, Singapore) consists of poly-lactic acid polymer on its abluminal surface, which is metabolised within 6–9 months to lactic acid, water and carbon dioxide. Drug delivery occurs over 30 days. The biodegradable polymer Yukon Choice PC showed comparable clinical outcomes at 5 years in a randomised trial against the permanent polymer XIENCE stent.[40] The SYNERGY System (Boston Scientific, Marlborough, Massachusetts) consists of a thin-strut (74 um), platinum chromium metal alloy stent with an ultrathin 4 um bioabsorbable poly (D,L-lactide-co-glycolide) polymer applied on the abluminal surface biodegrading as it elutes everolimus over 3 months. The bare luminal surface promotes earlier endothelialisation and less risk of inflammatory response. This system was non-inferior to the PROMUS Element Plus everolimus-eluting stent with respect to 1-year target lesion failure.[41] The ORSIRO Stent (Biotronik, Bulach, Switzerland) consists of ultra-thin cobalt-chromium L605 struts (60 um) covered with amorphous silicon carbide layer (applied via a plasma-enhanced chemical vapour deposition technique to reduce tissue reaction to metal) and a bio-degradable poly-L-lactic acid eluting sirolimus. The polymer degrades over 12-24 months. It proved to be non-inferior to Xience Prime in terms of late lumen loss at 9 months.[42] The ULTRAMASTER cobalt-chromium L605 Stent (Terumo Corp., Tokyo, Japan) consists of sirolimus bound to poly (D,L-lactide-co-caprolactone). Applied only on the abluminal side, it also is coated in a gradient fashion avoiding parts of

the stent with high physical stress, thereby reducing the chance of polymer cracking and delamination.[43] The BIO-RESORT study was the first to analyze all-comers, showing non-inferiority in patients treated with biodegradable polymer DES (Synergy, Boston Scientific and Orsiro, Biotronik) versus durable polymer DES (Resolute Integrity, Medtronic Inc.). The potential long-term benefits (e.g., of improved arterial healing) can next be assessed, given this pre-requisite early safety and efficacy of biodegradable polymer DES.[44] TRANSFORM-OCT compares in-stent neoatherosclerosis up to 18 months in follow-up between the Synergy and Resolute Integrity stents; early results report no difference but have lower overall event rates.[45] In contrast, early findings from PRISON IV show that the Orsiro stent does not meet non-inferiority against the Xience stent for in-segment late lumen loss but has higher binary restenosis (8% vs 2.1%; p=0.028). However, this is in the setting of chronic total occlusions (CTOs) and performance in a broader range of lesions remains to be determined.[46]

Delivery without polymer has been developed using ports on the abluminal surface, with gradual release from the intra-strut reservoir. This avoids exposure to potentially pro-inflammatory chemicals.[47] Medtronic (Minneapolis, Minnesota) has developed a polymer-free drug-filled stent. It is actually tri-layered with an outer cobalt-chromium shell, middle tantalum layer, and inner sirolimus nucleus. Laser drilled holes on the abluminal surface permit drug elution. The RevElution trial assessed 50 patients at 9 months following deployment illustrating very high rates of strut coverage by OCT (99%) and non-inferior late lumen loss compared to historical RESOLUTE data.[48]

3. **Anti-proliferative/immunosuppressive pharmacologic agents**
These agents are highly lipophilic and exert their effect on the smooth muscle cells of the arterial wall. Paclitaxel (TAXUS) binds to β-tubulin subunit of microtubules resulting in inhibition of microtubular assembly and arrest of cell replication in G_0–G_1 and mitotic phases. The *limus* analogues (everolimus, zotarolimus and biolimus) bind to FKBP12, inhibiting mTOR – mammalian target of rapamycin, upregulation of cyclin-dependent kinase inhibitor p27Kip1, blocking smooth muscle cell proliferation during G_1 phase of the cell cycle.

Commonly used agents include everolimus (e.g. XIENCE, Abbott Vascular, Santa Clara, California and PROMUS, Boston Scientific, Maple Grove, Minnesota), zotarolimus (e.g. RESOLUTE, Medtronic Inc., Minneapolis, Minnesota), sirolimus (e.g. ORSIRO, Biotrinik, Bulach, Switzerland), and biolimus-eluting stainless steel (e.g. BIOMATRIX-FLEX, Biosensors International, Singapore).[49,50]

12.4 Bioresorbable vascular scaffolds

The concept of a degradable stent has been a theoretically attractive concept to overcome some of the problems inherent with a permanent vascular metallic prosthesis. These include risks of late stent thrombosis, restenosis and neo-atherosclerosis, persistent inflammation, loss of normal vessel curvature and impaired vasomotion with potential for strut fracture. Fully bioresorbable stents must provide mechanical support to allow for remodelling (as well as a platform for elution of anti-proliferative agents to retard restenosis) over the first 3–6 months, with gradual bioreabsorption thereafter, often complete after 2 years.

The Igaki-Tamai poly-L-lactic acid coronary stent (Kyoto Medical Planning Co., Ltd., Kyoto, Japan) was the first bioabsorbable vascular scaffolds (BVS) used in humans.

The ABSORB bioresorbable vascular scaffold (Abbott Vascular) consists of a 150-µm thick bioresorbable poly-L-lactide scaffold with a 7-µm thick bioresorbable poly (D,L-lactide) coating facilitating elution of everolimus. The balloon-expandable frame consists of an architecture of circumferential in-phase hoops linked by straight bridges providing uniform vessel coverage and radial strength approaching the MultiLink stent. Though there is a crossing profile of 1.4 mm, it requires adequate vessel pre-dilatation prior to insertion. Radio-opaque platinum markers at each end aid in visibility. It is recommended to have a low threshold to utilise intravascular imaging to guide optimal placement, sizing and expansion, and there is a narrower post-dilation capacity compared to metallic stents. A large, multicentre trial, involving 2008 patients with stable or unstable angina, randomised in a 2:1 ratio to receive an everolimus-eluting bioresorbable vascular (ABSORB) scaffold or an everolimus-eluting cobalt–chromium (Xience) stent was recently reported. Noninferiority for target lesion failure at 1 year was confirmed in the statistical analysis (7.8% of patients in the Absorb group vs. 6.1% of patients in the Xience group, $p = .007$ for noninferiority). As treated analysis revealed target lesion failure rates of 8.0% and 6.0%, respectively, still statistically noninferior. Device thrombosis in the first year after implantation occurred in 1.5% of patients in the Absorb group versus 0.7% of patients in the Xience group ($p = .13$).[51] Event rates (including stent thrombosis) seem to be less when BVS is utilized for lesions with reference vessel diameters greater than 2.25 mm. Long-term outcomes of the Absorb scaffold are in progress: Absorb China shows ongoing noninferiority at two-years and ABSORB III long-term data are eagerly awaited. In the ABSORB II study, BVS did not meet non-inferiority with respect to vasomotion or late-lumen loss compared to Xience.[52,53,54]

The novolimus-eluting (a metabolite of sirolimus, macrocyclic lactone mTOR inhibitor with potent anti-proliferative properties) DESolve bioresorbable poly-L-lactic acid coronary scaffold system (Elixir Medical, Sunnyvale, California) showed an acceptable 0.20 ± 0.32 mm in-scaffold late lumen loss at 6 months when evaluated in 126 patients.[55]

Magnesium forms the base for another currently used BVS platform providing radial support for 9–12 months and potentially less risk of fracture. The electronegative charge that develops during degradation is potentially antithrombotic. There is higher inherent mechanical strength which allows for thinner struts (120 µm). DREAMS magnesium alloy (Biotronik, Berlin, Germany) combined with a limus anti-proliferative agent illustrates encouraging angiographic, IVUS and clinical results in a small clinical study involving 123 subjects.[56]

The ReZolve 2 BVS (Reva Medical, Inc., San Diego, CA) is produced on a desaminotyrosine polycarbonate platform (polycarbonate co-polymer of tyrosine analogues) offers radial support for 6 months followed a gradual resorption process over 1–2 years. Interestingly, water, ethanol and carbon dioxide are the degradation products. The device is combined with sirolimus. The Ideal BioStent (Xenogenics Corp., Canton, Massachusetts/MultiCell Technologies Inc., Woonsocket, Rhode Island), also combined with sirolimus, is composed of a poly-lactic anhydride containing two salicylic acid molecules linked to a sebacic acid molecule degrading to salicylate, water and carbon dioxide by 15 months.

12.5 Specialty stents

Though these will be more thoroughly discussed in later chapters, the following is a sample of the various derivatives and innovative designs beyond the traditional coronary stent frame, designed to address the many complexities of coronary artery disease.

1. **Biologically coated stents**
   The Genous bioengineered Cobalt Chromium (CoCr) stent is an example of a biologically coated stent. This structure combines thin stent struts (80 µm), dual helix design. The unique feature is the incorporation of endothelial progenitor cells (EPCs) capture technology utilising anti-CD34 antibodies on the stent surface. EPCs promote healing through accelerated endothelial regeneration. The new Combo stent combines an abluminal bioresorbable polymer combined with sirolimus and luminal EPC capturing technology mounted on a dual helical stent design. The REMEDEE Registry involving 1000 patients was reported at the Transcatheter Cardiovascular Therapeutics meeting in San Francisco on 11–15 October 2015. It was designed to evaluate the COMBO Dual Therapy Stent for the treatment of coronary lesions in the routine clinical care. One-year target lesion failure was 5.7%, including 1.7% cardiac death, 0.7% target vessel myocardial infarction and 4.4% ischemia-driven target lesion revascularisation. The stent thrombosis rate was low at 0.6%, which tended to occur early.

2. **Barrier devices – Embolic protection**
   Mesh stents were developed to reduce the embolisation of thrombotic debris in the setting of acute myocardial infarction and in diseased saphenous vein grafts

with friable atheroma. MGuard (InspireMD, Boston, Massachusetts) is an example, composed of 316L stainless steel bare metal balloon-expandable stent (100 μm strut thickness) covered with a biostable 20-μm polymer (polyethylene terephthalate) MICRONET mesh attached to the proximal and distal crowns of the stent. The MICRONET expands along with the stent resulting in a pore size of 150–180 μm. When compared with commercially available stents (40% of which were drug eluting), there was improved ST segment resolution and a trend towards improved mortality in the setting of acute myocardial infarction at the expense of increased target-lesion ischemic-driven revascularisation.[57] The MGuard Prime composed of CoCr with strut thickness of 80 μm enhances flexibility and deliverability.

3. **Barrier devices – Covered stents**

Covered stents are utilised for coronary arterial (or saphenous vein graft) rupture or perforation as a result of complications arising from interventional procedures or occasionally to exclude coronary fistulae or aneurysms. They are highly effective at covering and sealing the site of vessel perforation, halting the extravasation potentially leading to catastrophic haemopericardial tamponade. Poly-tetrafluoroethylene (PTFE) covered stents for coronary and saphenous vein graft use are available and examples include the Symbiot™ covered stent system (Boston Scientific), which consists of a double layer of expandable PTFE surrounding a self-expanding nitinol stent and the Jostent GraftMaster Coronary Stent Graft (Abbott, Abbott Park, Illinois) consisting of a single PTFE layer sandwiched between two coaxial 316L stainless steel balloon-expandable stents. They are less deliverable than simple stents due to the coating (and in the some cases, two concentric layers of stents) and usually require adequate lesion pre-dilatation. With its single-layer covered-stent design, the PK Papyrus (BIOTRONIK, Berlin) has greater flexibility and a 24% smaller crossing profile. Though highly effective to seal perforations, covered stents are not effective at reducing distal embolisation when utilised in degenerated saphenous vein grafts. Every interventional facility should carry an array of sizes and lengths of the covered stent, at arm's length availability for these rare but often unexpected complications (Figure 12.3).

4. **Bifurcation stents**

The challenge of bifurcation lesions will be addressed in a later chapter. Single- or two-stent techniques (e.g. crush, T-stent, culotte) utilising conventional stents will be described in this dedicated chapter. There are, however, broad categories of specialty stents designed for bifurcation lesions.

a. **Dedicated side branch stents**

Tryton Side Branch Stent (Tryton Medical, Durham, North Carolina) is an example of this technology utilising CoCr design with markers to indicate the transition zone. It is deployed in the side branch artery using a standard single-wire,

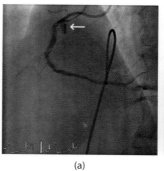 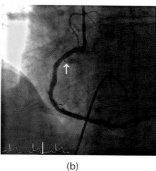

(a)   (b)

Figure 12.3 Covered stent. **(a)** Perforation in the proximal RCA following rotational atherectomy. A contained extravasation is evident (horizontal arrow). **(b)** A covered Jostent GraftMaster Coronary Stent Graft (Abbott, Abbott Park, Illinois) is implanted across the area of vessel perforation. Careful observation reveals a continued leak (vertical arrow), which was eventually sealed after high-pressure dilatation within the covered stent with a non-compliant balloon.

balloon-expandable stent delivery system. Subsequently, the main branch is rewired through the ostial gap in the open architecture of the Tryton stent allowing for placement and incorporation of a conventional drug-eluting stent for the main vessel, with complete lesion coverage. Recent studies have suggested this device combined with a DES in the main branch is safe with comparable outcomes for both the side branch and main branch when compared with a main vessel DES plus balloon angioplasty of the side branch strategy.[58]

b. **Stents to facilitate side branch access**

Stenting of the main branch by definition may cross the origin of a significant side branch. Access through the strut of a conventional stent (preferably closest to the carina) can be achieved with the guidewire with subsequent balloon dilatation of the stent strut. Balloon and/or stent access to the side branch is thus facilitated. The STENTYS nitinol-based stent (bare metal or drug-eluting varieties) is deployed in the main branch by a semi-compliant balloon catheter with resultant splitting of the retractable sheath in order to allow auto-expansion. With subsequent crossing and expansion of strut leading into the side branch with a balloon catheter, the small distinctive interconnectors are designed to fracture/cleave, enhancing side branch access for a conventional stent as well as facilitating coverage of the outer wall of the side branch opposite from the carina. This optimal flaring is dependent on crossing the side branch through struts adjacent to the carina such that the detached wing of stent can be lifted proximally to cover the wall opposite the carina.

The Axxess stent (BioSensors International, Singapore) is a dedicated self-expanding nitinol stent that is deployed in a flared, skirt-like fashion in the proximal vessel abutting the level of the carina. By optimising treatment of the proximal limb, it provides slight coverage of the ostia of two branches on the outer wall opposite from the carina. It is most appropriate if the angle of bifurcation is not excessive in order to ensure there is appropriate apposition to the side branch outer wall by this flared stent. Hence, the architecture of the bifurcation is preserved and allows separate stent access to each branch if needed. The stent is abluminally coated with a biodegradable poly-lactic acid (PLA) polymer releasing the immunosuppressive Biolimus A9 (BA9), to reduce restenosis.

The BIOSS stent (Balton Inc., Warsaw, Poland) consists of a tapered profiled balloon delivering a stent (bare metal or drug-eluting) with a large cell, in its mid segment, positioned across the side branch ostium, protecting the carina and permitting open and unopposed access to the opposite branch should an additional conventional stent be required. In comparison to standard DES bifurcation strategy, the sirolimus BIOSS LIM strategy resulted in less binary restenosis rates provided final kissing balloon inflation was undertaken (5.9% vs. 11.8%, $p < .05$).[59] A proximal to distal vessel angle <180° theoretically reduces the strut gap opposite the side branch and optimally opens the gap towards the side branch ostium.

The Nile stent (Minvasys, Gennevilliers, France) is a 6F compatible CoCr alloy stent bare metal (73-μm thickness) or with polymer-free abluminal paclitaxel elution (+5 μm). The stent has proximal, middle and distal zones, and designed such that the distal and middle segments are detached on one side to allow flaring into the side branch. The delivery system involves two independent monorail balloon catheters, one designed for main branch stent deployment in and the other for expansion of the stent towards the side branch. The stent is advanced over two guidewires (one through the main branch balloon catheter and the side branch guidewire exiting through the gap between the middle and distal stent segments). Occasionally, entanglement of guide wires requires system withdrawal to enable rewiring. Three radiopaque markers on the main balloon catheter ensure accurate positioning once the device reaches the desired position at the bifurcation. Sequential deployment of the main branch balloon is followed by advancement of a second balloon into the side branch. Guidewire access to the two branches is maintained. After kissing balloon inflation, proximal optimisation technique may be necessary to correct malapposition of the proximal segment.

References

1. Lincoff AM et al. Abrupt vessel closure complicating coronary angioplasty: Clinical, angiographic and therapeutic profile. *J Am Coll Cardiol* 1992; 19(5): 926–35.
2. King SB 3rd et al. Balloon angioplasty versus new device intervention: Clinical outcomes. A comparison of the NHLBI PTCA and NACI registries. *J Am Coll Cardiol* 1998; 31(3): 558–66.
3. Sigwart U et al. Emergency stenting for acute occlusion after coronary balloon angioplasty. *Circulation* 1988; 78: 1121–7.
4. Schatz RA et al. Clinical experience with the Palmaz-Schatz coronary stent. Initial results of a multicenter study. *Circulation* 1991; 83(1): 148–61.
5. Fischman DL et al. A randomized comparison of coronary-stent placement and balloon angioplasty in the treatment of coronary artery disease. Stent Restenosis Study Investigators. *N Engl J Med* 1994; 331(8): 496–501.
6. Serruys PW et al. A comparison of balloon-expandable-stent implantation with balloon angioplasty in patients with coronary artery disease. Benestent Study Group. *N Engl J Med* 1994; 331(8): 489–95.
7. Colombo A et al. Intracoronary stenting without anti-coagulation accomplished with intravascular ultrasound guidance. *Circulation* 1995; 91(6): 1676–88.
8. Karrillon GJ et al. Intracoronary stent implantation without ultrasound guidance and with replacement of conventional anticoagulation by antiplatelet therapy. 30-day clinical outcome of the French Multicenter Registry. *Circulation* 1996; 94(7): 1519–27.
9. Schömig A et al. A randomized comparison of antiplatelet and anticoagulant therapy after the placement of coronary-artery stents. *N Engl J Med* 1996; 334(17): 1084–9.
10. Colombo A et al. Selection of coronary stents. *J Am Coll Cardiol* 2002; 40(6): 1021–33.
11. Stoeckela D et al. A survey of stent designs. *Minim Invasive Ther Allied Technol* 2002; 11(4): 137–47.
12. Serruys P. (editors). *Handbook of Coronary Stents*, 1st Edition. London: Martin Dunitz Ltd, 1997.
13. Balcon R et al. Recommendations on stent manufacture, implantation and utilization. Study Group of the Working Group on Coronary Circulation. *Eur Heart J* 1997; 18(10): 1536–47.
14. Buchwald A et al. Initial clinical results with the Wiktor stent: A new balloon-expandable coronary stent. *Clin Cardiol* 1991; 14(5): 374–9.
15. Pentousis D et al. Preliminary clinical experience with the Bard XT coronary stent. *Am Heart J* 1998; 136(5): 786–91.
16. Sangiorgi G et al. Engineering aspects of stents design and their translation into clinical practice. *Ann Ist Super Sanita* 2007; 43(1): 89–100.
17. Schmidt W et al. Characteristic mechanical properties of balloon-expandable peripheral stent systems. *Rofo* 2002; 174(11): 1430–7.
18. Kastrati A et al. Intracoronary stenting and angiographic results: Strut thickness effect on restenosis outcome (ISAR-STEREO) trial. *Circulation* 2001; 103(23): 2816–21.

19. Pache J et al. Intracoronary stenting and angiographic results: Strut thickness effect on restenosis outcome (ISAR-STEREO-2) trial. *J Am Coll Cardiol* 2003; 41(8): 1283–8.

20. Kolandaivelu K et al. Stent thrombogenicity early in high-risk interventional settings is driven by stent design and deployment and protected by polymer-drug coatings. *Circulation* 2011 Apr 5;123(13): 1400-1409.

21. Schmitz KP et al. Interaction of radial strength and flexibility of coronary stents. *Biomed Tech (Berl)* 1998; 43 Suppl: 376–7.

22. Ormiston JA et al. Stent longitudinal integrity bench insights into a clinical problem. *JACC Cardiovasc Interv* 2011; 4(12): 1310–7.

23. Jorge C, and Dubois C. Clinical utility of platinum chromium bare-metal stents in coronary heart disease. *Med Devices (Auckl)* 2015; 8: 359–67.

24. Menown IB et al. The platinum chromium element stent platform: From alloy, to design, to clinical practice. *Adv Ther* 2010; 27(3): 129–41.

25. Bennett J, and Dubois C. A novel platinum chromium everolimus-eluting stent for the treatment of coronary artery disease. *Biologics* 2013; 7: 149–59.

26. O'Brien BJ et al. A platinum-chromium steel for cardiovascular stents. *Biomaterials* 2010; 31(14): 3755–61.

27. Duerig TW, and Wholey M. A comparison of balloon- and self-expanding stents. *Min Invas Ther & Allied Technol* 2002; 11(4): 173–8.

28. Foin N et al. Maximal expansion capacity with current DES platforms: A critical factor for stent selection in the treatment of left main bifurcations. *EuroIntervention* 2013; 8: 1315–25.

29. Choi G et al. Methods for quantifying three-dimensional deformation of arteries due to pulsatile and nonpulsatile forces: Implications for the design of stents and stent grafts. *Ann Biomed Eng* 2009; 37(1): 14–33.

30. Gomez-Lara J et al. A comparison of the conformability of everolimus-eluting bioresorbable vascular scaffolds to metal platform coronary stents. *JACC Cardiovasc Interv* 2010; 3(11): 1190–8.

31. Mortier, P et al. Comparison of drug-eluting stent cell size using micro-CT: important data for bifurcation stent selection. *EuroIntervention* 2008 Nov;4(3):391–396.

32. Ormiston JA et al. Stent deformation following simulated side-branch dilatation: a comparison of five stent designs. *Catheter Cardiovasc Interv.* 1999 Jun;47(2):258–264.

33. Yamada R et al. Impact of stent platform on longitudinal stent deformation: An in vivo frequency domain optical coherence tomography study. *Cardiovasc Interv Ther* 2016.

34. Kastrati A et al. Increased risk of restenosis after placement of gold-coated stents: Results of a randomized trial comparing gold-coated with uncoated steel stents in patients with coronary artery disease. *Circulation* 2000; 101(21): 2478–83.

35. Moses JW et al. Sirolimus-eluting stents versus standard stents in patients with stenosis in a native coronary artery. *N Engl J Med* 2003; 349(14): 1315–23.

36. Pendyala L et al. Passive and active polymer coatings for intracoronary stents: Novel devices to promote arterial healing. *J Interv Cardiol* 2009; 22(1): 37–48.

37. Kandzari DE et al. *BIONICS: A Prospective, Randomized Trial of a Ridaforolimus-Eluting Coronary Stent vs a Zotarolimus-Eluting Stent in a More-Comers Population of Patients With Coronary Artery Disease.* TCT2016. Oct 30, 2016. Washington, DC.

38. Smits PC et al. *The NIREUS Randomized Trial: One-Year Results of the BioNIR Ridaforolimus-Eluting Coronary Stent System (BioNIR) European Angiography Study.* TCT2016. Oct 31, 2016. Washington, DC.

39. Serruys PW et al. Improved safety and reduction in stent thrombosis associated with biodegradable polymer-based biolimus-eluting stents versus durable polymer-based sirolimus-eluting stents in patients with coronary artery disease: Final 5-year report of the LEADERS (Limus Eluted From A Durable Versus ERodable Stent Coating) randomized, noninferiority trial. *JACC Cardiovasc Interv* 2013; 6(8): 777–89.

40. Kufner S1 et al. Five-year outcomes from a trial of three limus-eluting stents with different polymer coatings in patients with coronary artery disease: Final results from the ISAR-TEST 4 randomised trial. *EuroIntervention* 2016; 11(12): 1372–9.

41. Kereiakes DJ, et al. Efficacy and safety of a novel bioabsorbable polymer-coated, everolimus-eluting coronary stent: The EVOLVE II Randomized Trial. *Circ Cardiovasc Interv.* 2015 Apr;8(4):e002372.

42. Windecker S et al. Comparison of a novel biodegradable polymer sirolimus-eluting stent with a durable polymer everolimus-eluting stent: results of the randomized BIOFLOW-II trial. *Circ Cardiovasc Interv.* 2015 Feb;8(2):e001441.

43. Saito N. et al. Drug diffusion and biological responses of arteries using a drug-eluting stent with nonuniform coating. *Medical Devices: Evidence and Research* 2016:9.

44. Von Birgelen C et al. Very thin strut biodegradable polymer everolimus-eluting and sirolimus-eluting stents versus durable polymer zotarolimus-eluting stents in allcomers with coronary artery disease (BIO-RESORT): a three-arm, randomized, non-inferiority trial. *Lancet* 2016 Nov 26;388(10060):2607-2617.

45. Guagliumi G et al. TRANSFORM-OCT: A prospective, randomized trial using OCT imaging to evaluate strut coverage at 3 months and neoatherosclerosis at 18 months in bioresorbable polymer-based and durable polymer-based drug-eluting stents. TCT2016. Nov 2, 2016. Washington, DC.

46. Teeuwen K et al. Randomized multicenter trial investigating angiographic outcomes of hybrid sirolimus-eluting stents with biodegradable polymer compared with everolimus-eluting stents with durable polymer in chronic total occlusions: The PRISON IV Trial. *JACC Cardiovasc Interv.* 2017 Jan 23; 10(2):133–143.

47. Abizaid A, and Costa JR. New drug-eluting stents: An overview on biodegradable and polymer-free next-generation stent systems. *Circ Cardiovasc Interv* 2010; 3(4): 384–93.

48. Worthley SG et al. First-in-Human Evaluation of a Novel Polymer-Free Drug-Filled Stent: Angiographic, IVUS, OCT, and Clinical Outcomes From the RevElution Study. *JACC Cardiovasc Interv* 2017 Jan 23;10(2):147–156.

49. Tsuchida K et al. One-year results of a durable polymer everolimus-eluting stent in de novo coronary narrowings (The SPIRIT FIRST Trial). *EuroIntervention* 2005; 1(3): 266–72.

50. Banerjee S. The resolute integrity zotarolimus-eluting stent in coronary artery disease: A review. *Cardiol Ther* 2013; 2(1): 17–25.

51. Ellis SG et al. Everolimus-Eluting bioresorbable scaffolds for coronary artery disease. *N Engl J Med* 2015; 373: 1905–15.

52. Gao R et al. *ABSORB China: Two-Year Clinical Results in Patients with Coronary Artery Disease Randomized to the Absorb Bioresorbable Vascular Scaffold Versus Metallic Drug-Eluting Stents*. TCT2016. Oct 30, 2016. Washington, DC.

53. Serruys PW et al. ABSORB II: Three-Year Clinical Outcomes from a Prospective, Randomized Trial of an Everoliumus-Eluting Bioresorbable Vascular Scaffold vs an Everolimus-Eluting Metallic Stent in Patients with Coronary Artery Disease. TCT2016. Oct 31, 2016. Washington, DC.

54. Serruys, PW et al. Comparison of an everolimus-eluting bioresorbable scaffold with an everolimus-eluting metallic stent for the treatment of coronary artery stenosis (ABSORB II): A 3-year, randomized, controlled, single-blind, multicenter trial. *Lancet* 2016.

55. Abizaid A et al. Serial multimodality imaging and 2 year clinical outcomes of the novel DESolve novolimus-eluting bioresorbable coronary scaffold system for the treatment of single de novo coronary lesions. *J Am Coll Cardiol Interv* 2016; 9(6): 565–74.

56. Haude M et al. Safety and performance of the second-generation drug-eluting absorbable metal scaffold in patients with de-novo coronary artery lesions (BIOSOLVE-II): 6 month results of a prospective, multicentre, non-randomised, first-in-man trial. *Lancet* 2016; 387(10013): 31–9.

57. Dudek D et al. Mesh-covered embolic protection stent implantation in ST-segment-elevation myocardial infarction: Final 1-year clinical and angiographic results from the MGUARD for acute ST elevation reperfusion trial. *Circ Cardiovasc Interv* 2015; 8(2): e001484.

58. Généreux P et al. A randomized trial of a dedicated bifurcation stent versus provisional stenting in the treatment of coronary bifurcation lesions. *J Am Coll Cardiol* 2015; 65(6): 533–43.

59. Gil RJ et al. Regular drug-eluting stents versus the dedicated coronary bifurcation sirolimus-eluting BiOSS LIM stent: The randomised, multicentre, open-label, controlled POLBOS II trial. *EuroIntervention* 2015; 11(7).

Coronary stenting II: New developments

SCOT GARG, HARRIET HURRELL

13.1 Introduction

Percutaneous coronary intervention (PCI) has evolved since the first metal devices were implanted into coronary arteries in the late 1980s.[1] These initial self-expanding devices were quickly replaced by balloon-expandable bare-metal stents (BMS)[2] and then at the turn of the twenty-first century by drug-eluting stents (DES).[3] These latter devices revolutionised interventional cardiology practice by dramatically reducing repeat revascularisations, and consequently there was renewed confidence in treating complex coronary artery.

Despite their benefits, these devices were not without their problems, and concerns were raised as to whether the price to pay for this improved efficacy was adverse safety following reports of increased rates of death and myocardial infarction (MI) due to stent thrombosis (ST) occurring many months after DES implantation.[4] Reassuringly, re-analyses of the pivotal randomised trials of the first-generation sirolimus-eluting and paclitaxel-eluting stents versus BMS using standardised outcomes as per the Academic Research Consortium definitions showed that the use of DES was not associated with any added risk of mortality or MI.[5] Notably, rates of ST, and in particular very-late (>1 year) ST, were non-significantly higher with DES, with particularly concern registry data reporting a continued ~0.4%–0.6% per year risk of very-late ST that persisted for at least 5 years after DES implantation.[6]

ST has always been a recognised undesirable complication of implanting intra-coronary devices (Figure 13.1)[7–11] with each event carrying a risk of mortality and MI of 33% and 70%–80%, respectively.[12] Early ST events are by

in large attributable to procedural factors such as stent under-deployment, or under-sizing.[13,14] The triggers for late/very-late ST are thought to be the pathological effects of delayed healing, impaired endothelialisation, inflammation, allergic reactions, neo-atherosclerosis, and vascular dysfunction within stented segments. The elution of cytotoxic and cytostatic drugs from the DES, together with the presence of permanent non-erodible polymers, has been cited as possibly mechanisms for these late events.[15] The lasting presence of the stent polymer, long after its effective function has ended, may also account for continued vascular healing which has been implicated in the phenomena of continual neointimal hyperplasia and the subsequent accrual of clinical events long after stent insertion.[16]

These safety concerns, particularly in relation to very-late ST, were a clear realisation that newer generations of DES were needed and provided the necessary stimulus for their development. These design modifications have centred on the three main components of the DES – the anti-proliferative coating, the polymer and the stent platform.

13.2 The anti-proliferative agent

The consistent benefits observed with DES over BMS in randomised and observational studies in all arrays of patient and lesion types have established that coronary stents should elute an anti-proliferative drug, whose purpose is to limit neointimal proliferation.[17,18] The first-generation DES eluted either the immunosuppressive macrocyclic lactone limus agent sirolimus or the anti-proliferative agent, paclitaxel (Figure 13.2). Notwithstanding the structural differences between these first-generation DES, comparative studies and

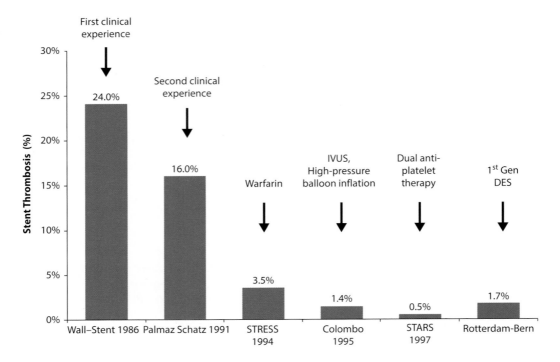

Figure 13.1 Temporal evolution in the incidence of definite stent thrombosis according to changes in adjunct pharmacotherapy, stent type (bare-metal or drug-eluting) and PCI technique. IVUS, intra-vascular ultrasound; DES, drug-eluting stent. The rate of acute (<24 hours) and subacute (1–14 days) stent thrombosis with the first coronary devices was 16%–24% despite using peri-procedural heparin, aspirin, dipyridamole and low-molecular-weight dextran.[7,8] To address this, warfarin was tried and successfully reduced stent thrombosis rates to 3.5%; however, its use lead to haemorrhagic complications in up to 10% of patients post-PCI.[9] Colombo et al. then showed that stent thrombosis could be reduced using IVUS, and high-pressure balloon inflation together with a combination of aspirin and ticlopidine instead of warfarin, dextran and dipyridamole.[10] Finally the randomised STARS study confirmed that DAPT with aspirin and ticlopidine was more effective at reducing stent thrombosis compared to aspirin monotherapy or aspirin and warfarin in combination.[11]

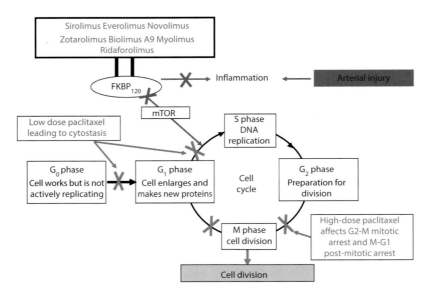

Figure 13.2 Mechanism of action of the two groups of anti-proliferative drugs used on drug-eluting stents. Macrocyclic lactones (biolimus A9, everolimus, myolimus, novolimus, sirolimus, ridaforolimus and zotarolimus) inhibit the mechanistic target of Rapamycin (mTOR) resulting in cell cycle arrest. Paclitaxel inhibits smooth muscle cell proliferation through the stabilisation of microtubules, thereby preventing cell division. FKBP, FK506-binding protein.

meta-analyses demonstrated significantly lower rates of late lumen loss, repeat revascularisation and ST with sirolimus-eluting stents (SES) compared to paclitaxel-eluting stents (PES).[18,19] Consequently, most contemporary DES elute limus agents, with paclitaxel largely being the anti-proliferative agent of choice to be released from drug-coated balloons.[20]

The array of contemporary limus agents, which have been developed through (1) modifications of the carbon atom 40 on the macrocyclic ring (zotarolimus, everolimus, biolimus and ridaforolimus); (2) removal of a methyl-group from carbon atom 16 (novolimus) or (3) replacement of the oxygen on carbon atom 32 of the macrocyclic ring (myolimus), offer differences in degrees of immunosuppression and liphophilicity, with the latter influencing the rate of drug absorption into the arterial wall.

Pre-clinical data exist to suggest that everolimus, sirolimus and zotarolimus have a comparable ability to suppress neointimal hyperplasia when controlling for stent platform, polymer, drug load and drug release kinetics.[21] In clinical practice, these variables differ considerably amongst stents making the direct link between these new agents and improved outcomes hard to determine. Setting these differences aside, DESs eluting sirolimus, everolimus, zotarolimus and biolimus have been compared with each other and BMS directly in randomised studies and their subsequent meta-analyses, and in-directly through network meta-analyses.[17,18,22–24] The fluoropolymer-coated thin-strut everolimus-eluting stent (EES, Abbott Vascular, Santa Clara, California) (Table 13.1) has the largest evidence base in terms of patient numbers and years of follow-up, and has consistently been shown to have the best combination of efficacy and safety.[17,18] For example, Palmerini's meta-analysis of over 51,000 patients at a median follow-up of 3.8 years concludes the following:[17]

1. EES is the only DES to show a significant reduction in all-cause mortality compared with BMS (HR 0.81, 95% CI 0.64–1.00, $p < .05$), SES (HR 0.86, 95% CI 0.70–1.00, $p < .05$) and PES (HR 0.81, 95% CI 0.68–1.00, $p < .05$), together with offering the greatest reduction in cardiac death versus BMS (HR 0.71, 95% CI 0.54–0.91, $p < .05$). No mortality reductions have been seen in the individual comparison of other DES with BMS or between DES.

2. EES significantly reduces the risk of MI compared with BMS (HR 0.66, 95% CI 0.52–0.85, $p < .05$), SES (HR 0.78, 95% CI 0.64–0.95, $p < .05$) and PES (HR 0.64, 95% CI 0.52–0.78, $p < .05$).

3. EES is the only DES to significantly reduce the rate of definite ST compared to BMS (HR 0.48, 95% CI 0.29–0.82, $p < .05$). Uniquely significant reductions have also been seen with EES versus PES (HR 0.42, 95% CI 0.27–0.64, $p < .05$) and EES versus biolimus-eluting stents (BES, HR 0.58, 95% CI 0.31–1.00, $p < .05$), whilst the significant reduction in ST compared with SES (HR 0.41, 95% CI 0.26–0.64 $p < .05$) was also seen with zotarolimus-eluting stents (ZES, Medtronic, Santa Rosa, California) versus SES (HR 0.55, 95% CI 0.36–0.93, $p < .05$).

4. EES offers the greatest reduction in target vessel revascularisation (TVR) compared to BMS (HR 0.34, 95% CI 0.19–0.57, $p < .05$). In comparison, other limus DES reduce the risk of TVR versus BMS with hazard ratios of 0.40–0.58 (all $p < .05$).

Factors behind these results with EES include the following:

- Elution of everolimus that is slightly more lipophilic than sirolimus, and therefore is more rapidly absorbed into the arterial wall.
- The stent platform has a strut thickness of 81 μm, and is coated with a 7.6-μm thick, non-erodible, co-polymer of polyvinylidene fluoride co-hexafluoropropylene (PVDF-HFP) and poly n-butyl methacrylate (PBMA), a combination that is potentially associated with less inflammation than SES and PES.[25]

Table 13.1 Specicifications of the second-generation permanet polymer DES

Stent	Drug (concentration)	Polymer	Polymer thickness (μm)	Release kinetics (days)	Metal	Geometry	Strut thickness (μm)
TAXUS Element	Paclitaxel (100 μg/cm²)	Poly(styrene-b-isobutylene-b-styrene)	15	<10% (90)	PtCr	Open cell	81
Endeavor	Zotarolimus (100 μg/cm²)	Phosphorylcholine	4.1	95% (14)	CoCr	Open cell	91
Endeavor RESOLUTE	Zotarolimus (10 μg/mm)	Biolinx	4.1	85% (60)	CoCr	Open cell	91
Xience V	Everolimus (100 μg/cm²)	PBMA and PVDF-HFP	7	80% (90)	CoCr	Open cell	81
PROMUS Element	Everolimus (100 μg/cm²)	PBMA and PVDF-HFP	7	80% (90)	PtCr	Open cell	81

CoCr, cobalt chromium; PBMA, poly-(n-butyl methacrylate); PtCr, platinum chromium; PVDF-HFP, poly-(vinylidene fluoride-co-hexafluoropropylene).

- The combination of thin-struts, the thrombo-resistant properties of the fluoropolymer and the reduced polymer and drug load may contribute to the low rates of ST with EES.[26]

13.3 The stent polymer

The stent polymer allows regulated release of anti-proliferative agents over a prescribed time period, with their function redundant once drug-elution has been completed. Polymers, in particular the non-biocompatible polymers utilised in the first-generation DES, have been shown to trigger hypersensitivity reactions, chronic inflammation, endothelial dysfunction and neo-atherosclerosis all of which have been implicated in delaying arterial healing, and thereby potentially causing late- and very-late ST.[12,25–27] In an effort to improve safety on the background of these accusations, together with a greater understanding of the polymer's function, efforts have been directed at improving polymer biocompatibility, reducing the polymer load, whilst new DES have been developed, which utilise polymers that biodegrade once their function (drug-elution) has been completed (Figure 13.3, Table 13.2), and DESs which do not use any polymer at all (Table 13.3).

13.3.1 Reducing polymer load

Historically, DES had a polymer coating on all sides (conformal); however, contemporary DESs now have polymer coatings just on their abluminal side (side away from the lumen). Whilst this reduces polymer 665 load which intuitively improves safety, data from studies comparing the Promus EES (Boston Scientific, Natick, Massachusetts) with a conformal polymer, to the Synergy EES (Boston Scientific) with an abluminal polymer show significantly greater endothelial

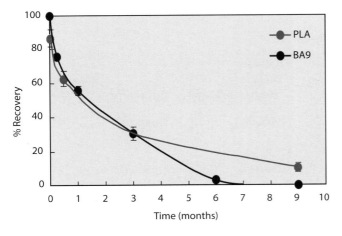

Figure 13.3 Temporal change in concentration of Biolimus A9 (BA9) and the poly-lactic acid (PLA) polymer on the BioMatrix stent (Biosensors, Morges, Switzerland). After 9 months, following drug elution and biodegradation of the PLA polymer, all that remains is the stainless steel stent platform.

coverage at 21 days with the abluminal polymer stent (72.5% coverage vs. 38.8%, $p < .001$). In addition, a greater concentration of VE-Cadherin was seen at cell junctions with the abluminal polymer stent, suggesting improved endothelial function.

13.3.2 Biodegradable polymers

The time-dependent need for stent polymers has led to the development of DES with biodegradable polymers. These devices offer the functions of a conventional DES at the time of deployment, whilst following polymer breakdown they offer the long-term safety benefits of a BMS. Establishing the optimal composition, biocompatibility, formulation and degradation time of the polymer has been a challenge. Of note, degradation times for contemporary biodegradable polymer DES vary for stents using, for example, poly-(DL-lactide/glycolide) co-polymer (PLGA), poly-lactic acid (PLA) and poly-caprolactone (PCL) to 2–3 months, 9 months and as long as 36 months, respectively (Table 13.2). Hand in hand with this is establishing the optimal pharmacokinetics of the anti-proliferative agent released by the degrading polymer. Finally, consideration is needed to deal with the acidic environment associated with the inflammatory reaction to polymer breakdown.

These conceptual challenges have not hindered the development of these devices, many of which have entered routine clinical use. As illustrated in Table 13.2, differences exist between these groups of devices in terms of stent platform, drug eluted and as mentioned previously drug elution kinetics and the polymer degradation time. The first generations of biodegradable polymer devices (BioMatrix BES, Biosensors, Morges, Switzerland, and Nobori BES, Terumo, Japan) have been in use for nearly a decade and have now been joined by a heterogeneous group of the second-generation biodegradable polymer devices which use a platform of cobalt or platinum chromium instead of stainless steel; elute other macrocyclic lactone inhibitors such as sirolimus, everolimus, novolimus and myolimus instead of biolimus have struts which are between 61 and 80 μm thick compared to 120–125 μm and have polymers with a thickness of 2–15 μm instead of 10–20 μm. These improvements have prompted development of a second iteration of the BioMatrix stent—BioMatrix alpha (Biosensors, Morges, Switzerland) that will be available in 2016, and whilst it utilises the same polymer and elutes biolimus, the platform will be made of cobalt chromium and have struts of 84 μm.

The only data comparing different biodegradable polymer devices comes from the SORT-OUT VII study, which randomised 2530 patients to treatment with the first-generation Nobori BES or the second-generation Orsiro SES (Biotronik, Germany).[28] The study met its primary endpoint of target lesion failure (TLF), a composite of cardiac death, target vessel MI and target-lesion revascularisation (TLR) with rates of 3.8% and 4.6% with the Orsiro and Nobori stent, respectively ($P_{non-inferior} < 0.001$).[29] No differences were

Table 13.2 Available metallic stents with a biodegradable polymer

Stent (manufacturer) (Ref)	Drug (dosage)	Drug release (%) Release (time in days)	Stent platform	Strut/Max. coating thickness, μm	Polymer type (duration of biodegradation, months)	In-stent late loss (mm)
First generation						
BioMatrix (Biosensors)	Biolimus A9 (15.6 μg/mm)	45% (30)	SS	112/10[a]	PLA[a] (6–9)	0.13[e]
NOBORI (Terumo)	Biolimus A9 (15.6 μg/mm)	45% (30)	SS	112/10[a]	PLA[a] (6–9)	0.11[e]
Axxess (Biosensors)	Biolimus A9 (22 μg/mm)	45% (30)	Nitinol	152/15[a]	PLA[a] (6–9)	0.29MB[e] 0.29SB[e]
Combo (OrbusNeich)	EPC + Sirolimus (5 μg/mm)	95% (35)	SS	100/3–5[a]	PLA, PLGA, CAP(< 3)[a]	0.39[e]
Excel stent (JW Medical System)	Sirolimus (195–376 μg)	NA	SS	119/15	PLA (6–9)	0.21[c]
Second generation						
BioMatrix Alpha (Biosensors)	Biolimus	45% (30)	CoCr	84/10[a]	PLA[a] (6–9)	NA
SYNERGY (Boston Scientific)	Everolimus (LD 56 μg/20 mm) (SD 113 μg/20 mm)	50% (60)	PtCr	71/3 (LD)4 (SD)	PLGA Rollcoat[a] (3)	0.13 (LD)[c] 0.10 (SD)[c]
Elixir Myolimus (Elixir Medical)	Myolimus (3 μg/mm)	90% (90)	CoCr	81/<3	PLA (6–9)	0.08[c]
DESyne BD (Elixir Medical)	Novolimus (5 μg/mm)	90% (90)	CoCr	81/<3	PLA (6–9)	0.16[c]
Infinnium (Sahajanand)	Paclitaxel (122 μg/19 mm)	50% (9–11)	SS	80/4–5	PLLA, PLGA, PLC, PVP (7)	0.54[e]
Ultimaster (Terumo)	Sirolimus (3.9 μg/mm)	100% (120)	CoCr	80/15	PLC (4)	0.04[c]
MiStent (Micell)	Crystalline Sirolimus (9–11 μg/mm)	100% (60)	CoCr	64/15	PLGA (3)	0.03[b]
Supralimus (Sahajanand Medical)	Sirolimus (125 μg/19 mm)	50% (9–11)	SS	80/4–5	PLLA, PLGA, PLC, PVP (7)	0.09[c]
FIREHAWK (MicroPort)	Sirolimus (55 μg /18 mm)	75% (30)	CoCr with grooves	NA	Abluminal groove filled PLA[a] (9)	0.13[b]
Svelte (Svelte Medical)	Sirolimus (220 μg/cm²)	80% (28)	CoCr	81/6	PLGA (12)	0.22[c]
BioMime (Meril Life Sciences)	Sirolimus (1.25 μg/mm²)	NA	CoCr	65/2	PLGA + PLLA	0.15[d]
Orsiro (Biotronik)	Sirolimus (1.4 μg/mm²)	100% (100)	CoCr	71/11	PLLA (15)	0.05[e]
BuMA (SinoMed)	Sirolimus	100% (30)	SS	100/10	PLGA + (3)	0.24[e]
Inspiron DES (Scitech)	Sirolimus (56 μg/13 mm)	NA	CoCr	75/5[a]	PLA + PLGA (6–8)	0.22[c]

CAP, e-caprolactone; CoCr, cobalt chromium; EPC, endothelial progenitor capture; LD, low dose; NA, not available; PES, paclitaxel eluting stent; PLC, 75/25 poly-L-lactide-co-caprolactone; PLGA, 50/50 poly-DL-lactide-co-glycolide; PLLA, poly-L-lactic acid; PtCr, platinum chromium; PVP, polyvinyl pyrrolidone; SD, standard dose; SES, sirolimus eluting stent; SS, stainless steel.

[a] Abluminal polymer.
[b] Angiographic follow-up at 4 months.
[c] Angiographic follow-up at 6 months.
[d] Angiographic follow-up at 8 months.
[e] Angiographic follow-up at 9 months.

Table 13.3 Polymer-free metallic stents which are either currently available, or undergoing clinical evaluation

Stent (manufacturer) (Ref)	Drug (dosage)	Drug release (%) Release time	Stent platform	Strut/coating thickness, µm	Surface modification	Study (no. of patients)	Angiographic follow-up, months	In-stent late loss, mm (vs. control)	Binary restenosis, % (vs. control)	Current status
AmazoniaPax (Minvasys)	Paclitaxel (2.5 µg/mm²)	98% 30 days	CoCr	73/5ᵃ	Abluminal micro-drop spray crystallisation process	FIM (Pax n = 16 vs. PES n = 15)	4	0.77 vs. 0.42	NA	C.E.
BioFREEDOM (Biosensors)	Biolimus A9 (SD[b] 15.6 µg/mm) (LD[c] 7.8 µg/mm)	90% 50 hours	SS	112	Micro-porous surface	FIM (SD[b] n = 25 vs. LD[c] n = 25 vs. PES n = 25)	4	0.08 vs. 0.37[b,d] 0.12 vs. 0.37[c,d]	NA	C.E
VESTAsync (MIV Therapeutics)	Sirolimus (total = 55 µg)	100% 3 months	SS	65/0.6	Nanoporous hydroxyapitate	FIM (n = 15)	9	0.36	0	Ongoing trials
Cre8 (CID)	Amphilimus (0.9 µg/mm²)	100% 3 months	CoCr	80/0.3	Carbon coating/Abluminal reservoir/	RCT (Cre8 n = 162 vs. PES n = 161)	6	0.14 vs. 0.34[d]	3.1 vs. 2.0	C.E
Yinyi (Liaoning Biomed. Mat.)	Paclitaxel	NA	SS	NA	NA	RCT (Yinyi n = 82) vs. EXCEL n = 85)	–	–	–	Ongoing trials
Bicare + (Lepu Medical)	Sirolimus (1.6 µg/mm²) & Probucol (0.8 µg/mm²)	80% sirolimus & 22% probucol 28 days	SS	NA	Nanoporous cavities	FIM (n = 32)	4	0.14	3.1	Ongoing trials
Focus NP (Envision Scientific)	Sirolimus	NA	SS	NA	Nanoparticles	FIM (n = 100)	6	–	–	Ongoing trials
Mitsu (Meril Medical)	Merilimus (45 µg/mm²)		CoCr	40/<2	Nanoparticles	–	–	–	–	Ongoing trials
Hollow-core DFS (Medtronic)	Sirolimus (1.1 µg/mm²)	68% 28 days	CoCr		Hollow wire	FIM (n = 00)	–	–	–	Ongoing trials
Yukon (Translumina)	Sirolimus (11.7–21.9 µg)	67%/7 days	SS	87	Micro-porous surface	RCT (Yukon n = 225 vs. PES n = 225)	9	0.48 vs. 0.48	12.6 vs.11.6	C.E.

All differences are not significant unless stated. BMS, bare-metal stent; C.E, Conformité Européene; CoCr, cobalt chromium; FIM, first-in-man; LD, low dose; NA, not available; PES, paclitaxel eluting stent; RCT, randomised controlled trial; SD, standard dose; SS, stainless steel.

ᵃ Abluminal.

ᵇ SD, standard dose 15.6 µg/mm.

ᶜ LD, low dose 7.8 µg/mm.

ᵈ <0.001

seen in any of the components of TLF. The secondary end-point of definite ST at 1 year was significantly lower with the Orsiro stent (0.4% vs. 1.2% p = .03), which was driven by significantly fewer early events. These differences can be hypothesised to be due to the between-stent differences in strut thickness, polymer degradation time, and drug release time, therefore suggesting that performances of biodegradable polymer DESs are not a class effect.

Individually, all biodegradable polymer DESs have been shown in randomised clinical studies against contemporary durable polymer devices to be largely non-inferior with regards angiographic and clinical outcomes.[30–37] In terms of proving the theory, porcine studies have shown less inflammation,[38] and clinical studies, improved vasomotion,[39] and fewer uncovered struts as assessed by optical coherency tomography (OCT) at 6–8 months follow-up[40] with biodegradable versus permanent polymer DES. Definitive proof of concept, however, remains lacking, as only data from a few studies all using the first-generation biodegradable polymer DES are available with long enough follow-up to examine whether these devices actually improve long-term

safety, and even these were not sufficiently powered for this endpoint. The most compelling data to date come from final analysis of the LEADERS study which showed significantly lower rates of very-late definite ST between 1 and 5 years in patients treated with the BioMatrix biodegradable polymer BES, compared with the Cypher SES.[30] As a caveat, the study enrolled 1707 patients and was only powered for clinical and angiographic outcomes at 9 months, and therefore these results whilst compelling are really only hypothesis generating. In contrast to these data, the NEXT study showed no significant differences in clinical outcomes including cardiac death, MI, TLR and ST at 3-year follow-up amongst 3235 patients treated with Nobori BES (n = 1576) or EES (n = 1582).[41] Moreover, landmark analysis showed similar risks of death, MI, TLR and definite ST between 1 and 3 years follow-up (Figure 13.4).

Numerous meta-analyses have been conducted comparing outcomes in patients treated with permanent versus biodegradable polymer DES.[17,18,22,24,42–44] As mentioned, the individual studies used in these meta-analyses are limited by the lack of long-term follow-up data, and

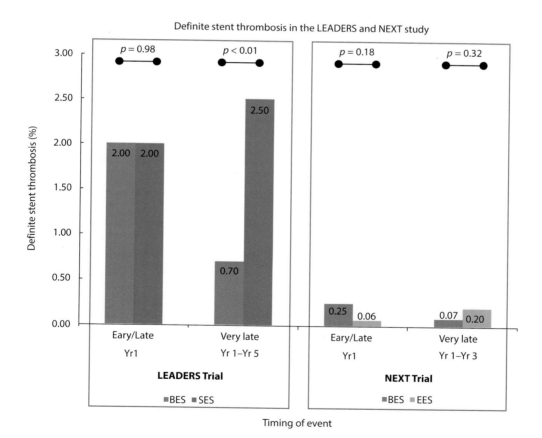

Figure 13.4 The rates of early/late and very-late definite stent thrombosis for patients receiving the biodegradable polymer biolimus-eluting stent versus the permanent polymer sirolimus-eluting and everolimus-eluting stents in the respective all-comers randomised LEADERS, and NEXT study.[30,41] There were no between-stent differences in rates of stent thrombosis at 1-year follow-up in either study. In the LEADERS study, rates of very-late stent thrombosis between 1- and 5-year follow-up were significantly lower with the biodegradable polymer stent, whilst in the NEXT study there were no between-stent differences in very-late stent thrombosis out to 3 years follow-up. Overall rates of stent thrombosis were markedly lower in the NEXT study. Of note, neither study was powered for stent thrombosis.

the absence of results from studies using the second-generation biodegradable polymer DES. Patient-level meta-analyses by Navarese et al. (median of 9 months, n = 7464)[43] and Stefanini et al. (4 years, n = 4062)[42] reported positive signals in favour of biodegradable polymer stents, albeit in modest populations, with significantly lower in-stent late loss (p = .004), definite ST (HR 0.56, p = .02) and very-late ST (HR 0.22, p = .004). The results from larger network meta-analyses differ, with no significant differences observed in safety or efficacy between the two groups.[17,18,22,24] Of note, Palmerini et al. reported significantly higher rates of definite ST with biodegradable polymer DES compared to EES at 1 year (OR 2.44, 95% CI 1.30–4.76), which was a consequence of early events.[22] More recently, a network meta-analysis with a median follow-up of 3.8 years demonstrated that use of EES resulted in a borderline, but significant, reduction in definite ST compared with the biodegradable polymer BES (HR 0.58, 95% CI 0.31–1.00, p < .05).[17] The same study also demonstrated that the only significant reductions in very-late definite ST with the biodegradable polymer BES were seen in studies where SES was the comparator stent; no advantage was seen in direct comparisons with EES and PES, or in indirect comparisons with ZES and BMS.

13.3.3 Polymer-free DES

Concerns that the stent polymer played a central role in triggering adverse events provided the impetus to develop DES that elute anti-proliferative drugs without a polymeric coating. Additional advantages of this physical absence include an improvement to the integrity and uniformity of the stent surface, as *in vitro* studies have demonstrated that polymers can crack and peel during stent deployment.[45] Without the polymer, drug elution has been achieved through either physical modifications to the stent's surface or using a non-polymeric biodegradable carrier with resulting elution times of between 50 hours and 90 days for contemporary devices (Figure 13.5, Table 13.3).

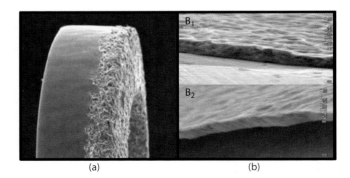

Figure 13.5 Scanning electron microscopy of the surface of the BioFreedom stent and of the VESTAsync stent. **(a)** The microporous surface of the BioFreedom stent and **(b)** the VESTAsync stent. The rough surface (B₁) of the VESTAsync stent is smoothed over (B₂) following the addition of a sirolimus coating that is 0.6 μm thick.

The evidence to support these perceived benefits comes predominantly from pre-clinical studies showing improved healing and reduced inflammation with polymer-free DES. For example, at 180 days in the porcine model, compared with a permanent polymer SES, use of the polymer-free BES was associated with decreased fibrin formation and less inflammation suggesting superior arterial healing.[46] Pre-clinical assessment of the polymer-free VESTAsync SES (MIV Therapeutics, Atlanta, Georgia) showed reduced signs of delayed vascular healing, suggesting less local toxicity and a faster healing response. Porcine pre-clinical studies of the amphilimus eluting Cre8 stent (CID, Italy) show the absence of a chronic inflammatory response as evidenced by reduced inflammatory scores and neointimal thickness when compared to permanent polymer SES controls.[47]

Clinical studies have largely been limited to first-in-man studies or randomised studies powered for angiographic endpoints in selective patient populations with low-risk coronary anatomy with the first-generation DES used as controls.[48–51] Angiographic follow-up of early iterations showed disappointing late loss values of up to 0.48 mm,[48] which was initially thought to be due to rapid drug elution; however, respective late loss values of 0.08 and 0.14 mm with contemporary devices eluting biolimus (over 50 hours)[51] and amphilimus (over 3 months)[49] have dispelled this theory and restored some confidence in these devices.

Despite these latter results, limited data and cost have prevented identification of a definitive role for these devices in routine clinical practice. Nevertheless, a potential area of use may be in patients who require the proven efficacy of a DES but are unable to comply with the required duration of dual anti-platelet therapy (DAPT) for reasons such as planned surgical procedures or drug intolerance etc. This novel role was recently assessed in the LEADERS FREE study, which randomised 2500 patients, who owing to comorbidity or a high-risk of bleeding were unable to receive DAPT for longer than 1 month, to treatment with the BioFreedom BES (Biosensors, Morges, Switzerland) or a BMS.[52] Disappointingly, the control arm was a BMS rather than a DES and commonest met inclusion criteria (in 64% of the study cohort) was age > 75 years old. Notwithstanding this, the study did report significantly lower rates of the composite primary safety endpoint of cardiac death, MI, ST (9.4% vs. 12.9%, p < .001 for non-inferiority and p = .005 for superiority) and the primary efficacy endpoint of clinically indicated TLR (5.1% vs. 9.8%, p < .001) with use of the BioFreedom DES compared to BMS.[52]

The study provides useful data and identifies a potential niche area for the use of polymer-free DES; however, continuing improvements in the safety of permanent and biodegradable polymer DES,[17,18] together with changes to the recommended duration of DAPT post-PCI, are likely to hamper their routine use. Post-elective PCI, the recommended duration of DAPT has already been shortened from 12 to 6 months, and guidance from the ESC suggests

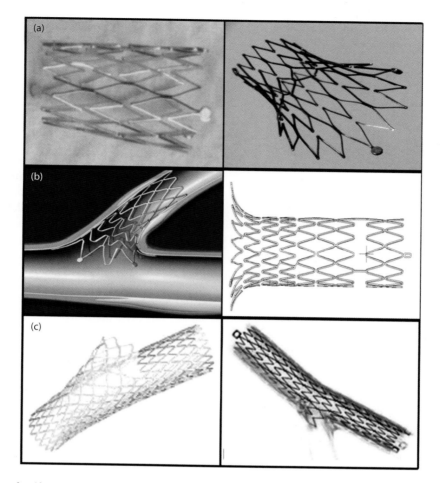

Figure 13.6 Examples of self-expanding bifurcation stents: (a) Axxes, (b) Capella and (c) Stentys.

3 months of DAPT can be used when a contemporary DES is implanted in a patient with high bleeding risk.[53] These guidelines may also change following studies, such as Global Leaders,[54] which has explored the use of 1 month of aspirin and ticagrelor, followed by 23 months of ticagrelor alone (i.e., no aspirin) in all-comers patients receiving a biodegradable polymer BES. The results are awaited; however, if the study confirms the safety of using only 1 month of DAPT, then the potential advantages of polymer-free DES may be nullified.

Other polymer-free technologies that remain in the early stages of development are as follows:

1. **Drug-filled stents (Medtronic)**
   These novel polymer-free DES are made from a tri-layer wire:
   - The outer layer is made of a cobalt alloy that provides radial strength.
   - The middle layer is made of tantalum that enables the device to be radio-opaque.
   - The core material of the inner layer of the wire is removed to produce hollow struts which function as the reservoir for sirolimus that is present at a dose of 1.1 µg/mm^2.

Drug release occurs through an average of five laser-drilled holes, each with a minimal bore diameter of 20 µm, on the abluminal side of each stent. Drug elution, which occurs with a profile similar to durable polymer DES, commences on stent deployment and is controlled and sustained through natural diffusions via direction interaction with the vessel wall. Pre-clinical data show 68% and 93% of the sirolimus is released at 28 and 90 days, respectively, with histology confirming that this drug release is effective at suppressing neointimal hyperplasia compared to BMS controls ($P < .001$), with minimal inflammation.[55] On the basis of these data, the RevElution clinical trial is being conducted which will enrol 100 patients. Preliminary OCT data from the first six patients show early healing and high rates of strut coverage at 1 month.[55]

2. **Nanotechnology**
   These stents have a standard platform that is coated with a nanomatrix made up of nanoparticles of anti-proliferative drug combined with stabilising excipients. The advantages of using these nanoparticles for drug delivery include
   - *In vivo* drug stability due to encapsulation
   - Reduced drug dosage

- Controlled and reproducible drug release kinetics, together with rapid drug release enabling rapid vessel healing
- Deep penetration into the vessel wall to improve efficacy
- Increased intracellular drug uptake with prolonged residence time at the target site

Contemporary examples of this technology are limited, and the FOCUS np® (Envision Scientific Private, Ltd. Corporation, Surat, India) DES system is the most studied. This polymer-free stent has a cobalt chromium stent platform and is coated with nanoparticles that have a mean diameter of 210 nm and contain sirolimus within two excipients, facilitating a two-phase programmed drug release. The first phase is a burst release occurring within 60 s of stent deployment followed by a second phase of programmed release over 40 days. Following successful preclinical studies of FOCUS np which, in the porcine model, demonstrated comparable efficacy and less fibrin deposition to the permanent polymer BES, a 100 patient first-in-man study has completed enrolment, and the results are awaited.

13.4 Stent platform

The stent platform provides the skeleton of the stent, and its purpose is twofold. At the time of stent deployment, its role is to provide enough radial force to prevent acute vessel recoil, which can occur following balloon-induced vessel dissection. Subacutely, it serves as a scaffold, which facilitates vessel healing and prevents plaque prolapse. It follows that once vessel healing is complete the skeleton serves no effective role, and consequently there has been interest in replacing the permanent metal skeleton of historical and most contemporary stents with fully bioresorbable materials.

13.4.1 Permanent stent platform

Since the deployment of the first coronary stent in 1986,[1] the stent platform has undergone many changes, which have been prompted through the realisation of the complex interaction between the material the stent is made from, the strut dimensions, the stent cell configuration and the degree of vessel wall injury sustained during stent deployment, the latter of which affects the resultant degree of neointimal hyperplasia. These factors also influence a stent's deliverability which is vitally important for procedural success particularly when considering the increasingly complex patients and lesions being treated with PCI in contemporary practice.

The physical properties of the stent material directly influence the strut dimensions and the stent's radio-opacity. The first coronary stent was the Wallstent (Boston Scientific), which was made of nitinol, an alloy of nickel and titanium which offered properties such as shape memory, biocompatibility, fatigue resistance and super elasticity, thereby enabling the stent to be self-expanding. This method of deployment offers advantages over balloon-expandable stents such as

prevention of immediate vessel wall injury, a lower incidence of edge dissections, reduced rates of side branch occlusion and no-reflow, and positive remodelling.[56] However, disadvantages include the need for a delivery catheter to ensure stent security, and thick struts to maintain radial force; hence, they have a poor delivery profile. Following the arrival of DES, nitinol self-expanding stents fell out of favour; however, there has been a revival of interest following new stent designs which have incorporated thinner struts, drug coatings and improved delivery systems. Currently these devices are being used for niche coronary settings such as bifurcation lesions (Figure 13.6), acute MI and small vessels. A full review of devices and current data are available elsewhere.[57]

The first-generation DESs were made of stainless steel; however, this alloy has been replaced in contemporary DES with alloys of cobalt or platinum chromium. These alloys offer greater radio-opacity, which assists with stent placement particularly when dealing with overlapping stents, and ostial lesions. Platinum alloys do tend to offer greater visibility; however, the newly developed Resolute Onyx stent (Medtronic) has increased its radio-opacity through the use of a layered wire that has a dense metal core of tantalum surrounded by a cobalt nickel alloy outer layer. Reassuringly, the PLATINUM trial reported no significant differences in clinical outcomes at 3-year follow-up between patients randomised to stents identical in all aspects other than one being a made of cobalt chromium (Xience EES, Abbott Vascular) and the other platinum chromium (Promus Element EES).[58]

Other advantages of the new alloys compared with stainless steel are greater tensile strength, such that sufficient radial strength to prevent vessel closure is attainable from struts as thin as 60 μm (Orsiro SES), which is more than 50% thinner than the stainless steel struts on the Cypher SES. Thinner struts increase procedural success through improved stent deliverability and potentially enhance clinical outcomes through reduced peri-stent inflammation and fibrin deposition; reduced thrombogencity; superior re-endothelialisation; less shear disturbance; and less vascular trauma to the elastic lamina and medial wall.[59–65] These peri-vascular benefits of thinner struts have been shown in studies of BMS and may not be entirely applicable to DES where drug elution appears to have a greater influence on outcomes.[66] In the PERSUS workhorse trial, angiographic outcomes at 9 months and clinical outcomes out to 5 years were comparable amongst 1262 patients randomised 3:1 to stents identical in all aspects other than one being a thin strut (81 μm) platinum chromium stent and other a thicker strut (132 μm) stainless steel stent.[67,68]

In addition to these new materials and resultant changes in strut thickness, changes have also occurred to the cell configuration and the number of cell connectors, both of which influence deliverability, and the unsupported circumferential sectional area. The closed-cell design of the Cypher SES activated fewer platelets, and reduced tissue prolapse, however, its lack of flexibility restricted deliverability and increased its risk of stent fracture, which was compounded by its visibility.[69,70] In contrast, open-cell designs, with minimal connectors ensure excellent deliverability and minimise arterial injury. Of note, a balance is necessary, however, between striving for excellent deliverability through design changes and thinner stent struts, and exposing stents through reduced axial strength to the risk of longitudinal deformation and its resultant clinical consequences.[71] Retrospective studies highlighted the platinum chromium Element EES (Boston Scientific) to be most prone to this phenomenon; however, this has not been confirmed in prospective studies,[72] and parallel with this to ease concerns, has been education and subtle design modifications, such as the introduction of additional connectors.

13.4.2 Biodegradable scaffolds

In recent times significant research has been directed towards developing biodegradable vascular scaffolds (BVS), which function to maintain vessel patency and prevent acute vessel closure following balloon angioplasty induced dissection; furthermore, once vessel healing has taken place they biodegrade into inert substances allowing the restoration of normal physiology (Figure 13.7), whilst removing any residual intra-vascular foreign material.[73-76] The primary stimulus for their development has been the professed disadvantages of permanent metal stents such as the absence of any functionality once vessel healing has taken place; the risk of neoatherosclerosis and adverse events; allergic reactions to metals; hypersensitivity to polymers and the inability to anastomose a stented segment with a bypass graft. As illustrated in Table 13.4 and Figure 13.8, numerous BVS have been developed many of which are still undergoing early clinical evaluation; however, several have already gained CE mark and have entered routine practice.

The most extensively studied scaffold to date is the ABSORB everolimus-eluting scaffold (ABBOTT Vascular) which was initially evaluated in the ABSORB Cohort A and B first-in-man studies, which helped verify that the theoretical advantages of BVS were a reality with multi-modality

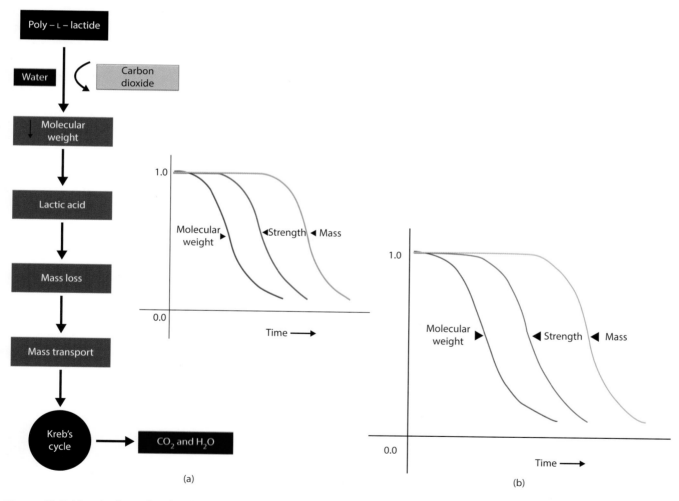

(a)

(b)

Figure 13.7 Metabolism of poly-L-lactide acid (PLLA) and bioabsorption curves for bioabsorbable materials. **(a)** The metabolism of PLLA biodegradable stents. Hydrolysis of PLLA results in the loss of molecular weight, and reduction in both strength and mass. Ultimately, PLLA is metabolised into lactic acid, CO_2 and H_2O. **(b)** Bioabsorption curves for a bioabsorbable material. Molecular weight is lost first, followed by strength, and then mass. Therefore, the stent loses its biomedical importance long before substantial loss of mass occurs.

Table 13.4 Specifications of bioresorbable scaffolds

Company	Strut material	Coating	Eluted drug	Radio-opacity	Strut thickness (µm)	Duration of radial support	Resorption time (months)	Angiographic late loss (mm)
Igaki-Tamai (Kyoto medical)	PLLA	Nil	Nil	Gold marker	170	6 months	24–36	0.48[b]
AMS (Biotronik)	Mg alloy	Nil	Nil	Nil	165	Days or months	<2	1.08[a]
DREAMS I (Biotronik)	Mg alloy	PLGA	Paclitaxel	Nil	120–130	NA	3–4	0.64[b]
DREAMS II (Biotronik)	Mg alloy	PLA	Sirolimus	Marker	120–150	NA	12	0.27[b]
BVS 1.0 (Abbott Vascular)	PLLA	PDLLA	Everolimus	Platinum marker	156	Weeks	24	0.44[b]
Absorb BVS 1.1 (Abbott Vascular)	PLLA	PDLLA	Everolimus	Platinum marker	156	6 months	24	0.19[b]
REVA (REVA Medical)	Tyrosine-derived polycarbonate polymer	Nil	None	Scaffold	200	3–6 months	24	1.81[b]
ReZolve (REVA Medical)	Tyrosine-derived polycarbonate polymer	Nil	Sirolimus	Scaffold	114–228	4–6 months	24	NA
Fantom (REVA Medical)	Des-aminotyrosine–derived Polycarbonate	NA	Sirolimus	Scaffold	<127	NA	36	NA
IDEAL BioStent (Xenogenics)	Polylactide anhydride mixed with a polymer of salicylic acid with a sebacic acid linker	Salicylate lined with adipic acid	Sirolimus	Scaffold	160–175	3 months	6	NA
DESolve (Elixir)	PLLA	PLLA	Novolimus	Marker	150	NA	12–24	0.19[c]
DESolve 100 (Elixir)	PLLA	PLLA	Novolimus	Marker	100	NA	12–24	NA
ART18Z (ART)	PLLA	Nil	Nil	Nil	170	3–6 months	18	NA
Amaranth PLLA (Amaranth)	PLLA	Nil	Nil	None	150–200	3–6 months	12	0.90[b]
Fortitude (Amaranth)	PLLA	NA	NA	NA	120	NA	NA	NA
Xinsorb (Huaan)	PLLA, PCL, PLGA	PDLLA	Sirolimus	Marker	160	NA	N/A	0.17[b]
On-ABS (OrbusNeich)	PLLA, PDLLA, PCL	EPC	Sirolimus	None	150	NA	N/A	NA
BIOLUTE-next	Magnesium alloy	PLA + nanocarriers	Sirolimus	Marker	120	NA	NA	NA

EPC, endothelial progenitor capture; Mg, magnesium; N/A, not applicable; PCL, poly-L-lactide-co- caprolactone; PDLLA, poly-D,L-lactide; PLGA, poly-lactide-co-glycolide; PLLA, poly-L-lactic acid.

[a] Angiographic follow-up at 4 months.
[b] Angiographic follow-up at 6 months.
[c] Angiographic follow-up at 8 months.

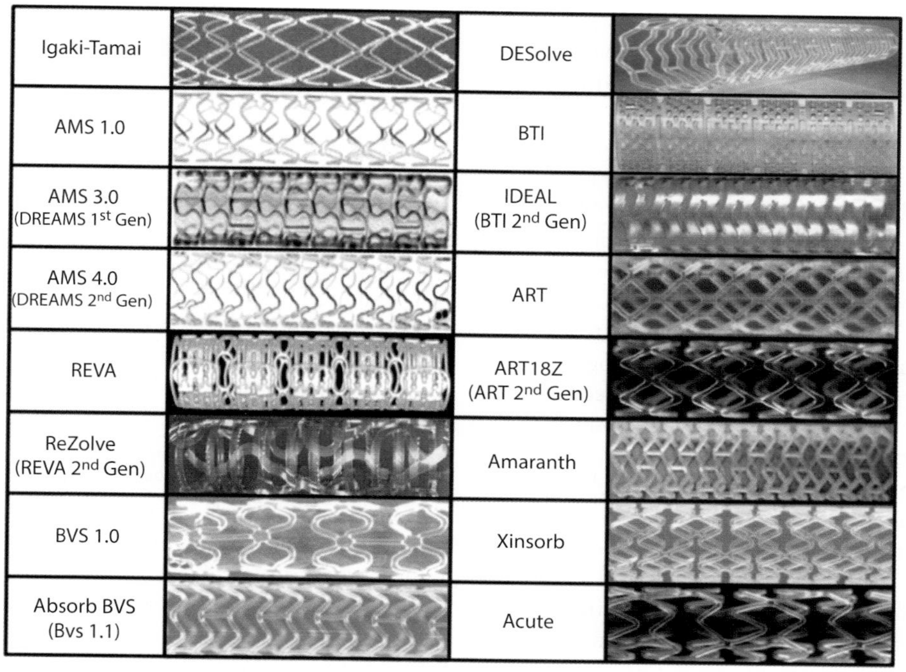

Figure 13.8 Bioresorbable scaffolds undergoing pre-clinical and clinical evaluation.

intra-coronary imagining confirming the bioresorption of the ABSORB BVS struts and the restoration of coronary vasomotion.[76,77] Other clinical data are derived from registries, and six completed randomised studies against permanent metal DES.[76,78–86] These six studies enrolled a total of 3820 predominantly stable patients (BVS n = 2339 vs. EES n = 1401 or BES n = 80) and all but ABSORB II have reported their primary endpoint. The EVERBIO II was the only one powered for superiority of DES over BVS, and failed to demonstrate any significant differences in the primary endpoint of in-stent late lumen loss at 9 months (BVS 0.28 mm vs. EES/BES 0.25 mm, p = .30).[82] The remaining four studies all achieved their pre-specified criteria for non-inferiority which were in-segment late loss at 12 months in ABSORB China (BVS 0.19 mm vs. EES 0.13 mm, $P_{non-inferiority}$= 0.01)[83] TLF at 12 months in ABSORB Japan (BVS 4.2% vs. EES 3.8%, $P_{non-inferiority}$ < 0.01)[84] and ABSORB III (BVS 7.8% vs. EES 6.1%, $P_{non-inferiority}$ = 0.07, $P_{superiority}$ = 0.16)[85] and optical frequency domain imaging healing score at 6 months based on the presence of uncovered and/or malapposed stent struts and intraluminal filling defects in the TROFI II trial (BVS 1.74 vs. EES 2.80; $P_{non-inferiority}$ < 0.01).[86] Notwithstanding these data, several challenges remain for this technology in regard to their design, efficacy and safety.

13.4.2.1 BVS design

The heterogeneous structural characteristics of current BVS are summarised in Table 13.4. The commonest BVS platform is PLLA; however, several other materials have also been tried such as magnesium, salicylic acid, and tyrosine-derived polycarbonate. All these materials have considerably less tensile strength compared with metal alloys, resulting in BVS devices needing to have struts that are 100–200 µm thick to ensure they provide sufficient radial support during deployment and prevent acute vessel recoil during vessel healing. These thicker struts have resulted in some devices requiring the use of 7F guiding catheters and can also cause difficulties when delivering and deploying BVS in challenging coronary anatomy. Despite these valid concerns, real-world data of the ABSORB BVS from single-centre registries of consecutive patients, and from the multi-centre GHOST-EU registry have shown high rates of device success, and good clinical outcomes when using BVS in patients with multiple co-morbidities or complex anatomy such as Type B2/C lesions, chronic total occlusions, ostial lesions, bifurcation lesions and long lesions requiring overlapping scaffolds.[87,88] In terms of performance, thicker struts result in more of the strut abutting into the lumen, and this can interfere with blood flow dynamics, potentially contributing to the risk of ST.[89–92] Currently, it is not clear whether thinner struts on scaffolds offers the same advantages that have been realised with metallic DES, not least because the healing response to these devices is different with continuing positive remodelling which can negate the effects of neointimal hyperplasia.[76,78,91]

Many scaffolds share the same platform, however, biodegradation times vary, and this can also directly influence outcomes. More rapid bioresorption can lead to loss of scaffold integrity prior to the completion of vessel healing, leading to scaffold fracture, restenosis and other adverse clinical events. There are several examples illustrating the intricate relationship between the performance of a BVS, its biodegradation time, and the elution of anti-proliferative drugs. As illustrated in Table 13.4, the magnesium absorbable scaffold has had three iterations all using a magnesium alloy that has been refined from that used in the initial AMS scaffold, resulting in prolongation of the absorption period from 1–2 months (AMS) to 3–4 months (DREAMS 1G) and then 12 months (DREAMS 2G), and a corresponding reduction in strut thickness. Furthermore whilst the AMS had no drug coating, the DREAMS 1G and 2G eluted paclitaxel and sirolimus, respectively. These changes resulted in the in-segment late loss falling from 0.83 mm at 4 months to 0.52 mm at 6 months and then 0.27 mm at 6 months for the AMS, DREAMS 1G and DREAMS 2G scaffolds, respectively.[93–95] Some of these improvements are no doubt due to the introduction of a drug coating; however, the majority is due to prolongation of the absorption period. In the Progress AMS study, intra-vascular ultrasound showed a 42% reduction in the external elastic membrane at 4 months follow-up, indicating that the primary reason for the poor performance of the AMS BVS was due to early vessel recoil. This vessel recoil was attributable to the loss of radial force from early rapid degradation, such that no stent support was available to oppose vessel contraction; a natural response of the vessel to injury.[96]

Similarly initial first-in-man studies of tyrosine-derived polycarbonate polymer REVA stent showed unacceptable late loss of up to 1.81 mm at 6 months follow-up.[97] Part of this was due to the absence of a drug coating together with failure to establish the optimal properties of the scaffold material.

13.4.2.2 BVS efficacy

The above discussion and the data presented in Table 13.4 confirm that similar to permanent metallic DES, the absence of drug elution leads to unacceptably high late loss with BVS. Reassuringly, first-in-man studies have shown acceptable late loss values of 0.19 mm with the CE marked ABSORB EES and DESolve novolimus-eluting scaffold (Elixir Medical, Sunnyvale, California)[98] despite concerns regarding their strut thicknesses of 157 and 150 μm, respectively.

Meta-analysis of randomised studies of the ABSORB EES compared to metallic DES have shown inferior angiographic performance with a greater in-device late lumen loss at a median of 10 months follow-up (weight mean difference 0·08 [95% CI 0.05–0.12]; $p < .0001$).[99] As a caveat, however, poorer angiographic performance was only noted in studies where angiographic follow-up took place at 6–9 months ($p = .02$), whilst it was comparable when angiographic follow-up took place at 12 months or beyond ($p = .12$). These data may reflect the difference in healing and adaptive responses of the coronary vessel to implantation of a metallic versus bioresorbable devices. Nevertheless, these differences did not affect clinical outcomes with comparable rates of TLR (OR 0.97, 95% CI 0.66–1.43, $p = .87$) and TLF (OR 1.20, 95% 0.90–1.60, $p = .21$) at a median of 12 months follow-up.[99]

13.4.2.3 BVS safety

One of the perceived benefits of a BVS is the long-term absence of any intra-vascular material, and consequently it was hoped that device thrombosis would become a thing of the past. Randomised studies, and their meta-analysis have all shown a consistent non-significant higher risk of MI at a median of 12 months follow-up in patients treated with the ABSORB BVS compared with a metal EES (OR 1·36, 95% CI 0·98–1·89, $p = .06$).[99] Furthermore, as expected considering the populations enrolled, the same meta-analysis has shown similar mortality between both groups (OR 0.95, 95% CI 0.45–2.00, $p = .89$); however, significant heterogeneity ($p = .02$) existed for this outcome amongst the six included studies. Unfortunately, the hope that BVS would be immune to the risk of thrombotic events has not come to fruition. Meta-analysis of randomised studies indicate a consistently higher risk of definite/probable ST with the ABSORB BVS compared with the metallic EES (OR 1.99, 95% CI 1.00–3.98, $p = .05$) with the risk being highest between 1 and 30 days after implantation (OR 3.11, 95% CI 1.24–7.82, $p = .02$).[99] The preponderance for these subacute events, despite rates of DAPT in excess of 80% and frequent post-dilatation, suggests the need for further optimisation of lesion selection and implantation techniques. Notably, the timing of these events is consistent with the GHOST-EU registry, which reported a rate of definite/probable ST of 3.4% (23 events), of which 65% (15 events) occurred within 30 days of the index procedure.[80] The majority of these cases had not had post-dilatation or intra-vascular imaging guidance during device implantation. As with metallic stents, outcomes were poor with death and non-fatal MI occurring in 3 (13%) and 15 (65%) patients, respectively. Randomised studies and registries do not yet have long-term follow-up data; however, examples of very-late definite scaffold thrombosis have been reported with one event occurring 22 months following BVS implantation.[100] Fortunately these events are scarce; however, they serve to increase vigilance, and indicate that no intra-coronary implant is exempt from thrombosis.

13.5 Conclusions

Safety concerns with the first generation of DES prompted welcome new developments in stent technology. Outcomes with contemporary permanent polymer DES, however, remain hard to surpass when compared to DES using biodegradable polymers, no polymers or bioresorbable scaffolds. Of note, however, are the improvements in the individual performance of all stents/scaffolds, such that detecting clinically meaningful differences in performance is increasingly difficult without the need to perform exorbitantly expensive mega-trials. Beneficially, clinicians now have a variety of stents to choose from, allowing stent choice to be tailored to the individual patient.

References

1. Sigwart U et al. Intravascular stents to prevent occlusion and restenosis after transluminal angioplasty. *N Engl J Med* 1987; 316(12): 701–6.
2. Serruys PW et al. A comparison of balloon-expandable-stent implantation with balloon angioplasty in patients with coronary artery disease. Benestent Study Group. *N Engl J Med* 1994; 331(8): 489–95.

3. Morice MC et al. A randomized comparison of a sirolimus-eluting stent with a standard stent for coronary revascularization. *N Engl J Med* 2002; 346(23): 1773–80.

4. Camenzind E et al. Stent thrombosis late after implantation of first-generation drug-eluting stents: A cause for concern. *Circulation* 2007; 115(11): 1440–55; discussion 55.

5. Stettler C et al. Outcomes associated with drug-eluting and bare-metal stents: A collaborative network meta-analysis. *Lancet* 2007; 370(9591): 937–48.

6. Daemen J et al. Early and late coronary stent thrombosis of sirolimus-eluting and paclitaxel-eluting stents in routine clinical practice: Data from a large two-institutional cohort study. *Lancet* 2007; 369(9562): 667–78.

7. Serruys PW et al. Angiographic follow-up after placement of a self-expanding coronary-artery stent. *N Engl J Med* 1991; 324(1): 13–7.

8. Schatz RA et al. Clinical experience with the Palmaz-Schatz coronary stent. Initial results of a multicenter study. *Circulation* 1991; 83(1): 148–61.

9. Fischman DL et al. A randomized comparison of coronary-stent placement and balloon angioplasty in the treatment of coronary artery disease. Stent Restenosis Study Investigators. *N Engl J Med* 1994; 331(8): 496–501.

10. Colombo A et al. Intracoronary stenting without anticoagulation accomplished with intravascular ultrasound guidance. *Circulation* 1995; 91(6): 1676–88.

11. Leon MB et al. A clinical trial comparing three antithrombotic-drug regimens after coronary-artery stenting. Stent Anticoagulation Restenosis Study Investigators. *N Engl J Med* 1998; 339(23): 1665–71.

12. Mauri L et al. Stent thrombosis in randomized clinical trials of drug-eluting stents. *N Engl J Med* 2007; 356(10): 1020–9.

13. Garg S, and Serruys P. Benefits of and safety concerns associated with drug-eluting coronary stents. *Expert Rev Cardiovasc Ther* 2010; 8(3): 449–70.

14. Holmes DR, Jr. et al. Stent thrombosis. *J Am Coll Cardiol* 2010; 56(17): 1357–65.

15. Nakazawa G et al. The pathology of neoatherosclerosis in human coronary implants bare-metal and drug-eluting stents. *J Am Coll Cardiol* 2011; 57(11): 1314–22.

16. Raber L et al. Five-year clinical and angiographic outcomes of a randomized comparison of sirolimus-eluting and paclitaxel-eluting stents: Results of the Sirolimus-Eluting Versus Paclitaxel-Eluting Stents for Coronary Revascularization LATE trial. *Circulation* 2011; 123(24): 2819–28, 6 p following 28.

17. Palmerini T et al. Long-term safety of drug-eluting and bare-metal stents: Evidence from a comprehensive network meta-analysis. *J Am Coll Cardiol* 2015; 65(23): 2496–507.

18. Bangalore S et al. Bare metal stents, durable polymer drug eluting stents, and biodegradable polymer drug eluting stents for coronary artery disease: Mixed treatment comparison meta-analysis. *BmJ* 2013; 347: f6625.

19. Schomig A et al. A meta-analysis of 16 randomized trials of sirolimus-eluting stents versus paclitaxel-eluting stents in patients with coronary artery disease. *J Am Coll Cardiol* 2007; 50(14): 1373–80.

20. Scheller B et al. Treatment of coronary in-stent restenosis with a paclitaxel-coated balloon catheter. *N Engl J Med* 2006; 355(20): 2113–24.

21. Steigerwald K et al. Vascular healing in drug-eluting stents: Differential drug-associated response of limus-eluting stents in a preclinical model of stent implantation. *EuroIntervention* 2012; 8(6): 752–9.

22. Palmerini T et al. Clinical outcomes with bioabsorbable polymer- versus durable polymer-based drug-eluting and bare-metal stents: Evidence from a comprehensive network meta-analysis. *J Am Coll Cardiol* 2014; 63(4): 299–307.

23. Palmerini T et al. Stent thrombosis with drug-eluting and bare-metal stents: Evidence from a comprehensive network meta-analysis. *Lancet* 2012; 379(9824): 1393–402.

24. Kang SH et al. Biodegradable-polymer drug-eluting stents vs. bare metal stents vs. durable-polymer drug-eluting stents: A systematic review and Bayesian approach network meta-analysis. *Eur Heart J* 2014; 35(17): 1147–58.

25. Joner M et al. Endothelial cell recovery between comparator polymer-based drug-eluting stents. *J Am Coll Cardiol* 2008; 52(5): 333–42.

26. Kolandaivelu K et al. Stent thrombogenicity early in high-risk interventional settings is driven by stent design and deployment and protected by polymer-drug coatings. *Circulation* 2011; 123(13): 1400–9.

27. Joner M et al. Pathology of drug-eluting stents in humans: Delayed healing and late thrombotic risk. *J Am Coll Cardiol* 2006; 48(1): 193–202.

28. Jensen LO et al. Randomized comparison of a sirolimus-eluting Orsiro stent with a biolimus-eluting Nobori stent in patients treated with percutaneous coronary intervention: Rationale and study design of the Scandinavian Organization for Randomized Trials with Clinical Outcome VII trial. *Am Heart J* 2015; 170(2): 210–5.

29. Jensen LO. Randomized comparison of a biodegradable polymer ultrathin strut sirolimus-eluting stent with a biodegradable polymer biolimus-eluting stent in patients treated with percutaneous coronary intervention: The SORT OUT VII trial. *Circ Cardiovasc Interv* 2016 Jul;9(7). pii: e003610. doi: 10.1161/CIRCINTERVENTIONS.115.003610.

30. Serruys PW et al. Improved safety and reduction in stent thrombosis associated with biodegradable polymer-based biolimus-eluting stents versus durable polymer-based sirolimus-eluting stents in patients with coronary artery disease: Final 5-year report of the LEADERS (Limus Eluted from a Durable Versus ERodable Stent Coating) Randomized, noninferiority trial. *JACC Cardiovasc Interv* 2013; 6(8): 777–89.

31. Smits PC et al. Abluminal biodegradable polymer biolimus-eluting stent versus durable polymer everolimus-eluting stent (COMPARE II): A randomised, controlled, non-inferiority trial. *Lancet* 2013; 381(9867): 651–60.

32. Christiansen EH et al. Biolimus-eluting biodegradable polymer-coated stent versus durable polymer-coated sirolimus-eluting stent in unselected patients receiving percutaneous coronary intervention (SORT OUT V): A randomised non-inferiority trial. *Lancet* 2013; 381(9867): 661–9.

33. Natsuaki M et al. Biodegradable polymer biolimus-eluting stent versus durable polymer everolimus-eluting stent: A randomized, controlled, noninferiority trial. *J Am Coll Cardiol* 2013; 62(3): 181–90.

34. Raungaard B et al. Zotarolimus-eluting durable-polymer-coated stent versus a biolimus-eluting biodegradable-polymer-coated stent in unselected patients undergoing percutaneous coronary intervention (SORT OUT VI): A

randomised non-inferiority trial. *Lancet* 2015; 385(9977): 1527–35.

35. Kereiakes DJ et al. Efficacy and safety of a novel bioabsorbable polymer-coated, everolimus-eluting coronary stent: The EVOLVE II randomized trial. *Circ Cardiovasc Interv* 2015; 8(4).

36. Windecker S et al. Comparison of a novel biodegradable polymer sirolimus-eluting stent with a durable polymer everolimus-eluting stent: Results of the randomized BIOFLOW-II trial. *Circ Cardiovasc Interv* 2015; 8(2): e001441.

37. Wijns W et al. Randomised study of a bioabsorbable polymer-coated sirolimus-eluting stent: Results of the DESSOLVE II trial. *EuroIntervention* 2015; 10(12): 1383–90.

38. Koppara T et al. Histopathological comparison of biodegradable polymer and permanent polymer based sirolimus eluting stents in a porcine model of coronary stent implantation. *Thromb Haemost* 2012; 107(6): 1161–71.

39. Rusinaru D et al. Bioabsorbable polymer-coated sirolimus-eluting stent implantation preserves coronary vasomotion: A DESSOLVE II trial sub-study. *Catheter Cardiovasc Interv* 2015; 86(7): 1141–50.

40. Barlis P et al. An optical coherence tomography study of a biodegradable vs. durable polymer-coated limus-eluting stent: A LEADERS trial sub-study. *Eur Heart J* 2010; 31(2): 165–76.

41. Natsuaki M et al. Final 3-year outcome of a randomized trial comparing second-generation drug-eluting stents using either biodegradable polymer or durable polymer: NOBORI biolimus-eluting versus XIENCE/PROMUS everolimus-eluting stent trial. *Circulation Cardiovasc Interv* 2015; 8(10).

42. Stefanini GG et al. Biodegradable polymer drug-eluting stents reduce the risk of stent thrombosis at 4 years in patients undergoing percutaneous coronary intervention: A pooled analysis of individual patient data from the ISAR-TEST 3, ISAR-TEST 4, and LEADERS randomized trials. *Eur Heart J* 2012; 33(10): 1214–22.

43. Navarese EP et al. Safety and efficacy of biodegradable vs. durable polymer drug-eluting stents: Evidence from a meta-analysis of randomised trials. *EuroIntervention* 2011; 7(8): 985–94.

44. Navarese EP et al. Safety and efficacy outcomes of first and second generation durable polymer drug eluting stents and biodegradable polymer biolimus eluting stents in clinical practice: Comprehensive network meta-analysis. *BMJ* 2013; 347: f6530.

45. Basalus MW et al. Scanning electron microscopic assessment of the biodegradable coating on expanded biolimus-eluting stents. *EuroIntervention* 2009; 5(4): 505–10.

46. Tada N et al. Polymer-free biolimus a9-coated stent demonstrates more sustained intimal inhibition, improved healing, and reduced inflammation compared with a polymer-coated sirolimus-eluting cypher stent in a porcine model. *Circ Cardiovasc Interv* 2010; 3(2): 174–83.

47. Moretti C et al. Cre8 coronary stent: Preclinical in vivo assessment of a new generation polymer-free DES with Amphilimus formulation. *EuroIntervention* 2012; 7(9): 1087–94.

48. Mehilli J et al. Randomized trial of a nonpolymer-based rapamycin-eluting stent versus a polymer-based paclitaxel-eluting stent for the reduction of late lumen loss. *Circulation* 2006; 113(2): 273–9.

49. Carrie D et al. A multicenter randomized trial comparing amphilimus- with paclitaxel-eluting stents in de novo native coronary artery lesions. *J Am Coll Cardiol* 2012; 59(15): 1371–6.

50. Costa JR, Jr. et al. 1-year results of the hydroxyapatite polymer-free sirolimus-eluting stent for the treatment of single de novo coronary lesions: The VESTASYNC I trial. *J Am Coll Cardiol Interv* 2009; 2(5): 422–7.

51. Costa R et al. Polymer-free biolimus A9-coated stents in the treatment of de novo coronary lesions: 4- and 12-month angiographic follow-up and final 5-year clinical outcomes of the prospective, multicenter BioFreedom FIM clinical trial. *J Am Coll Cardiol Interv* 2016; 9(1): 51–64.

52. Urban P et al. Polymer-free drug-coated coronary stents in patients at high bleeding risk. *N Engl J Med* 2015; 373(21): 2038–47.

53. Windecker S et al. 2014 ESC/EACTS guidelines on myocardial revascularization. *EuroIntervention* 2015; 10(9): 1024–94.

54. Vranckx P et al. Long-term ticagrelor monotherapy versus standard dual antiplatelet therapy followed by aspirin monotherapy in patients undergoing biolimus-eluting stent implantation: Rationale and design of the GLOBAL LEADERS trial. *EuroIntervention* 2015; 11(7).

55. Worthley S. Drug-filled stent: Concept, pre-clinical studies and early clinical observations. Presentation at Transcatheter Therapeutics 2015, San Francisco, CA, 2015.

56. Konig A et al. Stent design-related coronary artery remodeling and patterns of neointima formation following self-expanding and balloon-expandable stent implantation. *Catheter Cardiovasc Interv* 2002; 56(4): 478–86.

57. Garg S et al. In: Eeckhout E et al. (editors), Coronary Artery Stents, Chapter 3.3, PCR–EAPCI *Textbook of Percutaneous Interventional Cardiovascular Medicine*. Europa Publications, Paris, 2015.

58. Meredith IT et al. Three-year results comparing platinum-chromium PROMUS element and cobalt-chromium XIENCE V everolimus-eluting stents in de novo coronary artery narrowing (from the PLATINUM Trial). *Am J Cardiol* 2014; 113(7): 1117–23.

59. Garasic JM et al. Stent and artery geometry determine intimal thickening independent of arterial injury. *Circulation* 2000; 101(7): 812–8.

60. Sullivan TM et al. Effect of endovascular stent strut geometry on vascular injury, myointimal hyperplasia, and restenosis. *J Vasc Surg* 2002; 36(1): 143–9.

61. Kastrati A et al. Intracoronary stenting and angiographic results: Strut thickness effect on restenosis outcome (ISAR-STEREO) trial. *Circulation* 2001; 103(23): 2816–21.

62. Pache J et al. Intracoronary stenting and angiographic results: Strut thickness effect on restenosis outcome (ISAR-STEREO-2) trial. *J Am Coll Cardiol* 2003; 41(8): 1283–8.

63. Briguori C et al. In-stent restenosis in small coronary arteries: Impact of strut thickness. *J Am Coll Cardiol* 2002; 40(3): 403–9.

64. Timmins LH et al. Increased artery wall stress post-stenting leads to greater intimal thickening. *Lab Invest* 2011; 91(6): 955–67.

65. Koskinas KC et al. Role of endothelial shear stress in stent restenosis and thrombosis: Pathophysiologic mechanisms and implications for clinical translation. *J Am Coll Cardiol* 2012; 59(15): 1337–49.

66. Pache J et al. Drug-eluting stents compared with thin-strut bare stents for the reduction of restenosis: A prospective, randomized trial. *Eur Heart J* 2005; 26(13): 1262–8.

67. Kereiakes DJ et al. Clinical and angiographic outcomes after treatment of de novo coronary stenoses with a novel platinum chromium thin-strut stent: Primary results of the PERSEUS (Prospective Evaluation in a Randomized Trial of the Safety and Efficacy of the Use of the TAXUS Element Paclitaxel-Eluting Coronary Stent System) trial. *J Am Coll Cardiol* 2010; 56(4): 264–71.

68. Kereiakes DJ et al. Long-term follow-up of the platinum chromium TAXUS element (ION) stent: The PERSEUS workhorse and small vessel trial five-year results. *Catheter Cardiovasc Interv* 2015; 86(6): 994–1001.

69. Aoki J et al. Incidence and clinical impact of coronary stent fracture after sirolimus-eluting stent implantation. *Catheter Cardiovasc Interv* 2007; 69(3): 380–6.

70. Park MW et al. Incidence and clinical impact of fracture of drug-eluting stents widely used in current clinical practice: Comparison with initial platform of sirolimus-eluting stent. *J Cardiol* 2012; 60(3): 215–21.

71. Arnous S et al. Incidence and mechanisms of longitudinal stent deformation associated with Biomatrix, Resolute, Element, and Xience stents: Angiographic and case-by-case review of 1,800 PCIs. *Catheter Cardiovasc Interv* 2015; 86(6): 1002–11.

72. von Birgelen C et al. Third-generation zotarolimus-eluting and everolimus-eluting stents in all-comer patients requiring a percutaneous coronary intervention (DUTCH PEERS): A randomised, single-blind, multicentre, non-inferiority trial. *Lancet* 2014; 383(9915): 413–23.

73. Garg S, and Serruys PW. Coronary stents: Looking forward. *J Am Coll Cardiol* 2010; 56(Suppl 10): S43–78.

74. Serruys PW et al. Bioresorable scaffolds. In: Eeckhout E et al. (editors), *Percutaneous Interventional Cardiovascular Medicine*. Paris: Europa Edition Publishing. Part III, Chapter 4, 2012, pp. 145–177.

75. Serruys PW et al. Evaluation of the second generation of a bioresorbable everolimus-eluting vascular scaffold for the treatment of de novo coronary artery stenosis: 12-month clinical and imaging outcomes. *J Am Coll Cardiol* 2011; 58(15): 1578–88.

76. Serruys PW et al. A bioabsorbable everolimus-eluting coronary stent system (ABSORB): 2-year outcomes and results from multiple imaging methods. *Lancet* 2009; 373(9667): 897–910.

77. Serruys PW et al. Evaluation of the second generation of a bioresorbable everolimus drug-eluting vascular scaffold for treatment of de novo coronary artery stenosis: Six-month clinical and imaging outcomes. *Circulation* 2010; 122(22): 2301–12.

78. Ormiston JA et al. A bioabsorbable everolimus-eluting coronary stent system for patients with single de-novo coronary artery lesions (ABSORB): A prospective open-label trial. *Lancet* 2008; 371(9616): 899–907.

79. Abizaid A et al. The ABSORB EXTEND study: Preliminary report of the twelve-month clinical outcomes in the first 512 patients enrolled. *EuroIntervention* 2015; 10(12): 1396–401.

80. Capodanno D et al. Percutaneous coronary intervention with everolimus-eluting bioresorbable vascular scaffolds in routine clinical practice: Early and midterm outcomes from the European multicentre GHOST-EU registry. *EuroIntervention* 2015; 10(10): 1144–53.

81. Serruys PW et al. A bioresorbable everolimus-eluting scaffold versus a metallic everolimus-eluting stent for ischaemic heart disease caused by de-novo native coronary artery lesions (ABSORB II): An interim 1-year analysis of clinical and procedural secondary outcomes from a randomised controlled trial. *Lancet* 2015; 385(9962): 43–54.

82. Puricel S et al. Comparison of everolimus- and biolimus-eluting coronary stents with everolimus-eluting bioresorbable vascular scaffolds. *J Am Coll Cardiol* 2015; 65(8): 791–801.

83. Gao R et al. Bioresorbable vascular scaffolds versus metallic stents in patients with coronary artery disease: ABSORB china trial. *J Am Coll Cardiol* 2015; 66(21): 2298–309.

84. Kimura T et al. A randomized trial evaluating everolimus-eluting Absorb bioresorbable scaffolds vs. everolimus-eluting metallic stents in patients with coronary artery disease: ABSORB Japan. *Eur Heart J* 2015; 36(47): 3332–42.

85. Ellis SG et al. Everolimus-eluting bioresorbable scaffolds for coronary artery disease. *N Engl J Med* 2015; 373(20): 1905–15.

86. Sabate M et al. Everolimus-eluting bioresorbable stent vs. durable polymer everolimus-eluting metallic stent in patients with ST-segment elevation myocardial infarction: Results of the randomized ABSORB ST-segment elevation myocardial infarction-TROFI II trial. *Eur Heart J* 2015; 37(3): 229–40.

87. Grundeken MJ et al. Treatment of coronary bifurcation lesions with the Absorb bioresorbable vascular scaffold in combination with the Tryton dedicated coronary bifurcation stent: Evaluation using two- and three-dimensional optical coherence tomography. *EuroIntervention* 2015; 11(8): 877–84.

88. Mattesini A et al. ABSORB biodegradable stents versus second-generation metal stents: A comparison study of 100 complex lesions treated under OCT guidance. *JACC Cardiovasc Interv* 2014; 7(7): 741–50.

89. Ormiston JA et al. First serial assessment at 6 months and 2 years of the second generation of absorb everolimus-eluting bioresorbable vascular scaffold: A multi-imaging modality study. *Circ Cardiovasc Interv* 2012; 5(5): 620–32.

90. Bourantas CV et al. Effect of the endothelial shear stress patterns on neointimal proliferation following drug-eluting bioresorbable vascular scaffold implantation: An optical coherence tomography study. *JACC Cardiovasc Interv* 2014; 7(3): 315–24.

91. Serruys PW et al. Dynamics of vessel wall changes following the implantation of the absorb everolimus-eluting bioresorbable vascular scaffold: A multi-imaging modality study at 6, 12, 24 and 36 months. *EuroIntervention* 2014; 9(11): 1271–84.

92. Farooq V et al. Intracoronary optical coherence tomography and histology of overlapping everolimus-eluting bioresorbable vascular scaffolds in a porcine coronary artery model: The potential implications for clinical practice. *JACC Cardiovasc Interv* 2013; 6(5): 523–32.

93. Erbel R et al. Temporary scaffolding of coronary arteries with bioabsorbable magnesium stents: A prospective, non-randomised multicentre trial. *Lancet* 2007; 369(9576): 1869–75.

94. Haude M et al. Safety and performance of the drug-eluting absorbable metal scaffold (DREAMS) in patients with

de-novo coronary lesions: 12 month results of the prospective, multicentre, first-in-man BIOSOLVE-I trial. *Lancet* 2013; 381(9869): 836–44.

95. Haude M et al. Safety and performance of the second-generation drug-eluting absorbable metal scaffold in patients with de-novo coronary artery lesions (BIOSOLVE-II): 6 month results of a prospective, multi-centre, non-randomised, first-in-man trial. *Lancet* 2016; 387(10013): 31–9.

96. Waksman R et al. Early- and long-term intravascular ultrasound and angiographic findings after bioabsorbable magnesium stent implantation in human coronary arteries. *JACC Cardiovasc Interv* 2009; 2(4): 312–20.

97. Costa RA. *REVA ReZolve Clinical Program Update*. Miami Beach: Transcatheter Cardiovascular Therapeutics, FL2012.

98. Yan J, and Bhat VD. Elixir medical's bioresorbable drug eluting stent (BDES) programme: An overview. *EuroIntervention* 2009; 5(Suppl F): F80–2.

99. Cassese S et al. Everolimus-eluting bioresorbable vascular scaffolds versus everolimus-eluting metallic stents: A meta-analysis of randomised controlled trials. *Lancet* 2016; 387(10018): 537–44.

100. Sato T et al. Very late thrombosis observed on optical coherence tomography 22 months after the implantation of a polymer-based bioresorbable vascular scaffold. *Eur Heart J* 2015; 36(20): 1273.

Stent thrombosis and restenosis

S ANDREW MCCULLOUGH, GEORGE D DANGAS

14.1 Introduction

Since the evolution of coronary stenting, both stent thrombosis, the development of a platelet and fibrin clot on the endothelial metal prosthesis, in stent restenosis (ISR) and the variable neo-endothelialisation of the stent platform, have been observed. Much of the research in interventional cardiology has been to develop therapies and newer stents to prevent these unintended syndromes. We hereafter distinguish between both stent thrombosis and ISR, and discuss the prevalence, risk factors, pathophysiology and preventative measures we take to minimise the risk of their development.

14.2 Stent thrombosis

Stent thrombosis, as defined by the academic research consortium (ARC) in 2007, is the angiographic or pathological total or partial thrombotic occlusion within a stent that is associated with ischemic symptoms, electrocardiogram (ECG) changes or elevated cardiac biomarkers. Stent thrombosis (ST) can be classified as early (<30 days), late (>30 days), or very late (>1 year). The ARC also allows for defining probable stent thrombosis and possible stent thrombosis.[1]

14.2.1 Incidence

The incidence of ST has decreased as advances in anti-platelet therapy and stent technology have evolved.

Indeed, as stent technology has advanced a recent meta-analysis has revealed that 'second generation' drug eluting stents (DESs) significantly reduce the incidence of stent thrombosis compared with 'first generation' drug eluting and bare metal stents (BMSs), and this benefit has been shown out to 2 years.[2-4] That said, current rates of stent thrombosis for BMSs and 'second generation' DESs are similar, estimated at approximately 0.5%–3% depending on the clinical syndrome at the time of implantation (e.g., stable vs. acute infarction).[5] The incidence of very late stent thrombosis is estimated at approximately 0.6% annually for first generation DESs and nearly eliminated in second generation DESs. On the other hand, recurrent stent thrombosis has been documented at rates ranging from 6% to 19%. Published reports demonstrate variability in mortality rates after stent thrombosis, ranging from 11% to 42%, likely from the lack of a consensus definition until 2007. The exact mechanisms leading to such striking mortality rates are unknown; however, in a 2008 report on 86 patients with ST segment elevation myocardial infarction (STEMI) secondary to stent thrombosis compared to those without, rates of successful re-perfusion during percutaneous coronary intervention (PCI) were lower (80.4% vs. 96.9%) and rates of distal thrombus embolisation were higher (6.5% vs. 0%).[6] The most 'mortal' type of stent thrombosis is sub-acute sub-type, and most deaths occurred within 1 week of stent implantation.[7]

14.3 Clinical presentation and pathophysiology

Stent thrombosis can present in a variety of ways, though typically the patient will experience symptoms of ischemia, ECG changes and biomarker elevations consistent with an acute myocardial infarction. Akin to this, stent thrombosis can also present as sudden cardiac death. Various risk factors for stent thrombosis have been identified and are related to patient characteristics, procedural and post-procedural characteristics and lesion characteristics (Table 14.1). Pathophysiologically stent thrombosis generally occurs via of the following mechanisms: (1) exposure of blood to the prothrombotic stent components prior to re-endothelialisation, causing activation of the clotting cascade, (2) slow flow within the stent, (3) inadequate suppression of platelet activity (resistance to medications or non-adherence) and (4) the presence of a prothrombotic state (e.g., malignancy or an acute coronary syndrome). As such, it cannot be emphasised enough that an optimal procedural result is important to minimising the risk of stent thrombosis. When patients with stent thrombosis undergo coronary angiography, they are found to have a partially or completely occlusive thrombus in the stent scaffold.

Early stent thrombosis occurs within 30 days after stent implantation, and is usually secondary to technical and procedural factors. Sub-optimal angiographic results, including slow flow and residual dissection, have been associated with early stent thrombosis.[8] Anti-platelet therapy and anticoagulant therapy at the time of the procedure (discussed below) are also key in preventing early stent thrombosis as the thrombogenic stent scaffold is exposed to the blood surface as it is not yet re-endothelialised. Late stent thrombosis is associated with delayed re-endothelialisation (e.g., in first generation DES vs. BMS), ongoing vessel inflammation and fibrin deposition. Stent malapposition may also cause late stent thrombosis, usually from the arterial wall remodelling away from the stent struts over time.

The use of intravascular imaging, specifically intravascular ultrasound (IVUS) and optical coherence tomography (OCT), at the time of angiography is safe to explore the mechanisms of stent thrombosis once the patient is stable. These techniques have identified several stent-related factors that predispose patients to stent thrombosis, including stent underexpansion, stent malapposition, stent fracture, dissection, new plaque rupture, negative remodelling at the stent edge and neoatherosclerosis.[9,10]

Stent underexpansion occurs when an undersized stent is selected for the target vessel or when the arterial wall does not allow for full expansion of the stent at the time of initial implantation. Stent underexpansion should be treated with high-pressure balloon angioplasty, and should not be treated by placing a new stent, as rigid non-compliant arterial walls will generally not accommodate more stent layers. If balloon expansion is ineffective, subsequent treatment options include rotational atherectomy, excimer laser therapy and coronary artery bypass surgery (CABG). *Stent malapposition* occurs when a blood filled space is located between the stent and the vessel wall, and is ameliorated with balloon angioplasty. *Stent fracture* tends to occur in right coronary artery (RCA) lesions, tortuous lesions, overlapping stents, and can be treated with a small stent to cover the fracture. *Dissections* at the stent edge can lead to stent thrombosis, and can be easily covered with a new stent. *New plaque rupture* can cause stent thrombosis via a native adjacent plaque with thrombus extending into the previously placed stent. *Negative remodelling* distal to a stent causes slow flow within the stent, predisposing to stent thrombosis and lastly *neoatherosclerosis* within the stent lumen has been observed as a cause of plaque rupture in both BMSs and DESs.

14.4 Preventing stent thrombosis

Optimal stent implantation technique cannot be overemphasised in preventing stent thrombosis. Stents should be the appropriate length, as well as be appropriately expanded and apposed to the vessel wall. It is known that increasing stent length leads to increasing incidence of stent thrombosis; however, choosing too short of a stent can result in dissections near the stent edge, miss part of the lesion, and

Table 14.1 Predictors of stent thrombosis

Patient	Lesion	Procedural	Post-procedural
Early stent thrombosis			
Cancer, heart failure, PAD, DM, medication non-compliance, genetic mutations, thrombocytosis	Bifurcation, LAD, vessel size, lesion length, thrombus, SVG lesion	Stent undersizing, underexpansion, malapposition, lack of P@Y12 receptor antagonist, stent length	DAPT discontinuation
Late stent thrombosis			
ESRD, smoking, STEMI, medication non-compliance	LAD, incomplete endothelialisation, delayed healing, prior IVBT, SVG lesion	DES (compared with BMS), permanent polymer DES, overlapping DES	DAPT discontinuation, late stent malapposition

Source: Adapted from Claessen BE et al., *JACC Cardiovasc Interv*, 7, 10, 2014.

as a result predispose to stent thrombosis. One must weigh that bifurcations treated with two stents can notoriously take a longer time to re-endothelialise, further increasing the risk of stent thrombosis.[5] In addition to procedural technique, multiple pharmacologic therapies, including anti-thrombotic and anti-platelet agents, have been developed and tested in an effort to reduce stent thrombosis.

14.4.1 Anti-thrombotic therapy

At the time of PCI, parenteral anti-coagulation with unfractionated heparin, low molecular weight heparin, or bivalirudin, a direct thrombin inhibitor, can be administered to prevent acute stent thrombosis. The hallmark harmonising outcomes with revascularisation and stents in acute myocardial infarction (HORIZONS-AMI) trial randomised 3602 patients with STEMI undergoing primary PCI to receive either bivalirudin or the combination of heparin and a glycoprotein IIb/IIIa inhibitor. In this study, bivalirudin was associated with an increased incidence of acute stent thrombosis (1.3% vs. 0.3%, $p < .01$), however there was no difference in the incidence of stent thrombosis at 1 year. Also in this trial bivalirudin was shown to drastically reduce bleeding rates and mortality, and as such its use has been favoured during PCI since then.[11]

The question remained as to how bivalirudin compared to heparin without the concomitant use of GPIs. As such, the HEAT PPCI and MATRIX trials have both recently documented no differences between the incidence of stent thrombosis and bleeding between heparin and bivalirudin.[12,13] The bleeding risk with heparin has been attenuated in these trials likely as a result of transradial access site utilisation, adjunctive glycoprotein IIb/IIIa inhibitors and potent P2Y12 inhibitors, but these have had no effect on early stent thrombosis.[14]

14.4.2 Anti-platelet therapy

Dual anti-platelet therapy (DAPT) is the cornerstone of preventing stent thrombosis. This was initially observed in the STARS trial, which showed tremendous benefit of the combination of aspirin with ticlodipine versus aspirin and warfarin or aspirin alone, and has been re-affirmed with the development of each new anti-platelet agent.[15] Four agents are currently used (due to ticlodipine's haematological side effects) to inhibit the P2Y12-type platelet adenosine diphosphate receptor, thus inhibiting platelet activation. The four P2Y12 antagonists currently available for use are clopidogral, prasugrel, ticagrelor and cangrelor. Another anti-platelet agent vorapaxor is also available, however its use has not been widely adopted and it will not be discussed here.

Clopidogrel is a prodrug that binds and irreversibly inhibits the P2Y12 receptor. In addition to its importance after a myocardial infarction, clopidogrel was shown to be non-inferior to and better tolerated than ticlodipine in preventing stent thrombosis.[16] Clopidogrel is metabolised in the liver, where genetic variations in enzyme activity can dramatically alter a patient's response to the drug. As such, newer P2Y12 receptor antagonists have been developed to improve platelet inhibition.

Prasugrel is a thienopyridine that was developed to more quickly and effectively inhibit platelets than clopidogrel. Its use was validated in the TRITON trial, a trial which randomised 13,608 patients with moderate- to high-risk acute coronary syndromes undergoing PCI to 6–15 months of dual anti-platelets therapy. In this trial, prasugrel significantly reduced the rate of stent thrombosis as compared with clopidogrel (1.1% vs. 2.4%, $p < .001$) at the cost of increasing the rate of non-CABG related TIMI major bleeding ($p = .03$), major or minor bleeding ($p = .002$). Additionally, prasugrel increased mortality in patients with a prior stroke, and as such should not be given to patients with a history of transient ischemic attack or stroke.[17]

Ticagrelor is an oral non-thienodypyridine, and is a reversible inhibitor of the receptor. The efficacy of ticagrelor was tested in the PLATO trial, a randomised trial of 18,624 patients with an acute coronary syndrome, which compared ticagrelor against clopidogrel. Amongst patients in the study who received a stent, the rate of definite stent thrombosis was lower in patients treated with ticagrelor (1.3% vs. 1.9%, $p = .009$), and there were no differences in bleeding between the two groups. Additionally, it was noted that ticagrelor significantly reduced the rate of all-cause mortality (4.5% vs. 5.9%, $p < .001$).[18]

Most recently, cangrelor, the first intravenous P2Y12 receptor antagonist, has been validated for use after PCI. In the CHAMPION PHEONIX trial, 11,145 patients were randomised in a double-blinded double-dummy fashion to a 48-hour infusion of cangrelor followed by clopidogrel or clopidogrel alone. Patients treated with cangrelor had significantly less intraprocedural stent thrombosis (0.6% vs. 1.0%, $p = .04$), stent thrombosis at 48 hours (0.8% vs. 1.4%, $p = .01$) and stent thrombosis at 30 days (1.3% vs. 1.9%, $p = .01$).[19]

14.5 Duration of dual anti-platelet therapy

Currently the bulk of research being performed in interventional cardiology is geared towards determining the optimal duration of DAPT. Currently, the ACC/AHA recommends 1 year of DAPT after BMS or DES implantation; however the European guidelines now recommend 1 month of DAPT after BMS placement, 6 months of DAPT after DES and only 3 months after the uncomplicated use of second generation DESs. In both the United States and European guidelines, it is recommended that patients with and acute coronary syndrome receive either prasugrel or ticagrelor in favour of clopidogrel for 1 year following stent implantation.[5] Several clinical trials have recently been completed that show similar rates of stent thrombosis in low-risk patients who only receive 6 months of DAPT versus 24 months of DAPT.[20]

In 2014, the landmark DAPT trial was completed that compared 12 months with 30 months of DAPT after DES placement. 9961 patients were randomised to an additional

18 months of thienopyridine treatment or placebo in addition to aspirin. It was found that patients who received continued treatment with thienopyridines had significantly lower rates of stent thrombosis (0.4% vs. 1.4%, $p < .001$) and major adverse cardiovascular and cerebrovascular events (4.3% vs. 5.9%, $p < .001$) at the cost of increased moderate to severe bleeding (2.5% vs. 1.6%, $p = .001$). This trial demonstrates that for patients undergoing DES placement, continuing DAPT is beneficial, but must be continually weighed against the risk of bleeding. Subsequent meta-analyses have been performed on patients who continue DAPT beyond 1 year, and they all reinforce that continuation of DAPT reduces the risk of stent thrombosis, but increases the risk of major bleeding.[21] This balance favours long DAPT after first generation DESs, but not as much after the use of second generation DESs.

Patients must be educated regarding the risks of DAPT interruption and non-compliance. Studies show that the risk of stent thrombosis and DAPT non-compliance lasts for the first 6 months after stent implantation, and decreases thereafter.[5] Additionally, when considering patients for elective surgery or invasive testing after stent implantation, it is preferable to postpone the procedure until 1 year after stent implantation if possible, and aspirin should be continued throughout the procedure. Careful temporary observed discontinuation rather than unsupervised DAPT disruption might also be feasible when necessary.[22]

14.6 Triple therapy

In certain circumstances, patients may undergo or have recently undergone stent implantation and require systemic oral anticoagulation. The What is Optimal anti-platElet and anticoagulant therapy in patients with oral anticoagulation and coronary StenTing (WOEST) trial addressed the safety of triple anticoagulation, and found that 12 months of combination therapy consisting of oral anticoagulation with clopidogrel was superior to the combination of oral anticoagulation, clopidogrel and aspirin in terms of bleeding and mortality without any difference in the risk of stent thrombosis at 1 year.[23] Additionally, another form of triple therapy with the use of aspirin, clopidogrel and cilostazol has been reported in Asian populations with good safety and efficacy. Notably, Asian populations have high rates of genetically driven clopidogrel resistance.[24]

14.7 Risk stratification

To risk stratify patients with regard to the risk of stent thrombosis, it is important to remember to modify risk factors when feasible. Additionally, it may be prudent for physicians to choose BMSs in patients with a high bleeding risk in lesions with a low risk of restenosis. Two scores have been developed to assist in the risk assessment for the development of bleeding risk. The first can be useful in patients who present with acute coronary syndromes, and incorporates both patient and procedural characteristics (Table 14.2).[5] The second score used data from the DAPT study and also incorporates patient and procedural characteristics (Table 14.3, www.daptstudy.org).[21] Regardless of which risk stratification method practitioners use, judiciously administering DAPT whilst weighing a patient's risk of bleeding remains paramount.

14.8 Future directions

As stated above, patients must be *continually* assessed for the risk of stent thrombosis and the risk of bleeding whilst on DAPT. Currently, studies are underway to determine the efficacy of anti-platelet monotherapy versus DAPT in preventing stent thrombosis in the first 12 months after DES implantation in patients who have completed 3 months of DAPT with aspirin and ticagrelor. The results of the ongoing LEADERS-FREE and TWILIGHT studies could change the way we treat patients after PCI, and lower the risk of bleeding (NCT01623180 and NCT02270242).

Table 14.2 Risk score for probable or definite stent thrombosis in patients with acute coronary syndrome

Variable	Integer for risk score calculation		
Type of acute coronary syndrome	NSTE-ACS w/o ST changes +1	NSTE-ACS with ST Changes +2	
Current smoking	Yes: +1	No: +0	
Insulin-dependent diabetes mellitus	Yes: +2	No: +0	
History of PCI	Yes: +1	No: +0	
Platelet count	<250k: +0	250k–400k: +1	>400k: +2
Absence of pre-PCI heparin	Yes: +1	No: +0	
Aneurysm or ulceration	Yes: +2	No: +0	
Baseline TIMI flow 0/1	Yes: +1	No: +0	
Final TIMI flow <3	Yes: +1	No: +0	
Number of vessels treated	1 vessel +0	2 vessels +1	3 vessels: +2
Add to calculate ST risk score			

Source: Adapted from Claessen, B.E. et al., *JACC Cardiovasc Interv*, 7, 10, 2014.
A score >9 indicated patients at high risk of stent thrombosis.

Table 14.3 DAPT score for predicting risk of bleeding and stent thrombosis

Patient characteristics			
Age	<65	65–74 (−1)	>75 (−2)
Diabetes mellitus	Yes (+1)	No	
Smoking within 2 years	Yes (+1)	No	
Prior MI or PCI	Yes (+1)	No	
History of CHF or EF<30%	Yes (+1)	No	
Procedure characteristics			
MI at presentation	Yes (+1)	No	
Stenting of vein of graft	Yes (+1)	No	
Stent diameter <3 mm	Yes (+1)	No	

Source: Adapted from www.daptstudy.org.
A score of 2 or greater identifies patients in whom the risk of stent thrombosis outweighs the risk of bleeding on continued DAPT.

14.9 In stent restenosis

ISR after stent implantation is historically the most burdensome problem associated with coronary intervention. ISR is defined as an angiographic reduction in lumen diameter of >50% at follow-up angiography after stent implantation, and is thought to be secondary to arterial damage resulting in subsequent neointimal tissue proliferation.[25] ISRs can vary in their morphologic appearance, and these differences account for important differences in clinical, prognostic and therapeutic implications. The Mehran classification[26] is as follows:

- Class I, 'Focal ISR': Lesions <10 mm and
  - Type IA: at the unscaffolded segment of a stent (e.g., a gap)
  - Type IB: within the body of the stent
  - Type IC: at the proximal or distal stent margin
  - Type ID: a combination of these sites, or 'multi-focal ISR'
- Class II 'Diffuse ISR': Lesions are >10 mm in length and occupy the body of the stent, without extension to the outside margins
- Class III, 'Diffuse proliferative ISR': Lesions are >10 mm and extend beyond the body of the stent
- Class IV, 'ISR with total occlusion': lesions with a TIMI flow of 0

The most widely used definition of ISR has been proposed by the ARC, and is present when there is a need for ischemia-driven repeat revascularisation, which includes >70% luminal narrowing alone or >50% luminal narrowing accompanied by recurrent angina pectoris, objective signs of ischemia at rest or with exercise, or an abnormal invasive functional diagnostic test (e.g., FFR > 0.8).[1] As ISR is the result of cell proliferation, it usually takes time to develop as opposed to stent thrombosis, which generally occurs within the first 30 days after stent placement. It is possible that ISR and stent thrombosis can coexist, and at the time of angiography these patients have both neointimal hyperplasia as well as a focal thrombosis inside the stent.

14.9.1 Incidence

The initial incidence of ISR in trials comparing bare metal and DESs was 30% vs. <6%.[25] As DESs became more widely adopted, more complex percutaneous procedures were performed, and the incidence of ISR rose to the double digits, with rates of restenosis in more complex patients at >10%.[27] As the second generation of DESs has evolved, head to head trials of everolimus versus paclitaxel eluting stents have shown significantly lower rates of target vessel failure with the everolimus eluting stent.[28] Similar overall outcomes in ISR and target lesion re-vascularisation have been observed in trials of both sirolumus and zotarolimus eluting stents as well. Most recently, the TUXEDO-India trial (Taxus Element versus Xience Prime in a Diabetic Population) revealed low rates of target vessel failure overall, yet significantly lower rates of target vessel and target lesion re-vascularisation in patients treated with everolimus eluting stents,[29] expanding findings observed in the non-diabetic population to that with diabetes.

Lastly, fully bioabsorbable stents have been developed in recent years to limit stent-related mechanical complications, including persistent inflammation, strut fracture and ongoing intimal proliferation within the stent frame. Preliminary studies of the everolimus eluting bioabsorbable scaffold have shown non-inferior clinical outcomes compared to everolimus eluting stents, with respect to ischemia driven target lesion re-vascularisation (6%–8%).[30] This technology is expected to further evolve over time.

The average time until development of ISR and associated symptoms after stent implantation is approximately 5 months after BMS implantation and between 8 and 13 months after DES implantation.[25] In the TAXUS II study, comparing BMS and paclitaxel-eluting stents, patients underwent serial IVUS for 2 years after stent deployment. In patients treated with BMS had a decrease in neointimal hyperplasia, whilst patients treated with PES experienced an increase in neotintimal hyperplasia, though the total neointimal area was still significantly smaller in PES treated patients.[31] This finding has also been observed in patients treated with sirolimus and everolimus eluting stents.[28] The mechanism of the late increase in neointimal hyperplasia in DES treated patients remains unclear. Additionally, it should be noted that the earlier ISR develops, the worse its outcome is after PCI.

14.10 Clinical presentation

As the stent scaffold becomes progressively obstructed by neo-intimal hyperplasia, most patients experience recurrent angina, though some cases of ISR are clinically silent. Given the time frame it takes for restenosis to occur, most cases of ISR were believed to be clinically benign; however, data suggests that patients present anywhere on the spectrum of ischemia. Data in both the BMS population and DES population suggest that ISR can present as both unstable angina in up to 50%–60% of patients and as a myocardial infarction in up to 20% of patients.[25] The mechanism of myocardial infarction in patients with ISR is not entirely clear. Clinically silent completely occlusive restenosis can be difficult to distinguish from an old thrombotic event, and high-grade restenosis can cause slow flow, promote thrombosis and lead to an acute coronary syndrome. It was observed in a secondary analysis of the Prevention of Restenosis with Tranilast and its Outcomes (PRESTO) trial that patients who present with an acute coronary syndrome have a higher incidence of recurrent major adverse cardiac events and binary restenosis compared with patients who present with stable angina.[32]

14.11 Mechanisms of restenosis

The reasons why some patients experience ISR and the reasons only some segments in the same patient restenosis are unclear. Indeed the prevention of ISR in a DES depends upon the stent platform, agent delivered and the drug carrier. In addition to the initial arterial injury and resultant neointimal hyperplasia, it is thought that technical, mechanical and biologic mechanisms predispose DES patients to ISR.

14.11.1 Technical factors

As stated above with regard to stent thrombosis, it cannot be over emphasised that an optimal procedural result is necessary for the development of ISR. Technical factors that result in ISR include residual uncovered plaque, stent gap and uncovered barotrauma. Additionally, a short *stent gap* between two DES typically occurs in a zone of balloon injury, does not receive optimal drug delivery, and can result in ISR. Lastly, *barotrauma outside the stented segment* can result in restenosis. A subgroup analysis from an early sirolimus eluting stent study revealed that exposed margins of stent that did not cover the entire length of balloon injury were the primary sites of restenosis.[33] This has decreased as the use of predilation with shorter balloons, utilisation of longer stents to cover injury and post-dilation within stented regions has increased.

14.11.2 Mechanical factors

Mechanical factors that contribute to ISR include stent underexpansion and malapposition, non-uniform drug distribution and stent fracture. For a DES to most effectively protect against ISR, the drug must be delivered transmurally and circumferentially, and in areas of malapposition and underexpansion optimal drug delivery is compromised. As noted above, stent underexpansion results from choosing an inappropriately sized stent during implantation or failure to fully expand the stent. *Stent malapposition* occurs when the stent fails to fully articulate with the vessel wall (i.e., in a tortuous or calcific lesion), resulting in a blood filled space between the stent struts and the intima. Underexpansion and malapposition can be difficult to detect angiographically, and can be more easily identified with the use of IVUS. Additionally, *non-uniform drug distribution* may occur if the polymeric drug coating is stripped during stent delivery. In this case, focal areas within the stented segment less than optimal drug distribution, and increased risk of ISR. Lastly, stent fractures, areas within the stent that partially or completely separate after implantation, result in loss of the metal scaffolding at the site of the fracture and sub-optimal drug delivery. The need for target lesion re-vascularisation in cases of stent fracture has been reported from 15% to 60%.[25]

14.11.3 Biologic factors

Biologic factors, namely hypersensitivity to any of the stent components as well as non-response to the pharmacologic agent, can predispose to ISR. It has been reported that hypersensitivity to nickel and molybdenum in stainless steel BMSs potentially contributed to ISR, likely via local inflammation and neointimal proliferation.[34] In DESs, patients can have hypersensitivity to the metal scaffold, the polymer coating, or the pharmacologic agent. The Research on Adverse Drug/Device events and Reports (RADAR) project noted 261 hypersensitivity reactions after DES placement and 17 reactions to the DES itself.[35] In addition to hypersensitivity reactions, recent data suggest genetic predispositions or alterations can create resistance to the anti-proliferative drugs used in DESs.[25]

14.12 Treatment of restenosis

Guidelines recommend PCI with DES implantation for ISR in DESs. There are a variety of treatment options for drug eluting ISR, and these include: intravascular brachytherapy (IVBT), implantation of another DES, plain old balloon angioplasty (POBA), cutting (or scored) balloon angioplasty, drug eluting balloon (DEB) angioplasty and CABG. IVBT was formerly used with success in alleviating restenosis, however recent trials showed superiority of DES implantation to IVBT, and this technique is currently reserved as a palliative treatment.

DES implantation is the preferred modality for treating ISR of DESs, and has shown superiority to IVBT, POBA and cutting balloon angioplasty.[36,37] Given that one of the mechanisms of restenosis in DES treated patients in resistance to the agent delivered, several trials have sought to determine if different DESs are superior to implantation of the same DES. In the ISAR-DESIRE and ISAR-DESIRE 2 trials (Intracoronary Stenting and Angiographic Results:

DESs for ISR), there were no differences in late lumen loss or target lesion re-vascularisation if a different DES was implanted for the treatment of restenosis.[25,38] Limitations of repeat DES implantation are that conventionally no more than two layers of DES should be used in a single vessel, and as such treatment with POBA, cutting balloon angioplasty, drug-eluting balloon angioplasty and CABG remain valid therapeutic alternatives.

POBA with a larger high-pressure balloon can be useful for treating ISR, however the balloon will frequently slip. This technical problem has been subverted by the use of cutting, or scoring balloons. The addition of anti-proliferative agents to balloons for treatment of restenosis represents another technological advance. A recent meta-analysis of 11 trials that included 2059 patients with restenosis who underwent DEB, DES, or POBA revealed that both DES and DEB treatment for restenosis had less target lesions revascularization (TLR) and angiographic restenosis that patients who underwent POBA.[39] Additionally, the recently presented ISAR-DESIRE 4 trial revealed use of a cutting (or scored) balloon prior to DEB for treatment of restenosis had less angiographic restenosis, but no differences in TLR at 1 year.[40] Lastly, for patients who repeatedly experience restenosis or for those who have multi-vessel restenosis, coronary artery bypass grafting should be considered for treatment of restenosis. Additionally, any patient who experienced ISR in a DES should remain on DAPT as long as it is tolerated.

14.13 Conclusion

Stent thrombosis and ISR have both limited the results of PCI since the development of coronary stenting. We examined the differences in these two entities, as well as the risk factors, pathophysiologic mechanisms and treatment options for both. The judicious use of PCI, risk stratification and close follow-up are necessary in limiting these complications. Additionally, patients should be appropriately selected for and receive DAPT for at least 1 year, or even longer for high-risk patients. Many advances have been made in stent technology and anti-platelet therapy in an effort to attenuate both stent thrombosis and ISR.

References

1. Cutlip DE et al. Clinical end points in coronary stent trials: A case for standardized definitions. *Circulation* 2007; 115: 2344–51.
2. Philip F et al. Stent thrombosis with second-generation drug-eluting stents compared with bare-metal stents: Network meta-analysis of primary percutaneous coronary intervention trials in ST-segment–elevation myocardial infarction [corrected]. *Circ Cardiovasc Interv* 2014 Feb; 7(1): 49–61.
3. Mauri L et al. Stent thrombosis in randomized clinical trials of drug-eluting stents. *N Engl J Med* 2007 Mar 8; 356(10): 1020–9.
4. Palmerini T et al. Stent thrombosis with drug-eluting and bare-metal stents: Evidence from a comprehensive network meta-analysis. *Lancet* 2012 Apr 14; 379(9824): 1393–402.
5. Claessen BE et al. Stent thrombosis: A clinical perspective. *JACC Cardiovasc Interv* 2014 Oct; 7(10): 1081–92.
6. Chechi T et al. ST-segment elevation myocardial infarction due to early and late stent thrombosis a new group of high-risk patients. *J Am Coll Cardiol* 2008 June 24; 51(25): 2396–402.
7. Dangas GD et al. Clinical outcomes following stent thrombosis occurring in-hospital versus out-of-hospital: Results from the HORIZONS-AMI (Harmonizing Outcomes with Revascularization and Stents in Acute Myocardial Infarction) trial. *J Am Coll Cardiol* 2012 May 15; 59(20): 1752–9.
8. van Werkum JW et al. Predictors of coronary stent thrombosis: The Dutch Stent Thrombosis Registry. *J Am Coll Cardiol* 2009 Apr 21; 53(16): 1399–409.
9. Alfonso F et al. Findings of intravascular ultrasound during acute stent thrombosis. *Heart* 2004 Dec; 90(12): 1455–9.
10. Kubo T et al. Assessment of culprit lesion morphology in acute myocardial infarction: Ability of optical coherence tomography compared with intravascular ultrasound and coronary angioscopy. *J Am Coll Cardiol* 2007 Sep 4; 50(10): 933–9.
11. Stone GW et al. HORIZONS-AMI trial investigators. Bivalirudin during primary PCI in acute myocardial infarction. *N Engl J Med* 2008 May 22; 358(21): 2218–30.
12. Shahzad A et al. HEAT-PPCI trial investigators. Unfractionated heparin versus bivalirudin in primary percutaneous coronary intervention (HEAT-PPCI): An open-label, single centre, randomised controlled trial. *Lancet* 2014 Nov 22; 384(9957): 1849–58.
13. Valgimigli M et al. MATRIX investigators. Bivalirudin or Unfractionated Heparin in Acute Coronary Syndromes. *N Engl J Med* 2015 Sep 10; 373(11): 997–1009.
14. Bittl JA et al. Factors affecting bleeding and stent thrombosis in clinical trials comparing bivalirudin with heparin during percutaneous coronary intervention. *Circ Cardiovasc Interv* 2015; 8: e002789.
15. Leon MB et al. A clinical trial comparing three antithrombotic-drug regimens after coronary-artery stenting. Stent Anticoagulation Restenosis Study Investigators. *N Engl J Med* 1998 Dec 3; 339(23): 1665–71.
16. Taniuchi M et al. Randomized comparison of ticlopidine and clopidogrel after intracoronary stent implantation in a broad patient population. *Circulation* 2001 July 31; 104(5): 539–43.
17. Wiviott SD et al. TRITON-TIMI 38 investigators. Prasugrel versus clopidogrel in patients with acute coronary syndromes. *N Engl J Med* 2007 Nov 15; 357(20): 2001–15.
18. Wallentin L et al. PLATO investigators, Freij A, Thorsén M. Ticagrelor versus clopidogrel in patients with acute coronary syndromes. *N Engl J Med* 2009 Sep 10; 361(11): 1045–57.
19. Bhatt DL et al. CHAMPION PHOENIX investigators. Effect of platelet inhibition with cangrelor during PCI on ischemic events. *N Engl J Med* 2013 Apr 4; 368(14): 1303–13.
20. Valgimigli M et al. Prolonging dual antiplatelet treatment after grading stent-induced intimal hyperplasia study (PRODIGY) investigators. Short- versus long-term duration

of dual-antiplatelet therapy after coronary stenting: A randomized multicenter trial. *Circulation* 2012 Apr 24; 125(16): 2015–26.

21. Mauri L et al. DAPT study investigators. Twelve or 30 months of dual antiplatelet therapy after drug-eluting stents. *N Engl J Med* 2014 Dec 4; 371(23): 2155–66.

22. Mehran R et al. Cessation of dual antiplatelet treatment and cardiac events after percutaneous coronary intervention (PARIS): 2 year results from a prospective observational study. *Lancet* 2013 Nov 23; 382(9906): 1714–22.

23. Dewilde WJ et al. WOEST study investigators. Use of clopidogrel with or without aspirin in patients taking oral anticoagulant therapy and undergoing percutaneous coronary intervention: An open-label, randomised, controlled trial. *Lancet* 2013 Mar 30; 381(9872): 1107–15.

24. Park KH et al. Efficacy of triple anti-platelet therapy including cilostazol in acute myocardial infarction patients undergoing drug-eluting stent implantation. *Korean Circ J* 2009 May; 39(5): 190–7.

25. Dangas GD et al. In-stent restenosis in the drug-eluting stent era. *J Am Coll Cardiol* 2010 Nov 30; 56(23): 1897–907.

26. Mehran R et al. Angiographic patterns of in-stent restenosis: Classification and implications for long-term outcome. *Circulation* 1999; 100: 1872–8.

27. Morice MC et al. Sirolimus- vs paclitaxeleluting stents in de novo coronary artery lesions: The REALITY trial: A randomized controlled trial. *JAMA* 2006; 295: 895–904.

28. Kedhi E et al. Second-generation everolimus-eluting and paclitaxel-eluting stents in real-life practice (COMPARE): A randomised trial. *Lancet* 2010; 375: 201–9.

29. Kaul U et al. TUXEDO–India investigators. Paclitaxel-Eluting versus Everolimus-Eluting Coronary Stents in Diabetes. *N Engl J Med* 2015 Oct 29; 373(18): 1709–19.

30. Ellis SG et al. ABSORB III investigators. Everolimus-Eluting Bioresorbable Scaffolds for Coronary Artery Disease. *N Engl J Med* 2015 Nov 12; 373(20): 1905–15.

31. Tsuchida K et al. Two-year serial coronary angiographic and intravascular ultrasound analysis of in-stent angiographic late lumen loss and ultrasonic neointimal volume from the TAXUS II trial. *Am J Cardiol* 2007 Mar 1; 99(5): 607–15.

32. Assali AR et al. Acute coronary syndrome may occur with in-stent restenosis and is associated with adverse outcomes (the PRESTO trial). *Am J Cardiol* 2006; 98: 729–33.

33. Moses JW et al. Sirolimus-eluting stents versus standard stents in patients with stenosis in a native coronary artery. *N Engl J Med* 2003; 349: 1315–23.

34. Koster R et al. Nickel and molybdenum contact allergies in patients with coronary in-stent restenosis. *Lancet* 2000; 356:1895–7.

35. Nebeker JR et al. Hypersensitivity cases associated with drug-eluting coronary stents: A review of available cases from the Research on Adverse Drug Events and Reports (RADAR) project. *J Am Coll Cardiol* 2006; 47: 175–81.

36. Alfonso F et al. A randomized comparison of sirolimus-eluting stent with balloon angioplasty in patients with in-stent restenosis: Results of the Restenosis Intrastent: Balloon Angioplasty Versus Elective Sirolimus-Eluting Stenting (RIBS-II) trial. *J Am Coll Cardiol* 2006; 47: 2152–60.

37. Stone GW et al. Paclitaxel-eluting stents vs vascular brachytherapy for in-stent restenosis within baremetal stents: The TAXUS V ISR randomized trial. *JAMA* 2006; 295: 1253–63.

38. Mehilli J et al. Randomized trial of paclitaxel versus sirolimus-eluting stents for treatment of coronary restenosis in sirolimus-eluting stents: The ISAR-DESIRE 2 (Intracoronary Stenting and Angiographic Results: Drug Eluting Stents for In-Stent Restenosis 2) study. *J Am Coll Cardiol* 2010; 55: 2710–6.

39. Lee JM et al. Comparison among drug-eluting balloon, drug-eluting stent, and plain balloon angioplasty for the treatment of in-stent restenosis: A network meta-analysis of 11 randomized, controlled trials. *JACC Cardiovasc Interv* 2015; 8(3): 382–94.

40. Byrne R et al. ISAR-DESIRE 4: Intracoronary stenting and angiographic results: Optimizing treatment of drug eluting stent in-stent restenosis. Presented at TCT 2015. October 2015.

A practical approach to percutaneous interventions in chronic total occlusions

SANJOG KALRA, DIMITRI KARMPALIOTIS, JEFFREY W MOSES

Often referred to as the 'final frontier' in coronary intervention, chronic total occlusions (CTOs) are amongst the most challenging lesions treated by interventional cardiologists percutaneous coronary intervention (PCI) of these complex lesions, until recently, had been considered at relatively high risk of complications, of uncertain clinical benefit and with uncertain success rates. However, with the advent of specialised tools, treatment strategies, growing clinical experience and emerging evidence of clinical benefit, CTO PCI is steadily becoming a recognised subspecialty of coronary intervention. This chapter reviews the histopathologic features of CTOs, the rationale and benefits of CTO revascularisation and provides an overview of established technical strategies to facilitate success in these demanding procedures.

15.1 Background

Coronary CTOs are generally defined as the total obstruction of coronary blood flow for at least 3 months (and thus not due to an acute thrombotic event). In general, these vessels have antegrade native vessel thrombolysis in myocardial infarction (TIMI) grade 0 flow, but may have filling of the distal vessel by either antegrade (ipsilateral) or contralateral (retrograde) collaterals.[1] Functional CTOs or sub-total occlusions are similar disease segments with TIMI 1 antegrade flow, either luminal or via bridging collaterals and can be distinguished from segments of disease in which there is a residual lumen (termed *pseudo-occlusions*) by a subtle *to-and*-fro distal flow appearance of contrast (indicating retrograde non-opacified flow). Dual catheter angiography is vital to defining these lesion types and the recanalisation approach that is most likely to be successful.

CTOs are common. In 2012, Fefer and colleagues identified CTOs in 18% of patients presenting for cardiac catheterisation in whom coronary disease was found with electroencephalogram (ECG) evidence of infarction in only 25% of these cases and normal ejection fractions in over 50%. Interestingly, in the same study, the attempt rate for these lesions was only 10%, indicating that despite a high prevalence, patients with these lesions are often relegated to surgical or medical therapy. Barriers to more widespread adoption of CTO PCIs may include uncertainty regarding the clinical benefit of these procedures, their complexity and length, a perception of unacceptably high complication risks and overall operator discomfort with the specialised techniques and equipment necessary to achieve success.

15.2 Rationale, indications and clinical benefits of CTO PCI

Ultimately, the indications and rationale for CTO PCI are similar to those for non-CTO PCI: reduction in symptoms with improvement in quality of life, a reduction in ischaemia and possibly, a decrease in mortality and myocardial infarction. A growing body of evidence, mostly from large registry studies, supports the utility of CTO PCI in achieving these key clinical benefits, but there remains a reluctance to refer patients for these procedures. Indeed, the presence of a CTO is amongst the most common indications for referral to coronary artery bypass grafting (CABG),[2] despite evidence that revascularisation of CTOs in multi-vessel CABG is frequently suboptimal (68% in the Synergy between Percutaneous Coronary Intervention with TAXUS and Cardiac Surgery [SYNTAX] trial cohort).[3] Though there remains a need for randomised controlled trial evidence to pinpoint the exact clinical scenarios in which CTO PCI is most beneficial, there is a clear signal that these procedures are safe and effective in achieving the goals of revascularisation in the appropriately selected patient.

15.2.1 Role of ischaemia and collateral flow

Multiple observational studies have indicated increased cardiac risk with large ischaemic burden. One study of over 10,000 patients who underwent quantitative myocardial perfusion imaging revealed that revascularisation, when more than 10% of myocardium was at risk, was associated with a prognostic benefit.[4] Further insight was gained from the Clinical Outcomes Utilizing Revascularization and Aggressive Drug Evaluation (COURAGE) nuclear sub-study, which compared revascularisation plus optimal medical therapy (OMT) with OMT alone, in a cohort of stable coronary disease patients. Again, revascularisation plus OMT was superior to OMT alone with respect to reduction of both ischaemia and angina and was most useful in those with at least moderate ischaemic burden

(≥10%).[5] Further, in a study of patients who underwent CTO PCI with perfusion imaging, 1 year pre and post showed a large change in ischaemic burden post-procedure with a Summed Difference Score change of as over 16 in patients with severe ischaemia.[6] This evidence suggests that patients who will derive the most benefit from revascularisation are those with large ischaemic burdens.

Despite the common misconception that collateral flow beyond a CTO can provide adequate blood supply, evidence indicates that nearly all viable myocardium supplied by collaterals due the presence of a CTO is ischaemic. Werner and colleagues assessed both coronary flow reserve (CFR) and fractional flow reserve (FFR) patients with CTOs supplied by collaterals with greater than Rentrop grade 1 flow.[7] This study demonstrated a mean FFR of only 0.32 ± 0.13 with a range of 0.03–0.78 indicating ischaemia in all subjects. Similarly, Sachdeva and colleagues found ischaemia at rest in 78% of patients at maximal hyperaemia with no correlation between collateral grade and FFR result.[8] In essence, viable myocardium subtended by CTOs is largely ischaemic and as such, patients with these lesions and moderate-to-large ischaemic burden are likely to benefit from revascularisation.

15.2.2 Effect of CTO PCI on mortality

There is a strong association between successful CTO revascularisation and decreased mortality, particularly in the acute coronary syndrome setting.[9,10] In an evaluation of long-term outcomes of CTO PCI in 1791 patients, Mehran and colleagues found that successful CTO PCI was an independent predictor of lower cardiac mortality (hazard ratio [HR]: 0.40, 95% confidence interval [CI]: 0.21–0.75, $p < .01$) and correlated with lower all-cause mortality (HR: 0.63, 95% CI: 0.40–1.00, $p = .05$) at 5 years of follow-up.[11] Subsequently, two large meta-analyses reviewing the effects of successful CTO PCI using data from 13 to 23 observational studies, respectively, found a nearly 3.5% reduction in absolute mortality (with a relative risk reduction of 44%–46%) with a successful procedure versus those in whom CTO PCI had failed.[12,13] Further insight into this important area of CTO PCI outcomes will undoubtedly come from the results of DECISION-CTO and the Euro-CTO trial, though these results may be several years away.

15.2.3 Effect on left ventricular dysfunction

Both left ventricular dysfunction (due to myocardial ischaemia) and survival improve the following surgical revascularisation.[14–16] As such, it is not surprising that reperfusion of ischaemic myocardium following CTO PCI has similar effects. In studies by Van Belle and Sirnes, left ventricular function improved by 5%–8% on left ventriculography was observed at 6 months following successful CTO PCI.[17,18] Magnetic resonance imaging (MRI) studies have also demonstrated improvement in left ventricular (LV) dynamics (specifically segmental wall thickness [SWT]) following CTO

PCI. Baks and colleagues, in 27 patients, demonstrated that SWT improved in patients with viable myocardium (<50% transmural extent of infarction, measured by late gadolinium enhancement), with an association between left ventricular ejection fraction (LVEF) improvement and amount of viable myocardium.[19] Similarly, Kirschbaum and colleagues showed an improvement in SWT out to 3 years of follow-up in patients with less than 25% transmural infarction.[20] Improvement in LV dynamics *did not occur* in either study in patients with greater than 75% transmural infarction. Hence, improvement LV dynamics and LVEF do occur following CTO revascularisation and may continue long term but it only occurs in those with viable myocardium. Accordingly, viability in dysfunction myocardial segments subtended by CTOs should be confirmed prior to CTO PCI to ensure optimal results.

15.2.4 Effect on quality of life

Perhaps the most important benefit of CTO PCI is an improvement in quality of life. In the COURAGE trial, symptomatic benefit in patients with successful CTO revascularisation was significant.[21] Similarly, in the FlowCardia's Approach to Chronic Total Occlusion Recanalization (FACTOR) trial, successful CTO recanalisation was also associated with improvement in Seattle Angina Questionnaire (SAQ) scores in multiple domains including angina frequency, physical limitation and quality of life.[22] A meta-analysis of six observational studies reporting results from over 7000 patients found a relative reduction of over 50% in anginal symptoms following successful CTO PCI[12] though considerable heterogeneity ($I^2 = 65\%$) was noted in the angina group in this study and no analysis of the extent of anti-anginal medical therapy was included. Despite these caveats, it appears clear that successful CTO PCI does indeed lead to a reduction in symptoms and an improvement in quality of life.

15.3 CTO anatomy and histopathology

The histopathology of CTOs is an area of active study, utilizing traditional methods and modern technologies such as intravascular micro-CT, micro-MRI and intravascular ultrasound (IVUS). Studies have aimed to describe CTO histopathology to ultimately lend insight into the bases of procedural success and failure.

In CTOs, gross vessel architecture is preserved, where the intima and neointima remain distinct from the vascular media (muscularis layer) and adventitia with an intact external elastic lamina. This maintenance of vascular architecture forms the basis modern CTO recanalisation techniques that exploit these fundamental components of vascular anatomy, both as lesion-crossing routes and scaffolding in which specialised manoeuvres are performed (Figure 15.1).

Early necropsy studies examining human CTOs have shown that morphologic characteristics may predict histologic composition. Tapered-tip caps (a predictor of angioplasty success) contain areas of luminal recanalisation with micro-channels, which are comprised of loosely packed fibrous tissue and tend to be short.[23] Conversely, lesions with blunt tips are longer and composed of more densely packed fibrous material that is less amenable to guidewire passage. Blunt-tipped lesions also tend to be more mature (older) and composed of more fibrocalcific intimal plaque than younger occlusions.[24]

Utilising advanced imaging techniques, recent studies have systematically described the natural history of CTOs. Early experimental occlusions are composed of an inflammatory infiltrate containing neutrophils and mononuclear cells that penetrate an occlusive thrombus. The density of this infiltrate peaks at 2 weeks post-occlusion and declines thereafter as loosely packed collagen extracellular matrix (ECM) infiltrates the body of the thrombus. This process is accompanied by negative remodelling of the surrounding vessel and decay of the internal elastic lamina.[24,25] Proteoglycan-enriched ECM deposition occurs early between 2 and 6 weeks post-occlusion and is concentrated at proximal and distal ends of the lesion. Over time, these areas are replaced by densely packed collagen, creating the so-called *proximal and distal caps* that constitute a physical barrier to successful guidewire passage.[25]

Recanalisation micro-vascular channels (MCs) that extend throughout 80% of human and experimental CTOs speculate a potential proximal-to-distal tract through

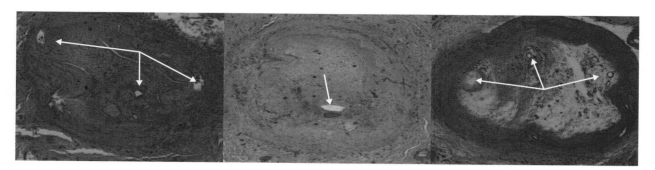

Figure 15.1 Histologic cross section of coronary chronic total occlusion (CTO). Histologic cross sections of CTOs of different ages demonstrating the presence of microchannels (arrows).

which guidewire passage may occur. MCs within human CTOs were first described by Katsuragawa and colleagues;[23] these small vascular channels were noted at both proximal and distal lesion segments, ranging from 160 to 230 μm in diameter. Srivatsa elaborated describing MC networks in all lesions regardless of age that extend into the vessel media and adventitia.[24] Most recently, micro-CT, micro-ultrasound and micro-MRI studies have confirmed that these tiny vascular channels extend both longitudinally and outward through CTOs, connecting with the *vasa vasorum* or intimal plaque neovasculature via a 'corkscrew' or 'crescent-shaped' route.[26] With respect to their utility as a translesional pathway for guidewire advancement, Munce and colleagues demonstrated that although MCs are indeed present longitudinally across 85% of CTOs, may be continuous and are largest in diameter at 2 weeks, they become discontinuous, fragmented and sharply angled by 6 weeks[25,27] and degenerate further by 12 weeks. As such, these discontinuous MCs are unlikely to provide a singular and continuous channel for guidewire passage; however, they may still alter local issue architecture rendering a 'path of least resistance' through a CTO.

Given the challenges inherent to human necropsy studies, experimental models have added a great deal to our understanding of CTO histopathology. It remains, however, important to recognise the limitations of experimental CTO models and the data derived from them. Both murine and rabbit CTOs have been created using intra-arterial thrombin injections or levo poly lactic acid (l-PLA) polymer arterial plug insertion.[28] The lesions formed in these models lack both the atherosclerotic substrate and the calcification typical of human CTO lesions.[25,26,29] Ongoing study in this area, using increasingly innovative imaging methods (e.g. intravascular ultrasound virtual histology [IVUS-VH]) are critical to improving our understanding of human CTO histopathology and thus, CTO revascularisation success rates.[30,31]

15.4 Peri-procedural considerations

15.4.1 Program development

Fundamentally, CTO PCI is a procedure that requires infrastructural and human resource input in excess of standard PCI in order to achieve success. Any successful CTO program requires a supportive administrative and clinical environment, with a dedicated maybe team of interventionalists, nurses, angiographic and haemodynamic specialists and administrators, all of whom are knowledgeable about the clinical, academic and economic benefits of CTO PCI. Further, a generalised commitment to teamwork, with procedures discussed amongst senior operators and a commitment to learning from national and international experts through courses and proctoring is key to successfully mastering the cognitive and technical aspects of CTO treatment. Increasing operator experience has been found to influence outcome[32] with many high-volume centres using

a model in which two experienced operators are involved in most procedures.[33]

15.4.2 Procedure planning and complication avoidance

Meticulous planning remains the most important non-technical aspect of CTO PCI. Careful pre-operative consultation in which an informed discussion regarding the potential benefits, local success rates, procedural length and potential for complications is critical. One should, of course, not use this discussion to dissuade patients from seeking treatment, particularly given that success rates rise and complications rates fall in CTO PCI with mounting operator experience.[34] For these reasons, *ad hoc* or *on-the table* CTO PCI is generally discouraged.

Following a careful review of the clinical presentation, physical examination and imaging data, several CTO specific assessments should be made, primarily to avoid complications during the procedure. A careful vascular assessment is necessary to ensure that large bore sheaths and catheters will be accommodated by the patient's vasculature without causing important limb ischaemia. Additionally, careful evaluation for bleeding risk factors and ability to adhere to dual antiplatelet therapy is also crucial to avoid both bleeding complications from procedural anticoagulation and, given the long stent lengths frequently used in CTO PCI,[11] stent thrombosis.

Contrast use in CTO PCI exceeds that of routine coronary interventional procedures.[35,36] As such an individualised assessment of the risks of contrast exposure key. An assessment of kidney function and measurement of left ventricular end diastolic pressure prior to commencement in pts with chronic kidney disease will allow operators to specify a reasonable *a priori* contrast limit for their procedure and institute appropriate peri-procedural hydration to minimise the risk of contrast-induced nephropathy (CIN).[37,38]

CTO PCI procedures can be prolonged and require the use of specialised equipment that can take considerable time to deliver. Hence, it is not surprising that radiation exposure during CTO PCI is also higher than in conventional PCI procedures.[39] As such operators should become accustomed to maintaining excellent radiation hygiene – using low frame rates (e.g. 7.5 f/s) for wiring, low-dose fluoroscopy, radiation optimizing equipment and imaging in shallow and sometimes atypical angiographic views to minimise radiation delivery.

Radiation-induced skin injury (RSI) comprises a major avoidable morbidity of CTO interventions. Below 5 Gray (Gy), clinically significant RSI is unlikely whereas at exposures greater than 10 Gy, there may be a need for surgical intervention.[40] As such, a key component of the peri-procedural physical examination is a careful skin survey, particularly of the back to ensure freedom from RSI caused during previous procedure attempts (Figure 15.2a); if evidence of radiation injury is detected, consideration

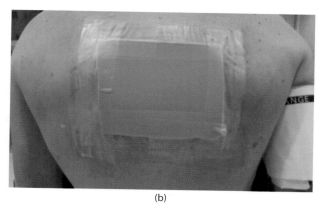

(a) (b)

Figure 15.2 Radiation-induced skin injury and shielding. Example of a radiation burn. **(a)** The square area of redness is a painless radiation burn in the shape of an image intensifier. This is a superficial injury requiring only observation and strict avoidance of further irradiation; more serious injuries can result in chronic pain and subdermal tissue necrosis. **(b)** A piece of lead shielding taped over the area of injury to protect it during a subsequent CTO percutaneous coronary intervention (PCI) procedure. Angles where the radiopaque shield were selected to complete the procedure, thereby ensuring no irradiation of the injured skin.

should be given to cancelling the procedure until expert consultation is achieved. Once cleared, or if the RSI is limited to only superficial tissues, then care must be taken to ensure no irradiation of the injured skin occurs. This can be accomplished by taping a radiation shield or radiopaque marker on top of the affected area so that fluoroscopic angles that image the target artery without irradiating the injured skin can be chosen (Figure 15.2b).

Protocols for follow-up and management of patients who have received radiation doses of greater than 6 Gy should be implemented. Notably, biopsy of areas of RSI may be detrimental to healing and should be avoided unless absolutely necessary.

15.4.3 Diagnostic angiography

Excellent pre-procedural diagnostic angiography is a key to successful CTO PCI. Once a CTO has been identified, efforts should be made to elucidate the following: (a) the length of the occlusion; (b) the nature of the proximal cap (blunt or tapered); (c) the course and quality of the occluded vessel (i.e. tortuous, calcified, diffusely diseased, small); (d) the source and direction of distal vessel flow, if any and (e) the course of collaterals supply the target vessel beyond the occlusion (Figure 15.3). As such, dual catheter angiography with injections that fully opacify both the donor and target vessels can be essential. Cine acquisitions must be sufficiently long to allow for collateral and distal vessel filling, identification of the distal cap and be free of panning, as the origin and course of small collateral channels are challenging to delineate with moving reference points. Finally, operators should become accustomed to imaging in 'non-standard' or atypical angiographic views, with shallow angles if necessary to image collaterals in as perpendicular a plane as possible to facilitate guide wire navigation. In

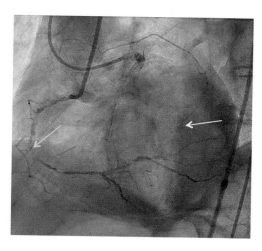

Figure 15.3 Dual injection with key features. Dual (right and left) coronary simultaneous angiography demonstrating a CTO of the right coronary artery. The occluded segment begins at the proximal cap (yellow arrow) and ends at the distal cap (red arrow). The distal vessel is supplied by retrograde collateral vessels (white arrow), arising here from the atrial branch of the left circumflex artery.

general, the entire area subtended by the vessel of interest must be visible prior to each acquisition. At minimum, two orthogonal images containing the key anatomic features should be obtained.

15.4.4 Predictors of success and strategy selection

An understanding of anatomical features and procedural complexity is germane to both case selection and procedure planning. An ideal scoring system would (a) facilitate procedural planning and efficiency for expert operators, (b) inform less experienced operators of the need for a proctor of referral to an expert and (c) more granularity in the informed consent discussion patient regarding success rates and potential complications.[41] Recently, several scoring mechanisms have been introduced to assist in this process.

15.4.4.1 J-CTO and progress CTO scores

The multicenter CTO registry of Japan (J-CTO) score, the most widely used of these prediction models, is based on angiographic CTO anatomy and the presence of a previously failed recanalisation attempt.[42] By awarding one point for each of a blunt proximal cap, lesion length over 20 mm, tortuosity within the CTO of more than 45°, *any* calcification and a failed previous attempt, a score out of 5 is computed to predict successful guidewire crossing into true lumen distal to the occluded segment within 30 minutes. This score also classifies a given procedure into one of four classes of difficulty: easy (J-CTO 0), intermediate (J-CTO 1), difficult (J-CTO 2) or very difficult (J-CTO 3 or more) (Figure 15.4 and Table 15.1).

Several limitations of the J-CTO score have become evident as operator experience with CTO PCI has grown. First, this score was derived using a relatively small patient

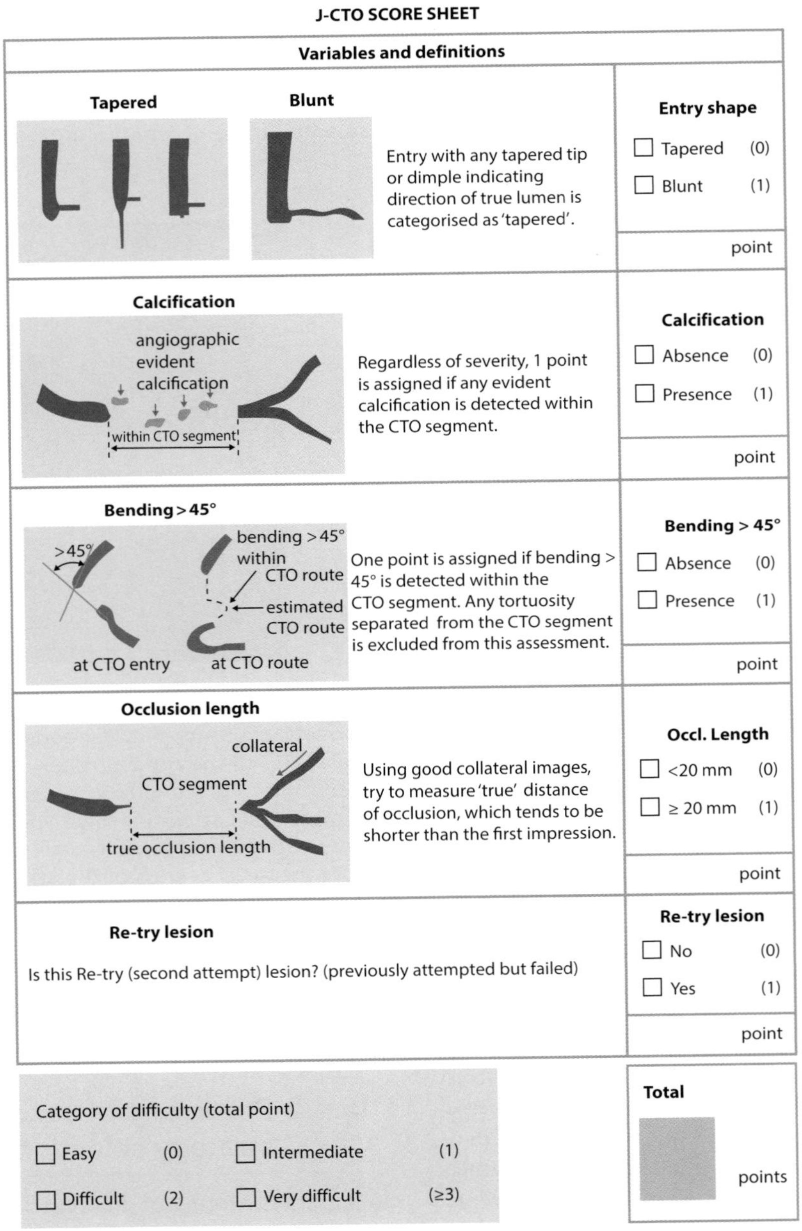

Figure 15.4 Japanese chronic total occlusion (J-CTO) scoring sheet. Scoring sheet for a four-point anatomic scoring system designed to predict likelihood of successful wire crossing of a CTO within 30 minutes. Scores are also correlated with case difficulty as indicated. (Reprinted from Morino Y et al., *JACC Cardiovasc Interv.*, 4, 213–221, 2011. With permission.)

Table 15.1 Commonly used CTO specific wires, classified by task

Guidewire	Manufacturer	Design features	Coating and tip	Tip load (gf)	Task categories
Fielder FC	Asahi	Non-tapered tip 0.014 in., 180/300 cm	Hydrophilic, full polymer jacket	0.8	■
Fielder XT	Asahi	Tapered tip 0.009 in., shaft 0.014 in., 190/300 cm	Hydrophilic, full polymer jacket	0.8	■ □
Fielder XT—A	Asahi	Tapered tip 0.009 in., Shaft 0.014 in., 180/300 cm	Hydrophilic, polymer jacket	1.0	■ □ ■
Fielder XT—R	Asahi	Tapered tip 0.009 in., Shaft 0.014 in., 180/300 cm	Hydrophilic, polymer jacket	0.6	■
Fighter	Boston Scientific	Tapered tip 0.009 in., Shaft 0.014 in., 190/300 cm	Hydrophilic, clear polymer jacket over spring coil and tip	1.5	■ □ □
Suoh	Asahi	Non-tapered tip 0.014 in., 180/300 cm	Hydrophilic, non-jacketed over spring and coil tip	0.3	■
Sion Black	Asahi	Non-tapered tip 0.014 in., 190/300 cm	Hydrophilic, polymer jacket on distal 20 cm	0.8	■
Pilot 50	Abbott	Non-tapered tip 0.014 in., 190/300 cm	Hydrophilic, polymer jacket	1.5	□ ■ ■ ■
Sion	Asahi	Non-Tapered tip 0.014 in., 180/300 cm	Hydrophilic, non-jacketed over spring coil and tip.	0.7	■ ■
Samurai RC	Boston Scientific	Non-tapered tip 0.014 in., 190/300 cm	Hydrophilic coating over distal 24 cm	1.2	■
HI-TORQUE Whisper MS	Abbott	Non-tapered tip 0.014 in., 180/300 cm	Hydrophilic, polymer jacket	1.0	■
Sion Blue	Asahi	Non-Tapered tip 0.014 in., 180/300 cm	Hydrophilic, non-jacketed over spring coil (distal 18.5 cm), Hydrophobic tip	0.5	■
Samurai	Boston Scientific	Non-Tapered tip 0.014 in., 190/300 cm	Hydrophilic, non-jacketed, reduced coating on distal 1 cm	0.5	■
HI-TORQUE BMW Universal II	Abbott Vascular	Non-tapered tip with shaping ribbon 0.014 in., 190/300 cm	Hydrophilic coating	0.7	■
Hornet	Boston Scientific	Tapered tip 0.008 in, 0.014 in shaft, 190/300 cm	Hydrophilic coating over spring coil and tip	1.0	□
Gaia First	Asahi	Tapered tip 0.010 in. Shaft 0.014 in., 190 cm	Hydrophilic, non-jacketed. Tip hydrophilic	1.5	□
Gaia Second	Asahi	Tapered tip 0.011 in. Shaft 0.014 in., 190 cm	Hydrophilic, non-jacketed. Tip hydrophilic	3.5	□
Gaia Third	Asahi	Tapered tip 0.011 in. Shaft 0.014 in., 190 cm	Hydrophilic, non-jacketed. Tip hydrophilic	4.5	■ □
Miracle 3/ MIRACLEbros 3	Asahi	Non-tapered tip. 0.014 in., 180 cm length	Hydrophobic (silicone)	3.0	■ □
Miracle 6/ MIRACLEbros 6	Asahi	Non-tapered tip. 0.014 in., 180 cm length	Hydrophobic (silicone)	6.0	■ □
Miracle 12/ MIRACLEbros 12	Asahi	Non-tapered tip 0.014 in., 180 cm length	Hydrophobic (silicone)	12.0	■
Pilot 150	Abbott	Non-tapered tip 0.014 in., 190 and300 cm length	Hydrophilic, polymer jacketed	2.7	■
Pilot 200	Abbott	Non-tapered tip 0.014 in., 190 and 300 cm length	Hydrophilic, polymer jacketed	4.1	■

(Continued)

Table 15.1 (Continued) Commonly used CTO specific wires, classified by task

Guidewire	Manufacturer	Design features	Coating and tip	Tip load (gf)	Task categories
Conquest/ Confianza	Asahi	Tapered tip 0.009 in. Shaft 0.014 in. 180 cm length. Spring coil length 20 cm	Hydrophobic (silicone)	9.0	■
Confianza Pro	Asahi	Tapered tip 0.009 in. Shaft 0.014 in., 180 cm length. Spring coil length 20 cm	Hydrophilic non-jacketed over spring coil. Hydrophobic tip and shaft	9.0	■
Hornet 10	Boston Scientific	Tapered tip 0.008 in. Shaft 0.014 in. 190/300 cm	Hydrophilic over spring coil and tip	10.0	■
Confianza Pro 12	Asahi	Tapered tip 0.009 in. Shaft 0.014 in., 180 cm length. Spring coil length 20 cm	Hydrophilic non-jacketed over spring coil. Hydrophobic over shaft and 1 mm tip	12.0	■ ■
Hornet 14	Boston Scientific	Tapered tip 0.008 in. Shaft 0.014 in. 190/300 cm	Hydrophilic over spring coil and tip	14.0	■ ■
Astato XS 20	Asahi	Tapered tip 0.009 in. Shaft 0.014 in., 180 cm length. Spring coil length 17 cm	Hydrophilic non-jacketed over spring coil. Hydrophobic tip and shaft	20.0	■ ■
Stingray Wire	Boston Scientific	Tapered tip, 0.009 in., Shaft 0.014 in. 185/300 cm	Hydrophilic over coil and tip	12.0	■
RG 3	Asahi	Non-tapered tip. Tip and shaft 0.010 in. 330 cm	Hydrophilic over spring coil and tip		■
R350	Vascular Solutions	Nitinol alloy. Non-tapered tip, 0.013 in shaft, 5 mm platinum coil, tapers to 0.006 in under coils, 350 cm length	Hydrophilic over distal 200 cm		■

gf, gram force.
■ Access (Workhorse)   ■ Collateral Crossing   □ Directed Navigation   ■ Fenestration Re-entry
■ Directed Penetration   ■ Knuckling   □ Micro-channel Crossing   ■ Externalisation

cohort of less than 500 patients, 10 years ago. Both operator experience and technology have grown since this score was introduced, with the introduction of the hybrid algorithm for CTO PCI being key amongst these innovations[43]; the use of the algorithm alone has increased success rates by almost 15% in contemporary registries[44,45] (see below for details) and has shown that the initial strategy is successful in only 44% of cases. Further, though guidewire passage through the CTO is generally the primary technical challenge of CTO PCI, it is often only one of several encountered. For example, 66% of CTO PCI procedures at our centre are performed on post-CABG patients, whose lesions are more calcified than non-post CABG patients[46] and in whom success rates are lower[47]; the J-CTO score fails to capture the gradation of calcification (and thus ability to ultimately dilate the target vessel) that exists in these patients. Further, with progression to increasingly sophisticated guidewire

technologies (such as the introduction of the Asahi Gaia wire family), an ability to deliver micro-catheters or other gear past the proximal cap after wire crossing has become a more common failure mode.

Several attempts have been made to define another effective scoring system for CTO PCI.[48,49] Unfortunately, many of these attempts have important limitations, including a lack of dual catheter angiography, lower overall success rates (60%–70% vs. >90% in contemporary US registries) and limited use of the hybrid algorithm.

Most recently, the progress CTO score, developed and validated using data from a large, multicentre, post-hybrid-algorithm-era registry has attempted to address these limitations.[50] This score, designed to predict technical failure (a more clinically useful endpoint than wire crossing within 30 minutes), is based on both angiographic and clinical features. Using multivariable analysis, independent predictors of technical failure were isolated within a derivation cohort of 521 lesions and validated on a second cohort of 260 lesions. Proximal cap ambiguity, a lack of interventional collaterals, moderate or severe vessel tortuosity and left circumflex target vessel were all found to independently predict technical failure with odds ratios of 2.40–3.86[50] (Figure 15.5). Of note, the progress CTO is observational and not equipped with angiographic core lab analysis or clinical events adjudication. Large, contemporary registries that include these adjudication mechanism and prospective consecutive enrolment (e.g. the OPEN-CTO database) will be instrumental refining both the JCTO and progress CTO scores, to the benefit of both operators and patients.

15.4.4.2 Hybrid algorithm for CTO PCI

Previously, the focus was on antegrade wire escalation techniques, regardless of anatomic features, lesions carrying high J-CTO scores, blunt proximal caps, heavy calcification and poor distal vessel visualisation portended high failure rates.[42,51–53] However, with the introduction of advanced antegrade strategies[54] and retrograde recanalisation techniques using septal collaterals by Surmely and colleagues in 2007,[55] success rates began to rise.[56] Given this rapidly growing body of techniques and technologies, a systematic, efficient and teachable algorithm designed to facilitate strategy selection and procedural efficiency was designed. Termed 'The Hybrid Algorithm' (Figure 15.6),[43] this method aimed to both predict the best initial revascularisation strategy and characterise factors that may necessitate a switch of strategies based on anatomic features of the CTO (ostial or blunt proximal cap morphology, lesion length, severe tortuosity

or calcification, side branch at the occlusion and the presence of interventional collaterals). The algorithm aims to facilitate constant advancement of the 'Base of

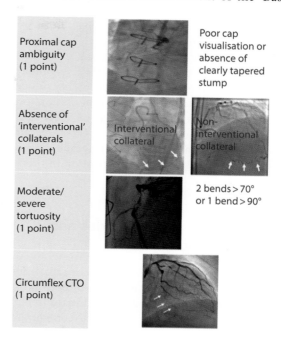

Figure 15.5 The PROGRESS CTO scoring sheet. Summary scoring sheet for the PROGRESS CTO score aimed at predicting technical success in CTO PCI using contemporary methods, such as the Hybrid Algorithm. The PROGRESS CTO score correlates with the J-CTO score with respect to technical success. (Reprinted from Christopoulos G et al., *JACC Cardiovasc Interv.*, 9, 1–9, 2016. With permission.)

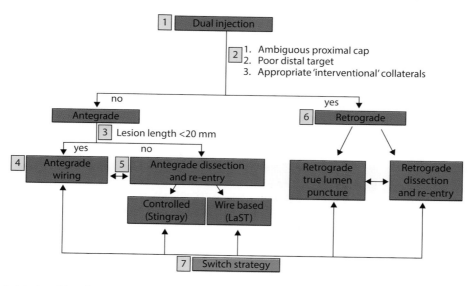

Figure 15.6 The hybrid algorithm for CTO PCI. Multistep, anatomically based procedural planning model to facilitate success in CTO PCI. Anatomical features of the target lesion and the presence of interventional collaterals are key to choosing an initial strategy. Strategy switch is recommended to avoid stalling of the progress, recognizing that the operator may switch back and forth between strategies to achieve technical success. (Reprinted from Brilakis ES et al., *JACC Cardiovasc Interv.*, 5, 367–379, 2012. With permission.)

Operations (BO)', defined as the point within the vessel from which the operator is working to recanalise the CTO. For example, in antegrade cases, the BO progresses from the proximal cap to just prior to the distal cap, beyond which, successful wire crossing can be declared (if in the true lumen).

Since its inception, important gains in success rates of CTO PCI have been achieved.[44,45,57] A fundamental underpinning of the algorithm is the ability of operators to switch between strategies without hesitation to ensure constant progress towards the goal of successful CTO recanalisation. As such, the modern CTO operator will need to hone both antegrade and retrograde skills equally to ensure optimal use of revascularisation in this patient subset.

15.4.5 Vascular access, guides and sheath selection

The choice of vascular access (femoral or radial) for CTO PCI rests in the careful consideration of both procedural and operator variables that must be addressed to maximise success. The most frequently employed configuration for coronary CTO procedures in high-volume centres includes large bore (8 Fr) bi-femoral access with long (45 cm), kink-resistant sheaths to overcome iliac tortuosity and two 8 Fr, coaxial guide catheters with aortic back-wall support to maximise system stability and ease gear delivery. With increasing experience and technical knowledge, a 'hybrid' radial (6 or 7 Fr) and femoral 8 Fr approach can be considered to minimise the risk of vascular complications.[58,59] Recently, the use of a bi-radial platform been described with success rates comparable to those of the bi-femoral approach,[60] however, given the need for smaller guides and active guide support using this configuration, its use should be limited to experienced operators.

As dual catheter angiography is critical to decision-making in CTO PCI, where possible, operators should use two guide catheters to ensure optimal opacification of both target and donor arteries. Retrograde guides, in general, should be short (90 cm) to allow for sufficient working length in cases of wire externalisation. Our practice is to routinely use short guides for both the antegrade and retrograde limbs, particularly when more than one vessel may be addressed during a given procedure. This approach allows all therapeutic options (e.g. contralateral as well as ipsilateral retrograde approaches) to remain available. The use of side holes should be avoided on the retrograde guide in the left main coronary artery as their presence may mask deep seating of the guide catheter and thus predispose to donor artery injury. Finally, care should be taken throughout the procedure to clear or 'back-bleed' both guide catheters at regular intervals to ensure the clearance of any debris or micro-thrombi that may develop especially when there are long intervals between injections.

15.4.6 Procedural anticoagulation and monitoring

Where possible, we feel that patients should be either loaded with or maintained on dual antiplatelet therapy (Aspirin plus a P_2Y_{12} inhibitor) prior to the commencement of the procedure.

The heparin is mainstay of anti-thrombotic therapy in CTO PCI. It is monitored throughout the procedure using activated clotting times (ACTs), with a goal of over 300 seconds for antegrade procedures and *at least* 350 seconds for retrograde procedures.[61] Experience with bivalirudin in CTO PCI is limited. In general, the use of this agent is not recommended as its pharmacokinetics requires constant blood exposure and ongoing flow to maintain efficacy and thus may predispose to catheter or equipment thrombosis. The use of glycoprotein (GP) IIb/IIIa has not been studied in CTO PCI and should be avoided given the higher risk of bleeding complications in these procedures.

ACT monitoring should be protocolised every 30 minutes and administered by the cath lab nursing staff. We believe that similar protocols should be in place for end-tidal CO_2, radiation dose and patient comfort monitoring. With each member of the team empowered in a defined, crucial role, the entire team will share in the gratification of a successful and safe procedure.

15.5 Technical strategies

15.5.1 The CTO toolbox

The 'CTO Toolbox' is comprised of both equipment (e.g. specialised wires, microcatheters, guide extensions, controlled dissection and re-entry devices, angled catheters) and specialised techniques (e.g. Bob Sled, Scratch and Go, Move the Cap, Dancing). A detailed knowledge of this armamentarium is fundamental to procedural success and requires an ongoing commitment to continual education and awareness of equipment refinements to understand its optimal use.

This section will endeavour to introduce the fundamentals of the CTO Toolbox as it pertains to the most commonly employed antegrade and retrograde CTO PCI strategies. For a detailed review of the toolbox and techniques, please see online resources at www.ctofundamentals.org.

15.5.1.1 Wires

A recent explosion of technology in the area of CTO PCI now affords access to a menu of highly sophisticated guidewires for these procedures. This myriad of choices, however, is not necessarily an asset, particularly to the nascent practitioner who aims to develop the intimate knowledge of wires necessary to become a safe, successful and *efficient* CTO operator.

CTO wires may be organised into eight classes, using a 'task-specific' approach, with wires fitting into one or several of these categories based on their unique structural and functional properties and their role in CTO PCI procedures. The eight task classes are as follows (summarised in Table 15.2):

Table 15.2 Commonly used microcatheters in CTO PCI, their dimensions and recommended uses

Microcatheter	Manufacturer	Catheter length	Tip ID	Tip OD	Distal shaft OD	Proximal (main) shaft OD	Design features	Special considerations and/or recommendations
Finecross	Terumo Interventional Systems	150 cm	0.018 in. (0.45 mm)	0.022 in. (0.57 mm)	1.8 Fr	2.6 Fr	Stainless steel braided shaft, hydrophilic coating	Very low profile and highly deliverable but limited pushability or ability to spin. Good for small but straight collaterals.
Corsair	Asahi Intecc	135/150 cm	0.015 in. (0.38 mm)	0.016 Fr (0.42 mm)	2.6 Fr	2.8 Fr	Dual layer braided stainless steel shaft, flexible, kink resistant tip	Can be used to traverse collaterals or as a channel dilator. Larger bore proximal shaft provides good wire backup for advancement and spinning.
TurnPike	Vascular Solutions	135/150 cm	0.015 in. (0.38 mm)	0.021 in. (0.53 mm)	2.6 Fr	3.1 Fr	Hybrid construction of braid and a dual-layer coil	Workhorse microcatheter that performs well in most CTO cases. Nylon coil on distal end of TP Spiral enhances trackability. Tip on TP Gold facilitates forward enhancement in particularly tough lesions.
TurnPike Spiral	Vascular Solutions	135/150 cm	0.015 in. (0.38 mm)	0.021 in. (0.53 mm)	2.6Fr	3.1 Fr	encapsulated between two polymer layers (five layers total)	
TurnPike Gold	Vascular Solutions	135 cm	0.016 in. (0.41 mm)	0.028 in. (0.71 mm)	3.2 Fr	3.1 Fr		
TurnPike LP	Vascular Solutions	135/150 cm	0.016 in. (0.41 mm)	0.021 in. (0.53 mm)	2.2 Fr	2.9 Fr	Similar construction with thinner tip braiding to given lower profile	Excellent for very tortuous or epicardial collateral crossing but low profile reduces backup support.
Micro14	Roxwood Medical	155 cm	0.016 in. (0.41 mm)	0.021 in. (0.53 mm)	1.9 Fr	2.5 Fr	Variable pitch braided shaft, torquable	Excellent low-profile microcatheter useful for fine and tortuous collaterals. Also available with extra-supportive tip profile (Micro14es) for enhanced pushability.
Caravel	Asahi Intecc	135 cm	0.016 in. (0.40 mm)	0.20 in. (0.48 mm)	1.9 Fr	2.6 Fr	ACT-one core precision braided shaft with very low crossing profile	Low profile and hydrophilic coating allows excellent navigation of tortuous collaterals. Can only torque this device in one direction.
Tornus * 2 sizes available	Asahi Intecc	135 cm 135 cm	0.41 mm 0.41 mm	0.60 mm 0.70 mm	Tapered 2.6 Fr	2.1 Fr 3.0 Fr	Stainless steel braided catheter	Available in 2.1 and 2.6 Fr. More useful as a support catheter given higher profile and risk of collateral vessel injury. Can also be used as a 'channel dilator'.

LP, low profile; Fr, French guage; CTO, chronic total occlusion; PCI, percutaneous coronary intervention.

1. Access (Workhorse) – low tip load, linear torque responsive, easily shaped, supportive and inexpensive wires designed to navigate large vessels, including those with high grade but not complete occlusions (e.g. Sion Blue, Samurai, BMW Universal II, Pro-Water)
2. Directed Navigation – flexible, intermediate tip load, highly torque responsive wires that are both stiff and flexible depending on the axis of the wire and are capable of navigating the body of an occlusion under careful, deliberate advancement (e.g. Gaia First, Gaia Second)
3. Directed Penetration – tapered tip or jacketed, high tip load wires with progressive torsional rigidity that are capable of *focal* penetration of very resistant tissue (e.g. proximal and distal caps, calcium) to allow progress of the BO but *not* for advancement through the coronary artery (e.g. Hornet 10, Hornet 14, Confianza Pro 12, Miracle Bros 12, Gaia Third)
4. Microchannel – polymer jacketed, low or very low tip load, tapered or low-profile wires designed to gently allow crossing of short occlusions with microchannel antegrade flow without injuring the residual true lumen (e.g. Fighter, Fielder XT, Gaia First)
5. Collateral Crossing – lubricious, low or very low tip load, atraumatic (bunt) tip wires designed to navigate tiny collateral channels while minimizing risk of perforation (e.g. Sion, Sion Black, Fielder FC, Samurai RC)
6. Fenestration Re-Entry – tapered or polymer jacketed, intermediate to high tip load wires capable of focused penetration of a tissue plane or navigation of multiple dissection planes to find the true lumen (e.g. Stingray wire, Confianza Pro 12)
7. Knuckling – polymer jacketed, low-to-intermediate tip load and moderate column strength wires with a natural tendency to prolapse and produce dissection planes with minimal trauma (e.g. Fielder XT, Pilot 200, Fighter)
8. Externalisation – core-to-tip designed, long length wires (>300 cm) with shaft flexibility, designed to be externalised once the CTO has been crossed and along which PCI procedure can be performed (e.g. RG3, R350)

Over time, operators should aim to become highly familiar with one to two wires in each task class to optimise success and keep inventory (and costs) manageable.

15.5.1.2 Microcatheters

Prior to the introduction of microcatheters, capable of dilating collateral channels and displacing friction to facilitate lesion passage, the BO was established using over-the-wire (OTW) balloon catheters or early, non-torquable microcatheters (e.g. Finecross, Terumo Medical Corporation, Tokyo, Japan). These catheters would provide support for antegrade wiring as well as a rapid exchange platform through which different CTO wires could be introduced into the lesion. The OTW balloon platform, however, was difficult to advance beyond the proximal cap and impaired optimal wire usage though adverse catheter–wire interactions. Accurate determination of the proximal and distal ends of the OTW balloon was also challenging as the 1.5 OTW balloons are equipped with mid-markers but lack proximal or distal markers.

In 2010, the Corsair microcatheter (Asahi Intec) was introduced as a channel dilator and exchange catheter to facilitate both antegrade and retrograde CTO PCI.[62] This sophisticated microcatheter composed of 10 tungsten wires braded into a metallic tube with a soft 2.8 Fr tip and hydrophilic polymer coating can be spun both clockwise and counterclockwise to allow *rotational displacement of friction* and thus advancement along a wire, through a tight lesion or resistant tissue.

Multiple specialised microcatheters have since been introduced to facilitate CTO crossing and navigation, unique properties that make them suitable for a variety of situations. See Table 15.3 for a summary of commonly used microcatheters and their features.

15.5.2 Antegrade strategies

The antegrade crossing strategy is well suited to short lesions with tapered proximal caps and good distal vessel visualisation as per the hybrid algorithm in Figure 15.6. New operators attempting to gain experience in CTO PCI should begin by attempting these lesions.

Table 15.3 Common collateral connections between native coronary arteries

Donor artery	Recipient artery	Collateral location/course	Collateral type
LAD	PDA	LAD to PDA septals	Septal, limited tortuosity
LAD	PDA	Apical LAD to PDA	Epicardial, generally tortuous
Circumflex	RCA	Atrial branch, AV groove circumflex	Epicardial, generally straight
Obtuse marginal	Diagonal	D1 or D2 to distal OM branches	Epicardial, highly mobile, tortuous

RCA-to-RCA and left (LAD or circumflex)-to-left not detailed above.
LAD, left anterior descending artery; PDA, posterior descending artery; RCA, right coronary artery; AV, atrioventricular; D1, first diagonal; D2, second diagonal branch.

15.5.2.1 Antegrade wire escalation

Access wire is loaded into a 135 cm microcatheter with a standard tip shape, advanced into the artery and advanced to the proximal cap. In rare instances, this wire may penetrate into or across the lesion. In most cases, where the wire prolapses at the occlusion, the microcatheter should be advanced along the wire to 1 mm from the proximal cap. It may be necessary to treat stenosis proximal to the occlusion to facilitate delivery of gear. If guide support is challenging, it may be necessary to place a guide extension (e.g. Guideliner or Guidezilla) or anchor balloon (Figure 15.7) at this stage to increase guide stability.

Once the microcatheter is placed at the proximal cap (or just prior to it in the case of Direct Navigation wires), a BO has been established and will be advanced distally as the procedure progresses. Next, an appropriate wire, selected from the Directed Penetration, Microchannel or Directed Navigation classes should be selected, based on the anatomic features of the lesion. A short, 1 mm, 30°–45° bend (Figure 15.8) should be placed on this wire (unless pre-shaped) and the wire should be lubricated generously with saline as it is introduced through the microcatheter to the BO. The wire should be carefully manipulated through the proximal cap and the body of the occlusion towards the distal true lumen. As steady progress is made, the microcatheter can be advanced up to 2 mm before the wire tip to facilitate wire advancement. Of paramount importance, however, is that position of the wire within the vessel architecture is verified in two orthogonal views using angiographic clues (e.g. calcification) and retrograde contrast injections prior to advancement of any gear, including the microcatheter. This penultimate rule of wire position confirmation before gear advancement holds for all strategies in CTO PCI, as sub-millimetre wire perforations within the body of a CTO are rarely concerning whereas their extension due to catheter penetration can have catastrophic consequences.

If wire progress stops, the operator must carefully determine the mechanism for stall-based wire position, behaviour, tactile feedback and angiographic appearance. The next choice of wire will be based on this determination (see Section 5.1.1 for details).

Once the wire achieves a position beyond the distal cap, the microcatheter can be advanced through the remainder of the occlusion. Once this manoeuvre is accomplished, the specialised CTO wire is changed for a standard Access wire, the microcatheter is withdrawn using a balloon-trap technique (see Figure 15.9) and balloon dilation of the target vessel can commence.

15.5.2.1.1 Parallel/seesaw wiring

If a sub-intimal wire position is achieved during an AWE attempt, a change in strategy to avoid further expansion of the sub-intimal space is advised as any expansion of this compartment will make re-entry more challenging. Used

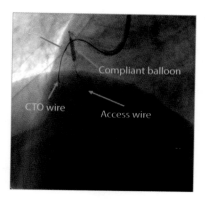

Figure 15.7 The anchor balloon technique. The anchor balloon technique is a manoeuvre undertaking to increase guide catheter support and stability. An Access wire is introduced into a proximal, *preferably disease-free* side branch of the target vessel. Along this wire a one-to-one or slightly undersized compliant balloon is introduced and inflated to low pressures (e.g. 8 atm). This inflated balloon will 'anchor' the guide into the ostium of the vessel to facilitate delivery of additional gear. Operators must be aware of developing ischaemia due to the transient occlusion of flow in the 'anchoring side branch' being used. MC, microcatheter; CTO, chronic total occlusion; atm, atmospheres.

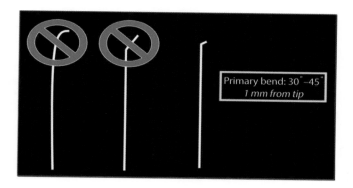

Figure 15.8 The PCI CTO Wire Bend. Typical 1 mm, 30°–45° bend should be used, unless the wire is pre-shaped. Care should be taken to avoid breakage of the wire tip. Long or sweeping bends should be avoided.

frequently by Japanese and European operators, the Parallel Wiring strategy entails leaving the sub-intimal wire in place (both as a marker and to obstruct entry into the sub-intimal track) while introducing a second microcatheter and Penetration wire. This second wire is then redirected towards the true lumen and away from the marked sub-intimal track.

A modification of this approach employs the Crusade Microcatheter (Kaneka Medical Products, Japan), a dual lumen catheter with one monorail port and a second OTW port. This catheter is introduced along the monorail port on the sub-intimal wire and advanced up to the entry point of the sub-intimal space. Next the Penetration wire is introduced through the OTW port for parallel wiring

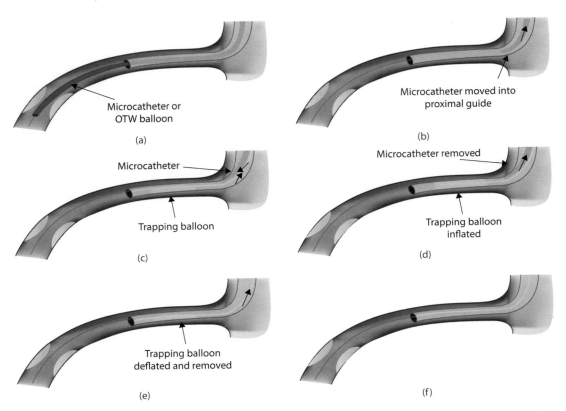

Figure 15.9 Balloon trap technique for maintenance of wire position. The balloon trap technique can be used to maintain wire position during equipment exchanges. (a) Removal of the microcatheter or OTW balloon is required; (b) the microcatheter is retracted out of the vessel and into the guide catheter along the wire; (c) a trapping balloon (3.0 mm for 8F guides, 2.5 mm for 7F guides, 2.0 mm for 6F guides) is introduced through the haemostatic valve *alongside* microcatheter, not on a wire, and advanced proximal to the tip of the microcatheter but not into the vessel; (d) the trapping balloon is inflated to 14 atm to hold the wire in place and the microcatheter is removed; (e) The trapping balloon is deflated and removed and the entire system is cleared of entrained air; (f) the wire remains in place as intended. (Adapted from Brilakis ES et al., *Catheter Cardiovasc Interv.*, 79, 3–19, 2012. With permission.)

as described above. This catheter allows the introduction of multiple wires while maintaining ideal BO position and without the need for a second microcatheter.

15.5.2.1.2 IVUS guided proximal cap puncture and directed wiring

At times, though the proximal cap may be blunt or ambiguous, other features of the CTO lend themselves best to an antegrade strategy. In such situations, IVUS can be used to resolve proximal cap ambiguity. In this technique, a standard workhorse wire is placed in a side branch that is immediately adjacent to the proximal cap of the CTO. Next, a forward imaging IVUS device (e.g. short tip Eagle Eye IVUS; Volcano Corporation, San Diego, CA) is advanced along the workhorse wire towards the ostium of the side branch until the proximal cap is visualised on the IVUS monitor. Next, the location of the cap is co-registered angiographically and then under real-time IVUS and angiographic guidance, the proximal cap is punctured with a stiff Direct Penetration wire. Once the position of the wire is confirmed, a microcatheter is carefully advanced into the aperture within the proximal cap (created by the Penetration wire) and

antegrade wire escalation or de-escalation techniques are followed (Figure 15.10a and b).

Similarly, in scenarios where the course of the vessel/occlusion is unclear, IVUS imaging from the side branch can be used to visualise the crossing wire to confirm its position within the vessel architecture, thereby facilitating wire advancement and enhancing the safety of the procedure.

15.5.2.2 Antegrade dissection re-entry

An alternative strategy for antegrade recanalisation, once a sub-intimal wire position is achieved, is controlled antegrade dissection re-entry (ADR). Once the decision to pursue ADR is made, antegrade injections should be assiduously avoided to prevent hydraulic extension of the dissection plane; all visualisation should be via retrograde collateral filling of the distal vessel and other angiographic cues. Further, care should be taken with wire tip control as any movement of the wire within the sub-intimal space (even intentional) may come at the cost of expanding intramural haematoma and a decrease in distal vessel visualisation.

The ADR technique is safe and effective in CTO PCI[54,63] and has eliminated sub-intimal wire position as an

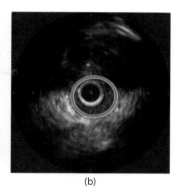

Figure 15.10 Intravascular ultrasound (IVUS) guided proximal cap localisation and puncture technique. This method can be used to solve location ambiguity associated with blunt proximal caps located at or near bifurcations. **(a)** Configuration for IVUS guided proximal cap puncture with forward imaging IVUS catheter position in a side branch near the proximal cap and base of operations in target vessel near start of the occlusion. **(b)** IVUS image demonstrating side branch (red circle) and proximal cap of CTO (yellow asterix).

automatic failure mode of these procedures. This method, however, does force the operator to deviate from traditional principles. In ADR, once the sub-intimal space is entered, the microcatheter is carefully advanced to the tip of the wire without allowing the wire to move forward (this is a challenging manoeuvre that requires considerable practice). Next, using a Kuckling wire (e.g. Fielder XT) with a 'J-tip', the wire is pushed into the sub-intimal space, where it will prolapse onto itself. Once this prolapse or 'knuckle' is created, the wire is pushed through the vessel architecture to create an intentional (but limited) dissection plane until a healthy area of horizontal vessel beyond the distal cap is reached. Ideally, the last few millimetres of the dissection should be completed with the CrossBoss (see Section 5.2.3) to minimise haematoma formation. In general, the sub-intimal space will provide considerably less resistance to wire advancement than the lesion itself. As such, meticulous wire control when transiting gear in and out of the BO is essential; in particular, care should be taken not to advance the knuckle beyond the origin of any important side branches, as these will be lost if controlled re-entry is performed distal to their origins. Once a landing zone (LZ) within the true lumen has been selected, the microcatheter is advanced to the sub-intimal space adjacent to it (the re-entry zone) and the knuckle wire is withdrawn. Upon completion of these steps, a controlled re-entry manoeuvre is possible (see below).

Of note, as the wires are withdrawn, microcatheters will have a tendency to be drawn further down the vessel; operators should be aware of this tendency and position their microcatheters accordingly to prevent inadvertent extension of the dissection plane.

15.5.2.2.1 The stingray – preparation

The Stingray (Boston Scientific Corporation, USA) is a controlled re-entry balloon catheter designed to facilitate wire transition from the sub-intimal space into the true lumen.

Fundamentally, the Stingray is an OTW flat headed balloon (comprised of two 1.5 mm balloons bound together) that, once inflated, necessarily wraps around the true lumen within the sub-intimal space. The device has three exits ports, of which one is at the end of the catheter and the remaining two are 180 apart from one another; the result of this configuration is that one of these two ports is directed towards the adventitia and the other towards the true lumen LZ (Figure 15.11).

As preparation of the Stingray prior to deployment is crucial, a 'double-prep method' is used. Herein, a three-way stopcock is attached to the balloon port and a dry 20 cc syringe is used to aspirate air from inside the balloon assembly with the goal of creating a vacuum within the device. The stopcock is turned off towards the balloon and this sequence is repeated. Next, a 3 cc syringe filled with pure contrast is connected to the stopcock and opened to allow contrast to be sucked into the balloon tip of the catheter. Once this preparation is complete, the device can be delivered to the re-entry zone.

15.5.2.2.2 Stingray deployment

A supportive wire, such as a Miracle Bros 12, is advanced through the microcatheter in the sub-intimal space 1–2 mm distal to the re-entry zone. The microcatheter is then carefully withdrawn using a balloon trap to ensure wire position in maintained. Next, the Stingray device is loaded on the support wire and advanced to the re-entry zone. Occasionally, the delivery of even the new lower profile Stingray device can be challenging; if this is the case, low pressure dilation of the delivery track with a 1.5 mm balloon may be necessary.

Once delivered to the re-entry zone, an insufflator is connected to the balloon port of the Stingray and the device is inflated to 6 atm. With the device deployed (inflated), the image intensifier is moved to an angle where the Stingray appears as a single contrast filled straight line; at this angle,

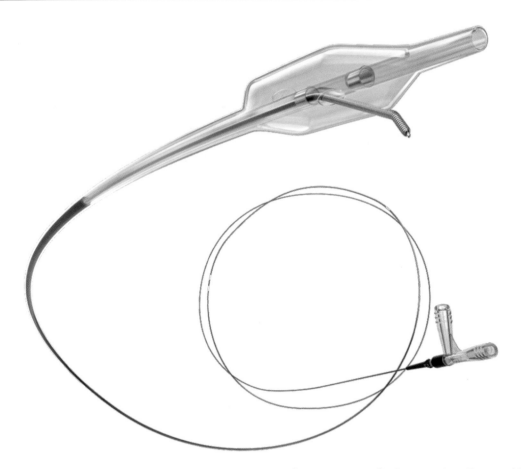

Figure 15.11 The stingray controlled re-entry catheter. (Courtesy of Boston Scientific Corporation, Boston, USA.)

one port is pointed upwards and the other port pointed downwards, with both ports perpendicular to the axis of visualisation and is the optimal view for the stick and swap re-entry procedure (see Section 5.2.2.3).

Prior to inflation, it may be useful to perform sub-intimal transcatheter withdrawal (STRAW) by aspirating at the balloon port with a 10 cc syringe to decompress any intramural haematoma that may have developed with sub-intimal dissection. This process may restore distal visualisation and facilitate stick and swap re-entry by collapsing the sub-intimal space to render the properly oriented Stingray exit port as close to the intima as possible.

15.5.2.2.3 The stick and swap procedure

In order to re-enter the true lumen using the Stingray device, a stick and swap must be performed. In this procedure, a Pilot 200 wire is prepared with an angled 1 mm bend similar to that of the pre-shaped Stingray Penetration wire (a stiff, high tip load wire provided for use with the Stingray balloon that is designed to puncture from the sub-intimal space, through the intima and into the true lumen). Next, the Stingray wire is advanced into the wire port of the device and manoeuvred out of the side port that appears adjacent to the intima (in the direction of the vessel). If re-entry is successful, a pop is often felt. Given this wire's tendency to cross tissue planes, once re-entry is performed, the

Stingray wire is 'swapped' for the Pilot 200 prepared earlier with the goal of manoeuvring the Pilot wire through the same port and track created by the Stingray wire into the distal true lumen. Once true lumen wire position is confirmed in orthogonal views by retrograde contrast injection, the Stingray is deflated and removed and the Pilot 200 is exchanged for a workhorse wire using a microcatheter and balloon trap technique.

If re-entry is unsuccessful, the Stingray balloon can be deflated and gently advanced forward within the sub-intimal space to a new re-entry zone where the stick and swap procedure can be re-attempted. This procedure, termed 'Bobsledding', must be performed with great care to maintain as controlled sub-intimal space as possible.

15.5.2.3 CrossBoss

The CrossBoss is an OTW catheter with a 3 Fr atraumatic metallic tip that is advanced, with or without wire guidance, through a CTO or in the sub-intimal space adjacent to it (Figure 15.12). Device can be placed at the proximal cap, ideally along a supportive Directed Penetration (e.g. Miracle Bros 12) wire that first establishes entry into the proximal cap. Once in place, the catheter is spun as rapidly as possible using the attached torqueing device with gentle forward pressure. As the device advances, care must be taken to ensure that it is progressing along the course of the vessel.

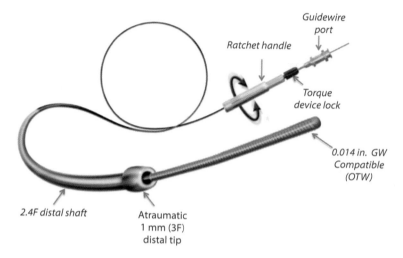

Figure 15.12 The CrossBoss catheter with key features. (Courtesy of Boston Scientific Corporation, Boston, USA.)

If the device appears to move offline, an angiogram must be performed to confirm its position; though this device is unlikely to exit the vessel, it does have a tendency to enter side branches and as such, may result in unwanted dissections or perforation in branch vessels. The CrossBoss can be redirected using a wire if desired. The device has a tension release mechanism within its torque tool that is activate when clicking is heard during advancement. The purpose of this mechanism is to dissipate torque that exceeds design limits but its activation may also suggest that the device is impacting a rigid structure (such as a stent strut or heavy calcification) and requires redirection.

Once the CrossBoss achieves a position beyond the distal cap, a retrograde injection angiogram is performed. Approximately 30% of the time, the device will be in the distal true lumen, in which case a workhorse wire can be advanced through it into the distal vessel. If the distal end of the device is in the sub-intimal space, a support wire can be delivered through it and positioned in a satisfactory re-entry zone. The CrossBoss can then be withdrawn and the Stingray Re-Entry system is introduced as described above.

15.5.2.4 Star technique

Now used primarily as a bailout manoeuvre, sub-intimal tracking and re-entry (STAR) was introduced by Colombo in 2005 as wire-based re-entry strategy.[64] In this STAR technique, a soft, polymer jacketed wire is introduced into a dissection plane with an 'umbrella tip' and advanced aggressively into the distal vessel with the goal of shearing the tissue intimal layer to create a common space between the sub-intimal space and the true lumen. Once performed, these vessels are often left for 6 weeks to allow healing to occur; following these 'investment' procedures, patients often return with antegrade flow rendering the intervention easier than the initial CTO.

15.5.3 Retrograde strategies

The retrograde technique, the domain of experienced operators, is a key component of the hybrid algorithm and has markedly increased success rates in CTO PCI.[65,66] Since the technique was described, success rates have increased to over 90% at experienced centres with acceptable complication rates.

Fundamentally, this strategy involves using intercoronary collaterals to establish a BO in the true lumen at the distal cap. With microcatheter back up, a Collateral Crossing wire is carefully advanced through an appropriately selected collateral to the distal cap in the target vessel. Thereafter, the microcatheter is carefully advanced along the Crossing wire to its tip to establish the retrograde BO in the target vessel. Finally, using one of the several techniques, a wire is advanced retrograde through the occlusion (but within the architecture of the vessel), manipulated into antegrade guide and externalised. The result is a long, full-body rail along which PCI can be performed. The specifics of these strategies and their unique considerations are discussed below.

15.5.3.1 Retrograde case selection

Retrograde recanalisation techniques are best employed as a primary approach in long lesions, with blunt proximal caps and suitable interventional collaterals (dependent on operator skill level); as such, predictors of primary antegrade failure are reasonable indications for a primary retrograde approach.[43] Further, the retrograde approach can be employed in lieu of converting to an investment procedure when antegrade strategies fail as an antegrade sub-intimal wire position is a prerequisite for success reverse controlled antegrade and retrograde sub-intimal tracking (R-CART) (see below for details).

Though morphology of coronary collaterals is highly varied, the location of these recruitable, pre-formed coronary-to-coronary connections[67] are somewhat predictable. Common collateral connections and locations (septal or epicardial) are summarised in Table 15.4.

Table 15.4 Cardiac and non-cardiac complications of CTO PCI

Complication	Common aetiologies	Clinical setting	Clinical manifestations	Cath Lab management	Frequency	Preventative measures and other recommendations
Cardiac complications						
Coronary perforation with or without tamponade	• Equipment exit through coronary artery • Coronary evulsion during MC advancement • Stent oversizing or over-dilation	• At any time during CTO PCI procedure	• Chest pain • Haemodyanmic instability • Decreased fluoroscopic motion of heart border • Contrast stain that clears on angiography	• Emergent echo • Haemodyanmic resuscitation (blood/fluids/ vasoactive meds) • Pericardiocentesis • Balloon tamponade • Bead or thrombin injection • Coiling of bleeding vessel • Covered stent placement	Coronary: 4.3% Collateral: 7.9% Tamponade: 1.4%	• Use of contralateral injections to visualise the distal vessel and artery course prior to equipment advancement • Use of intravascular imaging to guide stent sizing • AVOID reversal of anti-coagulation if possible due to risk of donor vessel thrombosis
Guide/donor vessel thrombosis or occlusion	• Lack of adequate anti-coagulation • Resistance to administered anti-coagulant • Administration of protamine or other reversal agent • Aortic dissection at level of vessel origin • Sub-intimal stenting with poor outflow	• At anytime during CTO PCI • Long procedures • Long periods without adequate flushing of guide catheters • Challenge guide engagements	• Chest pain • Heart failure • Arrhythmia (ischaemic) • Shock/sudden haemodynamic instability • Lack of vessel flow on angiography ± visible vessel thrombus	• Haemodynamic resuscitation • Restore systemic anti-coagulation to target levels • Manual thrombectomy ± intracoronary abciximab • Replace guide catheters (if indicated)	Extremely rare	• Catastrophic complication that carries high mortality • Ensure protocolised checks of anti-coagulation status • Antegrade ACT >300 • Retrograde ACT >350 • Avoid use of bivalirudin • Avoid anti-coagulation reversal agents unless absolutely necessary • Use intravascular imaging and/or collateral injections to confirm outflow prior to stenting

(Continued)

Table 15.4 (Continued) Cardiac and non-cardiac complications of CTO PCI

Complication	Common aetiologies	Clinical setting	Clinical manifestations	Cath Lab management	Frequency	Preventative measures and other recommendations
Ischaemia	• Occlusion of collateral supply with equipment • Injury to donor vessel with reduced flow • Injury to distal vessel bed due to embolization of atheromatous contents (e.g. in SVG) • Equipment entrapment in collateral	• Vein graft recanalization • Cases with ipsilateral/single conduit collateral flow • During donor vessel injury (e.g. coronary or aorto-ostial dissections) • Equipment transit through very tortuous or intra-myocardial collaterals	• Chest pain • Heart failure • Haemodynamic instability • Arrhythmia (ischaemic) • Silent	• If distal embolisation occurs, consider injection of nitroprusside or adenosine as tolerated • Rapid stenting of injured areas in donor vessel • Removal of equipment from collaterals (last resort)	MI: Upto 3% Q Wave MI: 0.6% Donor vessel Dissection: 2% Equipment Entrapment: 1.2%	• Minimise procedural time • Consider use of haemodynamic support where collateral flow is limited to small, single vessels and ventricular function is poor • Meticulous care with guide, micro-catheter and wire positioning (especially in donor vessel) • Avoid use of very small/tortuous/intra-myocardial collateral conduits
Non-cardiac complications						
Vascular access complications	• Challenging body habitus (e.g. obese patients) • Presence of important PAD • Vessel calcification at site of puncture • Large bore sheaths	• Potential in any CTO PCI procedure	• Overt bleeding • Unexplained hypotension • Back pain or other signs of retroperitoneal haemorrhage	• Manual pressure • Up-sizing of sheath to fully occlude arteriotomy • Balloon tamponade at site of bleeding • May need to place covered stent over arteriotomy if conservative measures fail • Surgical evacuation of retroperitoneal haematoma	Vascular access complications: 2%	• Meticulous care with vascular access • Use of ultrasound to localise location and healthy segment of vessel • Use of micro-puncture kits in obese patients for initial access • Clinical suspicion must be maintained till at least 24 hours post-procedure

(Continued)

Table 15.4 (Continued) Cardiac and non-cardiac complications of CTO PCI

Complication	Common aetiologies	Clinical setting	Clinical manifestations	Cath Lab management	Frequency	Preventative measures and other recommendations
Radiation skin injury	• Poor radiation hygiene • Prolonged procedures • Use of high magnification • Use of high frame rates • Use of steep angulations • Overuse of cine-acquisition imaging	• New CTO operators • Patients with previously failed procedures • Large patient body habitus	• Radiation skin injury, apparent days to weeks after the procedure • (Figure 2a and b)	N/A	Radiation skin injury: 1%	• Use low magnification • Cycle through multiple views during procedure • Use low frame rates and limit cine acquisition imaging • Use collimation • Decrease fluoroscopy time by not stepping on imaging pedal unless absolutely necessary • Use trapping techniques for exchanges • Avoid steep imaging angles • Pay careful attention to radiation dose monitoring parameters (e.g. air kerma) • Stop procedure if radiation dose exceeds safe limits and schedule second attempt
Contrast nephropathy	• Excessive contrast utilisation in a susceptible patient	• Patients with risk factors of contrast nephropathy: • Underlying CKD • Advanced age • Diabeteso Low LVEF • Heart failure	• Rise in serum creatinine by either 25% of baseline or 0.5 mg/dL within 24–48 hours of contrast administration	N/A	Contrast nephropathy in CTO PCI: 1.8%	• Correct hypovolaemia prior to procedure • Protocolised IV fluid administration during and post procedure • Careful monitoring in susceptible patients post-procedure is key to recognition • Perform procedures when serum creatinine at or close to patient's baseline

For a detailed discussion and meta-analysis of complications in CTO PCI, including frequency estimates, please see.
ACT, activated clotting time; CKD, chronic kidney disease; LVEF, Left ventricular ejection fraction; CTO PCI, chronic total occlusion percutaneous coronary interventions; MC, microcatheter; MI, myocardial infarction; PAD, peripheral arterial disease; SVG, saphenous vein graft.

In general, septal collaterals develop between the left anterior descending (LAD) artery and the posterior descending artery (PDA) branch of the right coronary artery (RCA). These collaterals can flow in either direction depending on the location of the occlusion. Virtually all other intracoronary collaterals are epicardial. Coronary collaterals are extremely fragile vessels, prone to both dissection and perforation. Predictably, the clinical consequences of injury to septal collaterals (which are by definition encased within the septum) are substantially less important than similar injuries to epicardial collaterals, which can result in rapid blood loss, tamponade and haemodynamic compromise. As such, early experience with retrograde CTO PCI should be limited to septal or bypass graft collaterals, be in the presence of an experienced proctor for at least the first 5–10 cases and should only be undertaken after considerable experience with antegrade CTO PCI techniques has been accrued. Given their high risk of perforation and generally tortuous morphology, epicardial collaterals should only be considered as 'suitable' by expert retrograde operators.

15.5.3.2 Retrograde CTO PCI platform

Selection of guide catheters for retrograde procedures should be based closely on the dual catheter angiogram findings. For the majority of cases, EBU or XB type guide catheters for the left system and Amplatz left guides for the right system will be optimal though, in cases of ostial RCA occlusion, the use of Judkins right catheters may be considered. As recommended above, both guide catheters should be 90 cm (though strictly speaking, only the retrograde guide necessitates this length to allow retrograde gear to reach the antegrade guide). In the retrograde limb, at least 6 Fr (but optimally 7 Fr) catheters should be used to allow for support and to ease gear delivery. To ensure the largest target possible, the antegrade guide should be an 8 Fr catheter. We recommend the use of side hole guides in the antegrade system to allow for some pressure dissipation with antegrade injections, particularly in the case of an accidently delivered injection after the creation of antegrade dissection planes. Finally, we recommend that the antegrade system be on a manual injection manifold to allow careful modulation of the force of contrast injections, should the need arise.

In general, long microcatheters must be used to advance retrograde wires though collaterals into the distal target vessel through the occlusion. In R-CART procedures, where an antegrade system (i.e. wire and microcatheter) is also required, short microcatheters may be used (see Tables 15.2 and 15.3 for a list and description of recommended Collateral Crossing wires and Microcatheters for retrograde procedures). Finally, great care should be taken to achieve and maintain ACTs of greater than 350 seconds (using heparin) throughout the procedure to prevent catheter or equipment thromboses.

15.5.3.3 Retrograde collateral crossing

As with all retrograde PCI, wire manipulation in these procedures begins with Access or Workhorse wire engagement of the target collateral vessel with careful microcatheter advancement to its origin. The Access wire is then withdrawn in favour of a blunt tip, low tip load, lubricious Collateral Crossing wire (e.g. Sion, Suoh) with a short, sub-millimetre tip bend. Of note, saline should be injected at introducer port of the microcatheter as any wire is removed to prevent air entrainment into the device. The Crossing wire is then gently advanced into the collateral and directly along the identified course towards the distal target vessel in a probing motion. Great care is taken to ensure free tip movement and to avoid knuckling of the Crossing wire in the collateral given the fragility of these vessels. If little or no progress is made after several minutes, the microcatheter may be advanced slightly into the collateral, followed by removal of the wire and selective injection of the collateral to delineate the precise connection with the target zone. The wiring procedure may be repeated until successful wire access to this zone is achieved and confirmed by retrograde angiography in two orthogonal views. Though occasional ventricular premature beats (VPBs) may be encountered as the crossing wire transitions from the collateral to the distal target vessel, frequent or runs of VPBs indicate suboptimal tip position, myocardial irritation and herald collateral injury.

Following confirmation of position, the microcatheter is carefully advanced through the collateral to the distal wire tip, thereby establishing the retrograde BO. During this manoeuvre, the operator must be keenly aware of the retrograde guide position (which will tend to push out of the coronary ostium), the distal wire tip (which will have a tendency to retract backwards) and the tip of the microcatheter as it advances through the collateral. With any manipulation of this system, all three of these components are affected, the changes to which must be anticipated by the operator and promptly rectified. Alternating clockwise and counterclockwise spinning of the microcatheter will facilitate its advancement along the wire; this one operator manoeuvre is a critical skill in CTO PCI and may take considerable time to master. Care must be taken to avoid over rotation of the microcatheter to avoid *microcatheter fatigue* (first encountered with the Corsair device); this phenomenon which presents as resistance to wire movement within the microcatheter must be recognised early and promptly remedied (by microcatheter replacement).

15.5.3.4 Retrograde true-to-true

Fundamentally, this strategy involves wire passage in the retrograde direction, through the distal cap, body of the occlusion and proximal cap into the true lumen of the antegrade vessel. Though this approach is successful in less than 30% of cases,[61] it is a useful strategy in short lesions without significant tortuosity where the location and course of the proximal vessel is unambiguous. In this strategy, a Directed Penetration or Directed Navigation wire is used to breach the distal cap and transit through the occlusion. If the true lumen proximal vessel wire position is achieved and confirmed, both the wire and retrograde microcatheter are advanced into the antegrade guide. At this stage, the retrograde wire is withdrawn and exchanged for a long externalisation wire (e.g. RG3 or R350) that is advanced until it exits the haemostatic valve of the antegrade guide.

Once the externalised wire is captured outside the body (to create a retrograde-to-antegrade rail), PCI of the target lesion can be performed. Prior to the introduction of equipment antegrade along the externalised wire, the retrograde microcatheter must be retracted into the distal target vessel. It is critical that *full microcatheter coverage* of the guidewire within the collateral vessel is maintained to prevent collateral laceration. Further, during the microcatheter retraction, the retrograde guide will invariably be drawn into the proximal donor vessel. It is crucial to anticipate this guide movement and *fully disengage* the retrograde guide while the microcatheter is retracted. Failure to do so may result is serious injury to the ostial or proximal donor vessel.

Once PCI is complete, the retrograde gear must be removed. The procedure for retrograde gear divestiture is described in Section 5.3.5.

15.5.3.5 Reverse controlled antegrade and retrograde subintimal tracking (R-CART)

During retrograde wiring, most commonly, the distal cap is crossed with an appropriate wire but a sub-intimal wire position is obtained. This is a fundamental component of the R-CART procedure.

Upon confirmation of position in the vessel architecture with vessel 'dancing', the retrograde microcatheter is advanced along the wire to its tip (several millimetres beyond the distal cap). An umbrella-type bend is placed on a Knuckling wire, which is then advanced via the retrograde microcatheter through the body of the occlusion within the sub-intimal space. This is followed by advancement of the microcatheter to advance the retrograde BO.

To establish an antegrade BO, a short microcatheter is placed at the proximal cap via the antegrade guide using an Access-group wire. This wire is then exchanged for a Penetration or Navigation wire to breach the proximal cap and enter the sub-intimal space in the antegrade direction. If suited, this wire can be knuckled and advanced in the sub-intimal space in an antegrade manner to several millimetres past the retrograde BO, thereby creating an antegrade and retrograde BO overlap zone. If the antegrade Penetration wire is not suited for knuckling, the microcatheter can be advanced into the sub-intimal space where a Knuckling wire can be introduced to achieve the overlap position.

With the antegrade and retrograde wires now in a common sub-intimal space, balloon angioplasty over the antegrade wire (at low to intermediate pressures) is performed at the overlap zone with goal of ablating the tissue separating the antegrade and retrograde wires. Balloon sizing for this

manoeuvre to the size of the vessel to ensure adequate tissue disruption should be considered. Following this manoeuvre, a new retrograde Penetration or Nagivation-group wire is used to traverse tissue planes to enter the same plane as the antegrade wire. If this is successful, the retrograde wire will advance into the antegrade guide or the aorta (see Figure 15.13a through d for a schematic representation of the R-CART procedure).[68] If, after several tissue ablation attempts, retrograde wire navigation into the antegrade guide is unsuccessful, a Guideliner or similar guide extension can be placed antegrade into the sub-intimal space to facilitate the process (Guideliner Assisted Reverse CART). Alternative strategies include the use of larger balloons to achieve greater tissue ablation, the use of slightly smaller

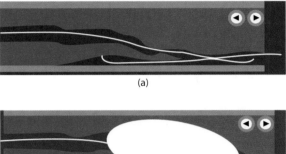

(a)

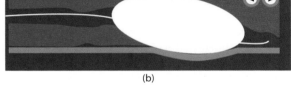

(b)

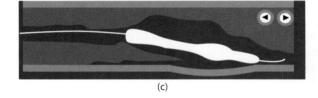

(c)

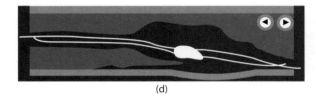

(d)

Figure 15.13 Reverse controlled antegrade and retrograde subintimal tracking. A schematic representation of the key steps in reverse controlled antegrade and retrograde sub-intimal tracking. **(a)** The antegrade and retrograde wires are positioned adjacent to one another within the sub-intimal space of the CTO. **(b)** An appropriately sized balloon is introduced along the anterograde wire and inflated to ablate the tissue planes separating the two wires to create a common space. **(c)** The antegrade balloon is deflated. **(d)** The retrograde wire is manoeuvred into the antegrade guide and externalised. Subsequent stenting can be performed over the externalized wire. (Adapted from Rathore S et al., *JACC Cardiovasc Interv.*, 3, 155–164, 2010.)

balloons (i.e. vessel size minus 0.5 mm) with retrograde advancement/tissue plane navigation using a higher-tip load Directed Navigation wire (e.g. Gaia 2), or movement of the antegrade and retrograde BO overlap to a different location within the CTO where the tissue ablation/retrograde wire navigation procedure can be repeated. Once the retrograde wire and microcatheter are successfully advanced into the antegrade guide, the retrograde wire is exchanged for a dedicated externalisation wire, which is fully externalised and over which PCI can be performed.

15.5.3.5.1 Snaring to complete externalisation

Once an aortic wire position is obtained and confirmed by wire behaviour (the wire should move and advance freely up the ascending aorta into the brachiocephalic artery), an alternative method to secure retrograde wire position within the antegrade guide is snaring. In this procedure, the retrograde microcatheter is advanced into the aorta long the retrograde wire, which is exchanged for a long Pilot 200 wire with exaggerated primary and secondary bends (10–20 mm). The Pilot wire is then placed in the ascending aorta or brachiocephalic artery. Next the antegrade guide is withdrawn into the ascending aorta and an 18–30 mm EnSnare is introduced through it to capture the Pilot wire. Capture must occur on the soft end of the wire to avoid wire entrapment within the snare. Finally, using a simultaneous push-pull technique, the antegrade guide is advanced along the snared wire to capture the retrograde microcatheter (resident in the aortic root) and seat the antegrade guide back into the ostium of the target vessel. The wire is then carefully liberated from the snare, withdrawn and changed for an externalisation-group wire as previously described.

15.5.3.6 Retrograde gear removal

Following the completion of PCI along the externalised wire, the retrograde gear must be withdrawn. This final component of the retrograde CTO PCI procedure is exceptionally important; if it is done improperly, severe injury to the patient may occur. There are three key aspects of retrograde gear divestiture: (1) microcatheter protection of collaterals; (2) retrograde guide disengagement and (3) collateral control (most important when epicardial collaterals are used).

Following PCI, the retrograde microcatheter is re-advanced into the antegrade guide and the externalisation wire is replaced with a Collateral Crossing wire to maintain collateral wire access in case of collateral injury hidden by the microcatheter. Next, the retrograde guide is *fully disengaged* and pulled out of the field of view. With the guide held in this position, the retrograde microcatheter is carefully retracted to the origin of the collaterals used for the procedure. A retrograde guide is re-engaged and an angiogram is performed to confirm collateral integrity and to exclude meaningful injury. Once integrity of these vessels is confirmed, the microcatheter is advanced into the stented segment of the target vessel. At this stage, the Collateral Crossing wire and retrograde microcatheter can be carefully withdrawn (the retrograde guide must again be disengaged during this process to prevent injury to the donor vessel ostium). Following the removal of all equipment, both antegrade and retrograde angiograms are performed to document final PCI results.

15.5.3.7 Vessel patency following CTO PCI

Once definitive wire access across the CTO has been obtained, standard PCI may be performed. The use of IVUS to define both stent size and length, facilitate positioning and ensure optimal deployment is key. However, beyond the use of optimal stenting technique, it is important to recognise that vessel patency following CTO PCI depends on multiple factors, including stent choice, crossing technique and patient co-morbidities.

Beginning with data from the Total Occlusion Study of Canada (TOSCA)-1 study, it is clear that stenting is superior to PTCA (provided satisfactory stent outflow is achieved) with respect to restenosis, re-occlusion and clinically driven target vessel revascularisation (TVR).[69,70] Following in the introduction of sirolimus eluting stents (SESs), considered a first generation DES, the PRISON II study demonstrated a decrease in major adverse cardiovascular events (MACE) at 12-month clinical follow-up, driven by a decrease in TVR, target lesion revascularisation (TLR) and target vessel failure (TVF) with the use of SES.[71] The GISSOC II – GISE trial, which examined bare metal stents (BMSs) versus SES in CTO PCI noted reduced binary restenosis and re-occlusion at 6-month angiographic follow-up and decreased TVR at 12-month clinical follow-up in the SES group.[72] The largest of the BMS versus first generation DES trials, the ACROSS-CYPHER study, demonstrated similar findings with a 33% absolute risk reduction (85% relative risk reduction) in treated segment re-stenosis as well as important reductions in in-stent restenosis in patients treated with SES versus BMS at 6-month angiographic follow-up.[73]

The introduction of second generation DES (everolimus and zotarolimus eluting stents) further decreased vessel re-occlusion[74] and stent thrombosis rates.[75] Most recently, the EXPERT CTO Trial studied 250 consecutively enrolled patients undergoing CTO PCI using contemporary methods and everolimus eluting stents (EESs).[76] Compared with data from previous CTO trials (12-month MACE of 24.4%), treatment with EES was associated with lower composite adverse events for both intent-to-treat (18.5%) and per-protocol populations (8.2%) with 1-year TLR similar to previous trials at 6.4%.[76]

Interestingly, the use of uncontrolled re-entry techniques with long areas of sub-intimal dissection is associated with an increase TLR, angiographic restenosis and stent re-occlusion in CTO PCI. In a study from the Florence PCI registry, Valenti and colleagues demonstrated a 57% long-term re-occlusion rate following the use of the STAR technique versus another contemporary dataset.[74] Finally, patient factors, most notably the presence of diabetes, may also influence vascular patency following CTO PCI; an absolute difference of 17.3% in binary restenosis in patients with diabetes was noted in the ACROSS-CYPHER study.[73]

15.6 Complications of CTO PCI

Critical to any successful CTO PCI program is comfort with the management procedural complications, which occur at rates higher than in normal PCI procedures.[34] These complications can be broadly classified into one of two groups: intracardiac and extracardiac.

15.7 Summary and conclusions

CTOs are commonly encountered lesions for which revascularisation is a safe and effective therapy. CTO PCI is a cognitively and technically challenging procedure that required a detailed understanding of both vascular architecture and the use of specialised equipment. These procedures are learned in an iterative fashion, with early experience best developed under the mentorship of expert operators. As with early angioplasty, our developing understanding of the techniques and tools used to tackle this challenging lesion subset is likely to result in increased success rates and further improvement in clinical outcomes for our patients.

References

1. Di Mario C et al. European perspective in the recanalisation of Chronic Total Occlusions (CTO): Consensus document from the EuroCTO Club. *EuroIntervention* 2007; 3(1): 30–43.
2. Christofferson RD et al. Effect of chronic total coronary occlusion on treatment strategy. *Am J Cardiol* 2005; 95(9): 1088–1091.
3. Farooq V et al. Quantification of incomplete revascularization and its association with five-year mortality in the synergy between percutaneous coronary intervention with taxus and cardiac surgery (SYNTAX) trial validation of the residual SYNTAX score. *Circulation* 2013; 128(2): 141–151.
4. Hachamovitch R et al. Comparison of the short-term survival benefit associated with revascularization compared with medical therapy in patients with no prior coronary artery disease undergoing stress myocardial perfusion single photon emission computed tomography. *Circulation* 2003; 107(23): 2900–2907.
5. Shaw LJ et al. Optimal medical therapy with or without percutaneous coronary intervention to reduce ischemic burden: Results from the Clinical Outcomes Utilizing Revascularization and Aggressive Drug Evaluation (COURAGE) trial nuclear substudy. *Circulation* 2008; 117(10): 1283–1291.
6. Safley DM et al. Changes in myocardial ischemic burden following percutaneous coronary intervention of chronic total occlusions. *Catheter Cardiovasc Interv* 2011; 78(3): 337–343.
7. Werner GS et al. Determinants of coronary steal in chronic total coronary occlusions donor artery, collateral, and microvascular resistance. *J Am Coll Cardiol* 2006; 48(1): 51–58.
8. Sachdeva R et al. The myocardium supplied by a chronic total occlusion is a persistently ischemic zone. *Catheter Cardiovasc Interv* 2014; 83(1): 9–16.
9. Valenti R et al. Impact of chronic total occlusion revascularization in patients with acute myocardial infarction treated by primary percutaneous coronary intervention. *Am J Cardiol* 2014; 114(12): 1794–1800.
10. George S et al. Long-term follow-up of elective chronic total coronary occlusion angioplasty: Analysis from the U.K. Central Cardiac Audit Database. *J Am Coll Cardiol* 2014; 64(3): 235–243.
11. Mehran R et al. Long-term outcome of percutaneous coronary intervention for chronic total occlusions. *JACC Cardiovasc Interv* 2011; 4(9): 952–961.
12. Joyal D et al. Effectiveness of recanalization of chronic total occlusions: A systematic review and meta-analysis. *Am Heart J* 2010; 160(1): 179–187.
13. Khan MF et al. Effects of percutaneous revascularization of chronic total occlusions on clinical outcomes: A meta-analysis comparing successful versus failed percutaneous intervention for chronic total occlusion. *Catheter Cardiovasc Interv* 2013; 82(1): 95–107.
14. Vanoverschelde JL et al. Time course of functional recovery after coronary artery bypass graft surgery in patients with chronic left ventricular ischemic dysfunction. *Am J Cardiol* 2000; 85(12): 1432–1439.
15. Haas F et al. Ischemically compromised myocardium displays different time-courses of functional recovery: Correlation with morphological alterations? *Eur J Cardiothorac Surg* 2001; 20(2): 290–298.
16. Velazquez EJ et al. Coronary-artery bypass surgery in patients with ischemic cardiomyopathy. *N Engl J Med* 2016; 374(16): 1511–1520.
17. Van Belle E et al. Effects of stenting of recent or chronic coronary occlusions on late vessel patency and left ventricular function. *Am J Cardiol* 1997; 80(9): 1150–1154.
18. Sirnes PA et al. Improvement in left ventricular ejection fraction and wall motion after successful recanalization of chronic coronary occlusions. *Eur Heart J* 1998; 19(2): 273–281.
19. Baks T et al. Prediction of left ventricular function after drug-eluting stent implantation for chronic total coronary occlusions. *J Am Coll Cardiol* 2006; 47(4): 721–725.
20. Kirschbaum SW et al. Evaluation of left ventricular function three years after percutaneous recanalization of chronic total occlusions. *Am J Cardiol* 2008; 101(2): 179–185.
21. Borgia F et al. Improved cardiac survival, freedom from MACE and angina-related quality of life after successful percutaneous recanalization of coronary artery chronic total occlusions. *Int J Cardiol* 2012; 161(1): 31–38.
22. Grantham JA et al. Quantifying the early health status benefits of successful chronic total occlusion recanalization: Results from the FlowCardia's Approach to Chronic Total Occlusion Recanalization (FACTOR) Trial. *Circ Cardiovasc Qual Outcomes* 2010; 3(3): 284–290.
23. Katsuragawa M et al. Histologic studies in percutaneous transluminal coronary angioplasty for chronic total

occlusion: Comparison of tapering and abrupt types of occlusion and short and long occluded segments. *J Am Coll Cardiol* 1993; 21(3): 604–611.

24. Srivatsa SS et al. Histologic correlates of angiographic chronic total coronary artery occlusions: Influence of occlusion duration on neovascular channel patterns and intimal plaque composition. *J Am Coll Cardiol* 1997; 29(5): 955–963.

25. Jaffe R et al. Natural history of experimental arterial chronic total occlusions. *J Am Coll Cardiol* 2009; 53(13): 1148–1158.

26. Thind AS et al. Investigation of micro-ultrasound for microvessel imaging in a model of chronic total occlusion. *Ultrason Imaging* 2007; 29(3): 167–181.

27. Munce NR et al. Intravascular and extravascular microvessel formation in chronic total occlusions a micro-CT imaging study. *JACC Cardiovasc Imaging* 2010; 3(8): 797–805.

28. Prosser L et al. Implantation of oxygen enhanced, three-dimensional microporous L-PLA polymers: A reproducible porcine model of chronic total coronary occlusion. *Catheter Cardiovasc Interv* 2006; 67(3): 412–416.

29. Finn AV et al. The differences between neovascularization of chronic total occlusion and intraplaque angiogenesis. *JACC Cardiovasc Imaging* 2010; 3(8): 806–810.

30. Guo J et al. A virtual histology intravascular ultrasound analysis of coronary chronic total occlusions. *Catheter Cardiovasc Interv* 2013; 81(3): 464–470.

31. Strauss BH et al. Microvessels in chronic total occlusions: Pathways for successful guidewire crossing? *J Interv Cardiol* 2005; 18(6): 425–436.

32. Thompson CA et al. Retrograde techniques and the impact of operator volume on percutaneous intervention for coronary chronic total occlusions an early U.S. experience. *JACC Cardiovasc Interv* 2009; 2(9): 834–842.

33. Karmpaliotis D et al. Development of a high-volume, multiple-operator program for percutaneous chronic total coronary occlusion revascularization: Procedural, clinical, and cost-utilization outcomes. *Catheter Cardiovasc Interv* 2013; 82(1): 1–8.

34. Brilakis ES et al. Procedural outcomes of chronic total occlusion percutaneous coronary intervention: A report from the NCDR (National Cardiovascular Data Registry). *JACC Cardiovasc Interv* 2015; 8(2): 245–253.

35. Kahn JK et al. High-dose contrast agent administration during complex coronary angioplasty. *Am Heart J* 1990; 120(3): 533–536.

36. Michael TT et al. Temporal trends of fluoroscopy time and contrast utilization in coronary chronic total occlusion revascularization: Insights from a multicenter united states registry. *Catheter Cardiovasc Interv* 2015; 85(3): 393–399.

37. Brown JR et al. Does safe dosing of iodinated contrast prevent contrast-induced acute kidney injury? *Circ Cardiovasc Interv* 2010; 3(4): 346–350.

38. Brar SS et al. Haemodynamic-guided fluid administration for the prevention of contrast-induced acute kidney injury: The POSEIDON randomised controlled trial. *Lancet* 2014; 383(9931): 1814–1823.

39. Suzuki S et al. Radiation exposure to patient's skin during percutaneous coronary intervention for various lesions, including chronic total occlusion. *Circ J* 2006; 70(1): 44–48.

40. Balter S et al. Fluoroscopically guided interventional procedures: A review of radiation effects on patients' skin and hair. *Radiology* 2010; 254(2): 326–341.

41. Wyman RM. Do we need another predictive scoring tool for chronic total occlusion percutaneous coronary intervention? *JACC Cardiovasc Interv* 2015; 8(12): 1549–1551.

42. Morino Y et al. Predicting successful guidewire crossing through chronic total occlusion of native coronary lesions within 30 minutes: The J-CTO (Multicenter CTO Registry in Japan) score as a difficulty grading and time assessment tool. *JACC Cardiovasc Interv* 2011; 4(2): 213–221.

43. Brilakis ES et al. A percutaneous treatment algorithm for crossing coronary chronic total occlusions. *JACC Cardiovasc Interv* 2012; 5(4): 367–379.

44. Pershad A et al. Validation and incremental value of the hybrid algorithm for CTO PCI. *Catheter Cardiovasc Interv* 2014; 84(4): 654–659.

45. Christopoulos G et al. The efficacy and safety of the 'hybrid' approach to coronary chronic total occlusions: Insights from a contemporary multicenter US registry and comparison with prior studies. *J Invasive Cardiol* 2014; 26(9): 427–432.

46. Sakakura K et al. Comparison of pathology of chronic total occlusion with and without coronary artery bypass graft. *Eur Heart J* 2014; 35(25): 1683–1693.

47. Teramoto T et al. Initial success rate of percutaneous coronary intervention for chronic total occlusion in a native coronary artery is decreased in patients who underwent previous coronary artery bypass graft surgery. *JACC Cardiovasc Interv* 2014; 7(1): 39–46.

48. Alessandrino G et al. A clinical and angiographic scoring system to predict the probability of successful first-attempt percutaneous coronary intervention in patients with total chronic coronary occlusion. *JACC Cardiovasc Interv* 2015; 8(12): 1540–1548.

49. Opolski MP et al. Coronary computed tomographic prediction rule for time-efficient guidewire crossing through chronic total occlusion: Insights from the CT-RECTOR multicenter registry (Computed Tomography Registry of Chronic Total Occlusion Revascularization). *JACC Cardiovasc Interv* 2015; 8(2): 257–267.

50. Christopoulos G et al. Development and validation of a novel scoring system for predicting technical success of chronic total occlusion percutaneous coronary interventions: The PROGRESS CTO (Prospective Global Registry for the Study of Chronic Total Occlusion Intervention) Score. *JACC Cardiovasc Interv* 2016; 9(1): 1–9.

51. Hsu JT et al. Impact of calcification length ratio on the intervention for chronic total occlusions. *Int J Cardiol* 2011; 150(2): 135–141.

52. Dong S et al. Predictors for successful angioplasty of chronic totally occluded coronary arteries. *J Interv Cardiol* 2005; 18(1): 1–7.

53. Stone GW et al. Procedural outcome of angioplasty for total coronary artery occlusion: An analysis of 971 lesions in 905 patients. *J Am Coll Cardiol* 1990; 15(4): 849–856.

54. Brilakis ES et al. Use of the stingray guidewire and the venture catheter for crossing flush coronary chronic total occlusions due to in-stent restenosis. *Catheter Cardiovasc Interv* 2010; 76(3): 391–394.

55. Surmely JF et al. Coronary septal collaterals as an access for the retrograde approach in the percutaneous treatment of coronary chronic total occlusions. *Catheter Cardiovasc Interv* 2007; 69(6): 826–832.

56. Hsu JT et al. Traditional antegrade approach versus combined antegrade and retrograde approach in the percutaneous treatment of coronary chronic total occlusions. *Catheter Cardiovasc Interv* 2009; 74(4): 555–563.

57. Christopoulos G et al. Application and outcomes of a hybrid approach to chronic total occlusion percutaneous coronary intervention in a contemporary multicenter US registry. *Int J Cardiol* 2015; 198: 222–228.

58. Jolly SS et al. Radial versus femoral access for coronary angiography or intervention and the impact on major bleeding and ischemic events: A systematic review and meta-analysis of randomized trials. *Am Heart J* 2009; 157(1): 132–140.

59. Nathan S, and Rao SV. Radial versus femoral access for percutaneous coronary intervention: Implications for vascular complications and bleeding. *Curr Cardiol Rep* 2012; 14(4): 502–509.

60. Rinfret S et al. Retrograde recanalization of chronic total occlusions from the transradial approach; early Canadian experience. *Catheter Cardiovasc Interv* 2011; 78(3): 366–374.

61. Brilakis ES et al. The retrograde approach to coronary artery chronic total occlusions: A practical approach. *Catheter Cardiovasc Interv* 2012; 79(1): 3–19.

62. Tsuchikane E et al. The first clinical experience with a novel catheter for collateral channel tracking in retrograde approach for chronic coronary total occlusions. *JACC Cardiovasc Interv* 2010; 3(2): 165–171.

63. Danek BA et al. Use of antegrade dissection re-entry in coronary chronic total occlusion percutaneous coronary intervention in a contemporary multicenter registry. *Int J Cardiol* 2016; 214: 428–437.

64. Colombo A et al. Treating chronic total occlusions using subintimal tracking and reentry: The STAR technique. *Catheter Cardiovasc Interv* 2005; 64(4): 407–411; discussion 412.

65. Karmpaliotis D et al. Retrograde coronary chronic total occlusion revascularization: Procedural and in-hospital outcomes from a multicenter registry in the United States. *JACC Cardiovasc Interv* 2012; 5(12): 1273–1279.

66. Karmpaliotis D et al. Outcomes with the use of the retrograde approach for coronary chronic total occlusion interventions in a contemporary multicenter US registry. *Circ Cardiovasc Interv* 2016; 9(6).

67. Werner GS. The role of coronary collaterals in chronic total occlusions. *Curr Cardiol Rev* 2014; 10(1): 57–64.

68. Rathore S et al. A novel modification of the retrograde approach for the recanalization of chronic total occlusion of the coronary arteries intravascular ultrasound-guided reverse controlled antegrade and retrograde tracking. *JACC Cardiovasc Interv* 2010; 3(2): 155–164.

69. Buller CE et al. Primary stenting versus balloon angioplasty in occluded coronary arteries: The Total Occlusion Study of Canada (TOSCA). *Circulation* 1999; 100(3): 236–242.

70. Agostoni P et al. Clinical effectiveness of bare-metal stenting compared with balloon angioplasty in total coronary occlusions: Insights from a systematic overview of randomized trials in light of the drug-eluting stent era. *Am Heart J* 2006; 151(3): 682–689.

71. Suttorp MJ et al. Primary Stenting of Totally Occluded Native Coronary Arteries II (PRISON II): A randomized comparison of bare metal stent implantation with sirolimus-eluting stent implantation for the treatment of total coronary occlusions. *Circulation* 2006; 114(9): 921–928.

72. Rubartelli P et al. Comparison of sirolimus-eluting and bare metal stent for treatment of patients with total coronary occlusions: Results of the GISSOC II-GISE multicentre randomized trial. *Eur Heart J* 2010; 31(16): 2014–2020.

73. Kandzari DE et al. Clinical and angiographic outcomes with sirolimus-eluting stents in total coronary occlusions: The ACROSS/TOSCA-4 (Approaches to Chronic Occlusions With Sirolimus-Eluting Stents/Total Occlusion Study of Coronary Arteries-4) trial. *JACC Cardiovasc Interv* 2009; 2(2): 97–106.

74. Valenti R et al. Predictors of reocclusion after successful drug-eluting stent-supported percutaneous coronary intervention of chronic total occlusion. *J Am Coll Cardiol* 2013; 61(5): 545–550.

75. Moreno R et al. Randomized comparison of sirolimus-eluting and everolimus-eluting coronary stents in the treatment of total coronary occlusions: Results from the chronic coronary occlusion treated by everolimus-eluting stent randomized trial. *Circ Cardiovasc Interv* 2013; 6(1): 21–28.

76. Kandzari DE et al. Safety and effectiveness of everolimus-eluting stents in chronic total coronary occlusion revascularization: Results from the EXPERT CTO Multicenter Trial (Evaluation of the XIENCE Coronary Stent, Performance, and Technique in Chronic Total Occlusions). *JACC Cardiovasc Interv* 2015; 8(6): 761–769.

16

PCI for bifurcation lesions

ANTONIO COLOMBO, GORAN STANKOVIC

16.1 Introduction

Approximately 15%–20% of percutaneous coronary interventions (PCI) are performed to treat coronary bifurcations and those procedures are recognised for being technically challenging and associated with lower procedural success rates and worse clinical outcomes compared with non-bifurcation lesions.[1,2] Morphologically, bifurcation lesions are complex, with differences in the severity and distribution of atherosclerotic disease in the main vessel (MV) and the side branch (SB), and variation in vessel diameters and bifurcation angle, which have all been identified as risk factors of restenosis and stent thrombosis following percutaneous intervention.[3]

The definition of coronary bifurcation lesion most widely adopted by interventional community is proposed by the European Bifurcation Club (EBC)[4] and describes a bifurcation lesion as *'a coronary artery narrowing occurring adjacent to, and/or involving, the origin of a significant side branch'*. A 'significant' SB is defined as *any* branch that 'you do not want to lose' in the global context of a particular patient (symptoms, location of ischaemia, branch responsible for symptoms or ischaemia, viability, collateralising role of the jeopardised branch, left ventricular ejection fraction).[4] Today, we have several bifurcation classifications proposed,[5-7] but the advantage of the classification proposed by Medina lies in its simplicity.[8] Each segment is assigned a value '0' in the absence of significant stenosis and '1' in the presence of disease. A value of 0 or 1 is, therefore, assigned to each of the

three segments separated in the following order: proximal MV, distal MV and SB, with numbers separated by comas.

Autopsy studies and in vivo intravascular ultrasound (IVUS) evaluation demonstrated that atherosclerosis occurs predominantly in low shear-stress regions at lateral walls of bifurcation in the MV and the SB, whilst the flow divider region (the carina) involvement by atherosclerosis is extremely uncommon.[9,10] As a result, MV stenting creates angiographic worsening of SB ostial lesion due to a combination of MV plaque and carina shift, which occurs even in absence of significant ostial disease of the SB.[11] Thus, the more important issue in bifurcation PCI is selecting an appropriate strategy for an individual bifurcation and optimising the performance of this technique.

MADS classification (Main - Across - Distal - Side) of bifurcation stenting techniques,[4] adopted by the EBC, is based on two principles: the final position of the stent(s) in the bifurcation and the implantation order. Limitation of MADS classification is that it does not incorporate information on balloon or wire manoeuvres, such as SB protection by wire or balloon. But whatever was the initial step and strategy, the decision whether to use one or two stents should be planned as early as possible.

16.2 The fractal geometry of coronary bifurcation

To understand the rationale of various bifurcation stenting strategies, we have to understand anatomical features of coronary bifurcation that resemble laws of branching systems found in nature.[2] Ramifications of the coronary tree follow the natural law of minimum energy expenditure in providing the underlying myocardium with the optimum amount of blood required.[3] As a consequence, all three segments in a bifurcation have the fractal geometry, with specific diameters and this constant relation between three segments was defined by Murray's law more than 90 years ago, and has been recently simplified by Finet.[12] The proximal 'mother' segment of the MV is consequently always larger in diameter, compared with the distal segments, and equals (according to fractal ratio equation) approximately two-thirds of the sum of two 'daughter' vessels diameters. This natural fractal law has to be kept in mind for optimal stent and balloon sizing in order to achieve adequate strut apposition. It is also true that atherosclerotic disease may affect in differently and unpredictably the proximal, the distal MV and the SB, therefore, assessment with specific imaging modalities such as intravascular ultrasound (IVUS) or optical coherence tomography (OCT) may be necessary.[13–16]

16.2.1 Approach to bifurcation treatment

16.2.1.1 The provisional approach

Several randomised trials and meta-analyses comparing one versus two stents in the treatment of coronary bifurcations demonstrated that stent implantation in the MV ('provisional' SB stenting strategy) remains the preferred strategy.[3,12,17–22] This strategy is quick, safe, easy to perform and associated with results that are comparable with a complex two-stent approach. The provisional strategy resulted in comparable efficacy outcomes (target vessel and lesion re-vascularisation rates) and lower rates of (periprocedural) myocardial infarction (MI), less contrast use, lower x-ray doses and a shorter procedural time.[3,23] The consensus from randomised trial data was that routine two-vessel stenting did not improve either angiographic or clinical outcomes for most patients with

coronary bifurcation lesions.[12,21,22] Furthermore, available two-stent techniques have some drawbacks caused by the limitations of the conventional drug-eluting stents, such as a limited expansion caused by the cell size through which the second stent is advanced in culotte stenting, or three layers of struts when using crush stenting variants. However, it could also be claimed that routine dual vessel stenting did not implicate a significant penalty either.[12] If necessary, second stent can be implanted in the SB utilising a T-stenting,[24] T and small protrusion (TAP stenting),[25] culotte[26] or reverse/internal mini-crush technique.[27] The choice is left to the operator preference, but technique selection will depend mainly on bifurcation angle. Recent improvement in two-stent techniques resulted in improved clinical results of bifurcation stenting and it has been demonstrated that 5-year clinical outcome following left main bifurcation stenting with 'double kissing crush' (DK-crush) was associated with a significantly decreased major adverse cardiovascular events (MACE) rates compared with the provisional approach, mainly because of reduction in target vessel re-ascularisation.[28]

Figure 16.1 summarises a proposed approach to bifurcation lesions with SB stenting strategy as intention to treat only in cases where disease on the SB extends outside the ostium and the SB has a significant area of distribution.[3]

16.2.1.2 Provisional SB stenting technique

A 6F guide catheter is generally used, although 7F guiding catheter may be preferred when complex two-stent strategies are planned. After wiring of both branches, the MV is pre-dilated when required (Figure 16.2, panel a). There is a general consensus that SB should be pre-dilated only if severely narrowed or diffusely diseased (>5 mm), or there is an unfavourable extreme angulation of the SB take off.[3,29,30] However, recent randomised study showed that SB pre-dilatation may improve the angiographic result of provisional stenting.[31] When there is uncertainty regarding the need for SB

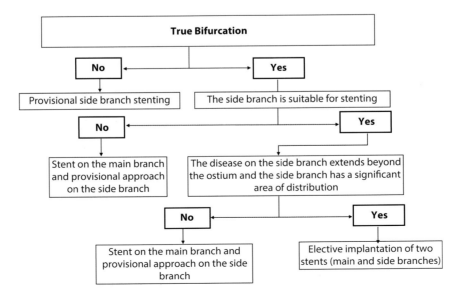

Figure 16.1 Our proposed algorithm for stenting bifurcation lesions.

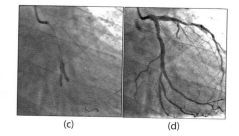

Figure 16.2 Provisional stenting technique. **(Panel a)** Baseline angiogram showing bifurcation lesion in left circumflex coronary artery (LCx) and obtuse marginal branch (OM) was considered a main vessel [MV] and distal LCx a side branch [SB]). **(Panel b)** Direct stenting of the MV. **(Panel c)** Final kissing balloon inflation. **(Panel d)** Final angiographic result.

dilatation an assessment of the SB ostium following myocardial bridging (MB) pre-dilatation may be helpful.

Next step is stent implantation in the MV across the SB, jailing wire in the SB (Figure 16.2, panel b). Stent selection for the MV is crucial and primary stent should be sized according to the distal MV diameter.[12] If the angiographic results in MV and SB are acceptable, the procedure is finished and jailed wire can be removed.[30]

Different criteria have been used in randomised trials for acceptable result in the SB following MV stenting.[3] If the result at SB ostium is not satisfactory, the SB is rewired with the MV wire (wire exchange) before removing jailed wire. Wire re-cross through the distal strut following MV stenting is strongly suggested because it creates better SB scaffolding than proximal crossing.[32] In order to enhance SB access through the 'carina strut', the proximal optimisation technique (POT technique) has been proposed, and relates to a method of expanding the stent at the carina, using a short oversized balloon.[2] Performance of POT technique adapts workhorse stents to fractal anatomy of bifurcation lesions, which is especially important in bifurcation lesions with a large SB because of a bigger difference between proximal and distal MV diameters. A short necrotic core (NC) balloon should be sized according to the proximal MV reference diameter and distal balloon marker should be positioned in front of the carina whilst the proximal marker is still inside the stent in order to avoid geographical miss.

The jailed wire in the SB should always be left in place as a marker until complete re-crossing has been done. In addition, jailed wire modifies favourably the angle between both branches and keeps the SB open. In case of difficulty in advancing the wire into the SB, beside POT, wire reshaping, exchange for a hydrophilic polymer-coated or a stiffer wire or even a micro-catheter may help to overcome the technical problems.[3]

There is still a debate regarding the use of routine final kissing inflation (FKI), with general agreement that in the absence of an angiographically tight lesion at the ostium of the SB, FKI may not be routinely required.[12] However, when a tight lesion (>75%) is present in the SB after MV stenting, it is known that a kissing balloon inflation will reduce its functional significance (Figure 16.2, panel c).[33] Therefore, two appropriate strategies are either to use a pressure wire to interrogate the significance of the SB lesion, or, simply

to do FKI knowing that this reduces the proportion that remain physiologically significant. This is also supported by the NORDIC III trial, which demonstrated that there is no penalty for performing FKI.[12]

After re-crossing the SB, balloon dilation of the SB ostium and FKI should be performed. FKI is proposed if the SB is dilated through the MV stent struts in order to correct MV stent distortion and facilitate future access to the SB[32,34] (Figure 16.2, panel d). Balloon selection for FKI is very important. The diameter of both balloons is based on diameters of distal branches. The length of the MV balloon must be sufficiently short (or the stent long enough) to avoid inflation outside the MB stent, and the SB balloon should also be short in order to decrease the damage of the SB.

The appropriate sequence of balloon inflation to achieve optimal results and minimise the proximal MB stent deformation is currently a subject of discussion. Recently, Foin et al.[35] proposed 'sequential balloon inflation' as an alternative method to FKI. The procedure starts by inflating the SB at 12 atm, then deflating the SB at 4 atm and inflating the MB at 12 atm. With this technique final elliptical deformation in the proximal MV is reduced and SB access is optimised by reduced ostial area stenosis, compared with simultaneous FKI.[36] The elliptical deformation after FKI can also be corrected by a second POT (re-POT), as described by Foin.[37]

16.2.1.3 A second stent in the SB following provisional approach

Stenting of the SB is clearly indicated in occasions of major SB dissections or compromised SB flow after FKI. However, the problem of residual stenosis is still controversial because angiographic assessment of the SB ostium is not easy. If the result remains unsatisfactory after FKI (>75% residual stenosis, dissection, TIMI flow grade < 3 in a SB ≥ 2.5 mm or FFR < 0.75),[3,33,38] SB stenting should be performed. According to randomised trials, a second stent in the SB may be necessary in 2%–51% of cases.[18–20,39,40] FFR or imaging techniques, such as IVUS and OCT, could be of value in SB assessment after balloon dilation.

When SB stenting is required, the T stenting technique is commonly used (Figure 16.3).[41] Stent is positioned at the ostium of the SB without protrusion inside the MV stent (Figure 16.3, panel c). In bifurcations with wide angles (close to 90°), T-stenting provides complete coverage of the SB ostium.

The T and small protrusion (TAP) technique is a modification of the T-stenting technique and is based on an intentional minimal protrusion of the SB stent inside the MV stent (Figure 16.4).[25] The advantages of the TAP-stenting technique are compatibility with 6F guiding catheters, full coverage of side-branch ostium and facilitation of FKI.[3] The main drawback is related with the creation of a 'metallic neocarina' of variable length.[3] FKI is performed to complete procedure.

If bifurcation angle is smaller (less than 70°), some operators prefer using the Culotte technique in order to improve SB ostial scaffolding. The Culotte technique leads to full coverage of the bifurcation but with two layers of struts in the proximal MV. The procedure starts with MV stenting, as in original description by Chevalier,[26] although the first stent can be deployed across the most angulated branch, which is usually the SB (technique named inverted Culotte technique and described below in a two-stent techniques as intention to treat).[2,3,42]

Another technique that was developed with the intent to abolish gap at SB ostium is a reverse or internal mini-crush.[43] In this technique first stent is implanted in the MV and balloon dilatation with kissing inflation towards the SB is performed.[3] Second stent is inserted in the SB and pulled-back to protrude minimally inside the MV stent. The reverse crush can be performed with a 6F guiding catheter since protruding segment of the SB stent is crushed with the balloon in the MV. After that SB is rewired and high-pressure balloon inflation is performed and procedure ended by FKI (two-step FKI).

16.2.1.4 Two stents as an 'intention to treat'

A meta-analysis of randomised studies demonstrated that a provisional approach was comparable with two-stent strategy in terms of mortality, repeat re-vascularisation and quality of life,[3,23,44] whilst provisional technique reduced the risk of periprocedural MI and stent thrombosis.[45,46] Current expert consensus is that large calibre true bifurcations with significant ostial SB length disease require a systematic two-stent strategy.[12,21]

If upfront two-stent strategy is planned, the size and territory of distribution of the SB and the angle between the MV and the SB should be analysed. The most frequently utilised two-stent techniques are culotte, mini-crush or DK-crush and V and simultaneous kissing stent technique.[3]

16.2.1.5 Inverted culotte technique

The procedure starts with pre-dilatation of both branches and stent implantation into the most angulated branch, which is usually the SB (Figure 16.5, panel b).[3,2,42] POT technique is performed and the MV is rewired through the struts of the SB stent. A second stent is advanced and expanded into the MV, followed by repeated POT (Figure 16.5, panel c). Procedure is completed after FKI (Figure 16.5, panel d). Important limitation of culotte technique is dependence on maximal stent cell diameter.[12] For this reason open

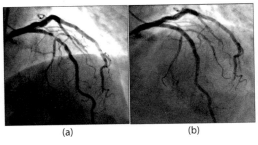
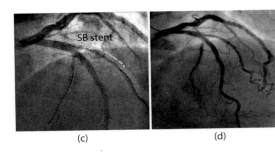

(a) (b) (c) (d)

Figure 16.3 T stenting technique. **(Panel a)** Baseline angiogram showing true bifurcation lesion left anterior descending (LAD)-D1. **(Panel b)** Result after main vessel (MV) stenting. **(Panel c)** Side branch (SB) stent positioning (dashed yellow line), proximal stent marker aligned with MV stent. **(Panel d)** Final angiographic result.

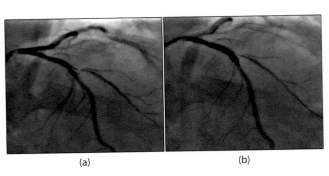
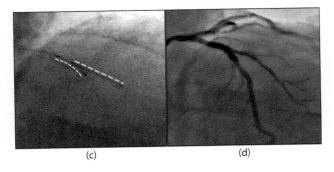

(a) (b) (c) (d)

Figure 16.4 T and small protrusion (TAP) technique. **(Panel a)** Baseline angiogram showing LAD-D1 bifurcation lesion. **(Panel b)** Angiogram after LAD stenting. **(Panel c)** Positioning of the side branch (SB) stent (dashed yellow line), with small protrusion inside the LAD stent, where a non-inflated balloon is placed (dashed white line). **(Panel d)** Final angiographic result.

cells stents are preferable. Other disadvantage is that rewiring both branches through the stent struts can be difficult.[3]

This technique is suitable for a narrow angle bifurcation with similar size of both branches.[3] Disadvantages are that the culotte technique creates a double-stent layer at the carina and in the proximal part of the MV.[3] To reduce excess of metal in the proximal MV, minimal overlap is suggested (mini-culotte).

16.2.1.6 The mini-crush technique

The classical crush technique[47] consists in partial protrusion of the SB stent in the MV, which is crushed by the MV stent. The main disadvantage of this technique is that it requires a 7F-guiding catheter. In order to use a 6Fr-guiding catheter a 'balloon step mini-crush' technique[3,48] is suggested (Figure 16.6). After pre-dilatation of the MV and the SB, stent is inserted in the SB with minimal protrusion inside the MV and deflated balloon in the MV (Figure 16.6, panel b). Stent in the SB is deployed and, after control angiogram, balloon and wire are removed into the guiding catheter. MV balloon is then inflated to crush protruding struts. After that stent is inserted in the MV and deployed at high pressure (Figure 16.6, panel d). SB is then rewired and procedure completed by FKI (Figure 16.6, panels e and f).

Clinical outcome of crush technique is improved by FKI inflation,[49] which is now strongly recommended.

The DK-crush technique differs from the classical crush technique because kissing balloon inflation is performed twice, first, after the part of the SB stent protruding into the MV is crushed with a balloon in the MV and, second, after MV stenting.[50]

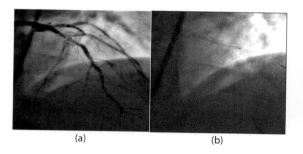
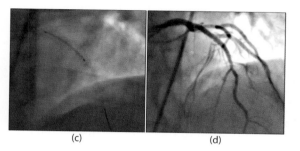

(a) (b) (c) (d)

Figure 16.5 Culotte stenting technique. **(Panel a)** Baseline angiography showing LAD-D1 true bifurcation lesion. **(Panel b)** Positioning of the diagonal stent. **(Panel c)** Positioning of the LAD stent after proximal optimisation technique (POT) and wire exchange. **(Panel d)** Final angiographic result.

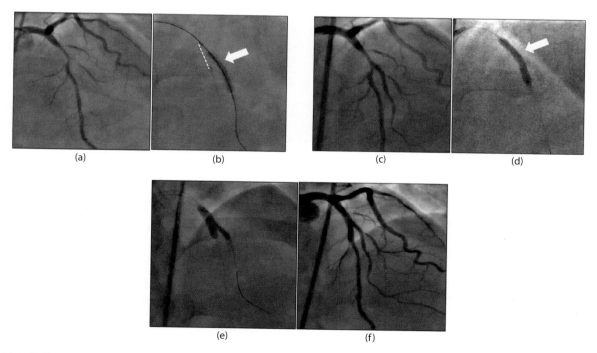

(a) (b) (c) (d)

(e) (f)

Figure 16.6 Balloon-step mini-crush stenting technique: **(Panel a)** Baseline angiography showing LAD-D1 bifurcation lesion, with occluded diagonal branch. **(Panel b)** SB stent deployment (white thick arrow), with non-inflated balloon in the LAD (dashed white line). **(Panel c)** Control angiogram after SB stent crush. **(Panel d)** MV stent inflated (white thick arrow). **(Panel e)** Final kissing inflation. **(Panel f)** Final angiographic result.

The main advantage of the crush technique is that immediate patency of both branches is secured, which is specifically important when the SB is large or difficult to wire.[3] The main disadvantage of this technique is the need to re-cross multiple layers of struts with guidewire and balloon.[3]

16.2.1.7 The V and the simultaneous kissing stent techniques

The V-stenting and the simultaneous kissing stent (SKS) techniques are performed by simultaneous implantation of two stents.[3,51,52] Both branches are wired and fully predilated. Stents are advanced in the MV and the SB. Stents are positioned with proximal stent markers overlapped and deployed with simultaneous inflation and deflation.[3] Stents are sized according to diameter of two daughter vessels (1:1) and stent length is selected to completely cover diseased segments. The main advantage of the V and SKS technique is permanent access to both branches.[3] In addition, a FKI is performed without need to re-cross through the stent struts. Main disadvantage is metallic 'double barrel' neocarina created in the proximal MV, which may increase the risk of restenosis or stent thrombosis.[2] Lesions most suitable for this technique are very proximal lesions, with the angle between the branches less than 70°. The V-stenting technique is also suitable for other bifurcations, provided that the vessel proximal to bifurcation is free of disease and that there is no need to deploy additional stent more proximally.[3]

16.2.1.8 Dedicated bifurcation stents

Multiple dedicated bifurcation systems have been developed, both to facilitate the provisional, single-stent, strategy and a more complex two-stent approach. These devices may potentially overcome limitations of conventional stents in coronary bifurcations (SB protection, multiple layers, distortion, SB access, crossing through side of the stent, gaps in scaffolding).[3,12] Ideal dedicated stent should have a brief learning curve, simplify PCI procedure (i.e. reduce procedural times, decrease contrast use), adjust to range of bifurcation anatomies (involving a variety of distal bifurcation angles), improve procedural success rates, have a predictable acute result of the SB and ensuring a long-term patency of the SB without compromising the acute and long-term results of the MV. However, although efforts to produce such dedicated bifurcation stents are advanced, most of these devices have not yet been compared in a randomised trial with either the provisional or the two-stent strategy using conventional DES, except for the Tryton stent (Tryton Medical, Durham, NC, USA), which was compared with the provisional approach in the Tryton Investigational Device Exemption (IDE) trial but the primary non-inferiority endpoint was not met.[21,53]

16.2.1.9 Bioresorbable scaffolds

Bioresorbable scaffolds (BRS) provide a new tool for percutaneous treatment of coronary bifurcation lesions. The recent GHOST-EU (Gauging coronary Healing with biOresorbable Scaffolding plaTforms in EUrope) registry, for example included patients with bifurcation lesions in 23.1% of the cases.[54] As a result, current recommendations[55] are based on limited expert opinion,[21] case reports[56-59] or on insights from bench studies performed on the bioresorbable vascular scaffold (Absorb BRS; Abbott Vascular, Santa Clara, CA).[60,61] The provisional strategy remains the default approach to bifurcation treatment with BRS. If correctly performed, SB dilatation, mini-kissing balloon inflation, crossover to SB stenting and elective double stenting are feasible without causing scaffold disruption.[21] There are several potential theoretical advantages of BRS use in this lesion subset, like a better future access to the SB due to disappearance of scaffold struts overhanging SB ostium and potential reduced risk of very-late scaffold thrombosis, which needs to be confirmed in future studies. Considering that currently available BRS have wide and thick struts, the strategy we propose when two stents are needed is to implant a metal stent on the SB.[62,63] Ideally, if new BRS platforms with thinner and stronger struts are developed, this will improve scaffold implantation in bifurcation lesions and permit the use of more complex implantation techniques.

16.3 Conclusions

Selection of appropriate strategy for individual bifurcation lesion and optimal procedural result ensure satisfactory early and long-term clinical outcome. Provisional strategy remains the gold standard technique for most bifurcation lesions since routine two-vessel stenting does not improve either angiographic or clinical outcomes. However, further studies are required to determine, which bifurcation lesions may particularly benefit from planned upfront two-stent strategy. Dedicated bifurcation stents may further improve procedural and clinical outcomes of percutaneous treatment of coronary bifurcation lesions. Despite the current technical limitations, BRS use in bifurcation lesions utilising provisional technique seems to be feasible and safe. Improved BRS designs, with thinner struts and more resistant to fracture, may become a new standard for percutaneous treatment of coronary bifurcation lesions.

References

1. Louvard Y et al. Percutaneous coronary intervention for bifurcation coronary disease. *Heart* 2004; 90: 713–22.
2. Stankovic G et al. Percutaneous coronary intervention for bifurcation lesions: 2008 consensus document from the fourth meeting of the European Bifurcation Club. *EuroIntervention* 2009; 5: 39–49.
3. Colombo A, and Stankovic G. Bifurcations and branch vessel stenting. In: Eric J. Topol et al. (editors), *Textbook of Interventional Cardiology*, 6th Edition. Philadelphia, PA: Saunders Elsevier, 2012, pp. 270–87.
4. Louvard Y et al. Classification of coronary artery bifurcation lesions and treatments: Time for a consensus! *Catheter Cardiovasc Interv* 2008; 71: 175–83.

5. Movahed MR, and Stinis CT. A new proposed simplified classification of coronary artery bifurcation lesions and bifurcation interventional techniques. *J Invasive Cardiol* 2006; 18: 199–204.

6. Movahed MR. Coronary artery bifurcation lesion classifications, interventional techniques and clinical outcome. *Expert Rev Cardiovasc Ther* 2008; 6: 261–74.

7. Y-Hassan S et al. A Novel Descriptive, Intelligible and Ordered (DINO) classification of coronary bifurcation lesions. Review of current classifications. *Circ J* 2011; 75: 299–305.

8. Medina A et al. A new classification of coronary bifurcation lesions. *Rev Esp Cardiol* 2006; 59: 183.

9. Nakazawa G et al. Pathological findings at bifurcation lesions: The impact of flow distribution on atherosclerosis and arterial healing after stent implantation. *J Am Coll Cardiol* 2010; 55: 1679–87.

10. Oviedo C et al. Intravascular ultrasound classification of plaque distribution in left main coronary artery bifurcations: Where is the plaque really located? *Circ Cardiovasc Interv* 2010; 3: 105–12.

11. Koo BK et al. Anatomic and functional evaluation of bifurcation lesions undergoing percutaneous coronary intervention. *Circ Cardiovasc Interv* 2010; 3: 113–9.

12. Hildick-Smith D et al. Consensus from the 5th European Bifurcation Club meeting. *EuroIntervention* 2010; 6: 34–8.

13. Fujino Y et al. Impact of main-branch calcified plaque on side-branch stenosis in bifurcation stenting: An optical coherence tomography study. *Int J Cardiol* 2014; 176: 1056–60.

14. Sakamoto N et al. Intravascular ultrasound predictors of acute side branch occlusion in coronary artery bifurcation lesions just after single stent crossover. *Catheter Cardiovasc Interv* 2016 Feb 1; 87(2): 243–50.

15. Costa RA et al. Bifurcation lesion morphology and intravascular ultrasound assessment. *Int J Cardiovasc Imaging* 2011; 27: 189–96.

16. Sato K et al. Calcification analysis by intravascular ultrasound to define a predictor of left circumflex narrowing after crossover stenting for unprotected left main bifurcation lesions. *Cardiovasc Revasc Med* 2014; 15: 80–5.

17. Colombo A et al. Randomized study of the crush technique versus provisional side-branch stenting in true coronary bifurcations: the CACTUS (Coronary Bifurcations: Application of the Crushing Technique Using Sirolimus-Eluting Stents) Study. *Circulation* 2009; 119: 71–8.

18. Colombo A et al. Randomized study to evaluate sirolimus-eluting stents implanted at coronary bifurcation lesions. *Circulation* 2004; 109: 1244–9.

19. Ferenc M et al. Randomized trial on routine vs. provisional T-stenting in the treatment of de novo coronary bifurcation lesions. *Eur Heart J* 2008; 29: 2859–67.

20. Pan M et al. Rapamycin-eluting stents for the treatment of bifurcated coronary lesions: A randomized comparison of a simple versus complex strategy. *Am Heart J* 2004; 148: 857–64.

21. Lassen JF et al. Percutaneous coronary intervention for coronary bifurcation disease: Consensus from the first 10 years of the European Bifurcation Club meetings. *EuroIntervention* 2014; 10: 545–60.

22. Stankovic G et al. Consensus from the 7th European Bifurcation Club meeting. *EuroIntervention* 2013; 9: 36–45.

23. Behan MW et al. Simple or complex stenting for bifurcation coronary lesions/clinical perspective. *Circ: Cardiovasc Interv* 2011; 4: 57–64.

24. Lefevre T et al. Stenting of bifurcation lesions: A rational approach. *J Interv Cardiol* 2001; 14: 573–85.

25. Burzotta F et al. Modified T-stenting with intentional protrusion of the side-branch stent within the main vessel stent to ensure ostial coverage and facilitate final kissing balloon: The T-stenting and small protrusion technique (TAP-stenting). Report of bench testing and first clinical Italian-Korean two-centre experience. *Catheter Cardiovasc Interv* 2007; 70: 75–82.

26. Chevalier B et al. Placement of coronary stents in bifurcation lesions by the 'culotte' technique. *Am J Cardiol* 1998; 82: 943–9.

27. Porto I et al. 'Crush' and 'reverse crush' technique to treat a complex left main stenosis. *Heart* 2006; 92: 1021.

28. Chen SL et al. Five-year clinical follow-up of unprotected left main bifurcation lesion stenting: One-stent versus two-stent techniques versus double-kissing crush technique. *EuroIntervention* 2012; 8: 803–14.

29. Pan M et al. Drug-eluting stents for the treatment of bifurcation lesions: A randomized comparison between paclitaxel and sirolimus stents. *Am Heart J* 2007; 153: 15 e1–7.

30. Pan M et al. A stepwise strategy for the stent treatment of bifurcated coronary lesions. *Catheter Cardiovasc Interv* 2002; 55: 50–7.

31. Pan M et al. Assessment of side branch predilation before a provisional T-stent strategy for bifurcation lesions. A randomized trial. *Am Heart J* 2014; 168: 374–80.

32. Ormiston JA et al. Drug-eluting stents for coronary bifurcations: bench testing of provisional side-branch strategies. *Catheter Cardiovasc Interv* 2006; 67: 49–55.

33. Koo BK et al. Physiological evaluation of the provisional side-branch intervention strategy for bifurcation lesions using fractional flow reserve. *Eur Heart J* 2008; 29: 726–32.

34. Brunel P et al. Provisional T-stenting and kissing balloon in the treatment of coronary bifurcation lesions: Results of the French multicenter 'TULIPE' study. *Catheter Cardiovasc Interv* 2006; 68: 67–73.

35. Foin N et al. Kissing balloon or sequential dilation of the side branch and main vessel for provisional stenting of bifurcations: Lessons from micro-computed tomography and computational simulations. *JACC Cardiovasc Interv* 2012; 5: 47–56.

36. Mortier P et al. Provisional stenting of coronary bifurcations: Insights into final kissing balloon post-dilation and stent design by computational modeling. *JACC Cardiovasc Interv* 2014; 7: 325–33.

37. Foin N et al. Tools & techniques clinical: Optimising stenting strategy in bifurcation lesions with insights from in vitro bifurcation models. *EuroIntervention* 2013; 9: 885–7.

38. Koo BK et al. Physiologic assessment of jailed side branch lesions using fractional flow reserve. *J Am Coll Cardiol* 2005; 46: 633–7.

39. Steigen TK et al. Randomized study on simple versus complex stenting of coronary artery bifurcation lesions: The Nordic bifurcation study. *Circulation* 2006; 114: 1955–61.

40. Colombo A et al. Randomized study of the crush technique versus provisional side-branch stenting in true coronary bifurcations: The CACTUS (Coronary Bifurcations: Application of the Crushing Technique Using Sirolimus-Eluting Stents) study. *Circulation* 2009; 119: 71–8.

41. Verheye S et al. 9-month clinical, angiographic, and intravascular ultrasound results of a prospective evaluation of the Axxess self-expanding biolimus A9-eluting stent in coronary bifurcation lesions: The DIVERGE (Drug-Eluting Stent Intervention for Treating Side Branches Effectively) study. *J Am Coll Cardiol* 2009; 53(12): 1031–9. doi:10.1016/j.jacc.2008.12.012.

42. Kaplan S et al. Culotte versus T-stenting in bifurcation lesions: Immediate clinical and angiographic results and midterm clinical follow-up. *Am Heart J* 2007; 154: 336–343.

43. Hussain F. Provisional reverse 'mini-crush' technique for bifurcation angioplasty. *J Invasive Cardiol* 2008; 20: E154–7.

44. Sirker A et al. The impact of coronary bifurcation stenting strategy on health-related functional status: A quality-of-life analysis from the BBC One (British Bifurcation Coronary; Old, New, and Evolving Strategies) study. *JACC: Cardiovascular Interventions* 2013; 6: 139–45.

45. Zimarino M et al. Late thrombosis after double versus single drug-eluting stent in the treatment of coronary bifurcations: A meta-analysis of randomized and observational studies. *JACC: Cardiovascular Interventions* 2013; 6: 687–95.

46. Maeng M et al. Long-term results after simple versus complex stenting of coronary artery bifurcation lesions: Nordic Bifurcation Study 5-year follow-up results. *J Am Coll Cardiol* 2013; 62: 30–4.

47. Colombo A et al. Modified T-stenting technique with crushing for bifurcation lesions: Immediate results and 30-day outcome. *Catheter Cardiovasc Interv* 2003; 60: 145–51.

48. Lim PO, and Dzavik V. Balloon crush: Treatment of bifurcation lesions using the crush stenting technique as adapted for transradial approach of percutaneous coronary intervention. *Catheter Cardiovasc Interv* 2004; 63: 412–6.

49. Ge L et al. Clinical and angiographic outcome after implantation of drug-eluting stents in bifurcation lesions with the crush stent technique: Importance of final kissing balloon post-dilation. *J Am Coll Cardiol* 2005; 46: 613–20.

50. Chen SL et al. Study comparing the double kissing (DK) crush with classical crush for the treatment of coronary bifurcation lesions: The DKCRUSH-1 Bifurcation Study with drug-eluting stents. *Eur J Clin Invest* 2008; 38: 361–71.

51. Schampaert E et al. The V-stent: A novel technique for coronary bifurcation stenting. *Cathet Cardiovasc Diagn* 1996; 39: 320–6.

52. Sharma SK. Simultaneous kissing drug-eluting stent technique for percutaneous treatment of bifurcation lesions in large-size vessels. *Catheter Cardiovasc Interv* 2005; 65: 10–6.

53. Généreux P et al. A randomized trial of a dedicated bifurcation stent versus provisional stenting in the treatment of coronary bifurcation lesions. *J Am Coll Cardiol* 2015; 65: 533–43.

54. Capodanno D et al. Percutaneous coronary intervention with everolimus-eluting bioresorbable vascular scaffolds in routine clinical practice: Early and midterm outcomes from the European multicentre GHOST-EU registry. *EuroIntervention* 2015 Feb;10(10):1144–53.

55. Tamburino C et al. Contemporary practice and technical aspects in coronary intervention with bioresorbable scaffolds: A European perspective. *EuroIntervention* 2015; 11(1):45–52.

56. Grundeken MJ et al. Three-dimensional optical coherence tomography evaluation of a left main bifurcation lesion treated with ABSORB(R) bioresorbable vascular scaffold including fenestration and dilatation of the side branch. *Int J Cardiol* 2013; 168: e107–8.

57. Dzavik V et al. Complex bifurcation percutaneous coronary intervention with the Absorb bioresorbable vascular scaffold. *EuroIntervention* 2013; 9: 888.

58. Gogas BD et al. Three-dimensional reconstruction of the post-dilated ABSORB everolimus-eluting bioresorbable vascular scaffold in a true bifurcation lesion for flow restoration. *JACC Cardiovasc Interv* 2011; 4: 1149–50.

59. van Geuns RJ et al. 3-Dimensional reconstruction of a bifurcation lesion with double wire after implantation of a second generation everolimus-eluting bioresorbable vascular scaffold. *Int J Cardiol* 2011; 153: e43–5.

60. Dzavik V, and Colombo A. The absorb bioresorbable vascular scaffold in coronary bifurcations: Insights from bench testing. *JACC Cardiovasc Interv* 2014; 7: 81–8.

61. Ormiston JA et al. Absorb everolimus-eluting bioresorbable scaffolds in coronary bifurcations: A bench study of deployment, side branch dilatation and post-dilatation strategies. *EuroIntervention* 2015 Feb;10(10):1169–77.

62. Kawamoto H et al. Clinical outcomes following bioresorbable scaffold implantation for bifurcation lesions: Overall outcomes and comparison between provisional and planned double stenting strategy. *Catheter Cardiovasc Interv* 2015; 86(4): 644–52.

63. Naganuma T et al. 1-year follow-up optical coherence tomography of a 'hybrid' neocarina after T-stenting with small protrusion technique using a bioresorbable vascular scaffold and a metallic stent. *JACC Cardiovasc Interv* 2015; 8: e101–3.

17

Percutaneous coronary intervention for left main stem disease

SEUNG-JUNG PARK, SE HUN KANG

17.1 Introduction

Since the first description of left main coronary artery (LMCA) disease in a patient who died from cardiogenic shock secondary to acute myocardial infarction by James Herrick in 1912,[1] there have been tremendous advancements in the treatment of LMCA disease. Patients with LMCA disease have been classified into two subgroups: protected (a previous patent coronary artery bypass graft [CABG] surgery to one or more major branches of the left coronary artery) and unprotected (without such bypasses). The increased efficacy and long-term survival benefits of CABG surgery compared with medical therapy mean that CABG has been the standard treatment for unprotected LMCA disease since the 1970s,[2-4] with the use of percutaneous coronary intervention (PCI) being confined to surgically high-risk patients and those with protected LMCA disease. However, rapid advancements in techniques, devices and adjunctive pharmacotherapies led PCI to extend its clinical application for patients with unprotected LMCA disease. The widespread availability of drug-eluting stents (DES) has improved outcomes and lowered the threshold required for performing PCI instead of CABG for LMCA disease. As a result, the prevalence of LMCA stenting has significantly increased worldwide during the last decade. Furthermore, several recent large registries and randomised controlled trials have demonstrated that LMCA stenting yields comparable mortality and morbidity rates with CABG, making unprotected left main intervention a potential alternative treatment to CABG.[5-9] This chapter will provide an overview of current concepts, techniques and outcomes of PCI with either bare metal stents (BMS) or DES based on the published literature.

17.2 Anatomy and pathology

The LMCA arises from the mid-portion of the left aortic sinus of Valsalva, below the sinotubular junction of the aortic root. The LMCA ends by bifurcating into the left anterior descending (LAD) and left circumflex (LCX) arteries in approximately two-thirds of patients and trifurcates into the LAD, LCX and ramus intermedius in the others. The LMCA is responsible for supplying flow to approximately 75% of the left ventricle. An autopsy study that examined 100 cases found that the LMCA had an average length of 10.8 ± 5.2 mm (range 2–23 mm), an average diameter of 4.9 ± 0.8 mm and an average angle of division of the terminal branches of 86.7 ± 28.8 (range, 40–165) and also found a positive correlation between LMCA length and the angles of its terminal branches.[10] The anatomic portion of the LMCA is divided into three regions: the ostium, mid-shaft and distal bifurcation. Atherosclerotic involvement in these regions varies depending on histology and haemodynamic mechanics. Histologically, the ostial portion resembles the aorta, as it is rich in aortic smooth muscle cells and elastic fibres. The distal bifurcation is the region's most susceptible to atherosclerosis due to blood flow disturbance and associated low shear stress. In particular, the lateral walls (opposite the flow divider) at the bifurcation are the most frequent site of atherosclerotic plaque accumulation, whilst the flow divider (bifurcation carina itself) is usually spared because of the relatively high shear stress.[11] Pathologic plaque composition of LMCA disease varies from pathologic intimal thickening to thin-cap fibroatheroma with or without plaque rupture.[12] In cases of mild LMCA disease, the most frequent underlying plaque type is pathologic intimal thickening (64%), followed by fibroatheroma with an early or late stage necrotic core (17%). However, most lesions with significant LMCA disease show more complex plaques, such as fibroatheromas with late core, thin-cap fibroatheroma, surface ruptures, fissures and intraplaque haemorrhage. A recent intravascular ultrasound (IVUS) analysis demonstrated the diffuse nature of atherosclerosis involving both the parent LMCA segment and both flow dividers (LAD and LCX). Atherosclerotic plaques extend from the LMCA to the LAD in 90% of patients and LCX in 62% of patients.[13]

17.3 Determination of significant LMCA disease

17.3.1 Coronary angiography

Traditionally, angiographic diameter stenosis of 50% has been considered a cut-off for significant LMCA disease. However, the conventional coronary angiogram is only a lumenogram and has critical limitations in assessing lesion morphology and plaque characteristics. The view of the left main trunk is often short in length and lacks the normal segment for comparison. In addition, contrast material in the aortic cusp sometimes obscures the ostium, and 'streaming' of the contrast material may result in a false impression of luminal narrowing. As a result, marked discrepancies in the interpretations of the degree of stenosis in LMCA narrowing have been documented.[14,15] More importantly, the degree of angiographic diameter stenosis alone is not sufficient to assess the actual functional severity of LMCA disease. One study demonstrated a considerable discrepancy between the coronary angiography and fractional flow reserve (FFR) in the evaluation of intermediate LMCA disease, where 29.1% of patients showed a 'visual functional mismatch' between angiographic and functional significance.[16] The majority (79.0%) of mismatched patients had 'reverse mismatch,' where there is an underestimation of the functional significance of the stenosis in cases where patients have angiographically insignificant but functionally significant stenosis. Because of the critical prognostic importance associated with functionally significant unprotected LMCA, the decision to revascularise the intermediate LMCA disease should not be determined by coronary angiogram alone.

17.3.2 Fractional flow reserve

FFR is a pressure wire-based index used to identify ischaemia-producing coronary stenosis and is simply expressed as the ratio between the mean pressure of the aorta and the mean pressure distal to the stenosis in the maximal coronary hyperaemic condition. FFR is unique because it is not affected by haemodynamic conditions (e.g. blood pressure, heart rate, or contractile state) and is lesion specific, which makes it ideally suited to the assessment of multiple lesions in patients with multi-vessel and left main disease. An FFR value of >0.75–0.80 has been suggested to be a strong predictor of favourable survival and low event rates in patients with intermediate LMCA disease, making it a useful cut-off value to determine significant LMCA disease. In a study involving 213 patients with intermediate LMCA disease, 5-year survival rates of 138 patients treated medically with an FFR ≥ 0.80 and 75 patients treated surgically with an FFR <0.80 were 89.8% and 85.4%, respectively ($p = .48$).[16] Several other studies using FFR cut-off values of 0.75–0.80 as a surrogate for revascularisation showed similar outcomes (Table 17.1) and, as a result, FFR-guided decision-making for the treatment of LMCA disease is generally accepted.[17–20] Practically, the FFR of LMCA disease should be interpreted with caution, as isolated LMCA disease is very rare with most disease-associated stenosis in the LAD and/or LCX, both of which tend to increase the FFR value measured across LMCA disease. Therefore, in these situations, the functional significance of intermediate LMCA disease should be reassessed after correction of the distal coronary artery stenosis (Figure 17.1).[21]

17.3.3 Intravascular ultrasound

As conventional angiography has several limitations, IVUS is often used to assess the severity of LMCA disease. For accurate assessment, it is important to keep the IVUS catheter coaxial with the LMCA and to disengage the guiding catheter from the ostium so that the guiding catheter is not mistaken for a calcific lesion with a lumen dimension equal to the inner lumen of the guiding catheter. The IVUS-derived minimal lumen area (MLA) has frequently been used to determine the functional significance of intermediate LMCA disease. Traditionally, an MLA cut-off value of 6.0 mm^2 has been considered to represent functionally significant LMCA disease. This value was derived primarily from Murray's law, with an MLA of 4.0 mm^2 considered to represent the ischaemic threshold of the LAD or LCX, and was supported by a clinical study.[20] However, recent studies reported that the IVUS MLA value corresponding to ischaemia-producing lesions of non-LM epicardial coronary arteries is <3 mm^2, and application of Murray's law to these values suggests that the IVUS MLA of a stenotic LMCA should be <5.0 mm^2.[22–24] Park et al. attempted to determine the IVUS-derived MLA criteria corresponding to an FFR < 0.80 in 112 patients with isolated intermediate LMCA disease who underwent pre-interventional IVUS

Table 17.1 Summary of key studies of FFR-guided decision-making in LMCA stenosis

Study	Treatment	FFR cut-off value	No. of patients	Mean follow-up (months)	Clinical outcomes		
					Death, n (%)	Myocardial infarction, n (%)	Revascularisation, n (%)
Hamilos et al.[16]	CABG	<0.80	75	35 ± 25	7 (9.6)	0	4 (5.5)
	medication[a]	≥0.80	138		9 (6.5)	1	17 (12.3)
Bech et al.[17]	CABG	<0.75	30	29 ± 15	1	1	2
	medication[a]	≥0.75	24		0	0	5
Courtis et al.[18]	CABG or PCI	<0.75[b]	60	13 ± 10	3 (5)	1 (2)	9 (11)
	medication	>0.80	82	14 ± 12	3 (4)	4 (5)	1 (3.7)
Lindstaedt et al.[19]	CABG	<0.75[b]	27	29 ± 18	4 (14.8)	1 (3.7)	1 (3.7)
	medication[a]	>0.80	24	29 ± 14	0	0	6 (25)*
Jasti et al.[20]	CABG or PCI	<0.75	14	38	0	0	0
	medication[a]	≥0.75	37		3 (NC)	0	4

NC, non-cardiac death; LMCA, left main coronary artery; FFR, fractional flow reserve; PCI, percutaneous coronary intervention; CABG, coronary artery bypass grafting.

[a] Individualised decision was recommended based on additional clinical data if the FFR was between 0.75 and 0.80.
[b] Medical treatment or PCI elsewhere in the coronary tree.
*p < .05.

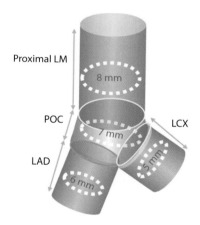

Figure 17.1 Cut-off values of minimal stent area for the prediction of angiographic in-stent restenosis on a segmental basis. LM, left main; POC, polygon of confluence; LAD, left anterior descending artery; LCX, left circumflex artery. (From Park, S.J. et al., J Am Heart Assoc., 1, 6, 2012.)

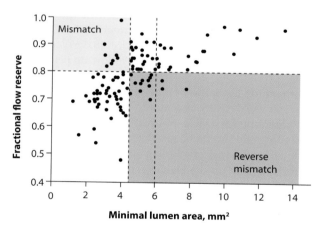

Figure 17.2 Scatter plot of intravascular ultrasound minimal lumen area versus fractional flow reserve. (From Park, S.J. et al., JACC Cardiovasc Interv, 7, 8, 2014.)

and FFR measurements (Figure 17.2)[25] and found that the IVUS-derived MLA value that best predicted FFR < 0.80 was <4.5 mm² (77% sensitivity, 82% specificity, 84% positive predictive value, 75% negative predictive value, area under the curve = 0.83, 95% confidence interval [CI] = 0.76–0.96, p < .001), similar to the theoretical cut-off of < 5.0 mm². Interestingly, the positive predictive value of IVUS-measured MLA was <4.5 mm², which was acceptably high, and the anatomical parameter provided by IVUS appeared to correlate well with the functional significance of LMCA

disease. Thus, in cases when FFR measurement is not feasible, IVUS-derived MLA criteria could possibly be used as a surrogate for the functional significance of LMCA disease.

17.4 Technical issues involved in LMCA intervention

17.4.1 Stenting procedures

Once the decision is made to perform revascularisation, careful evaluation of the lesion's complexity is required to assess the feasibility and ensure the success of PCI with stent implantation. During unprotected LMCA intervention, a femoral approach with large lumen-guiding catheters (7–8 Fr) is preferred. Coaxial alignment of the guiding catheter is important to minimise vessel injury and ensure proper positioning of the stent. With the refinement of stent technology came a marked reduction in restenosis rates, and with the large calibre and easy accessibility of most LMCAs, stenting of ostial and shaft LMCA lesions can be performed safely using careful haemodynamic monitoring and a meticulous guiding technique.

In ostial LMCA lesions the stent is generally deployed to protrude 1–2 mm into the aorta for full lesion coverage, whilst aorto-ostial coverage is not mandatory for treatment of disease that is limited to the shaft. Procedural and long-term outcomes in the DES era seem to be favourable. A brief and multiple balloon inflation procedure is required to avoid ischaemic complications. A multi-centre observational study demonstrated 99% procedural success after PCI with DES in the ostial and/or mid-shaft disease of unprotected LMCA, with no cases of in-hospital myocardial infarction (MI) or death, a mean late lumen < 0.01 mm at angiographic follow-up and favourable long-term outcomes (3.4% cumulative mortality and 4.7% target vessel revascularisation [TVR] at median 2.4 years).[26] Another study reported 4.1% cardiac deaths, 9.3% TVR and 19.1% major adverse cardiac events for ostial/mid-shaft interventions; these outcomes were better compared with the outcomes in distal bifurcation lesions in unprotected LMCA (19.1% vs. 28.5%; adjusted hazard ratio [HR], 1.48, 95% confidence interval [CI] 1.16–1.89; p = .001) at a follow-up period of 3.4 years.[27]

Bifurcation lesions are prone to lesion development due to greater shear stress and more frequent turbulent blood flow.[11] Stenting for LMCA bifurcation lesions is technically demanding and should be restricted to highly skilled interventionalists. The selection of an appropriate stenting strategy is dependent on the plaque configuration surrounding the LMCA, especially around the ostium of LCX. In general, the single-stent strategy has been more frequently used and showed more favourable long-term clinical outcomes compared with the two-stent strategy.[28] However, noticeable

rates of side branch (SB) occlusion have been reported from the real-world registry (8.4%), the majority of which occurred in true bifurcation lesions.[29] IVUS should be used to determine the accurate disease status for both the main and side branches and to determine the optimal stenting strategy (Table 17.2).[30] For provisional stenting in the LCX, wire insertion before stenting is generally needed in cases of narrowing at the LCX ostium, severe stenosis of the main branch due to large plaque burden at risk for plaque shifting, narrow angle of the LCX origination, or deterioration of the LCX ostium after pre-dilation of the main branch. Thus, IVUS use is strongly recommended to determine the appropriate stenting strategy, as it provides more accurate information of the disease status and degree of vascular remodelling relative to conventional angiograms. A number of two-stent techniques with various levels of complexities and indications, such as T-stenting, culotte stenting, crush stenting and simultaneous kissing stenting or Y-stenting are available. Currently, there is little consensus on which two-stent approach is better. Nevertheless, in either the single-stent or two-stent strategy, optimal stent expansion is very important for preventing restenosis and adverse clinical outcomes.[31]

17.4.2 IVUS-guided optimisation

IVUS is useful for determining anatomical configuration, selecting a treatment strategy and defining an optimal immediate stenting outcome during intervention. Although there is some controversy on the clinical impact of IVUS-guided stenting for unprotected LMCA, along with some cost–benefit concerns,[32] this adjuvant method has recently gained support from many interventional cardiologists. A sub-group analysis from the Revascularization Unprotected Left Main Coronary Artery Stenosis: Comparison of Percutaneous Coronary Angioplasty Versus Surgical Revascularization (MAIN-COMPARE) registry that included 201 propensity-score matched patient pairs demonstrated that there was a strong tendency towards a lower risk for 3-year mortality with IVUS guidance compared with angiography

Table 17.2 Anatomical features used to determine single-stent or two-stent strategies in the treatment of unprotected LMCA bifurcation

Strategy	Anatomical features
Single-stent	• Insignificant stenosis at the ostial LCX with Medina classification 1,1,0 or 1,0,0 • Small LCX with <2.5 mm in diameter • Diminutive LCX, right dominant coronary system • Wide angle with LAD • No concomitant disease or only focal disease in LCX
Two-stent	• Significant stenosis at the ostial LCX with Medina classification 1,1,1 or 1,0,1 or 0,1,1 • Large LCX with ≥2.5 mm in diameter • Diseased left dominant coronary system • Narrow angle with LAD • Concomitant diffuse disease in LCX

LMCA, left main coronary artery; LCX, left circumflex artery; LAD, left anterior descending artery.

guidance (6.3% vs. 13.6%, log-rank p = .063; HR, 0.54; 95% CI, 0.28–1.03).[33] In particular, for 145 matched pairs of patients receiving DES, the 3-year rate of mortality was significantly lower with IVUS guidance (4.7% vs. 16.0%, log-rank p = .048; HR, 0.39; 95% CI, 0.15–1.02). Mortality rates started to diverge 1 year after the procedure. Given that the IVUS guidance did not reduce the risk of mortality in 47 matched pairs of patients receiving BMS (8.6% versus 10.8%, log-rank p = .35; HR, 0.59), this study indicates that IVUS guidance may play a role in reducing very late stent thrombosis and subsequent long-term mortality. A recent IVUS-TRONCO-ICP Spanish study also demonstrated the importance of IVUS surveillance during LMCA stenting.[34] The IVUS-guided group was associated with lower incidences of composite cardiac death, MI and TLR and stent thrombosis at 3 years. A recent report from Kang et al. gave insights into the optimal minimal stent area (MSA) cut-off obtained from IVUS for prediction of restenosis and long-term clinical outcome after DES implantation for LMCA disease. After analysing 403 patients undergoing sirolimus-eluting stent implantation, the MSA criteria that best predicted angiographic in-stent restenosis on a segmental basis were 5.0 mm² for the LCX ostium, 6.3 mm² for the LAD ostium, 7.2 mm² for the polygon of confluence (POC) and 8.2 mm² for the proximal LMCA above the POC. Stent under-expansion was more frequent in the two-stent group than in the one-stent group (54% vs. 27%, p = .001). In addition, in the two-stent group, the LCX ostium was the most common site of under-expansion (37%), which may explain the greater risk of restenosis when LMCA bifurcation lesions are treated with a two-stent strategy. Overall, angiographic restenosis was more frequent in lesions with under-expansion than in those without under-expansion (24.1% vs. 5.4%, p = .001). Even in the two-stent group, lesions with complete expansion at all sites showed only 6% of the restenosis rate, which was similar to that of the one-stent group (6.3%) or in non-bifurcation LMCA lesions (4.5%).[31]

17.4.3 Haemodynamic support

Patients with normal left ventricular function are usually tolerant of brief global ischaemia during the balloon occlusion. But patients in an unstable haemodynamic condition need pharmacologic- or device-based haemodynamic support during the procedure for LMCA disease. Of the haemodynamic support devices (including intra-aortic balloon pumps, percutaneous haemodynamic support devices, or left ventricular assist devices), the intra-aortic balloon pump has been used most frequently. For provisional use, another femoral routine using a small sheath to enable rapid insertion of an intra-aortic balloon pump is recommended before PCI for high-risk patients. Although intra-aortic balloon support did not significantly reduce 30-day mortality in patients with cardiogenic shock complicating acute myocardial infarction,[35] a study surveying the prophylactic role of intra-aortic balloon pump in 219 elective LMCA interventions in patients with distal LMCA bifurcation lesions and a low ejection fraction of less than 40% showed that patients with elective intra-aortic

balloon pump support had lower procedural complications than those not receiving support (1.4% vs. 9.3%, p = .032).[36] Therefore, intra-aortic balloon pump support could be considered for patients with high-risk conditions, low ejection fraction or unstable presentations. The PROTECT (Prospective, Randomized Clinical Trial of Hemodynamic Support With Impella 2.5 Versus Intra-Aortic Balloon Pump in Patients Undergoing High-Risk Percutaneous Coronary Intervention) II study evaluated the feasibility of Impella 2.5 and intra-aortic balloon pump support in patients with complex three-vessel disease or unprotected LMCA disease and depressed ejection fraction. Although there was a trend for improved outcomes for Impella 2.5-supported patients at 90 days, no differences in 30-day incidence of major adverse events between intra-aortic balloon pump and Impella 2.5 support groups were found.[37] Further studies are required to determine the feasibility of new support devices such as Tandem-Heart or the Impella 2.5 in patients with LMCA disease.

17.5 Outcomes of unprotected left main intervention

17.5.1 Intervention using BMS

LMCA disease is an attractive target for percutaneous intervention due to its large vessel size, short lesion length and lack of tortuosity. Thus, LMCA intervention has shown its feasibility and acceptable short- and mid-term outcomes in the BMS era. Several studies have shown favourable short- or mid-term outcomes (in-hospital mortality, 0%–4.3%; mortality at 6–12 months, 2.5%–10.8%) in low-risk patients undergoing elective PCI using BMS for unprotected LMCA disease.[38–42] However, considerable risk of restenosis (18%–31%) and repeat revascularisation (7.3%–33.6%) that might lead to worst-case outcomes such as sudden death and acute MI have limited the durability of LMCA stenting with BMS. Therefore, LMCA stenting had to be reserved for selected patients who were not candidates for CABG or refused to receive CABG in the BMS era.

17.5.2 Intervention using DES

Compared with BMS, DES are associated with marked reductions in restenosis and the need for repeat revascularisation in unprotected LMCA disease. Several early observational studies have shown promising outcomes after PCI using DES compared with BMS, despite being limited by non-randomisation, small numbers of patients, and short follow-up periods.[43–45] In a subsequent meta-analysis comparing outcomes for DES and BMS after LMCA stenting, a total of 44 studies including 10,342 patients who received DES or BMS were analysed.[46] The respective cumulative event rates for DES and BMS at 3 years were 8.8% and 12.7% for death, 4.0% and 3.4% for MI, 8.0% and 16.4% for target vessel revascularisation/target lesion revascularisation and 21.4% and 31.6% for major adverse cardiovascular events (MACE). Adjusted outcomes at 3 years favoured DES, including the reduction of mortality. Regarding the differential benefit of DES for the prevention of restenosis, the two most widely applicable, first generation DES (sirolimus- and paclitaxel-eluting stents) were evaluated in previous studies. The studies showed a comparable result between the two DES.[47,48] Another study compared the safety and efficacy of the zotarolimus-eluting stent with the everoliumus-eluting stent for the treatment of unprotected LMCA disease, and both groups showed similar results in the occurrence of the primary endpoint and the safety endpoint at 1-year follow-up.[49]

17.5.3 Outcomes following treatments using PCI versus CABG

There are fundamental differences in the methodologies of PCI and CABG for treating coronary artery disease. In PCI, the lesion is directly relieved by stents whilst in bypass surgery and a graft is placed on the mid-coronary vessel, well beyond the lesion, where the epicardial vessel is relatively free of disease. Thus, one of the advantages of CABG over PCI is the achievement of more complete revascularisations, which leads to reductions in future revascularisation rates. However, the bypassed arteries have the potential to show accelerated atherosclerosis progression and chronic total occlusion lesions occur more frequently, which may be problematic when considering revascularisation after graft failure. The choice of PCI or CABG for treatment of unprotected LMCA disease should be based on the clinical and anatomical features of each case and with consideration of the advantages and disadvantages of each procedure. One study that allowed a comparison of the feasibility of PCI as an alternative to CABG used patients enrolled on the MAIN-COMPARE registry, which included 2240 patients with unprotected LMCA disease who underwent intervention (BMS, n = 318; DES, n = 784; CABG, n = 1138) at 12 major cardiac centres in South Korea (Figure 17.3).[5,50] The 3-year outcome report using propensity-score matching and the 5-year report using the inverse probability of treatment weighting method showed that the risk of death and the combined risk of death, Q-wave MI or stroke were not significantly different between patients undergoing PCI versus those undergoing CABG. A similar pattern was observed in patients treated with either DES or BMS. However, the risk of repeat revascularisation was significantly higher in the PCI group than in the CABG group, with HRs varying according to the type of implanted stent. Furthermore, the DES recipients were almost sixfold more likely to require repeated revascularisation compared with those who underwent surgery, whilst the BMS recipients were almost 10-fold more likely. Given that the recommendations for CABG for unprotected LMCA disease have been mostly based on the survival benefit it provides over medical therapy, the lack of statistically significant differences in mortality supports PCI as an alternative option to bypass surgery.

The Synergy between PCI with TAXUS drug-eluting stent and Cardiac Surgery (SYNTAX) trial compared the outcomes of PCI using paclitaxel-eluting stents versus

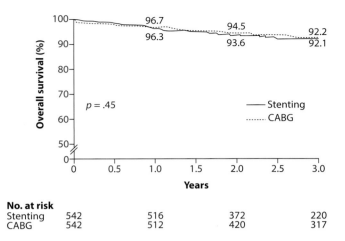

Figure 17.3 Kaplan–Meier curves for death in a cohort of patients matched for propensity scores who underwent stent implantation or bypass surgery. (From Seung, K.B. et al., *N Engl J Med*, 358, 17, 2008.)

CABG for unprotected LMCA disease in a subgroup analysis from a randomised cohort study.[6] In the subset of LMCA disease including 348 patients receiving CABG and 357 receiving PCI, PCI and CABG demonstrated equivalent 12-month rates of major adverse cardiovascular and cerebrovascular events (MACCE) (PCI vs. CABG, 15.8% vs. 13.7%). In these patients, the higher rate of repeat revascularisation after PCI (PCI vs. CABG, 11.8% vs. 6.5%; p = .01) was offset by a higher incidence of stroke after CABG (CABG vs. PCI, 2.7% vs. 0.3%; p = .01). Even after a 5-year follow-up period,[51] there were no significant differences in the rates of death (PCI vs. CABG, 12.8% vs. 14.6%, p = .53), MI (PCI vs. CABG, 8.2% vs. 4.8%, p = .1) or MACCE (PCI vs. CABG, 36.9% vs. 31.0%, p = .12) between patients who had received PCI and those who received CABG. The incidence of stroke was lower (PCI vs. CABG, 1.5% vs. 4.3%; p = .03), whilst the incidence of repeat revascularisation was higher (PCI vs. CABG, 26.7% vs. 15.5%; p < .01) in the PCI group. When patients were stratified according to SYNTAX score terciles, the MACCE incidence rates did not differ between the PCI and CABG groups in patients with low (0–22) and intermediate (23–32) scores. Although the SYNTAX trial results are favourable towards PCI, it should be noted that the LMCA disease analysis was carried out as a post hoc analysis and was not the primary objective of the study; these results should therefore be considered as hypothesis generating. Another small, randomised trial by Boudriot et al. compared sirolimus-eluting stenting (n = 100) with CABG (n = 101) for patients with unprotected LMCA disease.[52] The primary endpoint was non-inferiority in freedom from the composite of cardiac death, MI and the need for TVR at 12 months. The incidence of the primary endpoint was 13.9% in the CABG group and 19.0% in the PCI group (p = .19). The combined rates for death and MI were comparable (CABG vs. PCI, 7.9% vs. 5.0%), but PCI was inferior to CABG for repeat revascularisation rates (CABG vs. PCI, 5.9% vs. 14.0%; p = .35). Although cumulatively these data supported the efficacy and safety of LMCA stenting, these studies are limited in value because of their small sample sizes and exploratory natures. The Premier of Randomised Comparison of Bypass Surgery versus Angioplasty Using Sirolimus-Eluting Stent in Patients with Left Main Coronary Artery Disease (PRECOMBAT) trial LMCA-targeted randomised study was designed to provide more definitive insights into the safety and efficacy of LMCA stenting. This study randomised 600 patients with unprotected LMCA disease to treatment with either CABG or PCI with sirolimus-eluting stents (Figure 17.4).[7] At 1 year, PCI was non-inferior to CABG for the incidence of MACCE (absolute risk difference, 2%; upper margin of 95% CI, 5.6%; HR, 1.56; $p = .011$). By 2 years, the MACCE rate (PCI vs. CABG, 12.2% vs. 8.1%; HR, 1.5; 95% CI, 0.9–2.52; $p = .12$) and the composite rate of death, MI or stroke (PCI vs. CABG, 4.4% vs. 4.7%; HR, 0.92; 95% CI, 0.43–1.96; $p = .83$) remained comparable between the PCI and CABG groups. However, the 2-year rate of ischaemia-driven TVR was significantly higher in the PCI group than in the CABG group (PCI vs. CABG, 9% vs. 4.2%; HR, 2.18; 95% CI, 1.1–4.32; $p = .022$). Owing to these registries and randomised studies showing that PCI is feasible in the treatment of unprotected LMCA disease, the updated guidelines for the treatment of LMCA disease upgraded PCI as a reasonable or considerable treatment (level of evidence B) in pre-specified patients to improve survival.[9,53] A more global, large-scale randomised trial with long-term follow-up, the Evaluation of Xience Prime versus Coronary Artery Bypass Surgery for Effectiveness of Left Main Revascularisation (EXCEL) trial, is being performed to compare PCI and CABG in approximately 2500 patients with unprotected LMCA disease, and the final 5-year result of the PRECOMBAT trial might provide more strong evidence.

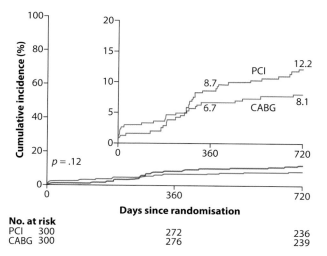

Figure 17.4 Cumulative incidence of the major adverse cardiac or cerebrovascular events in the percutaneous coronary intervention and coronary artery bypass graft surgery. (From Park, S.J. et al., *N Engl J Med*, 364, 18, 2011.)

17.6 Conclusions

Current evidence from observational and randomised clinical trials has demonstrated the procedural and long-term safety and efficacy of unprotected LMCA intervention. Thus, the guidelines for the treatment of LMCA disease should include PCI as a reasonable treatment in specified patient groups to improve clinical outcomes. An integrated approach that combines more advanced devices with specialised techniques, adjunctive imaging support and optimal pharmacotherapies has greatly improved the success rates of PCI and long-term clinical outcomes. Further randomised trials designed to compare PCI with new-generation DES and CABG are ongoing and will help clarify the differential effects of PCI versus CABG for the treatment of unprotected LMCA disease.

References

1. Herrick JB. Landmark article (JAMA 1912). Clinical features of sudden obstruction of the coronary arteries. By James B. Herrick. *JAMA* 1983; 250(13): 1757–65.
2. Takaro T et al. The VA cooperative randomized study of surgery for coronary arterial occlusive disease II. Subgroup with significant left main lesions. *Circulation* 1976; 54(Suppl 6): Iii107–17.
3. Chaitman BR et al. Effect of coronary bypass surgery on survival patterns in subsets of patients with left main coronary artery disease. Report of the Collaborative Study in Coronary Artery Surgery (CASS). *Am J Cardiol* 1981; 48(4): 765–77.
4. Caracciolo EA et al. Comparison of surgical and medical group survival in patients with left main coronary artery disease. Long-term CASS experience. *Circulation* 1995; 91(9): 2325–34.
5. Seung KB et al. Stents versus coronary-artery bypass grafting for left main coronary artery disease. *N Engl J Med* 2008; 358(17): 1781–92.
6. Morice MC et al. Outcomes in patients with de novo left main disease treated with either percutaneous coronary intervention using paclitaxel-eluting stents or coronary artery bypass graft treatment in the Synergy Between Percutaneous Coronary Intervention with TAXUS and Cardiac Surgery (SYNTAX) trial. *Circulation* 2010; 121(24): 2645–53.
7. Park SJ et al. Randomized trial of stents versus bypass surgery for left main coronary artery disease. *N Engl J Med* 2011; 364(18): 1718–27.
8. Fihn SD et al. 2012 ACCF/AHA/ACP/AATS/PCNA/SCAI/STS guideline for the diagnosis and management of patients with stable ischaemic heart disease: A report of the American College of Cardiology Foundation/American Heart Association task force on practice guidelines, and the American College of Physicians, American Association for Thoracic Surgery, Preventive Cardiovascular Nurses Association, Society for Cardiovascular Angiography and Interventions, and Society of Thoracic Surgeons. *Circulation* 2012; 126(25): e354–471.
9. Windecker S et al. 2014 ESC/EACTS Guidelines on myocardial revascularization: The Task Force on Myocardial Revascularization of the European Society of Cardiology

(ESC) and the European Association for Cardio-Thoracic Surgery (EACTS) Developed with the special contribution of the European Association of Percutaneous Cardiovascular Interventions (EAPCI). *Eur Heart J* 2014; 35(37): 2541–619.

10. Reig J, and Petit M. Main trunk of the left coronary artery: Anatomic study of the parameters of clinical interest. *Clin Anat* 2004; 17(1): 6–13.

11. Prosi M et al. Influence of curvature dynamics on pulsatile coronary artery flow in a realistic bifurcation model. *J Biomech* 2004; 37(11): 1767–75.

12. Virmani R et al. Lessons from sudden coronary death: A comprehensive morphological classification scheme for atherosclerotic lesions. *Arterioscler Thromb Vasc Biol* 2000; 20(5): 1262–75.

13. Oviedo C et al. Intravascular ultrasound classification of plaque distribution in left main coronary artery bifurcations: Where is the plaque really located? *Circ Cardiovasc Interv* 2010; 3(2): 105–12.

14. Fisher LD et al. Reproducibility of coronary arteriographic reading in the coronary artery surgery study (CASS). *Cathet Cardiovasc Diagn* 1982; 8(6): 565–75.

15. Isner JM et al. Accuracy of angiographic determination of left main coronary arterial narrowing. Angiographic-histologic correlative analysis in 28 patients. *Circulation* 1981; 63(5): 1056–64.

16. Hamilos M et al. Long-term clinical outcome after fractional flow reserve-guided treatment in patients with angiographically equivocal left main coronary artery stenosis. *Circulation* 2009; 120(15): 1505–12.

17. Bech GJ et al. Value of fractional flow reserve in making decisions about bypass surgery for equivocal left main coronary artery disease. *Heart* 2001; 86(5): 547–52.

18. Courtis J et al. Usefulness of coronary fractional flow reserve measurements in guiding clinical decisions in intermediate or equivocal left main coronary stenoses. *Am J Cardiol* 2009; 103(7): 943–9.

19. Lindstaedt M et al. Clinical outcome in patients with intermediate or equivocal left main coronary artery disease after deferral of surgical revascularization on the basis of fractional flow reserve measurements. *Am Heart J* 2006; 152(1): 156.e1–9.

20. Jasti V et al. Correlations between fractional flow reserve and intravascular ultrasound in patients with an ambiguous left main coronary artery stenosis. *Circulation* 2004; 110(18): 2831–6.

21. Park SJ et al. Unprotected left main percutaneous coronary intervention: Integrated use of fractional flow reserve and intravascular ultrasound. *J Am Heart Assoc* 2012; 1(6): e004556.

22. Lee CH et al. New set of intravascular ultrasound-derived anatomic criteria for defining functionally significant stenoses in small coronary arteries (results from Intravascular Ultrasound Diagnostic Evaluation of Atherosclerosis in Singapore [IDEAS] study). *Am J Cardiol* 2010; 105(10): 1378–84.

23. Kang SJ et al. Validation of intravascular ultrasound-derived parameters with fractional flow reserve for assessment of coronary stenosis severity. *Circ Cardiovasc Interv* 2011; 4(1): 65–71.

24. Waksman R et al. FIRST: Fractional Flow Reserve and Intravascular Ultrasound Relationship Study. *J Am Coll Cardiol* 2013; 61(9): 917–23.

25. Park SJ et al. Intravascular ultrasound-derived minimal lumen area criteria for functionally significant left main coronary artery stenosis. *JACC Cardiovasc Interv* 2014; 7(8): 868–74.

26. Chieffo A et al. Favorable long-term outcome after drug-eluting stent implantation in nonbifurcation lesions that involve unprotected left main coronary artery: A multicenter registry. *Circulation* 2007; 116(2): 158–62.

27. Naganuma T et al. Long-term clinical outcomes after percutaneous coronary intervention for ostial/mid-shaft lesions versus distal bifurcation lesions in unprotected left main coronary artery: The DELTA Registry (drug-eluting stent for left main coronary artery disease): A multicenter registry evaluating percutaneous coronary intervention versus coronary artery bypass grafting for left main treatment. *JACC Cardiovasc Interv* 2013; 6(12): 1242–9.

28. Kim WJ et al. Comparison of single- versus two-stent techniques in treatment of unprotected left main coronary bifurcation disease. *Catheter Cardiovasc Interv* 2011; 77(6): 775–82.

29. Gwon HC et al. Long-term clinical results and predictors of adverse outcomes after drug-eluting stent implantation for bifurcation lesions in a real-world practice: The COBIS (Coronary Bifurcation Stenting) registry. *Circ J* 2010; 74(11): 2322–8.

30. Moussa I, and Colombo A. *Tips and Tricks in Interventional Therapy of Coronary Bifurcation Lesions*. CRC Press, 2010.

31. Kang SJ et al. Comprehensive intravascular ultrasound assessment of stent area and its impact on restenosis and adverse cardiac events in 403 patients with unprotected left main disease. *Circ Cardiovasc Interv* 2011; 4(6): 562–9.

32. Agostoni P et al. Comparison of early outcome of percutaneous coronary intervention for unprotected left main coronary artery disease in the drug-eluting stent era with versus without intravascular ultrasonic guidance. *Am J Cardiol* 2005; 95(5): 644–47.

33. Park SJ et al. Impact of intravascular ultrasound guidance on long-term mortality in stenting for unprotected left main coronary artery stenosis. *Circ Cardiovasc Interv* 2009; 2(3): 167–77.

34. de la Torre Hernandez JM et al. Clinical impact of intravascular ultrasound guidance in drug-eluting stent implantation for unprotected left main coronary disease: Pooled analysis at the patient-level of 4 registries. *JACC Cardiovasc Interv* 2014; 7(3): 244–54.

35. Thiele H et al. Intraaortic balloon support for myocardial infarction with cardiogenic shock. *N Engl J Med* 2012; 367(14): 1287–96.

36. Briguori C et al. Elective versus provisional intraaortic balloon pumping in unprotected left main stenting. *Am Heart J* 2006; 152(3): 565–72.

37. O'Neill WW et al. A prospective, randomized clinical trial of hemodynamic support with Impella 2.5 versus intra-aortic balloon pump in patients undergoing high-risk percutaneous coronary intervention: The PROTECT II study. *Circulation* 2012; 126(14): 1717–27.

38. Park SJ et al. Elective stenting of unprotected left main coronary artery stenosis: Effect of debulking before stenting and intravascular ultrasound guidance. *J Am Coll Cardiol* 2001; 38(4): 1054–60.

39. Takagi T et al. Results and long-term predictors of adverse clinical events after elective percutaneous interventions on unprotected left main coronary artery. *Circulation* 2002; 106(6): 698–702.

40. Black A et al. Unprotected left main coronary artery stenting: Correlates of midterm survival and impact of patient selection. *J Am Coll Cardiol* 2001; 37(3): 832–8.

41. Silvestri M et al. Unprotected left main coronary artery stenting: Immediate and medium-term outcomes of 140 elective procedures. *J Am Coll Cardiol* 2000; 35(6): 1543–50.

42. Park SJ et al. Stenting of unprotected left main coronary artery stenoses: Immediate and late outcomes. *J Am Coll Cardiol* 1998; 31(1): 37–42.

43. Valgimigli M et al. Short- and long-term clinical outcome after drug-eluting stent implantation for the percutaneous treatment of left main coronary artery disease: Insights from the Rapamycin-Eluting and Taxus Stent Evaluated At Rotterdam Cardiology Hospital registries (RESEARCH and T-SEARCH). *Circulation* 2005; 111(11): 1383–9.

44. Chieffo A et al. Early and mid-term results of drug-eluting stent implantation in unprotected left main. *Circulation* 2005; 111(6): 791–95.

45. Park SJ et al. Sirolimus-eluting stent implantation for unprotected left main coronary artery stenosis: Comparison with bare metal stent implantation. *J Am Coll Cardiol* 2005; 45(3): 351–6.

46. Pandya SB et al. Drug-eluting versus bare-metal stents in unprotected left main coronary artery stenosis a meta-analysis. *JACC Cardiovasc Interv* 2010; 3(6): 602–11.

47. Valgimigli M et al. Sirolimus-eluting versus paclitaxel-eluting stent implantation for the percutaneous treatment of left main coronary artery disease: A combined RESEARCH and T-SEARCH long-term analysis. *J Am Coll Cardiol* 2006; 47(3): 507–14.

48. Mehilli J et al. Paclitaxel- versus sirolimus-eluting stents for unprotected left main coronary artery disease. *J Am Coll Cardiol* 2009; 53(19): 1760–8.

49. Mehilli J et al. Zotarolimus- versus everolimus-elutingstents for unprotected left main coronary artery disease. *J Am Coll Cardiol* 2013; 62(22): 2075–82.

50. Park DW et al. Long-term safety and efficacy of stenting versus coronary artery bypass grafting for unprotected left main coronary artery disease: 5-year results from the MAIN-COMPARE (Revascularization for Unprotected Left Main Coronary Artery Stenosis: Comparison of Percutaneous Coronary Angioplasty Versus Surgical Revascularization) registry. *J Am Coll Cardiol* 2010; 56(2): 117–24.

51. Morice MC et al. Five-year outcomes in patients with left main disease treated with either percutaneous coronary intervention or coronary artery bypass grafting in the synergy between percutaneous coronary intervention with taxus and cardiac surgery trial. *Circulation* 2014; 129(23): 2388–94.

52. Boudriot E et al. Randomized comparison of percutaneous coronary intervention with sirolimus-eluting stents versus coronary artery bypass grafting in unprotected left main stem stenosis. *J Am Coll Cardiol* 2011; 57(5): 538–45.

53. Levine GN et al. 2011 ACCF/AHA/SCAI Guideline for Percutaneous Coronary Intervention. A report of the American College of Cardiology Foundation/American Heart Association Task Force on Practice Guidelines and the Society for Cardiovascular Angiography and Interventions. *J Am Coll Cardiol* 2011; 58(24): e44–122.

Haemodynamic support for high-risk percutaneous intervention

JOHN M LASALA, ALEJANDRO AQUINO

18.1 Introduction

There has been a growth in a population of patients with coronary artery disease for which revascularisation has been precluded by the presence of significant co-morbidities. The use of haemodynamic support devices has helped provide an avenue of treatment for these patients. We aim in this chapter to summarise briefly the data that have driven the use of each device followed by a presentation of the practical application of each device.

18.2 Evidence supporting the use of haemodynamic support devices

18.2.1 Intra-aortic balloon pump

The first study for the intra-aortic balloon pump (IABP) was first published in 1962[1] and it has remained a mainstay treatment for cardiogenic shock despite inconclusive evidence[2] and only modest augmentation in cardiac output.[3]

There exists an abundance of studies that have sought to clarify the role of IABP in myocardial infarction (MI) complicated by cardiogenic shock as well as in high risk (HR)-percutaneous coronary intervention (PCI). One meta-analysis reviewed the cohort data for MI complicated by cardiogenic shock.[4] They found that while for patients treated with thrombolysis there was a mortality benefit (18%) at 30 days, this effect was not seen in the primary PCI group. Instead, IABP was associated with an increase in mortality of 6% at 30 days.[4] Another retrospective study sought to determine whether IABP support at the time of HR-PCI would provide any benefit. They retrospectively examined 48 patients with acute myocardial infarction (AMI) complicated by cardiogenic shock and found that IABP-supported PCI was associated with more favourable in-hospital outcomes including lower creatine kinase (CK)-MB levels and mortality.[5]

The ambiguity as to the benefit of IABP in this setting persists in the randomised trials that have been performed. The IABP-Shock II trial randomised 600 patients with MI and cardiogenic shock to either IABP or not. And while there was no difference in the secondary safety endpoints including major bleeding and stroke, there was no mortality benefit.[6] A second randomised trial (Balloon Pump-Assisted Coronary Intervention Study [BCIS]-1) also failed to demonstrate a reduction in major adverse cardiac and cerebral events (MACCE) at 6 months for routine and elective placement of IABP for HR-PCI.[7] However, when these patients were followed out to a median of 51 months, there was a 34% relative reduction in all-cause mortality for the IABP group.[8]

Overall, there is no consensus as to the role of IABP in HR-PCI; however, IABP remains a key tool for providing haemodynamic support. Despite this, in the most recent guidelines for ST-elevation myocardial infarction (STEMI), IABP carries a Class IIA indication for the treatment of STEMI complicated by cardiogenic shock.[9]

18.2.2 TandemHeart

The TandemHeart (CardiacAssist®) device transports oxygenated blood via a centrifugal pump from the left atrium to the femoral artery. It was approved for short-term haemodynamic support in 2005 with several early small series suggesting its safety and efficacy in improving haemodynamic parameters in cardiogenic shock, as well as its viability in supporting PCI.[10–12] A pair of small, randomised trials compared TandemHeart to the IABP with analogous results. In one of the aforementioned studies, 33 patients with cardiogenic shock (70% of which were secondary to MI) were randomised to either IABP or TandemHeart. TandemHeart provided significant improvement in haemodynamic measures including higher cardiac index (CI), higher mean arterial pressure and lower pulmonary capillary wedge pressure. Despite this, TandemHeart did not impart mortality benefit as 30-day survival rates were no different between the groups.[13] Similar findings were seen in a cohort of 40 patients with acute MI complicated by cardiogenic shock where TandemHeart imparted haemodynamic but no mortality benefit with an increased rate of severe bleeding and limb ischaemia.[14]

The use of TandemHeart has also been shown to be a viable support strategy in performing high-risk coronary interventions. Although no randomised trial exists for TandemHeart in HR-PCI, several series have reported high procedural success rates.[15,16] In a series of 54 HR-PCI patients (median ejection fraction [EF] 20%, median SYNTAX (Synergy between Percutaneous Coronary Intervention with Taxus and Cardiac Surgery) score 33, median Jeopardy score 10) who were deemed to be high surgical risk due to significant co-morbidities (Society of Thoracic Surgeons [STS] score of 13%), there was a procedural success rate of 97% with 6-month survival of 87%.[15] In accordance to previous experiences, TandemHeart provided improvement in haemodynamic parameters with decreased filling pressures and increased cardiac output (4.7→5.7 L/min, $p = .03$).

In summary, despite limited randomised data, there is ample evidence that TandemHeart improves haemodynamic parameters in patients presenting with cardiogenic shock and provides sufficient support to perform HR-PCI. These benefits may come at the cost of significant vascular complications.

18.2.3 Impella

Recent interest on haemodynamic support for high-risk PCI has centred on the Impella device. An early case report documented the ability of the Impella to unload the left ventricle and improve cardiac output in a patient with severe systolic dysfunction undergoing HR-PCI.[17] Subsequent small series helped to establish the safety and feasibility of Impella-supported HR-PCI.[18–20] One such study, PROTECT I (Feasibility Trial Investigating the Use of the Impella 2.5 System in Patients Undergoing High-Risk PCI), prospectively examined the capability of Impella to meet safety and efficacy endpoints in patients with low left ventricular (LV) ejection fraction (≤35%) undergoing unprotected left main or last remaining conduit intervention.[20] Twenty patients at various sites were followed for 30 days with the primary safety endpoint defined as incidence of MACCE, while the efficacy endpoint was the freedom from haemodynamic instability (mean arterial pressure < 60 mmHg for 10 minutes or need for pressor support). Favourable results (two deaths unrelated to device use and no incidence of haemodynamic compromise) helped further the role of Impella as a viable option for haemodynamic support in HR-PCI. The ISAR-SHOCK (Efficacy Study of LV Assist Device to Treat Patients With Cardiogenic Shock) trial compared the level of haemodynamic support provided by the Impella to the IABP for patients in cardiogenic shock. Impella was found to provide more support as evidenced by an increased CI and mean arterial pressure; however, there was no mortality benefit as it remained close to 50% in both groups.[21] It must be noted, however, that the study was not powered to show a mortality benefit.

Two large observational registries were formed in the United States (USPella)[22] and Europe (EuroPella)[23] to collect data on use for all Impella devices and provide insight into real-world clinical experience. Analysis from the HR-PCI subset of both registries demonstrated similar results, including comparable 30-day mortality rates (4%–5.5%) and an improvement in the ejection fraction. In addition, there was an improvement in the SYNTAX score that signalled the ability to allow the completion of complex revascularisation. These results helped to further solidify the feasibility of Impella in HR-PCI.

The next progression in establishing the role of Impella 2.5 in HR-PCI came in the form of a multicentre, randomised control trial comparing it to the IABP for patients undergoing non-emergent revascularisation (PROTECT II).[24] The study was stopped early for futility based on the composite endpoint of major adverse events (MAE) at 30 days (Table 18.1), this decision was based on the analysis on data at 50% enrolment (327 of planned

654 subjects). However, when the analysis included the additional subjects that had been enrolled at the time of the trial stoppage (total 452 subjects), there was a trend towards benefit for Impella with regards to MAE at 30 days that became significant at 90 days (Figure 18.1). Subgroup analysis demonstrate that for the patients not treated with atherectomy there was a significant reduction in MAE at 90 days (36.5% vs. 48.7%, p = .014). In the non-atherectomy group this was more.[25] Recently, a global registry has been initiated to accumulate more data on HR-PCI and other applications of Impella. The evidence accumulated from the USPella, EuroPella, PROTECT I and PROTECT II led to the approval by the Food and Drug Administration (FDA) in 2012 for the use of the Impella 2.5 for HR-PCI.

Table 18.1 Individual components of composite major adverse events for PROTECT II

Death

Stroke/transient ischaemia attack (TIA)

Myocardial infarction

Repeat revascularisation

Need for cardiac operation or thoracic or abdominal vascular operation or vascular operation for limb ischaemia

Acute renal dysfunction

Cardiopulmonary resuscitation or ventricular arrhythmia requiring cardioversion

Increase in aortic insufficiency by more than one grade

Severe hypotension defined as systolic blood pressure or augmented diastolic pressure (whichever is greater) <90 mmHg for ≥5 min requiring inotropic/pressor medications or intravenous fluid

Failure to achieve angiographic success defined as residual stenosis <30% after stent implantation

18.2.4 Extracorporeal membrane oxygenation

The role of venoarterial (VA) extracorporeal membrane oxygenation (ECMO) lies not as a tool for elective HR-PCI but rather as a measure for providing both respiratory and haemodynamic support for patients in various states of cardiac demise. VA ECMO can provide support for patients who are unable to wean from cardiopulmonary bypass (CPB) following cardiac surgery, as well as those in cardiogenic shock or suffering cardiac arrest.[26–28] Mortality remains high with the use of VA ECMO, however, there may be some benefit provided.[29–33] Sheu et al. found that early initiation of ECMO support may improve mortality at 30 days for those suffering STEMI with cardiogenic shock. Furthermore, ECMO may serve as a bridge to more definitive advanced therapies such as left ventricular assist device (LVAD) or transplant.

There are no randomised control trials evaluating the use of ECMO in HR-PCI; however, there has been abundant experience demonstrating its feasibility in the form of case reports and single-centre cohort studies.[31,34–39] Additionally, it was found to be a viable option for rapid support in coronary or structural cases complicated by cardiovascular collapse.[40]

18.3 Practical guide to haemodynamic support devices

18.3.1 Intra-aortic balloon pump

18.3.1.1 Introduction and components

The IABP has grown to be the most widely used haemodynamic support device since its introduction in the 1960s.[1] This device employs the counterpulsation of a balloon in the descending aorta to improve cardiac output and increase

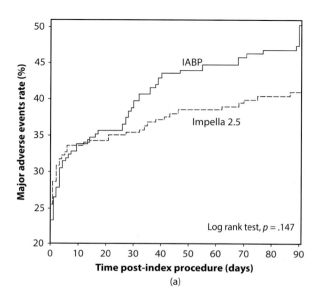

(a)

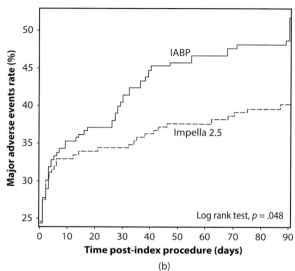

(b)

Figure 18.1 Kaplan–Meier curves for major adverse events in PROTECT II.

coronary perfusion. The system is comprised of a dual-lumen balloon catheter and the control console. The inner catheter lumen accepts the guidewire during placement and is then used to obtain pressure readings for monitoring. The gas lumen serves as the conduit for the exchange of helium in and out of the balloon.

18.3.1.2 Haemodynamic effects

The haemodynamic consequences of counterpulsation can be organised into those that occur during inflation and those during deflation. Inflation occurs at the onset of diastole and causes a displacement of blood that increases the diastolic pressure in the aorta. There is resulting increase in systemic mean arterial pressure and cardiac output as well as an improvement in coronary perfusion. Balloon deflation is timed to occur immediately prior to systole leading to an abrupt drop in aortic pressure just prior to ventricular ejection. This reduces the ventricular afterload and leads to decreased workload and improved cardiac output (Table 18.2).

18.3.1.3 Technical considerations and contraindications

As with other forms of haemodynamic support, the presence of aortic and ileo-femoral vascular disease is an important consideration. The femoral vasculature must be able to accept a 7 or 8 Fr sheath size. Calcified atherosclerotic plaque in the aorta may lead to abrasion of the balloon and eventual rupture.

Table 18.2 Haemodynamic effects of intra-aortic balloon pump

Inflation	Deflation
Increase in diastolic pressure	Decreases systemic resistance
Increase in mean arterial pressure	Decreases systolic blood pressure
Increase in systemic perfusion	Increases cardiac output
Increase in coronary perfusion	Decreases wedge

Proper balloon volume sizing can maximise the haemodynamic benefit for the patient. Increases in balloon volume (up to 50 cc) are accomplished by adding length to the balloon. Thus, sizing charts are based on patient height so as to avoid balloon obstruction of left subclavian and bilateral renal perfusion. Balloon position should be performed under fluoroscopy to avoid this potential complication. If the placement cannot be performed under live fluoroscopy then immediate verification via a chest plain film is warranted. The proper position of the distal tip is at 1–2 cm *distal* to left subclavian artery (second to third intercostal space). However, one study suggests that placing the tip 2 cm *above* the carina may be a more reliable landmark.[41] Additionally, serial monitoring of the left radial pulse and urine output can signal malposition or movement of the IABP.

18.3.1.4 Management

One of the most important functions of the console is to provide real-time information regarding the timing of balloon inflation and deflation. There are several modes to set balloon function including electroencephalocardiogram (ECG) and pressure triggering. ECG triggering is the most commonly used; however, it is susceptible to arrhythmias.

Recognition of mistimed balloon inflation and/or deflation is vital to ensure proper haemodynamic support. The correct IABP waveform consists of inflation in diastole at the dicrotic notch causing an augmentation of the diastolic pressure above the unassisted pressure (Figure 18.2). Deflation should occur just before systole and cause a decrease in the end diastolic pressure and peak systolic pressure. There are four scenarios to recognise: early inflation, late inflation, early deflation and late deflation. When early inflation is occurring the balloon is expanding prior to the dicrotic notch and can encroach onto the previous systolic phase (Figure 18.3). The detrimental effects can include premature closure of the aortic valve with resulting increased filling pressures and afterload that results in increased myocardial O_2 demand. Late inflation occurs after the dicrotic notch and can lead to poor diastolic augmentation and with it poor coronary perfusion

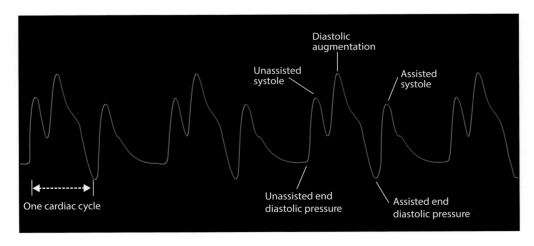

Figure 18.2 Normal intra-aortic balloon pump timing.

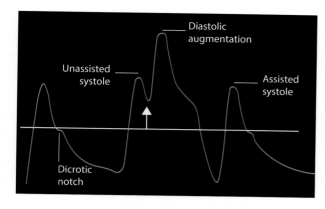

Figure 18.3 Early inflation.

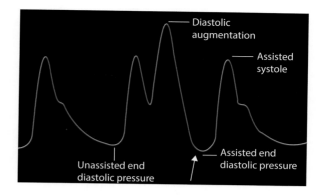

Figure 18.5 Early deflation.

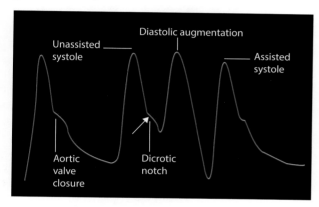

Figure 18.4 Late inflation.

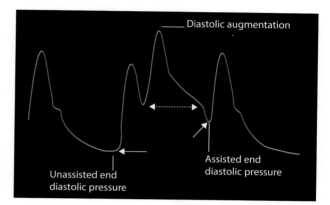

Figure 18.6 Late deflation.

(Figure 18.4). In addition, there is ineffective afterload reduction and increased mixed venous oxygen saturation (MVO2) demand. Early deflation leads to a sharp drop right in aortic pressure during the diastolic phase and limits pressure augmentation and coronary flow (Figure 18.5). It can also lead to poor afterload reduction and increased myocardial O_2 demand. Finally, late deflation causes the balloon to impede on the subsequent systolic phase and the work of the heart against and inflated balloon lead to increased afterload and increased myocardial O_2 demand (Figure 18.6).

Contraindications to the placement of the IABP include severe aortic insufficiency, aortic aneurysm and peripheral vascular disease. The IABP may also be inserted without a sheath; however, this technique is contraindicated if there is significant scar tissue or if the patient is obese. Potential complications include limb ischaemia, bleeding at the insertion site, thrombocytopenia, infection and aortic dissection. Rupture of the balloon may also occur and is signalled by the presence of blood within the tubing or with a 'gas loss' alarm. In this case, the device should be stopped immediately and removed.

Long-term IABP support can be safely accomplished via a subclavian approach that minimises infection and allows the patient to ambulate.[42] This approach is one possible option for the haemodynamic support of patients undergoing work-up for transplant or LVAD.

18.4 TandemHeart

18.4.1 Introduction and components

The TandemHeart® (CardiacAssist, Inc.) is a support device that delivers blood from the left atrium to the arterial system (femoral artery) utilising an extracorporeal centrifugal pump (Figure 18.7). The TandemHeart system is composed of (1) an inflow cannula (21 Fr) with trans-septal placement into the left atrium, (2) an outflow cannula (15 or 17 Fr) placed into the femoral artery, (3) centrifugal pump and (4) control console.

Inflow and Outflow Cannulae: The inflow cannula is placed from the femoral vein into the left atrium via a trans-septal puncture. The cannula is 21 Fr and comes in either 62 or 72 cm lengths and blood inflow comes through 14 side holes at the distal tip. The arterial outflow cannula is 17 cm in length and comes in either 15 or 17 Fr. Both cannulae contain three radio-opaque markings at the distal end allowing accurate fluoroscopic placement.

Centrifugal Pump: The centrifugal pump is hydrodynamic and utilises a fluid bearing system created by constant saline infusion into the lower housing that minimises friction. The pump itself has a maximum flow of 8.0 L/min, however, flow is also dependent on inflow and outflow cannula size with the variable in this system being

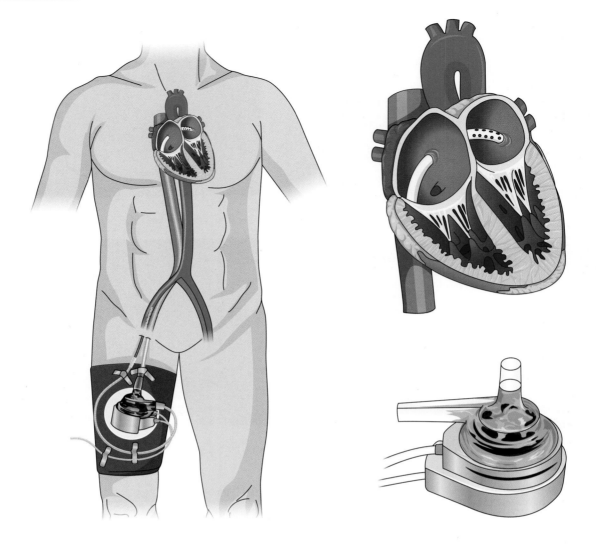

Figure 18.7 TandemHeart system.

the outflow arterial cannula (4.0 L/min with 15 Fr and 5.0 L/min with 17 Fr).

Console: The controller is designed for ease-of-use with onscreen step-by-step set-up guidance as well as self-diagnostic algorithms and alarms. The console provides power to the system and has a battery backup that can provide up to 1 hour of operation.

18.4.2 Haemodynamic effects

The haemodynamic result of the TandemHeart moving blood from the left atrium into the peripheral arterial system is two-fold. There is an unloading of the LV that reduces workload and myocardial oxygen demand. In addition, the delivery of blood to the peripheral arterial system leads to an increase of cardiac output and mean arterial pressure.[43] An important concept to consider is that this also increases the LV afterload that depending on the other haemodynamic parameters may lead to a net neutral effect on myocardial oxygen demand.

18.4.3 Technical considerations and contraindications

As with other types of haemodynamic support devices, the size of the peripheral vasculature can limit the use of the TandemHeart. The venous cannula is 21 Fr while the arterial cannula can be either 15 or 17 Fr. Serial assessment must be made of the access sites to assess for any possible complication or compromise of distal perfusion. Frequent examination of limb colour and temperature is need; however, it is important to keep in mind that the distal pulse may not be palpable due to the non-pulsatile flow from the device. Placement of a sheath to provide antegrade flow to the distal limb may help prevent ischaemia.

The placement of the TandemHeart venous cannula requires a trans-septal puncture. For an experienced operator, a trans-septal puncture is a relatively safe procedure. However, approximately 1% of cases develop complications[44] that include cardiac wall perforation, aortic root puncture, pericardial effusion or tamponade, stroke and death.[45] For those with less experience, methods to help delineate the atrial septal anatomy such as intra-cardiac echo (ICE) or trans-oesophageal echo (TEE) may be more costly but may minimise complications. The placement of a pigtail catheter to the aortic annulus will mark the structure and help avoid inadvertent puncture of the aortic root. An important consideration is that the fasting status of a patient may lead to reduced left atrial volume and administration of intravenous fluid may make LA puncture easier. Finally, it is vital to work under adequate anticoagulation once access is gained into the left atrium to minimise the risk of stroke.

Contraindications for the placement of the TandemHeart include any condition that prohibits anticoagulation. In addition, the presence of a ventricular septal defect or aortic insufficiency precludes placement.[46]

18.4.4 Management

The flow provided by the TandemHeart is dependent on several factors including the systemic and pulmonary resistance, cannula size and position, and fluid balance. Support is initiated at 5500 rpm and subsequently raised by 250–500 rpm until there is no long an increase in flow. This is the maximum flow for that particular set of aforementioned parameters. Should more flow be desired then the fluid balance, vascular resistance and right ventricular (RV) function should be assessed and addressed. This highlights the need for continued haemodynamic monitoring as well as the utility of a Swan–Ganz catheter to help assess total cardiac output and filling pressures.

The TandemHeart console provides alarms that are categorised into three settings: low, medium and high priority. The alarms are accompanied by the triggering conditions and associated causes that can guide troubleshooting (Figure 18.8).

Vibration in the system's tubing may signal inadequate filling of the left atrium and should trigger an evaluation for the root cause including hypovolaemia, pulmonary hypertension, cardiac tamponade, bleeding, RV failure or arrhythmias. Kinks in the tubing, cannula migration and thrombus in the circuit should also be assessed.

The importance of adequate anticoagulation has been previously mentioned. Although protocols may vary among centres, activated clotting time (ACT) should be maintained between 180 and 220 seconds. Additional heparin administration should be considered if the flow drops below 1 L/min or if the system is stopped for more than 5 minutes (not recommended).

Complications for this device have been mentioned but are summarised here and include bleeding, limb ischaemia, arrhythmias, tamponade, atrial perforation and residual ASD.[4]

Weaning from the TandemHeart should be performed when deemed clinically appropriate by the managing team.

Flow rate is decreased by 50% every hour but is not to be reduced below 1 L/min. If the patient remains stable then the device may be turned off and the arterial cannula immediately clamped followed by the venous cannula. The device is then retracted from the left atrium into the right atrium and the heparing is stopped. Once the ACT reaches appropriate levels (per hospital protocol), the femoral cannulae may be removed.

18.5 Impella

18.5.1 Introduction and components

The Impella® (Abiomed®) is a percutaneous ventricular support device that utilises a micro-axial pump to move blood from the left ventricle to the aorta. There are three classes available that provide increasing levels of support: Impella 2.5 (2.5 L/min), Impella CP (~3.5 L/min) and the Impella 5.0 (5.0 L/min). All three have been approved in the United States to provide haemodynamic support for up to 6 hours. Additionally, based on the data from trials such as PROTECT I and PROTECT II,[20,25] the Impella 2.5 has also been approved for use in haemodynamically stable patients undergoing elective or urgent HR-PCI.

The Impella support system is comprised of three major components: (1) catheter, (2) purge system and (3) automated controller (Figure 18.9). An impeller and its adjacent motor are located near the outlet area in the ascending aorta. As it rotates, negative pressure draws ventricular blood into the inlet area and through the cannula (Figure 18.10). The flow through the cannula is dependent on the rotation speed of the impeller for which there are nine settings: P0–P8. In order to protect the motor, the purge fluid (5% dextrose with heparin) forms a hydraulic pressure shield that prevents blood from migrating proximally past the impeller and into the motor housing.

18.5.2 Haemodynamic effects

There are two primary effects that the Impella imparts: (1) an unloading of the ventricle (lower end-diastolic volume and pressure) and (2) an increase in forward flow (higher mean arterial pressure). There is a reduction in LV end-diastolic pressure and volume that translates into decreased wall tension and myocardial oxygen demand.[17] Furthermore, there is evidence of improved coronary perfusion pressure and hyperaemic flow velocity with a decrease in micro-vascular resistance with Impella 2.5.[47]

An important concept to recognise with Impella, as with other forms of LV support, is the device's reliance on a functional right ventricle in providing left ventricle filling (unless there is concurrent RV support). And while transient arrhythmias can be tolerated, more sustained tachycardias or asystole will compromise the haemodynamic support.[48]

High Priority

Alarm	Condition	Causes
Low flow	Flow <1.0 LPM	Kinks or restrictions in cannulae or tubing Hypovolemia Right heart failure
Critically low battery	Less than 10 minutes of battery life remain AND controller is operating on battery power.	Hardware failure of battery backup. Operating on battery for an extended period of time
System overtemp	Controller electronics temp >65°C	Air inlet / exhaust obstructed Fan failure Controller near a heat source

Medium Priority

Alarm	Condition	Causes
Infusate pres error	Infusion pressure >600 or <50mmHg. >600 can occur within approximately 1 hour of start up with some pumps. <50: pump seal worn, increased risk of blood in lower housing.	Infusion set not properly laced. Kink or obstruction in infusion line. Stopcock not set properly. Leak in infusion set or pump infusion line.
Pres trndcr error	Pressure transducer disconnected or failed calibration.	Defective transducer Not open to atmosphere when connected

Low Priority

Alarm	Condition	Causes
System problem	Non-critical self-test failure was detected and acknowledged.	Call CardiacAssist, Inc. Technical Support.

Figure 18.8 TandemHeart alarms.

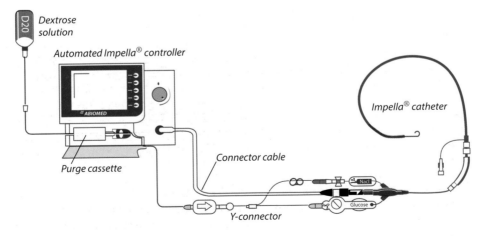

Figure 18.9 Impella system.

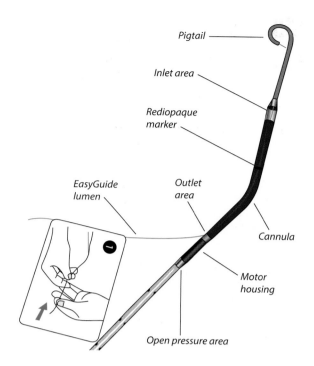

Figure 18.10 Impella catheter.

18.5.3 Technical considerations and contraindications

A common limitation to use of Impella support is the inadequacy of the peripheral vasculature in accommodating the large bore catheters. While the Impella 2.5 (12 Fr) and CP (14 Fr) can often be placed percutaneously via the femoral artery, the 5.0 device requires a surgical cut down of the femoral, axillary or subclavian artery. There is a need for anticoagulation (goal ACT > 250 seconds at placement, 160–180 seconds for maintenance), so the presence of a coagulopathy or recent haemorrhage may prohibit its use. The presence of a mechanical aortic valve or an LV mural thrombus preclude Impella use, as does significant aortic valve stenosis (valve area 0.6 cm^2 or less, except when performed with valvuloplasty) or insufficiency (2 + or greater by echo).

18.5.4 Management

Appropriate post-procedural management of the Impella system is paramount. The Impella controller is an important tool that allows continuous automated oversight of device parameters and function. While the device representative is an invaluable resource for help with troubleshooting, there are several scenarios with which the operator should be familiar.

18.5.4.1 Position monitoring

The automated Impella controller has two main displays that are useful in monitoring catheter position and function. The first is the Home Screen (Figure 18.11), which contains

an alarm window that can display up to three alarms simultaneously with troubleshooting suggestions. In addition, there is a central display area that displays an illustration of the determined Impella position with corresponding position indicator message. The Placement Screen displays two waveforms: placement signal waveform and motor current waveform (Figure 18.12). These waveforms signals can be used to determine the catheter position. If the catheter needs to be repositioned then imaging echocardiographic or fluoroscopic guidance is recommended.

One must keep in mind, that a severely dysfunctional left ventricle may be unable to generate a significant pressure difference across the aortic valve. This leads to dampening of the placement signal and motor current waveforms that limits their utility in determining catheter position. In this case, the operator must rely on patient haemodynamic parameter and imaging to monitor position.

During the initial placement of the Impella catheter, there is tendency for the catheter to dive forward into the ventricle that can be avoided by taking precautionary steps including placing the inlet area at approximately 3.5 cm below the aortic valve, removing the slack from the catheter over the aortic arch prior to starting the pump, tightening the Tuohy Borst valve and placing a leg immobiliser.

18.5.4.2 Suction alarm

Suction may occur with the Impella due to improper positioning or inadequate LV volume. The Impella position should always be confirmed with imaging and adjustments made in order to space the inlet from the ventricular wall. Inadequate LV volume may be secondary to overall volume depletion but can be seen when there is poor RV function leading to poor filling of the left side. Echocardiography or pulmonary artery catheter haemodynamics can help delineate the root cause of a suction alarm.

When encountered with suction, one can attempt to reposition the catheter, decrease the P-level, address disturbances in intravascular volume and minimise movement with the use of a leg immoboliser. It is paramount to recognise that a suction alarm at the initial placement of the catheter may signal the presence of thrombus. If correct position has been confirmed then the catheter may need to be removed and fully inspected while assuring that an appropriate ACT exists (>250 seconds). The presence of suction may lead to haemolysis.

18.5.4.3 Haemolysis

Patients must be monitored for signs of possible haemolysis such as new or worsening anaemia and the presence of dark-coloured urine. Laboratory testing may help confirm the presence of haemolysis including bilirubin, lactate dehydrogenase, haptoglobin and plasma free haemoglobin. Haemolysis usually indicates improper position but in general is due to three things (1) inlet obstruction (position or volume), (2) obstruction within the cannula (clot) and (3) outflow obstruction (AV or aortic wall close to outlet).

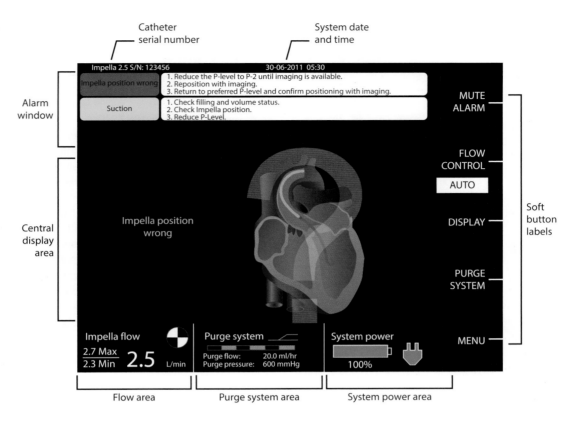

Figure 18.11 Home screen.

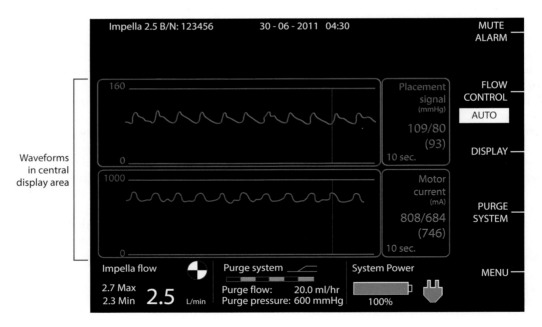

Figure 18.12 Placement screen.

18.5.4.4 Heparin-induced thrombocytopenia

If heparin-induced thrombocytopenia (HIT) is suspected then all heparin products should be stopped and confirmatory testing performed. The care team must then make a risk-benefit decision as to continue without heparin in the system. Direct thrombin inhibitors may be used for systemic anticoagulation or in the purge solution.[49]

18.5.4.5 Weaning

Once the decision has been made to wean the patient from support then the flow should be decreased 2 P-levels at a time as haemodynamically tolerated until reaching P2. If the patient tolerates P2, the catheter may be pulled completely into the aorta and systemic anticoagulation held. Once the ACT is less than 150 seconds, the flow is reduced to P-0 and the catheter and introducer may be removed. In general, the longer the Impella has been in place, the longer the weaning process will take. If utilised to support HR-PCI weaning should take 5–10 minutes; however, if it has been left in for several days then it may take hours.

18.6 Extracorporeal membrane oxygenation

18.6.1 Introduction and components

ECMO is a form of mechanical cardiopulmonary support that can be provided for a prolonged period. There are two general modes of ECMO support: (1) veno-venous (VV) and (2) VA (Figure 18.13). In VV ECMO, blood is taken from the right atrium then oxygenated and CO_2 removed prior to being returned to the right atrium. This form of ECMO provides only respiratory support with the patient still being dependent on his or her own haemodynamic condition. In contrast, VA ECMO provides both respiratory and haemodynamic support. In this case, blood is pulled from the venous system (right atrium or inferior vena cava [IVC]) and following gas exchange is delivered back to the arterial system at either central or peripheral cannulation sites.

There are a variety of configurations for an ECMO system, however, there are several fundamental components including (1) drainage and perfusion cannulae, (2) centrifugal (most common) or roller pump and (3) membrane oxygenator and heat exchanger.

Our discussion here will focus on VA ECMO and its role in haemodynamic support for patients with cardiogenic shock or requiring salvage during cardiac arrest.[50–52] There are a number of indications for VA ECMO summarised in Table 18.3.[53] ECMO is not initiated for the sole purpose of supporting HR-PCI. On the contrary, it is the pre-existing form of support for post-surgical or arrest patients who now require cardiac catheterisation and if need be intervention.

VA ECMO should be used in those thought to have a reversible course of cardiac failure; however, it may be utilised as bridge to advanced therapies.[54–56] Patients who fail to wean from CPB following cardiac surgery can also be transitioned to VA ECMO.[50,51]

18.6.2 Haemodynamic effects

There are two competing effects of ECMO on the left ventricle. As blood is pulled from the venous system, there is a decrease in preload and consequently the end-diastolic volume and end-diastolic pressure in the left ventricle, which reduces wall tension and work. In contrast, as blood returns to the arterial system, there is an increase in afterload and work.[57]

18.6.3 Technical considerations and contraindications

Contraindications to ECMO include the presence of an irreversible process, multi-organ failure, prolonged CPR (>60 minutes), aortic dissection and severe aortic regurgitation. In addition, patients with active bleeding or with contraindication to anti-coagulation are generally not candidates for ECMO support. Another factor to consider includes the presence of significant peripheral arterial disease.

Cannulae for VA ECMO can be placed either centrally or peripherally. Central access usually consists of the drainage cannula placed in the right atrium and the perfusion cannula in the ascending aorta. This approach requires a sternotomy or thoracotomy and is most often an option for those surgical patients who fail to wean from CPB. Peripheral cannulation may require a cut down but can often be performed percutaneously. The drainage cannula may access the venous circulation at the jugular or femoral vein. The perfusion cannular is most often placed in the femoral artery but may also utilise the axillary, subclavian or in rare circumstances the

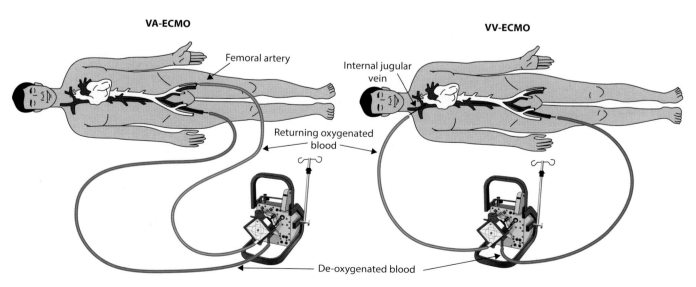

Figure 18.13 Venoarterial and veno-venous extracorporeal membrane oxygenation configuration.

Table 18.3 Indications for venoarterial extracorporeal membrane oxygenation

Cardiogenic shock: with or without myocardial infarction
Fulminant myocarditis
Pulmonary hypertension and right heart failure
Pulmonary embolus with haemodynamic compromise
Cardiac arrest (assisted cardiopulmonary resuscitation)
Medication overdose
Non-ischaemic cardiomyopathy including sepsis-induced cardiomyopathy
Bridge to decision for transplant or VAD
Support postcardiac surgery

Source: Mehta, H. et al., Indications and complications for VA-ECMO for cardiac failure. Latest in Cardiology @ ACC.org. July 14, 2015.
LVAD, left ventricular assist device.

carotid artery (although this site is more commonly used in infants). In femoral artery cannulation, especially in patients with peripheral vascular disease, there may be a need to place an additional cannula into the femoral artery directing blood flow anterograde down the ipsilateral limb in order to prevent ischaemia.

18.6.4 Management

The active management of ECMO can become quite complex and outside of the scope of this chapter. We aim to address several of the more practical aspects to management. A perfusionist is required to manage the ECMO circuits and should be present during any procedure in the cardiac cath lab. Anticoagulation is key in preventing the formation of thrombus in the system. Heparin is most commonly used with goal ACT of 180–250.

Common complications include bleeding, thrombosis, infection and limb ischaemia.[58] Haemorrhage is often seen and most commonly involves the access site but may occur in any organ and can be devastating when the central nervous system is involved.[58] The risk of thrombosis can range from 8% to 17%.[58] Managing the balance between the risks for haemorrhage and trombosis requires frequent monitoring. The risk of infection of any indwelling line must be recognised and appropriate aseptic procedures followed. Limb ischaemia can be secondary to a direct effect of the cannula interrupting distal flow or from an embolic phenomenon. Supplemental antegrade flow via a cannula placed in the femoral artery as previously mentioned may be help circumvent this problem. Other options include a cannula placed in the dorsalis pedis or posterior tibial arteries.[57]

References

1. Moulopoulos SD et al. Diastolic balloon pumping (with carbon dioxide) in the aorta – a mechanical assistance to the failing circulation. Am Heart J 1962; 63: 669–75.

2. Thiele H et al. Shock in acute myocardial infarction: The Cape Horn for trials? Eur Heart J 2010; 31: 1828–35.

3. Scheidt S et al. Intra-aortic balloon counterpulsation in cardiogenic shock. Report of a co-operative clinical trial. N Engl J Med 1973; 288: 979–84.

4. Sjauw KD et al. A systematic review and meta-analysis of intra-aortic balloon pump therapy in ST-elevation myocardial infarction: Should we change the guidelines? Eur Heart J 2009; 30: 459–68.

5. Abdel-Wahab M et al. Comparison of hospital mortality with intra-aortic balloon counterpulsation insertion before versus after primary percutaneous coronary intervention for cardiogenic shock complicating acute myocardial infarction. Am J Cardiol 2010; 105: 967–71.

6. Thiele H et al. Intraaortic balloon support for myocardial infarction with cardiogenic shock. N Engl J Med 2012; 367: 1287–96.

7. Perera D et al. Elective intra-aortic balloon counter pulsation during high-risk percutaneous coronary intervention: A randomized controlled trial. JAMA 2010; 304: 867–74.

8. Perera D et al. Long-term mortality data from the balloon pump-assisted coronary intervention study (BCIS-1): A randomized, controlled trial of elective balloon counterpulsation during high-risk percutaneous coronary intervention. Circulation 2013; 127: 207–12.

9. O'Gara PT et al. 2013 ACCF/AHA guideline for the management of ST-elevation myocardial infarction: A report of the American College of Cardiology Foundation/American Heart Association Task Force on Practice Guidelines. J Am Coll Cardiol 2013; 61: e78–e140.

10. Kar B et al. Use of the TandemHeart percutaneous ventricular assist device to support patients undergoing high-risk percutaneous coronary intervention. J Invasive Cardiol 2006; 18(4): A6.

11. Kar B et al. Clinical experience with the TandemHeart percutaneous ventricular assist device. Tex Heart Inst J. 2006; 33(2): 111–5.

12. Vranckx P et al. The TandemHeart, percutaneous transseptal left ventricular assist device: A safeguard in high-risk percutaneous coronary interventions. The six-year Rotterdam experience. EuroIntervention 2008; 4(3): 331–7.

13. Burkhoff D et al. A randomized multicenter clinical study to evaluate the safety and efficacy of the TandemHeart percutaneous ventricular assist device versus conventional therapy with intraaortic balloon pumping for treatment of cardiogenic shock. Am Heart J 2006; 152(3): 469.e1–e8.

14. Thiele H et al. Randomized comparison of intra-aortic balloon support with a percutaneous left ventricular assist device in patients with revascularized acute myocardial infarction complicated by cardiogenic shock. Eur Heart J 2005; 26(13): 1276–83.

15. Alli OO et al. Percutaneous left ventricular assist device with TandemHeart for high-risk percutaneous coronary intervention: The Mayo Clinic experience. Cathet Cardiovasc Interv 2012; 80(5): 728–34.

16. Thomas JL et al. Use of a percutaneous left ventricular assist device for high-risk cardiac interventions and cardiogenic shock. J Invasive Cardiol 2010; 22: 360–4.

17. Valgimigli M et al. Left ventricular unloading and concomitant total cardiac output increase by the use of percutaneous Impella Recover LP 2.5 assist device during high-risk coronary intervention. Cathet Cardiovasc Interv 2005; 65: 263–7.

18. Henriques JP et al. Safety and feasibility of elective high-risk percutaneous coronary intervention procedures with left ventricular support of the Impella Recover LP 2.5. *Am J Cardiol* 2006; 97: 990–92.

19. Burzotta F et al. Feasibility and long-term safety of elective Impella-assisted high-risk percutaneous coronary intervention: A pilot two-centre study. *Cardiovasc Med (Hagerstown)* 2008; 9(10): 1004–10.

20. Dixon SR et al. A prospective feasibility trial investigating the use of the Impella 2.5 system in patients undergoing high-risk percutaneous coronary intervention (The PROTECT I Trial): Initial U.S. experience. *J Am Coll Cardiol Interv* 2009; 2: 91–6.

21. Seyfarth M et al. A randomized clinical trial to evaluate the safety and efficacy of a percutaneous left ventricular assist device versus intra-aortic balloon pumping for treatment of cardiogenic shock caused by myocardial infarction. *J Am Coll Cardiol* 2008; 52: 1584–8.

22. Maini B et al. Real-world use of the Impella 2.5 circulatory support system in complex high-risk percutaneous coronary intervention: The USpella Registry. *Catheter Cardiovasc Interv* 2012; 80: 717–25.

23. Sjauw KD et al. Supported high-risk percutaneous coronary intervention with the Impella 2.5 device: The Europella registry. *J Am Coll Cardiol* 2009; 54: 2430–34.

24. O'Neill WW. The current use of Impella 2.5 in acute myocardial infarction complicated by cardiogenic shock: Results from the USpella Registry. *J Interv Cardiol* 2014; 27(1): 1–11.

25. Dangas GD et al. Impact of hemodynamic support with Impella 2.5 versus intra-aortic balloon pump on prognostically important clinical outcomes in patients undergoing high-risk percutaneous coronary intervention (from the PROTECT II randomized trial). *Am J Cardiol* 2014; 113: 222–8.

26. Myat A et al. Percutaneous circulatory assist devices for high-risk coronary intervention. *JACC Cardiovasc Interv* 2015; 8(2): 229–44.

27. Thiagarajan RR et al. Extracorporeal membrane oxygenation to support cardiopulmonary resuscitation in adults. *Ann Thorac Surg* 2009; 87: 778–85.

28. Grambow DW et al. Emergent percutaneous cardiopulmonary bypass in patients having cardiovascular collapse in the cardiac catheterization laboratory. *Am J Cardiol* 1994; 73: 872–5.

29. Chen JS et al. Analysis of the outcome for patients experiencing myocardial infarction and cardiopulmonary resuscitation refractory to conventional therapies necessitating extracorporeal life support rescue. *Crit Care Med* 2006; 34: 950–7.

30. Nichol G et al. Systematic review of percutaneous cardiopulmonary bypass for cardiac arrest or cardiogenic shock states. *Resuscitation* 2006; 70: 381–94.

31. Sheu JJ et al. Early extracorporeal membrane oxygenator-assisted primary percutaneous coronary intervention improved 30-day clinical outcomes in patients with ST-segment elevation myocardial infarction complicated with profound cardiogenic shock. *Crit Care Med* 2010; 38: 1810–17.

32. Koutouzis M et al. Percutaneous coronary intervention facilitated by extracorporeal membrane oxygenation support in a patient with cardiogenic shock. *Hellenic J Cardiol* 2010; 51(3): 271–4.

33. Tsao NW et al. Extracorporeal membrane oxygenation-assisted primary percutaneous coronary intervention may improve survival of patients with acute myocardial infarction complicated by profound cardiogenic shock. *J Crit Care* 2012; 27(5): 530.e1–e11.

34. Dardas P et al. ECMO as a bridge to high-risk rotablation of heavily calcified coronary arteries. *Herz* 2012; 37: 225–30.

35. Ricciardi M et al. Emergency extracorporeal membrane oxygenation (ECMO)-supported percutaneous coronary interventions in the fibrillating heart. *Catheter Cardiovasc Interv* 1999; 48: 402–5.

36. Vanzetto G et al. Percutaneous extracorporeal life support in acute severe hemodynamic collapses: Single centre experience in 100 consecutive patients. *Can J Cardiol* 2009; 25: e179–e186.

37. Kagawa E et al. Should we emergently revascularize occluded coronaries for cardiac arrest?: Rapid-response extracorporeal membrane oxygenation and intra-arrest percutaneous coronary intervention. *Circulation* 2012; 126(13): 1605–13.

38. Wu MY et al. Using extracorporeal membrane oxygenation to rescue acute myocardial infarction with cardiopulmonary collapse: The impact of early coronary revascularization. *Resuscitation* 2013; 84(7): 940–5.

39. Tomasello SD et al. Outcome of extracorporeal membrane oxygenation support for complex high-risk elective percutaneous coronary interventions: A single-center experience. *Heart Lung* 2015; 44(4): 309–13.

40. Arlt M et al. Early experiences with miniaturized extracorporeal life-support in the catheterization laboratory. *Eur J Cardiothorac Surg* 2012; 42: 858–63.

41. Kim JT et al. The carina as a useful radiographic landmark for positioning the intraaortic balloon pump. *Anesth Analg* 2007; 105(3): 735–8.

42. Raman J et al. Subclavian artery access for ambulatory balloon pump insertion. *Ann Thorac Surg* 2010; 90(3): 1032.

43. Thiele H et al. Reversal of cardiogenic shock by percutaneous left atrial-to-femoral arterial bypass assistance. *Circulation* 2001; 104(24): 2917–22.

44. De Ponti R et al. Trans-septal catheterization in the electrophysiology laboratory: Data from a multicenter survey spanning 12 years. *J Am Coll Cardiol* 2006; 47: 1037–42.

45. Earley MJ. How to perform a transseptal puncture. *Heart* 2009; 95(1): 85–92.

46. Naidu SS. Novel percutaneous cardiac assist devices: the science of and indications for hemodynamic support. *Circulation* 2011; 123(5): 533–43.

47. Remmelink M et al. Effects of left ventricular unloading by Impella Recover LP 2.5 on coronary hemodynamics. *Cathet Cardiovasc Interv* 2007; 70: 532–7.

48. Ostadal P et al. Direct comparison of percutaneous circulatory support systems in specific hemodynamic conditions in a porcine model. *Circ Arrhythm Electrophysiol* 2012; 5: 120.

49. Burzotta F et al. Impella ventricular support in clinical practice: Collaborative viewpoint from a European expert user group. *Int J Cardiol* 2015; 201: 684–91.

50. Mikus E et al. CentriMag venoarterial extracorporeal membrane oxygenation support as treatment for patients with refractory postcardiotomy cardiogenic shock. *ASAIO J* 2013; 59(1): 18–23.

51. Slottosch I et al. Outcomes after peripheral extracorporeal membrane oxygenation therapy for postcardiotomy cardiogenic shock: A single-center experience. *J Surg Res* 2013; 181(2): e47–e55.

52. Kim H et al. Efficacy of veno-arterial extracorporeal membrane oxygenation in acute myocardial infarction with cardiogenic shock. *Resuscitation* 2012; 83(8): 971–5.

53. Mehta H et al. Indications and complications for VA-ECMO for cardiac failure. *Latest in Cardiology @ ACC.org.* July 14, 2015.

54. John R et al. Experience with the Levitronix CentriMag circulatory support system as a bridge to decision in patients with refractory acute cardiogenic shock and multisystem organ failure. *J Thorac Cardiovasc Surg* 2007; 134(2): 351–8.

55. Russo CF et al. Veno-arterial extracorporeal membrane oxygenation using Levitronix centrifugal pump as bridge to decision for refractory cardiogenic shock. *J Thorac Cardiovasc Surg* 2010; 140(6): 1416–21.

56. Barth E et al. Extracorporeal life support as a bridge to high-urgency heart transplantation. *Clin Transplant* 2012; 26(3): 484–8.

57. Chung M et al. Monitoring of the adult patient on veno-arterial extracorporeal membrane oxygenation. *Scientific World Journal* 2014; 2014.

58. Gaffney AM et al. Extracorporeal life support. *BMJ* 2010; 341, Article ID c5317.

Acute coronary syndrome: PCI for unstable angina and non-ST elevation myocardial infarction

CLAIRE MCCUNE, IAN MENOWN

19.1 Introduction

Acute coronary syndrome (ACS) encompasses a spectrum of ischaemic conditions typically related to plaque rupture or erosion with subsequent thrombus formation and partial or complete coronary occlusion.[1] After further investigation including a 12-lead electrocardiogram (ECG) and biomarkers, the term ACS is usually subdivided into ST-elevation myocardial infarction (STEMI) and non-stent thrombosis (ST) elevation acute coronary syndrome (NSTEACS) the latter in turn being subdivided into non-ST-elevation myocardial infarction (NSTEMI) if biomarkers are elevated and unstable angina if biomarkers are normal (Figure 19.1). Older literature may use the terms Q wave myocardial infarction (MI) and non-Q wave MI, but these are best defined at discharge and are of limited practical value at acute presentation.

This chapter describes practical aspects of contemporary percutaneous coronary intervention (PCI) practice in unstable angina and NSTEMI (while PCI for STEMI is addressed later).

19.2 Epidemiology

The annual incidence of NSTEMI is higher than STEMI and this trend is increasing, likely due to ongoing improvements in primary and secondary prevention. Although STEMI may be associated with higher in-hospital mortality, NSTEMI is associated with higher long-term mortality.[2]

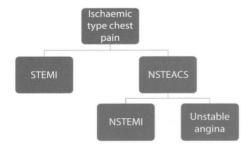

Figure 19.1 The spectrum of acute coronary syndrome.

19.3 Clinical assessment

Unlike STEMI, symptom presentation in NSTEACS is often vague or atypical leading to a delayed diagnosis. This symptom pattern is likely due to the pathophysiological findings of sub-occlusive plaque transiently occluding/reopening/re-occluding and may explain the frequently encountered stuttering presentation. The determination of event onset in NSTEMI is thus also less precise than in STEMI. In addition, some patients with an NSTEMI presentation may even be delayed STEMI in which the initial ST elevation has resolved. Understanding of this is important when considering the optimal PCI approach.

19.3.1 ECG

A 12-lead ECG is recommended within 10 minutes of first medical contact. While classic features include ST depression (Figure 19.2), T wave inversion or transient ST elevation, the initial ECG may be normal in up to half of patients. In patients with ongoing symptoms but normal 12-lead ECG, additional leads V7-V9 or V3R-V4R or by body surface map[3] may detect distal circumflex or right ventricular related ST elevation which is of practical relevance since they behave more like a conventional STEMI patient in the cath lab.

19.3.2 Biomarkers

Myocardial ischaemia leads to a dynamic elevation of cardiac troponin >99th percentile of healthy individual levels. However, troponin elevation must be interpreted within the context of the patient's clinical presentation and other investigations. Older troponin assays have typically required a repeat sample at 6 or 12 hours to rule in/rule out MI. The time interval to the second sample may be shortened by use of high-sensitivity troponin. The European Society of Cardiology (ESC) has recommended use of a 0-hour/3-hour pathway (Figure 19.3) which may enable earlier diagnosis and potentially earlier treatment, or if MI is ruled out, earlier discharge. A rapid rise on from the first to second sample

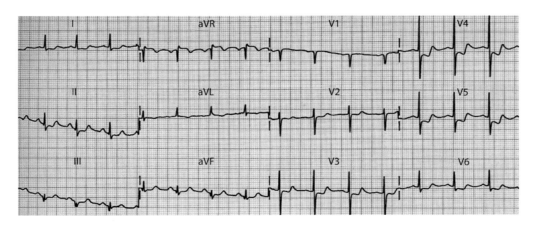

Figure 19.2 ECG illustrating ST depression. (Adapted from Menown, I.B., *Am J Cardiol.*, 85, 8, 2000.)

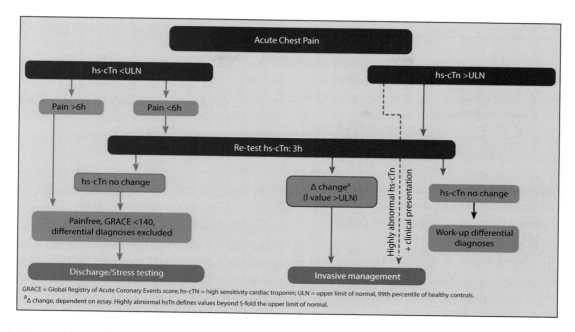

Figure 19.3 0-hour/3-hour rule-out algorithm of non-ST-elevation ACSs using high-sensitivity cardiac troponin assays. (From 2015 ESC Guidelines for the management of acute coronary syndromes in patents presenting without persistent ST-segment elevation.)

is a helpful marker of acute ischaemic insult although a high initial value is adequate for diagnosis, and delayed NSTEMI presentations >12–24 hours may not necessarily show further rise on repeat sample.

An even earlier 0-hour/1-hour pathway may be possible using high-sensitivity troponin with a validated algorithm.[4] Research is also ongoing for alternative biomarkers such as copeptin (C-terminal provasopressin) which is released earlier than troponin in MI and heart-type fatty acid binding protein which has been found to indicate risk across the ACS spectrum (including troponin-negative patients).[4]

19.3.3 Differential diagnosis of troponin elevation

While new high-sensitivity troponin assays improve sensitivity and specificity for myocardial necrosis they are frequently elevated with non-ACS causes of myocardial stress as described in the following box.

DIFFERENTIAL DIAGNOSIS OF CARDIAC TROPONIN ELEVATION

Cardiac causes
- Acute coronary syndromes
- Tachyarrhythmias
- Heart failure/Myocarditis/Tako-Tsubo cardiomyopathy/Infiltrative disease/Drug toxicity
- Structural heart disease (e.g. aortic stenosis)

- Coronary spasm
- Cardiac contusion or cardiac procedures

Extra-cardiac causes
- Aortic dissection
- Pulmonary embolism/Pulmonary hypertension
- Renal dysfunction
- Acute neurological events
- Hypo and hyperthyroidism
- Extreme physical endurance
- Rhabdomyolysis
- Critical illness
- Hypertensive emergencies

Thus, the universal definition of acute MI requires detection of a rise and/or fall of cardiac biomarkers (preferably troponin) with at least one value >99th percentile of the upper reference limit (URL) *plus* evidence of myocardial ischaemia as recognised by clinical symptoms of ischaemia and/or ECG changes.[5] Distinct subtypes are recognised. Type 1 MI, the major focus for this chapter, is a primary coronary event as evidenced by a raised biomarker (preferably troponin) in the setting of symptoms of ischaemia and new ECG changes. Type 2 MI, which may be seen with the differential diagnoses above, is secondary to ischaemia from an imbalance between oxygen supply and demand. Type 3 MI is sudden cardiac death, accompanied by new ECG change, or verified coronary thrombus by angiography or autopsy, but death occurring before blood samples could be taken. Type 4 MI is associated with PCI and type 5 associated with coronary artery bypass surgery.

19.4 Initial risk stratification

While pharmacological and revascularisation strategies can improve the prognosis, risks of treatment may outweigh benefit in some patients especially those at low cardiovascular (CV) risk or high bleeding risk[6] and thus early and accurate risk stratification is required.

While troponin contributes significantly to risk assessment in clinical practice, simply classifying patients as 'troponin positive' or 'troponin negative' is less predictive of patient outcome than well-validated scoring systems such as Global Registry of Acute Coronary Events (GRACE) or thrombolysis in myocardial infarction (TIMI) risk scores which use multiple risk components.[7] Indeed, many troponin-positive patients may be at low to medium risk, whereas some troponin-negative patient may be at high risk.

19.4.1 TIMI score

The TIMI risk score (below box) was developed from the TIMI-11B trial in the 1990s to predict the occurrence of all-cause mortality, MI or urgent revascularisation at 14 days.[8] It was validated in later trials including VANQWISH and ESSENCE, but is less commonly used in current practice.

TIMI RISK SCORE FOR NSTEMI

Each individual risk parameter scores 1 point:

- Age ≥65 years
- ≥3 Risk Factors for coronary heart disease (CAD)
- Known CAD (stenosis ≥50%)
- Aspirin use in past 7 days
- Severe angina (≥2 episodes w/in 24 hours)
- ST changes ≥0.5 mm
- Cardiac biomarker change[8]

19.4.2 GRACE score

The GRACE score was developed from the GRACE registry and may be used in all subtypes of ACS.[9] It has also been externally validated,[10] has a higher discriminatory power than the TIMI score (c-statistic = 0.81 vs. 0.68; p = .02) and is used in current ESC guidelines.[11] Although the GRACE score uses standard clinical variables, it is algorithm based and thus requires use of an online or downloaded calculator which enables prediction of in-hospital, 6 month, 1- and 3-year mortality.[11] GRACE 2.0 was developed utilising the 'Mini-GRACE' algorithm for use when serum creatinine and Killip class may not be available (Figure 19.4).[11]

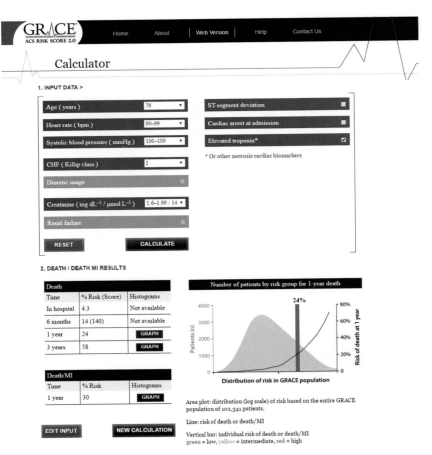

Figure 19.4 GRACE score variables and the Grace 2.0 risk calculator. http://gracescore.org/WebSite/WebVersion.aspx.

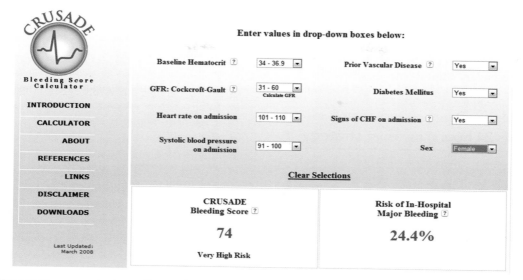

Figure 19.5 CRUSADE score calculator. (Reproduced with permission from Duke University.)

19.4.3 Bleeding risk

Bleeding risk is known to be associated with worse outcomes and is associated with factors such as advancing age, female gender, renal impairment and pre-existing anaemia.

The CRUSADE score has been developed and validated as a means of quantifying bleeding risk for individual NSTEMI patients.[12] Like GRACE, CRUSADE uses standard clinical variables entered into an online algorithm (Figure 19.5) (http://www.crusadebleedingscore.org/index .html) and may be considered in patients undergoing coronary angiography to quantify bleeding risk, Class IIb Level B.[4]

19.5 Invasive assessment

19.5.1 Routine invasive versus initial conservative strategies

Most patients with NSTEMI benefit from a routine invasive versus initial conservative strategy whereas in patients without NSTEMI whose symptoms settle and who have a GRACE score <140, an initially conservative approach may be reasonable (Figure 19.3). A meta-analysis of randomised NSTEACS trials showed significant reductions in composite death, MI or rehospitalisation for ACS at 1 year overall, but particularly in biomarker-positive patients and with no benefit in biomarker-negative women.[13] TACTICS TIMI 18 reported that the magnitude of ST segments deviation and troponin elevation in patients with NSTEACS predicted those who benefitted from an early invasive strategy.[14] A meta-analysis of NSTEACS patients from FRISC-II, ICTUS and RITA-3 reported a 19% reduction in CV death or nonfatal MI at 5 years with a routine invasive strategy (14.7% vs.

17.9%; hazard ratio [HR] 0.81, 95% confidence interval [CI] 0.71–0.93; p = .002) with patients at highest risk receiving greatest benefit.[15]

19.5.2 Timing of an invasive approach

Studies to date have shown conflicting results with regards to the optimal timing of the invasive approach in NSTEACS. Many older predate contemporary practice and are difficult to compare due to different procedural practices. Current guidelines thus take a relatively pragmatic approach.

19.5.3 Immediate invasive strategy (<2 hours)

Highest risk NSTEMI patients are not well represented in clinical studies. The consensus of both European and American guidelines is that patients at highest risk should have an immediate (<2 hours) invasive angiography regardless of ECG or biomarker findings.[6,16]

An immediate invasive strategy (<2 hour) is recommended in patients with at least one of the following very high-risk criteria:

- Haemodynamic instability or cardiogenic shock
- Recurrent or ongoing chest pain refractory to medical treatment
- Life-threatening arrhythmias or cardiac arrest
- Mechanical complications of MI
- Acute heart failure with refractory angina or ST deviation
- Recurrent dynamic ST or T wave changes, particularly intermittent ST elevation

Class I Level C[4]

However, for patients without one or more very-high-risk criteria (see previous page), an immediate <2 hours (primary PCI like) versus >2-hour strategy has not been found of benefit with respect to biomarker elevation after intervention or secondary clinical outcomes.[4]

19.5.4 Early (<24 hours) invasive strategy

An early (<24 hours) versus later invasive strategy was assessed in a meta-analysis of seven randomised studies [$n = 5,370$] and four observational studies [$n = 77,499$], including ISAR-COOL, ELISA, OPTIMA, LIPSIA-NSTEMI, ABOARD and TIMACS, and did not show any benefit with respect to death, MI or major bleeds. The early strategy was associated with a lower risk of refractory ischaemia (3.8% vs. 7.3%; OR 0.55 [95% CI 0.35, 0.86]; $p = .008$). A pre-specified analysis of TIMACS found that early intervention in patients with high GRACE score improved the primary endpoint (composite of death, MI or stroke at 6 months) (HR 0.65; 95% CI, 0.48–0.89) but not in patients with low-to-intermediate GRACE score (HR 1.12; 95% CI, 0.81–1.56; $p = .01$).[17]

Based on current evidence, the ESC recommend that patients who meet criteria for high risk (as detailed in the following box) should have an early invasive strategy.[6]

An early invasive strategy (<24 hour) is recommended in patients with at least one of the following high-risk criteria:

- Rise or fall in cardiac troponin compatible with MI
- Dynamic ST- or T-wave changes (symptomatic or silent)
- GRACE score >140

Class I Level A[4]

19.5.5 Routine (<72 hours) invasive strategy

Patients at lower risk (i.e., without relevant troponin rise, dynamic ECG change or GRACE > 140) but with a secondary high-risk criterion (see below) should be considered for invasive assessment during the hospital stay and preferably within 72 hours as per ESC guidelines.[6]

However, there is controversy over the interpretation of optimum timing of this approach due to variation in trial procedure. Current National Institute for Health and Care Excellence (NICE) UK guidance recommends invasive assessment within 96 hours for patients with a predicted 6-month mortality above 3.0%.[7]

An invasive strategy (<72 hour) is recommended in patients with at least one of the following intermediate-risk criteria:

- Diabetes mellitus
- Renal insufficiency (eGFR <60 mL/min/1.73 m2)
- LVEF <40% or congestive heart failure
- Early post-infarction angina
- Recent PCI
- Prior CABG
- GRACE risk score > 109 and <140
- Recurrent symptoms or known ischaemia on non-invasive testing

Class I Level A[4]

19.5.6 Non-invasive assessment prior to discharge

Low-risk patients who do not meet any secondary high-risk criteria should have a non-invasive ischaemia assessment before discharge with invasive management for positive ischaemia testing.[6,7]

In patients with none of the aforementioned risk criteria and no recurrent symptoms, non-invasive testing for ischaemia (preferably with imaging) is recommended before deciding on an invasive evaluation. Class I Level A[4]

19.6 Angiography

19.6.1 Access

Given the increased bleeding risk for ACS patients in the setting of potent antithrombotic therapy, the choice of access route is of practical relevance.

The MATRIX trial, which enrolled 8,404 ACS patients undergoing urgent angiography (80% with follow on PCI) reported radial versus femoral access was associated with a 33% reduction in non-coronary artery bypass graft (CABG) major bleeding (1·6% vs. 2·3%, relative risk [RR] 0·67; 95% CI 0·49–0·92; $p = .013$), a 14.6% trend towards reduced death, MI or stroke (8.8% vs. 10.3%).[18]

Radial access by experienced operators is thus recommended over the transfemoral access in ACS and is easily managed post procedure (Figure 19.6).

Since the femoral approach still has a role for procedures such as intra-aortic balloon counter pulsation implantation, it is important to maintain proficiency with femoral technique.[4] For patients with poor bilateral radial access, the ulnar route may be an alternative non-femoral option and is currently being evaluated in clinical studies.[19]

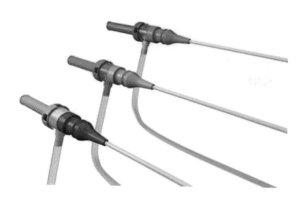

Figure 19.6 Radial artery access. (Reproduced with permission from Terumo.)

Radial over femoral access is recommended for coronary angiography and PCI. Class I Level A[4]

19.6.2 The culprit lesion

The culprit lesion in NSTEACS can be more difficult to characterise than in ST elevation acute coronary syndrome (STEACS) with many patients having multiple lesions that could fulfil the criteria for a culprit lesion. Regional ECG or echocardiographic findings may help with localisation and two of the following characteristics should be present to identify a lesion as a culprit lesion.[4]

Angiographic features of a culprit lesion (two or more suggestive):

- Intraluminal filling defects consistent with thrombus
- Plaque ulceration
- Plaque irregularity
- Dissection
- Impaired flow

Although fractional flow reserve has an established role with stable coronary disease, it has a more limited role in NSTEACS where microvascular dysfunction can lead to overestimation of fractional flow reserve (FFR) values and therefore underestimation of stenosis severity.[20] Intravascular imaging by intravascular ultrasound (IVUS) (Figure 19.7) or optical coherence tomography (OCT) (Figure 19.8) may help identify ruptured plaques or thrombus. On IVUS, typical features of AMI include plaque rupture, thrombus, positive remodelling, attenuated plaque, spotty calcification, and thin-cap fibroatheroma. IVUS may allow more appropriate stent sizing and has been associated with reduced in-hospital mortality post-MI.[21] However, with higher costs and procedural risks, intravascular imaging is not required routinely in NSTEMI.[22,23]

19.7 Pharmacological adjuncts and controversies

19.7.1 Timing of antiplatelet loading

It is generally accepted that NSTEMI patients should be loaded with aspirin at presentation, but optimum timing of P2Y12 initiation remains unclear. Whilst pre-treatment may lead to better levels of intra-procedural platelet inhibition, there are risks of overtreatment and bleeding as well as a potential delay to surgery for patients who require CABG.

Established and more recent studies have only partly addressed the question (Figures 19.8 and 19.9).

In the ACCOAST (A Comparison of Prasugrel at PCI or Time of Diagnosis of Non-ST-Elevation Myocardial Infarction) study, NSTEMI patients scheduled for early invasive strategy, prasugrel pre-treatment versus prasugrel delayed until after diagnostic angiography (mean time difference 4.3 hours) was not associated with reduction in the composite of CV death, MI, CVA (cerebrovascular accident), urgent revascularisation or bailout use of glycoprotein IIb/IIIa inhibition ($p = .81$) but was associated with an increase in TIMI major bleeding and life-threatening non-CABG bleeding.[24] Thus, pre-treatment with prasugrel prior to PCI is not recommended.

There are no prospective data regarding optimum timing of clopidogrel and ticagrelor. Expert opinion suggests avoiding clopidogrel and ticagrelor pre-treatment in patients with a shorter delay (<48 hours) until angiography, and considering pre-treating patients with longer waits (>48 hours) but further prospective research is required.[25] Intravenous Cangrelor enables rapid onset and offset of P2Y12 effect and may have a logical role in short-delay patients.

19.7.2 Duration of antiplatelet therapy after NSTEMI

The current recommendation is for 12 months of dual antiplatelet therapy (DAPT) following NSTEMI regardless of revascularisation strategy or stent type.[4] This is based on the practice within studies such as CURE, TRITON TIMI 38, PLATO and CREDO (unless there is a contraindication such as excessive bleeding) and then long-term monotherapy (with aspirin or P2Y12).

19.7.3 Shorter duration DAPT after PCI in NSTEMI

Shorter duration DAPT may be reasonable for patients deemed to be at high bleeding risk which is thought to outweigh their ischaemic risk (Class IIb Level A[4]). Already

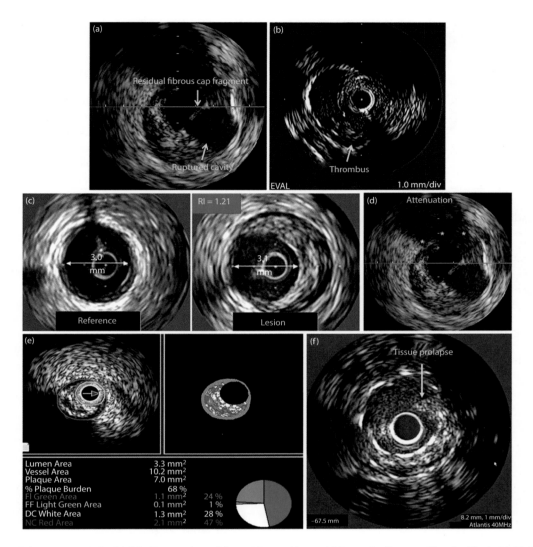

Figure 19.7 IVUS features in NSTEACS. (Reproduced from Young Hong, Y.J. et al., *Korean Circ J.*, 45, 4, 2015. With permission.)

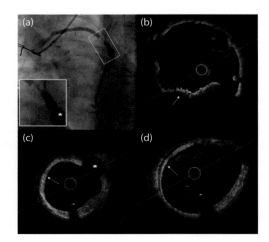

Figure 19.8 OCT appearance from a patient with lateral NSTEACS due to a vein graft culprit. (Reproduced from Davlouros, P. et al., *J Am Coll Cardiol Intv*, 4, 2011. With permission.)

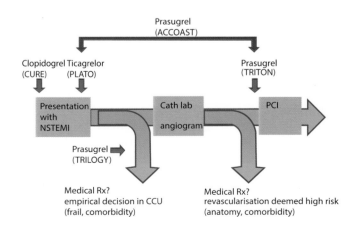

Figure 19.9 Variation in timing of P2Y12 administration during the NSTEMI pathway between different clinical trials.

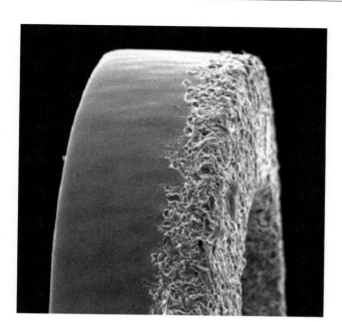

Figure 19.10 BioFreedom stainless steel stent incorporating a novel microporous abluminal surface. Reproduced with permission from Biosensors.

contemporary third generation stents with permanent polymer only require a 6-month course of DAPT, with a 3-month course thought reasonable in patients at high bleeding risk.

The BioFreedom stent has a novel microporous abluminal surface which enables controlled release of Biolimus A9, with therapeutic concentrations in local tissue sustained up to 28 days post-implantation (Figure 19.10). The absence of surface polymer may facilitate early stent healing and a shorter course of DAPT.

In the ACS sub-study of the LEADERS-FREE trial, BioFreedom versus bare metal stent was associated with a 57% reduction in the primary efficacy endpoint of clinically driven TLR (3.9 vs. 9.0%, $p = .009$), and a 50% reduction in the primary safety endpoint of CV death, stent thrombosis or MI (9.3 vs. 18.5%, $p = .001$), driven by lower rates of cardiac mortality (3.4 vs. 6.9%, $p = .049$) and MI (6.9 vs. 13.8%, $p = .005$). For patients at higher bleeding risk undergoing PCI following NSTEMI, use of newer rapidly healing stents such as BioFreedom appears logical (rather than bare metal stent or conventional DES) to allow flexibility for shorter course DAPT if required.

19.7.4 Extended duration DAPT?

The value of prolonged DAPT beyond 1 year in high-risk patients is a subject of ongoing research. The DAPT study randomised patients who had undergone PCI and tolerated an initial 12 months DAPT to an additional 18 months of DAPT versus discontinuation of DAPT. In the subgroup who presented with acute MI ($n = 3,576$), extended duration DAPT was associated with reduced stent thrombosis (0.5% vs. 1.9%, $p < .001$) and MACCE (3.9% vs. 6.8%; $p < .001$) but increased GUSTO moderate or severe

bleeding (1.9% vs. 0.8%, $p = .005$).[26] A 'DAPT score' has been developed from the DAPT study dataset to help identify high-risk patients who are most likely to benefit from prolonged duration therapy.

The PEGASUS-TIMI 54 trial randomised 21,162 patients with prior MI (<3 years) to ticagrelor for up to 3 years versus placebo.[27] Two doses of ticagrelor were tested with the lower 60 mg bd dose subsequently licenced for this indication. Ticagrelor 60 mg bd was associated with a significant reduction in CV death, MI or stroke versus placebo (7.77% vs. 9.04%; HR 0.84; $p = .004$). There was no difference in intracranial haemorrhage or fatal bleeding although TIMI major bleeding was twice as frequent.

> P2Y12 inhibitor administration in addition to aspirin beyond 1 year may be considered after careful assessment of the ischaemic and bleeding risks of the patient. Class IIb Level A[4]

19.7.5 Specific antithrombotic therapeutics in NSTEMI

Detailed descriptions of antithrombotic drugs for PCI are included in later chapters but considerations relevant to NSTEACS patients are described below.

19.7.6 Aspirin

Aspirin irreversibly inactivates cyclooxygenase, thereby inhibiting prostaglandin and thromboxane synthesis. In NSTEACS, an initial loading dose (300–325 mg) should be considered regardless of treatment strategy.[6] The CURRENT-OASIS 7 reported no benefit in aspirin doses higher than 75–150 mg in the long term.[28]

> Aspirin is recommended for all patients without contraindications at an initial oral loading dosed of 150–300 mg (in aspirin-naive patients) and a maintenance dose of 75–100 mg/day long-term regardless of treatment strategy. Class I Level A[4]

19.7.7 Clopidogrel

Clopidogrel, a thienopyridine, is an inactive prodrug which requires cytochrome P450 for activation and subsequent platelet P2Y12 inhibition.[4] The CURE study demonstrated the additional benefit of clopidogrel to aspirin in NSTEACS with or without PCI. CURRENT-OASIS 7 reported that enhanced dosing (600 mg loading, 150 mg daily for 7 days daily, then 75 mg daily) versus standard dosing (300 mg loading, then 75 mg daily) in NSTEMI patients undergoing PCI was associated with reduced CV death, MI or CVA at 30 days (3.9% vs. 4.5%; $p = .039$) and reduced definite stent thrombosis (0.7% vs. 1.3%; $p = .0001$) although more major bleeding (1.6% vs. 1.1%; $p = .009$).[28]

Even with a 600 mg pretreatment dose, some patients show high residual platelet reactivity (possibly related to gene polymorphisms). This variability in response, delay in onset of action and lower overall inhibition of platelet activation compared with prasugrel and ticagrelor has led to preference for the newer P2Y12 inhibitors in ESC guidelines.[4]

> Clopidogrel (300–600 mg loading dose, 75 mg daily dose) is recommended for patients who cannot receive ticagrelor or prasugrel or who require oral anticoagulation. Class 1 Level A[4]

19.7.8 Prasugrel

Prasugrel is a P2Y12 inhibitor and a prodrug with a more predictable and more rapid onset of action than clopidogrel. In the NSTEACS subgroup of TRITON-TIMI-38,[29] prasugrel versus clopidogrel was associated with an 18% reduction in the primary efficacy end point (CV death, non-fatal MI or non-fatal CVA) (HR 0.82; $p = .002$) although with higher non-CABG TIMI major bleeding (HR 1.40; $p = .02$). NSTEMI patients with diabetes and those with a stent thrombosis event on clopidogrel may derive particular benefit. Prasugrel is contraindicated in patients with prior TIA or stroke due to a finding of net harm. It is not generally recommended in those >75 years or with body weight <60 kg unless individual benefit is felt to outweigh risk (in which case a lower maintenance dose of 5 mg per day is recommended).

> - Prasugrel (60 mg loading dose, 10 mg daily dose) is recommended in patients who are proceeding to PCI if no contraindication. Class 1 Level B[4]
> - It is not recommended to administer prasugrel in patients in whom coronary anatomy is not known. Class III Level B[4]

19.7.9 Ticagrelor

Ticagrelor is a reversibly binding cyclopentyltriazolopyrimidine with a rapid onset of P2Y12 inhibition (30 minutes) but relatively faster offset of action and quicker platelet recovery.[4] In the NSTEACS subgroup of the PLATO study,[30] ticagrelor versus clopidogrel was associated with a 17% reduction in CV death, MI or CVA (10.0 vs. 12.3%; $p = .0013$) but increased non-CABG major bleeding (4.8 vs. 3.8%; HR 1.28; 95% CI = 1.05–1.56).

> Ticagrelor (180 mg loading dose, 90 mg twice daily) is recommended, in the absence of contraindications, for all patients at moderate-to-high risk of ischaemic events (e.g. elevated cardiac troponins), regardless of initial treatment strategy and including those pretreated with clopidogrel (which should be discontinued when ticagrelor is started). Class 1 Level B[4]

19.7.10 Cangrelor

Cangrelor is a potent intravenous nonthienopyridine adenosine triphosphate analogue with <10 minutes half-life. Prospective trial data in NSTEACS are awaited but intravenous P2Y12 inhibition could benefit patients undergoing urgent PCI instead of, or before full effectiveness of oral P2Y12 loading, and the fast offset could benefit those requiring early scheduling of CABG.

> Cangrelor may be considered in P2Y12 inhibitor–naïve patients undergoing PCI. Class IIb Level A[4]

19.7.11 Glycoprotein IIb/IIIa inhibitors

Control of platelet aggregation and binding to abnormal surfaces is mediated by GPIIb/IIIa receptors. While GP IIb/IIIa inhibitors had a strong position in older guidelines,[2] advances in PCI technique, stents and newer adjunctive pharmacotherapy has rendered their current position less certain and upstream (pre-cath lab) treatment is no longer recommended.[4]

> - GPIIb/IIIa inhibitors during PCI should be considered for bailout situations or thrombotic complications. Class IIa Level C[4]
> - It is not recommended to administer GPIIb/IIIa inhibitors in patients in whom coronary anatomy is not known. Class III Level A[4]

19.7.12 New antiplatelet drugs

Advances in understanding of platelet activation, amplification and aggregation has enabled identification of multiple potential therapeutic targets[31] such as direct thromboxane A2 antagonists (terutroban and picotamide), inhibition of collagen and ristocetin-mediated platelet function (DZ-697b), the phosphodiesterase III inhibitor (cilostazol) and inhibitors of the platelet thrombin receptor protease-activated receptor (PAR)-1 (e.g. vorapaxar and atopaxar). However, the additive benefit of any of these agents to current treatments for NSTEMI patients undergoing PCI remains to be established.

> Anticoagulation reduces the incidence of thrombus during instrumentation in PCI and is recommended for all patients in addition to antiplatelet therapy during PCI.[6]

19.8 Anticoagulation

19.8.1 Unfractionated heparin

Unfractionated heparin (UFH) has indirect anti-thrombin activity. Given its narrow therapeutic window it is often monitored in the lab using the activated clotting time (ACT) but due to the impracticalities of maintaining a therapeutic range over a longer period, it is now rarely used outside of the cardiac catheterisation lab.

- UFH prior to coronary angiography is recommended at a dose of 60–70 IU/kg i.v. (max 5000 IU) and infusion (12–15 IU/kg/h) (max 1000 IU/h), target aPTT 1.5–2.5× control.[6]
- During PCI according to ACT or 70–100 IU/kg i.v. in patients not anticoagulated (50–70 IU/kg if concomitant with GPIIb/IIIa inhibitors). Class I Level B[4]
- Additional ACT-guided i.v. boluses of UFH during PCI may be considered following initial UFH treatment. Class IIb Level B[4]

19.8.2 Bivalirudin

Bivalirudin is an intravenous direct antithrombin inhibitor. In the ACUITY trial with moderate to high-risk NSTEACS patients, in those who subsequently underwent PCI bivalirudin alone versus UFH plus GPIIb/IIIa was associated with less bleeding (4% vs. 7%, $p < .0001$) but increased rates of composite ischaemia (9% vs. 8%; $p = .45$).[32] In contrast, Bivalirudin plus GPIIb/IIIa versus UFH plus GPIIb/IIIa was not associated with any difference in outcomes.

Bivalirudin (0.75 mg/kg i.v. bolus, followed by 1.75 mg/kg/hour for up to 4 hours after the procedure) is recommended as an alternative to UFH plus GPIIb/IIIa inhibitors during PCI. Class 1 Level A[4]

19.8.3 Enoxaparin

Enoxaparin has several potential advantages over UFH including a more predictable dose-response, higher anti-factor Xa:IIa ratio, less inhibition by platelet factor 4, and helps inhibit the early rise in von Willebrand factor.[33,34] Use of 'stacked-on' UFH in subjects already receiving enoxaparin may result in excessive antithrombotic levels (over twice the therapeutic anti-Xa level and over three times the therapeutic anti-IIa level) despite ACT levels appearing acceptable.[35] Thus, in NSTEACS patients who have received recent enoxaparin and come for PCI, continuing anticoagulation with enoxaparin is preferred to 'stacked-on' UFH. No additional enoxaparin is required if the previous s.c. injection has been given within 8 hours. Between 8 and 12hours, to maintain optimum anti-Xa levels (0.5–1.2 IU/mL), enoxaparin i.v. (0.3 mg/kg) top-up should be given (Figure 19.11).[33]

Enoxaparin should be considered as an anticoagulant for PCI in patients pretreated with s.c. enoxaparin. Class IIa Level B[4]

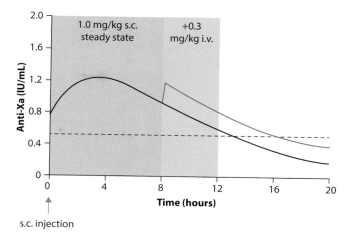

s.c. injection

Figure 19.11 Anti-Xa activity following subcutaneous injection of enoxaparin ±intravenous top-up. (Reproduced from Menown, I.B.A., *Br J Cardiol.*, 15, 2, 2008. With permission.)

19.8.4 Fondaparinux

While fondaparinux was found to have a favourable efficacy: bleeding profile in OASIS 5, it was associated with significantly higher incidence of catheter thrombosis even with use of a 100U UFH catheter flush. Thus, fondaparinux cannot be used to support patients undergoing PCI and full-dose UFH is recommended.

In patients on fondaparinux (2.5 mg s.c. daily) undergoing PCI, an (additional) i.v. bolus of UFH (70–85 IU/kg, or 50–60 IU/kg in the case of concomitant use of GPIIb/IIIa inhibitors) is recommended during the procedure. Class I Level B[4]

19.8.5 Invasive assessment

While some patients may have normal or non-obstructive coronary arteries, 40%–80% may have multivessel disease, including left main disease in up to 10%. Identification of the culprit lesion in NSTEACS is not always straightforward and OCT studies have shown that more than one culprit-like lesion is not uncommon. Acute plaque rupture may be suspected by intraluminal filling defects consistent with thrombus (such as contrast hold up or occlusion), plaque ulceration (i.e., contrast and hazy contour beyond the vessel lumen), plaque irregularity, dissection or impaired flow. Up to a quarter of patients present with a totally occluded artery of which two-thirds are already collateralised making differentiation between a culprit versus chronic occlusion difficult. In the absence of obstructive disease, OCT, if available, may be helpful to demonstrate superficial erosions of a non-obstructive thin-cap fibroatheroma. While fractional flow reserve is often helpful in stable patients, current techniques may underestimate the significance of a coronary stenosis in the acute setting and further prospective study is required.

19.8.6 Complete revascularisation

NSTEACS patients with (significant) multivessel disease should be considered for complete revascularisation because incomplete revascularisation has been associated with higher mortality and poorer CV outcomes. In SYNTAX, patients with complete revascularisation or residual SYNTAX scores ≤ 8 had comparable 5-year mortality (8.5% and 8.7%, respectively; p = .60). In contrast, a score > 8 was associated with 35.3% all-cause mortality at 5 years (p < .001).[36] However, pursuing complete revascularisation may carry increased procedural risk and this should be considered in context of the individual patient. As NSTEMI patients are often older and with poorer renal function, options to reduce risk include staged revascularisation of non-culprit disease to reduce procedural risk and contrast load.[36]

19.8.7 Revascularisation strategy in multivessel disease

There are a lack of prospective trials comparing PCI versus CABG in NSTEACS patients with multivessel CAD. PCI may allow faster revascularisation of the culprit lesion, a lower risk of stroke and avoidance of deleterious effects of cardiopulmonary bypass on the ischaemic myocardium. In contrast, CABG may facilitate more complete revascularisation in complex multivessel disease.

In ACUITY-PCI, where the decision to perform PCI or CABG was left to the discretion of the investigator, 78% underwent PCI (n = 4,412) versus only 22% CABG (n = 1,215). Patients with PCI had lower rates of peri-procedural stroke (0% vs. 1.1%; p = .03), MI (8.8% vs. 13.3%; p = .03), major bleeding and renal injury. There was no significant difference in mortality although PCI patients more frequently developed recurrent ischemia requiring repeat revascularisation.[37]

It is generally agreed that most NSTEACS patients with single-vessel disease are best managed by ad hoc PCI of the culprit lesion. In those with multivessel disease, especially with a syntax score of 22 or more, a Heart Team review is encouraged, although if ongoing ischaemia, haemodynamic instability, pulmonary oedema, recurrent ventricular arrhythmia or total culprit artery occlusion requiring urgent revascularisation, ad hoc culprit lesion PCI is often appropriate without Heart Team review.[6] In this situation, if the residual SYNTAX score is still elevated, a Heart Team review of the approach to the remaining lesions may be appropriate.[6]

19.9 PCI technical considerations in NSTEACS

19.9.1 Sheath

Radial access is preferred over femoral access in most NSTEACS patients to reduce bleeding risk. While larger radial sheaths can be used, a 6F sheath size is preferred to reduce risk of radial spasm which may be more common in the acute than elective setting. The recently available glidesheath (Terumo) enables use of a standard 7F guide through a 6F radial sheath. Alternatively, a sheathless 7F guide can be used although such guides tend to have stiffer tips which may increase risk of coronary trauma.

19.9.2 Guidewire

For non-occlusive lesions, a 'workhorse' wire is usually appropriate. For a thrombotic occlusive lesion, while a workhorse wire still often passes easily, some operators prefer a hydrophilic coated wire such as a Pilot 50 (Abbott) or Sion Black (Asahi) although care must be taken with such wires due to a higher risk of subintimal passage or perforation. Since NSTEMI patients are often older with longstanding coronary disease, wires suitable for diffuse, complex, tortuous or fibrocalcific disease may be required.

19.9.3 Lesion preparation

While direct stenting may be possible, adequate lesion preparation is prudent in most cases. Usually this can be achieved by a compliant pre-dilatation balloon (trying to avoid excessive pre-dilatation to reduce risk of distal embolism, no reflow or dissection). However, more complex anatomy may require non-compliant pre-dilatation balloons, scoring/cutting balloons or rotablation. Excessive thrombus can be debulked by thombectomy although this is rarely undertaken in NSTEMI.

19.9.4 Stent choice

Contemporary stents are characterised by thinner strut flexible platforms enabling improved trackability, conformability and reduced risk of side branch compromise (Figure 19.12)[38] – an important consideration in thrombotic or complex lesions. Practical knowledge of design advances may guide appropriate stent choice for different lesion anatomical scenarios.

Use of more biocompatible permanent polymers or biodegradable polymers for drug elution may be associated with improved clinical outcomes.[39,40]

In high bleeding risk patients, shorter courses of DAPT are now permissible with new generation permanent polymer stents and a only 1 month of DAPT is required after the polymer-free drug coated BioFreedom stent (which showed superior efficacy and superior safety vs. bare metal stent in ACS patients).

Fully bioresorbable vascular scaffolds may enable longer term restoration of vessel vasomotion and facilitate later bypass grafting to the segment if required. However, their role in NSTEMI is still under investigation, particularly in patients with more complex or calcific anatomy. At present, they still require an extended DAPT course of 2 years to reduce the risk of late stent thrombosis and thus are unsuitable for patients at high bleeding risk.

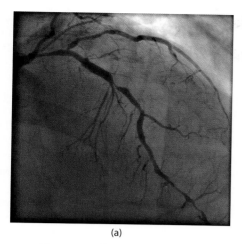

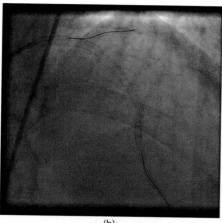

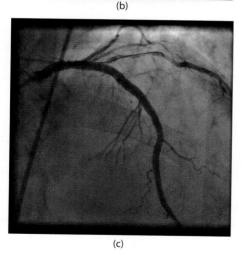

Figure 19.12 Continuous left main, proximal, mid and distal left anterior descending (LAD) stenting with overlapping Promus stents (2.5–>4.0 mm diameter) illustrating the high conformability of the stent platform. The patient had non-ST elevation myocardial infarction, not suitable for coronary artery bypass surgery due to distal LAD disease. The procedure was well tolerated with no post-PCI biomarker elevation despite the long stent length. (a) baseline (b) post stenting without contrast to illustrate conformability (c) post-stenting with contrast. (Reproduced from Menown, I.B. et al., *Adv Ther.*, 27, 3, 2010. With permission.)

19.9.5 Post-dilatation

Given the higher likelihood of resistant fibrocalcific disease, post-dilatation particularly with longer stent lengths is good practice to optimise stent expansion and vessel apposition. Intravascular imaging is strongly encouraged if size is uncertain and particularly encouraged in left main intervention where vessel size can frequently underestimated by angiography alone.[41]

19.9.6 Discharge

Once the culprit lesion (±non-culprit disease) is revascularised and access site haemostasis is secured, the patient may be discharged, provided their echocardiography has been done, their rhythm is stable and no additional investigation or drug treatment titration is required. Same day discharge may be undertaken safely for most NSTEMI patients.[42]

19.10 Special groups

19.10.1 Atrial fibrillation

Patients with atrial fibrillation (AF) requiring oral anticoagulation (OAC), but also NSTEACS requiring antiplatelet therapy represent a challenging group in whom to optimise the balance of coronary/stent protection, stroke prevention and reduction in bleeding.

19.10.2 Peri-procedural management

In AFCAS (management of patients with AF undergoing coronary artery stenting) patients who received PCI and were discharged on triple therapy including low molecular weight heparin (LMWH) had a significantly higher bleeding risk compared to warfarin-based triple therapy.[43] Thus for patients undergoing angiography and already receiving warfarin, *continuation of warfarin may be preferable rather than bridging* (which may increase the risk of thromboembolism or bleeding) and no parenteral anticoagulation is needed if the international normalised ratio (INR) is > 2.5.[4]

Non vitamin K oral anticoagulants (NOACs) do not appear to prevent contact/catheter thrombus activation and thus should not be used as the sole anticoagulant to support PCI. For non-urgent PCI, NOACs should be stopped 24 hours beforehand then heparin or bivalirudin used during the procedure.[44] In emergency PCI, additional heparin or bivalirudin should be used although bleeding risks may be higher.[45] Idarucizumab (Figure 19.13) has been approved as a dabigatran reversal agent based on the REVERSE-AD trial in which Idarucizumab was shown to reverse the anticoagulant effect of dabigatran within minutes.[46] Andexanet alfa, a recombinant engineered version of human factor Xa with the ability to bind factor Xa inhibitors is undergoing evaluation for reversal of factor Xa inhibitors.

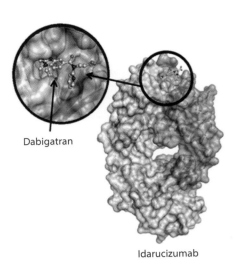

Dabigatran

Idarucizumab

Figure 19.13 Idarucizumab bound to dabigatran. (Reproduced with permission from Boehringer Ingelheim.)

- An early invasive coronary angiography (within 24 hour) should be considered in moderate-high risk patients irrespective of OAC exposure, to expedite treatment allocation (medical vs. PCI vs. CABG) and to determine the optimal antithrombotic regimen. Class IIa Level C[4]
- During PCI, additional parenteral anticoagulation is recommended for warfarin-treated patients if INR is <2.5 and for all NOAC patients irrespective of the timing of the last NOAC dose. Class I Level C[4]
- Uninterrupted therapeutic anticoagulation with warfarin or NOACs should be considered during the periprocedural phase. Class IIa Level C[4]

19.10.3 Post-PCI: Double or triple therapy?

Compared with OAC alone, double therapy (OAC plus single therapy) increases bleeding risk two- to threefold and triple therapy (OAC plus DAPT) increases bleeding risk three- to fivefold. Thus, choice of therapy is of importance particularly in higher bleeding risk groups. The CHA_2DS_2VASc score allows calculation of stroke risk and the HAS-BLED score aids bleeding risk estimation. As the risks/benefits of triple therapy are based on clopidogrel, substitution with other P2Y12 inhibitors is best avoided until prospective data are available. To minimise bleeding risk addition it is recommended to commence a proton pump inhibitor and close monitoring of INR if warfarin is used.

WOEST randomised patients undergoing mainly elective PCI to dual therapy with OAC and clopidogrel versus triple therapy with combination OAC, clopidogrel and aspirin. Double therapy was associated with a 64% reduction in bleeding events (19.4% vs. 44.4%; HR 0.36, $p < .0001$) but without difference in thrombotic or thromboembolic

events.[47] However, WOEST was a relatively small trial, underpowered for efficacy endpoints, mostly in an elective PCI setting and the bleeding endpoint was mainly driven by minor bleeding events.

ISAR-TRIPLE trial studied 614 PCI patients (1/3 ACS) who required anticoagulation. Patients were assigned to 6 weeks versus 6 months of triple therapy (short-term clopidogrel with continued aspirin and warfarin use). There was no significant difference in the rates of death, MI, stent thrombosis, ischaemic stroke or TIMI major bleeding at 9 months, or in the combined incidence of death, MI, stent thrombosis and ischaemic stroke.

While prospective trials are ongoing, the following ESC pragmatic guidance has been recommended (although this predates the LEADERS FREE trial data).

- Following coronary stenting, DAPT including new P2Y12 inhibitors should be considered as an alternative to triple therapy for patients with NSTEACS and AF with a CHA_2DS_2VASc score of 1 (in males) or 2 (in females). Class IIa Level C[4]
- If at low bleeding risk (HAS-BLED ≤ 2), triple therapy with OAC, aspirin (75–100 mg/day) and clopidogrel 75 mg/day should be considered for 6 months, followed by OAC and aspirin 75–100 mg/day or clopidogrel (75 mg/ day) continued up to 12 months. Class IIa Level C[4]
- If at high bleeding risk (HAS-BLED ≥ 3), triple therapy with OAC, aspirin (75–100 mg/day) and clopidogrel 75 mg/day should be considered for a duration of 1 month, followed by OAC and aspirin 75–100 mg/day or clopidogrel (75 mg/ day) continued up to 12 months irrespective of the stent type (BMS or new-generation DES). Class IIa Level C[4]

19.11 Elderly

In contemporary practice, up to a third of ACS patients are >75 years of age and the number >85 years is expected to triple by 2035.[48]

However, elderly patients remain under-studied in clinical trials, are less likely to receive guideline-directed treatment and are at risk of having treatment decisions made based on their chronological rather than biological age.[49] Inherently, bleeding risk increases with age and the elderly are more likely to have multiple comorbidities including chronic kidney disease (CKD). It is therefore recommended to fully evaluate patient specific risk and treat on a case-by-case basis.

19.11.1 Drugs in the elderly

Antiplatelets are often inappropriately under-prescribed in the elderly due to misperceptions of risk versus benefit despite post hoc analysis showing greater reduction in

30-day mortality, and a greater absolute risk reduction in vascular endpoints versus younger patients.[49]

While use of clopidogrel in PCI CURE among patients ≥65 years showed smaller absolute (3.5% vs. 3.9%) and relative (20.7% vs. 39.8%) reduction in CV death/MI at 1 year, those with high TIMI risk score (which is strongly driven by age) or prior revascularisation, were more likely to benefit.[49]

While the PLATelet inhibition and patient Outcomes (PLATO) study showed that absolute incidences of vascular events and bleeding events were higher in the elderly, there was heterogeneity in the benefit of ticagrelor over clopidogrel in patients ≥75 years (n = 2,878) for reduction in CV death/MI/stroke, definite stent thrombosis or all-cause mortality (Figure 19.14) and no heterogeneity in the small excess of PLATO-defined non-CABG major bleeding (Figure 19.15).[49,50]

Conversely, prasugrel-based DAPT is associated with an excess bleeding in elderly patients, particularly those with a history of CVA/transient ischemic attack (TIA) and low body weight (issues common in elderly patients). Routine use of this drug is not generally recommended in elderly patients, and if, after careful consideration, it is used, a lower 5 mg dose is recommended.[4,49]

Regarding parenteral anticoagulation, increasing age may be associated with higher APTT after heparin and higher anti-Xa levels after LMWH.[49,51] While LMWH has a more predictable dose-response than UFH, it should still be dose adjusted according to body weight and renal function (which typically decline with age).

19.11.2 Revascularisation in the elderly

Although trial data regarding revascularisation in the elderly are relatively limited and suggest increased bleeding risk, they do support consideration of an early invasive strategy in most elderly patients where clinically appropriate.

In FRISC II, the beneficial reduction in death/MI with an early invasive versus conservative strategy was more marked in those >65 versus <65 years old.[52] In TACTICS TIMI 18, NSTEACS patients >75 years old showed a marked reduction in death/MI with an early invasive versus conservative strategy (10.8% vs. 21.6%; p = .016) although with high rates of major bleeding.[53]

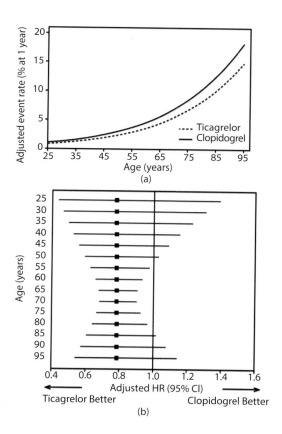

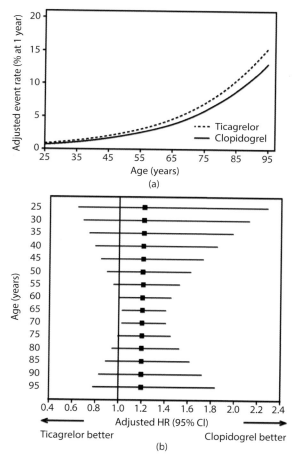

Figure 19.14 All-cause mortality according to age. (a) Estimated event rate at 12 months, ticagrelor vs clopidogrel. (b) Treatment effect by patient age. HR, hazard ratio, CI confidence interval. (Reproduced from Husted, S. et al., *Cir Cardiovasc Qual Outcomes.*, 5, 5, 2012. With permission.)

Figure 19.15 Overall non-coronary artery bypass graft-related bleeding according to age. (a) Estimated event rate at 12 months, ticagrelor vs clopidogrel. (b) Treatment effect by age. HR hazard ratio, CI confidence interval. (Reproduced from Husted, S. et al., *Cir Cardiovasc Qual Outcomes.*, 5, 5, 2012. With permission.)

In patients with multivessel or left main stem disease, CABG may offer complete revascularisation but with longer recovery times. Current CABG versus PCI trial data are limited in the elderly and tend to include those with more favourable profiles but suggest higher early mortality then improved survival beyond this.[49,54] Effects beyond mortality must however be considered. Patients >80 years have twice the risk of developing cognitive, neurological and renal impairment and significantly lower discharge to home rates.[55] Consideration of the patient as an individual is key regarding both their comorbid state and their revascularisation preferences.

> Elderly patients should be considered for an invasive strategy and, if appropriate, revascularisation after careful evaluation of potential risks and benefits, estimated life expectancy, comorbidities, quality of life, frailty and patient values and preferences. Class IIa Level A[4]

19.12 Diabetes

Diabetes is an independent predictor of mortality in NSTEACS patients and is included within multiple calculators of CV risk. Furthermore, it is becoming more frequent and is often associated with other risk factors such as hypertension, obesity and renal failure.

NSTEACS patients with diabetes are more likely to develop complications and have two to three times higher rates of mortality.[56] An early invasive strategy may be of particular benefit in patients with diabetes.[52] Selection of the most appropriate revascularisation method should take account of clinical presentation (e.g. ongoing ischaemia, arrhythmia), pattern and complexity of coronary disease, ease of stenting/grafting, ischaemic burden, presence of heart failure and co-morbid state.[4] Diabetic patients with complex anatomy should be discussed with the Heart Team and clinical scores should be used to assess lesion complexity (SYNTAX) and surgical mortality (EuroSCORE II/STS).[4]

Future Revascularisation Evaluation in Patients with Diabetes Mellitus (FREEDOM) compared CABG versus PCI in elective diabetic patients with multivessel disease (without left main involvement). Death, non-fatal MI or stroke was lower with CABG compared to PCI but with higher rates of stroke.[57] The SYNTAX and CARDia trials demonstrated no difference in death, MI or CVA for diabetic patients but repeat revascularisation was more common with patients treated with PCI.[58,59] A meta-analysis of eight trials found that patients with diabetes who received CABG had lower all-cause mortality than those receiving PCI (RR 0·67, 95% CI 0·52–0·86; p = .002).[60] CABG is thus preferred in moderate to higher risk multivessel disease patients with diabetes. However, PCI may be considered in patients with a SYNTAX score ≤22.[1]

Newer P2Y12s may be of particular benefit in diabetic patients undergoing PCI for NSTEACS.

Renal function should be closely monitored post-PCI, particularly in patients receiving metformin (which should be held for at least 48 hours, and longer if renal function is found to have declined at 48 hours).[4]

> - It is recommended to screen all patients with NSTE-ACS for diabetes and to monitor blood glucose levels frequently in patients with known diabetes or admission hyperglycaemia. Class I Level C[4]
> - Glucose-lowering therapy should be considered in ACS patients with blood glucose >10 mmol/L (>180 mg/dL), with the target adapted to comorbidities, while episodes of hypoglycaemia should be avoided. Class IIa Level C[4]
> - Less stringent glucose control should be considered both in the acute phase and at follow-up in patients with more advanced CV disease, older age, longer diabetes duration and more comorbidities. Class IIa Level C[4]
> - Renal function should be monitored for 2–3 days after coronary angiography or PCI in patients with baseline renal impairment or who are taking metformin. Class I Level C[4]
> - In patients undergoing PCI, new-generation drug eluting stents are recommended over bare metal stents. Class I Level A[4]
> - In patients with stabilised multivessel CAD and acceptable surgical risk, CABG is recommended over PCI. Class I Level A[4]
> - In patients with stabilised multivessel CAD and a SYNTAX score ≤ 22, PCI should be considered as an alternative to CABG. Class IIa Level B[4]

19.13 Chronic kidney disease

NSTEACS patients with CKD have worse outcomes and are at high risk of complications from NSTEACS therapies. Estimated creatinine clearance should be checked in all NSTEACS patients. Pre-hydration prior to angiography and caution with contrast volume is recommended.[4]

Despite the risk of contrast-induced nephropathy with PCI, registry data has shown CABG is associated with higher postoperative haemodialysis dependence than PCI (OR 3.2, 95% CI 1.1–9.3; p < .001).[61]

Survival for CKD patients is poor regardless of the revascularisation strategy used with a 5-year survival of 22%–25%.[62] While CABG may be associated with lower long-term mortality versus PCI patients in CKD patients with triple vessel CAD, mortality risk for CABG versus PCI was similar in CKD and double vessel CAD (HR 1.12, 95% CI 0.52–2.34; p = .7).[61]

P2Y12 inhibitors may be used without dose adjustment in most renal patients but greater caution is required in patients with eGFR < 15 mL/min/1.73 m². Parenteral anticoagulation may require dose adjustment.[4]

- Assess kidney function by eGFR in all patients. Class I Level C[4]
- Administer the same first-line antithrombotic treatment as in patients with normal kidney function, with appropriate dose adjustment if indicated. Class I Level B[4]
- In patients undergoing an invasive strategy, hydration with isotonic saline and low- or iso-osmolar contrast media (at lowest possible volume) is recommended. Class I Level A[4]
- Coronary angiography and, if needed, revascularization are recommended after careful assessment of the risk – benefit ratio, in particular with respect to the severity of renal dysfunction. Class I Level B[4]
- In patients undergoing PCI, new-generation drug eluting stents are recommended over bare metal stents. Class I Level B[4]
- In patients with multivessel CAD, revascularisation strategy (e.g. ad hoc culprit-lesion PCI, multivessel PCI, CABG) should be based on clinical status comorbidities and disease severity (including distribution, angiographic lesion characteristics, SYNTAX score) according to the local Heart Team protocol. Class I Level C[4]

19.14 Secondary prevention

Use of secondary prevention remains suboptimal, yet is of central importance to long-term outcome. Key elements are summarised below.

Antiplatelet therapy post NTEACS: DAPT is usually recommended for 1 year (although with evolving indications for shorter or longer courses).

Lipid lowering: A high-intensity statin therapy should be started as early as possible post-MI, unless contraindicated, and should be maintained long-term Class I Level A.[4] In patients with low-density lipoprotein (LDL) cholesterol ≥70 mg/dL (≥1.8 mmol/L) despite a maximally tolerated statin dose, further reduction in LDL cholesterol with a non-statin agent should be considered. Class IIa Level B.[4]

ACE Inhibitors and Angiotensin Receptor Blockers: Following NSTEACS, NICE recommends an ACE inhibitor for all patients as soon as they are haemodynamically stable which should be continued indefinitely.[63,64] ESC guidelines assign a Class I Level A recommendation for ACE inhibitors in patients with left ventricular ejection fraction (LVEF) ≤40% or heart failure, hypertension or diabetes, unless contraindicated.[4] Angiotensin receptor blockers may be used as alternatives to ACE inhibitors, particularly if ACE inhibitors are not tolerated.[4]

Beta-Blockers: Consensus opinion recommends beta-blockers indefinitely after MI with the strongest evidence in patients with LV dysfunction. For patients with genuine beta-blockade intolerance, the rate-lowering calcium channel blockers verapamil or diltiazem may be considered, although are contraindicated in patients with impaired LV function. NICE recommends a beta-blocker for at least 12 months in all patients post-MI, and indefinitely in patients with LV systolic dysfunction.[64] ESC guidelines assign a Class I Level A recommendation for beta-blocker therapy in patients with LVEF ≤40%, unless contraindicated.[4]

Mineralocorticoid Receptor Antagonist (MRA) Therapy: NICE recommends initiation of MRA therapy 3–14 days post-MI for patients with symptoms and/or signs of heart failure and left ventricular systolic dysfunction.[64] ESC guidelines assign a Class I Level A recommendation for MRA use, preferably eplerenone, in patients with LVEF ≤35% and either heart failure or diabetes after NSTEACS but without significant renal dysfunction or hyperkalaemia.[4]

General Measures: Smoking cessation is potentially the most effective of all secondary prevention measures. Those who stop smoking have a subsequent mortality of less than half of those who continue to smoke.[65] Patients should adopt a Mediterranean-type diet, and eat regular fruit and vegetables but avoid vitamin supplements. Weight reduction in overweight patients is encouraged. Cardiac rehabilitation and moderate exercise (to the point of slight breathlessness) for 20–30 minutes on most days are associated with improved outcome. Participation in a formal cardiac rehabilitation programme is also associated with significant reduction in mortality rates.[66]

To optimise long-term patient outcomes following contemporary PCI for unstable angina or NSTEMI, the interventionist should thus ensure appropriate initiation and monitoring of secondary prevention medication, risk factor modification and provision of cardiac rehabilitation.

List of Abbreviation

ISAR-COOL	Intracoronary Stenting With Antithrombotic Regimen Cooling Off
OPTIMA	Observational Prospective study to esTIMAte the rates of outcomes in patients undergoing PCI with drug-eluting stent implantation who take statins
LIPSIA-NSTEMI	Leipzig Immediate versus early and late Percutaneou Scoronary Intervention triAl in NSTEMI
ABOARD	Angioplasty to Blunt the Rise of Troponin in Acute Coronary Syndromes Randomized for an Immediate or Delayed Intervention
TIMACS	Timing of Intervention in Acute Coronary Syndromes

References

1. Amsterdam EA et al. 2014 AHA/ACC Guideline for the management of patients with non-ST-elevation acute coronary syndromes. *J Am Coll Cardiol* 2014; 64(24): e139–e228.

2. Hamm CW et al. ESC Guidelines for the management of acute coronary syndromes in patients presenting without persistent ST-segment elevation: The Task Force for the management of acute coronary syndromes (ACS) in patients presenting without persistent ST-segment elevation of the European Society of Cardiology (ESC). *Eur Heart J* 2011; 32(23): 2999–3054.

3. Menown IB et al. Early diagnosis of right ventricular or posterior infarction associated with inferior wall left ventricular acute myocardial infarction. *Am J Cardiol* 2000; 85(8): 934–38.

4. Roffi M et al. 2015 ESC guidelines for the management of acute coronary syndromes in patients presenting without persistent ST-segment elevation. Task Force for the management of acute coronary syndromes in patients presenting without persistent ST-segment elevation of the European Society of Cardiology (ESC). *Eur Heart J* 2016;37(3):267–315

5. Alpert JS et al. The universal definition of myocardial infarction: A consensus document: Ischaemic heart disease. *Heart (British Cardiac Society)* 2008; 94(10): 1335–41.

6. Windecker S et al. 2014 ESC/EACTS guidelines on myocardial revascularization. The Task Force on Myocardial Revascularization of the European Society of Cardiology (ESC) and the European Association for Cardio-Thoracic Surgery (EACTS) developed with the special contribution of the European Association of Percutaneous Cardiovascular. *Eur J Cardiothorac Surg* 2014; 46(4): 517–92.

7. NICE. Unstable Angina and NSTEMI: Early Management. 2010. https://www.nice.org.uk/guidance/cg94

8. Antman EM et al. The TIMI risk score for unstable angina/non-ST elevation MI: A method for prognostication and therapeutic decision making. *JAMA* 2000; 284(7): 835–42.

9. Fox KA et al. Prediction of risk of death and myocardial infarction in the six months after presentation with acute coronary syndrome: Prospective multinational observational study (GRACE). *BMJ* 2006; 333(7578): 1091.

10. Bradshaw PJ et al. Validity of the GRACE (Global Registry of Acute Coronary Events) acute coronary syndrome prediction model for six month post-discharge death in an independent data set. *Heart (British Cardiac Society)* 2006; 92(7): 905–9.

11. Center for Outcomes Research UoMMS. Global Registry of Acute Coronary Events (GRACE). 2016. Available at http://www.outcomes-umassmed.org/grace/ (Accessed 16 April 2016).

12. Subherwal S et al. Baseline risk of major bleeding in non-ST-segment-elevation myocardial infarction: The CRUSADE (Can Rapid risk stratification of Unstable angina patients Suppress ADverse outcomes with Early implementation of the ACC/AHA Guidelines) Bleeding Score. *Circulation* 2009; 119(14): 1873–82.

13. O'Donoghue M et al. Early invasive vs conservative treatment strategies in women and men with unstable angina and non-ST-segment elevation myocardial infarction: A meta-analysis. *JAMA* 2008; 300(1): 71–80.

14. Sabatine MS et al. Combination of quantitative ST deviation and troponin elevation provides independent prognostic and therapeutic information in unstable angina and non-ST-elevation myocardial infarction. *Am Heart J* 2006; 151(1): 25–31.

15. Fox KA et al. Long-term outcome of a routine versus selective invasive strategy in patients with non-ST-segment elevation acute coronary syndrome a meta-analysis of individual patient data. *J Am Coll Cardiol* 2010; 55(22): 2435–45.

16. Writing Committee Members, Jneid H et al. 2012 ACCF/AHA focused update of the guideline for the management of patients with unstable angina/Non-ST-elevation myocardial infarction (updating the 2007 guideline and replacing the 2011 focused update): A report of the American College of Cardiology Foundation/American Heart Association Task Force on practice guidelines. *Circulation* 2012; 126(7): 875–910.

17. Mehta SR et al. Early versus delayed invasive intervention in acute coronary syndromes. *N Engl J Med* 2009; 360(21): 2165–75.

18. Valgimigli M et al. Radial versus femoral access in patients with acute coronary syndromes undergoing invasive management: A randomised multicentre trial. *Lancet* 2015; 385(9986): 2465–76.

19. McCune C et al. A review of the key clinical trials of 2015: Results and implications. *Cardiol Ther* 2016; 5(2): 109–132.

20. Pijls NH et al. Functional assessment of coronary stenoses: Can we live without it? *Eur Heart J* 2013; 34(18): 1335–44.

21. Singh V et al. Comparison of inhospital mortality, length of hospitalization, costs, and vascular complications of percutaneous coronary interventions guided by ultrasound versus angiography. *Am J Cardiol* 2015; 115(10): 1357–66.

22. Young Hong YJ et al. Role of intravascular ultrasound in patients with acute myocardial infarction. *Korean Circ J* 2015; 45(4): 259–65. https://doi.org/10.4070/kcj.2015.45.4.259.

23. Davlouros P et al. Evaluation of culprit saphenous vein graft lesions with optical coherence tomography in patients with acute coronary syndromes. *J Am Coll Cardiol Intv* 2011; 4: 683–93.

24. Montalescot G et al. Pretreatment with prasugrel in non-ST-segment elevation acute coronary syndromes. *N Engl J Med* 2013; 369(11): 999–1010.

25. Collet JB. The ACCOAST TRIAL. 2014. Available at http://www.escardio.org/Guidelines-&-Education/Journals-and-publications/Recommended-readings/Acute-Cardiovascular-Care/ACCA-Top-Stories/The-ACCOAST-trial.

26. Yeh RW et al. Benefits and risks of extended duration dual antiplatelet Therapy after PCI in patients with and without acute myocardial infarction. *J Am Coll Cardiol* 2015; 65(20): 2211–21.

27. Bonaca MP et al. Long-term use of ticagrelor in patients with prior myocardial infarction. *N Engl J Med* 2015; 372(19): 1791–800.

28. Mehta SR et al. Double-dose versus standard-dose clopidogrel and high-dose versus low-dose aspirin in individuals undergoing percutaneous coronary intervention for acute coronary syndromes (CURRENT-OASIS 7): A randomised factorial trial. *Lancet* 2010; 376(9748): 1233–43.

29. De Servi S et al. Clinical outcomes for prasugrel versus clopidogrel in patients with unstable angina or non-ST-elevation myocardial infarction: An analysis from the TRITON-TIMI 38 trial. *Eur Heart J Acute Cardiovasc Care* 2014; 3(4): 363–72.

30. Lindholm D et al. Ticagrelor vs. clopidogrel in patients with non-ST-elevation acute coronary syndrome with or without revascularization: Results from the PLATO trial. *Eur Heart J* 2014; 35(31): 2083–93.

31. Menown IB. Aspirin, P2Y12 blockers, cilostazol, PAR-1 blockers and emerging antiplatelet therapies: Can biomarkers guide clinical development and practice? *Biomark Med* 2011; 5(1): 1–3.

32. Stone GW et al. Bivalirudin in patients with acute coronary syndromes undergoing percutaneous coronary intervention: A subgroup analysis from the Acute Catheterization and Urgent Intervention Triage strategy (ACUITY) trial. *Lancet* 2007; 369(9565): 907–19.

33. Menown IBA. New anticoagulant strategies. *Br J Cardiol* 2008; 15(2): 87–94.

34. Murphy SA et al. Efficacy and safety of the low-molecular weight heparin enoxaparin compared with unfractionated heparin across the acute coronary syndrome spectrum: A meta-analysis. *Eur Heart J* 2007; 28(17): 2077–86.

35. Drouet L et al. Adding intravenous unfractionated heparin to standard enoxaparin causes excessive anticoagulation not detected by activated clotting time: Results of the STACK-on to ENOXaparin (STACKENOX) study. *Am Heart J* 2009; 158(2): 177–84.

36. Farooq V et al. Quantification of incomplete revascularization and its association with five-year mortality in the synergy between percutaneous coronary intervention with taxus and cardiac surgery (SYNTAX) trial validation of the residual SYNTAX score. *Circulation* 2013; 128(2): 141–51.

37. Ben-Gal Y et al. Surgical versus percutaneous revascularization for multivessel disease in patients with acute coronary syndromes: Analysis from the ACUITY (Acute Catheterization and Urgent Intervention Triage Strategy) trial. *JACC Cardiovasc Interv* 2010; 3(10): 1059–67.

38. Menown IB et al. The platinum chromium element stent platform: From alloy, to design, to clinical practice. *Adv Ther* 2010; 27(3): 129–41.

39. Shand JA, and Menown IBA. Drug eluting stents—The next generation. *Interv Cardiol* 2010; 2(3): 341–50.

40. Shand J et al. Novel stent and drug elution technologies: An update on bioabsorbable polymer stents, polymer free drug delivery and drug eluting balloons. *Interv Cardiol* 2011; 3(4): 473–81.

41. Shand JA et al. A prospective intravascular ultrasound investigation of the necessity for and efficacy of postdilation beyond nominal diameter of 3 current generation DES platforms for the percutaneous treatment of the left main coronary artery. *Catheter Cardiovasc Interv* 2014; 84(3): 351–8.

42. Hodkinson EC et al. An audit of outcomes after same-day discharge post-PCI in acute coronary syndrome and elective patients. *J Interv Cardiol* 2013; 26(6): 570–7.

43. Kiviniemi T et al. Bridging therapy with low molecular weight heparin in patients with atrial fibrillation undergoing percutaneous coronary intervention with stent implantation: The AFCAS study. *Int J Cardiol* 2015; 183: 105–10.

44. Lip GYH et al. Management of antithrombotic therapy in atrial fibrillation patients presenting with acute coronary syndrome and/or undergoing percutaneous coronary or valve interventions. *Eur Heart J* 2014; 35(45): 3155–79.

45. Vos GJA et al. Management of the patient with an acute coronary syndrome using oral anticoagulation. *Neth Heart J* 2015; 23(9): 407–14.

46. Pollack CV, Jr. et al. Idarucizumab for Dabigatran Reversal. *N Engl J Med* 2015; 373(6): 511–20.

47. Dewilde WJ et al. Use of clopidogrel with or without aspirin in patients taking oral anticoagulant therapy and undergoing percutaneous coronary intervention: An open-label, randomised, controlled trial. *Lancet* 2013; 381(9872): 1107–15.

48. Omar Rana RM et al. Percutaneous coronary intervention in the very elderly (≥ 85 years): Trends and outcomes. *Br J Cardiol* 2013; (20): 27–31.

49. McCune C et al. A review of current diagnosis, investigation, and management of acute coronary syndromes in elderly patients. *Cardiol Ther* 2015; 4(2): 95–116.

50. Husted S et al. Ticagrelor versus clopidogrel in elderly patients with acute coronary syndromes: A substudy from the prospective randomized PLATelet inhibition and patient Outcomes (PLATO) trial. *Cir Cardiovasc Qual Outcomes* 2012; 5(5): 680–8.

51. Campbell NR et al. Aging and heparin-related bleeding. *Arch Intern Med* 1996; 156(8): 857–60.

52. Lagerqvist B et al. 5-year outcomes in the FRISC-II randomised trial of an invasive versus a non-invasive strategy in non-ST-elevation acute coronary syndrome: A follow-up study. *Lancet* 2006; 368(9540): 998–1004.

53. Bach RG et al. The effect of routine, early invasive management on outcome for elderly patients with non-ST-segment elevation acute coronary syndromes. *Ann Intern Med* 2004; 141(3): 186–95.

54. Weintraub WS et al. Comparative effectiveness of revascularization strategies. *N Engl J Med* 2012; 366(16): 1467–76.

55. Bardakci H et al. Discharge to home rates are significantly lower for octogenarians undergoing coronary artery bypass graft surgery. *Ann Thorac Surg* 2007; 83(2): 483–9.

56. O'Donoghue ML et al. An invasive or conservative strategy in patients with diabetes mellitus and Non-ST-segment elevation acute coronary syndromes: A collaborative meta-analysis of randomized trials. *J Am Coll Cardiol* 2012; 60(2): 106–11.

57. Farkouh ME et al. Strategies for multivessel revascularization in patients with diabetes. *N Engl J Med* 2012; 367(25): 2375–84.

58. Kappetein AP et al. Treatment of complex coronary artery disease in patients with diabetes: 5-year results comparing outcomes of bypass surgery and percutaneous coronary intervention in the SYNTAX trial. *Eur J Cardio-Thorac Surg* 2013; 43(5): 1006–13.

59. Kapur A et al. Randomized comparison of percutaneous coronary intervention with coronary artery bypass grafting in diabetic patients. 1-year results of the CARDia (Coronary Artery Revascularization in Diabetes) trial. *J Am Coll Cardiol* 2010; 55(5): 432–40.

60. Verma S et al. Comparison of coronary artery bypass surgery and percutaneous coronary intervention in patients with diabetes: A meta-analysis of randomised controlled trials. *Lancet Diabetes Endocrinol* 2013; 1(4): 317–28.

61. Ashrith G et al. Short- and long-term outcomes of coronary artery bypass grafting or drug-eluting stent implantation for multivessel coronary artery disease in patients with chronic kidney disease. *Am J Cardiol* 2010; 106(3): 348–53.

62. Chang TI et al. Multivessel coronary artery bypass grafting versus percutaneous coronary intervention in ESRD. *J Am Soc Nephrol* 2012; 23(12): 2042–9.

63. NICE. MI—Secondary Prevention. 2015. Available at http://cks.nice.org.uk/mi-secondary-prevention#!scenario.

64. NICE. Myocardial Infarction: Cardiac Rehabilitation and Prevention of Further MI. NICE Guidelines [CG172]. 2013. https://www.nice.org.uk/guidance/cg172

65. Menown IB. Contemporary management of coronary heart disease. *J R Coll Physicians Edinb* 2010; 40(1): 44–7; quiz 8.

66. de Vries H et al. Cardiac rehabilitation and survival in a large representative community cohort of Dutch patients. *Eur Heart J* 2015; 36(24): 1519–28.

20

Acute coronary syndrome: Acute ST-segment elevation myocardial infarction

CHRIS SAWH, SHABNAM RASHID, JAMES PALMER, EVER D GRECH

The term 'acute coronary syndrome' (ACS) refers to a range of acute myocardial ischaemic states. It encompasses unstable angina, non-ST segment elevation myocardial infarction (NSTEMI) and ST segment elevation myocardial infarction (STEMI). These three entities are distinguished by recognisable electrocardiogram (ECG) changes and alterations in biochemical markers.[1]

The last decade has seen a massive increase in percutaneous coronary intervention (PCI) procedures for ACS, which has positively impacted patient survival and morbidity. In 2014, approximately two-thirds of all PCI procedures in the United Kingdom were for ACS patients with just over a quarter for acute STEMI.[2] This chapter addresses the role of PCI, which has largely replaced thrombolytic therapy, in the management of acute STEMI.

20.1 Pathophysiology of STEMI

Rupture of an inflamed, thin-capped atherosclerotic plaque containing a lipid-rich necrotic core within an epicardial coronary artery, triggering platelet aggregation, thrombin

generation and thrombus formation, has been identified as the common underlying event in ACS. It characterises the key clinical transition from stable coronary disease (which by itself runs a relatively benign course), into the subsequent major cause of the overall morbidity and mortality (including sudden cardiac death) of coronary artery disease. This in turn has been identified as the largest single cause of mortality in most developed nations. Acute STEMI usually occurs when plaque thrombus occludes the epicardial coronary artery resulting in distal myocardial ischaemia and infarction (Figure 20.1).

20.2 Reperfusion

The myocardium can tolerate and recover from around 15 minutes of total ischaemia without resultant myocyte death (infarction). Longer durations result in a progressive wavefront of myocyte death moving from the sub-endocardial to the sub-epicardial layers. Myocardium salvaged by reperfusion is time-dependent and largely located in the sub-epicardium and mid-myocardium (Figure 20.2).

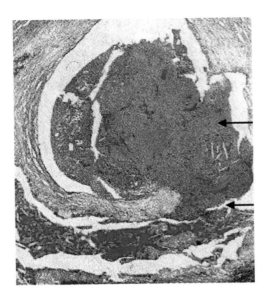

Figure 20.1 Histology of ruptured atheromatous plaque (lower arrow) and occlusive thrombus (top arrow) resulting in acute STEMI.

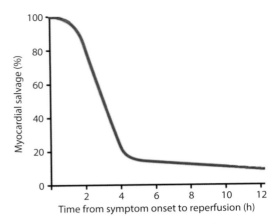

Figure 20.3 Impact of time delay to reperfusion on myocardial salvage and preservation of ventricular function, which in turn affects mortality. The highest salvage potential of reperfusion is seen within the first 3 hours after symptom onset. Patients presenting later are more likely to sustain a larger infarct and a higher mortality.

20.3 Recanalisation modalities

There are two main methods of re-opening an acutely thrombosed coronary artery: intravenous administration of a thrombolytic agent or primary PCI (Figure 20.4). Although thrombolytic therapy is easy to administer, both in hospital and the community, it has important limitations: the rate of racanalisation resulting in brisk (thrombolysis in myocardial infarction 3) flow at 90 minutes is only 55% with streptokinase or 60% with accelerated alteplase; a 5%–15% incidence of early or late re-occlusion leading to re-infarction, worsening ventricular function or death; a 1%–2% risk of intracranial haemorrhage associated with a high mortality and 15%–20% of patients with a contraindication to thrombolytic therapy.

Primary PCI mechanically disrupts and compresses the occlusive athero-thrombus, rapidly restoring antegrade blood flow. It offers a superior alternative to thrombolytic therapy in the immediate management of acute STEMI. This differs from sequential PCI, which is performed after thrombolytic therapy. After the early trials of thrombolytic drugs, there was much interest in *facilitated* PCI which was performed as a supplement to successful thrombolytic recanalisation. However, initial studies not only failed to show any advantage, but also found increased rates of major haemorrhage and emergency bypass surgery. Newer studies have shown conflicting results. In contrast rescue PCI refers to PCI within 12 hours of fibrinolysis for ongoing myocardial ischaemia/failed fibrinolysis (Table 20.1). The success of fibrinolysis is defined as >50% resolution of the ST segments on the ECG at 90 minutes after the administration of fibrinolysis. After successful fibrinolysis early angiography is recommended between 3 and 24 hours with/without PCI as this is associated with a reduction in re-infarction and recurrent ischaemia.[4]

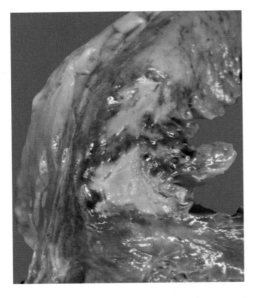

Figure 20.2 Transverse slice across the left ventricle 18 hours after acute STEMI, which was initially treated by thrombolytic therapy and then percutaneous coronary intervention (PCI). The patient died from uncontrolled cardiac dysrhythmias. There is pale infarcted myocardium as well as pronounced haemorrhage into the antero-lateral left ventricle, in keeping with reperfusion after thrombolytic therapy. (Image courtesy of Dr. S. K. Suvarna, Northern General Hospital, Sheffield.)

Patient survival depends on several factors, the most important being the restoration of brisk antegrade coronary flow, the time taken to achieve this ('time is muscle' is a well-known adage) and the sustained patency of the affected artery. The benefits of reperfusion are largely confined to the first 3 hours after the symptom onset, with only much smaller benefit likely up to 12 hours (Figure 20.3).[3]

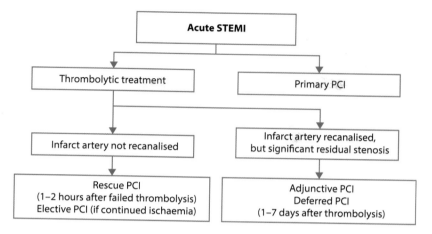

Figure 20.4 Methods of recanalisation in acute STEMI.

Table 20.1 Comparison of methods of recanalisation

	Thrombolysis	Rescue PCI	Primary PCI
Time from admission to recanalisation	1–3 hours after start of thrombolysis	Time to start of thrombolysis plus 2 hours	20–60 minutes
Recanalisation with brisk antegrade flow	55%–60%	85%	95%
Systemic fibrinolysis	+++	+++	–
Staff and catheter laboratory 'burden'	–	+	+++
Cost of procedure	+	+++	+++

20.4 Advantages of primary PCI

Large randomised studies have shown that thrombolytic therapy significantly reduces mortality compared to placebo, and this effect is maintained in the long term. Primary PCI confers additional short and long-term benefits by way of substantial reductions in mortality, cerebrovascular events, re-infarction and recurrent ischaemia (Figure 20.5).[3,5]

The immediate information provided by coronary angiography is valuable in determining subsequent management. Patients with severe and prognostically significant three-vessel coronary disease and/or left main stem disease can be referred for bypass surgery. It may also assist in the diagnosis of acute pericarditis, coronary spasm, type A aortic dissection and takotsubo cardiomyopathy, which may all present with ST segment elevation and where thromboytic therapy may be both unnecessary and harmful.

The morbidity and mortality associated with primary PCI is operator dependant, varying with the skill and experience of the interventionalist. It should be mainly considered for patients presenting early (<12 hours after the onset of symptoms). Procedural complications are significantly more common than with elective PCI, and patients often present with acute haemodynamic and electrophysiological instability. Some may have already undergone cardio-pulmonary resuscitation, cardioversion and may be ventilated prior to entering the cath lab. Even though it is usual to undertake primary PCI to the culprit occlusive lesion alone, procedures may be prolonged and complex. Prior knowledge of a patient's relevant medical history such as previous cerebral or systemic haemorrhagic events should not be overlooked in the urgency of cath lab transfer.

Ischaemic and reperfusion ventricular tachy- and brady-arrhythmias are common which may cause severe haemodynamic disturbance and can be promptly treated by intravenous drugs or electrical cardioversion. Reperfusion idioventricular arrhythmias are, however, often transient and managed conservatively. Right coronary artery procedures are often associated with sinus arrest, atrioventricular block, idioventricular rhythm and severe hypotension. The interventionalist must be ready to recognise and promptly correct these sudden aberrations, whilst simultaneously carrying out the procedure. Although surgical backup may be available, emergency bypass is now a rare event as even the most serious complications can be more rapidly addressed within the cath lab itself. Rare surgical indications include coronary anatomy unsuitable for PCI, post-infarction ventricular septal defect, acute papillary muscle rupture or ventricular free wall rupture causing haemopericardium and tamponade (Figure 20.6). The rapid availability of portable echocardiography in the cath lab has made this a valuable diagnostic tool in managing such problems.

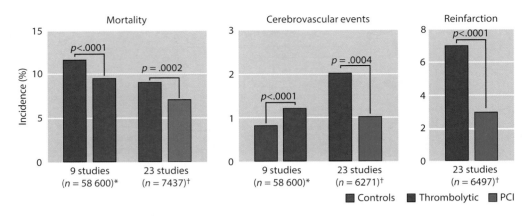

Figure 20.5 Short-term effects of treatment with placebo, thrombolytic therapy or primary PCI on mortality, incidence of cerebrovascular events and non-fatal re-infarction, following acute STEMI in randomised studies. Of the 1% incidence of cerebrovascular events in patients undergoing primary PCI, only 0.05% was haemorrhagic. In contrast, patients receiving thrombolytic therapy had a 1% incidence of haemorrhagic cerebrovascular events ($p < .001$) and an overall 2% incidence of cerebrovascular events ($p = .0004$).[3,5]

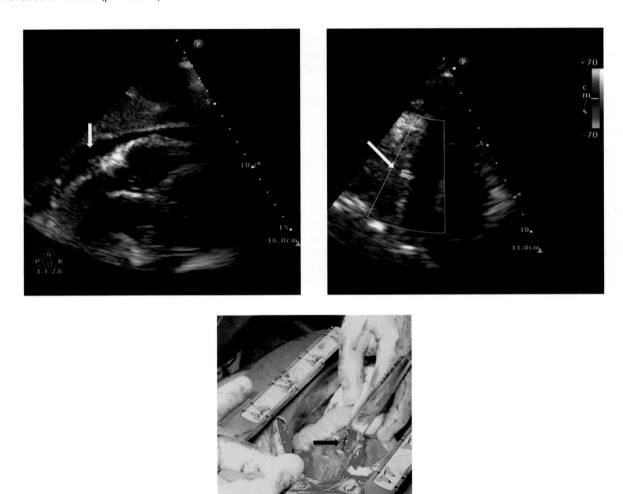

Figure 20.6 Following acute infero-lateral STEMI and successful primary PCI to the culprit right coronary artery (RCA), this patient became severely hypotensive and arrested in the cath lab. Suspected acute tamponade due to haemopericadium was confirmed on echocardiography (arrows) which showed lateral left ventricular free wall rupture. Emergency pericardio-centesis and auto-transfusion of aspirated blood (approximately 24 L) into the femoral vein allowed restoration of cardiac output prior to emergency surgery and successful patch application over the ventricular free wall rupture. This patient was discharged 10 days later.

20.5 Logistical hurdles

There are major logistical hurdles that need to be addressed in delivering an efficient and full 24–7 primary PCI service. Primary PCI can only be performed where there are adequate facilities, motivated and experienced cath lab staff who are available within 30 minutes of call-out, rapid emergency ambulance transport to the cath lab and skilled paramedics. Time delays to reperfusion are associated with significantly higher hospital and longer-term patient mortality and must be avoided where possible.[3]

The total ischaemic time can be sub-divided into the delay that can occur between patient symptom onset and first medical contact (patient related), and between first medical contact and reperfusion (health-care system related). The former may account for up to two-thirds of the total ischaemic time. Health-care system delays include two important performance time measures. The first is the *call-to-balloon time* (C2B) which is the time from patient first call for medical help to reperfusion and the current recommendation is less than 120 minutes. It is an important performance measure of the overall system of care and requires a swift and coordinated response between the emergency ambulance service and admitting hospitals. This can be difficult to achieve as patient transfer times, poor management strategies or other factors can lead to long delays. The other is the *door-to-balloon time* (D2B) which is the time from hospital admission to reperfusion, and should be less than 90 minutes.[6] This may also include the time for inter-hospital transfer when a patient presents to a centre without PPCI facilities.

20.6 Thrombolytic therapy as the alternative

Although PPCI within 120 minutes of first call or 90 minutes of hospital admission is recommended, this may not always be feasible as other factors come into play. In patients presenting to a non-PCI centre the decision about PPCI versus thrombolytic therapy may depend on time of onset of symptoms, risk of thrombolytic bleeding, presence of cardiogenic shock, heart failure and the time required to transfer the patient to a PPCI centre. Patients admitted to a PPCI centre may also be delayed if the cath lab is unavailable due to the simultaneous arrival of other PPCI patients. In circumstances when PPCI cannot be delivered within evidence-based guidelines, thrombolytic therapy can be considered.[7]

The DANish trial in Acute Myocardial Infarction-2 (DANAMI-2, Danish multicentre randomised study on thrombolytic therapy vs. acute coronary angioplasty in acute myocardial infarction) study demonstrated that STEMI patients who were transferred from a non-PCI centre had a reduction in the rate of re-infarction, compared to those patients treated with thrombolytic therapy.[8] The recent STREAM trial, an international multi-centre randomised study compared outcomes in patients with STEMI treated with thrombolytic therapy or PPCI. Patients who presented within 3 hours of symptom onset but unable to undergo PPCI within 1 hour of first medical contact were randomised to either early thrombolytic therapy (median time 100 minutes) with coronary angiography in 6–24 hours versus conventional PPCI. In the thrombolytic therapy group, patients received aspirin, clopidogrel, enoxaparin and tenecteplase. In this group thrombolysis in myocardial infarction (TIMI) 3 flow was 58.8% versus 20.7% in the PPCI group. Complete occlusion of an artery was higher in the PPCI group of 59.3% versus 16.0% in the thrombolytic therapy group. Coronary artery bypass surgery (CABG) rates were twice as high in the early thrombolytic therapy group. The composite primary end point including death from any cause, shock, congestive heart failure and re-infarction at 30 days occurred in 12.4% of the patients in the early thrombolytic therapy group and 14.3% in the PPCI group ($p = .24$, CI .68). However, a large proportion of patients (36.3%) in the thrombolytic therapy group required urgent angiography for failed thrombolysis. It is also important to note that intracranial haemorrhage was significantly higher in the early thrombolytic therapy group which has been reported in several other trials. In patients who present with STEMI within 3 hours of symptoms who are unable to undergo PPCI within 1 hour of first medical contact, thrombolytic therapy may be a potential alternative.[9] However, this has not yet been supported by the European Society of Cardiology (ESC) guidelines. The ongoing GRACIA-4 trial will provide further information about treatment of STEMI patients with PPCI versus immediate thrombolytic therapy with aspirin, clopidogrel and enoxaparin followed by cardiac catheterisation.[10]

20.7 Cardiogenic shock

If more than 40% of left ventricular (LV) myocardium becomes ischaemic, cardiogenic shock may ensue, with organ hypoperfusion and circulatory collapse. Signs include cool peripheries, cyanosis, hypotension, oliguria and reduced mental state. Hospital mortality is high and patients need to be managed quickly and aggressively. Inotropes and an intra-aortic balloon pump may be used for hypotension as this improves coronary perfusion. If there is sufficient blood pressure then agents to lower the afterload can be added to decrease cardiac work and pulmonary congestion. However, these measures have no impact on mortality which is principally dependent on prompt coronary artery recanalisation and myocyte reperfusion.[11]

Cardiogenic shock mortality is significantly higher in patients receiving thrombolytic therapy when primary PCI is the favourable option. The SHOCK PPCI trial demonstrated a reduction in mortality in patients with STEMI and cardiogenic shock who underwent PPCI compared to those who had medical therapy. Six months mortality was 50.3% in those who had PPCI and 63.1% who were treated medically.[12] Differences in mortality rates were apparent amongst the young and elderly patients with the latter experiencing higher mortality. There was a significant 30-day mortality reduction in patients <75 years of age, but no mortality benefit when revascularising those >75 years of age with STEMI and cardiogenic shock. However, there was a small number of patients >75 years in this trial. Data from registries have also demonstrated a survival benefit of revascularisation by PPCI in STEMI patients and cardiogenic shock regardless of age.[13,14] At present it is unclear as to whether patients with STEMI and cardiogenic shock with multi-vessel disease should have multi-vessel PCI at the time of PPCI to the culprit vessel, or whether this should be performed as a staged procedure. However, instinctively many interventionalists perform multi-vessel PCI in this setting. Currently, the CULPRIT-SHOCK trial is in progress to address this issue.[15]

20.8 The intra-aortic balloon pump (IABP)

The IABP improves myocardial oxygen supply by facilitating diastolic coronary blood flow. Therefore in myocardial ischaemia the IABP may improve myocardial blood flow in the presence of impaired left ventricular dysfunction.

Studies have shown improved haemodynamics in patients with acute MI and cardiogenic shock. There is an increase in mean arterial pressure and a reduction in systemic vascular resistance. In the SHOCK trial registry there was a mortality reduction at 6 months and 1 year after IABP.[16]

In a meta-analysis of STEMI patients with cardiogenic shock, IABP did not improve 30 day mortality or left ventricular ejection fraction. In another study patients with STEMI and cardiogenic shock who were treated by thrombolysis and had IABP inserted were found to have lower rates of revascularisation compared to those who did not have IABP. However, in patients with STEMI and cardiogenic shock who had revascularisation by PPCI, IABP was associated with a 6% increase in mortality. Confounding factors may have hampered any benefits that may have been seen with IABP. The study was not randomised, so it is unclear if the most unwell patients were assigned to the PPCI group.[17]

The largest trial to date of STEMI patients and cardiogenic shock (IABP-SHOCK II trial) showed that mortality rate at 30 days was 52% in those who had IABP and 51% mortality in those who did not have IABP. In the two groups, there was no difference in the rates of re-infarction, repeat revascularisation or stroke. However, other studies demonstrated mortality benefits with IABP in STEMI patients and cardiogenic shock when the follow up period was beyond 30 days. Based on registry data, the ESC and American guidelines have downgraded the use of IABP in STEMI patients with cardiogenic shock from class I to class IIa and IIb recommendation. At present there is no evidence that IV fluids, inotropes or left ventricular assist devices lead to improved survival rates in STEMI patients with cardiogenic shock.[18] Although no mortality benefit has been demonstrated for the use of IABP in STEMI patients and cardiogenic shock, IABP continues to be used for haemodynamic support in such patients.

20.9 Pharmacological agents

20.9.1 Nitroglycerin

Nitroglycerin may be administered to relieve chest pain and is a useful preload vasodilator in patients with acute pulmonary oedema. However, it should be avoided in hypotensive patients and those who have sustained right ventricular infarction[19] who are preload dependent and are therefore sensitive to such agents.

20.9.2 Aspirin

Aspirin irreversibly inhibits cyclo-oxygenase and thereby blocks production of thromboxane A2, a vasoconstrictor and highly potent platelet aggregation stimulant. It produces a rapid anti-thrombotic effect in an oral dose of 150–300 mg and should be given immediately in all patients with acute STEMI. It should be continued at a dose of 75–81 mg daily.[6] Rapid absorption occurs with non-enteric coated formulations.[20]

20.9.3 P2Y$_{12}$ receptor antagonists

These agents block platelet surface adenosine diphosphate (ADP) receptors of subtype P2Y$_{12}$, which is responsible for the initiation of platelet activation. They include clopidogrel, prasugrel and ticagrelor. Patients diagnosed with a STEMI should be commenced on a loading dose of aspirin and a P2Y$_{12}$ receptor antagonist immediately, unless contraindicated.

Clopidogrel, a thienopyridine, selectively and irreversibly binds to P2Y$_{12}$ platelet receptors. It is a pro-drug and requires a two-step hepatic bioactivation to be converted to its active metabolite via several cytochrome P450 enzymes, including CYP2C19. This is genetically determined by CYP2C19 alleles as well as age, weight, co-medication which inhibits relevant CYP enzymes and certain disease states. Any loss of function may result in reduced formation of clopidogrel's active metabolite and lower clopidogrel-induced platelet inhibition.[21] Clopidogrel has now been largely superseded by prasugrel or ticagrelor.

Prasugrel is also a thienopyridine pro-drug causing irreversible P2Y$_{12}$ receptor inhibition. Unlike clopidogrel it only needs one oxidative step to form its active moiety which is generated much more efficiently and in much higher concentration. It is prescribed as a loading dose of 60 mg followed by 10 mg daily. In the TRITON TIMI 38 trial, the primary end point of death from cardiovascular causes, non-fatal myocardial infarction or non-fatal stroke occurred in 12.1% of patients receiving clopidogrel and 9.9% of patients receiving prasugrel ($p < .001$). The rate of myocardial infarction was significantly reduced in the prasugrel group versus clopidogrel (7.4% vs. 9.7% respectively). Urgent target vessel revascularisation and stent thrombosis was also significantly lower in the prasugrel group. However, major bleeding was more common in the prasugrel group; 2.4% versus 1.8% in the clopidogrel group. Life threatening bleeding was 1.4% in the prasugrel group and 0.9% taking clopidogrel.[22] Prasugrel is not recommended in patients >75 years, <60 kg in body weight, previous stroke or transient ischaemic attack.

Ticagrelor is a reversibly binding non-thienopyridine oral $P2Y_{12}$-inhibitor which does not require hepatic biotransformation for activity. It is prescribed as a loading dose of 180 mg followed by 90 mg twice daily. In the PLATO trial, the primary end point at 12 months, a composite of death from vascular causes, myocardial infarction or stroke occurred in 9.8% of patients receiving ticagrelor compared with 11.7% of those receiving clopidogrel ($p < .001$). Major bleeding not related to coronary artery bypass grafting was significantly higher in the ticagrelor arm (4.5% vs. 3.8%, $p = 0.03$). The mortality rate, a pre-specified secondary end-point, was also significantly lower in the ticagrelor group. Side effects of ticagrelor include dyspnoea and ventricular pauses. Dyspnoea was present in 13.8% of patients with no compromise of pulmonary function, due to adenosine deaminase inhibition causing higher levels of adenosine. There was also a higher incidence of ventricular pauses in the first week which resolved at 30 days. There was no significant increase in syncope or pacemaker implantation in patients receiving clopidogrel or ticagrelor.[23]

More recently, interest has focused on the absorption delay with prasugrel and ticagrelor in the first few hours after oral administration, and the associated 2% incidence of acute stent thrombosis. The immediate action of intravenous glycoprotein IIb/IIa inhibitors may help to prevent this in a subset of STEMI patients, although this may increase bleeding complications. There is also increasing interest in the potent intravenous $P2Y_{12}$ platelet inhibitor, cangrelor, which has rapid onset and offset in the peri-PPCI period. This could be administered until the oral $P2Y_{12}$ inhibitor has been sufficiently absorbed, thus avoiding the problem of acute stent thrombosis.

20.9.4 Glycoprotein IIb/IIIa inhibitors (GPI)

GPI's are the most pharmacodynamically potent inhibitors of platelet function. The three available intravenous agents are abciximab, tirofiban eptifibitide. Their benefit in primary PCI have been evaluated and shown to be important agents. The first study (CADILLAC) showed that abciximab significantly reduced early recurrent ischaemia and reocclusion due to thrombus formation. There was no additional effect on restenosis or late outcomes compared with stenting alone. The slightly reduced rate of normal coronary flow that had been seen in other studies was again confirmed, but did not translate into a significant effect on mortality. Another study (ADMIRAL) examined the potential benefit of abciximab when given before (rather than during) primary stenting. Both at 30 days and 6 months follow up, abciximab significantly reduced the composite rate of reinfarction, the need for further revascularisation, and mortality. In addition, abciximab significantly improved coronary flow rates immediately after stenting, which persisted up to 6 months

with a significant improvement in residual left ventricular function. Abciximab seems to improve flow characteristics, prevents distal thrombo-embolisation and reduces the need for repeat angioplasty. It may also be administered as an intra-coronary bolus. A pooled analysis by Topol et al. showed a significant 30-day mortality benefit with abciximab.[24] The On-TIME 2 study ($n = 984$) compared high-dose tirofiban administered early in the ambulance before primary PCI with placebo. Patients also received aspirin and clopidogrel 600 mg. At one year the tirofiban group had significant lower mortality over placebo.[25]

However, in the last few years, the routine use of GPI's in PPCI has been questioned due to the increased use of newer and more efficient $P2Y_{12}$ inhibitors (prasugrel and ticagrelor), or bilvarudin. Current guidelines recommend their use mainly in patients with large amount of visible intra-coronary thrombus, or in bailout situations.

20.9.5 Anti-coagulants

Anti-coagulants are associated with a reduction in adverse outcomes but an increased risk of bleeding. The warfarin, aspirin, re-infarction study (WARIS II) demonstrated positive outcomes in individuals with myocardial infarction (MI) including STEMI, treated with warfarin alone. There was a significant reduction in death, non-fatal re-infarction and ischaemic stroke when compared to aspirin (16.7% vs. 20% respectively). Indeed there was a small number of major non-fatal bleeds with warfarin compared to aspirin alone (0.62% vs. 0.17%).[26] Warfarin may therefore be an alternative especially in patients with an aspirin allergy.

Anti-thrombotics that can be used during PPCI include unfractionated heparin, enoxaparin and bivalirudin. In the OASIS-6 trial, there was no mortality benefit in the factor Xa inhibitor fondaparinux, in patients with STEMI undergoing PPCI. However, fondaparinux reduced mortality and re-infarction rates in patients with STEMI not undergoing an invasive strategy without increased bleeding or stroke risk.[27]

The dosing for unfractionated heparin is 70–100 units/kg when no glycoprotein IIb/IIIa inhibitor is used, when the dose should be reduced to 50–60 units per kilogram. The activated partial thromboplastin time (APTT) is commonly checked during the PCI procedure since there is a relationship between the APTT and patient outcomes.

Enoxaparin is superior to unfractionated heparin in PPCI for patients with STEMI as there is a reduction in mortality and bleeding rates. In the FINESSE trial the rates of mortality, myocardial infarction, urgent revascularisation and refractory ischaemia was 5.3% in the enoxaparin arm and 8.0% in the unfractionated heparin arm. Enoxaparin was therefore associated with lower risks of cardiovascular events compared to unfractionated heparin.[28]

In the HEAT PPCI trial, intravenous heparin with bailout glycoprotein IIb/IIIa inhibitor was compared to bivalirudin with bailout glycoprotein IIb/IIIa inhibitor in STEMI patients. The primary outcome of mortality, stroke, reinfarction and revascularisation of a target vessel was assessed at

28 days. This occurred in 8.7% of patients in the bivalirudin group and 5.7% of patients in the heparin group ($p = .01$). The outcomes were mainly driven by a higher reinfarction rate in the bivalirudin group due to acute stent thrombosis. Major bleeding was similar in both groups.[29]

20.10 Primary PCI dilemmas

20.10.1 Bystander lesions

Approximately 40% of patients with STEMI have significant bystander disease in non-infarct arteries. An ongoing controversy is whether severely stenosed lesions in the non-infarct vessels should also be considered for PCI, once the culprit vessel has been opened. Current ESC and American College of Cardiology (ACC)/American Heart Association (AHA) guidelines recommend PPCI to the culprit vessel only during a STEMI. Moreover, until recently ACC/AHA guidelines categorised the performance of routine non-infarct artery PCI at the time of primary PCI as Class III – potentially harmful. However, recent randomised controlled trials suggest that PCI of a non-infarct artery may be safe and possibly beneficial. This should be considered in patients with multi-vessel disease who are hemodynamically stable, either at the time of primary PCI or as a planned staged procedure (Class IIb).

Two randomised trials compared outcomes in STEMI patients who had PCI to the culprit vessel versus PCI to the culprit vessel and bystander lesions. In the latter group favourable outcomes were seen. In the PRAMI trial cardiac death, non-fatal MI or refractory angina was reduced by 65% over a 23-month follow up period in the complete revascularisation group.[30] The CvLPRIT study showed a 55% reduction in major adverse cardiac events (MACE) in those who underwent complete revascularisation versus those who had PCI to the culprit vessel alone.[31] The main limitations with these studies was the small number of patients that were recruited in each arm. Furthermore, it is unclear as to the exact timing of PCI to the bystander lesions, that is, should this be done at the time of PPCI to the culprit vessel, as a staged procedure during inpatient stay or as an outpatient. The COMPLETE TRIAL is currently in progress and is recruiting the largest number of patients[32] and will provide further information as to whether patients should have culprit vessel PCI for STEMI or complete revascularisation.

20.10.2 Bare metal stents versus drug eluting stents

The mechanical scaffolding properties of coronary stents have largely addressed the previous problems of acute dissection and residual luminal narrowing, which resulted in early or late re-occlusion, or restenosis within the culprit vessel.

The use of drug eluting stents (DES) compared to bare metal stent (BMS) for PPCI has also been evaluated in a number of randomised studies and their main advantage has been the significant reduction in restenosis rates.[33]

However, there is an increased risk of late stent thrombosis with DES due to delayed endothelialisation of the stent. In a meta-analysis of 15 randomised controlled trials comparing the use of first generation DES with BMS in STEMI patients showed that target vessel revascularisation up to 1 year was significantly lower in patients who had DES than those who had BMS (4.5% vs. 9.8%). This was still predominant after a 5-year follow up period. One year stent thrombosis rates were lower in patients who received DES than those who had BMS (1.6% vs. 2.0%). However, in subsequent years stent thrombosis was higher for the DES group. There was no significant difference in the rates of death or myocardial infarction regardless of the type of stent that was used.[34] In the PASSION trial paclitaxel a first generation DES was compared with a BMS in STEMI patients. The rate of cardiac death, recurrent MI or target vessel revascularisation at 5 years was 18.6% in those who had a paclitaxel DES compared to 21.8% in the BMS group. Stent thrombosis was seen in 4.2% in those who had DES versus 3.4% in BMS group. There was no significant difference in adverse outcomes although very late stent thrombosis was more frequent in patients who had a DES.[35] Second generation stents with thinner struts have shown improved outcomes compared to first generation DES. The everolimus DES (a second generation stent) was compared to BMS in patients with STEMI. At 2-year follow up the rates of target vessel revascularisation was significantly lower in those who had everolimus DES; 2.9% versus 5.6% in BMS group. Stent thrombosis was also lower in the everolimus DES group. However, there was no difference in the combined end point of MI, death or target vessel revascularisation.[36] The 2012 ESC guidelines recommend the use of DES over BMS in STEMI patients.

20.10.3 Radial versus femoral route

Access to the coronary circulation can be achieved by either the radial or femoral route. Bleeding is a more common complication after PPCI due to the use of anti-platelet and anti-thrombotic agents. This is associated with adverse outcomes including stroke and death.[37] A meta-analysis assessing the safety and efficacy of the radial route and femoral route during PPCI for STEMI patients showed that the radial route was superior with lower death and major bleeding. Mortality rates were significantly lower in the radial access group at 2.7% versus 4.7% in the femoral access group. Stroke risk was similar in both groups. However, procedure time was on average 1.5 minutes longer in the radial access group[38] which delays timely reperfusion of the vessel. Anatomic differences in the course of the radial artery as well as engagement of the coronaries contribute to the length of the procedure. At present there are no guidelines recommending the preferred access route.

Advantages of the radial route include the ability to achieve haemostasis easily since the radial artery is superficial and easily compressible. This is particularly important during PPCI as the use of anti-thrombotics such as heparin and glycoprotein IIb/IIIa inhibitors increases the risk of bleeding especially when using the femoral route. There is also unlikely to be damage to adjacent structures in comparison to the femoral route. These features may make the radial route more attractive for PPCI.[39]

For patients in cardiogenic shock it is not entirely clear if the radial route is preferred. The intra-aortic balloon pumps can be delivered by the radial or femoral artery. In the RADIAL PUMP UP registry patients undergoing transfemoral intra-aortic balloon pump insertion had greater adverse outcomes when compared to the transradial route. In the transfemoral group, 30-day composite of post-procedural bleeding, cardiac death, myocardial infarction, target lesion revascularisation and stroke was 54.7% compared to 36.6% in patients who underwent the procedure radially. This was driven by access related bleeding from the femoral route.[40] Further studies are required to support the above findings as these patients were high-risk patients and may have had other confounders affecting reported outcomes.

20.10.4 Thrombus aspiration

One of the commonly encountered problems is distal embolisation of thrombus which may affect microvascular blood flow, myocardial perfusion and subsequent mortality.[41] Thrombus aspiration can prevent distal embolisation thereby improving microvascular tissue perfusion (Figure 20.7). The TAPAS trial investigated the frequency of myocardial blush grade of 0 or 1 in STEMI patients who underwent thrombus aspiration and PCI versus PCI alone. A myocardial blush grade of 0 or 1 occurred in 17.1% in the thrombus aspiration group versus 26.3% in the PCI only group. At 30 days the rate of death in those with myocardial blush of 0 or 1 was 5.2%, blush of 2 was 2.9% and blush of 3 was 1%. Therefore those individuals who had thrombus aspiration had better reperfusion and clinical outcomes compared to those who had conventional PCI without thrombus aspiration.[42]

More recently the TASTE trial studied mortality rates in STEMI patients who underwent thrombus aspiration

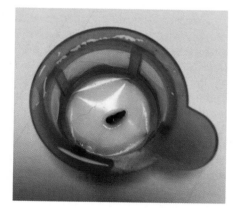

Figure 20.7 Thrombus successfully aspirated from the left anterior descending (LAD) artery using an aspiration catheter, in a patient with acute anterior STEMI.

and PPCI versus PPCI alone. There was no reduction in 30-day mortality and no significant difference with regards to stroke or neurological complications.[43] The subsequent TOTAL trial which recruited 10,063 patients found that routine thrombectomy did not reduce risk of cardiovascular death, recurrent MI, cardiogenic shock or New York Heart Association (NYHA) class IV heart failure. There was, however, an increase in the rate of stroke in the thrombus aspiration group of 0.7% versus 0.3% in the PCI alone group at 30 days.[44] Therefore, the routine use of thrombus aspiration is no longer generally recommended.

20.10.5 Massive thrombus and intra-coronary fibrinolysis

The presence of a large amount of luminal thrombi are an additional challenge as these readily fragment and embolise with balloon and/or stent deployment, causing no-reflow, a depressingly difficult complication which is frequently irreversible and carries a high mortality. There are a number of techniques in avoiding such problems and one is illustrated in Figure 20.8.

There is a paucity of data regarding the use of intra-coronary fibrinolysis in patients with STEMI and massive thrombus. Large thrombus is often very difficult to aspirate through a relatively narrow catheter, which may cause dislodgment downstream. In the present literature the use of intra-coronary fibrinolysis appears to be favourable in STEMI patients with massive thrombus who have failed thrombus aspiration. In one observational study, 30 STEMI patients received low-dose intra-coronary fibrinolysis for large thrombus and failed thrombus aspiration. Thrombolysis in Myocardial Infarction (TIMI) flow improved from 0 to 1 in 93% of patients to TIMI flow ≥2 in 97% of patients. Resolution of ST segment elevation of >50% occurred in 82% of patients. In hospital mortality was 10% and occurred in patients with cardiogenic shock. At a median of 14-month follow up 1 patient required target vessel revascularisation.[45] In a further case series of 12 patients with STEMI and failed thrombus aspiration for massive thrombus, intra-coronary fibrinolysis demonstrated significant improvements in TIMI flow grade and ST segment resolution. TIMI flow was 0–1 in 84% of patients pre-thrombolysis and 75% of patients had TIMI flow of 3 post-thrombolysis. The remaining patients had a TIMI flow of 2. ST segment resolution of >50% occurred in 85% of patients. The in-hospital MACE was 16%.[46]

20.10.6 Late STEMI presentation

A few patients may present later than 12 hours of initial symptom onset but have ongoing chest pain with evidence of ischaemia on their ECG. They can still be considered for PPCI if symptom onset is unclear and stuttering. In patients who present with a very late STEMI (more than 3 days after the onset of pain), PCI was not found to be superior to medical

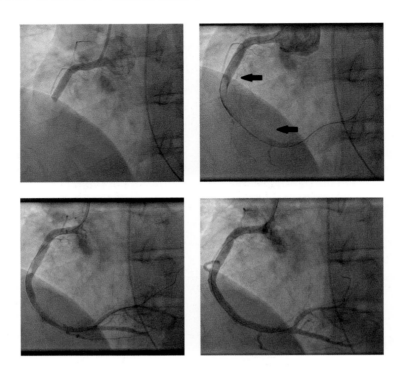

Figure 20.8 Top left: total proximal RCA occlusion in a patient with acute inferior STEMI. Top right: initial guidewire crossing revealed the presence of massive intra-luminal thrombus (between two arrows). Bottom left: Intermittent intra-coronary administration of a thrombolytic agent over 30 minutes resulted in significant dissolution and 'debulking' of the fresh thrombus. Bottom right: This was followed by successful stent deployment without thrombus embolisation or 'no-flow'.

therapy. The occluded artery trial (OAT) trial randomised stable patients who were 3–28 days after their STEMI with an ejection fraction of <50% or proximal coronary occlusion to receive either PCI with optimal medical therapy versus optimal medical therapy alone. The study found that PCI was not superior to patients that were treated with optimal medical therapy alone. PCI did not reduce mortality rates, re-infarction or heart failure. Furthermore, at 4-year follow up there was a trend towards excess of re-infarction in the PCI group.[47]

20.11 Indicators of reperfusion and no-reflow

20.11.1 Thrombolysis in myocardial infarction (TIMI flow)

Although resolution of ST segment elevation on the ECG is frequently used to indirectly determine reperfusion, this does have limitations. Angiographic assessment of antegrade flow using the TIMI scale may be useful. TIMI flow is graded from 0 to 3. 0 is defined as no flow beyond the occlusion. Grade 1 is incomplete perfusion around the point of occlusion. Grade 2 is complete perfusion but delayed perfusion of the distal coronary circulation. Grade 3 is complete perfusion at the normal expected rate.[48]

In a retrospective analysis of STEMI patients post-PPCI, TIMI 3 flow was associated with better outcomes compared to those with ≤TIMI 2 flow. In hospital mortality was 6.4% in those with TIMI 3 flow versus 32.9% in those ≤TIMI 2 flow. Cardiogenic shock was present in 10.9% of patients with

TIMI 3 flow and 24.3% in patients with ≤TIMI 2 flow. The use of IABP was lower in patients with TIMI 3 flow; 5.8% versus 11.4%. If TIMI flow did not improve after 6 months, patients had worse NYHA class and tended to undergo repeat coronary angiography. Therefore adverse outcomes are seen in patients who have ≤TIMI 2 flow post-PPCI for STEMI.[49]

20.11.2 Myocardial blush grade

Myocardial blush grade (MBG) measures myocardial perfusion and is assessed by angiography. MBG is graded from 0 to 3. No myocardial blush is graded as 0 and this is due to leakage of contrast into the extracellular space. Minimal myocardial blush is 1, moderate myocardial blush is graded as 2, normal myocardial blush is graded as 3. Acquisition runs by fluoroscopy need to be long enough to see the venous phase of contrast passage.[50] Despite achieving TIMI 3 flow after PPCI for STEMI patients some may have reduced perfusion at the myocardial tissue. Distal embolisation of thrombus and no reflow may account for this.

In STEMI patients who achieved TIMI 3 flow post-PPCI, MBG was assessed and outcomes including MACE, infarct size and left ventricular ejection fraction were analysed. MACE, infarct size and mortality rates were higher in patients with MBG of 0/1 compared to those who had MBG of 2 or 3. Left ventricular ejection fraction was lower with a MBG of 0 or 1 versus those with MBG of 2 or 3. Therefore MBG was found to be an independent predictor for outcomes in STEMI patients.[51] Other studies have also confirmed similar findings. Another study in which patients achieved TIMI 3 flow

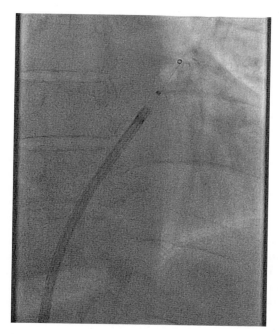

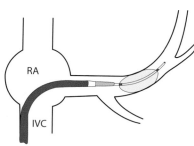

Figure 20.9 PICSO balloon catheter positioning within main coronary sinus (RA: right atrium; IVC: inferior vena cava).

post-PPCI for STEMI found that 1 year all cause mortality was 17% if a patient had a MBG of 0, 10% for MBG of 1, 6% for MBG of 2 and 4% for MBG of 3. In routine clinical practice both TIMI flow and MBG can be readily documented.[52]

20.11.3 No-reflow

The no-reflow (also referred to as low-flow) phenomenon is the partial or complete failure of blood to re-perfuse an ischaemic area despite alleviation of the physical obstruction. It occurs in 0.6%–3.2% of PPCI cases and may result in persisting ECG abnormalities, arrhythmias, hypotension and cardiogenic shock.[53] It has been shown to be a strong predictor of mortality and in one study was associated with a 5-year mortality of 18.2%, compared to 9.5% of patients who had normal flow. The precise pathophysiology is not understood and it has been proposed that structural damage to the microvasculature causing vasoconstriction, calcium overload, myocardial oedema and endothelial dysfunction,[54] restrict normal blood flow to the myocytes. Distal embolisation of disrupted athero-thrombus after balloon inflation may also be a contributing factor. Pharmacological treatment of no-reflow includes intra-coronary nitrate, adenosine, verapamil, a glycoprotein IIb/IIIa inhibitor as well as an intra-aortic balloon pump, which may improve target vessel blood flow.

20.12 Future developments to enhance reperfusion

Although the early and sustained recanalisation of the culprit thrombotic occlusion is a prerequisite for myocardial salvage and limitation of infarct size, this does not necessarily

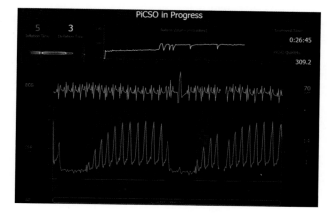

Figure 20.10 PICSO console showing ECG synchronised intermittent balloon inflations.

result in complete myocardial tissue perfusion. Distal microvascular dysfunction and reperfusion injury are known to occur, which may limit expected benefits. Unfortunately, several pharmacological interventions designed to limit reperfusion dysfunction have all been disappointing and may reflect the complexity of this phenomenon. Recently, a new Pressure-controlled Intermittent Coronary Sinus Occlusion (PICSO) device appears to show some early promise and is currently undergoing clinical trial evaluation with a prospective randomised study planned for 2017. It consists of a soft balloon catheter which is positioned within the coronary sinus via the femoral vein (Figure 20.9). After successful PCI recanalisation, ECG-synchronised intermittent helium balloon inflations and deflations based on coronary sinus pressure are carried over a period of approximately 20 minutes (Figure 20.10). The intermittent increase of venous pressure in the coronary sinus induces a continuous rise and fall of pressure gradients in the microcirculatory bed, clearing debris and eliminating metabolic waste. In doing so, it improves microvascular reperfusion potentially reducing reperfusion injury and reducing final infarct size.

20.13 Cardiac rehabilitation and prevention

The importance of cardiac rehabilitation and preventative drug therapy has been detailed in Chapter 19 and these are equally applicable to STEMI patients. One area that is frequently overlooked is the impact of cigarette smoke and cessation. Although recognised as an independent risk factor since the Framingham Heart study in the 1950's[55] the magnitude of this risk has been undefined. However, recent data has indicated that smokers presented with acute STEMI around 10 years younger than non-smokers and that almost a half of all acute STEMI's were attributable to smoking alone.[56] Furthermore, although all age groups were at much greater (threefold) risk of an acute STEMI, younger smokers were particularly vulnerable and were eight times more likely to suffer an acute STEMI than their non-smoking peers. This risk is even higher in female smokers whose risk is twelvefold. An interesting windfall is that the risk in those who do give up smoking is similar to those who have never smoked.[57] Therefore an awareness of this higher risk is an essential public health message.

References

1. Menown IB et al. Optimizing the initial 12-lead electrocardiographic diagnosis of acute myocardial infarction. *Eur Heart J* 2000; 21: 275–83.
2. Ludman P. BCIS Audit Returns. Adult Interventional Procedures. 2014. Available at http://www.bcis.org.uk/documents/BCIS_Audit_2014_20012016_for_web.pdf.
3. Fibrinolytic Therapy Trialists' (FTT) Collaborative Group. Indications for fibrinolytic therapy in suspected acute myocardial infarction. Collaborative overview of early mortality and major morbidity results from all randomised trials of more than 1000 patients. *Lancet* 1994; 343: 311–22.
4. Di Mario C et al. Immediate angioplasty versus standard therapy with rescue angioplasty after thrombolysis in the Combined Abciximab REteplase Stent Study in Acute Myocardial Infarction (CARESS-in-AMI): An open, prospective, randomised, multicentre trial. *Lancet* 2008; 371: 559–68.
5. Keeley EC et al. Primary angioplasty versus intravenous thrombolytic therapy for acute myocardial infarction: A quantitative review of 23 randomised trials. *Lancet* 2003; 361: 13–20.
6. Gara PT et al. 2013 ACCF/AHA Guideline for the management of ST elevation myocardial infarction. A report of the American College of Cardiology Foundation/American Heart Association task force on practise guidelines. *J Am Coll Cardiol* 2013; 60: 485–510.
7. Pinto DS et al. Benefit of transferring ST segment elevation myocardial infarction for percutaneous coronary intervention compared with administration of onsite fibrinolytic declines as delay increase. *Circulation* 2011; 124: 2512–21.
8. Anderson HR et al. Danish multicenter randomised study on fibrinolytic therapy versus acute coronary angioplasty in acute myocardial infarction-2 (DANAMI-2). *Am Heart J* 2003; 146: 234–41.
9. Armstrong PW et al. Fibrinolysis or primary percutaneous coronary intervention in ST segment elevation myocardial infarction. *N Engl J Med* 2013; 368: 1379–87.
10. Sanchez PL, GRACIA group. Comparison of primary PCI Vs post-thrombolysis PCI as reperfusion strategies in STEMI (GRACIA4). NCT02268669.
11. Webb JG et al. Percutaneous coronary intervention for cardiogenic shock in the SHOCK trial registry. *Am Heart J* 2001; 141: 964–70.
12. Hochman JS et al. Should we emergently revascularize occluded coronaries for cardiogenic shock: One-year survival following early revascularization for cardiogenic shock. *JAMA* 2001; 285: 190–2.
13. Dauerman HL et al. Outcomes and early revascularization for patients greater than or equal to 65 years of age with cardiogenic shock. *Am J Cardiol* 2001; 87: 844–8.
14. Dauerman HL et al. Outcomes of percutaneous coronary intervention among elderly patients in cardiogenic shock: A multicenter, decade-long experience. *J Invasive Cardiol* 2003; 15: 380–4.
15. Culprit lesion only PCI versus multivessel PCI in cardiogenic shock (CULPRIT-SHOCK). Thiele H. University of Luebeck. NCT01927549.
16. Sanborn TA et al. Impact of thrombolysis, intra-aortic balloon pump counterpulsation, and their combination in cardiogenic shock complicating acute myocardial infarction: A report from the SHOCK trial registry. Should we emergently revascularize Occluded Coronaries for cardiogenic shocK? *J Am Coll Cardiol* 2000; 36: 1123–9.
17. Sjauw KD et al. A systematic review and meta-analysis of intra-aortic balloon pump therapy in ST-elevation myocardial infarction: Should we change the guidelines? *Eur Heart J* 2009; 30(4): 459–68.
18. Thiele H et al. Intra-aortic balloon counterpulsation in acute myocardial infarction complicated by cardiogenic shock (IABP-SHOCK II): Final 12 month results of a randomised, open-label trial. Intraaortic Balloon Pump in cardiogenic shock II (IABP-SHOCK II) trial investigators. *Lancet* 2013; 382(9905): 1638–45.
19. Come PC, and Pitt B. Nitroglycerin-induced severe hypotension and bradycardia in patients with acute myocardial infarction. *Circulation* 1976; 54: 624–8.
20. Antithrombotic Trialists' Collaboration. Collaborative meta-analysis of randomised trials of antiplatelet therapy for prevention of death, myocardial infarction, and stroke in high risk patients. *Br Med J* 2002; 324: 71–86.
21. Collet JP et al. Dose effect of clopidogrel reloading in patients already on 75-mg maintenance dose: The Reload with Clopidogrel Before Coronary Angioplasty in Subjects Treated Long Term with Dual Antiplatelet Therapy (RELOAD) study. *Circulation* 2008; 118: 1225–33.
22. Wiviott SD et al. Prasugrel versus clopidogrel in patients with acute coronary syndromes. *N Engl J Med* 2007; 357: 2001–15.
23. Wallentin L et al. Ticagrelor versus clopidogrel in patients with acute coronary syndromes. *N Engl J Med* 2009; 361: 1045–57.

24. Topol EJ et al. A preferred reperfusion strategy for acute myocardial infarction. *J Am Coll Cardiol* 2003; 42: 1886–9.

25. Van't Hof AW et al. Prehospital initiation of tirofiban in patients with ST-elevation myocardial infarction undergoing primary angioplasty (On-TIME 2): A multicentre, double-blind, randomised controlled trial. *Lancet* 2008; 372: 537–46.

26. Hurlen M et al. Effects of warfarin, aspirin and the two combined, on mortality and thromboembolic morbidity after myocardial infarction: The WARIS-II (Warfarin–Aspirin Reinfarction Study) design. *Scand Cardiovasc J* 2000; 34: 168–71.

27. Yusuf S et al. Effects of fondaparinux on mortality and reinfarction in patients with acute ST-segment elevation myocardial infarction: The OASIS-6 randomized trial. *JAMA* 2006; 295: 1519–30.

28. Montalescot G et al. Enoxaparin in primary and facilitated percutaneous coronary intervention. A formal prospective non randomized substudy of the FINESSE trial (Facilitated intervention with Enhanced Reperfusion Speed to Stop Events). *JACC Cardiovasc Interv* 2010; 3(2): 203–12.

29. Shahzad A et al. Unfractionated heparin versus bivalirudin in primary percutaneous coronary intervention (HEAT-PPCI): An open-label, single centre, randomised controlled trial. *Lancet* 2014; 384:1849–58.

30. Wald DS et al. Randomized trial of preventive angioplasty in myocardial infarction. *N Engl J Med* 2013; 369: 1115–23.

31. Gershlick AH et al. Randomized trial of complete versus lesion-only revascularization in patients undergoing primary percutaneous coronary intervention for STEMI and multivessel disease: The CvLPRIT trial. *J Am Coll Cardiol* 2015; 65(10): 963–72.

32. Mehta S. Complete Vs culprit-only revascularization to treat multi-vessel disease after primary PCI for STEMI (COMPLETE). NCT01740479.

33. Pasceri V et al. Meta-analysis of clinical trials on use of drug-eluting stents for treatment of acute myocardial infarction. *Am Heart J* 2007; 153: 749–54.

34. Kalesan B et al. Comparison of drug-eluting stents with bare metal stents in patients with ST-segment elevation myocardial infarction. *Eur Heart J* 2012; 33(8): 977–87.

35. Vink MA et al. Five year follow-up after primary percutaneous coronary intervention with a paclitaxel-eluting stent versus a bare-metal stent in acute ST-segment elevation myocardial infarction: A follow-up study of the PASSION (Paclitaxel-Eluting Versus Conventional Stent in Myocardial Infarction with ST-Segment Elevation) trial. *JACC Cardiovasc Interv* 2011; 4(1): 24–9.

36. Sabaté M et al. The EXAMINATION trial (Everolimus-Eluting Stents Versus Bare-Metal Stents in ST-Segment Elevation Myocardial Infarction): 2-year results from a multicenter randomized controlled trial. *JACC Cardiovasc Interv* 2014; 7(1): 64–71.

37. Ndrepepa G et al. Periprocedural bleeding and 1-year outcome after percutaneous coronary interventions: Appropriateness of including bleeding as a component of a quadruple endpoint. *J Am Coll Cardiol* 2008; 51: 690–7.

38. Karrowni W et al. Radial versus femoral access for primary percutaneous interventions in ST-segment elevation myocardial infarction patients: A meta-analysis of randomized controlled trials. *J Am Coll Cardiol Interv* 2013; 6(8): 814–23.

39. Rao SV et al. The transradial approach to percutaneous coronary intervention: Historical perspective, current concepts, and future directions. *J Am Coll Cardiol* 2010; 55: 2187–95.

40. Romagnoli E et al. Radial versus femoral approach comparison in percutaneous coronary intervention with intraaortic balloon pump support: The RADIAL PUMP UP registry. *Am Heart J* 2013; 166(6): 1019–26.

41. Stone GW et al. Impact of normalized myocardial perfusion after successful angioplasty in acute myocardial infarction. *J Am Coll Cardiol* 2002; 39: 591–7.

42. Svilaas T et al. Thrombus aspiration during primary percutaneous coronary intervention. *N Engl J Med* 2008; 358: 557–67.

43. Fröbert O et al. Thrombus aspiration during ST-segment elevation myocardial infarction. *N Engl J Med* 2013; 369: 1587–97.

44. Jolly SS et al. Randomized trial of primary PCI with or without routine manual thrombectomy. *N Engl J Med* 2015; 372: 1389–98.

45. Boscarelli D et al. Intracoronary thrombolysis in patients with ST-segment elevation myocardial infarction presenting with massive intraluminal thrombus and failed aspiration. *Eur Heart J Acute Cardiovasc Care* 2014; 3: 229–36.

46. Vaquerizo B et al. Intracoronary massive thrombosis treated with local fibrinolysis during percutaneous coronary intervention after failed aspiration: E-poster abstract presentation, TCTAP 2012, www.summitmd.com/angioplasty/summitmd_eposter.

47. Hochman JS et al. Occluded Artery Trial Investigators. Coronary intervention for persistent occlusion after myocardial infarction. *N Engl J Med* 2006; 355: 2395–407.

48. The TIMI Study Group. The thrombolysis in myocardial infarction (TIMI) trial. *N Engl J Med* 1985; 312: 932–6.

49. Kammler J et al. TIMI 3 flow after primary angioplasty is an important predictor for outcome in patients with acute myocardial infarction. *Clin Res Cardiol* 2009; 98(3): 165–70.

50. Van't Hof AWJ et al. Angiographic assessment of myocardial reperfusion in patients treated with primary angioplasty for acute myocardial infarction: Myocardial blush grade: Zwolle Myocardial Infarction Study Group. *Circulation* 1998; 97: 2302–6.

51. Henriques JPS et al. Angiographic assessment of reperfusion in acute myocardial infarction by myocardial blush grade. *Circulation* 2003; 107: 2115–9.

52. Kampinga MA et al. Is the myocardial blush grade scored by the operator during primary percutaneous coronary intervention of prognostic value in patients with ST-elevation myocardial infarction in routine clinical practice? *Circ Cardiovasc Interv* 2010; 3(3): 216–23.

53. Ramjane K et al. The diagnosis and treatment of the no-reflow phenomenon in patients with myocardial infarction undergoing percutaneous coronary intervention. *Exp Clin Cardiol* 2008; 13(3): 121–8.

54. Ndrepepa G et al. 5-year prognostic value of no-reflow phenomenon after percutaneous coronary intervention in patients with acute myocardial infarction. *J Am Coll Cardiol* 2010; 55(21): 2383–9.

55. Dawber TR et al. The epidemiology of coronary heart disease – the Framingham enquiry. *Proc R Soc Med* 1962;55:265–71.

56. Steele L et al. A retrospective cross-sectional study on the association between tobacco smoking and incidence of ST-segment elevation myocardial infarction and cardiovascular risk factors. *Postgrad Med J* 2015;92:492–6.

57. Lloyd A et al. Pronounced increase in risk of acute ST-segment elevation myocardial infarction in younger smokers. *Heart* 2017;103:586–91. Doi: 10.1136/heartjnl-2016-309595.

Percutaneous treatment of cardiogenic shock after myocardial infarction

JAYAN PARAMESHWAR, STEPHEN PETTIT, ALAIN VUYLSTEKE

Cardiogenic shock develops in up to 8% of patients following ST segment elevation myocardial infarction (STEMI) and up to 2.5% of patients after non-ST segment elevation myocardial infarction (non-STEMI).[1,2] The natural history of cardiogenic shock is a downward spiral of ischaemic left ventricular (LV) systolic dysfunction and worsening end-organ perfusion, leading to death. Mortality rates have decreased from 77% in the early 1990s to 47.9% by 2004.[3] This decrease may reflect the progress in the treatment of myocardial infarction (MI).

The initial diagnosis of cardiogenic shock is based on clinical criteria (Table 21.1).[4,5] The SHOCK trial demonstrated that emergency re-vascularisation for acute MI complicated by cardiogenic shock reduced mortality at one year by 13% when compared with a strategy of conservative therapy.[6] The survival benefit is maintained at 10 years. Emergency re-vascularisation is usually delivered by primary percutaneous coronary intervention (PPCI).

Most patients who undergo PPCI have a rapid improvement in their haemodynamic state with restoration of flow in the infarct-related coronary artery and resolution of acute ischaemic LV systolic dysfunction. The incidence of cardiogenic shock following initial treatment of MI has fallen substantially since the widespread availability of PPCI.

Risk factors for shock include: older age, anterior MI, hypertension, diabetes mellitus, multi-vessel coronary artery disease, prior MI and history of heart failure.[7]

21.1 Assessment and initial management of cardiogenic shock

A detailed assessment is required in any patient with ongoing clinical evidence of cardiogenic shock. Vital signs should be measured continuously. Clinical examination is essential to assess central venous pressure, peripheral perfusion, detect important heart murmurs and signs of pulmonary oedema. An arterial blood sample should be taken to determine the acid-base balance, to evaluate the adequacy of oxygenation and ventilation and to measure the serum lactate level. Echocardiography is vital to identify pathology that requires immediate surgical intervention such as rupture of a papillary muscle, the ventricular septum or the ventricular free wall.

Haemodynamic confirmation of cardiogenic shock requires measurement of intra-cardiac filling pressures and cardiac output (Table 21.1). This is usually achieved with a pulmonary artery flotation catheter, but it is possible to derive similar information by echocardiographic assessment. Intra-cardiac filling pressures and vasomotor tone will vary between patients with cardiogenic shock and this will alter the approach to treatment. The overall goal of therapy is restoration of adequate blood pressure and cardiac output. The strongest predictor of survival in the SHOCK trial was cardiac power output,[8] the product of mean arterial pressure and cardiac output, and 73% patients survived if their cardiac power output was more than 0.54 W. This equates roughly to a mean arterial pressure of 70 mmHg and a cardiac

Table 21.1   Diagnostic Criteria for Cardiogenic Shock

Clinical criteria	Systolic blood pressure <90 mmHg for >30 min
	Heart rate greater than 100 bpm
	Impaired end organ perfusion (oliguria, altered consciousness, elevated lactate)
Haemodynamic criteria	Cardiac index <1.8 L/min/m² without haemodynamic support
	Cardiac index <2.2 L/min/m² with support
	PCWP >15 mmHg
	Absence of low left and right sided intra-cardiac filling pressures

output of 4 L/min. Stroke work index also predicts short-term outcome. In patients who present with RV dysfunction post-MI, optimising the RV filling pressure is important and a right atrial pressure of 10–15 mmHg is probably ideal. Aggressive fluid resuscitation without measuring filling pressure is dangerous and should be avoided.

21.2 Medical treatment

Many drugs are given during the initial treatment of acute MI that have the potential to cause harm in patients who are developing cardiogenic shock.[9,10] Drugs that can precipitate shock include nitrates as they cause systemic vasodilatation; verapamil that causes systemic vasodilatation, bradycardia and reduced cardiac contractility; and beta-blockers that reduce cardiac output.[11,12] Intravenous fluids are frequently administered to patients with low blood pressure and may increase intra-cardiac filling pressures, ventricular stretch and exacerbate ventricular dysfunction.

Abnormalities of vasomotor tone may represent a target for drug treatment. MI may cause a systemic inflammatory response and vasodilatation. If mean arterial pressure is low and cardiac output is reasonable, then a vasoconstrictor such as noradrenaline or vasopressin may be used with care. Excessive use of vasoconstrictors is counter-productive and will only increase blood pressure at the cost of reduced cardiac output. Occasionally mean arterial pressure is high and cardiac output is low. In this situation, a vasodilator such as hydralazine, a phosphodiesterase inhibitor (milrinone, enoximone) or levosimendan may be administered. Inotropic agents may be given to increase cardiac contractility. All inotropic and vasoactive drugs may be harmful, particularly in higher doses. There is no definite evidence to support using one rather than the other. High levels of circulating endogenous catecholamines are inevitable in cardiogenic shock. One major benefit of monitoring the cardiac output is that it may enable the clinician to select the most physiologically appropriate agent and use this at the lowest necessary dose. A pulmonary artery flotation catheter is probably the most accurate method of achieving this in patients with very low cardiac output. Care should be given to the interpretation of the numbers issued from measurement with a PA catheter and no number should be evaluated in isolation.

21.3 Intra-aortic balloon pump

An intra-aortic balloon pump (IABP) is the simplest form of percutaneous mechanical circulatory support (MCS) and can be rapidly placed via the femoral artery. It has been the mainstay of cardiac support since the late 1960s and works on the principle of aortic counterpulsation.[13] A 7.5–8.0 Fr catheter is attached at its distal end to a polyethylene balloon. One lumen is attached to the pump and is used to inflate the balloon with gas. Helium is used because its low viscosity facilitates rapid transfer. Helium is rapidly absorbed from the blood if the balloon ruptures. The second lumen of the IABP is used for guidewire insertion and to transduce aortic pressure. Timing of balloon inflation and deflation is usually based on electrocardiogram or pressure triggers. The balloon inflates with the onset of diastole (middle of the T wave on surface ECG) and deflates at the onset of LV systole (peak of the R wave on surface ECG).

Inflation of the IABP augments mean arterial blood pressure, improving coronary and end-organ perfusion. Deflation of the IABP reduces LV afterload, improves LV ejection fraction and reduces LV end diastolic pressure. This is particularly helpful in patients with acute cardiogenic pulmonary oedema. IABP may be used for several weeks or months if required to reach definitive treatment such as heart transplantation. Optimal haemodynamic effect from the IABP depends on the balloon's position in the aorta, the blood displacement volume, balloon diameter in relation to aortic diameter, the timing of balloon inflation and deflation, and the patient's own heart rate, blood pressure and vascular resistance.

However, IABP requires anticoagulation if used for prolonged periods of time, restricts patients to bed and is associated with vascular access complications, infection and thrombocytopenia.[14] Aortic valve regurgitation greater than mild in degree is usually considered a contraindication to the use of IABP as balloon inflation in diastole may increase the regurgitation. The augmentation of cardiac output is rarely more than 0.5 L/min which may not be sufficient to meet the needs of the sickest patients. The IABP is also limited by its dependence on residual cardiac function and electrical stability.[15]

The safety and effectiveness of IABP counter-pulsation was assessed in the IABP-SHOCK II trial.[16,17] Six hundred patients with acute MI complicated by cardiogenic shock were randomised to IABP versus conventional therapy. All patients were expected to undergo early re-vascularisation and to receive 'best medical therapy'. IABP insertion was either just before or after re-vascularisation, at the investigator's discretion. There was no difference in the primary endpoint of all-cause mortality at 30 days (39.7% IABP arm and 41.3% in control arm). There was no difference in length of intensive care unit stay or time to haemodynamic stabilisation. There was no difference in major adverse events between the two groups (bleeding, peripheral vascular complications, sepsis and stroke). At the point of randomisation, the median heart rate was 92/min and the median systolic blood pressure was 90 mmHg. The median support duration was only 3 days. Patients in IABP SHOCK may have been a moderate risk group (40% mortality at 30 days), but this trial population derived no survival benefit from routine placement of an IABP.

21.4 Advanced percutaneous MCS

Many patients deteriorate despite conventional management and their outlook is bleak. There are several advanced percutaneous MCS options in this situation (Table 21.2). They may benefit patients by increasing cardiac output and decreasing oxygen consumption by unloading the heart. Delivering a good long-term outcome requires the right MCS option to be deployed at the right time. Clinician and institutional experience with the chosen form of percutaneous MCS is essential. There must be a clear long-term treatment strategy because percutaneous MCS can support patients for days or weeks, but rarely for months. In the absence of recovery, the only chance of survival to discharge from hospital is implantation of a durable LV assist device (LVAD) or heart transplantation. Careful patient selection is vital from the outset and difficult decisions will have to be made.[18, 19]

There are common problems associated with all advanced MCS devices. All devices utilise large intra-vascular cannulae. These are associated with a risk of vascular access complications including bleeding at the access site or obstruction to either arterial flow and/or venous return. All devices pose a risk of thrombosis and require anticoagulation. In turn, anticoagulation is associated with an increased risk of bleeding at any site. All devices are a potential source of infection and may become colonised during bloodstream infection.

The available percutaneous devices fall into three main categories:

Axial flow devices (e.g. Impella)
Left atrium (LA) to femoral/iliac artery bypass pumps (e.g. TandemHeart)
Veno-Arterial Extra Corporeal Membrane Oxygenation (V-A ECMO)

21.4.1 Trans-valvular percutaneous devices

Two types of trans-valvular percutaneous LVAD are commercially available, the Impella family of devices (Abiomed) and the Percutaneous Heart Pump (Thoratec). Both devices are placed via the femoral artery and sit across the aortic valve. Both are miniature axial continuous flow blood pumps which drain blood from the LV cavity and eject blood into the ascending aorta. The Impella family includes pumps which may be placed by a cardiologist (Impella 2.5, CP and RP) and pumps that require surgical cut-down to the femoral artery (Impella 5). The tip of the catheter is a pigtail loop that stabilises the device in the LV. The pigtail connects to a 12F (2.5 device), 14F (CP device) or 21F cannula (5.0 device). The proximal catheter shaft houses the motor power leads and purge and pressure measurement lumens. The proximal end has a hub which attaches to the console cable and side arms for attachment of purge solution and pressure measurement.

Supporting the circulation with such a pump reduces myocardial oxygen consumption, increases mean arterial pressure and reduce LV end-diastolic pressure. Adequate RV function or concomitant RVAD support is required as for the TandemHeart. The Impella 2.5 provides greater increase in cardiac output than the IABP (but less than the TandemHeart). The Impella CP and 5.0 devices provide comparable haemodynamic support to the TandemHeart. The device has FDA approval for 6 hours support and is CE marked for 5 days use.

The major advantage of this type of pump is ease of placement. However, these pumps require regular echocardiographic assessment because the pump is prone to displacement. Presence of a mechanical aortic valve or LV thrombus is a contraindication to this device. Aortic stenosis and regurgitation are relative contraindications. Haemolysis due to shearing is a problem in 5%–10% of patients in the first 24 hours, it may respond to repositioning the device. Persistent haemolysis can lead to acute kidney injury and requires the device to be removed.

The safety and effectiveness of the Impella 2.5 pump was assessed in the ISAR-SHOCK trial.[20] Twenty-six patients with cardiogenic shock were randomised to support with an Impella 2.5 or an IABP. Whilst cardiac index and blood pressure increased more in the Impella group, and lactate level was lower, no difference in mortality (30-day mortality 46% in both groups), major bleeding, distal limb ischaemia, arrhythmias and infection were found. The

Table 21.2   Comparison of commonly used Devices for Percutaneous Support

Device	Ease of placement	Flow	Afterload	Common problems
IABP	High	Around 0.5 L/min	Reduced	Vascular complications
Impella CP	Medium	Up to 4 L/min	Neutral	Catheter displacement, vascular complications
Tandem Heart	Low	Up to 5 L/min	Neutral	Need for trans-septal puncture, bleeding, vascular complications
V-A ECMO	Medium	Up to 5 L/min	Increased	Vascular complications, LV distension, Harlequin syndrome

Impella-EUROSHOCK Registry reported on 120 patients with cardiogenic shock after acute MI who were supported with the Impella 2.5 device.[21] Thirty-day mortality remained high at 64.2%, major adverse cardiac and cerebrovascular events occurred in 15%. Major bleeding at the vascular access site was seen in 28.6% of patients. After 317 ± 526 days of follow-up, survival was 28.3%. The USpella Registry reported on the use of this device in 38 US hospitals. Patients in whom the device was placed before PCI had a survival to discharge rate of 65% versus 40.1% for those patients who were supported post-PCI.[22] Complications of this device include haemolysis, peripheral vascular complications and aortic regurgitation. The European Society of Cardiology guidelines give a class IIb/level C recommendation for the use of LVADs in refractory cardiogenic shock post-MI.

The Impella RP is the first percutaneous miniature continuous flow right ventricular (RV) assist device and is attractive for use in patients with RV dysfunction after durable LVAD implantation or heart transplantation as well as shock due to RV dysfunction.[23] This device obtained a CE mark in 2014 and is approved for up to 14 days use in selected patients with right heart failure. A recent study reported its use in 30 patients with RV failure post-LVAD implantation and in patients post-cardiotomy and MI. The device was successfully deployed in all but one patient. There was a marked increase in cardiac index and fall in right atrial pressure as expected with an overall 30 day survival of 73%.[24]

21.4.2 Tandem Heart

The TandemHeart is an external continuous flow blood pump which drains blood from the LA and returns blood into the ascending aorta. The Tandem Heart has a complex drainage cannula (21F) which is placed via the femoral vein and passed through the inter-atrial septum to enter the LA. The return cannula is placed in the iliac artery via the femoral artery. Both cannulae are percutaneous but must be placed using fluoroscopic guidance by an operator who is familiar with trans-septal puncture. Other components of the device include a centrifugal pump and a control console. The trans-septal cannula is made of wire-reinforced polyurethane with a large end-hole and 14 side holes that allow left atrial blood to be aspirated. The return cannula is available in sizes from 15 to 19F and is the main determinant of maximal flow. The centrifugal blood pump contains a spinning impeller powered by an electromagnetic motor rotating between 3000 and 7500 rpm. The external console controls the pump and provides battery back-up in case of power failure. Anticoagulation with activated clotting time of 300 seconds or greater is required. The device is CE marked for use up to 30 days and FDA approved for up to 6 hours.

During support, both the LV and the pump contribute flow to the aorta simultaneously working in parallel (or tandem). Redirection of blood from the LA reduces LV preload, wall stress and myocardial oxygen demand. The increase in cardiac output and blood pressure improves systemic perfusion. The pump delivers 3.5 L (15 Fr cannula) to 5 L (19 Fr cannula) flow and this may be additive to LV output. Often LV contraction is minimal with a flat mean arterial pressure curve. Adequate RV function is required to fill the LA.

Thiele et al. randomised 41 patients to support with IABP or TandemHeart.[25] Although there was marked improvement in haemodynamic parameters with the latter, there was no difference in mortality (45% vs. 43%); bleeding requiring transfusion was reported in 95% of patients (median 8 units) and limb ischaemia in 35%. Burkhoff et al. compared IABP and TandemHeart in 42 patients with cardiogenic shock (70% post-MI). Median duration of support was 2.5 days. There was no difference in 30-day survival (64% in the IABP group and 54% in the TandemHeart group) but the study was discontinued because of slow recruitment. No difference in adverse effects was reported.[26] In a retrospective study of 117 patients supported with the TandemHeart, 30-day and 6-month mortality were 40.2% and 45.3%, respectively.[27]

The need for trans-septal puncture in a critically ill cohort who are usually coagulopathic limits the use of this device. Displacement of the cannula during patient transport or if the leg is moved is to be guarded against; displacement into the right atrium results in massive right to left shunting. The cannula can also migrate into the pulmonary vein leading to pump malfunction.

21.4.2.1 The Heartmate PHP

The HeartMate PHP is an axial flow pump which is positioned in the LV across the aortic valve like the Impella. It is introduced into the femoral artery via a 14F introducer sheath. Once in the LV, the outer sheath of the PHP is retracted fully expanding the cannula to 24F. As the integrated three-blade impeller spins, blood is pulled into the cannula from the LV and is pumped into the ascending aorta. It is hoped that the wide 24F expandable cannula and low operating speeds of 16,000–20,500 rpm will minimise shear stress on the blood. The device is said to deliver flow of 4–5 L/min. It has been used to support high-risk PCI and trials in cardiogenic shock are planned. It received a CE mark in July 2015.

21.4.3 Peripheral V-A ECMO

V-A ECMO provides cardiopulmonary support for patients whose hearts no longer provide adequate flow for tissue oxygenation.

Peripheral V-A ECMO requires an external centrifugal continuous flow blood pump and a membrane oxygenator for gas exchange. A venous cannula drains blood from the right atrium and oxygenated blood is returned to the aorta. In peripheral V-A ECMO, the drainage cannula is typically inserted in the femoral vein and pushed up to the right atrium. The return cannula is inserted in the femoral artery (see Figure 21.1). Percutaneous cannulation of other vessels, such as the axillary artery, is possible but used infrequently.

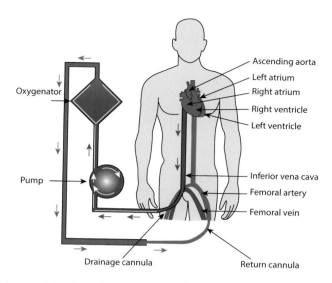

Figure 21.1 Peripheral veno-arterial extra-corporeal membrane oxygenation (V-A ECMO).

Cannulation of the femoral artery requires that a second, antegrade perfusion cannula is placed to perfuse the limb distal to the ECMO femoral cannula. Whilst the arterial cannula may be placed in a truly percutaneous fashion, surgical removal is typically required in order to repair the vascular access site. Anticoagulation is required, usually with unfractionated heparin.

Peripheral V-A ECMO may provide flow of 2.5–6 L/min depending on cannula size. It is the MCS of choice in patients with biventricular failure with impaired oxygenation. In an emergency, it can be placed without fluoroscopy at the patient's bedside, or even in the community. It allows rapid restoration of the circulation and safe transport of patients in severe acute cardiogenic shock.

However, peripheral V-A ECMO increases LV afterload thereby increasing oxygen demand and impeding myocardial protection. It does not unload the left ventricle and may actually increase filling pressure and volume. If the afterload is too high, the aortic valve may not open and stagnating blood in the LV significantly increases the risk of thrombus formation. The LV may need unloading with IABP, Impella, atrial septostomy or venting to treat pulmonary oedema.[28] Significant aortic regurgitation may worsen with ECMO and increase wall stress unless the ventricle is vented.

Cannulation complications are frequent particularly with prolonged use (>7 days) and include venous thrombosis and distal limb ischaemia. Patients with severe peripheral vascular disease are not suitable for peripheral V-A ECMO. Thromboembolic events may occur in the circuit or the patient. Haemorrhage is an important complication, around the cannula and retroperitoneally. The 'Harlequin syndrome' is a recognised complication of peripheral V-A ECMO; deoxygenated blood from the LV supplies the upper body and limbs (including the coronary circulation) whilst oxygenated blood via the ECMO circuit supplies the lower body and limbs with competing flow in the aorta.

There are no RCTs or meta-analyses with mortality as an endpoint. A single-centre retrospective comparison of 219 patients with cardiogenic shock post-MI treated with PCI and adjunctive ECMO with a historical control group of 115 patients without ECMO showed 60% 30-day survival in the former group and 35% in the latter.[29] Nicol et al. reviewed 84 studies of ECMO instituted for cardiogenic shock or cardiac arrest and showed an overall survival of 50%.[30] Recent reports found a 49% survival in patients supported with MCS or ECMO in cardiogenic shock[31] or 54% in a group receiving ECMO as part of their CPR management.[32]

21.5 Conclusion

The results of the few trials that have been carried out in this field show that currently available devices are effective in improving haemodynamic endpoints but have not increased survival. There are several possible reasons for this paradox. Cardiogenic shock post-MI is often associated with a systemic inflammatory response syndrome (SIRS) and with multi-organ failure (MOF). Once established these responses may progress despite restoration of coronary blood flow and cardiac output. Some of the devices (e.g. Impella 2.5) may not provide enough flow to support the circulation. Peripheral V-A ECMO does not unload the failing LV and, on its own, may not provide optimal support. All percutaneous devices are associated with significant complications that affect survival and limit the duration of support. For short-term mechanical devices to alter survival, there must be sufficient residual myocardium to allow weaning from support. Many patients with cardiogenic shock will only survive if short-term support can be followed by support with a durable, implantable ventricular assist device or heart transplantation. These therapies are only appropriate and available for a minority of patients. Difficult decisions will therefore need to be made when it is apparent that continued therapy is futile.

References

1. Goldberg RJ et al. Temporal trends in cardiogenic shock complicating acute myocardial infarction. *N Engl J Med* 1999; 340(15): 1162–8.
2. Hasdai D et al. Platelet glycoprotein IIb/IIIa blockade and outcome of cardiogenic shock complicating acute coronary syndromes without persistent ST-segment elevation. *J Am Coll Cardiol* 2000; 36(3): 685–92.
3. Babaev A et al. Trends in management and outcomes of patients with acute myocardial infarction complicated by cardiogenic shock. *JAMA* 2005; 294(4): 448–54.
4. Reynolds HR, and Hochman JS. Cardiogenic shock: Current concepts and improving outcomes. *Circulation* 2008; 117(5): 686–97.
5. Werdan K et al. Mechanical circulatory support in cardiogenic shock. *Eur Heart J* 2014; 35(3): 156–67.
6. Hochman JS et al. SHould we emergently revascularize Occluded Coronaries for cardiogenic shocK: An international randomized trial of emergency PTCA/CABG-trial design. The SHOCK Trial Study Group. *Am Heart J* 1999; 137(2): 313–21.

7. Lindholm MG et al. Cardiogenic shock complicating acute myocardial infarction; prognostic impact of early and late shock development. *Eur Heart J* 2003; 24(3): 258–65.

8. Fincke R et al. Cardiac power is the strongest hemodynamic correlate of mortality in cardiogenic shock: A report from the SHOCK trial registry. *J Am Coll Cardiol* 2004; 44(2): 340–8.

9. Meine TJ et al. Association of intravenous morphine use and outcomes in acute coronary syndromes: Results from the CRUSADE Quality Improvement Initiative. *Am Heart J* 2005; 149(6): 1043–9.

10. Indications for ACE inhibitors in the early treatment of acute myocardial infarction: Systematic overview of individual data from 100,000 patients in randomized trials. ACE Inhibitor Myocardial Infarction Collaborative Group. *Circulation* 1998; 97(22): 2202–12.

11. ISIS-4: A randomised factorial trial assessing early oral captopril, oral mononitrate, and intravenous magnesium sulphate in 58,050 patients with suspected acute myocardial infarction. ISIS-4 (Fourth International Study of Infarct Survival) Collaborative Group. *Lancet* 1995; 345(8951): 669–85.

12. Chen ZM et al. Early intravenous then oral metoprolol in 45,852 patients with acute myocardial infarction: Randomised placebo-controlled trial. *Lancet* 2005; 366(9497): 1622–32.

13. Papaioannou TG, and Stefanadis C. Basic principles of the intraaortic balloon pump and mechanisms affecting its performance. *ASAIO J* 2005; 51(3): 296–300.

14. Rastan AJ et al. Visceral arterial compromise during intra-aortic balloon counterpulsation therapy. *Circulation* 2010; 122(Suppl 11): S92–9.

15. Sjauw KD et al. A systematic review and meta-analysis of intra-aortic balloon pump therapy in ST-elevation myocardial infarction: Should we change the guidelines? *Eur Heart J* 2009; 30(4): 459–68.

16. Thiele H et al. Intraaortic balloon support for myocardial infarction with cardiogenic shock. *N Engl J Med* 2012; 367(14): 1287–96.

17. O'Connor CM, and Rogers JG. Evidence for overturning the guidelines in cardiogenic shock. *N Engl J Med* 2012; 367(14): 1349–50.

18. Basra SS et al. Current status of percutaneous ventricular assist devices for cardiogenic shock. *Curr Opin Cardiol* 2011; 26(6): 548–54.

19. Rihal CS et al. 2015 SCAI/ACC/HFSA/STS Clinical Expert Consensus Statement on the Use of Percutaneous Mechanical Circulatory Support Devices in Cardiovascular Care: Endorsed by the American Heart Association, the Cardiological Society of India, and Sociedad Latino Americana de Cardiologia Intervencion; Affirmation of Value by the Canadian Association of Interventional Cardiology-Association Canadienne de Cardiologie d'intervention. *J Am Coll Cardiol* 2015; 65(19): e7–e26.

20. Seyfarth M et al. A randomized clinical trial to evaluate the safety and efficacy of a percutaneous left ventricular assist device versus intra-aortic balloon pumping for treatment of cardiogenic shock caused by myocardial infarction. *J Am Coll Cardiol* 2008; 52(19): 1584–8.

21. Lauten A et al. Percutaneous left-ventricular support with the Impella-2.5-assist device in acute cardiogenic shock: Results of the Impella-EUROSHOCK-registry. *Circ Heart Fail* 2013; 6(1): 23–30.

22. Maini B et al. Real-world use of the Impella 2.5 circulatory support system in complex high-risk percutaneous coronary intervention: The USpella Registry. *Catheter Cardiovasc Interv* 2012; 80(5): 717–25.

23. Cheung AW et al. Short-term mechanical circulatory support for recovery from acute right ventricular failure: Clinical outcomes. *J Heart Lung Transplant* 2014; 33(8): 794–9.

24. Anderson MB et al. Benefits of a novel percutaneous ventricular assist device for right heart failure: The prospective RECOVER RIGHT study of the Impella RP device. *J Heart Lung Transplant* 2015; 34(12): 1549–60.

25. Thiele H et al. Randomized comparison of intra-aortic balloon support with a percutaneous left ventricular assist device in patients with revascularized acute myocardial infarction complicated by cardiogenic shock. *Eur Heart J* 2005; 26(13): 1276–83.

26. Burkhoff D et al. A randomized multicenter clinical study to evaluate the safety and efficacy of the TandemHeart percutaneous ventricular assist device versus conventional therapy with intraaortic balloon pumping for treatment of cardiogenic shock. *Am Heart J* 2006; 152(3): 469 e1–8.

27. Kar B et al. The percutaneous ventricular assist device in severe refractory cardiogenic shock. *J Am Coll Cardiol* 2011; 57(6): 688–96.

28. Koeckert MS et al. Impella LP 2.5 for left ventricular unloading during venoarterial extracorporeal membrane oxygenation support. *J Card Surg* 2011; 26(6): 666–8.

29. Sheu JJ et al. Early extracorporeal membrane oxygenator-assisted primary percutaneous coronary intervention improved 30-day clinical outcomes in patients with ST-segment elevation myocardial infarction complicated with profound cardiogenic shock. *Crit Care Med* 2010; 38(9): 1810–7.

30. Nichol G et al. Systematic review of percutaneous cardiopulmonary bypass for cardiac arrest or cardiogenic shock states. *Resuscitation* 2006; 70(3): 381–94.

31. Takayama H et al. Clinical outcome of mechanical circulatory support for refractory cardiogenic shock in the current era. *J Heart Lung Transplant* 2013; 32(1): 106–11.

32. Stub D et al. Refractory cardiac arrest treated with mechanical CPR, hypothermia, ECMO and early reperfusion (the CHEER trial). *Resuscitation* 2015; 86: 88–94.

Rotational coronary atherectomy

STEPHEN FORT

22.1 Introduction

Successful percutaneous coronary intervention (PCI) by balloon angioplasty (BA) and stenting relies on the expansion of the atheromatous vessel and/or plaque fissuring.

Calcified and fibrous atheromas resist balloon and stent dilatation, resulting in non-uniform expansion of eccentric lesions and under- or non-expansion in concentric lesions. Rotablation, or rotational atherectomy (RA) is a unique PCI technique that facilitates balloon and stent expansion in non-compliant fibrous and calcified lesions. A diamond tip burr, rotating at high speed, is advanced along a guide-wire selectively cutting hard or calcified plaque, while soft plaque and normal vessel wall are deflected away from the burr, minimising damage ('differential cutting'). Debrided micro-particles from the atheroma are flushed downstream and eventually removed by the reticulo-endothelial system. Unlike BA, lumen enlargement by RA is not achieved by vessel expansion.[1]

Rotablation was developed by Auth in the early 1980's as an alternative to BA.[2] While early clinical experience was encouraging, subsequent studies demonstrated increased procedural complications and restenosis when used as a stand-alone device.[3–5] The current utilisation of RA in PCI is 0.8%–3.1%.[6] As a consequence of PCI being attempted in more complex lesions, including chronic total occlusions (CTO) and elderly patients with more extensive coronary calcification however, interest in RA has recently increased.

This chapter will concentrate on the current role of RA as a complimentary device used to facilitate PCI in complex coronary lesions, as well as pharmacological and technical advances, avoidance and management of potential complications.

22.2 Device description and set-up

The Rotablator™ system is comprised of the following:

- Console
- Advancer unit
- DynaGlide foot pedal
- Rota-Link catheter
- RotaWire
- Flush/lubricant
- Gas supply

22.2.1 Console

The console controls and monitors the rotational speed of the burr and the turbine's gas supply (Figure 22.1). The compressed gas, foot pedal and advancer are all connect to the console. The ablation times are recorded, with warnings lights for DynaGlide setting and burr stalling. The console needs to be positioned so that the operator can visually monitor Rotablator function at all times but be accessible by the circulating cath lab staff for adjustment.

22.2.2 Advancer unit

The black fibre optic cable from the advancer (Figure 22.1) is connected to the front of the console. The advancers compressed gas supply line connects directly to the turbine port on the front of the console, adjacent to the DynaGlide (pink line) port. The advancer is also connected to the irrigation/flush system.

22.2.3 DynaGlide foot pedal

This unit is operated concurrently with fluoroscopy during rotablation. The foot pedal (Figure 22.1) is attached to the console by three colour-coordinated lines. Depressing the foot pedal activates the turbine. DynaGlide is selected by an 'on–off' switch on the side of the foot pedal, and confirmed by a light on front of the console.

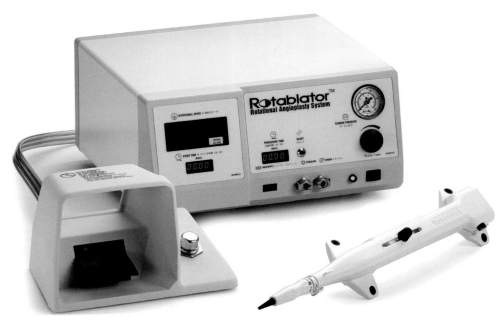

Figure 22.1 Rotablator™ system (L to R: foot pedal, console and advancer unit with attached burr catheter body). (Courtesy of Boston Scientific Corporation.)

22.2.4 Rota-Link catheter

The burr catheter (Figure 22.2) is rotated, irrigated and controlled by the advancer unit. Connecting the drive shaft of the burr to the advancer requires the advancers drive shaft is exposed, by unlocking and fully sliding forward the black advancer knob. The advancer knob is then relocked. The 'jaws' of the burr's drive shaft are exposed by withdrawing the copper sheath. Holding the drive shaft, away from the copper sheath, the interlocking 'jaws' of the advancer's drive shaft and burr are then snapped together. Test the connection by applying light pressure to pull the two apart. Once connected, advance the copper sheath back over the inter-locked 'jaws'. The catheter body of the burr is then slotted into the advancer by firstly unlocking and withdrawing the advancer knob, then clicking the burr into place. The irrigation port is then opened. Flush should be seen dripping form the end of the burr's catheter before the foot pedal is activated. The flush can be left on at all times, except when disconnecting the burr. The Rota-Link Plus system comprises an advancer unit and pre-connected burr. This burr can also be disconnected if upsizing is required.

22.2.5 Rotablator guidewires

Rotablator wires are unique to the Rotablator system. Conventional guidewires cannot be used. The Rotablator wires are 330 cm long with a stainless steel 0.009″ shaft and a 15 mm 0.014″ radio-opaque tip. There are two versions: RotaWire Floppy and RotaWire Extra Support guidewires. The Extra Support wire aids advancement of the burr into the vessel but at the expense of increased vessel straightening. The performance of both wires is markedly inferior when compared to modern, conventional guidewires.

22.2.6 Flush/lubricant

Pressurised heparinised saline or Rotaglide is essential for burr performance and prevention of damage from heat generation. Rotaglide is an emulsion of olive oil, glycerine, egg yolk phospholipids, sodium deoxycholate, L-histidine, disodium ethylenediaminetetraacetic acid (EDTA), sodium hydroxide and water. One 20 mL vial is added to 1 L bag of saline flush. Vasodilators can also be added to the flush. The flush needs to be pressurised to > 200 mmHg for effective irrigation.

22.2.7 Gas supply

Air or nitrogen cylinder is required. Oxygen should not be used. There needs to be a minimum of 500 psi in the tank with 90–110 psi delivered to the rear of the console.

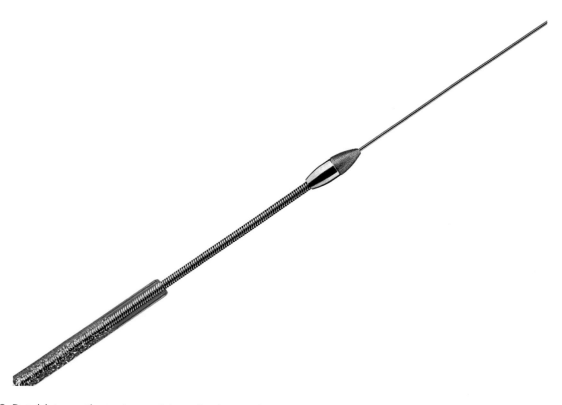

Figure 22.2 Rotablator catheter (comprising of a diamond-tipped burr, helical drive shaft and Teflon-coated sheath) on a Rotablator guidewire. (Courtesy of Boston Scientific Corporation.)

22.3 RA procedure

22.3.1 Guide catheter selection and vascular access

The full range of burr sizes requires use of guide catheters between 5 and 8 Fr. (Table 22.1). In practice, however, a 5 or 6 Fr. guide is usually sufficient for the vast majority of RA procedures, thus facilitating a trans-radial approach. Use of 5 or 6 Fr. guides also avoids the need for guide catheters with side holes. Since the majority of vessels and lesions preferentially treated by RA are high-risk complex lesions, requiring intracoronary stent insertion, good guide support is essential. There are no specific guides for RA and choice of guide catheter can be left at the operator's discretion.

22.3.2 Guidewire passage

Unlike modern 0.014″ guidewires, the Rotablator wires are difficult to torque and advance into tortuous vessels and across complex lesions. Additionally, the wire clip torquer is more difficult to use than those supplied for conventional 0.014″ guidewires. Most operators favour the use of a conventional guidewire and then exchange, via a micro-catheter or 'over-the-wire' balloon, to the Rotablator guidewire. The tip of the wire should be positioned as distally as possible in the largest diameter vessel.

22.3.3 Burr selection

Since many of the complications of RA are related to the use of large burrs, initial use of the smallest burr (1.25 mm) and then upsizing, is strongly recommended. The downsides of this approach are the need for burr exchange and higher procedural costs. Only in aorto-ostial lesions can use of a large initial burr (>0.7 burr/artery ratio) be considered.

22.3.4 Burr activation

Once the burr is connected to the advancer unit, and the irrigation system opened, the burr can be backloaded onto the wire. The turbine is activated via the foot

Table 22.1 Introducer/guide catheter sizing for RA

Burr size (mm)	Diameter (inches)	Minimum guide size (French)
1.25	0.049	5
1.50	0.059	5
1.75	0.069	6
2.0	0.079	6/7
2.25	0.089	7
2.5	0.098	7/8

pedal. The burr speed should be set outside the patient at 160,000–180,000 rpm for burrs 1.25–2.0 mm in diameter and 140,000–160,000 rpm for burrs >2.25 mm using the turbine pressure control knob on the console. After back loading, the wire clip torquer can be attached to the end of the wire to aid burr advancement to the lesion. Considerable back tension on the end of the wire may be required due to resistance within the guide and vessel. The brake button on the rear of the advancer should also be depressed during burr advancement to minimise friction.

Once the burr is positioned proximal to the lesion, administration of intracoronary vasodilators, fluids and inotrope infusion should be considered to reduce no-reflow. Begin rotablating by firstly loosening the black advancer knob, depressing the foot pedal and then gently advancing the burr into the lesion under full fluoroscopic guidance. Check that the initial burr speed is similar to that initially set outside the patient. Rotation speeds significantly below that set would indicate friction within the guide catheter, perhaps due to kinking, and will impair burr performance. The burr should be advanced in a pecking-like motion, with advancement and retraction of the burr to allow intermittent coronary perfusion. It is recommended that the initial ablation is brief (5–20 seconds), being careful not to advance the burr too fast or too forcibly.[7] Reductions in the burr rotation speed of > 5000 rpm are to be avoided. After each ablation, withdraw the burr to the starting position and check the patient's heart rate, blood pressure, ST segments and clinical status. Until the first burr has fully crossed the lesion and coronary flow is optimised, there is always the risk of no-reflow. Once the burr has fully crossed the lesion, the burr can be advanced for longer periods of time and over longer distances for final lesion 'polishing'.

After rotablating, the burr can be withdrawn using the DynaGlide function. DynaGlide rotates the burr at a slower speed (60,000–90,000 rpm) reducing resistance within the guide/vessel. It is activated via a button on the side of the foot pedal and visually confirmed on the control console. During this procedure, the wire clip torquer on the end of the wire can be inserted into the docking port at rear of the advancer, to deactivate the brake. Dynagliding can also be used to facilitate initial advancement of the burr to the lesion. However, this use of DynaGlide is controversial as it has been suggested that it may damage the lumen of the guide catheter and create debris. If DynaGlide is used before rotablation, it is important that the brake is activated, by removing the wire clip torquer from the docking port of the advancer once the burr has reached the lesion.

Additional atherectomy can be performed by increasing burr size. Fully debulking lesions, however, is often unnecessary as successful balloon inflation, even at low inflation pressure, is often achieved after successful use of a single small burr. Complications such as chest pain, vessel dissection, no-flow or abrupt vessel occlusion are all contraindications to further RA.

22.4 Adjunctive therapies

22.4.1 Vasodilators

Coronary vasodilators reduce the incidence of vasospasm and no-reflow in RA. Drugs used include intracoronary nitroglycerine (100–300 µg), verapamil (100–300 µg), diltiazem (100–300 µg), nitroprusside (50–100 µg) or adenosine (18–30 µg). Such agents should be administered prophylactically, and therapeutically, to improve coronary perfusion during RA. Use of intracoronary adenosine prior to RA in complex lesions has been shown to reduce the incidence of no-reflow.[8] Selective intracoronary administration of these agents via a micro-catheter can facilitate the administration of large doses in cases of severe spasm or no-reflow, while reducing the incidence of systemic side effects. Alternatively, vasodilators can be added to the flush system attached to the advancer unit.[9]

22.4.2 Glycoprotein IIb/IIIa inhibitors and bivalirudin

Increased platelet aggregability is associated with reduced coronary perfusion and symptomatic ischaemia. RA-induced platelet aggregability can be inhibited by apiximab infusion, with documented reductions in perfusion defects on sestamibi single-photon emission computed tomography, peri-procedural morbidity and cardiac enzyme elevation.[10-13] However, sub-group analysis of the ROTATE Registry failed to demonstrate any clinical benefit of apiximab in RA.[14] Sub-group analysis of the ROTAXUS study demonstrated that bivalirudin in RA significantly reduced peri-procedural myocardial infarctions, with a trend towards less access site bleeding.[15] Most operators favour the use of the more potent anticoagulation in RA than heparin alone.

22.4.3 New oral anti-platelet inhibitors

The use with the newer oral anti-platelet agents (ticagrelor and parsugrel) in RA has not been investigated.

22.4.4 Mechanical circulatory support

High-risk patients with multi-vessel disease, last remaining vessel and/or impaired left ventricular function undergoing RA are at particularly risk of hypotension, impaired coronary perfusion, no-reflow, arrhythmias, myocardial ischaemia and/or infarction. Insertion of an intra-aortic balloon pump (IABP) counter-pulsation or left ventricular assist device may prevent such complications.[16,17] The risk of access site complications is, however, increased.

22.5 Contraindications to RA

Contraindications to RA include

- Unable to cross with wire
- Saphenous vein by-pass grafts
- Lesions with thrombus
- Lesions with dissection
- Last remaining vessel with impaired left ventricular function

With the exception of un-crossable lesions, most of the above contraindications can be viewed as relative ones. RA has been used in such complex lesions and patients as a bail-out procedure, particularly if other PCI interventions have failed and as an alternative to by-pass surgery. For example, RA has been used in saphenous vein graft lesions, acute ST-segment elevation MI, coronary dissection and patients with impaired left ventricular function.[16-22] Figures 22.3 through 22.5 illustrate successful RA, followed by stent insertion, in a left circumflex artery dissected by previous high-pressure BA and unsuccessful stent insertion.

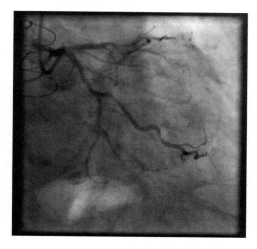

Figure 22.3 Right anterior oblique coronary angiographic view of sequential left mid circumflex and second obtuse marginal artery stenoses in a patient with prior by-pass surgery.

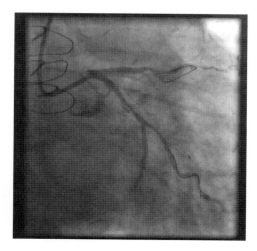

Figure 22.4 Right anterior oblique view of left mid circumflex artery dissection following high-pressure, non-compliant balloon dilatation and failed intracoronary stent insertion.

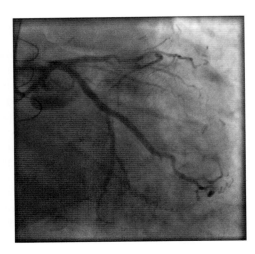

Figure 22.5 Right anterior oblique view following successful RA to facilitate intracoronary stent insertion and deployment of two overlapping DES in the left mid circumflex and second obtuse marginal arteries.

22.6 Clinical applications of RA

Increased operator experience with RA has decreased procedural complication rates despite use in complex, high-risk lesions and patients. Combination of RA with drug-eluting stents (DES) has also reduced restenosis.[23,24] However, the routine use of RA in PCI of moderately long calcified lesions has not been shown to be superior to BA and stenting without debulking.[25] RA has therefore become a complementary technique, facilitating procedural success in complex lesions subsets which respond poorly to BA and intracoronary stenting alone (Videos 22.1 and 22.2).

22.6.1 Failure to successfully cross lesions with a balloon and/or achieve optimal balloon expansion

Advances in modern guidewire technology has allowed increased success in lesion crossing, including CTO. Despite advances in balloon and guide technology, however, failure

to advance, or fully expand, balloons across heavily calcified lesions is still experienced. In such lesions, when extra guide catheter support and other adjunctive technologies and techniques have failed, RA or Tornus micro-catheter (Figure 22.6) can considered.[26–29] RA and Tornus can also be used synergistically.[30]

22.6.2 In-stent restenosis

RA is an option for treating in-stent restenosis (IRS), particularly if the neo-intimal hyperplasia is diffuse, intravascular imaging demonstrates the original stent to be optimally expanded and repeat stent insertion is to be avoided, for example, in small diameter vessels. If pre-PCI intravascular imaging is not used to assess stent geometry in ISR, high-pressure BA is recommended post-RA to ensure full stent expansion. The routine use of RA in diffuse ISR is not supported by the clinical trials, due to higher re-restenosis compared to BA and repeat stenting.[31,32] The routine use of low rather than high-pressure BA following RA has not been shown to reduce recurrent neo-intimal hyperplasia in IRS.

RA has a role in focal ISR that fails to respond to high-pressure BA. However, incomplete ISR dilatation secondary to lesion recoil should preferentially be treated with repeat DES insertion rather than debulking by RA. Final dilatation with drug-eluting balloons (DEB) can be considered in an attempt to reduce re-restenosis in ISR lesions post-RA when further stent insertion would be problematic.

22.6.3 Aorto-ostial lesions

Balloon dilation of aorto-ostial stenoses is often complicated by incomplete balloon dilation and/or vessel recoil, particularly in calcified or fibrotic lesions. RA is ideal at debulking such lesions but can be a technically challenging procedure. Coaxial guide catheter positioning is essential to achieve optimal lesion debridement and reduce complications in aorto-ostial lesions. Use of the RotaWire Extra Support guidewire may be beneficial to facilitate coaxial guide

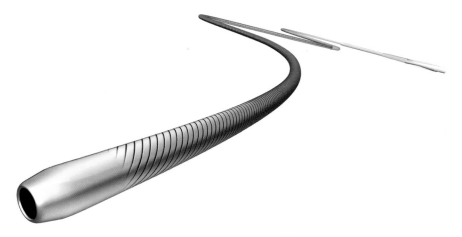

Figure 22.6 Tornus micro-catheter. (Courtesy of ASAHI INTECC Co. Ltd.)

support and to reduce the possibility of the burr transecting the guidewire. Large diameter proximal coronary vessels require the use of large burrs and large diameter guide catheters for effective debridement, thus potentially increasing vascular access site complications. Aorto-ostial lesions debulked by RA should be complimented by high-pressure balloon, cutting or 'scoring' balloon dilatation to maximise luminal expansion prior to final stent implantation.[33]

22.6.4 Side branch lesions

Similar to aorto-ostial lesions, balloon dilatation of side branch ostial lesions is frequently complicated by vessel recoil, with the additional risk of plaque shift into the parent vessel ('snow-ploughing'). RA of ostial side branch lesions is limited by the inability to use a second guidewire to protect the parent vessel. Therefore a 'stepped' approach, starting with a small burr, is highly recommended with gradual advancement of the burr at the lesion site to avoid burr and guidewire displacement, guidewire transection and damage to the unprotected parent vessel. While several studies have shown RA to be safe and effective in such lesions, there is a high-risk of restenosis. As such, final DES insertion, or perhaps DEB dilatation, should be considered in such lesions to improve long-term outcomes.[34-37]

22.6.5 Jailed side branches

RA can be used to treat side branch ostial lesions 'jailed' by a stent in the parent vessel. In addition to the above advantages of RA in 'un-jailed' ostial stenoses, RA also ablates the overlapping stent struts, thus facilitating balloon or stent insertion into the side branch.[38] Adjunctive or final balloon dilatation is still recommended post-RA. A high procedural success rate and low risk of complications has been reported, although the restenosis rate is high.[39] Consideration should therefore be given to adjunctive DEB dilatation or additional DES insertion once optimal debulking and dilation of the ostial stenosis has been achieved.

22.6.6 Stent ablation

RA has been successfully used to treat under-expanded stents deployed in heavily calcified plaques, allowing balloon dilatation to fully expand of the remaining stent, or to facilitate the insertion of additional stents.[40-42] The possible mechanisms of action of RA in stent ablation are fourfold: (1) removal of the underexpanded stent struts, (2) abrasion of the heavily calcified plaque, (3) thermal injury to the struts and plaque and (4) mechanical compression of the burr against the stent struts. All potentially contribute to increasing lesion compliance.[43-45]

RA of underexpanded stents (with or without overlaying neo-intimal hyperplasia) is a technically challenging procedure, particularly if long stents are involved. Complications include risk of heat generation and thermal injury (and hence increased restenosis) and entanglement of the struts with the burr leading to burr entrapment. It is strongly recommended that a 'stepped' approach is used starting with the smallest burr, with short (20–30 seconds) runs. Once completed, high-pressure balloon dilatation with non-compliant balloons is recommended to achieve optimal lesion/stent expansion prior to additional stent insertion or DEB dilatation.

22.6.7 Unprotected left main stenoses

RA has been shown to be both feasible and effective in treating heavily calcified left main stenoses in high surgical risk patients, particularly if a balloon fails to cross the lesion or fully expand.[46,47] Left ventricular support for these patients should be considered to prevent or reduce the haemodynamic consequences of no-reflow.

22.6.8 Chronic total occlusions

RA may be of benefit in CTO prior to stent insertion, given the high plaque and calcium burden in these lesions.[48]

22.7 Complications of RA and potential remedies

22.7.1 Non-spinning burr

If there is no noise from the turbine when the foot pedal is depressed, check the gas cylinder and its connections. If the turbine is spinning but not the burr, check the connection between burr drive shaft and the turbine in the Rota-Link advancer unit. Connecting the 'jaws' of the helical drive shaft in the Rota-Link advancer unit to the burr catheter can be challenging. The copper sheath covering the connection, can still be retracted over the coupling, without the 'jaws' being interlocked. To check if the two are not interlocked, disconnect the burr from the advancer and pull the two lightly in opposite directions. If the jaws are not interlocked within the copper sheath, the burr will disconnect from the coupling. Once reconnected, confirm interconnection of the 'jaws' by applying light counter traction between the burr and Rota-Link advancer unit before replacing the copper sheath.

22.7.2 Over-heating

Adequate cooling is essential before the burr is activated, both outside and inside the patient. Ensure the flush is running as evidenced by the drip chamber and fluid exiting the distal portion of the burr's sheath. The amount of heat generated by plaque debridement depends upon the technique used.[44] As thermal injury may increase the risk of peri-procedural myocardial infarction and restenosis, initial use of a small burr in a pecking-like motion is strongly recommended. Up-sizing burrs require the flush to be discontinued but must be restarted before activating the burr.

22.7.3 Retraction of the wire when rotablating

The guidewire brake in the advancer unit may not be engaged. Once the burr is in position the wire clip torquer must be removed from the advancer unit to engage the brake on the guidewire.

22.7.4 No-reflow

The majority of micro-particles created by RA are <100 microns in diameter and smaller than mature erythrocytes.[49] No- or slow-reflow can be caused by excessive lesion debridement and poor perfusion pressure to wash out the debris and/or associated thrombus. It occurs in approximately 7%–8% of cases.[50] No-reflow can be prevented, or reduced, by ensuring a good systemic blood pressure prior to burr advancement, frequent use of vasodilators, limiting duration of burr runs and length of burr advancement and allowing intermittent coronary flow using a pecking-like motion during burr advancement. Treatment of established no-reflow is similar to that complicating non-Rotablator cases.[51,52] In multi-vessel PCI with a high risk of RA-induced no-reflow, it is often beneficial to PCI the other lesions/vessels first before RA, in a bid to improve collateral perfusion and thus reduce the haemodynamic impact of no-reflow.

22.7.5 Heart block/hypotension

RA of dominant vessels has an additional, potential complication of heart block and associated hypotension. The underlying causes are identical to those described with no-reflow. Previous practice was to insert a temporary trans-venous pacing wire. Additional vascular access, however, increases the risk of vascular complications. Maintenance of the heart rate by temporary pacing often does not prevent associated hypotension. Prevention is best achieved by those measures described in avoiding no-reflow. If the starting heart rate and blood pressure are low, fluid boluses and/or inotropes should be considered before RA, including the administration of bolus atropine during the rotablation.

22.7.6 Burr stalling when rotablating

Resistance to burr rotation is demonstrated by a decline in the rotation speed displayed on the console and an audible reduction in burr noise. Excessive reduction in burr speed of > 5000 rpm is best managed by retracting the burr from the lesion and advancing more slowly or less forceful in a pecking-like motion. If it recurs, check the guide catheter is coaxial and not kinked. A higher burr speed or preferably a smaller burr can be tried if the above measures are not successful.

22.7.7 Burr entrapment

The distal portion of the elliptical burr is coated with 10-μm diamond microchips, but the proximal portion is smooth. If excessive force is applied to the advancing burr it can become stuck in the lesion or across the lesion but be unable to be withdrawn. This occurs in approximately 0.5% of cases.[53] Risk factors for burr entrapment include eccentric calcification, recently implanted stents and use of a large burr/artery ratio. If resistance is encountered retracting the burr, excessive traction is to be avoided or risk guide catheter-induced vessel dissection. When the burr cannot be withdrawn, there are number of options: (1) Cannulate the vessel with a second guide catheter and insert another guidewire into the vessel. Once effective balloon dilatation of the lesion has been achieved, reattempt burr withdrawal.[54] Figures 22.7 through 22.9 illustrate an example of burr entrapment during stent ablation with successful recovery of the burr using balloon dilation via a second guide catheter. (2) The Rotablator sheath can be removed to facilitate the insertion of additional wires and balloons by transecting the shaft near the advancer and withdrawing the Teflon-coated sheath. Extra guide catheter support for increased traction can then be gained by inserting a 'mother-and-child' catheter over the exposed Rotablator drive shaft, once the burr sheath has been removed.[55,56] (3) When using large diameter guide catheters, removal of the burr sheath may allow balloon dilatation via the same guide catheter. (4) Use a snare to encircle the burr to provide extra traction.[55]

If endovascular manoeuvres fail, surgical removal with bypass grafting is the last resort. For a review and suggested algorithm for management of Rotablator burr entrapment, see Sulimov et al.[57]

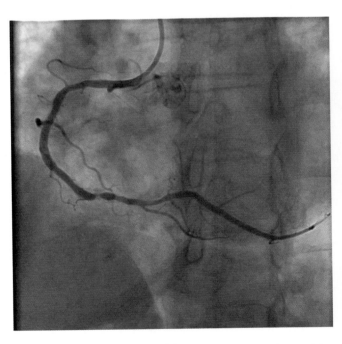

Figures 22.7 Left anterior oblique coronary angiographic view of distal right coronary artery IRS due to an underexpanded stent, using a trans-radial 6 Fr. Amplatzer Left-1 guide catheter.

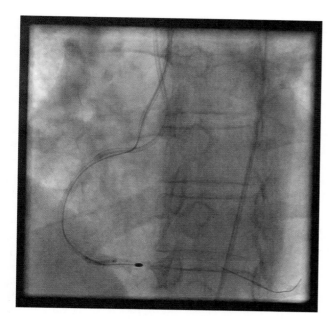

Figure 22.8 Left anterior oblique view of high-pressure, non-compliant balloon dilation in the distal right coronary artery IRS, with an entrapped Rotablator burr, via a transfemoral 6 Fr. Amplatzer Left-1 guide catheter.

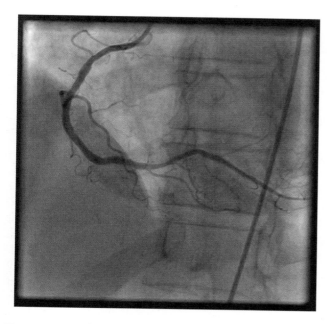

Figure 22.9 Left anterior oblique view following successful balloon dilatation of the distal right coronary artery IRS and Rotablator burr retrieval.

22.7.8 Rotawire entrapment

If a buddy wire is required to deliver a stent post-RA and the stent is advanced on the conventional guidewire, the Rotablator wire must be withdrawn before stent deployment. The shaft of the Rotawire is 0.09″ and the tip 0.014″, thus a 'jailed' Rotablator wire is difficult to retract. Should a Rotablator wire be 'jailed', it should be retrieved using an OTW balloon or micro-catheter, advanced on the Rotablator wire and tunnelled outside the expanded stent to facilitate traction and wire removal. In such cases, the stent should be post-dilated to ensure full apposition to the vessel wall.

22.7.9 Rotablator guidewire fracture

The thin 0.009″ guidewire and its 0.014″ radio-opaque tip can both be damaged by the rotating burr. Rapid advancement of the burr along an angulated wire can transect the guidewire. As only the 15 mm tip of the Rotablator wire is radio-opaque, it is difficult angiographically to appreciate when the Rotablator wire is transected. Guidewire fracture should be suspected when the advanced burr deviates offline. Imaging techniques such as intravascular ultrasound (IVUS) or optical coherence tomography (OCT) are often required to confirm the fractured guidewire and locate the proximal end. Attempts to remove the distal wire fragment using a snare device is difficult but should be attempted. Use a bioptome device is limited to wires in large proximal vessels. Should all attempts fail, and the wire left *in situ*, the stent length chosen should be long enough to cover the lesion and as much of the fractured guidewire as technically possible.

If the 0.014″ tip of the wire is not placed sufficiently distal to the lesion, it can be damaged directly by the burr. In such cases, retrieval of the wire tip from the distal vessel, or inserting a covering stent, is near impossible. Use of prolonged dual anticoagulant therapy should be considered in such cases to reduce wire-induced vessel thrombosis.

22.7.10 Vessel dissection

RA in the presence of known artery dissection is contraindicated. It is advised to wait 4 weeks for the dissection to heal, before attempting RA. However, RA has been used as a 'bail out' procedure in cases complicated by artery dissection.[21,22] RA can occasionally dissect coronary arteries. In such RA-induced dissections, the lesion should be fully dilated by high-pressure BA prior to attempted stent insertion, in preference to further RA.

22.7.11 Vessel perforation

Vessel perforation is a rare, but dreaded, potential complication of RA, although this may reflect the high-risks associated with complex lesion PCI, rather than any specific intervention.[58] Risk factors for RA-induced vessel perforation include the use of over-sized burrs, tortuous vessels and inadequate wire support. Treatment is similar to that of artery rupture secondary to balloon or stent inflation. Given that RA is preferentially used in complex vessels and lesions, emergency cardiac surgery is often required.

22.8 Randomised clinical trials

22.8.1 Excimer laser, rotational atherectomy, and balloon angioplasty comparison (ERBAC) study

Single-centre randomised study demonstrated that RA improved procedural success rates in complex lesion PCI but at the expense of higher clinical and angiographic restenosis and repeat revascularisation.[5]

22.8.2 Comparison of balloon angioplasty versus rotational atherectomy in complex lesions

Comparison of balloon angioplasty versus rotational atherectomy in complex lesions (COBRA) is the first randomised, prospective, multi-centre trial of RA versus BA in complex lesions. RA improved procedural results, with less bail-out stenting but was not associated with any long-term clinical or angiographic benefits.[59]

22.8.3 Study to determine rotablator and transluminal angioplasty strategy

Results of the randomised study to determine rotablator and transluminal angioplasty strategy (STRATAS) demonstrated the use of a large burr/artery ratio (>0.7) with very low-pressure BA in PCI of calcified or complex coronary stenoses offers no clinical or angiographic benefits compared to RA with a small burr/artery ratio (<0.7) followed by higher pressure BA.[60]

22.8.4 Coronary angioplasty and rotablator atherectomy trial

Coronary angioplasty and rotablator atherectomy trial (CARAT) is a multi-centre, randomised control trial of RA, which compared large and small burr/artery ratios (>0.7 vs. <0.7). No differences in procedural success, initial angiographic or long-term clinical benefit were found, although the larger burr approach was associated with greater procedural complications.[61]

22.8.5 Dilatation versus ablation revascularization trial

Dilatation vs. ablation revascularisation trial (DART) is a multi-centre, randomised control trial of RA in small vessels with non-calcified short stenoses (<20 mm in length) in a population with a high incidence of diabetes. No procedural or follow-up angiographic benefits were found when compared to BA alone.[62]

22.8.6 Atherectomy for treatment of diffuse in-stent restenosis trial

Atherectomy for treatment of diffuse in-stent restenosis trial (ARTIST) is a European, multicentre, randomised control trial of RA with low-pressure balloon dilatation versus high-pressure BA in PCI of diffuse ISR. There was no difference in the short-term outcomes but higher restenosis in the RA group. An IVUS sub-study demonstrated greater stent re-expansion in the high-pressure BA arm. RA with low-pressure BA was not shown to reduce recurrent neo-intimal hyperplasia.[31,63]

22.8.7 Rotational atherectomy versus balloon angioplasty for diffuse in-stent restenosis (ROSTER)

Rotational atherectomy versus balloon angioplasty for diffuse in-stent restenosis (ROSTER) is an IVUS-guided, single-centre, randomised trial of RA (burr/artery ratio >0.7) with low-pressure BA versus 'optimised' high-pressure BA in diffuse IRS. Procedural and angiographic success rates were similar, although repeat stent insertion was higher in the BA arm (31% vs. 10% resp.). Long-term clinical results were superior in the RA arm.[32]

22.8.8 Meta-analysis

Combined results from 16 trials (9222 patients) indicate that routine use of RA does not appear to improve long-term clinical results but is associated with higher complication rates, when compared to BA and stenting.[64]

22.8.9 Rotational atherectomy prior to taxus stent treatment for complex native coronary artery disease

Rotational atherectomy prior to Taxus stent treatment for complex native coronary artery disease (ROTAXUS) trial is a randomised control trial of RA versus BA in long calcified lesions prior to DES insertion. Routine RA did not influence long-term outcomes, although 12% crossed over to RA from the BA group.[65] DES implantation in complex coronary lesions can therefore be performed with BA alone, with RA as backup.

22.9 Conclusions

The European Association of Percutaneous Cardiovascular Interventions (EAPCI) has issued a consensus document with recommendations for the current and future practice of RA.[6] RA is a challenging technique with a steep learning curve and potentially high risk of complications. There is no compelling randomised controlled clinical data to justify the routine use of RA in PCI. However, the unique mechanism of action of RA, the selective debridement of non-compliant fibrotic and calcified atheromatous plaques make it an invaluable tool in the cardiac catheterisation laboratory. Used selectively in complex, highly calcified lesions, RA increases procedural success by facilitating DES insertion and expansion. In experienced hands, with a meticulous technique, RA can safely and effectively be performed without the need for on-site surgical backup.

References

1. Kovach JA et al. Sequential intravascular ultrasound haracterization of the mechanisms of rotational atherectomy and adjunct balloon angioplasty. *J Am Coll Cardiol* 1993; 22(4): 1024–32.

2. Ritchie JL et al. Rotational approaches to atherectomy and thrombectomy. *Z Kardiol* 1987; 76(Suppl 6): 59–65.

3. Warth DC et al. Rotational atherectomy multicenter registry: Acute results, complications and 6-month angiographic follow-up in 709 patients. *J Am Coll Cardiol* 1994; 24(3): 641–8.

4. Bertrand ME et al. Percutaneous transluminal coronary rotary ablation with Rotablator (European experience). *Am J Cardiol* 1992; 69: 470–4.

5. Reifart N et al. Randomized comparison of angioplasty of complex coronary lesions at a single center - excimer laser, rotational atherectomy, and balloon angioplasty comparison (ERBAC) study. *Circulation* 1997; 19: 91–8.

6. Barbato E et al. European expert consensus on rotational atherectomy. *EuroIntervention* 2015; 11(1): 30–6.

7. Stertzer SH et al. Effects of technique modification on immediate results of high speed rotational atherectomy in 710 procedures on 656 patients. *Cathet Cardiovasc Diagn* 1995; 36: 304–10.

8. Hanna GP et al. Intracoronary adenosine administered during rotational atherectomy of complex lesions in native coronary arteries reduces the incidence of no-reflow phenomenon. *Cathet Cardiovasc Intervent* 1999; 48: 275–8.

9. Cohen BM et al. Cocktail attenuation of rotational ablation flow effects (CARAFE) study: Pilot. *Cathet Cardiovasc Diagn* 1996; S3: 69–72.

10. Reisman M et al. Analysis of low-speed rotational atherectomy for the reduction of platelet aggregation. *Cathet Cardiovasc Diagn* 1998; 45: 208–14.

11. Williams MS et al. Activation of platelets in platelet-rich plasma by rotablation is speed-dependent and can be inhibited by abciximab (c7E3 Fab; ReoPro). *Circulation* 1998; 98: 742–8.

12. Koch KC et al. Influence of a platelet GPIIb/IIIa receptor antagonist on myocardial hypoperfusion during rotational atherectomy as assessed by myocardial Tc-99 m sestamibi scintigraphy. *J Am Coll Cardiol* 1999; 33: 998–1004.

13. Kini A et al. Reduction in periprocedural enzyme elevation by abciximab after rotational atherectomy of type B$_2$ lesions: Results of the Rota ReoPro randomized trial. *Am Heart J* 2001; 142(6): 965–9.

14. Vercellino M et al. Role of glycoprotein IIb/IIIa inhibitors for PCI with rotational atherectomy: A propensity score adjusted analysis from ROTATE registry. *EuroIntervention* 2014; 14A: Poster 163 (abstract).

15. Akin I et al. Comparison of bivalirudin and heparin in patients undergoing rotational atherectomy: A subanalysis of the randomised ROTAXUS trial. *EuroIntervention* 2014; 10: 458–65.

16. O'Murchu B et al. Role of intra-aortic balloon pump counterpulsation in high risk coronary rotational atherectomy. *J Am Coll Cardiol* 1995; 26: 1270–5.

17. O'Neill WW et al. A prospective, randomized clinical trial of hemodynamic support with Impella 2.5 versus intra-aortic balloon pump in patients undergoing high-risk percutaneous coronary intervention: The PROTECT II study. *Circulation* 2012; 126: 1717–27.

18. Cardenas JR et al. Rotational atherectomy in restenotic lesions at the distal saphenous vein graft anastomosis. *Cathet Cardiovasc Diagn* 1995; 36: 53–7.

19. Don CW et al. Use of rotational atherectomy in the body of a saphenous vein coronary graft. *J Inv Cardiol* 2009; 21(9): E168–70.

20. Mokabberi R, and Blankenship JC. Rotational atherectomy to facilitate stent expansion after deployment in ST-segment-elevation myocardial infarction. *Am Heart Hosp J* 2010; 8(1): 66–9.

21. Pedersen WR et al. Successful rotational atherectomy in the setting of extensive coronary dissection: A case of failed balloon angioplasty in a nondilatable calcified lesion complicated by balloon rupture and extensive dissection. *Cathet Cardiovasc Intervent* 2003; 59: 329–32.

22. Ho PC. Rotational atherectomy in coronary dissection. *J Invas Cardiol* 2010; 22(10): E204–7.

23. Meziliz N et al. Rotablation in the drug eluting era: Immediate and long-term results from a single center experience. *J Interv Cardiol* 2010; 23: 249–53.

24. Vaquerizo B et al. Aggressive plaque modification with rotational atherectomy and/or cutting balloon before drug-eluting stent implantation for the treatment of calcified coronary lesions. *J Interv Cardiol* 2010; 23: 240–8.

25. Buchbinder M et al. Debulking prior to stenting improves acute outcomes: early results from the SPORT trial. *J Am Coll Cardiol* 2000; 35(Suppl A): 9A (abstract).

26. Pagnotta P et al. Rotational atherectomy in resistant chronic total occlusions. *Cathet Cardiovasc Intervent* 2010; 76(3): 366–71.

27. Reifart N et al. A novel penetration catheter (Tornus) as bail-out device after balloon failure to recanalise long, old calcified chronic occlusions. *EuroIntervention* 2008; 3: 617–21.

28. Fang HY et al. Can a penetration catheter (Tornus) substitute traditional rotational atherectomy for recanalising chronic total occlusions? *Int Heart J* 2010; 51(3): 147–52.

29. Martin-Yuste V et al. Usefulness of the Tornus catheter in nondilatable coronary chronic total occlusion. *Rev Esp Cardiol* 2011; 64(10): 935–8.

30. Pagnotta P et al. Tornus catheter and rotational atherectomy in resistant chronic total occlusions. *Int J Cardiol* 2013: 167(6): 2653–6.

31. vom Dahl J et al. Rotational atherectomy does not reduce recurrent in-stent restenosis: Results of the angioplasty versus rotational atherectomy for treatment of diffuse in-stent restenosis trial (ARTIST). *Circulation* 2002; 105: 583–8.

32. Sharma SK et al. Randomized trial of rotational atherectomy versus balloon angioplasty for diffuse in-stent restenosis (ROSTER). *Am Heart J* 2004; 147(1): 16–22.

33. Jain SP et al. Comparison of balloon angioplasty versus debulking devices versus stenting in right coronary ostial lesions. *Am J Cardiol* 1997; 79: 1334–8.

34. Zimarino M et al. Rotational coronary atherectomy with adjunctive balloon angioplasty for the treatment of ostial lesions. *Cathet Cardiovasc Diagn* 1994; 33: 22–7.

35. Koller PT et al. Success, complications and restenosis following rotational and transluminal extraction atherectomy of ostial stenoses. *Cathet Cardiovasc Diagn* 1994; 31: 255–60.

36. Sabri MN et al. Immediate results of interventional devices for coronary ostial narrowing with angina pectoris. *Am J Cardiol* 1994; 73: 122–5.

37. Tan RP et al. Optimal treatment of non aorto-ostial coronary lesions in large vessels: Acute and long-term results. *Cathet Cardiovasc Intervent* 2001; 54(3): 283–8.

38. Abdelmeguid AE. New technique for stent jail: Another niche for the Rotablator. *Cathet Cardiovasc Diagn* 1997; 42: 321–4.

39. Sperling RT et al. Treatment of stent-jailed side branch stenoses with rotational atherectomy. *J Inv Cardiol* 2006; 18(8): 254–8.

40. Kobayashi Y et al. Rotational atherectomy (stentablation) in a lesion with stent underexpansion due to heavily calcified plaque. *Cathet Cardiovasc Intervent* 2001; 52(2): 208–11.

41. Medina A et al. Successful stent ablation with rotational atherectomy. *Cathet Cardiovasc Intervent* 2003; 60(4): 501–4.

42. Vales L et al. Successful expansion of an underexpanded stent by rotational atherectomy. *Int J Angiol* 2013; 22: 63–8.

43. Feldman T. Rotational ablation of stent metal components: The intersection between coronary intervention and auto body repair. *Cathet Cardiovasc Intervent* 2001; 52(2): 212–3.

44. Reisman M et al. Analysis of heat generation during rotational atherectomy using different operational techniques. *Cathet Cardiovasc Diagn* 1998; 44(4): 453–5.

45. Ho PC et al. Burr erosion in rotational ablation of metallic coronary stent: An electron microscopic study. *J Interv Cardiol* 2010; 23(3): 233–9.

46. Garcia-Lara J et al. Percutaneous coronary intervention with rotational atherectomy for severely calcified unprotected left main: Immediate and two-years follow-up results. *Cathet Cardiovasc Intervent* 2012; 80(2): 215–20.

47. Dahdouh Z et al. Rotational atherectomy for left main coronary artery disease in octogenarians: Transradial approach in a tertiary center and literature review. *J Interv Cardiol* 2013; 26: 173–82.

48. Tsuchikane E et al. Debulking of chronic coronary total occlusions with rotational or directional atherectomy before stenting: Final results of DOCTORS study. *Int J Cardiol* 2008; 125(3): 397–403.

49. Hansen DD et al. Rotational atherectomy in atherosclerotic rabbit iliac arteries. *Am Heart J* 1988; 115: 160–5.

50. Abbo KM et al. Features and outcome of no-reflow after percutaneous coronary intervention. *Am J Cardiol* 1995; 75(12): 778–82.

51. Eeckhout E, and Kern MJ. The coronary no-reflow phenomenon: A review of mechanisms and therapies. *Eur Heart J* 2001; 22: 729–39.

52. Jaffe R et al. Prevention and treatment of microvascular obstruction-related myocardial injury and coronary no-reflow following percutaneous coronary intervention: A systematic approach. *J Am Coll Cardiol Interv* 2010; 3(7): 695–704.

53. Yokoi H et al. A discussion of trapped rotablator cases. *Jpn J Interv Cardiol* 1999; 14: MC009.

54. De Vroey F et al. How should I treat an entrapped rotational atherectomy burr? *EuroIntervention* 2012; 7: 1238–44.

55. Cunnington M, and Egred M. GuideLiner, a child-in-a-mother catheter for successful retrieval of an entrapped rotablator burr. *Cathet Cardiovasc Intervent* 2012; 79(2): 271–3.

56. Kimura M et al. Successful retrieval of an entrapped rotablator burr using 5 Fr guiding catheter. *Cathet Cardiovasc Intervent* 2011; 78: 558–64.

57. Sulimov DS et al. Stuck rotablator: The nightmare of rotational atherectomy. *EuroIntervention* 2013; 9: 251–8.

58. Ajluni SC et al. Perforations after percutaneous coronary interventions: Clinical, angiographic, and therapeutic observations. *Cathet Cardiovasc Intervent* 1994; 32(3): 206–12.

59. Dill T et al. A randomized comparison of balloon angioplasty versus rotational atherectomy in complex coronary lesions (COBRA Study). *Eur Heart J* 2000; 21: 1759–66.

60. Whitlow PL et al. Results of the study to determine rotablator and transluminal angioplasty strategy (STRATAS). *Am J Cardiol* 2001; 87(6): 699–705.

61. Safian RD et al. Coronary angioplasty and rotablator atherectomy trial (CARAT): Immediate and late results of a prospective multicenter randomized trial. *Cathet Cardiovas Intervent* 2001; 53: 213–20.

62. Mauri L et al. Comparison of rotational atherectomy with conventional balloon angioplasty in the prevention of restenosis of small coronary arteries: Results of the dilatation vs. ablation revascularization trial targeting restenosis (DART). *Am Heart J* 2003; 145(5): 847–54.

63. Haager PK et al. Insufficient tissue ablation by rotational atherectomy leads to worse long-term results in comparison with balloon angioplasty alone for the treatment of diffuse in-stent restenosis: Insights from the intravascular ultrasound substudy of the ARTIST randomized multicenter trial. *Cathet Cardiovasc Intervent* 2003; 60: 25–31.

64. Bittl JA et al. Meta-analysis of randomized trials of percutaneous transluminal coronary angioplasty versus atherectomy, cutting balloon atherectomy, or laser angioplasty. *J Am Coll Cardiol* 2004; 43(6): 936–42.

65. Abdel-Wahab M et al. High-speed rotational atherectomy before paclitaxel-eluting stent implantation in complex calcified coronary lesions. The randomized ROTAXUS (rotational atherectomy prior to Taxus stent treatment for complex native coronary artery disease) trial. *J Am Coll Cardiol Intervent* 2013; 6(1): 10–19.

Excimer laser coronary angioplasty

ZULFIQUAR ADAM, MOHANED EGRED

23.1 Introduction

A decade after its introduction, the limitations of balloon angioplasty included both acute and longer term consequences of vessel injury related to barotrauma at the time of the procedure namely intimal dissection and restenosis respectively. This led to the development of devices that removed atherosclerotic plaque rather than just displacing it. Amongst these was laser coronary angioplasty.[1] The hope was that this technology would overcome the limitations of balloon angioplasty especially treating lesions considered not ideal for balloon angioplasty.[2] But there were disappointing results in randomised studies especially with regards to restenosis.[3,4] in addition, the development and widespread uptake of coronary stents coupled with the high costs of laser systems meant that there was lack of development of catheter technology and therefore limited uptake.

In recent years, there has been renewed interest with improved understanding of the laser tissue interface, better technique and equipment and a realisation that its use is best suited to specific circumstances. This chapter outlines the scientific background, experimental data, practical procedural techniques and clinical applications of excimer laser coronary angioplasty (ELCA) in the treatment of coronary artery disease.

23.2 Historical aspects

The use of argon laser angioplasty was first described in animals in 1982.[5] In humans, it was first performed in the context of salvaging an ischaemic limb in 1983.[6] These early applications of argon or Nd:YAG laser technology converted laser light to thermal energy in a continuous wave form to achieve tissue vaporisation. This laser thermal angioplasty was met with unsatisfactory results as a result of excessive thermal injury and vessel damage. ELCA was developed to avoid this. In contrast to continuous wave laser, pulses lasting nanoseconds of short wavelength ultraviolet (UV) energy are produced. These can precisely ablate a localised area of an atherosclerotic plaque without significant thermal injury.[7] After initial laboratory testing the first successful human ELCA was performed at Cedars-Sinai Medical Center in Los Angeles in 1988.[8] In the 1990s, there was an improvement in catheter design from early metal tipped probes to newer fibreoptic catheters with increased procedural success and lower complication rates.[9] Feasibility of a laser guidewire for chronic total occlusions (CTOs) was also shown[10] but later comparison with conventional wires did not show any significant clinical or procedural advantage[11] and due to limited use it is no longer available. Current generation catheters have either a concentric or an eccentric array of a high concentration of laser fibres. Furthermore, operator technique has also evolved with improved safety.

23.3 Excimer laser fundamentals

Laser is an acronym for Light Amplification by Stimulated Emission of Radiation. It refers to the process of creating a highly directional beam of monochromatic (single wavelength) light with high energy. The term excimer is an acronym for excited dimer. Excimer lasers release energy in the UV range (10–400 nm) in very short pulses rather than in a continuous wave form. The advantage of this as compared with lasers that emit in the infrared ranges is that the absorption depth is less (<100 µm) which reduces the risk of collateral tissue damage when ablating plaque. The precise wavelength of emission depends on the exact nature of the gas mixture from which the photons are generated. Experience in the cardiovascular field has involved the xenon chloride (XeCl) 308 nm laser, which became available in 1983 for research and was approved by the FDA for its first clinical indications in 1992. The laser beam is formed as a result of high-voltage electrical discharge across a mixture of the xenon gas and a highly diluted (0.1%) hydrogen chloride solution. An excited state molecule of XeCl (the excited dimer) is produced, which subsequently drops to its ground state of XeCl, a weakly covalent molecule, which liberates a photon with a wavelength of 308 nm (Figure 23.1). The photon can then interact with another excited electron and produce two photons of the same wavelength and phase. Mirrors are used to amplify this process by reflecting the photons but also permit emission of the photons and these will result in the formation of the laser beam.

23.3.1 Mechanisms of action

Excimer laser ablates vascular tissue by three mechanisms:

1. Photochemical (fracture of molecular bonds) – The UV light pulse hits the plaque and is highly absorbed with each photon generated carrying sufficient energy to break molecular bonds. The duration of the laser pulse is 125 billionths of a second (125 ns), that is, the time that UV light pulse hits the tissue/plaque.
2. Photothermal (tissue vaporisation) – The molecular bonds are also vibrated during the absorption process resulting in heat. Intracellular water is vaporised leading to cell rupture and the creation of a vapour bubble. This lasts 100 millionths of a second (100 µs).
3. Photokinetic (clearance of by-products) – The rapid expansion and collapse of the vapour bubble further breaks down plaque but also assists in clearing by-products of ablation (water, gases and small particles). The entire process is completed in 400 µs. The vast majority of these particles are minute enough to be cleared by the reticuloendothelial system minimising the risk of distal microembolisation (Figure 23.2).

Regardless of the mechanism(s), the excimer laser theoretically possesses three unique characteristics: it ablates tissue without thermal effect; it ablates on a pulse-by-pulse basis leaving smooth incision margins, at least during in vitro study; and it is the only laser capable of ablating calcified material.

23.4 Laser equipment

Modern ELCA equipment is manufactured by Spectranetics (Colorado, CO). The system consists of a laser unit that generates the laser beam, and a series of catheters of various sizes, 0.9, 1.4, 1.7 and 2.0 mm, which transmit this energy by fibre optics to the tip of the catheter, delivering the energy to the intended lesions.

The latest version of the Spectranetics laser unit, the CVX-300® system, is a portable unit, which is 35 in. (89 cm) high, 49 in. long (124 cm) and 24 in. (61 cm) wide, and weighs about 650 pounds (295 kg) (Figure 23.3). It emits laser energy with a catheter output flow range between 30 and 80 mJ/mm², a repetition rate of 25–80 pulses/s and a

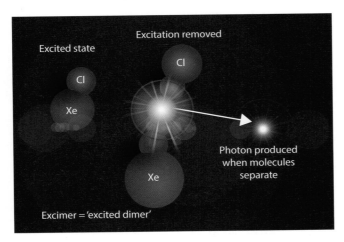

Figure 23.1 Generation of a photon. (Courtesy of The Spectranetics Corporation.)

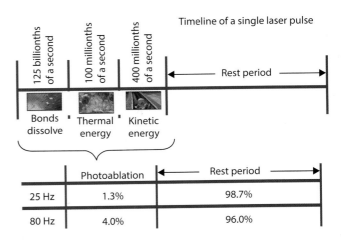

Figure 23.2 Schematic presentation of the mechanisms of action of laser and the pulsed nature of the waves. (Courtesy of The Spectranetics Corporation.)

pulse width of 125–200 ns (nominal 135 ns). This unit is also the energy source for other ELCA applications such as pacemaker lead extraction using the Spectranetics laser sheath (SLS) and peripheral excimer laser angioplasty (PELA).

Available laser catheters include conventional over-the-wire laser catheters, much less used currently, as well as the rapid exchange or monorail catheters. The rapid exchange version of the co-axial catheter (Vitesse C® and Vitesse Cos®) (Spectranetics Corp, Colorado, CO) produces a more axial force transmission and tip control than the earlier over-the-wire systems. Each coaxial catheter (Vitesse C and Vitesse Cos) consists of 65–250 individual 61-μm fibres concentrically arranged around the guidewire lumen. A radio-opaque marker is located at the distal end of the catheter to aid localisation of the laser tip within the coronary vasculature. The

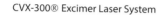

CVX-300® Excimer Laser System

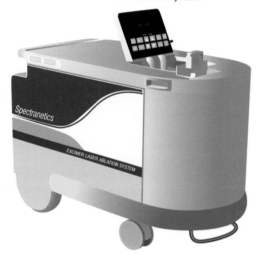

Figure 23.3 The new version of the Spectranetics laser unit, the CVX 300. This portable system generates 'cool' ultraviolet (UV) light with a 308 nm wavelength in controlled energy pulses. The excimer laser energy is delivered by means of laser catheters from this unit to the target tissue. (Courtesy of The Spectranetics Corporation.)

guidewire lumen begins at the tip of the catheter and exits the laser catheter 9 cm from the distal tip (Figure 23.4). The Vitesse Cos system is an improved version of the Vitesse C. It consists of a redesigned outer marker band, a smaller guidewire lumen and optimal spacing of fibres, thereby helping to increase the ablative area as well have more trackability. The concentric catheters were limited primarily to treat concentric lesions and are not suitable for treating highly eccentric plaques. In particular, treatment of lesions on the inner curve of an angulated segment of an artery results in less tissue ablation, and may cause disruption of the normal arterial wall opposite the plaque at the angulated segment of the artery.

To overcome this limitation, the Vitesse E® series (Spectranetics Corp, Colorado, CO) of eccentric excimer laser catheters were developed. The catheter shaft consists of an eccentric fibre optic bundle opposite the guidewire lumen, which runs through a tip with an eccentrically placed guidewire lumen. A radio-opaque marker with a radiolucent window is situated at the tip of the catheter. The window aids in directing the tip properly. There is a torque knob, which enables the catheter to be rotated so that the fibre optic bundle is in contact with the plaque. Currently, the majority of catheters used in practice are concentric. The eccentric catheters are recommended for in-stent restenosis and bifurcation lesions due to the ability to direct the laser beam using the torque knob.

The abovementioned catheters available for clinical use (Table 23.1), as are suggested guiding catheters for the various laser catheters and recommended laser catheter sizes for various vessel sizes.

23.5 Procedure

The laser machine requires 5 minutes of start-up time from the time it is turned on. Prior to the introduction of the laser catheter, it should be calibrated. This starts first by using a calibration catheter that is part of the machine then the sterile catheter that has been chosen for clinical use. The calibration is performed by pointing the tip of the catheter towards the energy detector on the CVX

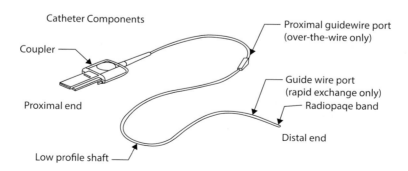

Figure 23.4 Schematic diagram of the components of a concentric laser catheter (Vitesse C® and Vitesse Cos®) (Spectranetics, Colorado, CO). At the distal end, the catheter consists of multiple concentrically or eccentrically arranged fibres around a guidewire lumen. At the proximal end, the laser fibres are held in a bundle to receive the laser beam from the unit. (Courtesy of The Spectranetics Corporation.)

Table 23.1 Coronary excimer laser catheters

Product description and size	Maximum settings (mJ/mm²/Hz)	Maximum timings	Guide compatibility	Approximate vessel size (mm)
Vitesse C 0.9 mm	60/40	5 s On 10 s Off	5F	>1.4
Vitesse X80 0.9 mm	80/80	10 s On 5 s Off	5F	>1.4
Vitesse Cos 1.4 mm	60/40	5 s On 10 s Off	7F	>2.1
Vitesse Cos 1.7 mm	60/40	5 s On 10 s Off	7F	>2.6
Vitesse Cos 2.0 mm	60/40	5 s On 10 s Off	8F	>3.0
Vitesse E 1.7 mm	60/40	5 s On 10 s Off	7F	>2.6
Vitesse E 2.0 mm	60/40	5 s On 10 s Off	8F	>3.0

300 unit and activating the laser, by pressing on the foot pedal. The laser will calibrate automatically and enter into a standby mode. Appropriately sized guiding catheters (see Table 23.1) should be used. For most cases, it is preferable to use a well-supported large bore guiding catheter with an adequate lumen that is needed to help flush saline using the 'saline flush protocol' (see Section 23.5.4) and guide catheters without side holes improve saline infusion.

Once the lesion is crossed with a guidewire, the tip of the guidewire is placed as distal as possible in order to help tracking of the laser catheter along the stiffer part of the wire. All laser catheters are compatible with 0.014-in. guidewires.

ELCA procedural success can be enhanced by using key techniques that are categorised into the 'Five S's of successful laser ablation'.

Selection of patient
Size of the laser catheter
Settings, fluence and pulse rate
Saline infusion
Slow advancement

23.5.1 Selection of patient

As discussed earlier, ELCA was initially developed as an alternative to balloon angioplasty but this has now evolved and is seen as an adjunct to conventional PCI. Table 23.2 lists the current recommended indications and contraindications for the use of ELCA. Case selection is paramount to achieving positive outcomes and this has been demonstrated with ELCA, where selective use has led to revival in its use. In fact, more recently further niche applications such as use in cases where there has been stent under expansion have also been described[12] and we now use it routinely for this indication. Similarly, it has been used in CTO PCI to help in softening then penetrating the proximal cap. We have also described a technique we labelled as RASER PCI where both laser and rotablation were used particularly when the rota wire would not pass to perform the rotational atherectomy and a normal PCI wire has. Laser is used to create a channel where the rotablation wire is introduced as laser is less effective in heavy calcification.[13]

Table 23.2 Indications and contraindications for ELCA

Current indications for the use of ELCA

Non-dilatable rigid lesions, i.e. failure to cross or dilate with balloon
Under-expanded and under-deployed stents
Chronic total occlusions (CTOs) crossable by a guidewire
Aorta-ostial lesions
Moderately calcified lesions
Saphenous vein grafts (SVG)
Long lesions and diffuse disease (>20 mm length)
Diffuse in-stent restenosis, as a 'debulking' technique prior to definitive re-dilatation
These are arranged in order of current frequency and relevance. The first three indications being the most common in practice.

Contraindication for the use of ELCA

Unprotected left main coronary artery
Acute angulation (>45°)
Coronary dissection
Lesions in vessels with diameter smaller than the catheter
With increased operator experience and use of ELCA, many of these can be done when laser is the only available option. In the author's experience, these cases can be done safely and successfully.

23.5.2 Size of catheter

The maximum diameter of a laser catheter should not exceed two-thirds of the diameter of the artery as highlighted in Table 23.1. When selecting the appropriate size catheter, it is best to consider the severity of the lesion in addition to vessel size. Given that the majority of cases are for uncrossable, undilatable lesions, a 0.9 mm catheter is usually used to great effect. Other instances, when it is wise to size conservatively, include tortuous vessels (should not attempt ELCA in >60° bends as laser light will not bend and may lead to perforation), poor visualisation and in calcified vessels. More aggressive sizing can be considered in large vessels with straight segments and in SVG.

Eccentric catheters can be used in cases of highly eccentric plaques, especially when they are situated at the bend of a vessel, in bifurcation lesions and in-stent restenosis.

23.5.3 Settings

The laser catheter is advanced so that the tip is in direct contact with the proximal end of the lesion to minimise the blood interface between the laser tip and the lesion. The fluence, amount of energy (mJ) at the catheter tip per unit (mm²) usually has a range between 30 and 80 mJ/mm². The repetition rate (frequency) range is between 25 and 80 Hz (pulses per second). The system calibrates at 45 mJ/mm² at 25 Hz. The first pass can be made at this setting and increased to maximum settings (see Table 23.1) if there is resistance. The manufacturer recommends increasing the fluence first then the frequency if the first activation is not successful. Starting at higher energy and repetition rate may lead to complications such as dissection and perforation. We now start at 40/40 and increase to 60/60 then 80/80 if resistance remains (when using a 0.9 mm catheter that is the most commonly used).

23.5.4 Saline flush protocol

The purpose of using a saline infusion is to remove contrast from the system as well as eliminate blood from the lasing field. The 308 nm wavelength photon beam is avidly absorbed by blood and contrast media, leading to the production of insoluble gas and rapidly expanding cavitation bubbles. These bubbles generate intense pressure wave pulses, which are in part responsible for complications such as dissections and perforations. Knowledge of this deleterious interaction led to the development of the saline flushing technique, which has substantially reduced the severity of coronary dissections, and is now a routine part of the procedure.

A 1 L bag of 0.9% normal saline is attached by means of a sterile intravenous line to one of the ports of a triple manifold via a three-way tap. Residual contrast is injected back into the contrast bottle. A fresh 20 mL Luer-lock control syringe is attached to another port and is used to flush all traces of blood and contrast from the entire system including the manifold, Y-connector, guiding catheter and the target coronary artery with normal saline. Just prior to activation of the laser, the assistant operator injects a 10 mL bolus of normal saline through the guiding catheter, and then continues to inject saline at a rate of 1–3 mL/s during the lasing procedure. Lasing is commenced immediately after the 10 mL bolus of saline. The saline injection is terminated at the end of a lasing sequence. The system will allow lasing for a maximum of 5 or 10 seconds at a time, then automatically enters a 10- or 5-second standby mode depending on the catheter size. The end of the standby period is marked by an audible signal indicating that the operator can continue. The time of activation can be adjusted, as some operators believe that shorter activation time leads to less complication. We mostly use 0.9 mm catheter, which is activated for 10 seconds and a standby for 5 seconds.

We have used laser with contrast in certain circumstances such as under-expanded stents or heavily calcified lesions where a rotablation wire would not pass but a normal PCI wire can.

23.5.5 Slow advancement

Slow advancement results in larger, 'cleaner', lumens and less likelihood of coronary dissection. The catheter is advanced at <1 mm/second for optimal results. Advancing faster than this defeats the intended purpose of debulking lesions and instead results in less dilatation (Figure 23.5).

In the early ELCA experience, only one pass would generally be performed through the entire lesion. With the improvement in catheter design and the proper use of saline infusion, operators have been able to optimise results, making additional laser passes when lesion contact can still be made.

Whilst using the eccentric laser catheters, there are two methods employed to ablate tissue. The first method involves simply advancing the catheter through the target

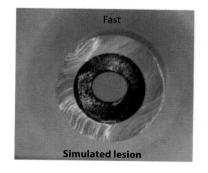 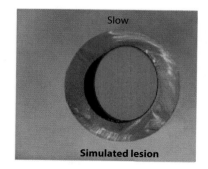

Figure 23.5 Lumen diameter after lasing with fast advancement (>1 mm/s) compared to slow advancement (<1 mm/s) in simulated lesions. (Courtesy of The Spectranetics Corporation.)

tissue, withdrawing the catheter and then repositioning the catheter tip using the torque knob, and then re-advancing the catheter again. The second method, which has not been used as commonly, involves actively torquing the catheter at the proximal part of the target lesion, in an attempt to ablate as much tissue as possible. The operator only advances the catheter when tissue has been removed in a 360° pattern. This method may limit the catheter from slipping into the lumen, which sometimes occurs when using the more commonly applied first method. Good short and long-term results are ensured by adjunctive balloon angioplasty and stent placement after the lasing procedure.

23.6 Laser safety

All operators must be trained in the use of laser. It should only be performed in a secure environment with measures taken to warn and prevent unauthorised access during lasing. In addition to these, all of the catheter lab staff present and the patient must wear eye protection (CVX-300® safety glasses) to protect against harm from mainly the therapeutic (invisible) which can be absorbed by the cornea. The aiming (red) coherent beam of the laser system can also potentially harm if there is exposure for prolonged periods. The required glasses must be labelled with optical density (OD) at laser wavelength. OD = 4 at 308 nanometers (CVX-300 Safety Glasses).

23.7 Avoiding and managing complications

ELCA is a procedure that requires careful attention to case selection and technical details. Improved procedural technique as detailed in Section 23.5 had led to a reduction in the major complications, which threatened to limit this procedure during the early experience. The incidence of coronary perforations and major flow limiting dissections has decreased significantly due to improved catheter design and better operator techniques, including the routine use of saline infusion.

Even with these technical improvements and appropriate case selection, it is important to recognise when ELCA should be abandoned. This is the case when there is failure to pass the catheter when other factors such as guide catheter selection and guidewire position have been optimised and laser energy is maximised. From a practical point of view, we have had success in many balloon uncrossable lesions even if the laser catheter did not pass through the lesion and was only activated at the entrance, as following the activation to the high energy, the balloon would pass and the procedure can be performed and finished successfully. This is the concept for using laser for modifying the proximal cap of CTOs.

The incidence of ELCA-induced major coronary dissections and abrupt vessel closure, once considered the Achilles' heel of this procedure, has been considerably reduced with the advent of the saline infusion technique in 1995.[14] Other measures used to prevent dissections include avoiding excessive force or over sizing the laser catheter and starting from a low energy and increasing that slowly. If a flow limiting dissection develops, the laser part of the procedure should be discontinued, and the dissection should be treated by balloon angioplasty and stent placement.

Perforation is also a serious complication. It has been reported to occur in 0.3%–2% of cases.[15,16] Perforations are more likely to occur in the following situations: (a) use of a catheter that is equal to or greater than the vessel diameter, (b) use of a concentric catheter on a very eccentric lesion, particularly if on a tight bend and (c) applying laser energy in a previously dissected vascular segment. Once a perforation is diagnosed, the laser catheter is removed without altering the guidewire position and the perforation treated in the described conventional manner.

23.8 Clinical studies

Most of the literature comes from the old era in the 1990s. The early experience involving the use of ELCA were mainly recorded in registries. In 1994, Litvack et al. published the results of the first 3000 patients (3592 lesions) treated with ELCA at 33 different sites.[16] These patients were treated by equipment manufactured by Advanced Interventional Systems (AIS). In this prospective registry, procedural success was 84% increasing to 90% with adjunctive balloon angioplasty. Procedural complications included significant dissection in 13%, perforation in 1% of lesions. Major ischaemic complications were defined as in-hospital mortality (0.5%), Q-wave myocardial infarction (2.1%) and in-hospital bypass surgery (3.8%). Coronary dissection (in 13% of lesions) was associated with major ischaemic complications in approximately 15% of the patients they occurred in. There was no difference in procedural success or in-hospital complications when the results were analysed according to ACC/AHA lesion type (32% were Type C lesions). It is also noteworthy that the use of adjunctive balloon angioplasty went up from 71% in the first 2000 patients compared with 95% in the last 1000 patients. These latter observations are particularly relevant to current practice as even with this early experience, there was recognition that ELCA procedural success was improved when used adjunctively with conventional PCI and there was a role for it in complex lesions.

The other main manufacturer of laser equipment at the time was Spectranetics. In 1997, results of the New Approaches to Coronary Intervention (NACI) registry were published.[17] In this series, 4429 patients were enrolled from 39 sites between 1990 and 1994. Of these, 887 patients (1000 lesions) received laser therapy with either the AIS system (487 cases) or the Spectranetics system (400 cases). Sixty percent of patients had unstable angina, ACC/AHA type C lesions were treated in 32% of cases. Procedural success (<50% residual lumen) was 84%. In-hospital mortality was 1.2%, MI occured in 4.5% of cases (Q wave 0.7%), 4.5% required CABG (2.7% as emergency) with a cumulative death/CABG/MI rate of 9.0%. At one year, the incidence of death, Q-wave MI or target vessel re-vascularisation was 42.3%. From core laboratory analysis of 839 lesions (752 patients), post-laser perforations occurred in 2.6% and dissection in 23.4% (22.0% grades B, C, D and 1.4% grades E, F).

Randomised studies comparing ELCA with balloon angioplasty involved only small numbers of patients. The Amsterdam-Rotterdam Trial (AMRO) randomised 308 patients with stable angina to either ELCA (with or without adjunctive balloon angioplasty) or balloon angioplasty.[3] Procedural success was 80% compared to 79% for balloon angioplasty. Six-month rates of the primary endpoint (death, MI, repeat re-vascularisation) were similar (33% for ELCA vs. 30% for balloon angioplasty). Restenosis rates were also similar (52% for ELCA vs. 41% for balloon angioplasty, $p = .13$).

The Excimer laser versus Rotational atherectomy versus Balloon Angioplasty Comparison (ERBAC) trial was a single-centre study conducted in Germany.[18] This trial randomised 685 patients with stable angina and complex lesions (native type B or C lesions) to either ELCA ($n = 232$), rotational atherectomy ($n = 231$) or balloon angioplasty ($n = 222$). Procedural success was highest in patients who underwent rotational atherectomy (89% vs. 77% for ELCA and 80% for balloon angioplasty, $p = .0019$). There was no difference in major in-hospital complications: death, Q-wave myocardial infarction or coronary artery bypass surgery (3.2% for rotational atherectomy vs. 4.3% for ELCA vs. 3.1% for balloon angioplasty, $p = .71$). However, at 6 months, target lesion re-vascularisation was higher in the rotational atherectomy group (42.4%) and the excimer laser group (46.0%) than in the angioplasty group (31.9%, $p = .013$).

Overall, these early trials demonstrated a failure of ELCA to achieve better clinical outcomes than PTCA with increased risk of vessel dissection and perforation from the formation of intraluminal vapour bubbles in blood. It is worth noting that current techniques, particularly saline infusion, as described earlier in this chapter are different to those used in these early trials. Additionally, some applications of ELCA such as in saphenous venous grafts, in-stent restenosis and total occlusions were not included.

23.9 Clinical examples

23.9.1 Undilatable or uncrossable lesions

Nowadays, PCI is performed increasingly in patients with complex calcified disease, many of whom are elderly and/or unsuitable for CABG. In moderately calcified lesions or tortuous anatomy where passage of a Rota Wire or suitable microcatheters for wire exchange is not possible, ELCA can provide the debulking needed to increase the likelihood of success. This was tested with the X80 0.9 mm catheter, which allows operation of higher energy (80 mJ/mm²/80 Hz) compared with standard catheters (60 mJ/mm²/40 Hz) in 100 calcified and/or balloon-resistant lesions ($n = 95$ patients).[19] The procedural success rate was 93% and a clinical success rate of 86%, with a low rate of procedural complications (five laser related dissections and one non-Q-wave MI). In the setting of total occlusions, ELCA can be used to facilitate balloon and stent advancement in fibrotic or calcific lesions.

ELCA provides an excellent tool for overcoming these difficult cases with its advantage of being suitable with any PCI guide wire and even in the presence of another buddy wire. Important to know that even when the catheter does not pass through the lesion, lasing at the proximal area with increasing settings will, in our experience, on many occasions, allow the passage of the predilatation balloons.

The figures below show a severely calcified and eccentric lesion in the LAD which could not be crossed with a rotawire or a normal PCI wire and was only crossed with difficulty with a stiff CTO/PCI wire, however, a microcatheter would not pass for rota wire exchange and similarly the smallest PCI balloon would not pass despite using a GuideLiner extension catheter. A LASER 0.9 mm catheter was used and a channel was created that allowed the passage of predilatation balloon then the delivery of stents with successful outcome.

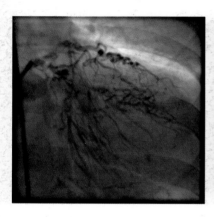
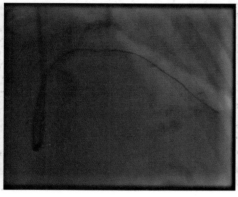
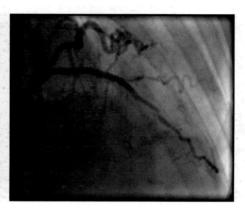

23.9.2 Under-expanded stents

Once deployed, it is often difficult to expand stents in under prepared lesions (mainly due to fibrocalcific atheroma). Techniques as cutting balloon and rotational atherectomy may be ineffective and possibly harmful in this setting. The use of ELCA through ablation of tissue and therefore de-bulking can assist in balloon expansion within a vessel that has proved resistant to dilatation after stent deployment.

This is our current approach to under-expanded stents and we have used ELCA for this indication for the last few years with excellent results and success. The laser is used in the normal fashion in saline flush and with increasing energy and frequency as required. We have described the successful use of concurrent contrast during laser for old under-expanded stent.[12]

This is a case of a patient treated with a drug eluting stent that was under-deployed and under-expanded despite using a high-pressure post-dilatation up to 30 atm. He returned with severe symptoms and severe in-stent restenosis, which was undilatatble with high-pressure non-compliant balloons. A 1.4 mm LASER catheter did not pass originally in saline medium but then by using a contrast medium whilst lasing, the restenosis was crossed and the stent expanded with insertion of a new stent with excellent final results.

23.9.3 Chronic total occlusion

The images below are an example of a CTO case of short occlusion at the ostial RCA which was crossed with a Pilot 200 wire but with the inability to cross it with any low profile balloons, Corsair or Turnpike Gold microcatheters. A 0.9 mm LASER catheter was used with diluted contrast medium and this passed at 80/80 setting and allowed the successful completion of the procedure. There has been some experiment in using laser at the proximal cap of a CTO where it was difficult to puncture through the cap, and using laser without a wire by just activating it at the cap resulted in modification and allowed the passage of a CTO/PCI wire and the successful completion of the procedure (personal communication).

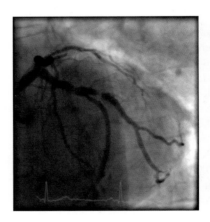
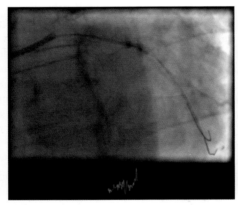
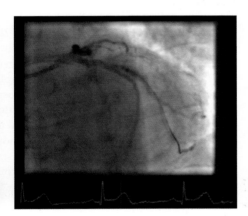
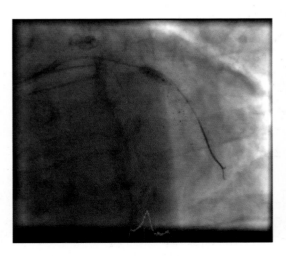
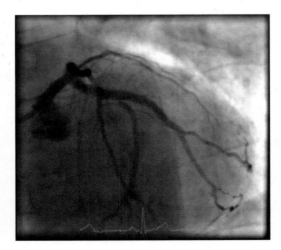

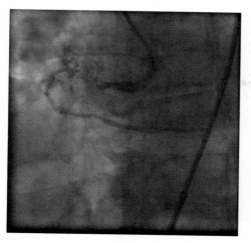

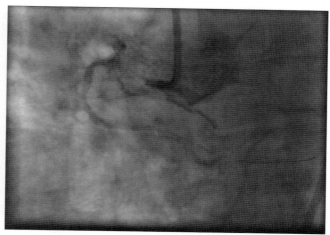

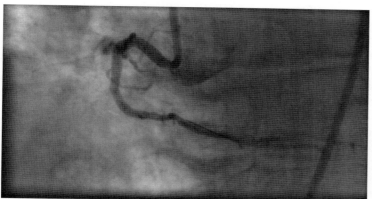

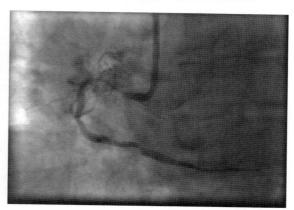

23.9.4 RSER PCI

In cases of heavy calcification, where rotablation may be the preferred approach, and the inability to pass a rotablation wire, we have used the combination of laser and rotablation where a normal PCI wire is passed then the laser catheter is used to create a channel that allows the delivery of the thin rotablation wire to allow for maximum debulking of heavy calcium. We use the term RASER PCI for these cases which allowed us to achieve a successful procedural outcome.[13] This is one of the main advantages of laser with the ability to use it on normal PCI wire in comparison to rotablation that can only be performed on its special thin wire with its difficult delivery in calcified and severe lesions. The images below are such a case. The rotablation wire could not be delivered distally and a normal PCI wire was used but a microcatheter could not be delivered for exchange either. RASER PCI was used where 0.9 mm laser catheter was used and created a channel and the rotablation wire was then delivered and rotablation performed with successful procedure that otherwise could have been undoable.

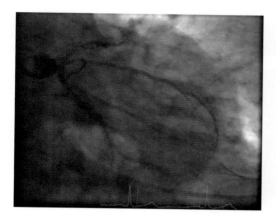

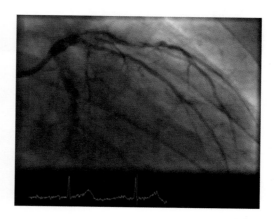

(Continued)

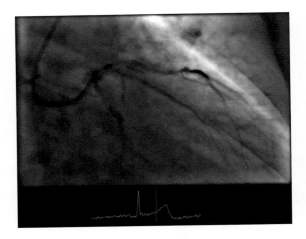

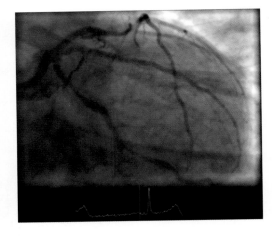

23.9.5 Saphenous vein graft

PCI to SVG remains a frequent practice. However, in the author opinion and practice this, and due to the poor outcome and the higher procedural complication rate with SVG PCI in addition to advances in CTO/PCI, has been replaced by native vessel CTO/PCI with great success. LASER, however remains a useful tool for PCI to SVG lesions that are usually multi-focal, diffuse and degenerative with tendency to distal and possibly proximal embolisation. LASER is particularly useful for acute thrombotic lesions.

In a small retrospective study of 31 patients, Ebersole et al. found that ELCA is associated with a high rate of success in acute occlusion of SVG.[20] Laser success was 87%, angiographic success was 97% and overall procedural success was 84%. Non-Q-wave MI (resurge in creatine kinase-MB [CK-MB] post-procedure) occurred in two patients (6%), in-hospital death in one patient (3%), and one repeat target vessel intervention in another patient (3%). There were three (10%) significant dissections (two laser induced, one guidewire induced). There were no episodes of acute closure or distal embolisation. In one of the original laser registries, data for the 545 stenoses treated by ELCA were analyzed.[21] Distal embolisation occurred in only 18 (3%) and ostial lesions and lesions in the body of small SVG had more favourable outcomes after treatment with ELCA. Based on very limited current data, ELCA may be used in SVG when filters cannot be utilised.

The images below are from an acutely occluded SVG in which normal ballooning did not establish any flow due to a heavy thrombus burden and laser use establish antegrade flow and allowed a successful completion on the procedure.

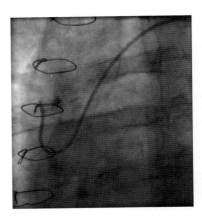

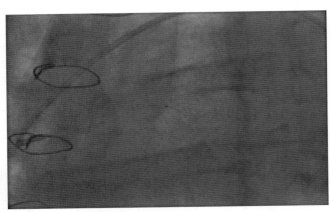

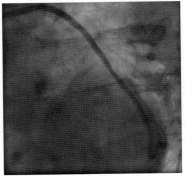

23.9.6 Future direction

The use of ELCA has regained its momentum due to improved safety and performance with the advanced and new catheters and the use of saline medium to deliver the energy.

There has been some work done into the development of laser catheter which can be used to ablate through heavily calcified plaques. This will be advancement as currently laser is not as effective in heavily calcified lesions.

Laser will remain an important tool for uncrossable, undilatable lesions as the most common indication with emerging uses in other clinical scenarios.

Laser use in under-expanded stents is a new approach in managing these difficult and clinically important cases. In addition, the use of laser with contrast for dealing with resistant lesions will gain momentum although should remain restricted to experienced laser users and in limited situations and saline flush should remain the normal practice.

Laser has also been tried for modifying and penetrating a resistant proximal CTO cap and with the increased and advanced CTO PCI, there is no doubt that laser is an important part in the treatment algorithm. RASER PCI with the combined use of LASER and rotablation is a useful, albeit expensive, approach for a subset of highly resistant and heavily calcified lesions.

23.10 Summary

Excimer laser debulks the tissue with its photochemical, photothermal and photokinetic property without causing significant injury. With important refinements and advancement, it has regained a renewed place in treating complex and resistant coronary lesions after a disappointing start.

When used in line with the instructions, it is an important tool that allows the completion of many difficult and complicated cases.

It is a useful tool in the catheterisation laboratory to treat lesions that are uncrossable or undilatable, a subset that is on the increase with the aging population we are treating on a daily basis, and will help achieve successful PCI results.

It is also helpful in cases where a stent was deployed but remains under-expanded with accumulating evidence of its efficacy in this group. In addition, laser is increasingly used for CTO PCI to facilitate modifying and affecting the proximal CTO cap to allow penetration and the completeness of the procedure. Laser has been used in certain circumstances and by experienced operators in a contrast rather than saline medium to increase its effect and allow a successful completion of complex PCI and even in heavily calcified lesions.

Laser has, in comparison to rotablation, the advantage of being usable on a normal PCI guide wire and in the presence of a second buddy wire that is frequently used in difficult lesions. Rotablation cannot be used with a second wire in place and requires a special thin wire that is on occasion difficult to deliver.

ELCA is an important tool in the interventionalists' armamentarium that, when used appropriately, allows the successful completion of complex coronary interventions and provides most patients with a non-surgical treatment and important symptomatic relief, where without its use these cases would be abandoned and frequently referred for surgery.

References

1. Waller BF. Crackers, breakers, stretchers, drillers, scrapers, shavers, burners, welders and melters—The future treatment of atherosclerotic coronary artery disease? A clinical-morphologic assessment. *J Am Coll Cardiol* 1989; 13(5): 969–87.
2. Cook SL et al. Percutaneous excimer laser coronary angioplasty of lesions not ideal for balloon angioplasty. *Circulation* 1991; 84(2): 632–43.
3. Appelman YE et al. Randomised trial of excimer laser angioplasty versus balloon angioplasty for treatment of obstructive coronary artery disease. *Lancet* 1996; 347(8994): 79–84.
4. Reifart N et al. Randomized comparison of angioplasty of complex coronary lesions at a single center. Excimer Laser, Rotational Atherectomy, and Balloon Angioplasty Comparison (ERBAC) Study. *Circulation* 1997; 96(1): 91–8.
5. Choy DS et al. Transluminal laser catheter angioplasty. *Am J Cardiol* 1982; 50(6): 1206–8.
6. Ginsburg R et al. Salvage of an ischemic limb by laser angioplasty: Description of a new technique. *Clin Cardiol* 1984; 7(1): 54–8.
7. Grundfest WS et al. Laser ablation of human atherosclerotic plaque without adjacent tissue injury. *J Am Coll Cardiol* 1985; 5(4): 929–33.
8. Litvack F et al. Percutaneous excimer laser coronary angioplasty. *Lancet* 1989; 2(8654): 102–3.
9. Bittl JA et al. The changing profile of patient selection, procedural techniques, and outcomes in excimer laser coronary angioplasty. Participating Investigators of the Percutaneous Excimer Laser Coronary Angioplasty Registry. *J Interv Cardiol* 1995; 8(6): 653–60.
10. Oesterle SN et al. Laser wire for crossing chronic total occlusions: 'learning phase' results from the U.S. TOTAL trial. Total Occlusion Trial With Angioplasty by Using a Laser Wire. *Cathet Cardiovasc Diagn* 1998; 44(2): 235–43.
11. Serruys PW et al. Total occlusion trial with angioplasty by using laser guidewire. The TOTAL trial. *Eur Heart J* 2000; 21(21): 1797–805.
12. Egred M. A novel approach for under-expanded stent: Excimer laser in contrast medium. *J Invasive Cardiol* 2012; 24(8):E161–3.
13. Egred M. RASER Angioplasty. *Catheter Cadriovasc Interv* 2012 May 1; 79 (6): 1009–12
14. Deckelbaum LI et al. Effect of intracoronary saline infusion on dissection during excimer laser coronary angioplasty: A randomized trial. The Percutaneous Excimer Laser Coronary Angioplasty (PELCA) Investigators. *J Am Coll Cardiol* 1995; 26(5): 1264–9.
15. Ghazzal ZM et al. Morphological predictors of acute complications after percutaneous excimer laser coronary angioplasty. Results of a comprehensive angiographic

analysis: Importance of the eccentricity index. *Circulation* 1992; 86(3): 820–7.

16. Litvack F et al. Percutaneous excimer laser coronary angioplasty: Results in the first consecutive 3,000 patients. The ELCA Investigators. *J Am Coll Cardiol* 1994; 23(2): 323–9.

17. Holmes DR, Jr et al. Excimer laser coronary angioplasty: The New Approaches to Coronary Intervention (NACI) experience. *Am J Cardiol* 1997; 80(10A): 99K–105K.

18. Vandormael M et al. Six months follow-up results following excimer laser angioplasty, rotational atherectomy and balloon angioplasty for complex lesions: ERBAC study. *Circulation* 1994; 90:I–213A

19. Bilodeau L et al. Novel use of a high-energy excimer laser catheter for calcified and complex coronary artery lesions. *Catheter Cardiovasc Interv* 2004; 62(2): 155–61.

20. Ebersole D et al. Excimer laser revascularization of saphenous vein grafts in acute myocardial infarction. *J Invasive Cardiol* 2004; 16(4): 177–80.

21. Bittl JA et al. Predictors of outcome of percutaneous excimer laser coronary angioplasty of saphenous vein bypass graft lesions. The Percutaneous Excimer Laser Coronary Angioplasty Registry. *Am J Cardiol* 1994; 74(2): 144–8.

24

Advantages and disadvantages in radial and femoral arterial access

RUBÉN RODRÍGUEZ, ALESSANDRA GIAVARINI, ISABELLE VANDORMAEL,
GIOVANNNI LONGO, CARLO DI MARIO

24.1 Introduction

In the early 1960s, Mason Sones, the father of selective coronary angiography, described and introduced 'brachial artery cut down' as the access site method to perform coronary angiography. Soon afterwards, the femoral approach using the percutaneous Seldinger technique started to spread amongst interventionists, thanks to its straightforwardness and lower complication rate in comparison to the brachial surgical approach.

Melvin Judkins designed a pre-shaped catheter for left and right coronary selective injection. When in 1977 Andreas Gruentzig reported the first successful balloon coronary angioplasty, 9 Fr guiding catheters became the standard and femoral access, was the only possible vascular approach. Along with the miniaturisation of angioplasty devices and the increasing use of 6 Fr guiding catheters, Kiemeneij was able to perform angioplasty using a method already established by Campeau et al., the radial approach.[1] The first report, which included 100 stenting procedures, demonstrated the growing popularity towards the radial approach as it clearly reduced the risk of bleeding and ultimately eliminated vascular complications. These complications were often seen as a result of combining aspirin, dipyridamole, dextran, heparin and subsequently warfarin

to prevent high in-stent thrombotic events. The advantages and disadvantages of femoral versus radial vascular approach for coronary angiography/interventions have been investigated in several studies based on which recommendations have been drawn. In this chapter, we review the radiological anatomy of the femoral and radial arteries, the most effective techniques to puncture and close the vascular access site, the most frequent complications following their instrumentation, the respective short-midterm outcome after coronary intervention and the differences in patient satisfaction, cath lab organisation and procedural cost.

24.2 The basics of femoral and radial access

24.2.1 Femoral artery access

The common femoral artery (FA) is an elastic artery extending from the inguinal ligament to the femoral bifurcation. Its normal lumen diameter ranges between 6 and 10 mm (Table 24.1).[2] It is palpable midway between the anterior superior iliac spine and pubic symphysis. It separates into the superficial and profunda femoral arteries.[3] Above the bifurcation, the common FA is part of the neurovascular fasciculus, which also includes the common femoral vein

Table 24.1 Anatomical, procedural and outcome aspects of the femoral and radial artery access for coronary angiography and percutaneous intervention

	Artery	
	Femoral	**Radial**
Anatomical Characteristics		
Mean vessel size in men, mm	9.8[a]	2.69 ± 0.40
Mean vessel size in women, mm	8.2[a]	2.43 ± 0.38
Anatomic variability and tortuosity	Less common	More common
Spasm	Not reported	Frequent
Adjacent neurovascular structures	Femoral vein and femoral nerve	No
Procedural Characteristics		
Max. sheath size supported, Fr	25	6–7
Catheter guide support	Usually stable	Sometimes unstable
Procedural and fluoroscopy times	Slightly lower	Slightly higher[b]
Access site crossover and procedural failure	Marginally lower	Marginally higher[b]
Learning curve	Shorter	Longer
Time to ambulation	(Variable) up to 6 hours	Immediate
Length of hospital stay	Longer	Shorter
Outcomes		
Access site complications	Higher	Significantly lower
Access artery occlusion	Rare	Up to 10%
Non-CABG major bleeds, %	2.1[c]	1.2 (HR 0.58; 0.46–0.72; $p < .001$)[c]
MACE after PCI for ACS, %	6.66[c]	5.99 (HR 0.86; 0.77–0.95; $p = .0051$)[c]

Source: From Sandgren, T et al., *J Vasc Surg*, 29, 503–10, 1999.
[a] Variability of the diameter of the common FA related to age and body size.
[b] Markedly influenced by operator's expertise.
[c] From the updated meta-analyses of the MATRIX trial
ACS, acute coronary syndrome; CABG, coronary artery by-pass graft; MACE, major adverse cardiovascular events; PCI, percutaneous coronary intervention; STEMI, ST-elevation myocardial infarction.

(medially) and the femoral nerve (laterally). In order to avoid some of the most common complications, it is essential to determine the right anatomical landmark for femoral puncture, which is ideally performed 1–2 cm below the inguinal ligament. These anatomical landmarks may not be as easily identifiable in overweight patients. A lower puncture site below the inguinal ligament increases the chance of puncturing the FA at the bifurcation or the superficial profunda branches. A puncture at this level more easily causes a pseudoaneurysm, a thrombus or even a dissection, as both vessels taper distally.

Punctures above the inguinal ligament, where the artery becomes deep into the pelvic cavity and is more difficult to compress due to the absence of a bone plane, have greater risk of bleedings that may cause retroperitoneal haematomas.

The femoral vein crosses over at the arterial bifurcation with the potential risk for arteriovenous communication.

Both fluoroscopy and ultrasound can be useful to gain access point, especially in higher risk groups (raised body mass indexes, women) as reported by several studies.[4–6] When using fluoroscopy, the operator can determine a safe puncture zone between the centre of the femoral head and a 14 mm inferior limit as seen on the image (Figure 24.1).

FA percutaneous access is gained through the Seldinger technique. After shaving and sterilisation, the groin is infiltrated with local anaesthetic. The puncture site must be recognised through anatomical landmarks and pulse palpation: the Seldinger needle is inserted where the strongest femoral pulse is noticed with an inclination angle between 30° and 45°. When stable back flow is observed, the dedicated guidewire is advanced into the needle which can then be removed. Finally, the sheath is inserted in the lumen through the wire.

At the end of the endovascular catheterisation and after sheath removal, adequate haemostasis achievement is a key step to avoid complications.

Manual compression should be applied for 15–30 minutes depending on the sheath size, followed by a compressive bandage for at least 6 hours. In case of enhanced bleeding risk, mechanical clamps can be used: they reduce the time of personnel requirement, ensure a more stable, constant compression and may reduce the incidence of complications.[7] Closure devices do not require further mechanical compression and have been found useful in reducing hospital stay and patients' bed rest period as compared to manual compression. Two different types of devices are available, either collagen haemostatic puncture or suture-mediated

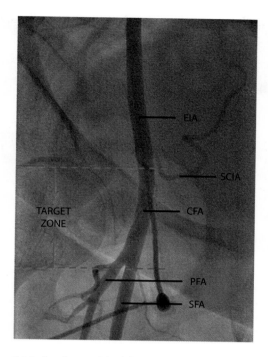

Figure 24.1 Angiographical femoral marks. The Common Femoral Artery (CFA) represents the target of a correct femoral puncture. Femoral head between red lines mark the limits for a safe puncture. Beyond the lower line, the risk of puncturing the bifurcation increases. Above the upper line, the risk of retroperitoneal hematoma rises markedly. The origin of the Superficial Circumflex Iliac Artery (SCIA) is the angiographic and vascular marker for the retroperitoneal cavity.
EIA: External Iliac Artery; CFA: Common Femoral Artery; PFA: Profunda Femoral Artery; SFA: Superficial Femoral Artery; SCIA: Superficial Circumflex Iliac Artery.

devices and will be discussed at greater length in a dedicated chapter.[7,8]

24.2.2 Radial artery access

The radial artery (RA) arises at the bifurcation of the brachial artery in the cubital fossa. It runs distally along the radial side of the forearm and joins the ulnar artery through the palmar arch, creating the dual circulation system in the hand. The anatomical features of RA confer advantages in terms of vascular access, compared to FA. Its small diameter (1.8–2.5 mm)[9] combined with its superficial location and the presence of a bone plane allow better haemostatic control after percutaneous coronary intervention (PCI) (Table 24.1). Together with the absence of nearby neurovascular structures, these characteristics explain the marked reduction of access site complications.[10–12] In contrast, its smaller calibre (one/sixth of the femoral)[9] means that the radial access can hardly accommodate devices larger than 6 Fr. This may become a limitation when performing PCI (especially in complex lesions such as left main, bifurcation, chronic total occlusion [CTO]). Furthermore, itstortuous

path, the relative frequency of radial spasm (it is a muscular artery) and the presence of unfavourable angles with the ascending aorta and aortic arch, especially in elderly patients with type 3 arch pattern, make this access more challenging for the operators. It is worth noting that these conditions increase patient discomfort as well as the risk of complications.

Before undertaking a procedure through the RA, careful revision of patient's medical history as well as examining both arms is crucial in order to exclude both relative and absolute contraindications. For example, arteriovenous fistula (as for haemodialysis), Raynaud syndrome (prone to spasm), impalpable or weak radial pulses (very small diameter, more challenging cannulation, harder navigation) and inadequate contribution of the ulnar artery to the palmar arch (assessed by Allen test with or without oximetry) represent some of these contraindications.

The actual importance of evaluating the 'dual hand circulation' prior to RA puncture has been recently questioned.[13] The Modified Allen test is the most common method to establish hand perfusion and consists of the following steps: simultaneous application of sustained pressure over the ulnar and the radial arteries; patient clinching of his fist until the palm appears pale; opening of patient's hand and releasing of the pressure over the ulnar artery. An effective 'dual hand circulation' is present if the hand's colour normalise within 3–15 seconds.[14] Other authors prefer using oximetry or plethysmography which might be less subjective than the conventional Allen test.[13,15] Although the choice between right or left RA is mainly a matter of operator's preference, he should be able to foresee potential difficulties. Elderly might have extreme tortuosity of the subclavian and anonymous trunk so that a left RA approach can be preferable. On the other hand, extreme type 3 aortic arches would make a left RA more challenging. The need to engage a left internal mammary graft forces the operator to use a left radial approach.[16]

Given the RA propensity for spasm, it is important that the procedure is held in a quiet environment, the patient is reassured and is given anxiolytic pre-medication. Particularly in women, the operators may expect that due to their smaller radial calibre, the frequency of spasm is higher.[17] Most operators prefer the use of lytic cocktails immediately after sheath insertion.

The optimal puncture site is 1 cm proximal to the styloid apophysis (Figure 24.2), where good compression after sheath removal is easily achieved. Several micropuncture kits are available for RA puncture. There are two ways to cannulate the RA. In the 'anterior technique', a single anterior wall puncture is performed with a 19-21-gauge needle and when back flow is visible, a short wire (0.018"–0.035") is introduced. This modified Seldinger technique may avoid puncture of the posterior arterial wall but, occasionally and in smaller arteries or for non-central punctures, the compression of the artery during insertion prevents back bleeding, observed only during needle withdrawal. Another limitation is the need of adjusting the position

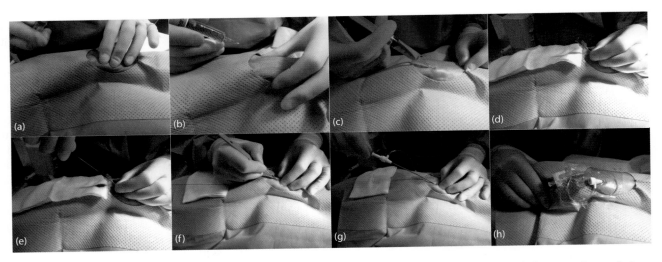

Figure 24.2 Radial artery puncture. Anatomical review of wrist joined to the palpation of the radial artery almost 1–2 cm proximal the styloid process, represent the primary steps for a correct puncture **(a, b)**. Subcutaneous infiltration, with 1–2 mL of local anaesthesia, is enough to reduce pain without impairing the pulse **(c)**. After the puncture of the anterior vessel wall, a pulsatile back flow appears **(d)**; thus, a 0.018″ wire is advanced through the artery **(e)**. Skin incision, made with a surgical blade parallel to the skin, is advisable to promote an easier and less traumatic sheath insertion **(f)**. After that the wire reach the rear of the sheath, it could be advanced **(g)** to achieve the final position **(h)**, securely fixed using a Tegaderm sheet.

of the needle with gentle rotation or change of angulation to allow a coaxial position of the needle and avoid dissections of the wall with the guide wire that should never be advanced if there the slightest resistance. With the 'tranfixive method' (or dual wall technique), the arterial lumen is entered with a cannula needle. Once back flow is observed in the reservoir, the needle is advanced through the posterior wall until back flow stops. The needle is then removed and the cannula is slowly withdrawn until back flow is seen again. At this moment, the wire can be inserted. For most diagnostic coronary angiography, 4–5 Fr sheaths are usually employed, whilst 5–6 Fr sheaths or bigger are required for PCI.

24.3 Access site complications

Both transfemoral and transradial catheterisations may lead to access site and vascular complications. The goal of an individual and procedure-based selection of the most suitable arterial access aims at reducing the rate of access site complications and at improving procedural success.

24.3.1 Femoral artery complications

The most frequent access site complications are bleeding, pseudoaneurysm/thrombus formation, distal embolisation and the creation of arteriovenous fistula.

Bleeding can occur at the beginning or during the procedure, more commonly after unsuccessful attempts have caused vessel trauma or around the sheath entry point, especially in calcified arteries. Most of the times, however, complications develop after sheath removal because of inadequate compression.

Female sex and the antithrombotic regimen are additional risk factors. Small arterial leakages may be clinically silent and resolve spontaneously with local compression at the end of the procedure or cause superficial bruising, with no major patient discomfort. More important bleeding may give rise to the formation of deep hard haematomas that can infiltrate the soft tissue below the inguinal ligament with slow spontaneous resolution or extend into the retroperitoneal space (Figure 24.3). Major blood loss can lead to hypotension (up to haemorrhagic shock) and may require blood transfusions. The rate of hematomas requiring either blood transfusion or surgical management is estimated at 2%–5%. Haematomas are associated with increase morbidity/hospital stay, patient distress and enhance costs.

Pseudoaneurysms, haematomas limited by surrounding planes and in communication with the arterial lumen, are reported in up to 3.7% of patient after femoral puncture, when systematic ultrasound is performed.[18] They develop more commonly when the femoral puncture is performed below the bifurcation. They are diagnosed as a pulsatile mass and produce a bruit at auscultation but diagnosis must be confirmed by ultrasound. Whilst in the past blind or echo-guided prolonged compression was the only alternative to surgical repair, treatment options now include ultrasound-guided injection of thrombin or collagen into the pseudoaneurysm cavity followed by prolonged compression and bed rest.

An arteriovenous fistula (0.1%–0.4%) originates either following accidental transfixion of vein and artery or secondary to the rupture of an arterial aneurysm into the adjacent vein. If spontaneous healing does not occur and the communication has haemodynamic relevance, endovascular or surgical treatment may be necessary.

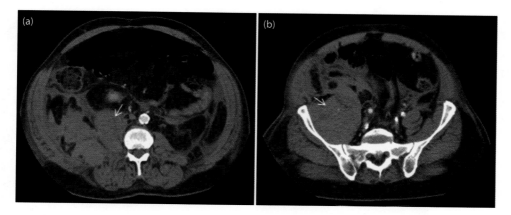

Figure 24.3 Retroperitoneal haematoma. Example of right retroperitoneal haematoma with involvement of the right Psoas muscle (white arrows) complicating right femoral artery puncture for PCI. **(a)** Cross section below the descending aorta bifurcation. **(b)** Cross section below the common iliac artery bifurcation. LEGENDS arrow.

FA dissection is also frequent, but often underestimated. In cases of flow-limiting dissections, treatment with balloon angioplasty with subsequent stenting may be required. Most of the times, however, dissections caused by retrograde puncture of the vessel with flap entry directed against the bloodstream will not extend distally and therefore resolve spontaneously thanks to centripetal flow splinting the intimal flap against the tunica media. Finally, arterial occlusion/thrombosis with limb ischemia is a life-threatening condition for which emergent endovascular or surgical intervention is needed. These events are rare but may develop in patients with pre-existing severe peripheral vascular disease.

24.3.2 Radial artery complications

The RA is a muscular vessel with high reactivity and propensity for spasms. In addition to unfavourable vascular anatomy, RA spasms have been described as the main cause of procedural failure.[19] Vasodilators can be used in this instance. However, the optimal pharmacological agent to minimise the incidence of radial spasms still remains unclear. In the SPASM trial, a combination of 2.5 mg of verapamil and 1 mg of molsidomine was associated with an incidence of radial spasms of 4.9% compared to 13.3% with verapamil only and 22.2% with placebo.[20] Shorter and hydrophilic sheaths can also reduce the incidence of radial spasms[21] (Figure 24.4 – panel a). It has also been described that RA wall protection from trauma using a long hydrophilic-coated sheath can reduce radial spasms.[22]

When the spasm occurs, the arterial lumen could collapse preventing the advancement of catheters and wires. When this happens, it is important to avoid forcing material through the spasm because catheters may become unmanoeuvrable. Generous sedation and the addition of a further dose of vasodilators may solve the problem. If the spasm persists, it is recommended to avoid subsequent contrast injection so as not to injure the wall vessel and try to withdraw slowly the blocked devices (Figure 24.5). Very

unusual cases of RA avulsion have been described after a forced removal of a catheter entrapped into a severe RA spasm.

Procedural failure can also be the consequence of vessel tortuosity (bend > 45°, incidence close to 6%) and anatomical variations. The latter has an incidence close to 10% and can be found at the radio-brachial (high origin of the RA from brachial-axillary artery, 3.4%; arterial loops), axillary-subclavian (retro-oesophageal right subclavian artery) or aortic level (aortic elongation) (Figure 24.4 – panels b through d). This is suspected when the guiding wire or catheter progression is difficult.[23] In most cases, operators manage to negotiate these variations by utilising hydrophilic wires (Figure 24.4 – panel b), smaller catheters, deep inspiration during catheter advancement and torquing. However, if the resistance persists, it is advisable to stop and check the anatomy with upper limb angiography, which would also exclude the occurrence of spasm. Navigation under fluoroscopy in the subclavian region is mandatory, since wire advancement into supra-aortic branches increases the risk of stroke. Even at this site, tortuosity and stenosis may be present, especially in elderly patients. Here again, it is essential not to force the wire and try to navigate gently.

Access site bleeding is a relatively rare complication of RA access (1%–3%).[24] It is usually managed easily with local measures such as increasing the external compression, often provided by dedicated inflatable pressure bandages. Large haematoma infiltrating the forearm are dangerous not much for the blood loss as for the risk of development of compartment syndrome. This complication is considered a medical emergency and needs surgical approach. If left untreated or treated too late the blood supply impairment may lead to permanent muscle and nerve damage. However, the incidence of compartment syndrome is extremely low, <0.01% in current registries.[25]

The occlusion of RA is more frequent and usually asymptomatic thanks to the double blood supply of the hand, having been reported in up to 10% of cases.[26] Systemic anticoagulation after sheath insertion is mandatory to avoid this

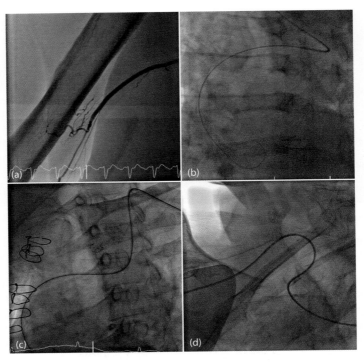

Figure 24.4 Radial challenges. **(a)** Severe spasm of the right radial artery extending to the brachial artery. **(b)** Anomalous course of the left subclavian artery (retroesophageal): aortic root as finally successfully reached through the employment of an Amplatz catheter and a hydrophilic wire. **(c, d)** Example of marked curvature and tortuosity at the level of the right subclavian artery.

complication. The recommended dose of heparin is 50 UI/kg and 70–100 UI/kg for diagnostic procedures and PCI, respectively.[27] Sheath removal with a non-occlusive technique has also been shown to improve arterial patency. This method consists of using the minimal amount of pressure to achieve haemostasis whilst still maintaining flow through the artery. Several studies have demonstrated a significant reduction in the rate of RA occlusion with this technique.[28,29] To check the presence of radial flow, oximetry is used during ulnar artery compression and simultaneous non-occlusive RA compression. After sheath removal, haemostasis is obtained by prolonged non-occlusive compression, using a folded gauze kept over the puncture site by an elastic bandage or via a dedicated plastic and air-based bracelet, the latter method gaining in popularity and use.[30]

Complications such as arteriovenous fistula or development of pseudoaneurysm are rare and usually managed with prolonged external compression.[31,32] During all procedures, intravenous analgesia can be given to reduce patients' discomfort.

24.4 Appropriateness of radial or femoral access

24.4.1 Femoral versus radial approach: Feasibility and access site crossover

Several factors influence the feasibility of a procedure through the RA. First, the inability to puncture or cannulate it due to operator skills, vessel tortuosity or radial spasms. Second, the selective engagement of the coronary ostia is challenged by the difficulty in catheter manipulation through the aortic arch (especially in the presence of vascular anomalies), since this can alter the catheter torsion response and its final angulation over the aortic plane. Dedicated radial catheters exist, but their use is not widespread. Finally, inadequate catheter support to perform PCI is more common when using radial access. These mentioned challenges to radial puncture may dictate the need to switch to alternative arterial access. Access site 'crossover' has significantly reduced with operator volume and experience.

Early studies showed higher procedural failure with transradial access as compared to femoral approach (7.2% vs. 2.4%, respectively, $p < .001$)[33] but these differences were not confirmed by the more recent trials reporting a trend towards similar procedural failure rates. In the RIVAL trial, the overall rate of access site crossover was 7.6% in the radial and 2% in the femoral group ($p < .01$). In patients randomised to radial approach ($n = 1594$), the most frequent reason for crossover was radial spasm (5.0%), followed by subclavian tortuosity (1.9%) and RA loop (1.3%). At centres undertaking a high proportion of radial procedures, the crossover gap was narrower (4.4% radial vs. 2.3% femoral, $p = .007$).[10] The recent MATRIX trial carried on by experienced radial operators ('radialists') reported similar results (4.1% vs. 2.3%, respectively), although the overall procedural success rate (defined as post-procedure TIMI 3 flow

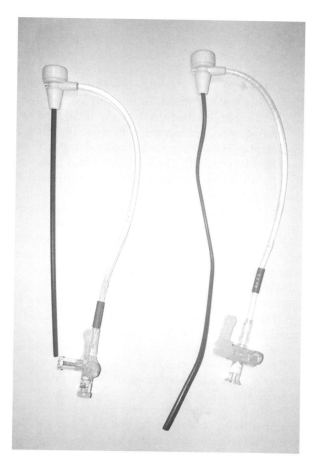

Figure 24.5 Sheath alterations after marked radial spasm. Two 5 Fr sheaths removed after transradial procedures. Left: normal sheath with no modification in structure. Right: sheath elongated and thinner in the proximal segment due to severe radial artery spasm.

and <30% coronary stenosis) was comparable between groups (92.7% vs. 92.8% p = .88).[34] Registries confirmed the progressive reduction in the need of access site crossover and suggest this trend was driven by the improvement in materials, technique and operators' expertise over recent years.[11,35] Sub-analysis of the PREVAIL study showed failure rates below 4% when transradial access was used (over 85% of cases).[19]

24.4.2 Procedural time and radiation exposure

The comparison of transradial and transfemoral approach must take into consideration procedure times and radiation exposure, both closely connected to operator's experience. For years, the perception that radial access has a 'steep learning curve', is time consuming and is associated with higher fluoroscopy time, has limited its wider utilisation.

Older registries[36–38] revealed up to 25%–50% increase in a variety of indirect measures of radiation exposure[39] with the worst results observed amongst inexperienced operators. In the RIVAL study, transradial approach was associated with significant longer fluoroscopy time (9.8 vs. 8.0 minutes, p < .0001).[10] The right radial route has been associated with a significantly higher radiation exposure than the left radial approach, regardless of the operator's proficiency.[40,41] Leaning forward with the operator's head beyond the protection shield has become a real concern in light of a recent reports of left brain hemisphere gliomas amongst interventional cardiologists/radiologists.[42] Nevertheless, several studies have demonstrated a reduction in radial–femoral radiation exposure difference after completion of the learning curve.[43–45] This data highlight that radial access know-how lowers procedure time and radiation exposure, whilst maintaining safety and procedural success.

The alleged delay in gaining arterial access and entering coronary arteries may play a crucial role in the setting of acute myocardial infarction (AMI), which has been addressed in several trials. In the RIFLE-STEACS trial, door-to-balloon time was 60 minutes (35–99 minutes) for radial and 53 minutes (31–91 minutes) for femoral access (p = .175).[46] Despite taking slightly longer, radial approach allowed to perform reperfusion within the guideline-recommended time.[47] In the RADIAL-STEMI trial, radial and femoral door-to-balloon times were equivalent (32 vs. 31 minutes, respectively; p = .31).[48] Access site crossover, a particular concern in PCI for STEMI, was reported only in 3.7% of the patients in the RADIAL-STEMI trial and did not affect the analysis of door-to-balloon time done on an intention to treat basis.

24.4.3 Expertise requirement and learning curve

Transfemoral access, although increasingly replaced by the transradial approach, is a well-established technique for cardiac catheterisation, and remains the default access site in some centres, due to its familiarity and feasibility. The radial approach is a demanding technique, whose above-mentioned drawbacks are minimised by operators' experience and centres' volume. A body of evidence suggests that access site and procedural success and time are strongly and positively influenced by radialists' volume and expertise.[49] In the RIVAL trial, centres with radial PCI volumes in the upper third (>146 radial PCI per year per operator) reported a benefit of radial versus femoral access for the primary outcome (HR 0.46, 95% CI 0.28–0.87; p = .015). In the PREVAIL study, a 10-fold lower rate of procedural failure was observed amongst operators who performed radial approach in 85% of their cases compared to those who used it less frequently (3.8% vs. 33%, respectively).[19] Similarly, the MATRIX trial showed primary endpoint improvement in patients undergoing radial PCI in high-volume centres (>80% of radial PCI).

The European Society of Cardiology Consensus Document recommends that institutional teams should aim at maintaining the highest feasible rate of radial approach, in order to achieve the greatest benefit: a reasonable objective of over 50% radial access in routine practice is proposed, amongst a minimum of 80 procedures/year per operator, including diagnostic and interventional procedures. This document also encourages the development of a 'radial access' programme based on a stepwise approach: after the first 50 cases, the feasibility of radial and femoral access should equalise; at this stage, it is important to attempt radial approach in consecutive patients and gradually, more complex procedures can be performed.[50] Nonetheless, femoral approach proficiency should be maintained in parallel to radial training. New interventional cardiologists must be equally competent in both accesses.

Radial Approach in Elective Patients: Over the past two decades, the number of PCIs performed worldwide has increased exponentially. This increased activity entails a significant burden for hospital bed turnover and a great interest in shortening the hospital stay. Many centres plan elective PCI as an outpatient procedure with early discharge. In that respect, the radial approach is optimal as it has the advantages of early ambulation, rapid haemostasis and decreasing access site complications. Several studies have proved the safety and feasibility of patient discharge after 6 hours of observation following elective, transradial PCI.[51-53]

Transradial approach seems to be promising in certain high-risk subgroups such as women, the elderly and STEMI presentation. Recent publications have focused on these subgroups (Table 24.2).

24.4.4 Radial approach in acute coronary syndrome: Safety, outcomes and effectiveness

A growing body of evidence suggests that post-PCI bleeding is an independent predictor of adverse events including death[55,56]: in the combined analysis of over 17,000 patients undergoing PCI (81% ACS), bleeding occurred in 2.1% of cases at the access site, whilst 3.3% were non access-site related. All TIMI-severity bleedings cause a greater than threefold increase in 1-year mortality, with non-access site bleeding associated to a risk twice as high compared to access-site bleeding.[57] Therefore, the overall patient/procedural bleeding risk must be carefully considered in the selection of the most appropriate arterial access. Radial approach significantly reduces access site-related bleeding in comparison to femoral access, as reported by a meta-analysis of randomised studies (2.1% vs. 5.6%, respectively; OR: 0.35; $p < .001$) as well as by large observational registries.[24,58,59] Importantly, the initial fear of a greater risk of cerebrovascular complication during transradial procedures was never observed in large trials.[34,60]

In terms of hard events, observational studies and a 2009 meta-analysis supported the hypothesis of improved patients' outcomes thanks to lower radial access-site bleedings.[11,61-63] The RIVAL study, a large multicentre trial ($n = 7021$) compared radial and femoral approach in ACS, in high-volume radialists centres. Despite a 60% reduction

in major vascular complications with radial access, no significant differences were reported in the primary composite endpoint (death, MI, stroke or major bleeding) compared to transfemoral PCIs (3.7% vs. 4.0%, respectively; HR: 0.92; $p = .5$) with a similar overall rate of bleeding and mortality.[54] Nevertheless, in the subgroup analysis of STEMI PCIs (roughly one-third of the total), the radial approach was associated to significant reduction in the primary outcome (HR 0.60, $p = .026$) and a decrease in mortality (HR 0.39, $p < .001$). The RIFLE-STEACS trial, which included 1001 STEMI patients undergoing primary PCI, reported a reduction in the incidence of NACE (death, MI, stroke or bleeding) (13.6 vs. 21%, radial vs. femoral, respectively; $p = .003$) and in cardiac mortality (5.3% vs. 9.2%; $p = .020$).[46] The authors attributed these differences to lower bleeding (7.8 vs. 12.2%; $p = .026$), particularly access-related, which, nonetheless, should be interpreted cautiously due to the overall high use of IIb/IIIa (nearly 70%), low use of bivalirudin and the recourse of larger sheath in the femoral group. The STEMI-RADIAL trial found a lower incidence of major bleedings in the radial compared to the femoral arm (1.4% vs. 7.2%, respectively; $p = .001$) with a significant MACE reduction (4.6% vs. 11%; $p < .001$), although mortality advantages were not confirmed (mortality rate 2.3% vs. 3.1%, respectively; $p = .64$).[48]

Different designs, exclusion criteria and endpoints make the comparison of the above-mentioned studies difficult: however, the reduction in radial access site complications was similar throughout all studies. Notably, radial access was not associated to a decrease in the overall bleeding risk in these studies, due to similar incidence of non-access site bleeding (50% of overall major bleeding) in the radial and femoral groups.

The MATRIX trial ($n = 8404$), the largest and most recent trial to date, found a significant reduction in the co-primary outcome of NACE in the transradial group (9.8% vs. 11.7%, radial vs. femoral, respectively; $p = .0092$). However, the reduction of the co-primary outcome of MACE did not meet the two-sided pre-specified $\alpha = 0.025$ statistical significance (8.8% vs. 10.3%; $p = .03$).[34]

24.4.5 Radial approach in unstable patients

A recent meta-analysis assessed the benefit of radial versus femoral approach in patients presenting with cardiogenic shock. Radial access was associated with significantly reduced risk of all-cause mortality and MACE (death, MI or stroke) at 30 days.[64]

In the RADIAL PUMP UP registry of patients receiving intra-aortic balloon pump, those undergoing transfemoral PCI ($n = 229$) had higher 30-day rate of net adverse clinical events than those ($n = 112$) undergoing radial PCI (57.4% vs. 36.6%, respectively; $p < .01$). Nevertheless, evidence in unstable patients is still lacking so that strong recommendation cannot be drawn yet.[65]

Table 24.2 Largest multicentre randomised trials on radial versus femoral approach in ACS: outcomes at a 30-day follow-up

Trial (year)	N	Mean age, y	Female, %	IIb/IIIa inhibitor FA/RA, %	Sheath size ≥ 7 Fr	Access site crossover	Primary endpoint	Bleeding definition and occurrence	Access site bleeding	Death	MI	Stroke
RIFLE-STEACS (2012)[46]	1001 STEMI	65	26.7	70/67.4	9.2% RA 18.6% FA (p < .01)	6.1% RA 2.8% FA (p = NA)	NACE 13.6% RA 21% FA (p = .003)	TIMI 7.8% RA 12.2% FA (p = .026)	2.6% RA 6.8% FA (p = .002)	5.2% RA 9.2% FA (p = .020)	1.2% RA 1.4% FA (p = 1)	0.8% RA 0.6% FA (p = .7)
RIVAL (2012)[54]	1958 STEMI GROUP	59	20.9	31/34.5	1.4% RA 4.5% FA (p < .01)	5.3% RA 1.6% FA (p < .01)	MACE 3.14% RA 5.19% FA (p = .026)	TIMI 0.84% RA 0.91% FA (p = .8)	1.26% RA 3.49% FA (p < .002)	1.26% RA 3.19% FA (p = .006)	1.16% RA 1.82% FA (p = .2)	0.5% RA 0.4% FA (p = .6)
RIVAL (2012)[54]	5063 NSTEMI GROUP	63	28.6	21.2/21.9	0.9% RA 6.7% FA (p < .01)	8.4% RA 2.2% FA (p < .01)	MACE 3.84% RA 3.46% FA (p = .49)	TIMI 0.63% RA 0.96% FA (p = .190)	1.45% RA 3.82% FA (p < .001)	1.25% RA 0.76% FA (p = .08)	1.92% RA 1.87% FA (p = .9)	0.6% RA 0.4% FA (p = .3)
STEMI-RADIAL (2014)[48]	707 STEMI	62	33	45/45	0% RA 0.4% FA (p = .2)	3.7% RA 0.6% FA (p = .003)	MACE 4.6% RA 11% FA (p < .001)	horizons-AMI 1.4% RA 7.2% FA (p = .001)	0.3% RA 0.8% FA (p = .62)	2.3% RA 3.1% FA (p = .64)	1.2% RA 0.8% FA (p = .72)	0.3% RA 0.3% FA (p = 1)
MATRIX (2015)[34]	8404 (STEMI= 4010; NSTEMI= 4394)	66	26	0.2/0.2	Not reported	Not reported	NACE 9.8% RA 11.7% FA (p < .001)	BARC 3–5 1.6% RA 2.3% FA (p = .0128)	1.7% RA 4.8% FA (p < .01)	1.6% RA 2.2% FA (p = .04)	7.2% RA 7.9% FA (p = .2)	0.4% RA 0.4% FA (p = 1)

(Continued)

Table 24.2 (*Continued*) Largest multicentre randomised trials on radial versus femoral approach in ACS: outcomes at a 30-day follow-up

Trial (year)	N	Mean age, y	Female, %	IIb/IIIa inhibitor FA/RA, %	Sheath size ≥ 7 Fr	Access site crossover	Primary endpoint	Bleeding definition and occurrence	Access site bleeding	Death	MI	Stroke
Meta-analysis (2015)[34]	19328 ACS	NA	NA	NA	NA	NA	MACE RR 0.86 (0.77–0.95) (p = .0051)	Non-CABG Major Bleeds RR 0.58 (0.46–0.72) (p < .001)	NA	RR 0.72 (0.60–0.88) (p = .001)	RR 0.91 (0.79–1.04) (p = .16)	RR 1.05 (0.69–1.60) (p = .80)

Meta-analysis reported in the MATRIX Trial.

ACS, acute coronary syndrome; BARC, bleeding academic research consortium; CABG, coronary artery bypass graft; FA, femoral approach; MACE, Major adverse cardiovascular events (death, stroke, myocardial infarction); MI, myocardial infarction); NACE, net adverse cardiovascular events (death, stroke, myocardial infarction and bleeding); RA, radial approach; RR, risk ratio; TIMI, Thrombolysis In Myocardial Infarction – major non-CABG related bleeding.

24.4.6 Radial approach in complex cases: Suitability for specific devices

Large catheters inserted via a FA can easily accommodate multiple wires, balloons, Rotablation burrs and microcatheters required for complex PCI (left main and bifurcation stenting, tight calcific lesions, CTO). The RA allows 6 Fr sheath in most patients with 7 Fr sheaths in taller subjects.[66] Two balloons, a stent delivery balloon and a second balloon, a balloon and a thin microcatheter (Finecross), a 1.50 mm – and with some effort a 1.75 mm – Rotablator burr, intravascular ultrasounds/optical coherence tomography catheters, 6 Fr guide extensions (Guideliner, Godzilla) are all 6 Fr compatible. With the exception of the most complex procedures requiring thicker microcatheters (Corsair, Turnpikes, Tornus, two stent delivery systems) the radial approach can be used for very complex procedures. Furthermore, the introduction of Sheathless guiding catheters (8.5 Fr with external diameter comparable to a 7 Fr Sheath) have expanded the spectrum of radial intervention feasibility.

Several case series reported similar success rates and no more vascular complications when rotational atherectomy was performed through the radial versus FA.[67,68]

Small studies have shown that bifurcation PCI can be achieved via radial approach with comparable results compared to the femoral access.[69]

In CTO, most operators prefer the stability and large catheter size allowed by 7 and 8 Fr catheters supported by 45 cm sheaths. Because dual arterial instrumentation for contralateral injection is required in more than two-third of cases, a radial access for the catheter in the donor vessel can reduce the bleeding risk with limited drawbacks (stability during long procedures can be enhanced by inserting an intracoronary wire), especially if no retrograde collaterals are present. In observational studies, transradial CTO PCI have shown similar success rate to transfemoral procedures, with less access site complications (<1%) but more frequent access site crossover (up to 6% when starting with bi-radial approach, due to insufficient support).[70–72]

24.4.7 Overall health system impact: Cost and in-hospital stay

The earlier ambulation and discharge allowed by a transradial approach translate into significant savings. Bleeding and vascular complications, more frequent with FA, also cause additional costs due to prolonged bed occupation, transfer to high dependency units and transfusions. Closure devices add a small additional cost for FA procedures, with some improvement in patient comfort but no reduction in major complications.[73] A 2009 meta-analysis reported a 0.5-day decline in hospital stay with radial approach.[11] A recent observational study evaluated the expenses of transradial and transfemoral PCI in 7121 patients from five different US hospitals: the former represented a total cost savings of $830, of which $705 was linked to shorter post-procedural in-patient stay.[74]

24.5 Guidelines recommendations and consensus

The 2013 Consensus Document on Radial Approach in Percutaneous Cardiovascular Interventions states that a default radial approach is acceptable in routine clinical practice and recommended in acute coronary syndromes as long as the operator has been properly trained. Nevertheless, proficiency in the femoral approach needs to be acquired and maintained for those cases requiring transfemoral access. Stable patients undergoing transradial diagnostic coronary angiography or PCI without complications can be considered for early discharge.[50] The European 2014 Revascularisation Guidelines and the 2015 NSTEMI Guidelines recommend radial approach as the preferred strategy to reduce PCI-related bleeding risk in primary PCI for STEMI as well as in the setting of NSTEMI (Class/Level of Recommendation II/A and I/A, respectively), provided that operator skills respect the required standards.[75]

However, whilst the European Society of Cardiology task force has given the highest level of recommendation to radial approach for PCIs, based on improved outcome, equivalent American Heart Association guidelines simply label the transradial access as a useful alternative to decrease vascular complications.

The differing interpretation of trials and registries is reflected in clinical practice. Great Britain moved from 10% to 71% of radial use in the last 10 years, but the increasing number of radialists across Europe is only partially mirrored by a similar phenomenon in the United States, where operators are adopting the radial approach at a slower pace.[76] They will, however, eventually be encouraged to increase their level of expertise to deal with new evidence-based data, not only suggesting better outcome for patients, but also a better cost/benefit ratio.[34]

References

1. Kiemeneij F, and Laarman GJ. Percutaneous transradial artery approach for coronary Palmaz-Schatz stent implantation. *Am Heart J* 1994; 128: 167–74.
2. Sandgren T et al. The diameter of the common femoral artery in healthy human: Influence of sex, age, and body size. *J Vasc Surg* 1999; 29: 503–10.
3. Grier D, and Hartnell G. Percutaneous femoral artery puncture: Practice and anatomy. *Br J Radiol* 1990; 63: 602–4.
4. Abu-Fadel MS et al. Fluoroscopy vs. traditional guided femoral arterial access and the use of closure devices: A randomized controlled trial. *Catheter Cardiovasc Interv* 2009; 74: 533–9.
5. Fitts J et al. Fluoroscopy-guided femoral artery puncture reduces the risk of PCI-related vascular complications. *J Interv Cardiol* 2008; 21: 273–8.

6. Seto AH et al. Real-time ultrasound guidance facilitates femoral arterial access and reduces vascular complications: FAUST (Femoral Arterial Access With Ultrasound Trial). *JACC Cardiovasc Interv* 2010; 3: 751–8.

7. Pracyk JB et al. A randomized trial of vascular hemostasis techniques to reduce femoral vascular complications after coronary intervention. *Am J Cardiol* 1998; 81: 970–6.

8. Baim DS et al. Suture-mediated closure of the femoral access site after cardiac catheterization: Results of the suture to ambulate aNd discharge (STAND I and STAND II) trials. *Am J Cardiol* 2000; 85: 864–9.

9. Yoo BS et al. Anatomical consideration of the radial artery for transradial coronary procedures: Arterial diameter, branching anomaly and vessel tortuosity. *Int J Cardiol* 2005; 101: 421–7.

10. Jolly SS et al. Radial versus femoral access for coronary angiography and intervention in patients with acute coronary syndromes (RIVAL): A randomised, parallel group, multicentre trial. *Lancet* 2011; 377: 1409–20.

11. Jolly SS et al. Radial versus femoral access for coronary angiography or intervention and the impact on major bleeding and ischemic events: A systematic review and meta-analysis of randomized trials. *Am Heart J* 2009; 157: 132–40.

12. Rao SV et al. The transradial approach to percutaneous coronary intervention: Historical perspective, current concepts, and future directions. *J Am Coll Cardiol* 2010; 55: 2187–95.

13. Greenwood MJ et al. Vascular communications of the hand in patients being considered for transradial coronary angiography: Is the Allen's test accurate? *J Am Coll Cardiol* 2005; 46: 2013–7.

14. Brzezinski M et al. Radial artery cannulation: A comprehensive review of recent anatomic and physiologic investigations. *Anesth Analg* 2009; 109: 1763–81.

15. Barbeau GR et al. Evaluation of the ulnopalmar arterial arches with pulse oximetry and plethysmography: Comparison with the Allen's test in 1010 patients. *Am Heart J* 2004; 147: 489–93.

16. Sciahbasi A et al. Transradial approach (left vs right) and procedural times during percutaneous coronary procedures: TALENT study. *Am Heart J* 2011; 161: 172–9.

17. Ercan S et al. Anxiety score as a risk factor for radial artery vasospasm during radial interventions: A pilot study. *Angiology* 2014; 65: 67–70.

18. Kacila M et al. The frequency of complications of pseudoaneurysms after cardiac interventional diagnostic and therapeutic interventions. *Med Arh* 2011; 65: 78–81.

19. Pristipino C et al. Identifying factors that predict the choice and success rate of radial artery catheterisation in contemporary real world cardiology practice: A sub-analysis of the PREVAIL study data. *EuroIntervention* 2010; 6: 240–6.

20. Kiemeneij F et al. Evaluation of a spasmolytic cocktail to prevent radial artery spasm during coronary procedures. *Catheter Cardiovasc Interv* 2003; 58: 281–4.

21. Rathore S et al. Impact of length and hydrophilic coating of the introducer sheath on radial artery spasm during transradial coronary intervention: A randomized study. *JACC Cardiovasc Interv* 2010; 3: 475–83.

22. Caussin C et al. Reduction in spasm with a long hydrophylic transradial sheath. *Catheter Cardiovasc Interv* 2010; 76: 668–72.

23. Lo TS et al. Radial artery anomaly and its influence on transradial coronary procedural outcome. *Heart* 2009; 95: 410–5.

24. Feldman DN et al. Adoption of radial access and comparison of outcomes to femoral access in percutaneous coronary intervention: An updated report from the national cardiovascular data registry (2007–2012). *Circulation* 2013; 127: 2295–306.

25. Tizon-Marcos H, and Barbeau GR. Incidence of compartment syndrome of the arm in a large series of transradial approach for coronary procedures. *J Interv Cardiol* 2008; 21: 380–4.

26. Kotowycz MA, and Dzavik V. Radial artery patency after transradial catheterization. *Circ Cardiovasc Interv* 2012; 5: 127–33.

27. Aykan AC et al. Comparison of low dose versus standard dose heparin for radial approach in elective coronary angiography? *Int J Cardiol* 2015; 187: 389–92.

28. Pancholy S et al. Prevention of radial artery occlusion-patent hemostasis evaluation trial (PROPHET study): A randomized comparison of traditional versus patency documented hemostasis after transradial catheterization. *Catheter Cardiovasc Interv* 2008; 72: 335–40.

29. Lerch S et al. Cerebral formation in situ of S-carboxymethylcysteine after ifosfamide administration to mice: A further clue to the mechanism of ifosfamide encephalopathy. *Toxicol Lett* 2006; 161: 188–94.

30. Bertrand OF et al. Transradial approach for coronary angiography and interventions: Results of the first international transradial practice survey. *JACC Cardiovasc Interv* 2010; 3: 1022–31.

31. Zegri I et al. Radial artery pseudoaneurysm following cardiac catheterization: Clinical features and nonsurgical treatment results. *Revista espanola de cardiologia* 2015; 68: 349–51.

32. Cauchi MP et al. Radial artery pseudoaneurysm: A simplified treatment method. *J Ultrasound Med* 2014; 33: 1505–9.

33. Agostoni P et al. Radial versus femoral approach for percutaneous coronary diagnostic and interventional procedures: Systematic overview and meta-analysis of randomized trials. *J Am Coll Cardiol* 2004; 44: 349–56.

34. Valgimigli M et al. Radial versus femoral access in patients with acute coronary syndromes undergoing invasive management: A randomised multicentre trial. *Lancet* 2015; 385: 2465–76.

35. Burzotta F et al. Vascular complications and access cross-over in 10,676 transradial percutaneous coronary procedures. *Am Heart J* 2012; 163: 230–8.

36. Ratib K et al. Operator experience and radiation exposure during transradial and transfemoral procedures. *JACC Cardiovasc Interv* 2011; 4: 936–7; author reply 7–8.

37. Lo TS et al. Comparison of operator radiation exposure with optimized radiation protection devices during coronary angiograms and ad hoc percutaneous coronary interventions by radial and femoral routes. *Eur Heart J* 2008; 29: 2180.

38. Bhatia GS et al. Transradial cardiac procedures and increased radiation exposure: Is it a real phenomenon? *Heart* 2009; 95: 1879–80.

39. Mercuri M et al. Radial artery access as a predictor of increased radiation exposure during a diagnostic cardiac catheterization procedure. *JACC Cardiovasc Interv* 2011; 4: 347–52.

40. Pancholy SB et al. Effect of vascular access site choice on radiation exposure during coronary angiography: The REVERE rrial (Randomized Evaluation of Vascular Entry Site and Radiation Exposure). *JACC Cardiovasc Interv* 2015; 8: 1189–96.

41. Pelliccia F et al. Comparison of the feasibility and effectiveness of transradial coronary angiography via right versus left radial artery approaches (from the PREVAIL Study). *Am J Cardiol* 2012; 110: 771–5.

42. Roguin A et al. Brain tumours among interventional cardiologists: A cause for alarm? Report of four new cases from two cities and a review of the literature. *EuroIntervention* 2012; 7: 1081–6.

43. Neill J et al. Comparison of radiation dose and the effect of operator experience in femoral and radial arterial access for coronary procedures. *Am J Cardiol* 2010; 106: 936–40.

44. Bertrand OF et al. Operator vs. patient radiation exposure in transradial and transfemoral coronary interventions. *Eur Heart J* 2008; 29: 2577–8.

45. Jang JS et al. The transradial versus the transfemoral approach for primary percutaneous coronary intervention in patients with acute myocardial infarction: A systematic review and meta-analysis. *EuroIntervention* 2012; 8: 501–10.

46. Romagnoli E et al. Radial versus femoral randomized investigation in ST-segment elevation acute coronary syndrome: The RIFLE-STEACS (Radial Versus Femoral Randomized Investigation in ST-Elevation Acute Coronary Syndrome) study. *J Am Coll Cardiol* 2012; 60: 2481–9.

47. Task Force on the management of ST-seamiot ESoC et al. ESC Guidelines for the management of acute myocardial infarction in patients presenting with ST-segment elevation. *Eur Heart J* 2012; 33: 2569–619.

48. Bernat I et al. ST-segment elevation myocardial infarction treated by radial or femoral approach in a multicenter randomized clinical trial: The STEMI-RADIAL trial. *J Am Coll Cardiol* 2014; 63: 964–72.

49. Jolly SS et al. Procedural volume and outcomes with radial or femoral access for coronary angiography and intervention. *J Am Coll Cardiol* 2014; 63: 954–63.

50. Hamon M et al. Consensus document on the radial approach in percutaneous cardiovascular interventions: Position paper by the European Association of Percutaneous Cardiovascular Interventions and Working Groups on Acute Cardiac Care** and Thrombosis of the European Society of Cardiology. *EuroIntervention* 2013; 8: 1242–51.

51. Wiper A et al. Day case transradial coronary angioplasty: A four-year single-center experience. *Catheter Cardiovasc Interv* 2006; 68: 549–53.

52. Small A et al. Day procedure intervention is safe and complication free in higher risk patients undergoing transradial angioplasty and stenting. The discharge study. *Catheter Cardiovasc Interv* 2007; 70: 907–12.

53. Jabara R et al. Ambulatory discharge after transradial coronary intervention: Preliminary US single-center experience (Same-day TransRadial Intervention and Discharge Evaluation, the STRIDE Study). *Am Heart J* 2008; 156: 1141–6.

54. Mehta SR et al. Effects of radial versus femoral artery access in patients with acute coronary syndromes with or without ST-segment elevation. *J Am Coll Cardiol* 2012; 60: 2490–9.

55. Rao SV et al. Impact of bleeding severity on clinical outcomes among patients with acute coronary syndromes. *Am J Cardiol* 2005; 96: 1200–6.

56. Rao SV et al. Bleeding and blood transfusion issues in patients with non-ST-segment elevation acute coronary syndromes. *Eur Heart J* 2007; 28: 1193–204.

57. Verheugt FW et al. Incidence, prognostic impact, and influence of antithrombotic therapy on access and nonaccess site bleeding in percutaneous coronary intervention. *JACC Cardiovasc Interv* 2011; 4: 191–7.

58. Karrowni W et al. Radial versus femoral access for primary percutaneous interventions in ST-segment elevation myocardial infarction patients: A meta-analysis of randomized controlled trials. *JACC Cardiovasc Interv* 2013; 6: 814–23.

59. Baklanov DV et al. The prevalence and outcomes of transradial percutaneous coronary intervention for ST-segment elevation myocardial infarction: Analysis from the National Cardiovascular Data Registry (2007 to 2011). *J Am Coll Cardiol* 2013; 61: 420–6.

60. Ratib K et al. Influence of access site choice on incidence of neurologic complications after percutaneous coronary intervention. *Am Heart J* 2013; 165: 317–24.

61. Wang YB et al. Randomized comparison of radial versus femoral approach for patients with STEMI undergoing early PCI following intravenous thrombolysis. *J Invasive Cardiol* 2012; 24: 412–6.

62. Montalescot G et al. Predictors of outcome in patients undergoing PCI. Results of the RIVIERA study. *Int J Cardiol* 2008; 129: 379–87.

63. Pristipino C et al. Major improvement of percutaneous cardiovascular procedure outcomes with radial artery catheterisation: Results from the PREVAIL study. *Heart* 2009; 95: 476–82.

64. Pancholy SB et al. Impact of access site choice on outcomes of patients with cardiogenic shock undergoing percutaneous coronary intervention: A systematic review and meta-analysis. *Am Heart J* 2015; 170: 353–61.

65. Romagnoli E et al. Radial versus femoral approach comparison in percutaneous coronary intervention with intraaortic balloon pump support: The RADIAL PUMP UP registry. *Am Heart J* 2013; 166: 1019–26.

66. Elgharib NZ et al. Transradial cardiac catheterization and percutaneous coronary intervention: A review. *Coron Artery Dis* 2009; 20: 487–93.

67. Egred M et al. High-speed rotational atherectomy during transradial percutaneous coronary intervention. *J Invasive Cardiol* 2008; 20: 219–21.

68. Gioia G et al. Coronary rotational atherectomy via transradial approach: A study using radial artery intravascular ultrasound. *Catheter Cardiovasc Interv* 2000; 51: 234–8.

69. Niccoli G et al. Coronary bifurcation lesions: To stent one branch or both? A meta-analysis of patients treated with drug eluting stents. *Int J Cardiol* 2010; 139: 80–91.

70. Sianos G et al. Recanalisation of chronic total coronary occlusions: 2012 consensus document from the EuroCTO club. *EuroIntervention* 2012; 8: 139–45.

72. Burzotta F et al. Radial approach for percutaneous coronary interventions on chronic total occlusions: Technical issues and data review. *Catheter Cardiovasc Interv* 2014; 83: 47–57.

73. Chase AJ et al. Association of the arterial access site at angioplasty with transfusion and mortality: The

M.O.R.T.A.L study (Mortality benefit Of Reduced Transfusion after percutaneous coronary intervention via the Arm or Leg). *Heart* 2008; 94: 1019–25.

74. Amin AP et al. Costs of transradial percutaneous coronary intervention. *JACC Cardiovasc Interv* 2013; 6: 827–34.

75. Roffi M et al. 2015 ESC Guidelines for the management of acute coronary syndromes in patients presenting without persistent ST-segment elevation: The Task Force for the management of acute coronary syndromes in patients presenting without persistent ST-segment elevation of the European Society of Cardiology (ESC). *Eur Heart J* 2015.

76. National Audit of Percutaneous Coronary Interventions. *Annual Public Report* January 2013, December 2013; www.bcis.org.uk.

Devices for femoral and radial haemostasis

TAWFIQ R CHOUDHURY, DOUGLAS G FRASER

25.1 Introduction

Percutaneous techniques to treat coronary artery disease, and more recently valvular heart disease, have revolutionised the field of cardiology. These procedures involve arterial access with the inherent risk of access site bleeding. According to Rao et al., 30%–70% of bleeding complications after percutaneous coronary intervention (PCI) is attributable to the vascular access site.[1] Hence, meticulous care to achieve adequate vascular haemostasis is essential. This is especially important in the current practice of interventional cardiology with the advent of more potent anti-platelet agents, the use of high doses of heparin, the performance of increasingly complex interventions and the use of large-sized sheaths in valvular interventions. For femoral access, manual compression still remains a commonly used method of achieving haemostasis.[2] However, several femoral haemostasis adjuncts to manual compression exist, including mechanical compression assist devices and haemostasis pads as well as dedicated, standalone vascular closure devices (VCDs). Radial access has now been widely adopted in most parts of the world including Europe, Canada and Australia and is gradually being taken up in the United States. Radial haemostasis is most commonly achieved by using radial compression devices. The aims of any such device would be to safely and efficiently achieve adequate haemostasis. The former would include a low rate of access site bleeding as well as a low rate of device-related complications. The latter would include a reduced time to haemostasis and ambulation, low preparation time and ease of use, patient comfort and satisfaction and financial savings, in terms of staff hours saved and reduced hospital stay. In this chapter, we review the currently available devices in the market, which are commonly used to achieve femoral and radial haemostasis.

25.2 Femoral VCDs

The rate of vascular complications associated with trans-femoral access ranges from 0.3% to 1% in diagnostic catheterisation and 1%–5% in PCIs.[3] Bleeding complications from femoral access are associated with increased morbidity and mortality.[4] Manual compression was the mainstay of achieving haemostasis and still is the default strategy when not suitable for VCDs. VCDs were introduced in the 1990s and can be classified as either passive or active devices. Passive devices augment the natural haemostatic process by applying procoagulant material, mechanical compression or deploying haemostatic plugs, which are extravascular and not directly or 'mechanically' fixed to the arterial wall. Examples of passive VCDs include mechanical compression assist devices such as Femostop™ (St. Jude Medical, St. Paul, MN), haemostatic pads such as Chito-seal (Abbott Vascular Devices, Redwood City, CA) and passive plug-based closure devices such as Exoseal™ (Cordis, Warren, NJ). Active devices, in contrast, directly 'seal' the arteriotomy site by apposing the arteriotomy edges or mechanically securing a haemostatic plug to the vessel wall with the aim of achieving immediate haemostasis. Active VCDs are based on sutures, collagen plugs or clips. The following section discusses active and passive VCDs in more detail.

25.3 Passive VCD

25.3.1 Mechanical compression

Mechanical compression devices are passive VCDs. The concept of mechanical compression devices is similar to manual compression, that is to apply pressure over the arterial puncture site. The disadvantage of these devices is that they are applied by an estimation of the site of arteriotomy and apply pressure over the artery proximal to the puncture site. Thus, these devices do not directly seal the point of entry into the vessel. Furthermore, the mechanical compressive force can be quite uncomfortable for patients and the patient has to lie still whilst the device is in place. The key advantage of these devices is that they are entirely external to the body and can save physician/nursing time by being substituted for manual compression. Furthermore, the data from studies using mechanical compression devices have shown that they are safe.[5] The data on whether these devices shorten the time to haemostasis or result in early ambulation as compared with manual compression have been mixed. In a comparison of the Femostop mechanical compression device with manual compression, the time to haemostasis was significantly longer in the Femostop group (35.2 minutes) compared with the manual compression group (12.9 minutes).[6] However, in a prospective study on 1000 patients undergoing elective coronary angiography via the femoral route, early ambulation after 90 minutes was achieved safely in the majority of patients after using the Femostop device.[7] Although mechanical compression devices have been used after sheath removal immediately after PCI and without manual compression, in our experience, mechanical compression devices are best not used as the sole means of achieving haemostasis after sheath removal but rather as an adjunct to manual compression (assisted manual compression).[8]

A host of mechanical compression assist devices are available in the market. An example is the widely used Femostop device. It has a pneumatic dome that is attached to the patient by means of a belt that goes round the patient's hips. The dome is placed over the femoral puncture site and inflated to above 20 mmHg above systolic pressure. The dome is then gradually deflated following set protocol. The puncture site is visible through the dome (Figure 25.1). The patient has to lie flat whilst the device is on. Other available devices in the market include ExpressAR (Advanced Vascular Dynamics, Portland, OR), CompressAR (Advanced Vascular Dynamics), SafeGuard (Merit Medical Inc., South Jordan, UT) and ClampEase (Semler Technologies, Portland, OR). Most devices consist of a pneumatic ball or a disc that is applied slightly proximal to the puncture site. A detailed description of each of these devices is beyond the scope of this chapter.

25.3.2 Haemostasis pads

Haemostatic pads are adjuncts to manual or mechanical compression. They contain procoagulant material embedded in them. They accelerate the thrombotic process and have been

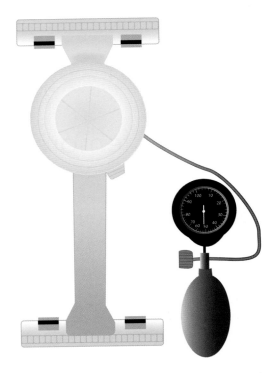

Figure 25.1 Femostop compression device (St. Jude Medical). The femostop compression device consists of a pneumatic compression dome that is inflated to supra-systolic pressures and the pressure in the dome then reduced over set times. (Courtesy of St. Jude Medical. All rights reserved.)

shown, when used in combination with manual compression, to be safe and to offer greater comfort to patients in comparison to manual compression and compression bandage. In a randomised controlled trial comparing two different haemostatic pads (Clos-Sur and Chito-Seal) versus manual compression, use of haemostasis pads shortened the time to haemostasis marginally but made no difference to the required bed rest time before ambulation.[9] Mleksuch compared Clo-Sur pad (Scion Cardiovascular, Miami, FL) versus manual compression in a randomised controlled trial. Although a shorter time to haemostasis (13.6 vs. 20.3 minutes; $p < .001$) and greater patient comfort were observed with the use of haemostatic pads, a higher rate of technical failure (19%) was also noted in the same group.[10] In the VIPER (Gore VIabahn Endoprosthesis with Heparin Bioactive Surface for SuPERficial Femoral Artery Endoluminal Bypass)-2 trial, a haemostatic dressing D-Stat (Vascular Solutions, Minneapolis, MN) was compared with active VCDs (Angioseal and Starclose). The rate of minor and major complications was higher in the haemostatic dressing group compared with the closure device groups.[11] Overall, although haemostatic pads provide greater patient comfort when compared with manual compression, the lack of significant reduction in time to ambulation, the technical failure rates observed and the availability of active closure devices with greater efficacy have meant that haemostatic pads are not widely used. A wide range of haemostatic pads are available in the market, including Celox Vascular™

(Celox Vascular, Medtrade Products, UK), D-stat, Syvek patch (Marine Polymer Technologies, Inc.), Clo-sur PAD, Chitoseal and Neptune Pad (TZ Medical, Portland, OR).

25.3.3 Wire-stimulated track thrombosis

Apart from haemostatic pads and mechanical compression devices, passive arteriotomy closure devices exist that enhance the haemostatic process via wire-stimulated track thrombosis (Figure 25.2). The Cardiva Catalyst® II and III (Cardiva Medical, Inc., Sunnyvale, CA) are passive VCDs that consist of a nitinol-braided mesh collapsible disc. The disc is attached to the end of a 0.035" wire, which is coated with procoagulant drugs chitosan and kaolin. The Catalyst III has in addition protamine sulphate coating to reverse the effects of heparin. The wire is inserted through the femoral sheath (up to 7F) and the sheath removed. The disc then expands and is pulled back against the intima. The procoagulant drugs in the wire coating then stimulate the physiological coagulation process. The disc is left to dwell for 15 minutes for diagnostic procedures and 120 minutes for interventional procedures. The disc and wire are then removed leaving nothing behind in the patient. However, a short period of manual compression is then necessary following disc and wire removal due to the re-bleeding risk at the time of removing the wire and disc through the arteriotomy track and is applied till complete haemostasis is achieved.

25.3.4 Exoseal

The Exoseal device (Cordis) is a passive closure device (Figure 25.3). It consists of a synthetic, bioabsorbable plug, composed of polyglycolic acid (PGA) and a plug delivery system. The device is inserted via the femoral sheath (up to 7F) and the PGA plug deployed extra-vascularly over the arteriotomy site. Following deployment, a further short duration of manual pressure is advised. The device cannot be used in vessels <5 mm diameter and through sheaths longer than 12 cm. The PGA plug gets completely absorbed within 60–90 days. In the randomised, single-centre study from Germany, the Exoseal was no different in terms of complications (haematoma > 5 cm, significant groin bleeding [thrombolysis in myocardial infarction {TIMI} major bleed], false aneurysm, and device failure) when compared with the commonly used Angioseal device (St. Jude Medical) (although there was a trend towards higher device failure in the Exoseal group).[12] However, in a larger, prospective, observational study comparing Exoseal with Angioseal and Proglide (Abbott Vascular Inc., Redwood City, CA), the Exoseal device had a higher complication rate compared with the other devices (3.6% vs. 1.2%, $p = .012$).[13]

25.3.5 Mynx

The Mynx device (AccessClosure, Inc., Mountain View, CA) is a passive VCD that deploys a synthetic, sealant plug composed of polyethylene glycol (Figure 25.4). The device is deployed through the procedural femoral sheath and consists

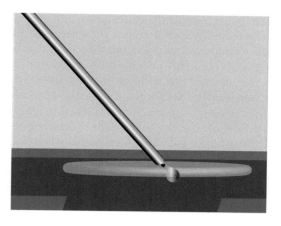

Figure 25.2 Cardiva Catalyst™ (Cardiva Medical, Inc.). The device consists of a nitinol disc loaded on a wire coated with procoagulant drug. The disc is placed inside the artery and placed under tension against the arterial wall whilst the wire track exposes the procoagulant drugs and facilitates haemostasis. (Courtesy of Dr Z Turi in Overview of Vascular Closure, May 2010, *Endovascular Today*.)

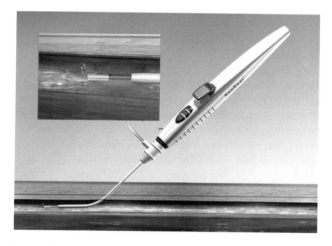

Figure 25.3 Exoseal™ (Cordis). A passive closure device consisting of a synthetic, bioabsorbable plug and a delivery system. The plug is delivered over the arteriotomy site. (Courtesy of Cardinal Health. © 2013 Cardinal Health. All Rights Reserved.)

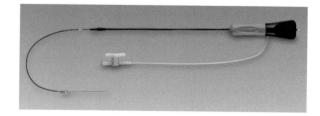

Figure 25.4 MYNXGRIP™ device (AccessClosure, Inc., Mountain View, CA). The Mynx™ passive closure device consists of a sealant plug which is deployed extra-vascularly over the arteriotomy site. A balloon inside the vessel is used for temporary tamponade whilst the sealant plug is deployed. (Courtesy of Cardinal Health. © 2013 Cardinal Health. All Rights Reserved.)

of a small balloon inside the vessel lumen and the plug. The balloon is pulled to anchor against the vessel wall allowing temporary tamponade and accurate positioning of the sealant plug extra-vascularly over the arteriotomy site. The balloon is then deflated and withdrawn and sealant expansion allows haemostasis. The plug gets resorbed within 30 days via hydrolysis. The Mynx device is deployable through a 5F, 6F and 7F procedural sheaths. In the study by Azmoon et al., the rate of device failure with Mynx was higher when compared with Angioseal.[14] In a report by Baker et al., they looked at the safety and efficacy of the Mynx device against Angioseal in 4074 patients undergoing PCI and found both devices to be similar in safety and efficacy.[15]

25.4 Active VCD

25.4.1 Angioseal

The Angioseal™ (St. Jude Medical) is one of the most widely used VCD and is a mixed active and passive closure device (Figure 25.5). The Angioseal consists of a polymer anchor, a collagen plug and a suture deployed via a dedicated sheath delivered over a guidewire. The sheaths are available in 6F and 8F sizes. Once the procedural sheath is removed over the guidewire, the Angioseal sheath is advanced over the wire. The sheath has a special arteriotomy locator and once position is confirmed within the arterial lumen, the wire and arteriotomy locator are removed. The polymer anchor is then deployed against the arterial wall intra-luminally and the collagen plug is pushed extra-vascularly against the arteriotomy site. A suture holds the anchor and the collagen plug together sandwiching the vessel wall in between. The suture is then cut below the level of the skin. These three components (anchor, collagen plug and suture) which remain in the body are bioabsorbable and dissolve within 90 days. A few versions of the Angioseal exist (STS, VIP) but they are based on the same principle. The Angioseal device has shown persistently high device success rates of >95% and a reduced time to haemostasis and ambulation compared with manual compression as well as other contemporary VCDs.[16,17,11,18] A similar device, the FemoSeal (St. Jude Medical, Uppsala, Sweden) consists of a bioabsorbable polymer anchor plate, which is deployed intra-arterially and an extra-arterial disc, between which the arteriotomy site is sandwiched. The FemoSeal device and the Exoseal were compared with manual compression in the ISAR-CLOSURE (Instrumental sealing of arterial puncture site closure device versus manual compression trial) randomised trial and both devices showed non-inferiority to manual compression in terms of access site-related complications and haemostasis time.[19]

25.4.2 Starclose

The Starclose device (Abbott Vascular Inc.) is a clip-based VCD, consisting of a 4-mm disc shaped nitinol clip that is deployed, through the procedural sheath, just outside the vessel wall over the arteriotomy site. The clip apposes the

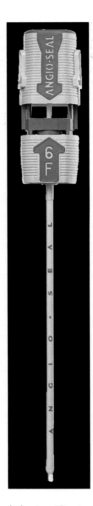

Figure 25.5 Angioseal device (St. Jude Medical). The Angioseal is an active closure device that delivers a bioabsorbable polymer anchor intra-arterially and a collagen plug extra-arterially and sandwiches the arteriotomy site in between, thus achieving haemostasis. (Courtesy of St. Jude Medical, All rights reserved.)

edge of the arteriotomy site, thus aiding in haemostasis. The disadvantage with the Starclose device is that this clip is left behind in the body permanently. However, the manufacturer states that the clip is MRI conditional. The device can be used with 5 and 6F procedural sheaths. The Starclose device was compared with the Angioseal device in a randomised, single-centre study and found to have similar efficacy in achieving haemostasis and no difference in complication rates and patient comfort.[20] Another randomised, single centre study by Ratnam et al. also showed no significant difference in complication rates between Angioseal and Starclose devices.[21]

25.4.3 Perclose proglide and prostar XL

The Perclose Proglide and Prostar XL (Abbott Vascular Inc.) are both suture-mediated VCDs. The Perclose device consists of a complex delivery system that drives two needles simultaneously into an intra-arterial footplate (Figure 25.6). This delivers a non-biodegradable polypropylene suture that is

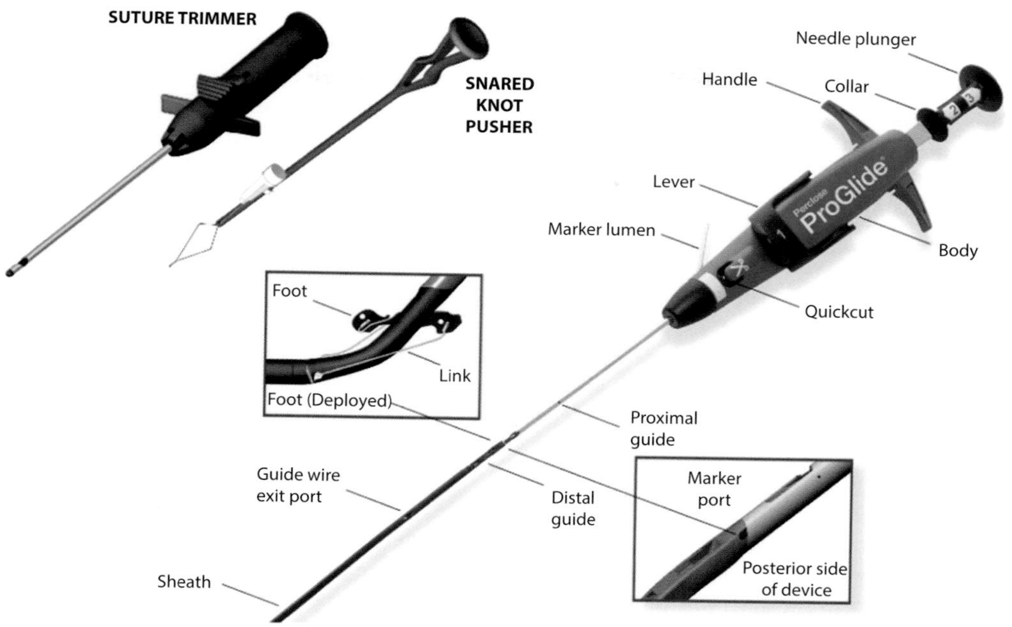

Figure 25.6 Perclose™ technology (Abbott Vascular Inc.). The Perclose system relies on using suture mediated apposition of the arteriotomy edges. (Courtesy of Abbott Vascular. ©2012 Abbott. All Rights Reserved.)

then pulled back through the arterial wall forming a suture loop. The part of the device with the needles is then withdrawn and the suture ends are now ready for deployment. At the end of the procedure, haemostasis is achieved by means of pushing a slipknot down to the arteriotomy site, thus causing apposition of the arteriotomy edges and achieving active haemostasis. The Prostar device uses four needles and delivers two sutures. The 6F Perclose Proglide is specified for use with 5–8F sheaths and the Prostar XL is designed for 8–10.5F sheaths. A number of studies have compared the Perclose Proglide to the Angioseal. Results have suggested a superiority of the Angioseal in achieving faster haemostasis. The safety data in terms of vascular complications have been mixed with some studies suggesting higher access site complications with the Perclose whereas others have failed to demonstrate a difference.[18,22,23] However, device deployment might be a factor in explaining these safety observations as the deployment of a Perclose is more complex than other commonly use VCDs, for example, Angioseal. In the study by Martin et al., they noticed a higher rate of device deployment failure in the Perclose group ($n = 10$) compared with the Angioseal group ($n = 0$).[18] The pre-closure technique with the Perclose Proglide can effectively be used for much larger sheaths. This is an advantage of the pre-closure technique. This is done by initially deploying a 6F sheath and then removing the sheath and deploying two Perclose Proglide devices at an angle to each other to create two suture loops ready for pre-closure. Next, a larger sheath is deployed as required for the procedure and at the end of the procedure the sheath is removed and the slipknots deployed. At our institution, we regularly use the Perclose Proglide device vascular closure in our trans-femoral

transcatheter aortic valve implantation (TAVI) procedures. The Prostar XL when compared with the Perclose Proglide device in trans-femoral TAVI showed a higher rate of major vascular complications in a multicentre study.[24]

25.4.4 Fish

The Femoral Introducer Sheath and Haemostasis (FISH) device (Morris Innovative Inc., Bloomington, IN) consists of a delivery sheath and a porcine intestinal mucosa derived patch loaded at the end of the sheath. The patch is delivered across the arteriotomy track and acts as a re-absorbable plug in the artery wall. The device is available in 5–8F sizes and is currently approved for diagnostic catheterisation purposes only. However, more data are needed to clarify the safety profile of the device before widespread adoption of its use. No study has yet compared the FISH device with the Angioseal device.

25.4.5 Axera

The Axera Arstasis device uses micro-needle technology to create a controlled, shallow angle, long arteriotomy that self-seals by utilising the intrinsic arterial pressure and tissue overlap. This device has to be deployed pre-procedurally and is currently approved in the United States for diagnostic procedures only for 5 and 6F sheaths.

25.5 Radial access compression devices

The superficial location of the radial artery, the lack of any overlying neurovascular structures, the dual arterial supply of the hand and the presence of the radial bone underneath the artery all make the radial artery easy to compress and thus achieve haemostasis. Patients undergoing procedures via a radial approach can be mobilised early after the procedure and discharged home sooner than patients undergoing procedures via a femoral approach.[25] The satisfaction of patients is also in general higher with the radial approach and the complication rate is lower than with femoral access.[26,27] As a result, the radial arterial approach to coronary interventions has been gaining increasing popularity across the globe.

Several haemostatic devices and adjuncts exist in the market for radial haemostasis. The aim of all such devices is to compress the radial artery. One of the most commonly used devices is the TR Band™ (Terumo IS, Somerset, NJ). This consists of a plastic band with an inflatable bladder that is inflated using air from a syringe (comes in pack) via a one way valve (Figure 25.7). The bladder is positioned precisely over the area of interest and then inflated. The transparent bladder and plastic band allow for accurate positioning and identification of any residual bleeding. Air is let out of the bladder in small decrements until just enough inflation of the balloon to achieve haemostasis is present whilst maintaining antegrade flow in the artery. A pulse oximeter can aid in detecting the latter. The reason why it is so important to achieve 'patent' haemostasis is because of the risk of radial artery occlusion (RAO). Excessive pressure over the radial artery to completely obliterate flow increases the risk of RAO. Once permanently occluded, the artery becomes unusable in the future for any further procedures or as a bypass graft. Furthermore, a lot of the time cardiologists do not check the ipsilateral ulnar arterial flow, but a pre-existing diseased ulnar artery together with new RAO can result in hand ischaemia. The Prevention of RAO-patent haemostasis

evaluation (PROPHET) randomised trial by Pancholy et al. compared patent haemostasis versus conventional compression.[28] A radial compression device Hemoband (Hemoband Corp., Portland, OR) was used with one arm receiving conventional compression pressures (control) whilst the other arm received pressures compatible with an arterial tracing on pulse oximetry (intervention). The intervention arm had a lower rate of RAO at 1 day (5% vs. 12%; $p < .05$) and 1 month (1.8% vs. 7%; $p < .05$). Pancholy then compared the Hemoband with the TR Band in another randomised study and found that the TR Band had significantly reduced RAO compared with the Hemoband.[29]

A number of other devices exist in the market for radial haemostasis. These include the Finale (Merit Medical Systems Inc.), Helix (Vascular Perspectives, UK), AirBand (Maquet Cardiovascular), Seal One (Perouse Medical), Radistop (St. Jude Medical, St. Paul, MN), Safeguard (Merit Medical Systems Inc.), R-Band (Vascular Solutions), RA-band (Atlantic World), RADStat (Merit Medical Systems Inc.) and RadAR (Advanced Vascular Dynamics) to name a few. These devices are virtually all based on the same concept of pressure application over the radial arteriotomy site. Haemostatic pads (discussed earlier) either with manual compression or in combination with compression devices and bandages have also been tested in radial artery haemostasis with encouraging results.[30]

25.6 Summary

Haemostatic devices for both radial and femoral arterial access have come a long way. A huge range of products now exist in the market. Meticulous attention during deployment is the key to avoid vascular access site complications. Radial haemostasis should always be obtained bearing in mind the concept of patent haemostasis. Where adequate haemostasis is not satisfactorily achieved with the use of a VCD, reverting to the default strategy of good quality manual compression is important.

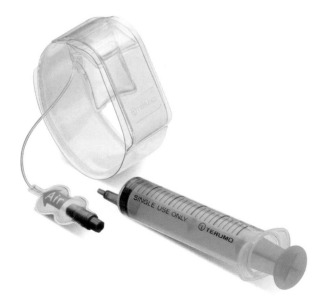

Figure 25.7 TR Band™ – Radial artery compression device. The TR Band consists of an inflatable bladder that is inflated over the arteriotomy site using a syringe via a one-way valve. (Courtesy of Terumo Europe NV. All rights reserved.)

References

1. Rao SV et al. The transradial approach to percutaneous coronary intervention: Historical perspective, current concepts, and future directions. *J Am Coll Cardiol* 2010; 55(20): 2187–95.
2. Schwartz BG et al. Review of vascular closure devices. *J Invasive Cardiol* 2010; 22(12): 599–607.
3. Alonso M et al. Complications with femoral access in cardiac cathetization. Impact of previous systematic femoral angiography and hemostasis with VasoSeal-ES collagen plug. *Rev Esp Cardiol* 2003; 56(6): 569–77.
4. Byrne RA et al. Vascular access and closure in coronary angiography and percutaneous intervention. *Nat Rev Cardiol* 2013; 10(1): 27–40.
5. Pracyk JB et al. A randomized trial of vascular hemostasis techniques to reduce femoral vascular complications after coronary intervention. *Am J Cardiol* 1998; 81(8): 970–6.

6. Walker SB et al. Comparison of the FemoStop device and manual pressure in reducing groin puncture site complications following coronary angioplasty and coronary stent placement. *Int J Nurs Pract* 2001; 7(6): 366–75.

7. Gall S et al. Rapid ambulation after coronary angiography via femoral artery access: A prospective study of 1,000 patients. *J Invasive Cardiol* 2006; 18(3): 106–8.

8. Jaspers L, and Benit E. Immediate sheath removal after PCI using a Femostop is feasible and safe. Results of a registry. *Acta Cardiol* 2003; 58(6): 535–7.

9. Nguyen N et al. Randomized controlled trial of topical hemostasis pad use for achieving vascular hemostasis following percutaneous coronary intervention. *Catheter Cardiovasc Interv* 2007; 69(6): 801–7.

10. Mlekusch W et al. Arterial puncture site management after percutaneous transluminal procedures using a hemostatic wound dressing (Clo-Sur P.A.D.) versus conventional manual compression: A randomized controlled trial. *J Endovasc Ther* 2006; 13(1): 23–31.

11. Rastan A et al. VIPER-2: A prospective, randomized single-center comparison of 2 different closure devices with a hemostatic wound dressing for closure of femoral artery access sites. *J Endovasc Ther* 2008; 15(1): 83–90.

12. Ketterle J et al. Comparison of Exo-Seal® and Angio-Seal® for arterial puncture site closure: A randomized, multi-center, single-blind trial. *Herz* 2015; 40(5): 809–16.

13. Kara K et al. Safety and effectiveness of a novel vascular closure devices following percutaneous coronary intervention: A prospective study of the ExoSeal compared to the Angio-Seal and ProGlide. *J Interv Cardiol* 2016; 29(1): 108–12, doi: 10.1111/joic.12264[published Online First: Epub Date].

14. Azmoon S et al. Vascular complications after percutaneous coronary intervention following hemostasis with the Mynx vascular closure device versus the AngioSeal vascular closure device. *J Invasive Cardiol* 2010; 22(4): 175–8.

15. Baker NC et al. Active versus passive anchoring vascular closure devices following percutaneous coronary intervention: A safety and efficacy comparative analysis. *J Interv Cardiol* 2016;29(1):108–12, doi: 10.1111/joic.12264[published Online First: Epub Date].

16. Applegate RJ et al. Vascular closure devices in patients treated with anticoagulation and IIb/IIIa receptor inhibitors during percutaneous revascularization. *J Am Coll Cardiol* 2002; 40(1): 78–83.

17. Ward SR et al. Efficacy and safety of a hemostatic puncture closure device with early ambulation after coronary angiography. Angio-Seal Investigators. *Am J Cardiol* 1998; 81(5): 569–72.

18. Martin JL et al. A randomized trial comparing compression, Perclose Proglide and Angio-Seal VIP for arterial closure following percutaneous coronary intervention: The CAP trial. *Catheter Cardiovasc Interv* 2008; 71(1): 1–5.

19. Schulz-Schupke S et al. Comparison of vascular closure devices vs manual compression after femoral artery puncture: The ISAR-CLOSURE randomized clinical trial. *JAMA* 2014; 312(19): 1981–7.

20. Veasey RA et al. A randomised controlled trial comparing StarClose and AngioSeal vascular closure devices in a district general hospital—The SCOAST study. *Int J Clin Prac* 2008; 62(6): 912–8.

21. Ratnam LA et al. Prospective nonrandomized trial of manual compression and Angio-Seal and Starclose arterial closure devices in common femoral punctures. *Cardiovasc Interv Radiol* 2007; 30(2): 182–8.

22. Zhou ZJ et al. Evaluation of two arterial closure devices, Angioseal and Perclose, in coronary catheter interventions. *Nan Fang Yi Ke Da Xue Xue Bao* 2011; 31(10): 1767–70.

23. Duffin DC et al. Femoral arterial puncture management after percutaneous coronary procedures: A comparison of clinical outcomes and patient satisfaction between manual compression and two different vascular closure devices. *J Invasive Cardiol* 2001; 13(5): 354–62.

24. Barbash IM et al. Comparison of vascular closure devices for access site closure after transfemoral aortic valve implantation. *Eur Heart J* 2015; 36(47): 3370–79.

25. Cooper CJ et al. Effect of transradial access on quality of life and cost of cardiac catheterization: A randomized comparison. *Am Heart J* 1999; 138(3 Pt 1): 430–6.

26. Valgimigli M et al. Radial versus femoral access in patients with acute coronary syndromes undergoing invasive management: A randomised multicentre trial. *Lancet* 2015; 385(9986): 2465–76.

27. Jolly SS et al. Radial versus femoral access for coronary angiography and intervention in patients with acute coronary syndromes (RIVAL): A randomised, parallel group, multicentre trial. *Lancet* 2011; 377(9775): 1409–20.

28. Pancholy S et al. Prevention of radial artery occlusion-patent hemostasis evaluation trial (PROPHET study): A randomized comparison of traditional versus patency documented hemostasis after transradial catheterization. *Catheter Cardiovasc Interv* 2008; 72(3): 335–40.

29. Pancholy SB. Impact of two different hemostatic devices on radial artery outcomes after transradial catheterization. *J Invasive Cardiol* 2009; 21(3): 101–4.

30. Dai N et al. A comparison of 2 devices for radial artery hemostasis after transradial coronary intervention. *J Cardiovasc Nurs* 2015; 30(3): 192–6.

Percutaneous removal of retained intravascular foreign bodies

SETHUMADHAVAN VIJAYAN, EVER D GRECH

26.1 Introduction

Percutaneous diagnostic and therapeutic procedures involving the heart and the circulation have become increasingly common and with new developments, this increase has become exponential. The past decade alone has seen a surge not only in the number of cardiovascular procedures undertaken but also in their complexity. Despite marked improvements in the safety of devices and procedural techniques, interventional cardiologists are occasionally faced with the complication of an unwanted intravascular foreign body. Although not common, such complications may pose a unique and difficult challenge, often requiring innovative and tailored approaches. It is therefore necessary for the practicing interventional cardiologist to be familiar with techniques for safe retrieval of unwanted foreign bodies to prevent potential adverse outcomes.

Turner and Sommers first reported a fatality from an intra-cardiac foreign body in 1954, involving a polyethylene catheter, which had embolised from the cubital vein into the right atrium.[1] In 1964, Thomas et al. described the first case of percutaneous retrieval of a foreign body from the right atrium and inferior vena cava (IVC).[2] A wide range of retained foreign objects have since been reported including stents, IVC filters, catheters, guidewires, coils, pacemaker lead fragments, septal and atrial appendage occluder devices and prosthetic heart valves. The majority have been associated with percutaneous

procedures, while a few have been reported as a complication of cardiac surgery.[3,4] This chapter provides an overview of some of the more commonly encountered retained foreign objects and management techniques.

26.1.1 Coronary stents

Unquestionably, the most common intravascular foreign body that adult cardiologists are likely to come across is the coronary stent. With advances in technology allowing greater stent deliverability, safety and effectiveness, the numbers deployed have risen exponentially over the past decade. Despite this, stents may become separated from the balloon catheter on which it is mounted and may end up being deployed in an area not originally intended.

Undeployed detached stents can lead to severe problems depending on their anatomical site. The most severe is coronary stent thrombosis resulting in acute occlusion and myocardial infarction, which is associated with significant morbidity and mortality.[5] Risk factors for detachment include vessel calcification, excessive coronary tortuosity and poor lesion preparation by way of limited balloon pre-dilatation. Historically, when stents were first introduced in the early 1990s, such events were much more common, as manual crimping of the stent onto the balloon by the operator was both necessary and not always as effective as intended.[6,7] Thankfully, this has been superseded by stents, which are now very firmly and effectively crimped onto the balloon catheter as part of the manufacturing process.

Modern stents are now so well applied that it is actually difficult to manually remove them off the balloon catheter. Despite this, there is one common procedural instance when a stent can be stripped off the balloon – with relative ease. This may occur when an undeployed stent is being withdrawn back into a guide catheter, which is not well aligned with the artery (such as the right coronary artery). The proximal stent edge may then be forcibly caught on the guide catheter 'lip' and they become wedged. The operator, who may be unaware that stent wedging has occurred, may feel some resistance and may exert even more traction on the stent catheter. The resulting longitudinal force exerted on the proximal edge of the stent by the guide catheter lip then strips the stent off the balloon with relative ease[7] (Figure 26.1). Recognising the cause of this initial resistance is essential in avoiding the consequence of stent loss. The operator can gently advance the stent catheter, realign the guide catheter and attempt again to retract the stent into the guide catheter. If resistance is again present, the only option may be to disengage the guide catheter from the coronary ostium, then remove the guide catheter, stent catheter and guidewire together from the patient. The stent catheter can be inspected and should be discarded if there is any proximal stent edge distortion. Guide support extension catheters can also cause the stent to be stripped off the balloon.[8]

Various techniques have been described to retrieve lost stents. The choice will be dependent on the anatomical site, whether the stent is still on the guidewire and the degree of stent expansion. Most will be unexpanded stents; those that have been expanded within a coronary artery cannot safely be retrieved percutaneously and may be left in situ or require surgical removal if deemed necessary.

Ensuring the guidewire position through the lumen of the stent is very important and the 'small balloon technique' can be initially considered. This involves passage of a small diameter balloon through the stent and then inflating the balloon distal to the stent allowing stent retrieval into the guide catheter by gently pulling back. If guidewire position is lost, occasionally attempting to rewire the stent with a suitable guidewire can be successful.

Other techniques using various devices have been described to retrieve the detached stent. These include the use of loop micro-snare (Figure 26.2), which may be used in one of two ways. In the 'proximal wire grab' method, the balloon catheter is removed and the loop of the micro-snare is placed over the proximal end of the guidewire. The snare is advanced until the distal end of the micro-catheter is positioned just proximal to the stent. The loop is then opened and advanced around the end of the stent. The loop is then closed to grab the stent and removed into the guide catheter. In the 'distal wire grab' method, a second guidewire is positioned adjacent to the stent and distal to the original guidewire. The micro-snare is looped over the proximal end of the second guidewire and advanced until the distal end of the micro-catheter is positioned distal to the stent and original guidewire. The loop is opened to snare the distal end of the original guidewire. The micro-snare, both guidewires and the stent can then be withdrawn together into the guide catheter.

Another technique that has been employed is using a second guidewire and twisting the wires together to trap the stent and then retrieving the entire system including the guiding catheter. Other devices such as biliary forceps, Cook retained fragment retriever and basket retrieval device can cautiously be used only if the stent is protruding out of the coronary artery into the aortic root.[9,10]

If retrieval is difficult then the stent may be deployed at the site of displacement by inflating an appropriately sized balloon to maintain lumen patency and reduce the risk of thrombosis (Figure 26.3). However, this may not always be an option if the site of displaced stent involves the left main stem or other large bifurcation, or if the stent is not suitably sized to be deployed at that site. In such cases, deployment of another suitably sized stent alongside the displaced stent, to the displaced stent from the lumen has been successful (Figure 26.4). In cases of partial displacement of the stent from the balloon, inflation of the balloon to a low pressure (two to four atmospheres) to fix the stent and retrieving it along with the entire system including the guiding catheter can be successful.[5]

There are reports of successfully managing un-deployed lost stents within the coronary arteries with regimes including long-term dual anti-platelet therapy and anti-coagulation therapy.[11] However, the risk of thrombosis is much higher in such cases.

Stent loss in the infrarenal peripheral arterial circulation does not usually lead to any clinical sequelae.[5] Trying to locate the lost stent with computed tomography (CT) scan may not always be successful and is of dubious clinical value

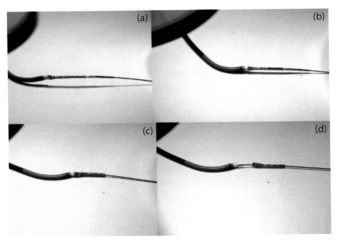

Figure 26.1 Mechanism by which a stent can be stripped off the balloon with relative ease. Attempting to retrieve the stent-balloon catheter when the guide catheter is not coaxial to the artery can lead to the proximal stent edge catching and wedging on the lip of the guide catheter (a). Continued traction (b) leads to the balloon being withdrawn into the guide catheter (c) leaving the stent loose on the guidewire (d).

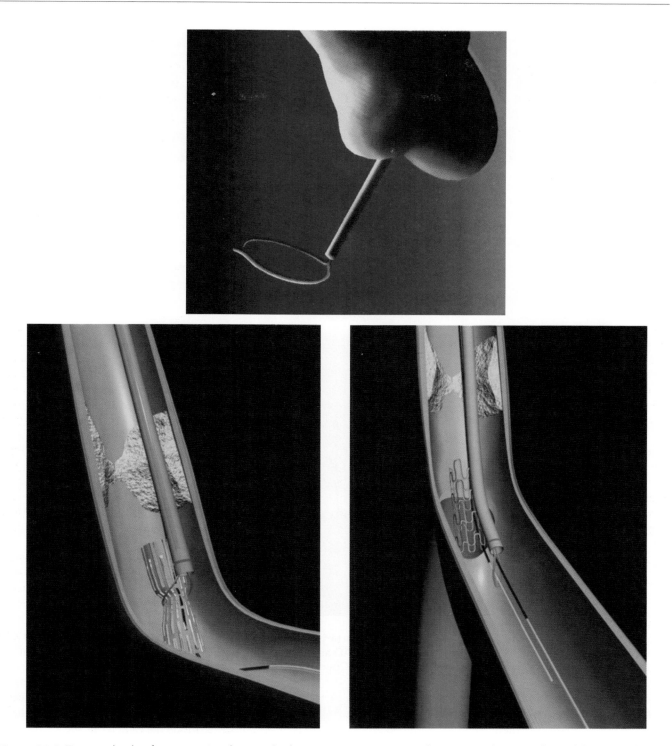

Figure 26.2 Two methods of stent retrieval using the loop micro-snare. (Top) The 'proximal wire grab' and (bottom) the 'distal wire grab'.

especially in the absence of symptoms. In reported case series, stents embolised to unknown locations, the clinical course was uneventful.[12,13] Embolisation of stent to the head and neck vessels can lead to disastrous complications. Use of snaring techniques to retrieve stents from cerebral arteries has been described.[14]

26.1.2 Guidewires

Guidewires of various widths and lengths are used widely for vascular access as well as for interventional procedures. Loss of guidewires is a rare complication[15] and has been reported in relation to a variety of procedures (Figure 26.5).[16–19] Coronary

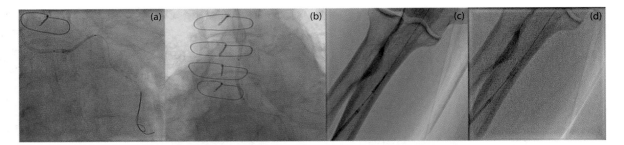

Figure 26.3 A stent could not be advanced across the intended coronary lesion and was withdrawn back into the guide catheter. In doing so, the stent became partially detached from the balloon (a) and (b). The stent and the balloon along with the guide catheter and the guidewire were gently withdrawn back to the radial artery (c). As the stent could not be externalised it was deployed within the radial artery (d). The percutaneous coronary intervention (PCI) was then completed without further complications. (Courtesy of Dr. KP Morgan, Northern General Hospital, Sheffield.)

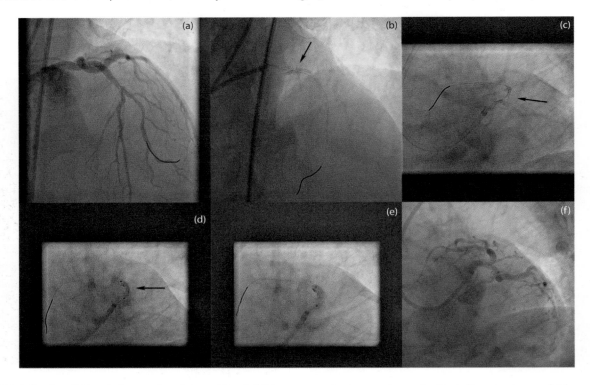

Figure 26.4 During PCI to left anterior descending (LAD) artery, a stent came loose in the left main stem, which could not be retrieved (arrow) (a–c). The stent was moved into the LAD and excluded from the lumen by deploying another stent to crush the un-deployed stent against the vessel wall (d–f). (Courtesy of Prof RF Storey, Northern General Hospital.)

guidewires are much smaller in width and can fracture. There are several reports of guidewire transection and loss with the use of rotational atherectomy.[20,21] Retained guidewire fragments have been managed conservatively without any serious complications.[19,22,23] However, the clinical course may not always be benign as retained wire fragments may act as a nidus for endothelial injury and platelet aggregation.[24,25]

Guidewire fragments are often long and can often be removed with snares and other retrieval devices without much difficulty[26]. However, firm entrapment of guidewire between an expanded stent and coronary wall (often used for side branch protection in bifurcation PCI) may be impossible to retrieve, and a surgical opinion is recommended.

If the proximal end of the guidewire is within the catheter or the arterial sheath, inflating a suitably sized balloon to trap the guidewire inside the catheter or sheath and then removing the guidewire along with the sheath or catheter as one unit can be successful. If it is causing symptoms and percutaneous attempts at retrieval of the fragments are unsuccessful, surgical intervention must be considered. Another option is to isolate the guidewire from coronary circulation by stenting and apposing the fragments to the vessel wall. Intensive anti-platelet and anti-coagulant regimes have been tried, but there is no convincing evidence regarding their effectiveness in preventing complications. Alexiou et al. in their series of nine patients report excellent results from surgery for retained guidewires and other foreign objects.[27]

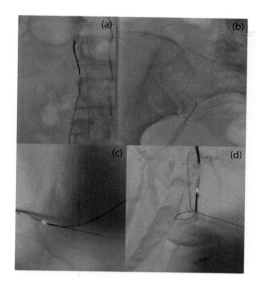

Figure 26.5 A lost guidewire extending down into the inferior vena cava after permanent pacemaker implantation. The right femoral vein was cannulated and a goose neck snare was used with a multipurpose guide catheter to successfully snare the wire and retrieve it. (Courtesy of Prof UM Sivananthan, Leeds General Infirmary.)

26.1.3 Septal/duct occluder devices

Embolisation of septal and duct occluder devices is relatively uncommon.[28,29] In a large meta-analysis of over 28,000 cases who underwent percutaneous closure of atrial septal defect (ASD) or patent foramen ovale (PFO), device embolisation requiring surgery was reported as the most common complication, which occurred in 0.4% of cases.[30] In addition, a further 0.3% of patients suffered embolisation of the devices successfully retrieved percutaneously. In another series of 3824 patients with Amplatzer septal occluders, an overall device embolisation rate of 0.55% was reported.[31] The most common reason cited for embolisation is under-sizing of the device. Repositioning the displaced device using snares or other equipment may be possible in select cases.[32]

In general, for devices that embolise into the atria, attempts should be made to pull the device into the IVC below the entry of the hepatic veins in preparation for retrieval. A stiff guidewire placed through the device can help to prevent migration and stabilise the device simplifying the retrieval process.[31] To avoid the possibility of entangling the device in either the mitral or the tricuspid valve apparatus, devices that have embolised to the ventricles may be safely moved antegradely across the semilunar valves prior to retrieval from aorta or pulmonary artery. Retrieval of the device is usually possible by pulling the device using a snare into a sheath using the screw on the right atrial disk and not the left atrial disk. Kim and Lee reported the retrieval of embolised duct occluder using a myocardial biopsy forceps[33] from the pulmonary artery. They also used a balloon as an adjunct to stabilise the device in order to help its retrieval. An example is shown on Figure 26.6. In a similar case, Goel et al.

reported the use of a goose neck snare to retrieve the device into the sheath and a pigtail catheter to stabilise the device.[34]

There are reports of late embolisation of Amplatzer ASD closure device leading to late complications.[35,36] Embolisation of duct occluder device to the thoracic aorta has been reported to lead to ischaemic injury to spinal cord[37].

26.1.4 Left atrial appendage closure devices

Left atrial appendage (LAA) closure devices have gained popularity in the past decade as an option to prevent thromboembolic strokes, especially in people who cannot tolerate oral anti-coagulation therapy. The embolisation rates of these devices are generally low.[35] In the multi-centre European Percutaneous Left Atrial Appendage Transcatheter Occlusion (PLAATO) study two patients out of 180 patients who received LAA occluder device had embolised.[36] One of these was thought to have occurred during resuscitation after cardiac tamponade. The other was due to inadequate sizing of the device, which was successfully retrieved by snaring.

Careful follow-up with echocardiography is necessary after implantation of LAA occluder devices as the displacement and embolisation can be completely asymptomatic or catastrophic depending on the site of embolisation.[37,38]

26.1.5 Trans-catheter aortic valve implantation valves

The accidental dislocation of valves used for trans-catheter aortic valve implantations (TAVIs) procedures is rare.[39] The migration of prosthesis during TAVI can often be managed by implanting a second device[40] (Figure 26.7). The CoreValve™ (Medtronic) device can sometimes be pulled back into position by catching one of the hooks. If this is not possible a technique of moving the valve to the descending aorta and crushing it against the aortic wall has been described.[39] The most common reason cited for embolisation is placing the valve too much towards the aortic side, followed by inadequate visualisation of the valve plane and failure to recognise the new valve was not coaxial to the valve plane. Inadequate ventricular pacing and previous mitral valve replacement where the mitral bioprosthesis struts causing displacement of the TAVI valve have also been cited as causes. Displaced valves are often positioned in the aorta with good prognosis on follow up.[41] Interestingly CT follow-up showed that the leaflets of the embolised TAVI valve in aorta remain open in all phases of the cardiac cycle.

In a review of published 71 cases of valve embolisations, Ibebuogu et al. described an overall incidence of 0.02%.[42] Most cases (>90%) occurred intraoperatively or within 1 hour. The common sites of embolisation were ascending aorta (38%), left ventricle (31%), descending aorta (23%) and aortic arch (8%). Late embolisations occurred mostly into the ventricle and was associated with high mortality (43%).

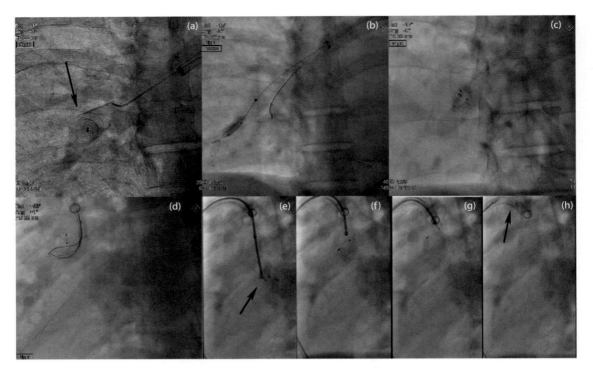

Figure 26.6 A duct occluder device that embolised (arrow) into the right pulmonary artery during attempted percutaneous closure of an arteriovenous malformation (a). Attempts at retrieving the device using a snare with stabilisation using a balloon (b). Mobilisation of the device using a pigtail catheter (c). Failed attempt at snaring the device (d). The plug was grabbed using a myocardial biopsy forceps (arrow) (e) and withdrawn into the sheath (f–h). (Courtesy of Dr. J Thomson, Leeds General Infirmary.)

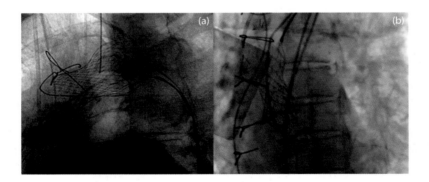

Figure 26.7 (a) A displaced TAVI valve (CoreValve) that has been snared by two goose neck snares being moved along the aorta to be left in a safe position distal to the origin of the left subclavian artery. (b) A displaced CoreValve in the aortic root and a second vale is deployed in the correct position. This procedure was performed inside a surgically placed bio-prosthetic valve. (Courtesy of Dr. C Malkin, Leeds General infirmary.)

26.1.6 Permanent pacemaker and related foreign objects

Permanent pacemaker implantation is a relatively safe procedure with very low reported rates of embolisation complications. There have been reports of the anchoring sleeve being embolised accidentally to the pulmonary arteries requiring percutaneous retrieval.[43] In a series of 45 patients referred for retrieval of foreign bodies in relation to device implantations or extractions over 10 years, there were 25 distal portions of introducer sheaths and 18 pacing lead fragments, one guidewire and one anchoring sleeve.[44] Percutaneous retrieval was successful in 93% of the cases.

Planned extraction of pacemaker systems is increasing every year. Non-functioning or redundant pacemaker leads can either be capped and left in situ or be extracted. The strategy depends on the experience of the operator and the dwell time of the leads. In their review, Rijal et al. did not find any difference between either strategy.[45] With the growing number of device implantations, the number of leads that need to be extracted is also increasing. Infectious complications such

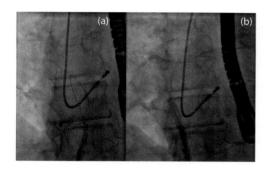

Figure 26.8 Trans-femoral approach for extraction of pacemaker leads using a snare device. (Courtesy of Dr. N Lewis, Northern General Hospital, Sheffield.)

as endocarditis affecting the pacemaker system, pacemaker pocket infection and pocket erosions are the most common indications for pacemaker system and lead extraction. A stepwise approach and escalation strategy have been suggested to be effective.[46] Simple traction is often the first technique employed and has good success rates in leads with short dwell time.[46,47] Over time, the leads can become adherent to the myocardium or vessel wall, due to encapsulating fibrotic tissue and simple traction alone will not be sufficient for extraction. The use of locking stylets, which are specialised tools designed to slide into the lumen of a lead and advanced to the tip of the lead where they are locked into position, can help with retrieval. A common third step in the stepwise approach of lead extraction is the use of a mechanical dilator sheath, which is advanced along the lead to disrupt and dilate the encapsulating fibrotic tissue. A trans-femoral approach with use of snares commonly the needle's eye snare (Cook medical) is another step that can be tried and has been reported to have good success rates (Figure 26.8).[48]

If these steps are not successful, powered traction tools that use an energy source to disrupt the adhesions and free the leads can be employed. The excimer laser sheath slides over the implanted lead and utilises a pulsed ultraviolet laser to vaporise adhesions that come into contact with the tip of the sheath. The penetration depth of the laser is only 100 μm and therefore, the vessel wall is not damaged by the sheath as it is advanced over the lead (Figure 26.9). The electrosurgical dissection sheath uses radiofrequency energy and permits localised application of energy unlike the circumferential dissection offered by laser. A rotating threaded tip sheath (Evolution, Cook medical) can be employed and is especially advantageous in disrupting calcified fibrosis.[49] Sometimes, leads can become fragmented during attempts to extract and other devices may need to be used to extract the fragments safely.[50,51]

26.1.7 Central venous catheter fragments

Fragments of central venous catheters may become embolised within the venous system and the heart.[52–54] In their review of published cases of central venous catheter embolisation, Surov et al. identified 215 cases over a 23-year period up to 2007. Of these, 143 were totally implanted venous devices (TIVDs) or port catheters and 72 percutaneous venous catheters (PVDs).[53] The majority of catheters were placed in the subclavian vein (56%). The most common sites of embolisation were the superior vena cava or peripheral veins (15%), right atrium (28%), right ventricle (22%) and pulmonary arteries (35%). A quarter of these were asymptomatic while most presented with catheter malfunction (56%). Arrhythmias were reported in 13% and pulmonary symptoms occurred in 4.7% of patients. Septic symptoms were rare at 1.8%. Mortality rate was also low at 1.8%. Catheter fracture in the infraclavicular region (known as the pinch-off syndrome) was described in 41% of the cases as the cause of fracture and embolisation and occurred more commonly in TIVDs. Catheter damage during explantation or catheter exchange was documented in 18% of cases and was more frequent with PVDs. Historically, the mortality rate was significantly higher with embolised catheter fragments, but most recent studies have shown that mortality rates are low. Most can be managed using percutaneous retrieval techniques.

26.1.8 Vena cava filters

Vena cava filters have been used as an alternative therapy for patients who have contraindications to anti-coagulation or in patients with continued emboli despite anti-coagulation. It has been reported that 6% of IVC filters migrate more than 1 cm and are usually asymptomatic. They are commonly retrieved after the desired duration of treatment through the jugular veins using snares. However, embolisation can occur during retrieval.[55,56] Fracture of IVC filter struts is a common complication of IVC filter placement with a reported incidence of 12%–25%.[57,58] There are several reports of fractured IVC filter fragments being embolised to the heart causing serious complications such as arrhythmias, tamponade and death.[59–62] Reports of migration and fragmentation have led to the removal of a model of IVC filter (model G1; C. R. Bard, Tempe, Arizona) from the medical device market and re-engineering of the filter to improve its stability and integrity. Filter surveillance with x-ray or CT to monitor filter integrity and stability has been recommended as a precaution until long-term follow-up data are available.[63] There are several reports of using conventional devices successfully to retrieve the filter fragments. Hannawa et al. described the use of intra-cardiac echocardiography (ICE) and three-dimensional (3D) electroanatomic (EA) mapping to safely retrieve intra-cardiac embolised filter struts.[57]

26.1.9 Miscellaneous objects

Adjunct devices used in coronary intervention such as intravascular ultrasound catheters, dilatation balloons and rotational atherectomy catheters have all been known to fracture and embolise.[64–66] They can often be removed percutaneously. Retained post-surgical epicardial pacing leads have also been reported to cause coronary artery

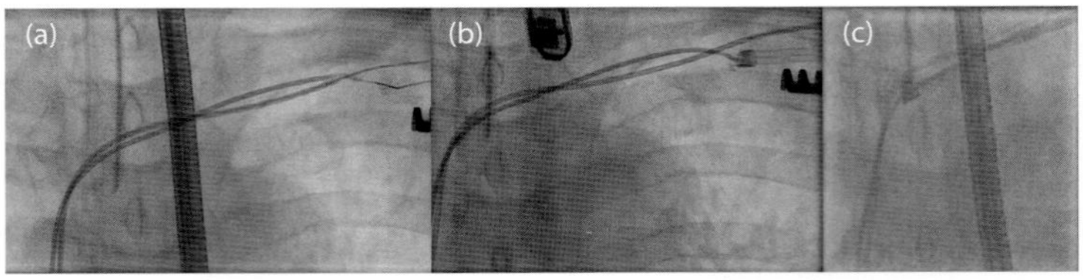

Figure 26.9 A patient with damaged pacemaker leads due to subclavian crush syndrome. The pacemaker system became infected and extraction was attempted. **(a)** The damaged lead during a failed attempt to introduce a locking stylet. **(b and c)** Use of an excimer laser sheath successfully released the adhesions. (Courtesy of Dr. N Lewis, Northern General Hospital, Sheffield.)

compression and out-of-hospital cardiac arrest.[67] Embolised needles have been reported especially in intravenous drug users.[68,69] Fracture and embolisation of metallic prosthetic valves leaflets have been reported. The Bjork–Shiley valve was particularly noted to suffer such complications.[70] Penetrating firearm injuries can sometimes lead to intravascular migration of objects such as shotgun pellets or bullet fragments away from the site of injury.[71,72] In one reported case, a shotgun pellet migrated to the coronary artery causing coronary occlusion and myocardial infarction.[73] There are also reports of foreign bodies from penetrating injuries migrating to the heart and remaining in situ without causing any complications.[74]

26.2 Devices used for retrieval

A variety of trans-catheter devices for retrieval of components are available. Some of the more commonly used devices and their use are described below.

26.2.1 Loop-snare retrieval systems

The loop-snare device is often the first choice in view of its safety and ease of use. There are several reports of various types of loop-snare retrieval systems to retrieve various intravascular foreign bodies.[75–77] A loop snare consists of a movable wire in the shape of a loop that is attached to or pulled through an outer catheter. The wire loop is advanced around the foreign body. Then the snare is tightened by advancing the sheathing catheter while keeping the wire loop still. There are several design variants of the loop snare system, which has enhanced its ease of use and success rate over the years such as the goose neck snare, which has a nitinol 90° snare loop to shaft orientation and remains coaxial to the vessel lumen, and Welter retrieval loop catheter, which permits the orientation of the loop at right angles to its shaft, enabling access to free floating foreign bodies. The EN Snare system is designed with three interlaced loops[4] (Figure 26.7). Several techniques such as proximal grab, distal grab, coaxial snare and lateral grasp techniques have been described each with its own pre-requisites, pros and cons.[78] If a dedicated loop retrieval system is not available, an effective 'home-made' snare can be fashioned using a guidewire and a guiding catheter.[79–81] Loop snares have

the advantage that they are simple to use, provide good perceptual feedback and yield good success rates even in less experienced hands. They are also flexible and follow the intravascular course more easily.

26.2.2 Retrieval baskets

Retrieval baskets have the advantage of being able to encircle the foreign body. The Cook® Dotter Intravascular Retrieval basket has a helical loop basket that is loaded into the hub of a catheter that expands upon emergence from the distal tip. It is normally used to retrieve renal calculi but has been used effectively to remove intravascular foreign bodies.[82] The Dormia basket (Gemini, Microvasive, Boston Scientific, USA) is commonly used in the biliary system for stone retrievals but it can also be used for endovascular retrievals.[83] The Dormia basket has a paired nitinol wire configuration that has a helical shape when opened up. It has a low delivery profile (2.4 Fr) with a round-wire construction that facilitates atraumatic manipulation.

Baskets have a powerful grasp and are capable of withdrawing relatively large foreign bodies. The disadvantage of baskets is that they can be difficult to guide and some types may have a rigid tip that poses a risk of vessel damage or perforation. Retrieval basket devices are particularly useful in retrieving objects in the great veins or intra-cardiac chambers or larger calibre arteries. To deploy the device, the basket is placed beyond the fragment and then opened. It is then withdrawn, allowing entrapment of the foreign body, at which time the basket is pulled shut and removed as a single unit.

26.2.3 Bioptome/grasping forceps

Snares are often not effective when the free end of the foreign body is not presenting. Intravascular grasping forceps can overcome this difficulty. Although there are several reports of employing these devices successfully, it must be borne in mind that these devices can be traumatic and should be handled by experienced operators. The rigid body, large diameter shaft inadequate catheter length have them not conducive for intravascular foreign body retrieval.[84] Myocardial biopsy forceps such as the flexible myocardial biopsy forceps and the Cordis biopsy forceps are available in various sizes and lengths and have been used for intravascular foreign body retrieval.[85] However, they are generally too rigid and large and are unsuitable to be used in coronary arteries except in the very proximal segments in the hands of experienced operators.

26.2.4 Miscellaneous techniques

Tip deflecting wires have been used successfully to hook and retrieve or reposition intravascular foreign bodies.[86] As mentioned previously, a simple, handmade snare may be fashioned using single or twin guidewires. The snare is created by doubling over an exchange-length wire at its mid-section and inserting it down a 4 Fr probing catheter. Alternatively, a snare may be created by looping the distal 5 cm of a standard-length wire,[87] or tying together the flexible ends of two 0.014-inch wires. The probing catheter is then passed through the guide catheter and positioned just proximal to the retained fragment. The loop is front-loaded through the probing catheter and gently passed over the object. Ideally, the loop should have a moderate bend to help encompass the fragment. Once the object is trapped, the wire ends are pulled firmly to secure the object against the catheter tip. The whole assembly is then withdrawn until it passes through the femoral sheath.

If the snare device cannot be steered into a tortuous or acutely angled coronary artery, twin 0.014-inch guidewires may be used. The wires are advanced separately into the coronary artery and positioned beside the fragment. The proximal wire ends are inserted into a torquer and clamped firmly together. The torquer is then rotated in a clockwise direction to form a helix of the two wires. With the Y-connector partially open, the double helix is propagated distally into the coronary artery, ensnaring the object, which can then be withdrawn into the guiding catheter and removed.[88,89]

A pigtail ventriculography catheter has been used to snare a catheter fragment in the venous system[90] and a broken guidewire in a coronary artery.[91] Distal embolic protection filter has been used successfully in a vein graft to remove a detached stent in the proximal portion of the vein graft.[85,92]

26.3 Management

There are reports of foreign bodies being lodged within the heart or vasculature remaining asymptomatic over several years.[52,93] The clinical significance of a retained foreign body is related to several factors such as nature and size of the foreign body, site of embolisation, potential to cause complications such as thrombosis or vascular occlusion, infection, perforation and arrhythmias. So, the management decision should be tailored to individual patients taking into consideration these factors as well as the relative ease of percutaneous or surgical retrieval. The relative merits and demerits of adopting a 'watchful wait' strategy should also be considered and weighed against the risks related to the additional procedure and its complications, need for anaesthesia, patient factors such as frailty and comorbidities. A heart team or multidisciplinary approach can be helpful in decision-making.

The first step towards decision making is to accurately identify the site of embolisation. For embolisations identified during the procedure in the cath lab, using fluoroscopy to locate the foreign body can be helpful. High frame rate imaging can be helpful in identifying small objects. Digital subtraction angiography technique is often helpful especially in the case of smaller and radiolucent objects.[94]

A chest radiograph may often be helpful in identifying even non-metallic foreign bodies and fragments. Echocardiography can be helpful in identifying intracardiac foreign bodies. In the case of a lost coronary stent, especially if embolism to important areas such as the cerebral circulation is suspected CT scanning can be helpful. However, routine full-body CT scanning cannot be advocated.

Magnetic resonance (MR) scans can be helpful in identifying foreign objects without the risk of ionising radiation. However, it must be borne in mind that interaction can occur between a metal foreign body and the MR environment causing other complications. Burns may result from MR-related heating. When the implant is made of a weakly magnetic material, it may be necessary to wait for 4–6 weeks until the device is fixed by tissue growth[95].

When considering percutaneous retrieval, the potential for further embolisation to other areas should be considered. There are reports of objects in the vena cavae migrating to the pulmonary arteries and even being embolised paradoxically through a PFO.[96,97]

The choice of the access and device for retrieval is again dictated by the location and orientation of the foreign body and the relative merits and demerits of each device, local availability of particular device and operator experience. Percutaneous retrieval is now the preferred option in most cases due to the excellent rates of success and relatively low rate of complications.[98–100]

Large fragments that are difficult to be removed may be mobilised to the peripheral veins/arteries and removed by surgical cut down.[101] Devices such as coronary stents can occasionally be moved away from the coronary arteries to the radial artery and if retrieval is not feasible, the stent can be deployed there with excellent results (Figure 26.2).

The common causes of failure of percutaneous retrieval include large size of foreign body, foreign body without a free edge, embolisation to small peripheral vessels, firmly adherent foreign body (e.g. thrombus formation, organised thrombus, straying into surrounding tissue and vessel wall, or entrapment by another medical device) and risk of severe complication during retrieval (e.g. arrhythmias, perforation of vessel wall and ventricles, artery spasm, thromboembolism or vessel damage).[102]

Complications from retrieval procedures although rare can sometimes be worse than the consequences of the embolised foreign body itself. There are reports of injury to femoral artery causing retroperitoneal haematoma during attempts to retrieve a lost stent.[9]

Retrieval and analysis of implanted medical devices, intact or failed, by autopsy is of critical importance in identifying problems that can help prevent such complications, improve safety of medical devices and improve care of patients.

26.4 Conclusion

The morbidity and mortality associated with retained intravascular foreign bodies are varied and difficult to assess. The management of patients with intravascular foreign bodies should be individualised. Percutaneous retrieval is often the preferred strategy and where it can be executed successfully; it should substantially diminish the clinical risk. To achieve this, operators should have a selection of retrieval devices and equipment available, and be familiar with their use.

References

1. Turner DD and Sommers SC. Accidental passage of a polyethylene catheter from cubital vein to right atrium; report of a fatal case. *N Engl J Med* 1954; 251(18): 744–745.
2. Thomas J et al. Non-surgical retrieval of a broken segment of steel spring guide from the right atrium and inferior vena cava. *Circulation* 1964; 30: 106–108.
3. Meyers JE et al. Carotid cutdown for surgical retrieval of a guidewire introducer: An unusual complication after mitral valve repair. *J Neurosurg* 2014; 121(4): 999–1003.
4. Thomas BK et al. Endovascular retrieval of an irrigation cannula from the thoracic aorta following cardiac surgery: A case report. *Int J Surg Case Rep* 2015; 16: 195–197.
5. Kammler J et al. Long-term follow-up in patients with lost coronary stents during interventional procedures. *Am J Cardiol* 2006; 98(3): 367–369.
6. Lohavanichbutr K et al. Mechanisms, management, and outcome of failure of delivery of coronary stents. *Am J Cardiol* 1999; 83(5): 779–781.
7. Bolte J et al. Incidence, management, and outcome of stent loss during intracoronary stenting. *Am J Cardiol* 2001; 88(5): 565–567.
8. Waggoner T et al. A unique complication of the GuideZilla guide extension support catheter and the risk of stent stripping in interventional & endovascular interventions. *Indian Heart J* 2015; 67(4): 381–384.
9. Brilakis ES et al. Incidence, retrieval methods, and outcomes of stent loss during percutaneous coronary intervention: A large single-center experience. *Catheter Cardiovasc Interv* 2005; 66(3): 333–340.
10. Chu CS et al. Successful retrieval of dislodged paclitaxel-eluting stent with a nitinol loop snare: A case report. *Kaohsiung J Med Sci* 2005; 21(12): 566–570.
11. Saleh L and Movahed MR. Successful conservative treatment of an undeployed embolized intracoronary stent with dual antiplatelet and warfarin therapy. *Exp Clin Cardiol* 2010; 15(3): e70–e72.
12. Colkesen AY et al. Coronary and systemic stent embolization during percutaneous coronary interventions: A single center experience. *Int Heart J* 2007; 48(2): 129–136.
13. Dunning DW et al. The long-term consequences of lost intracoronary stents. *J Interv Cardiol* 2002; 15(5): 345–348.
14. Oh Y et al. Foreign body removal by snare loop: During intracranial stent procedure. *Neurointervention* 2012; 7(1): 50–53.
15. Hartzler GO et al. Retained percutaneous transluminal coronary angioplasty equipment components and their management. *Am J Cardiol* 1987; 60(16): 1260–1264.
16. Hekmat M et al. Loss of guide wire: A rare complication of intra-aortic balloon pump insertion. *J Tehran Heart Cent* 2015; 10(1): 68.
17. Pokharel K et al. Missed central venous guide wires: A systematic analysis of published case reports. *Crit Care Med* 2015; 43(8): 1745–1756.
18. Abuhasna S et al. The forgotten guide wire: A rare complication of hemodialysis catheter insertion. *J Clin Imaging Sci* 2011; 1(40): 2156–7514.
19. Hong YM and Lee SR. A case of guide wire fracture with remnant filaments in the left anterior descending coronary artery and aorta. *Korean Circ J* 2010; 40(9): 475–477.
20. Woodfield SL et al. Fracture of coronary guidewire during rotational atherectomy with coronary perforation and tamponade. *Cathet Cardiovasc Diagn* 1998; 44(2): 220–223.
21. Foster-Smith K et al. Guidewire transection during rotational coronary atherectomy due to guide catheter dislodgement and wire kinking. *Cathet Cardiovasc Diagn* 1995; 35(3): 224–227.
22. van Gaal WJ et al. Guide wire fracture with retained filament in the LAD and aorta. *Int J Cardiol* 2006; 112(2): E9–E11.
23. Alomari I et al. Entrapped devices after PCI. *Cardiovasc Revasc Med* 2014; 15(3): 182–185.
24. Modi A et al. Delayed surgical retrieval of retained guidewire following percutaneous coronary intervention. *J Card Surg* 2011; 26(1): 46–48.
25. Kim TJ et al. Fatal subacute stent thrombosis induced by guidewire fracture with retained filaments in the coronary artery. *Korean Circ J* 2013; 43(11): 761–765.
26. Goyal V et al. Successful transradial retrieval of an embolized guidewire during transradial vascular access. *Catheter Cardiovasc Interv* 2014; 83(7): 1089–1092.
27. Alexiou K et al. Entrapped coronary catheter remnants and stents: Must they be surgically removed? *Tex Heart Inst J* 2006; 33(2): 139–142.
28. Pass RH et al. Multicenter USA Amplatzer patent ductus arteriosus occlusion device trial: Initial and one-year results. *J Am Coll Cardiol* 2004; 44(3): 513–519.
29. Chessa M et al. Early and late complications associated with transcatheter occlusion of secundum atrial septal defect. *J Am Coll Cardiol* 2002; 39(6): 1061–1065.
30. Abaci A et al. Short and long term complications of device closure of atrial septal defect and patent foramen ovale: Meta-analysis of 28,142 patients from 203 studies. *Catheter Cardiovasc Interv* 2013; 82(7): 1123–1138.
31. Levi DS and Moore JW. Embolization and retrieval of the Amplatzer septal occluder. *Catheter Cardiovasc Interv* 2004; 61(4): 543–547.
32. Peuster M et al. Transcatheter retrieval and repositioning of an Amplatzer device embolized into the left atrium. *Catheter Cardiovasc Interv* 2000; 51(3): 297–300.
33. Kim YS, and Lee SR. Percutaneous forceps retrieval of an embolized Amplatzer duct occluder. *Chonnam Med J* 2015; 51(2): 106–108.
34. Goel PK et al. Transcatheter retrieval of embolized AMPLATZER Septal Occluder. *Tex Heart Inst J* 2012; 39(5): 653–656.

35. Urena M et al. Percutaneous left atrial appendage closure with the AMPLATZER cardiac plug device in patients with nonvalvular atrial fibrillation and contraindications to anticoagulation therapy. *J Am Coll Cardiol* 2013; 62(2): 96–102.

36. Bayard YL et al. PLAATO (Percutaneous Left Atrial Appendage Transcatheter Occlusion) for prevention of cardioembolic stroke in non-anticoagulation eligible atrial fibrillation patients: Results from the European PLAATO study. *EuroIntervention*. 2010; 6(2): 220–226.

37. Obeid S et al. Percutaneous retrieval of an endothelialized AMPLATZER cardiac plug from the abdominal aorta 6 months after embolization. *Eur Heart J* 2014; 35(47): 19.

38. Schroeter MR et al. Uncommon delayed and late complications after percutaneous left atrial appendage closure with Amplatzer((R)) Cardiac Plug. *Clin Res Cardiol* 2014; 103(4): 285–290.

39. Ussia GP et al. Transcatheter aortic bioprosthesis dislocation: Technical aspects and midterm follow-up. *EuroIntervention* 2012; 7(11): 1285–1292.

40. Neragi-Miandoab S, and Michler RE. A review of most relevant complications of transcatheter aortic valve implantation. *ISRN Cardiol* 2013; 12(956252).

41. Tay EL et al. Outcome of patients after transcatheter aortic valve embolization. *JACC Cardiovasc Interv* 2011; 4(2): 228–234.

42. Ibebuogu UN et al. Review of reported causes of device embolization following trans-catheter aortic valve implantation. *Am J Cardiol* 2015; 115(12): 1767–1772.

43. Tokuda M et al. Percutaneous retrieval of a radiolucent anchoring sleeve embolized in pulmonary artery during pacemaker implantation. *Heart Vessels* 2015; 21: 21.

44. Calvagna GM et al. Transvenous retrieval of foreign objects lost during cardiac device implantation or revision: A 10-year experience. *Pacing Clin Electrophysiol* 2013; 36(7): 892–897.

45. Rijal S et al. Extracting versus abandoning sterile pacemaker and defibrillator leads. *Am J Cardiol* 2015; 115(8): 1107–1110.

46. Buiten MS et al. How adequate are the current methods of lead extraction? A review of the efficiency and safety of transvenous lead extraction methods. *Europace* 2015; 17(5): 689–700.

47. de Bie MK et al. Trans-venous lead removal without the use of extraction sheaths, results of > 250 removal procedures. *Europace* 2012; 14(1): 112–116.

48. Bordachar P et al. Extraction of old pacemaker or cardioverter-defibrillator leads by laser sheath versus femoral approach. *Circ Arrhythm Electrophysiol* 2010; 3(4): 319–323.

49. Oto A et al. Percutaneous extraction of cardiac pacemaker and implantable cardioverter defibrillator leads with evolution mechanical dilator sheath: A single-centre experience. *Europace* 2011; 13(4): 543–547.

50. Calvagna GM and Patanè S. Intravascular recovery of electrode fragments as a possible complication of transvenous removal intervention. *Int J Cardiol* 2014; 177(2): 560–563.

51. Ji SY et al. Use of an endoscopic bioptome for extraction of a retained pacemaker lead tip. *Arch Med Sci* 2014; 10(4): 853–854.

52. Holley CT et al. Retained catheter dilator in right ventricular outflow tract for 22 years. *J Card Surg* 2013; 28(6): 679–681.

53. Surov A et al. Intravascular embolization of venous catheter – causes, clinical signs, and management: A systematic review. *JPEN J Parenter Enteral Nutr* 2009; 33(6): 677–685.

54. Harrison E, and Lal S. Central venous catheter embolisation. *BMJ Case Rep* 2012; 21(10): 2012–007249.

55. Nakamura H et al. Percutaneous removal of inferior vena cava filter after migration to pulmonary artery using an 8-Fr multipurpose catheter. *Heart, Lung Circ* 2015; 24(8): e127–e129.

56. Bengali R and Vazquez R. Inferior vena cava filter embolus to the right ventricle: Anesthesia and high-risk percutaneous procedures. *J Cardiothorac Vasc Anesth* 2015; 29(5): 1322–1327.

57. Hannawa KK et al. Percutaneous extraction of embolized intracardiac inferior vena cava filter struts using fused intracardiac ultrasound and electroanatomic mapping. *J Vasc Interv Radiol* 2015; 26(9): 1368–1374.

58. Ferris EJ et al. Percutaneous inferior vena caval filters: Follow-up of seven designs in 320 patients. *Radiology* 1993; 188(3): 851–856.

59. Saeed I et al. Right ventricular migration of a recovery IVC filter's fractured wire with subsequent pericardial tamponade. *Cardiovasc Intervent Radiol* 2006; 29(4): 685–686.

60. Kumar SP et al. Fractured inferior vena cava filter strut presenting as a penetrating foreign body in the right ventricle: Report of a case. *J Card Surg* 2008; 23(4): 378–381.

61. Nicholson W et al. Prevalence of fracture and fragment embolization of Bard retrievable vena cava filters and clinical implications including cardiac perforation and tamponade. *Arch Intern Med* 2010; 170(20): 1827–1831.

62. Rossi P et al. Fatal outcome in atrial migration of the Tempofilter. *Cardiovasc Intervent Radiol* 1999; 22(3): 227–231.

63. Desjardins B et al. Fragmentation, embolization, and left ventricular perforation of a recovery filter. *J Vasc Interv Radiol* 2010; 21(8): 1293–1296.

64. Miyashita Y et al. Novel microsnare successfully used to remove small debris from the right coronary artery. *J Invasive Cardiol* 2011; 23(7): E161–E163.

65. Funatsu A et al. Successful retrieval of a broken intravascular ultrasound catheter tip in the coronary artery. *J Invasive Cardiol* 2010; 22(10): E197–E200.

66. Endo GJ et al. Emergent coronary artery bypass grafting after a broken Rotablator drive-shaft. *Interact Cardiovasc Thorac Surg* 2010; 11(5): 614–616.

67. Sultan A et al. The first reported case of a retained epicardial pacing wire causing coronary artery compression and out-of-hospital cardiac arrest. *Eur Heart J* 2014; 35(47): 3386.

68. Ngaage DL and Cowen ME. Right ventricular needle embolus in an injecting drug user: The need for early removal. *Emerg Med J* 2001; 18(6): 500–501.

69. LeMaire SA et al. Needle embolus causing cardiac puncture and chronic constrictive pericarditis. *Ann Thorac Surg* 1998; 65(6): 1786–1787.

70. Blot WJ et al. Twenty-five–year experience with the Björk-Shiley convexoconcave heart valve: A continuing clinical concern. *Circulation* 2005; 111(21): 2850–2857.

71. Vedelago J et al. Look away: Arterial and venous intravascular embolisation following shotgun injury. *J Trauma Manag Outcomes* 2014; 8(19): 1752–2897.

72. Huebner S, and Ali S. Bilateral shotgun pellet pulmonary emboli. *J Radiol Case Rep* 2012; 6(4): 1–10.

73. Hopkins HR, and Pecirep DP. Bullet embolization to a coronary artery. *Ann Thorac Surg* 1993; 56(2): 370–372.

74. Lundy JB et al. Conservative management of retained cardiac missiles: Case report and literature review. *J Surg Educ* 2009; 66(4): 228–235.

75. Golzio PG et al. Retrieval of pacemaker lead tip embolized into the distal pulmonary arterial bed during extraction procedure. *Pacing Clin Electrophysiol* 2007; 30(12): 1558–1561.

76. Rafie IM et al. Transfemoral contralateral technique to retrieve knotted coronary artery catheter using Amplatz Goose Neck snare catheter. *BMJ Case Rep* 2010.

77. Cahill AM et al. Percutaneous retrieval of intravascular venous foreign bodies in children. *Pediatr Radiol* 2012; 42(1): 24–31.

78. Woodhouse JB and Uberoi R. Techniques for intravascular foreign body retrieval. *Cardiovasc Intervent Radiol* 2013; 36(4): 888–897.

79. Mallmann CV et al. Retrieval of vascular foreign bodies using a self-made wire snare. *Acta Radiol* 2008; 49(10): 1124–1128.

80. Lee CY. Use of wire as a snare for endovascular retrieval of displaced or stretched coils: Rescue from a technical complication. *Neuroradiology* 2011; 53(1): 31–35.

81. Deftereos S et al. Successful retrieval of a coronary stent dislodged in the brachial artery by means of improvised snare and guiding catheter. *Int J Angiol* 2011; 20(1): 55–58.

82. Bellamy CM and Ramsdale DR. Removal of a knotted Swan-Ganz balloon catheter using a Dotter basket. *Postgrad Med J* 1988; 64(752): 475–476.

83. Sheth R et al. Percutaneous retrieval of misplaced intravascular foreign objects with the Dormia basket: An effective solution. *Cardiovasc Intervent Radiol* 2007; 30(1): 48–53.

84. Paulus BM and Fischell TA. Retrieval devices and techniques for the extraction of intravascular foreign bodies in the coronary arteries. *J Interv Cardiol* 2010; 23(3): 271–276. doi:10.1111/j.1540-8183.2010.00560.x.

85. Eggebrecht H et al. Nonsurgical retrieval of embolized coronary stents. *Catheter Cardiovasc Interv* 2000; 51(4): 432–440.

86. Nemcek AA, and Vogelzang RL. Modified use of the tip-deflecting wire in manipulation of foreign bodies. *Am J Roentgenol* 1987; 149(4): 777–779.

87. Brilakis ES et al. Hairpin-trap: A novel stent retrieval technique. *Catheter Cardiovasc Interv* 2011; 77(2): 213–216.

88. Gurley JC et al. Removal of retained intracoronary percutaneous transluminal coronary angioplasty equipment by a percutaneous twin guidewire method. *Cathet Cardiovasc Diagn* 1990; 19(4): 251–6.

89. Veldhuijzen FL et al. Retrieval of undeployed stents from the right coronary artery: Report of two cases. *Cathet Cardiovasc Diagn* 1993; 30(3): 245–248.

90. Auge JM et al. The use of pigtail catheters for retrieval of foreign bodies from the cardiovascular system. *Cathet Cardiovasc Diagn* 1984; 10(6): 625–628.

91. Krone RJ. Successful percutaneous removal of retained broken coronary angioplasty guidewire. *Cathet Cardiovasc Diagn* 1986; 12(6): 409–410.

92. Guigauri P, and Dauerman HL. A novel use for a distal embolic protection device: Stent retrieval. *J Invasive Cardiol* 2005; 17(3): 183–184.

93. Cimen T et al. Catheter inside the right heart for 22 years: To intervene or not to intervene? *Postepy Kardiol Interwencyjnej* 2015; 11(1): 62–63.

94. Barbiero G et al. Percutaneous retrieval of a radiolucent foreign body from an EVAR device by combining different image modalities. *Cardiovasc Intervent Radiol* 2009; 32(4): 785–788.

95. Shellock FG, and Crues JV. MR procedures: Biologic effects, safety, and patient care. *Radiology* 2004; 232(3): 635–652.

96. Casserly IP et al. Paradoxical embolization of a fractured guidewire: Successful retrieval from left atrium using a snare device. *Catheter Cardiovasc Interv* 2002; 57(1): 34–38.

97. Massin M et al. Percutaneous retrieval of broken silastic catheter from the left atrium in a critically Ill premature infant. *Cathet Cardiovasc Diagn* 1997; 42(4): 409–411.

98. Wolf F et al. Endovascular management of lost or misplaced intravascular objects: Experiences of 12 years. *Cardiovasc Intervent Radiol* 2008; 31(3): 563–568.

99. Liu JC et al. Percutaneous retrieval of intravascular foreign bodies: Experience with 19 cases. *Kaohsiung J Med Sci* 2002; 18(10): 492–499.

100. Gabelmann A et al. Percutaneous retrieval of lost or misplaced intravascular objects. *AJR Am J Roentgenol* 2001; 176(6): 1509–1513.

101. Egglin TK et al. Retrieval of intravascular foreign bodies: Experience in 32 cases. *AJR Am J Roentgenol* 1995; 164(5): 1259–1264.

102. Tateishi M and Tomizawa Y. Intravascular foreign bodies: Danger of unretrieved fragmented medical devices. *J Artif Organs* 2009; 12(2): 80–89.

PCI and the cardiac surgeon: A hybrid approach

MICHAEL W CAMMARATA, DAVID X M ZHAO

27.1 Introduction to hybrid revascularisation

The term 'hybrid coronary procedures' refers to a combination of procedures which brings together treatments traditionally available only in the operating room with those offered in the cardiac catheterisation laboratory to offer patients the benefits of all available technology. Hybrid procedures have been performed since the mid-1990s[1,2] and initially referred to the use of small thoracotomy to perform off-pump left internal mammary artery (LIMA) to left anterior descending (LAD) bypass in patients for whom the risk of being placed in circulatory arrest for traditional multi-vessel coronary artery bypass grafting (CABG) was too high and then performing multi-vessel percutaneous coronary intervention (PCI) in a staged fashion either immediately or up to a few days later to achieve complete revascularisation.[3]

As the tools that an interventional cardiologist has at his or her disposal improve (e.g. drug-eluting stents [DESs] vs. bare metal stents), the promise of a minimally invasive hybrid approach leading to improved short- and long-term outcomes may become reality. As the patient population referred to both the cardiac catheterisation laboratory and to surgery become more complex, a team approach combining the knowledge and expertise of multi-disciplines is appealing to minimise the procedural risk and improve the outcomes of patients. In the realm of interventional cardiology today, there are two major areas of hybrid procedures involving coronary revascularisation: combined CABG and PCI and valve replacement combined with PCI.

27.2 Hybrid PCI/CABG

Hybrid coronary revascularisation (HCR) is a treatment-strategy for coronary artery disease (CAD), which offers an alternative to either traditional CABG or PCI alone, with the goal being to completely re-vascularise the patient although reducing risk and maximising the benefits of the procedure. Since its inception in 1996,[1] advances in both surgical- and catheter-based techniques have made hybrid therapy a more attractive option for the treatment of multi-vessel CAD. The indications for such a procedure range from PCI of a culprit vessel during a stent thrombosis (ST)-elevation myocardial infarction with subsequent CABG of non-culprit lesions to planned interventions through a minimally invasive, off-pump technique to minimise surgical complications during CABG operation in a more stable patient.

27.2.1 DESs versus coronary artery bypass grafting

The traditional options for coronary reperfusion mainly centred around standard CABG with a median sternotomy and use of a variety of different vessel conduits to bypass multiple coronary arteries at once or the use over PCI and implantation of either a bare metal or DES. The use of PCI was typically reserved for single- or double-vessel disease in patients with low-to-intermediate risk. In a 2007 review of CAGB versus PCI, Bravata et al. demonstrated similar survival between PCI and CABG at 10 years. There was no difference between groups even when stratified by the presence of diabetes. There was a higher rate of revascularisation and a lower rate of relief of angina with PCI than with CABG. This study was quite limited in the modern day, however, due to the lack of studies using DESs that were not introduced to the market until 2003.[4] Initial enthusiasm over the use of DESs was very positive due to their decreased rates of in-stent restenosis when compared with bare-metal stent (BMS) at 1 year (5% vs. 30%).[5,6]

The synergy between percutaneous coronary intervention with Taxus and cardiac surgery (SYNTAX) trial has been the largest comparison trial of PCI versus CABG and has shown a net improvement in major adverse cardiac and cerebrovascular events (MACCEs) in patients with SYNTAX scores greater than or equal to 33, or with intermediate scores (23–33) when there is three-vessel CAD. For lower scores or patients with isolated left main CAD and intermediate scores, there was no statistically significant difference in the groups. This trial, however, is also somewhat limited in its findings in that the patients were randomised to first generation DESs (paclitaxel).[7] Recent data suggest improved outcomes with newer generation DESs. The newer everolimus-eluting stent has been shown in the SPIRIT IV trial to have a significant reduction in target lesion failure when compared with prior first generation DESs (relative risk 0.62) except in diabetic patients.[8]

In 2015, however, there was further evidence to suggest that CABG was superior in reducing MACCE events when the BEST trial was published and showed an overall reduction in MACCE when compared with everolimus-eluting stents at 5 years (15.3% vs. 10.6%).[9]

27.2.2 Patency of reperfusion therapy

The long-term patency rates of coronary bypass grafts are quite variable depending on the vessel used in the graft. Internal mammary arteries (IMAs) tend to have the highest patency rates of all graft types and have reported 5-year patency rate between 92% and 99%[10–12] and 10-year rates between 95% and 98%.[13,14] This correlates with increased event-free survival. Saphenous vein grafts (SVGs) have a poorer patency rate with the majority of grafts having lost patency at the 10-year mark.[4,15] For these reasons, it has become common practice to use the LIMA graft to bypass the LAD and use other grafts for smaller or less critical coronary arteries.

The second conduit used after the LIMA and used to bypass non-LAD vessels is the SVG. The radial artery and right IMA can also be used as alternative conduits in selected patients when the vasculature of the lower extremity is unsuitable for use in grafting. Failure rates for SVGs have been reported between 1.6% and 30%, with an average

of 20% at 1 year[10,16] and 40%–50% at 10 years.[14] The patency rate of free radial grafts tends to be closer to that of free IMA grafts with 4-year patency rates around 89%. In addition, the patency rates of all grafts are dependent on the anatomy of the grafted coronary artery with higher degrees of stenosis having higher rates of graft patency regardless of the type of graft used.[14]

Head-to-head comparison of SVGs to stents has not been performed; however, the patency rates of vein grafts can be compared with the rate of target lesion revascularisation (TLR) in non-LAD vessels for stents. In the era of BMS, the TLR for proximal right/circumflex coronary artery stents has been reported to be 13.8% at 1 year.[17] The sirolimus-eluting stent implantation (SIRIUS) trial has reported a TLR rate at 2-year follow-up of 5.8%, compared with 21.3% in the control group (BMS).[18] Newer generation DES has been found to be more efficacious in reducing ischaemia-driven target-lesion revascularisation;[19] however, the data have been mixed with TLR rates of between 2.0% and 9.2% at 1 year.[19–21] Therefore, it is believed that that PCI with DES is a better treatment for non-LAD CAD than an SVG.

Indications for hybrid CABG/PCI (minimally invasive direct CABG [MIDCAB] and totally endoscopic coronary artery bypass [TECAB]) include patients with multi-vessel disease who have high-grade proximal disease of the LAD along with favourable lesions for PCI in the left circumflex and right coronary artery territories. Other areas where PCI may represent a superior alternative to SVG conduit include the lack of or a poor quality of the conduit, a non-graftable but stentable vessel (e.g. left circumflex lesions in the atrioventricular groove with small, diffuse, obtuse margin), repeat operations in which PCI is preferable to avoid full cardiac dissection or in patients with concomitant pre-existing organ dysfunction, recent myocardial infarction or severe atherosclerotic aortic disease.

27.2.3 Hybrid procedures

Hybrid CABG/PCI is the combination of traditional surgical methods with PCIs. Examples include everything from the common scenario PCI of a culprit coronary lesion during a ST segment elevation myocardial infarction (STEMI) followed by conventional CABG during the same hospitalisation, to elective minimally invasive LIMA to the LAD with PCI to non-LAD lesions. The latter strategy attempts to combine the best aspects of CABG (the LIMA–LAD graft) with the best aspects of PCI (better patency rate than SVG). Several different methods exist to accomplish this goal; however, only the surgical arm of the treatment differs although the PCI part of the procedure remains constant.

In MIDCAB, the LIMA is harvested through a small left anterior thoracotomy incision or lower hemisternotomy. The LIMA–LAD bypass is then grafted to the beating heart (off-pump). The first published series of the MIDCAB patient was in 1996. Angelini et al.[1] reported on six patients who underwent MIDCAB LIMA–LAD combined with percutaneous trans-luminal coronary angioplasty/ stent to non-LAD vessels. Another method of harvesting and grafting the LIMA–LAD is closed-chest CABG surgery in which robotic systems allow for the manipulation of the graft vessel and target vessel within thoracic ports using fine instrument. In this case, however, there is the peripheral institution of cardiopulmonary bypass (CPB). At a separate operating console, the surgeon controls the instruments although the operation is viewed stereoscopically (three-dimensional view). This is also sometimes referred to as TECAB. In 1999, Loulmet et al.[22] introduced this technique. Later in 2000, Farhat et al.[15] performed the first TECAB with LIMA–LAD and PCI to the left circumflex system.

27.2.4 Hybrid PCI/CABG compared with conventional CABG

Large trials comparing the efficacy and graft patency of hybrid procedure versus traditional CABG procedures have not been performed; however, many series have been and continue to be published comparing the two approaches. In 2015, Phan et al. published a review of the majority of these retrospective studies. They were able to show no difference in all cause 30-day mortality or peri-procedural strokes. They did, however, show a significant reduction in myocardial infarctions (repeat revascularisation [rr] 0.67), blood transfusions (rr 0.54), length of stay in the intensive care unit (ICU) (–0.64 days) and length of hospital stay (–1.4 days) in the hybrid PCI/CABG group. These benefits were seen in the setting of an increased risk for rr 3.58.[23] Halkos et al. published the first prospective multicentre observational study comparing hybrid PCI with off-pump CABG. They found no difference in the survival of patients undergoing these procedures (Figure 27.1) and concluded that, although there was an increased rate of revascularisation in the hybrid procedure group, hybrid revascularisation is a reasonable minimally invasive alternative with comparable mid-term and long-term outcomes to off-pump CABG.[24] Using risk

stratification scores such as SYNTAX and European System for Cardiac Operative Risk Evaluation (euroSCORE), Leacche et al. reported that HCR is a safe alternative to CAGB in many patients with multi-vessel CAD. However, in high-risk patients with complex CAD (≥33 SYNTAX/>5 euroSCORE), CABG is superior to HCR (Figure 27.2).[25]

An additional recent systematic review performed by Gosain et al.[26] in 2015 combined 20 studies of at least 10 hybrid revascularisation procedures comparing traditional CABG results. They concluded that hybrid revascularisation may be beneficial in patients with multi-vessel CAD with LAD, which is amenable to bypass grafting and other (non-LAD) vessels which are amenable to PCI. They were unable to find any differences in mortality or MACCE in the cohort as a whole.

In addition to the multiple observational studies listed, there has been one randomised clinical trial comparing hybrid revascularisation (MIDCAB) with traditional CABG procedure – the POL-MIDES (HYBRID) trial.[27] The study team randomised 200 patients with multi-vessel CAD and at least one critical (>70%) lesion in the LAD to either MIDCAB hybrid revascularisation or conventional CABG. In an intent-to-treat analysis, they concluded that there was no difference in MACCE at 12 months. There were similar rates of blood transfusion, perioperative myocardial infarction and death. This study, however, was a pilot study designed to test feasibility and was not powered to detect mortality benefit.

27.2.5 One-stop or staged approach

Hybrid revascularisation by definition is a staged procedure with the period between LIMA–LAD bypass and coronary artery stenting being the main difference. In a one-stop approach to hybrid CABG/PCI, the procedure is completed on the same date in the same hybrid operating room with the surgical team completing the LIMA–LAD bypass first,

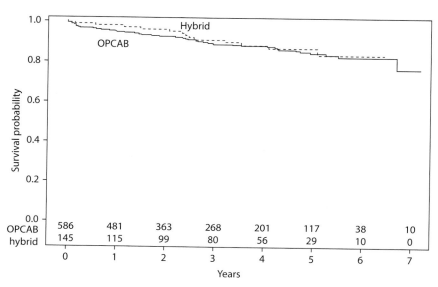

Figure 27.1 Kaplan–Meier 5-year survival estimates according to hybrid coronary revascularisation (HCR) or off-pump coronary artery bypass grafting (OPCAB) (*p* = .61). (From Halkos ME et al., *Ann Thorac Surg*, 92, 1695–1701, 2011.)

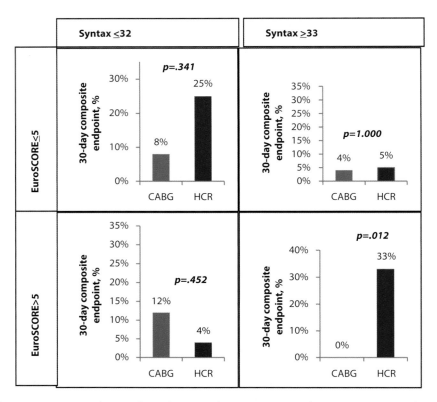

Figure 27.2 The 30-day composite cardiac and cerebrovascular outcomes in the coronary artery bypass grafting (CABG) group and HCR stratified by the synergy between percutaneous coronary intervention with Taxus and cardiac surgery (SYNTAX) and European system for cardiac operative risk evaluation (euroSCORE). (From Leacche M et al., *J Thorac Cardiovasc Surg*, 145, 1004–1112, 2013.)

then the interventional cardiology team performing PCI on the non-LAD vessels immediately thereafter. In a staged approach, the procedures are performed in different rooms separated in time by hours to weeks. In general, the one-step technique has been the goal given improved efficiency, patient satisfaction and cost.

Several concerns have arisen when planning a hybrid revascularisation procedure. First, when to perform PCI (before or after the bypass portion of the procedure)? On the one hand, if performed prior to the bypass procedure, more aggressive revascularisation can occur due to the ability to perform bypass on vessels, which cannot adequately be re-vascularised or if there is a complication of the stenting procedure. Unfortunately, however, this does mean performing unprotected PCI and performing the bypass operation under the influence of anti-platelet agents, increasing the risk for major bleeding. Also, when performing PCI prior to the surgical portion of the procedure, the surgical team is unable to perform immediate diagnostic angiography of the LIMA graft to confirm patency. Completion angiography may help to ensure graft patency, particularly in various minimally invasive and off-pump CABG.[28] Another concern is that of performing bypass surgery on patients taking anti-platelet agents. The risk of bleeding increases dramatically when patients are on these medications (even within 5 days). There is also a known increase in chest tube outputs, surgical intensive care length of stays and secular operation

for bleeding.[29] In addition, questions remain as to the effect of heparin reversal on stent patency, and this may lead to a higher rate of stent thrombosis, though no investigative trials or large observational studies have been performed.[30]

If PCI is performed after the surgical portion, the interventional cardiologist operator has the advantage of a protected environment with a LIMA–LAD bypass having been already performed and the ability to confirm LIMA patency immediately post-operatively, and potentially has a reduced risk of intraoperative bleeding. However, if unable to stent non-LAD vessels, a second higher risk operation may be required, though this is quite rare (<1%).[3] For all of these reasons, operators who perform two-step hybrid procedures generally use the CABG first approach. The American College of Cardiology Foundation/American Heart Association (ACCF/AHA) favour performing the CABG component initially as they view the ability to angio-graphically visualise the LIMA–LAD graft, the ability to use full anti-platelet therapy and having a protected anterior wall to be of the utmost benefit to patients undergoing hybrid revascularisation.[31]

In a one-step procedure, one can avoid the limitations of two-step hybrid procedures (potential risks of surgical/interventional procedures and the need for sedation/anaesthesia, inconvenient and generally less favourable for patients than the one-step procedure, logistic challenges and cost), but picks up a whole new set of issues. All one-step procedures would involve the use of an anti-platelet agent prior to completing the bypass portion of surgery and thus could significantly increase the risk for bleeding associated with this procedure. The true effect of anti-platelet agents on bleeding in hybrid cases is unknown and, to date, the data are mixed with some series showing an increase in bleeding risk and some showing no difference between the two. More observational studies are needed to make any definitive conclusions on the matter.

No head-to-head trials have been performed comparing the efficacy and safety of one-step and two-step hybrid revascularisation procedures. However, due to the current data, a one-step approach would be preferred for stable patients due to improved logistics, cost and preference. A staged approach may be more conducive to the situation for patients with STEMI having to undergo culprit vessel revascularisation with subsequent LIMA–LAD bypass.

27.2.6 Current standard of practice

In 1995, the MIDCAB procedure was introduced into the literature. It was usually performed through anterolateral thoracotomies and could be performed without CPB (off-pump coronary artery bypass [OPCAB]).[32] Although the benefits of OPCAB remain controversial and the outcomes of such procedures are more dependent on factors such as experience of the surgeon performing the procedure and[33] when performed by an experienced surgeon, the outcomes can be excellent. It is the current recommendation of the ACCF/AHA that hybrid revascularisation is reasonable in patients with limitations to traditional CABG (i.e. heavily calcified aorta or poor CABG targets), lack of suitable graft conduits or an unfavourable LAD for PCI due to excessive tortuosity or chronic total occlusion. Furthermore, they state that a hybrid approach may be reasonable as an alternative to multi-vessel PCI or CABG in an attempt to improve the overall risk–benefit ratio of the procedures.[31]

27.3 Hybrid valve/PCI

The other of the two main hybrid procedures is the hybrid valve plus PCI. This has been proposed to reduce operative morbidity and mortality, improve recovery time and improve cosmetic results of surgery when compared with surgery utilizing the conventional sternotomy approach. Minimally invasive valve procedures have been described using either a partial sternotomy[34] or a mini-thoracotomy.[35] Minimally invasive valve procedures had previously been contraindicated in patients with CAD, as revascularisation would require a different approach and a larger procedure that can be performed through the conventional mini thoracotomy or hemi-sternotomy.

27.3.1 Minimally invasive valve replacement

Minimally invasive valve surgery refers to techniques in which several alternative approaches to conventional

sternotomy can be used. Depending on the valve being replaced, the approach varies. In aortic valve surgeries, an upper hemi-sternotomy would be utilised, whereas, for mitral replacements, a right mini-thoracotomy or lower hemi-sternotomy could be utilised.[34,35] The rationale behind the smaller incision is improvement in patient healing and reduction in complications typically associated with a large sternotomy.[36]

Due to the intra-cardiac location of valves, CPB must be implemented for all valve replacement surgeries. Due to the limited approach in minimally invasive procedures, this can present some challenges to the cardiac surgeon. Specialised arterial, venous and endovascular cannulas and aortic occlusion devices are needed to institute cardioplegia, aortic cross clamping and implement external CPB.[37]

Several large series have compared the efficacy of minimally invasive valve replacement.[34,35,38–40] These series have shown reduced post-operative pain, faster recovery and fewer blood transfusions. Despite these results, the minimally invasive valve replacement was approached with trepidation due to high complexity of the operation and potential for prolonged operative time and patient safety. In addition, there was a much higher learning curve for performing the minimally invasive surgeries, and there were many limitations including certain comorbidities such as obesity, previous cardiac surgeries or pulmonary disease that precluded the use of this technique broadly. The ability to perform these operations had been relegated to large academic institutions with surgeons specialised in these procedures.[36] In addition, there was a significant selection bias in the study selection of relatively healthier patients and, despite statistical correction, it was felt that the selection bias could not be completely overcome.[41] These concerns, however, have been relatively tempered and minimally invasive valve surgery is felt to be a viable option for valve replacement with the possibility for lower complication rates and higher patient satisfaction.[42] Due to the benefits of minimally invasive surgery, it has been felt that combination with PCI may be a viable approach for the much broader population of patients with CAD and concomitant valve disease.

27.3.2 The hybrid valve/PCI procedure

Hybrid valve/PCI procedures are intended to minimise the operative and on-pump time of a surgical valve replacement surgery and to minimise the risk associated with a large sternotomy procedure by replacing access with a minimally invasive approach. This technique could be potentially helpful in patients with a poor conduit for bypass surgery in order to convert a high-risk valve/CABG into a lower risk isolated surgical valve replacement, or to convert a re-operative valve/CABG into a re-operative isolated valve surgery.

As has already been discussed, SVG patency rates at 1 year are likely lower than stent patency at 1 year. In addition, CABG/valve surgery carries a much higher risk than isolated valve surgery.[43] It would be reasonable to approach these procedures with a lower risk strategy when an IMA graft is not available or suitable for bypass surgery. In these cases, use of DES likely portends at least as good a prognosis as concomitant SVG grafting with reduced intra-operative mortality risk.

Given the increased overall mortality with combination CABG and valve surgery, it would be reasonable to warrant additional modalities of performing revascularisation and valve surgery without the increased operative and on-pump time that occurs during combination procedure (9.9% perioperative mortality).[43] Combining low-risk procedures, including single- or multi-vessel PCI, with a peri-procedural mortality rate of 1.27%[44] and lower risk, minimally invasive valve replacement (mortality rate 1%–2%) is a very appealing option in comparison with open procedure. In fact, in a review of 65 hybrid valve cases compared with 52 conventional cases, there was a statistically significant improvement in the perioperative morbidity, without showing a significant decrease in overall mortality, with low numbers and a trend towards significance for mortality.[45] Further review of the literature shows that the few studies which compare hybrid valve versus open procedure show at least comparable outcomes, if not superiority, at 30 days and 6 months. Part of the risk involved in these procedures is the performance of valve replacement in patients taking dual anti-platelet agents and the need for DAPT for some time after the procedure. There has been an increase in blood transfusions associated with the hybrid approach.[46] Additionally, when patients with known severe valvular disease present as an acute coronary syndrome, it can also be reasonable to perform PCI on culprit lesion and then perform minimally invasive valve surgery during the same hospitalisation or shortly thereafter. Byrne et al. published a series in 2005, including the patient with acute coronary syndromes. When they compared their outcomes with those predicted by the Society of Thoracic Surgeons mortality, they showed a significant reduction in mortality (3.8% vs. 22%).[47] No randomised clinical trials have yet been performed to evaluate the utility of hybrid approach in these situations. There continues to be (although decreasing) logistical barriers to routine use of this procedure broadly, and difficult surgical techniques demand a surgeon who specialises in a minimally invasive approach.

The use of hybrid revascularisation has also been reported in patients undergoing re-do sternotomy for combined valve diseases and CAD. Hybrid approach transforms a high-risk complex re-do valve surgery and CABG to an isolated valve surgery with concomitant stenting using a minimally invasive approach. The recent advent of trans-catheter valve replacement (TAVR) has made the use of this approach much less appealing given the broad data on the use of trans-catheter valves and the ability to perform valve-in-valve procedures[48] to reduce operative risk of re-do sternotomy. Reported mortality at 30 days with these procedures does remains high (17%), probably because of a combination of

multiple co-morbidities and advanced age leading to a very high surgical risk and selection bias in the outcome.

27.3.3 Limitations in hybrid valve approach

Valve/PCI hybrid procedures are somewhat limited. The impact that dual anti-platelet therapy has on the surgical bleeding risk during these procedures has yet to be determined. Although it would theoretically be possible to perform the valve replacement portion of this procedure prior to the PCI, it makes sense to correct haemodynamically significant CAD prior to higher risk valve replacement surgery; however, there are no published clinical trials determining which approach is better. Conflicting evidence in retrospective analyses leaves significant clinical equipoise.[46,47,49] In addition, the learning curve is quite steep for minimally invasive procedures and during this learning curve, reduced graft patency, increased operative times and possibly increased neurological events could significantly impair the utility of this procedure.[50] With the advent of TAVR, we could begin to see a dramatic decline in the already limited use of hybrid valve revascularisation; however, limited data exist on whether coronary artery revascularisation preceding TAVR has any proven benefit.

27.3.4 TAVR and the 'Heart Team'

TAVR is a novel and evolving cardiac intervention initially approved by the Food and Drug Administration (FDA) in 2011. The current standard of care and the most recent multi-disciplinary recommendations[51] require that a team approach to TAVR be employed. In addition, CMS NCD dictates that there be surgical and interventional cardiology co-operators making this a hybrid procedure. Surgeons play an integral role in the evaluation and management of patients with valvular heart disease, and their contribution in TAVR procedures is invaluable.

A large proportion of the adverse events associated with a TAVR involve the access site and haemostasis.[52,53] In addition, the current target population has a high prevalence of peripheral arterial disease making percutaneous access via a femoral arterial approach possible in only a certain sub-segment of the population. The direct aortic, trans-apical and subclavian approaches all require skilled surgical technique to facilitate valve placement. Although surgical involvement for percutaneous approaches is quite limited, the heart team is critical in case selection, procedural planning and complication management.

27.4 Conclusions

Hybrid valve/PCI and CABG/PCI procedures have been performed for over 20 years with origins in the 1990s. Despite evidence suggesting an overall benefit in terms of mortality, length of hospital stay and peri-procedural complications, these procedures are still only performed in a few centres where the surgical volume is high enough to support a specialised minimally invasive surgeon. Because of the great difficulty associated with these procedures and learning curve complications, there is likely to be limited utility in the near future. With the advent of percutaneous aortic valve implantation, the use of hybrid valve/PCI procedures will likely drop as the indications for percutaneous procedures become more inclusive of lower risk populations.

The use of CABG/PCI procedures remains promising, again with several setbacks to be expected in the use of minimally invasive cardiac surgical procedures. To date, the primary benefit of CABG over PCI is the use of an IMA graft to the LAD artery and this being performed in a less invasive setting without extracorporeal bypass has much promise. Further studies and training of cardiothoracic surgeons would be necessary to make this a more widely utilised technique.

References

1. Angelini GD et al. Integrated left small thoracotomy and angioplasty for multivessel coronary artery revascularisation. *Lancet* 1996; 347(9003): 757–758.

2. Lloyd CT et al. Integrated left anterior small thoracotomy and angioplasty for coronary artery revascularization. *Ann Thorac Surg* 1999; 68(3): 908–911; discussion 11–12.

3. Byrne JG et al. Hybrid cardiovascular procedures. *JACC Cardiovasc Interv* 2008; 1(5): 459–468.

4. Bravata DM et al. Systematic review: The comparative effectiveness of percutaneous coronary interventions and coronary artery bypass graft surgery. *Ann Intern Med* 2007; 147(10): 703–716.

5. Holmes DR, Jr et al. Analysis of 1-year clinical outcomes in the SIRIUS trial: A randomized trial of a sirolimus-eluting stent versus a standard stent in patients at high risk for coronary restenosis. *Circulation* 2004; 109(5): 634–640.

6. Stone GW et al. One-year clinical results with the slow-release, polymer-based, paclitaxel-eluting TAXUS stent: The TAXUS-IV trial. *Circulation* 2004; 109(16): 1942–1947.

7. Mohr FW et al. Coronary artery bypass graft surgery versus percutaneous coronary intervention in patients with three-vessel disease and left main coronary disease: 5-year follow-up of the randomised, clinical SYNTAX trial. *Lancet* 2013; 381(9867): 629–638.

8. Stone GW et al. Everolimus-eluting versus paclitaxel-eluting stents in coronary artery disease. *N Engl J Med* 2010; 362(18): 1663–1674.

9. Park SJ et al. Trial of everolimus-eluting stents or bypass surgery for coronary disease. *N Engl J Med* 2015; 372(13): 1204–1212.

10. Alexander JH et al. Efficacy and safety of edifoligide, an E2F transcription factor decoy, for prevention of vein graft failure following coronary artery bypass graft surgery: PREVENT IV: A randomized controlled trial. *JAMA* 2005; 294(19): 2446–2454.

11. Investigators B. The final 10-year follow-up results from the BARI randomized trial. *J Am Coll Cardiol* 2007; 49(15): 1600–1666.

12. Kim KB et al. Midterm angiographic follow-up after off-pump coronary artery bypass: Serial comparison using early, 1-year, and 5-year postoperative angiograms. *J Thorac Cardiovasc Surg* 2008; 135(2): 300–307.

13. Hayward PA, and Buxton BF. Contemporary coronary graft patency: 5-year observational data from a randomized trial of conduits. *Ann Thorac Surg* 2007; 84(3): 795–799.

14. Tatoulis J et al. Patencies of 2127 arterial to coronary conduits over 15 years. *Ann Thorac Surg* 2004; 77(1): 93–101.

15. Farhat F et al. Hybrid cardiac revascularization using a totally closed-chest robotic technology and a percutaneous transluminal coronary dilatation. *Heart Surg Forum* 2000; 3(2): 119–120; discussion 20–2.

16. Puskas JD et al. Off-pump vs conventional coronary artery bypass grafting: Early and 1-year graft patency, cost, and quality-of-life outcomes: A randomized trial. *JAMA* 2004; 291(15): 1841–1849.

17. Ashby DT et al. Comparison of clinical outcomes using stents versus no stents after percutaneous coronary intervention for proximal left anterior descending versus proximal right and left circumflex coronary arteries. *Am J Cardiol* 2002; 89(10): 1162–1166.

18. Weisz G et al. Two-year outcomes after sirolimus-eluting stent implantation: Results from the Sirolimus-Eluting Stent in de Novo Native Coronary Lesions (SIRIUS) trial. *J Am Coll Cardiol* 2006; 47(7): 1350–1355.

19. Kereiakes DJ et al. Comparison of everolimus-eluting and paclitaxel-eluting coronary stents in patients undergoing multilesion and multivessel intervention: The SPIRIT III (A Clinical Evaluation of the Investigational Device XIENCE V Everolimus Eluting Coronary Stent System [EECSS] in the Treatment of Subjects with De Novo Native Coronary Artery Lesions) and SPIRIT IV (Clinical Evaluation of the XIENCE V Everolimus Eluting Coronary Stent System in the Treatment of Subjects with De Novo Native Coronary Artery Lesions) randomized trials. *JACC Cardiovasc Interv* 2010; 3(12): 1229–1239.

20. Kedhi E et al. Second-generation everolimus-eluting and paclitaxel-eluting stents in real-life practice (COMPARE): A randomised trial. *Lancet* 2010; 375(9710): 201–209.

21. Brener SJ et al. Everolimus-eluting stents in patients undergoing percutaneous coronary intervention: Final 3-year results of the Clinical Evaluation of the XIENCE V Everolimus Eluting Coronary Stent System in the Treatment of Subjects with de Novo Native Coronary Artery Lesions trial. *Am Heart J* 2013; 166(6): 1035–1042.

22. Loulmet D et al. Endoscopic coronary artery bypass grafting with the aid of robotic assisted instruments. *J Thorac Cardiovasc Surg* 1999; 118(1): 4–10.

23. Phan K et al. Hybrid coronary revascularization versus coronary artery bypass surgery: Systematic review and meta-analysis. *Int J Cardiol* 2015; 179: 484–488.

24. Halkos ME et al. Hybrid coronary revascularization versus off-pump coronary artery bypass grafting for the treatment of multivessel coronary artery disease. *Ann Thorac Surg* 2011; 92(5): 1695–1701; discussion 701–702.

25. Leacche M et al. Comparison of 30-day outcomes of coronary artery bypass grafting surgery versus hybrid coronary revascularization stratified by SYNTAX and euroSCORE. *J Thorac Cardiovasc Surg* 2013; 145(4): 1004–1112.

26. Gosain P et al. Hybrid coronary revascularization: A systematic review. *Cardiol Rev* 2015; 23(2): 87–93.

27. Gasior M et al. Hybrid revascularization for multivessel coronary artery disease. *JACC Cardiovasc Interv* 2014; 7(11): 1277–1283.

28. Zhao DX et al. Routine intraoperative completion angiography after coronary artery bypass grafting and 1-stop hybrid revascularization results from a fully integrated hybrid catheterization laboratory/operating room. *J Am Coll Cardiol* 2009; 53(3): 232–241.

29. Cruden NL et al. Clopidogrel loading dose and bleeding outcomes in patients undergoing urgent coronary artery bypass grafting. *Am Heart J* 2011; 161(2): 404–410.

30. Cosgrave J et al. Protamine usage following implantation of drug-eluting stents: A word of caution. *Catheter Cardiovasc Interv* 2008; 71(7): 913–914.

31. Hillis LD et al. 2011 ACCF/AHA Guideline for Coronary Artery Bypass Graft Surgery. A report of the American College of Cardiology Foundation/American Heart Association Task Force on Practice Guidelines. Developed in collaboration with the American Association for Thoracic Surgery, Society of Cardiovascular Anesthesiologists, and Society of Thoracic Surgeons. *J Am Coll Cardiol* 2011; 58(24): e123–e210.

32. Atluri P et al. Off-pump, minimally invasive and robotic coronary revascularization yield improved outcomes over traditional on-pump CABG. *Int J Med Robot* 2009; 5(1): 1–12.

33. Sellke FW et al. Comparing on-pump and off-pump coronary artery bypass grafting: Numerous studies but few conclusions: A scientific statement from the American Heart Association council on cardiovascular surgery and anesthesia in collaboration with the interdisciplinary working group on quality of care and outcomes research. *Circulation* 2005; 111(21): 2858–2864.

34. Soltesz EG, and Cohn LH. Minimally invasive valve surgery. *Cardiol Rev* 2007; 15(3): 109–115.

35. Grossi EA et al. Minimally invasive mitral valve surgery: A 6-year experience with 714 patients. *Ann Thorac Surg* 2002; 74(3): 660–663; discussion 3–4.

36. Iribarne A et al. The golden age of minimally invasive cardiothoracic surgery: Current and future perspectives. *Future Cardiol* 2011; 7(3): 333–346.

37. Stevens JH et al. Port-access coronary artery bypass grafting: A proposed surgical method. *J Thorac Cardiovasc Surg* 1996; 111(3): 567–573.

38. Dogan S et al. Minimally invasive versus conventional aortic valve replacement: A prospective randomized trial. *J Heart Valve Dis* 2003; 12(1): 76–80.

39. Tabata M et al. Early and late outcomes of 1000 minimally invasive aortic valve operations. *Eur J Cardio-Thorac Surg* 2008; 33(4): 537–541.

40. Umakanthan R et al. Safety of minimally invasive mitral valve surgery without aortic cross-clamp. *Ann Thorac Surg* 2008; 85(5): 1544–1549; discussion 9–50.

41. Blackstone EH. Comparing apples and oranges. *J Thorac Cardiovasc Surg* 2002; 123(1): 8–15.

42. Wong MC et al. Advances in percutaneous treatment for adult valvular heart disease. *Intern Med J* 2009; 39(7): 465–474.

43. Hannan EL et al. Risk index for predicting in-hospital mortality for cardiac valve surgery. *Ann Thorac Surg* 2007; 83(3): 921–929.

44. Peterson ED et al. Contemporary mortality risk prediction for percutaneous coronary intervention: Results from 588,398 procedures in the National Cardiovascular Data Registry. *J Am Coll Cardiol* 2010; 55(18): 1923–1932.

45. Santana O et al. Staged percutaneous coronary intervention and minimally invasive valve surgery: Results of a hybrid approach to concomitant coronary and valvular disease. *J Thorac Cardiovasc Surg* 2012; 144(3): 634–639.

46. Shannon J et al. Do hybrid procedures have proven clinical utility and are they the wave of the future?: Hybrid procedures have proven clinical utility and are the wave of the future. *Circulation* 2012; 125(20): 2492–2503; discussion 503.

47. Byrne JG et al. Staged initial percutaneous coronary intervention followed by valve surgery ("hybrid approach") for patients with complex coronary and valve disease. *J Am Coll Cardiol* 2005; 45(1): 14–18.

48. Eggebrecht H et al. Valve-in-valve transcatheter aortic valve implantation for degenerated bioprosthetic heart valves. *JACC Cardiovasc Interv* 2011; 4(11): 1218–1227.

49. Brinster DR et al. Effectiveness of same day percutaneous coronary intervention followed by minimally invasive aortic valve replacement for aortic stenosis and moderate coronary disease ("hybrid approach"). *Am J Cardiol* 2006; 98(11): 1501–1503.

50. Svensson LG et al. Does right thoracotomy increase the risk of mitral valve reoperation? *J Thorac Cardiovasc Surg* 2007; 134(3): 677–682.

51. Holmes DR, Jr. et al. 2012 ACCF/AATS/SCAI/STS expert consensus document on transcatheter aortic valve replacement. *J Am Coll Cardiol* 2012; 59(13): 1200–1254.

52. Leon MB et al. Transcatheter aortic-valve implantation for aortic stenosis in patients who cannot undergo surgery. *N Engl J Med* 2010; 363(17): 1597–1607.

53. Popma JJ et al. Transcatheter aortic valve replacement using a self-expanding bioprosthesis in patients with severe aortic stenosis at extreme risk for surgery. *J Am Coll Cardiol* 2014; 63(19): 1972–1981.

28

PCI in centres without on-site cardiac surgery

KRISTEL LONGMAN, JEHANGIR DIN, SUNEEL TALWAR, PETER O'KANE

28.1 Introduction

The evolution of percutaneous coronary intervention (PCI) has resulted from many significant advances in operator technical skill, available equipment and increasing clinical applicability. The first human PCI was performed as a balloon only procedure (plain old balloon angioplasty [POBA]) to dilate a single coronary artery stenosis in 1977. The remarkable story of the first POBA by Andreas Gruentzig resulted in at least 23 years of vessel patency when followed up in 2001 and forms the basis of contemporary coronary interventional practice.[1] The early problems with access-site complications and high rates of restenosis which were such important limiting factors in the early years have been overcome in the last four decades to enable PCI to become a safe and durable therapy and additionally become the predominant strategy for coronary re-vascularisation.

The evolution of PCI equipment has been dramatic. In 1982, over-the-wire coaxial balloon systems were introduced, followed by the development of brachial guiding catheters and steerable guide wires. By 1986, Jacques Puel and Ulrich Sigwart implanted the first coronary Wallstents in Toulouse, France.[2] These reduced the need for repeated balloon angioplasty and from 1984, stents become commonplace. However, in the 1980s, abrupt and sub-acute closure of a coronary artery at the angioplasty site due to dissection and associated thrombus, were not uncommon and 5%–10% of patients required immediate emergency coronary artery bypass graft surgery (CABG) within 24 hours.

At this time, it seemed inconceivable that PCI could ever be performed without a waiting cardiothoracic theatre.[3] Indeed, the suggestion that PCI would one day be performed safely in a non-surgical centre would have been ridiculed. However, the continued evolutionary improvements in bare metal stent design resulted in increased deliverability to improve PCI safety by permitting bailout coronary stenting, (for which stents are used to treat a dissection or abrupt closure after balloon angioplasty), lower the occurrence of peri-procedural myocardial infarction (MI) and reduce the need for emergency CABG surgery. Subsequent randomised trials showed that primary stenting (stenting as a primary strategy) offered greater procedural success and lower rates of restenosis than balloon angioplasty with bailout stenting, but in-stent restenosis rates unfortunately remained high at around 30%, precluding the effective treatment of multivessel coronary artery disease.[4,5] Moreover, in some studies, peripheral vascular complications necessitating surgery, blood transfusion or both were more frequent after stenting than after balloon angioplasty and the mean hospital stay was long at just over 8 days on average.[5] Despite the advances in the technical and safety aspects of PCI, this remained a therapy largely only delivered in cardiothoracic surgical centres up until the end of the twenty-first century.

In a United Kingdom Government White Paper, from 2000, the National Health Service (NHS) was set a specific target to reduce mortality from coronary heart disease (CHD) and there was a corresponding expansion in re-vascularisation by both elective PCI for angina and emergency PCI for MI – primary PCI (PPCI). This national strategy led to an increase in detection of CHD by diagnostic angiography and an increased need for re-vascularisation by both PCI and CABG.

Shortly after this, in 2003 the first drug-eluting stent (DES), the Cypher, manufactured by Johnson & Johnson/Cordis, was approved by the U.S. Food and Drug Administration (FDA). This device had a durable polymer adherent to the metallic stent eluting sirolimus (rapamycin), which inhibited the proliferation of lymphocytes and smooth-muscle cells to restrict neointimal hyperplasia and reduce the restenosis phenomena. This major advance in metallic stent technology provided the concept that target lesion failure (TLF) would be confined to history opening up opportunity to treat more patients with PCI. Indeed, loud applause from the audience greeted the first public presentation of the RAVEL study where half of the 238 patients who had been randomised to the Cypher DES arm showed a complete absence of restenosis at 6 months.[6] The improved efficacy, procedural safety and durability of PCI with DES as expected led to an expansion in the indication and uptake PCI across the globe and for the first time selected patients with multi-vessel disease could be offered complete re-vascularisation without the need for general anaesthesia or extracorporeal circulation. With competitor DES development and innovation, PCI for multi-vessel CHD was born.

Although there was a growing demand and enthusiasm for PCI therapy, delivering the service in a timely and efficient manner was proving more challenging. In the United Kingdom, the typical network model was 'hub and spoke' where the large tertiary cardiac centre with on-site cardiothoracic surgery would perform all of the PCI procedures on patients referred in from district hospitals which were often many hours away by road. The advantage of this model was a centralisation of expertise for future PCI innovation amongst operators within the centre. But many cardiologists who worked in the district hospital had variable access to the tertiary unit and less opportunity for involvement in the PCI itself. Patients would of course receive excellent quality care once they arrived in the surgical centre but capacity was woefully inadequate and it was not uncommon for patients to wait 3 weeks for transfer after they had presented to the district hospital with an acute coronary syndrome (ACS).

Patients needed more local services and momentum was now gathering amongst cardiology departments within district hospitals without on-site cardiac surgery to develop a PCI service. Such ambitions met with mixed response amongst regional networks and naturally, many surgical

centres were resistant to the concept because of lost activity and subsequent financial downturn. The NHS central commissioning tariff structure of 'payment by results' meant that the revenue streams for PCI were high, particularly for non-emergent work, which encouraged many district hospitals further to develop a program for financial benefits. So began the rapid development of non-surgical PCI centres with the ethos of offering a local service to patients at the heart of the discussions.

Data continued to support the adoption of PCI for the majority of patients with CHD. In 2007, a meta-analysis of 23 randomised trials comparing PCI with CABG showed that after 10 years of follow-up, mortality was no different between the groups.[7] CABG was actually found to cause more procedure-related strokes (1.2% vs. 0.6%) but did still offer greater freedom from angina at 5 years. Notably, within this meta-analysis, nine of these trials were made up of PCI cohorts in which only POBA was performed and yet despite this, the results for a percutaneous approach were already seen to be non-inferior to bypass grafting.[7]

A subsequent analysis of individual patient data from 10 randomised trials showed that in non-diabetic patients, there was no difference in mortality whether treated by CABG or PCI. However, CABG offered a mortality advantage in diabetic and older patient subgroups.[8] This distinction between diabetic and non-diabetic patients has been replicated subsequently and has become a major decision-making variable when selecting the re-vascularisation technique.

Deciding on the most optimal re-vascularisation technique became the focus of several large randomised trials with the landmark SYNTAX trial the most cited.[9] This study compared re-vascularisation with TAXUS DES versus CABG for multi-vessel disease and is notable as the largest randomised study of PCI versus CABG with 1800 patients from 85 centres in Europe and the United States. It included all multi-vessel disease with the only exclusions being prior re-vascularisation, acute MI and need for concomitant cardiac surgery. The composite of all-cause death, MI and stroke was no different between the groups at 12 months (7.6% with PCI and 7.7% with CABG). When separated, the individual components of death and MI were also no different between the groups. Perhaps, the most important finding was the statistically significant excess of strokes after CABG compared with PCI (2.2% vs. 0.6%). This reproducible higher risk of stroke with cardiac surgery has since become one of the most important considerations for both clinicians and patients when evaluating the balance of risk and benefits of PCI versus CABG in multi-vessel disease.[9]

The notable variation in outcomes seen in diabetics and the increased risk of stroke evident with CABG surgery led to the concept of an individualised risk assessment and forms the basis of the multidisciplinary 'heart team' which has become integral to decision-making as part of the wider governance processes for CHD re-vascularisation options. The requirement for involvement of cardiac surgeons in these multidisciplinary meetings to determine the best therapy for CHD has represented a challenge for non-surgical

PCI centres. This has been overcome in many cases by close networking arrangements with the local cardiothoracic centre. The use of newer technologies such as telecardiology links with 'real-time' imaging transfer has made this feasible, practical and sustainable in non-surgical centres.

Non-surgical PCI centre development was further driven by the need to provide emergency PPCI for ST-elevation myocardial infarction (STEMI) since early opening of the infarct-related artery was highlighted by the original PPCI studies demonstrating a benefit over thrombolysis and later supported by larger meta-analysis of PPCI versus thrombolytic therapy studies.[10] Further research demonstrated clearly that 'time is myocardium' and there is now an established and clear association of interaction amongst risk-time and benefits of PPCI.[11] This is obviously a key factor in determining where interventional cardiac centres should be located and meant that non-surgical cardiac interventional centres have become integral to providing the time dependent PPCI component of coronary interventional services. This has been shown to be safe and effective with almost no requirement for emergency surgery in the setting.[12] In the United Kingdom, there has been a resultant increase in the number of PCI operators and centres (the majority without cardiac surgery on-site) to meet the demands of PPCI within strategic networks. The debate on whether centres should provide either a full 24/7 PPCI service or none at all in preference to offering simply a 9–5 PM PPCI service has not been resolved. There is also the general concept that all PCI consultant operators provide a share of 24/7 PPCI even if this is not in their own centre.

This expansion in interventional cardiology procedures and units has allowed the role of both the individual coronary interventionist and the wider multidisciplinary catheter lab team to develop to accommodate the needs of increasing patient and procedural complexity. Throughout Europe, United States and United Kingdom, increasing numbers of both emergency and elective percutaneous interventions are now being performed in non-surgical centres in a safe and effective way and with increasing published data to validate this approach.[13]

This chapter outlines the current position of non-surgical cardiac intervention centres, examines the available data pertaining to this practice and looks at the current recommendations for the systems, people and processes for the provision of a safe and effective percutaneous interventional service without on-site cardiac surgery.

28.2 Non-surgical PCI centres – data to support their existence

In the United Kingdom, the number and proportion of centres performing PCI without on-site surgery has increased year-on-year. Indeed, it is now the case that non-surgical PCI centres represent the majority with 69 non-surgical PCI centres and 48 surgical centres. From the 2013 UK national data, there were 37,008 PCI procedures undertaken in units without on-site cardiac surgery, representing 40% of the activity in the whole of United Kingdom. This continues to rise slightly year–on-year with 43% of angioplasty procedures in the United Kingdom being performed in a centre without on-site cardiac surgery in 2014.[14] As expected, the mean PCI volume is lower in non-surgical PCI centres compared to the surgical counterpart.

When analysing the guidance from a worldwide perspective, it is apparent that provision of PCI services should focus more on validated quality and safety outcomes than the type of the centre performing them. There are, however, some important considerations within this statement. For example, centre volume remains an important surrogate marker for these standards, although an exact cut off at which the volume effect is significant on quality remains unclear.[15]

Despite the high rate of development of non-surgical PCI centres in the last decade, there has been less support within the guidelines. For instance, current AHA/American College of Cardiology PCI guidelines, published in 2011, state that there is a Class IIa recommendation for PPCI in hospitals without on-site surgery, whereas the guidelines give only Class IIb support for non-PPCI. The authors state 'Elective PCI might be considered in hospitals without on-site cardiac surgery, provided that appropriate planning for programme development has been accomplished and rigorous clinical and angiographic criteria are used for proper patient selection'.[16]

This guidance may be explained by carefully reviewing the evidence base from which it was produced. When examining the practice of PCI in centres without on-site cardiac surgery, a distinction has previously been made between emergency (primary) angioplasty and elective interventions. There are separate datasets with specific considerations for each, which explains the difference in level of recommendation within the guidelines. The time-dependent nature of providing PPCI for an occluded artery shifts the balance of risks and benefits towards a more localised service provided that it is of adequate quality and has good outcomes monitored by a rigorous audit and outcome reporting system. This concept challenges the guidelines, but proponents consider that a higher volume and level of expertise improves outcome in STEMI patients who are at high risk of major adverse events. The provision of elective services has, in the past, been more debatable and is perhaps open to a more in-depth critical analysis pertaining to individual lesion, patient and centre details. There is also more of an opportunity for the patient to be worked up in the centre that provides the optimal therapy even if this is not the local service. Overall, the infrastructure and skill set required for both urgent and elective percutaneous interventions are, however, common to both and thus it is intuitive that increasing volume and safety of both types of procedure coexist.

Interestingly, since the most recent guidelines were written there has been two major multicentre randomised controlled trials comparing non-PPCI performed in surgical and non-surgical centres. In the CPORT-E trial, 18,867 patients were randomised 3:1 to undergo PCI in centres with off-site surgery versus on-site surgery.[17] There was no difference in the primary safety end point of 6-week mortality

(0.9% vs. 1.0%), nor in the incidence of emergency CABG (0.1% vs. 0.2%). Mortality in those patients who underwent emergency surgery was also no different between the non-surgical (2/13, 15.4%) and surgical (2/10, 20%) centres, implying that existent surgical transfer systems worked effectively. However, procedural success was lower in non-surgical centres (90.7% vs. 91.4%, p = .007) and target lesion re-vascularisation (TLR) was higher after 12 months (6.5% vs. 5.4%, p = .01). This may have been due to a more subtle difference in technical expertise or perhaps a lower threshold for an interventional cardiologist operating in a non-surgical centre to terminate a procedure before achieving success rather than persisting in a potentially more 'risky' procedural strategy, which could risk bailout CABG.

In the more recently published MASS COM trial, 3691 patients were randomised to undergo non-PPCI 3:1 to be treated in non-surgical or surgical centres.[18] Again, there was no difference in the primary safety end point of 30-day major adverse cardiac events (MACE) (9.2% vs. 9.1%), nor in the need for emergency CABG (0.3% vs. 0.1%). In contrast to the CPORT-E trial, there was also no difference in procedural success or in 12-month outcomes including target vessel re-vascularisation (TVR).

Clearly both studies support the safety of non-PPCI in hospitals without on-site cardiac surgery but it remains difficult to translate their findings directly to UK practice given the substantial differences in the organisation of services. For instance, the institutional non-surgical centre volumes are much higher in the United Kingdom (an average of just over 600 procedures/unit/year) compared with the very low-volume non-surgical centres that were studied in these trials (117/year in MASS COM, 150/year in CPORT-E). However, at least in the CPORT-E study, operators who also practiced in surgical centres staffed these very low-volume centres and so had individual PCI volumes, which were identical to those of the surgical centre interventionists. This may explain the difference in procedural success rates compared to MASS COM. Whilst the debate of minimal institutional versus individual operator volume is therefore difficult to resolve, these studies clearly support a role for non-surgical PCI centres to perform non-emergent PCI safely.

A subsequent randomised US study examined outcomes between surgical and non-surgical centres performing non-emergent PCI. There was again no difference in the co-primary end point which included the rates of major adverse cardiac events – a composite of death, MI, TLR/TVR or stroke – at 30 days (safety end point) and at 12 months (effectiveness end point).[18]

A very large meta-analysis including 914, 288 patients undergoing non-PPCI in a number of European as well as North American centres also supports the practice of PCI in non-surgical centres. This showed no difference in crude rates of in-hospital mortality or emergency CABG between patients treated in hospitals with off-site surgery and on-site surgery for both non-emergent or PPCI groups, suggesting that in real-world practice (which may include lower volume centres) there seem to be good signals of both safety and quality.[19]

The examination of the data presented from these studies collectively must also be considered within the context of there being significant safety advances in PCI technique within the study timeframes. For instance, current UK practice (along with European colleagues) has adopted radial artery access as the predominant route for PCI with penetration of over 75% of coronary intervention cases and this has led to a lower rate of bleeding complications, a reduced need for an overnight hospital stay and a coexistent upwards trend in day case PCI (with 25% of all PCI procedures performed as a day case in the United Kingdom 2014).[14]

Improved safety and feasibility of PCI through technical developments can only serve to improve the existing patient related outcome and enhance the case for performing non-urgent coronary interventions in non-surgical centres that have adopted such good practice.

28.3 Non-surgical centres – current extent and scope

In 2014, there were a total of 100 UK NHS interventional centres with a further 19 centres which performed a private commercial service. These centres provided close to a 100,000 PCI procedures annually, and the thorough, rigorously collected audit data provide a valuable insight into contemporary UK practice.[14]

These national audit data indicate that PCI in non-surgical centres can provide a high-quality and safe service to local populations avoiding the need to travel to surgical centres with comparable low emergent bypass, stroke, bleeding and access-site complications as seen between in-surgical PCI centres. The increase in PCI centres has now plateaued after a phase of rapid expansion from the early 2000s. In contrast, the number of non-interventional (angiography only) centres has been seen to decline as these have either adapted to provide intervention, closed or relocated to provide diagnostic angiography services in a neighbouring interventional centre. Only performing diagnostic coronary angiography in PCI-capable centres is intuitive and permits the option to perform essential emergent-PCI for diagnostic complications such as catheter-induced left main stem dissection. It also permits multidisciplinary discussion between PCI operators and cardiac surgeons as to the best re-vascularisation strategy and avoids direct referral of multi-vessel CHD for cardiac surgery by diagnostic operators who are less familiar with what PCI techniques can provide. Furthermore, current audit data show an approximate 1:3 ratio of interventions to diagnostic angiograms indicating that a critical review of all angiographic images by an trained interventionist is likely to be of value as a high proportion of these cases require more than just optimal medical therapy for angina.[14]

In order to provide this expertise, it is therefore essential to have interventional cardiologist placed in all centres in which significant volumes of angiography are being performed so that a local multidisciplinary review of re-vascularisation options is available. This multidisciplinary review should obviously include the input of a cardiothoracic surgeon, either by visits to the non-surgical centre or by remote telecardiology links.

Within the United Kingdom, the ratio of CABG:PCI has shifted dramatically in the last decade and the ratio now stands at nearly 1:5. A significant proportion of the growth in PCI is attributable to increasingly complex lesion therapy and multi-vessel re-vascularisations, now being performed routinely, made possible by a workforce of young enthusiastic interventional operators and technical equipment advancement making PCI safer and more durable. It is rare for multi-vessel CHD to be treated in one sitting and staging PCI is common meaning that the patient ratio of CABG:PCI is less than 1:5. However, the sheer number of PCI performed supports a practical need for the increased number of coronary interventional centres to provide for these patients, with the majority not having surgery on site (Figure 28.1).

The need for emergency surgery following PCI will always persist but is now very infrequent (Figure 28.2).[20] Situations during PCI that would have previously necessitated the need for emergent-CABG can now be safely and effectively managed in the PCI catheter lab (Table 28.1).[21] For example, the use of intra-coronary imaging to assist guide catheter dissections, covered stents for coronary vessel perforation and intra-vascular micro coils to address distal guide wire perforations (Figures 28.3 and 28.4). Indeed, the development of newer technologies to cope with unpredictable complications has meant that a modern coronary interventionist can now successfully treat all but the most catastrophic complications of PCI without the need for cardiac surgery.

This observation is supported by large datasets. In one registry of 24,188 PCI and 4768 CABG procedures over 14 years between 2000 and 2014 in the Netherlands, it was actually more common to perform bailout PCI rather than bailout CABG following PCI. Bailout PCI after unsuccessful CABG occurred in 0.77% (36/4768) versus bailout CABG after unsuccessful PCI in 0.25% (59/24,188). This is the first series to highlight this 'inverse' pattern and it demonstrates the importance of a collaborative approach between both highly skilled interventionists and highly skilled cardiac surgeons. Within this Dutch registry, coronary dissection and perforation were the main causes sited for emergent CABG but the rates of both these were actually seen to fall over the duration of the 10-year period studied. In fact, when considering data of the study from the last 3 years, the rate of CABG following PCI was only 0.15%, which is similar to current UK national data.[22]

These registry data are similar to that found previously in a US large registry which included all PCI procedures from 1992 to 2000. A total of 18,593 PCIs were performed with a need for emergency CABG in only 0.61% of cases. Again, the prevalence of emergency surgery was seen to decline from 1.5% of all PCIs in 1992 to 0.14% in 2000. It is, however, important to note that the morbidity and mortality of these patients remain high, with an in-hospital mortality rate of 15% following emergency bailout CABG after PCI.[22]

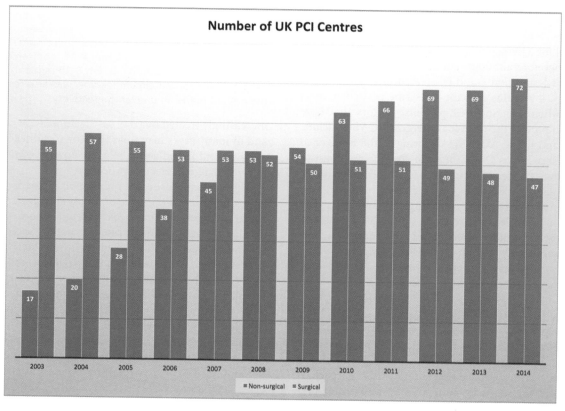

Figure 28.1 Number of surgical (red bars) and non-surgical centres (blue bars) in the United Kingdom over the last 13 years.

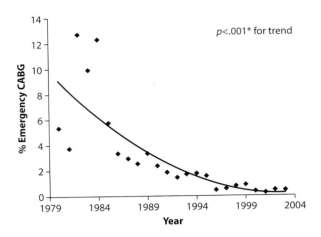

Figure 28.2 Percentage of patients requiring emergency coronary artery bypass grafting (CABG) after percutaneous coronary intervention (PCI) from 1979 to 2003 (n = 23,097) * Armitage test for trend.

Table 28.1 Indications for emergency cardiac surgery following PCI

Extensive coronary dissection	54%
Perforation/tamponade	20%
Recurrent acute vessel closure	20%
Haemodynamic instability	3%
Aortic dissection	2%
Guidewire fracture	1%

Source: Everaert B et al., Abstracts EuroPCR 2015 Euro15A-POS209.

The need for emergency surgery appears to be unpredictable, and therefore although guidance relating to the type of patient or lesion that could be treated in a non-surgical centre exists, it remains difficult to ascribe particular characteristics when selecting PCI patients. Factors that have been seen to predict the need for emergency CABG include female sex and worse ACC/AHA scoring of the intervened lesion, whilst previous CABG or prior stenting are negative and may reduce the need for emergent CABG.[21] Interestingly, although higher grade lesions – type B2 or C – may have a greater relative risk of emergency surgical bailout the data suggest that type A lesions comprise up to 15% of cases in which emergency surgery is performed.[23] Research into computational models to attempt to predict patients in whom emergency surgery may be more likely has been reported but these systems are not currently in widespread use.[24]

28.4 The impact of the radial approach

Increasingly, all cardiac units are moving towards a predominant radial approach for arterial access for PCI. High levels of patient service and satisfaction support this approach. It is a consistent finding from patient surveys that they prefer to be treated both locally and radially, provided there is sufficient expertise and safety data. In Europe, patients are

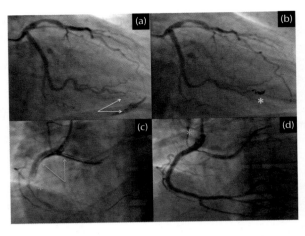

Figure 28.3 Distal guide wire perforation and guide catheter dissection during PCI. (a) and (b) A 67-year-old female patient who underwent intravascular ultrasound (IVUS)-guided PCI to the mid-LCx with lesion preparation and implantation of a single Absorb 3.0 mm × 23 mm BRS. After post-dilatation, it became clear that there was a distal guidewire perforation (a) with contrast extravasation (yellow arrows). This was treated with initial balloon tamponade and then deployment of three micro-coils (yellow *) to the distal vessel with successful resolution of the haemorrhage and avoidance of the need of a pericardial drain. (c) and (d) A 41-year-old gentleman presenting with inferior STEMI at 3 AM and treated with primary PCI (PPCI). Initial intubation of the aberrant right coronary artery (RCA) by a multi-purpose guide catheter was uneventful. However, after IVUS-guided 3.5 mm × 32 mm stent to the mid-vessel and post-dilatation with a 4.0 mm × 15 mm NC balloon, the guide was pulled inwards by balloon retraction which led to a very extensive and occlusive ostial and proximal vessel dissection (green arrows). The situation was treated with further DES back to the proximal vessel and a 5.5 mm × 18 mm Herculink BMS (green *) post-dilated with 6.0 mm × 15 mm balloon at the ostium. The aberrant circumflex flow was also restored and the patient made an uneventful recovery.

increasingly treated in a day case fashion, with radial access and in many cases may wear their own clothes leading to a more patient friendly and 'relaxed' environment for a low-/intermediate-risk elective procedure.

The increasing use of the radial approach as default has not only strengthened the safety data for all coronary interventional units but also has been seen to support non-surgical cardiac centres. Although rapid access to vascular surgical services is ideal for all PCI centres, it may be less critical to have it on-site when most PCI can be performed radially. In a recent analysis of over 46,000 patients undergoing PPCI for STEMI, transradial access was independently associated with a lower 30-day mortality (hazard ratio [HR]: 0.71, 95% confidence interval [CI]: 0.52–0.97; p < .05), in-hospital major adverse and cardiovascular events (MACCE) (HR: 0.73, 95% CI: 0.57–0.93; p < .05), major bleeding (HR: 0.37, 95% CI: 0.18–0.74; p < .01) and access-site complications (HR: 0.38, 95% CI: 0.19–0.75; p < .01).[25] Whilst this study did not explicitly examine the frequency of CABG after PCI for each route, the absolute rates of complications were seen

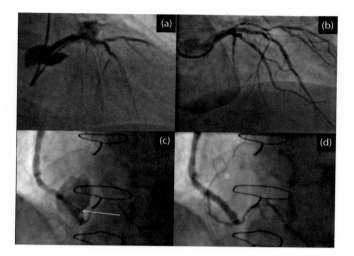

Figure 28.4 Covered stents deployed during PCI. **(a)** and **(b)** A 51-year-old female patient who underwent PCI to mid-left anterior descending artery (LAD) severe restenosis with lesion preparation. During delivery of a cutting balloon, deeper guide catheter position was undertaken which led to a proximal LAD dissection and perforation (red arrow) and subsequent no flow in the distal LAD and circumflex. This was managed with initial balloon tamponade and then deployment of a 3.5 mm × 15 mm covered stent carefully positioned between diagonal and circumflex ostia (red arrow) to avoid side branch occlusion. Further, DES was deployed further back to the left main stem and post-dilated with IVUS guidance. Despite the large contrast extravasation, there was no the need of a pericardial drain and the patient made a full recovery. **(c)** and **(d)** A 58-year-old gentleman who had previous CABG 10 years before and presenting with chest pain. An echocardiogram had shown a subcostal collection outside the pericardium and a cardiac CT showed a saccular aneurysm with apparent bleeding. He came to the catheter lab an emergency and when the right coronary artery saphenous vein graft was engaged with an AL1 guide catheter and guideliner, it was clear there was a narrowed neck aneurysm on IVUS with active contrast filling of the aneurysm (blue arrow). After on-table discussion with the local cardiac surgical centre the vein graft was treated with a 4.0 mm × 20 mm covered stent which was successful at sealing the leaking aneurysm. The native occluded RCA is now readily visible and could be a focus for future PCI (blue *).

to be low with a notably low rate of re-intervention of 0.5% in the radial group indicating that a low number of patients required a second PCI procedure (Table 28.2).[25]

28.5 The importance of physiological lesion assessment in non-surgical centres

The increasing importance of performing a comprehensive invasive physiological or imaging assessment with pressure wire assessment at the time of initial diagnostic procedure has been clearly demonstrated to improve clinical outcomes and cost-effectiveness in both the FAME and FAME II studies.[26–28] This approach has the benefit of selecting lesions for re-vascularisation based on physiology rather than anatomy alone. Studies have demonstrated that when considering re-vascularisation based on this type of physiological assessment, lesions may be down- or upgraded to be included or excluded in the SYNTAX score.[29]

Current data evaluating the impact of a physiologically driven re-vascularisation strategy can be extracted from the UK RIPCORD study which compared angiographic lesion assessment alone with pressure wire-guided re-vascularisation. This demonstrated that clinical management decisions for medical therapy, PCI or coronary artery bypass surgery were altered in a third of cases. A significant proportion of patients who had multi-vessel disease and would have been previously referred for coronary artery bypass surgery had their lesions downgraded and fell into lower SYNTAX score groups meaning the option of percutaneous intervention became appropriate.[29]

These patients could therefore not only have PCI as their re-vascularisation therapy but also increasingly could potentially have this performed in the same non-surgical centre conducting the physiological assessment in order to increase local treatment and cost-effectiveness.

Intravascular imaging with intravascular ultrasound (IVUS), optical coherence tomography (OCT) or optical frequency domain imaging (OFDI) provides insight into vulnerable plaques and assists in lesion-specific risk assessment together with the strategic planning of interventions either at the time or in future staged procedures.[30] IVUS-guided implantation of stents has been shown to be associated with a significantly reduced incidence of death, major adverse cardiac events and stent thrombosis and forms part

Table 28.2 Radial versus femoral access during STEMI – Insights from BCIS audit data

Variable	Radial (n = 18,037)	Femoral (n = 28,091)	p Value
MACCE	616 (3.4%)	2158 (7.7%)	<.001
Death at 30 days	456 (2.5%)	1875 (6.7%)	<.001
Re-infarction	60 (0.3%)	131 (0.5%)	.10
Re-intervention	87 (0.5%)	169 (0.6%)	.09
TIA/Stroke	47 (0.3%)	92 (0.3%)	.20

MACCE, major adverse and cardiovascular events; TIA, transient ischaemic attack.
Source: Mamas M et al., *J Am Coll Cardiol Intv*, 6, 7, 2013.

of contemporary PCI practice.[31] IVUS can be utilised as either a portable unit or integrated as part of catheter lab hardware, which makes this technology readily available in most non-surgical units. This permits more complex lesion subsets to undergo PCI and should allow high-quality interventions to be performed routinely.

The importance of individual lesion assessment both physiologically and anatomically is increasingly recognised as correlating to individual lesion treatment outcomes. For instance, insights from intra-coronary imaging have led to a more structured approach to lesion preparation for the implantation of contemporary devices such as bioresorbable scaffolds (BRS) and it has now become incorporated into the guidance for the implantation of these devices.[32]

Providing this type of lesion-specific assessment and therapy therefore requires a certain level of infrastructure within the catheter lab and non-surgical centres wishing to expand their therapeutic portfolio need to consider this. This work is in addition to standard diagnostic angiography and represents an increasing workload for many centres contributing to the appropriate use criteria (AUC) for performing subsequent PCI. As standards of physiological assessment are set, the larger numbers of patients who require this physiological/imaging assessment will mandate that these are performed in local non-surgical centres for practical purposes. The follow on from this is that those centres may then also provide the subsequent coronary intervention as long as the local catheter laboratory infrastructure and local expertise allow. Where specific procedural techniques are required, for example; rotational atherectomy, a subset of patients may be transferred to another centre with specific expertise and a track record of audited outcomes for the technique, although increasing data are emerging to support the safety of specific techniques such as rotablation and excimer laser coronary atherectomy (ELCA) use in non-surgical centres.[33–35]

28.6 Non-surgical PCI centre start up and quality standards

Within the United Kingdom, the British Cardiovascular Intervention Society (BCIS) mandates specific regulations for individual centre volume, operator experience, catheter lab personal training and surgical network requirements. Site accreditation is dependent on these factors and minimal requirements before new centres can commence a PCI program. There are also specific criteria regarding the responsibility to contribute to national audit datasets allowing analysis of every single procedure performed in the United Kingdom, through more than 100 data entry fields.[36]

In the United States, there exists a specific WSCC/ACC/AHA 2014 update on PCI without on-site surgical backup for Northern America.[37] This US guideline is specific not only about catheter lab facility, personnel, operator and structural standards but also provides case selection criteria including exclusion recommendations regarding specific patient and lesion characteristic, the utility of which has been discussed in Section 28.3.

Similar regulatory requirements exist in mainland Europe, under the auspices of the European Society for Cardiology/EAPCI. Mandates common to all national guidelines suggest that all centres worldwide must fulfil the requirements of the relevant professional regulatory body and participate in contemporaneous review of clinical outcomes and maintenance of standards.

The European ESC/EACTS guidelines for re-vascularisation interestingly do not discriminate between surgical and non-surgical centres but focus instead on networking between the two centre types to provide adequate surgical back up.[38] They are more specific regarding the provision of PPCI services, however, and do not advocate the use of a 'partial' PPCI programme, instead recommending that if a centre is planning to provide a PPCI service this should be a complete 24/7 operational program and not one which provides only daytime PPCI cover.[39]

Despite this, clear guidance there are a number of non-surgical centres in the United Kingdom, which only provide a 9AM–5PM service for PPCI and so have a low volume for such cases. Operator PPCI experience can be supplemented by their contribution to a larger networked service which appears to be a good compromise in that patient outcome is more liable to be dependent on operator experience of PPCI rather than the centre itself and 9AM–5PM service locally means door-to-balloon times may be much shorter for a selected group of patients who would otherwise have to travel further afield. It is unlikely to be feasible that a lower volume non-surgical PCI centre would have the infrastructure to offer a 24/7 service. Conversely, there are operators who provide a 9AM–5PM PPCI service who do not contribute to a 24/7 service within the network and this results in low-volume experience of PPCI overall and is less ideal for patient outcome. Currently, there is no legislation to prevent this.

The Australian and New Zealand guidelines are similar to the European guidance stating the importance of operator and institutional standards rather than division between non-surgical and surgical capability.

28.6.1 Surgical cover arrangements

In all of the country-specific guidance there exist detailed timeframes within which an urgent surgical transfer should occur in the event of a PCI complication. It is reassuring that emergency transfer for surgical intervention has come down significantly since the advent of intra-coronary stents but it remains necessary to maintain this link even if utilised very infrequently. In the United Kingdom, the 1991 data analysis showed that 2.6% of patients undergoing PCI required emergency CABG.[40] By 2007, this has come down to 1.1% and in the latest UK BCIS audit data presentation, emergency CABG only occurred in 0.05% of PCI cases.[14] Outcome analysis of this patient cohort demonstrates that emergency CABG in this situation does improve survival and indicates that the patients selected for surgical transfer were appropriate.

Therefore, it is essential that PCI centres without on-site surgical cover should have a viable protocol for emergency transfer to the nearest surgical centre. All stakeholders, including the relevant parties in the non-surgical centre and the surgical centre, must agree with the protocol. This protocol needs to be specific regarding training and availability of staff for emergency surgical transfers and should include an anaesthetist. Emergency transfer of patients should occur within a maximum timeframe of 1 h, with the ability to start cardiopulmonary bypass within 2 h of the call for surgical intervention.[37] The provision of specific equipment should also be considered, including a transportable intra-aortic balloon counter-pulsation pump (IABP). UK BCIS guidance makes the additional recommendation that the feasibility of ambulance transfer with the IABP be tested to confirm it can be achieved within the required 120-minute timeline.

A good working relationship with the cardiac surgical team in the surgical centre is essential for all non-surgical PCI centres. Collaborative working to derive local policies and protocols is recommended. It is also suggested that there should be at least annual reviews of the surgical transfer arrangements and that ongoing education is provided for all multidisciplinary catheter lab personnel. An auditable record of cases transferred for surgery should exist allowing contemporaneous analysis and reflection of the process.

28.6.2 Catheter lab PCI volume and operator PCI volume

In terms of catheter lab volume, this should be enough to maintain quality and safety standards, together with staff training and ongoing professional development. Non-surgical centre PCI volume should be enough to allow adequate experience for individual multidisciplinary staff hence enabling them to cope with emergencies and complications.

There has been an observation of better outcomes in higher volume centres with higher volume operators.[41] Based on these data, the existence of catheter labs performing less than 200 PCIs/year (not serving isolated populations) has be questioned, although exceptions to this may exist. For example, exclusion to this would be if the operators at that site also performed PCI at another site and had acceptable personal operator numbers and outcomes. American guidelines suggest that the minimum cases/operator should be greater than 50 PCIs (including a minimum of 11 PPCIs) annually whilst in the United Kingdom, this is set at 75 with no specific detail on case type. (The current mean number of PCIs/operator in the United Kingdom is 123/annum in 2014.) It is strongly recommended that PCI operators who offer training to fellows should complete 150 PCI cases/year as a minimum standard.[36]

Competency for individual operators in the United Kingdom is also assessed based on lifetime experience, other interventions (such as peripheral/TAVI work) and

ongoing professional development and operator outcome data. The UK revalidation process through the General Medical Council (GMC) every 5 years based on annual appraisal of the individual should serve to ensure PCI operators maintain sufficient high standards to provide optimal PCI provision.

The UK BCIS minimum centre volume standard is 400 cases/year with a minimum of three interventional cardiologists/centre. PPCI centres have been given guidance that they should perform an absolute minimum of a 100 STEMI cases/year, although there are many UK PCI centres who do not meet this standard, particularly those that provide only a 9AM–5PM service.

The mean number of PCI procedures/UK centre is 617 in non-surgical centres versus 1540 with surgery on site. From this, it can be seen that there are fewer surgical centres but generally these have both the highest number of interventional cardiologists and the highest volume of interventions. Even allowing for this, the majority of centres perform greater than 400 cases/year and therefore meet the minimum standard volume criteria. This is not necessarily the case in other countries, and there is likely to be ongoing debate as to what constitutes the specific volume of interventional practice, which supports basic safety standards.

28.7 Minimum requirements for safe PCI practice in United Kingdom

28.7.1 Catheter lab

At least one catheter lab should be available for elective and non-emergency cases but given potential faults or need for servicing then two are essential in order to guarantee an uninterrupted service. This is obviously mandatory in centres offering a comprehensive emergency PCI service. If no second cardiac catheter laboratory is available, then a second radiology (fluoroscopy enabled) laboratory is a possible alternative and depends on local arrangements.[36]

Contemporary archiving in a Digital Imaging and Communications in Medicine (DICOM) compatible format is mandatory and in the United Kingdom this should be stored and accessible for a minimum of 8 years. Non-surgical PCI centres should have facilities for real-time image transfer to facilitate discussion about individual patients' cases with either PCI colleagues or cardiac surgeons. Ideally, clinical strategic networks should exist within a given region and there should be investment in secure information technology to allow neighbouring sites to view archived patient data and facilitate optimal emergency care.

Patients undergoing coronary interventions need to have physiological monitoring of ECG, oxygen saturations and both non-invasive and invasive blood pressure monitoring. Staff should be trained in safe administration of sedatives. In the United Kingdom, they should be familiar with the guidelines from the Royal College of Anaesthetists for sedation for healthcare procedures and have a local policy and competency standard which has been achieved and signed off before administering conscious sedation.[42] Patients who have received sedation and/or analgesia should have their heart rate and oxygen saturation monitored continuously throughout the procedure. Given that carbon dioxide levels may rise under conscious sedation, capnography and/or anaesthetic support should be available, particularly when procedures are prolonged or supplementary oxygen is required.[42]

It is mandatory to have full resuscitation facilities including a defibrillator, anaesthetic ventilator, intra-aortic balloon counter pulsation equipment plus staff trained in line with current national and local guidelines available as a designated 'Resuscitation Team'. This should comprise at least one anaesthetist or intensive care doctor in addition to catheter lab personnel. The facility for urgent pericardial drainage, temporary pacing and echocardiography is also considered mandatory.

It is recommended, although not mandated, that devices to assist in chest compressions during which PCI can be performed are available, for two reasons (Figure 28.5). First, to improve the chances of procedural success in a patient who is in cardiac arrest, an automated chest compression device permits uninterrupted cardiac compression, thereby minimising catheter displacement and reducing procedural difficulty. Second, to reduce the radiation exposure to catheter laboratory personnel who would be otherwise near the ionising radiation source in the course of performing chest compressions. It is worth noting here that visualisation of coronary anatomy during PCI when these devices are in use is more limited and familiarisation with these limitations is very important within a training environment.

The need to continue performing PCI procedures in the face of ongoing cardiopulmonary resuscitation is enhanced in non-surgical centres as the traditional indications for a 'surgical bail out' procedure (perforation, dissection) are exactly those which will need to be dealt with by the coronary interventionist in these centres. Attendance at educational meetings that include discussion of complications in using newer techniques and technology (e.g. covered stents/coils) is encouraged so if and when these complications arise they can be dealt with expediently.

Monitoring of anticoagulation with activated clotting time (ACT) monitoring is paramount to procedure safety and should be available in the catheter lab. This is particularly important during longer PCI cases, such as chronic total occlusion (CTO) PCI where drops in ACT to subtherapeutic levels can be catastrophic.

28.7.2 Staff standards

The number of non-medical trained staff involved in a PCI procedure will depend on skill mix, complexity of the procedure and the number of medical staff involved and will vary worldwide amongst catheter labs, whether surgical or non-surgical. It is considered that good medical practice and optimising outcome for patients undergoing PCI is dependent on effective teamwork and multidisciplinary approach from non-medical staff.

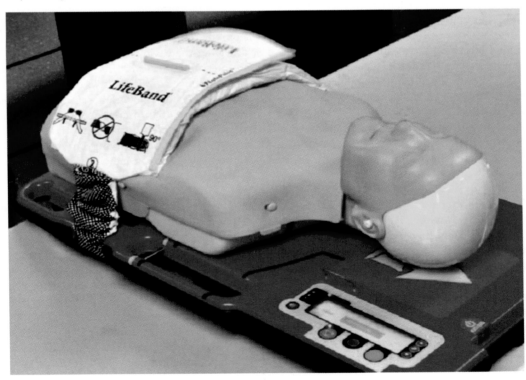

Figure 28.5 Automated chest compression device can be helpful in cardiac arrest situation, particularly out of hours when less staff are available to support the patient. Superior cardiac output can be delivered compared to manual chest compressions and PCI can continue whilst this is delivering therapy.

In the United Kingdom, it is recommended that there is a minimum of two nurses/catheter lab and one 'runner' nurse (one nurse at least band 5 and above)/shift for PCI procedures. In addition, one radiographer and one physiologist/catheter lab (usually band 6 and above) would be considered normal practice. Although multi-skilled practitioners or generic workers who may have a more complete set of skills may substitute team members, the absolute number should remain the same. For units with more than one catheter lab, a separate additional coordinator should be considered (band 6 and above). Outside the United Kingdom, the number of catheter lab staff can vary and may only consist of one nurse, physiologist and physician.

All staff should have a period of supervision and fulfil a competency-based training scheme within their hospital. Within the United Kingdom, there are currently no national competency guidelines for PCI specifically but documentation of completion of specified local training should be accessible. All senior members of the catheter lab team should hold an advanced life support certificate. All other members of the team should hold a minimum of an intermediate life support (ILS) certificate and be versed in emergencies within the catheter lab environment. The various roles of catheter lab staff working are summarised in Table 28.3.[36]

28.7.3 Radiation protection

Radiation protection in a non-surgical centre should be in line with that of a surgical centre. The same stringent standards to reduce the dose to both the patient and catheter lab personnel apply to all centres. Individual dose monitoring is mandatory.

All catheter lab staff should be aware of the latest guidelines on radiation protection. A representative of the radiation protection officer, who is usually a radiographer should ensure that all staff comply with appropriate monitoring and that lead screens, aprons, glasses and other methods of radiation shielding are available and used appropriately. Monitoring of individual dose exposure is mandatory all along. Cumulative dose measurement should be undertaken and appropriate steps taken to share this information with the individual staff member together with providing regular training updates to reduce individual exposure to a minimum.

Radiation risks from cardiac procedures should be discussed with the patient as part of the pre-procedure consent process. It is good practice to include the hazards associated with radiation exposure on the consent form for PCIs. Almost all the current catheter lab radiography sources are equipped with methods to calculate and record peak skin dose and dose area product. Recording of the patient's dose exposure is mandatory. There should also be systems in place to measure and recognise those patients requiring multiple high-dose exposures (e.g. computed tomography pulmonary angiogram [CTPA] followed by PCI). In the United Kingdom, it is the radiographer's responsibility to notify the operator where radiation exposure is above the notification threshold (2000 mGy for first notification and subsequent notifications at every 500 mGy increments).[43]

The patient should be informed if the peak skin dose exceeds 3000 mGy in order to highlight awareness of potential physical consequences such as erythema or skin blistering. To facilitate this transmission of information, many PCI centres have adopted a skin dose card or patient dose

Table 28.3 Catheter lab staffing roles in United Kindom; suggestions for good practice

Cardiac catheter lab team	Catheter lab role
Physician	Obtain consent and perform angioplasty procedures
	Responsible for radiation safety of entire team
	Lead catheter lab team in emergencies
	Document procedure and communication with patient
	Responsible for patient safety and governance, e.g. audit
Nurses (a minimum of two recommended)	Scrub to assist in angioplasty procedures
	Administer medication/conscious sedation
	Prepare equipment and document nursing care
Physiologist	Haemodynamic and electrocardiogram (ECG) monitoring
	Role in physiological assessment by pressure wire
	Documentation of physiological parameters during procedure
	May have role in audit/safety data recording
Radiographer	Responsible for fluoroscopic imaging and contrast
	Role in monitoring and reporting high doses/anomalies
	Involvement in the maintenance and safety of x-ray equipment
Runner/generic catheter lab worker	May be responsible for collecting angioplasty equipment, giving drugs, documentation and checklists
	Stock-taking and equipment maintenance

Source: Ludman P, BCIS Audit Returns 2012: Adult Interventional Procedures. 2014. Available at http://www.bcis.org.uk/pages/page_box_contents.asp?pageid=697&navcatid=11.

passport to record high-dose exposure and provide details of the warning symptoms and contact details for further advice.[36]

Of particular consideration in a centre with off-site surgery is the availability and expertise of local interventional radiologists and vascular interventional surgeons. A local interventional radiology service can provide useful support with peripheral stenting solutions and therapeutic options for vascular complications, which may have previously meant, a patient would not have a suitable coronary PCI option and a default surgical strategy would have been adopted. In addition, peripheral vascular interventionists to correct vascular complications rather than needing an open surgical procedure may provide an additional solution for vascular access-site complications.

28.7.4 PCI basic kit requirements

Angioplasty equipment should include a range of wires, balloon and stents including devices to treat coronary perforation if this occurs. There should be a robust method of inventory and stock control to prevent occasions where a kit is missing. As coronary dissection and perforation have been previously the main indications for emergency surgery, covered stents and coils are considered mandatory in a non-surgical centre (Figure 28.3). The improvements in covered stent technology and coils with coil pushing delivery systems may now be able to replace the traditional need of surgery for these complications. As these are used infrequently, careful record of expiry dates is advisable and it is advisable for operators in non-surgical centres to be regularly trained and updated in their use.

28.7.5 Diagnostic and PCI optimisation devices

The ability to perform physiological assessment with pressure wire, intra-coronary imaging with ultrasound or OCT is now becoming commonplace and constitutes evidence-based practice in whichever type of PCI centre the procedure is undertaken.[44] Pressure wire studies are now indicated in line with AUC. Not only do these techniques provide improved patient outcome but also are more cost-effective, as discussed earlier. Despite the overwhelming data, the uptake of pressure wire-guided PCI remains relatively conservative (e.g. 15% in the United Kingdom from 2014).[14] It is expected, in line with the emerging evidence to support ischaemia driven re-vascularisation, that all modern PCI centres (either surgical or non-surgical) will, in the near future, have pressure wire availability for the majority of routine cases.

Perhaps more debatable but certainly expected in a contemporary PCI lab is the availability of intra-coronary imaging. The use of invasive imaging with IVUS, OCT or OFDI enables complex PCI to be performed in a more predictable manner, for example, the use of IVUS to guide left main coronary artery stenting.[45] There are a variety of IVUS devices ranging from solid-state to rotational transducers. These provide high-quality ultrasound images with systems that can be permanently installed into the catheter lab or from a mobile cart. The 2015 UK guidelines for PCI state that both pressure wire and IVUS technology should form an essential part of interventional diagnostic procedures and should be available in all catheter laboratories performing coronary interventions.[36]

Higher resolution intra-coronary imaging with OCT or OFDI is also available in a number of non-surgical catheter labs, although the clinical utility outside of research for these techniques is less certain. OCT/OFDI is now considered the optimal imaging tool in stent failure cases as it usually provides a better understanding of the mechanism and subsequent guiding of the best therapeutic strategy.[46]

28.7.6 Complex lesions and high-risk patients

With an increasing age of patients presenting to cardiac catheter labs, the ability to effectively deal with calcific coronary lesions in paramount. Over the last decade, there has been a resurgence of the use of rotational atherectomy (RA) with equipment that has remained largely unchanged over the last 20 years. RA was historically considered a device used only in surgical PCI centres but with the clinical demand for effective lesion preparation, the device has seen its greatest uptake in non-surgical centres. This has been possible through training of operators and ancillary catheter lab staff through a combination of courses and on-site proctorships. The ability of offering a safe and sustainable RA program is dependent on individual operator experience and volume and it may be necessary in lower volume PCI units for consultant operators to work together during these cases.[33,34]

ELCA has also seen resurgence in utilisation in the last 10 years for a number of clinical indications including the non-crossable, non-expansible coronary lesions, acute thrombosis and under-expanded stents. This technology can safely be applied in non-surgical centres and is associated with a low rate of complications less than 1% perforation and <4% coronary dissection.[47] Unlike RA however, the frequency of ELCA use is much lower in practice and ideally the PCI centre whether surgical or non-surgical requires a PCI volume of at least 1000 cases/year to make ELCA a viable device to maintain.

28.7.7 Monitoring standards through audit

In the United Kingdom, all PCI centres are expected to collect comprehensive and accurate data that relate to the interventional treatment they provide for their patients. This includes information pertaining to the structure of service provision, the appropriateness of intervention and the process and outcomes of PCI. The data are expected to relate to each PCI centre. In the United States, the American College of Cardiology (ACC) ACC's National Cardiovascular Data Registry (NCDR) reports the outcomes of PCI procedures and these data are utilised to provide insights into contemporary practice and to set standards.[48]

The British Cardiovascular Interventional Society (BCIS) provides a clinical data set to allow a national comparison of results of interventional techniques and comparative audit. BCIS oversees and guides the collection and analysis of these data, which is currently hosted by the National Institute for Cardiovascular Outcomes Research (NICOR).

It is recommended that every cardiac interventional centre should provide the name of a designated clinician to lead the audit process and ensure that the infrastructure is in place. However, the ultimate responsibility for data completeness and accuracy should rest with the consultant PCI operator responsible for each PCI procedure.

External or internal data validation should be sought. It is therefore recommended that regular internal validation of case ascertainment, data completeness and data accuracy is

performed. An annual internal review of cardiogenic shock outcomes and data entry is recommended in this group of higher risk patients.[36]

28.8 What level of service can be developed in a non-surgical centre?

The PCI service at the Royal Bournemouth Hospital in the United Kingdom started in April 2005, with the local cardiac surgical centre approximately 30 miles East. The early set up and strategies have been published before.[49] Over the last decade, our centre has developed dramatically to provide a complete 24/7 PPCI provision amongst offering a complex array of lesion therapy utilising a variety of adjunctive devices and full intra-coronary imaging (Figure 28.6). Over 2000 PCI procedures are performed annually and include a full range of techniques for CTO lesion treatment (anterograde wire escalation, anterograde dissection re-entry using Crossboss and Sting Ray devices and retrograde skill set).

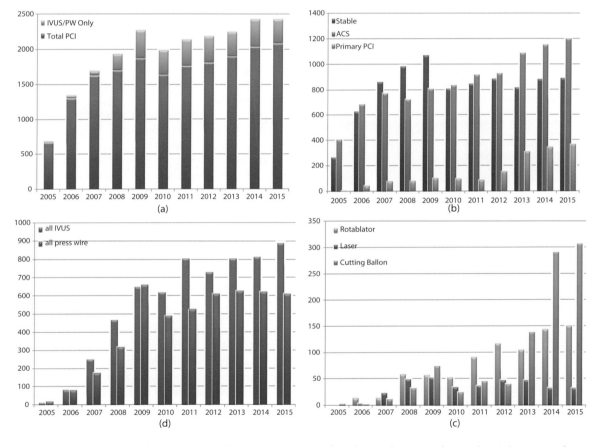

Figure 28.6 Ten-year activity profile at the Royal Bournemouth Hospital, UK, the United Kingdom's largest volume non-surgical centre. (a) The volume of total PCI (stent cases, red bars) and IVUS or pressure wire only cases (green bars) over a 10-year period. (b) The breakdown of PCI according to patient presentation with elective stable cases (purple bars), NSTEMI/unstable angina cases (blue bars) and STEMI with PPCI (orange bars). The centre started 24/7 PPCI in October 2012. (c) The volume of total IVUS cases (blue bars) and pressure wire cases (red bars) over a 10-year period. (d) The volume of adjunctive devices for lesion preparation with rotational atherectomy cases (green bars), laser atherectomy (purple bars) and cutting/scoring balloons (blue bars). The development of a dedicated bifurcation programme in March 2012 and bioresorbable vascular scaffold programme in March 2013 explains the extra use in cutting/scoring balloons over this period given the importance of lesion preparation for these contemporary devices.

Given the more elderly population on the South Coast of England, there is a high volume of rotational atherectomy cases performed (>150/year) and we perform the United Kingdom's largest volume of excimer laser coronary interventions. Left main coronary PCI occurs in up to 10% of all cases undertaken with dataset presented at International meetings. The PCI service is also supported by integrated IVUS with penetration of up to 50% of cases and an increasing number of high-resolution imaging performed with OCT and OFDI. We have also been forwards thinking in adopting early technology such as dedicated bifurcations stents and bioresorbable vascular scaffolds. These programs have been developed with rigorous data collection to support both acute procedure outcome and also longer term follow-up and results have been presented at international meetings. The BRS program has largely developed within the national UK registry and further within randomised control trials before this technology is used in a routine fashion. The early adoption of new devices and a commitment to high-quality service and outcome for patients has enabled the centre to develop multiple teaching courses with advanced training workshops aimed at consultant operators in addition to fellow courses to train future generations of interventionists. Participation in international trials and registries is a daily activity in the PCI catheter lab with many patients in complex PCI studies including those with poor left ventricular function, left main stem disease and those at high-bleeding risk (Figure 28.7).

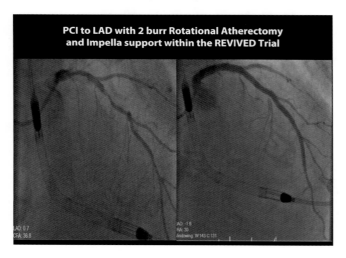

Figure 28.7 Complex PCI performed in a non-surgical PCI centre. This is an example of complex PCI undertaken in a 65-year-old man. He had previously presented with inferior STEMI and had PPCI to RCA. The LAD had diffuse calcified disease and on MRI 6 weeks later the left ventricular ejection fraction (LVEF) was only 20% with full LAD viability and dysfunctional anterior wall. The patient was therefore randomised within the REVIVED trial (comparing optimal medical therapy versus OMT + PCI) and was treated in the latter group. With Impella haemodynamic support the LAD was treated with 1.5 and 2.0 mm burrs for lesion preparation and subsequent reconstruction with 4 DES. One year after the PCI, the patient remains well with an ICD and has an LVEF of 35%.

The link with our local surgical centre has remained strong and we host a weekly Heart Team meeting with Consultant cardiothoracic surgeons using Lifestream.[50] This technology permits real-time sharing of non-degraded images of angiography, echocardiography, computed tomography (CT) and magnetic resonance imaging (MRI) and permits valuable efficient discussion to guide patient therapy. This system can also be linked to other PCI centres to permit network wide discussion of cases and allow transfer of patients to our centre for more complex PCI, for example, CTO or laser atherectomy. Our catheter labs also have a fully integrated audiovisual system which permits live case demonstrates and facilitates teaching workshops.

28.9 The future for non-surgical PCI centres

There is increasing data to support the existence and indeed value of non-surgical coronary interventional centres in providing high-quality safe interventions with an often lower than predicted MACCE rates observed. The rate of complication from all PCI is seen to be still reducing and the uptake of radial access will see this reduce even further. Emergency CABG rates remain low and when transfer for surgery is required, information from current literature suggest that this be performed in a timely and effective way, supported by local collaborative pathways and processes.

The close networking arrangements that have been formed between surgeons and coronary interventionists only serves to strengthen this system with the modern 'heart team' allowing high-level multidisciplinary discussion between physicians and surgeons within both surgical and non-surgical centres to optimise decision-making.

The national audit data from United Kingdom and European registries demonstrates good outcome data with no perceptible difference between surgical and non-surgical units. Clear guidance from national governing cardiac interventional organisations and the ongoing mandatory audit data analysis will ensure that the burgeoning need for PCI will be provided in a safe and sustainable way.

The next challenge for non-surgical PCI centres will be to develop structural interventional cardiology procedure programs such as transcatheter aortic valve implantation (TAVI), which currently are generally only performed in surgical centres. Many cardiologists believe that these types of therapies will always remain in the surgical centre but isn't that what was said about PCI 30 years ago?

References

1. Meier B. The first patient to undergo coronary angioplasty – 23-year follow-up. *N Engl J Med* 2001; 344: 144–5.
2. Sigwart U et al. Intravascular stents to prevent occlusion and restenosis after transluminal angioplasty. *N Engl J Med* 1987; 316: 701–6.
3. Cowley MJ et al. Emergency coronary bypass surgery after coronary angioplasty: The National Heart, Lung,

and Blood Institute's Percutaneous Transluminal Coronary Angioplasty Registry experience. *Am J Cardiol* 1984; 53(12): 22C–6C.

4. Fischman DL et al. Stent Restenosis Study Investigators. A randomized comparison of coronary-stent placement and balloon angioplasty in the treatment of coronary artery disease. *N Engl J Med* 1994; 331(8): 496–501.

5. Serruys PW et al. Benestent Study Group. A comparison of balloon-expandable-stent implantation with balloon angioplasty in patients with coronary artery disease. *N Engl J Med* 1994; 331(8): 489–95.

6. Morice MC et al. A randomized comparison of a sirolimus-eluting stent with a standard stent for coronary revascularization. *N Engl J Med* 2002; 346(23): 1773–80.

7. Bravata DM et al. Systematic review: The comparative effectiveness of percutaneous coronary interventions and coronary artery bypass graft surgery. *Ann Intern Med* 2007; 147: 703–16.

8. Hlatky MA et al. Coronary artery bypass surgery compared with percutaneous coronary interventions for multivessel disease: A collaborative analysis of individual patient data from ten randomised trials. *Lancet* 2009; 373: 1190–7.

9. Serruys PW et al. Percutaneous coronary intervention versus coronary-artery bypass grafting for severe coronary artery disease. *N Engl J Med* 2009; 360: 961–72.

10. Grines CL et al. Primary coronary angioplasty compared with intravenous thrombolytic therapy for acute myocardial infarction: Six-month follow up and analysis of individual patient data from randomized trials. *Am Heart J* 2003; 145(1): 47–57.

11. Tarantini G et al. Explanation for the survival benefit of primary angioplasty over thrombolytic therapy in patients with ST-elevation acute myocardial infarction. *Am J Cardiol* 2005; 96(11): 1503–5.

12. Peels HO et al. Percutaneous coronary intervention with off-site cardiac surgery backup for acute myocardial infarction as a strategy to reduce door to balloon time. *Am J Cardiol* 2005; 100(9): 1353–8.

13. Bommer WJ et al. The 4-year percutaneous coronary intervention California audit monitored pilot with offsite surgery (PCI-CAMPOS) outcomes in 205,052 patients in hospitals with and without onsite cardiac surgery. *J Am Coll Cardiol Conference* 2015; 65(10 Suppl 1): A1687.

14. Ludman P. BCIS Audit Returns 2012: Adult Interventional Procedures. 2014. Available at http://www.bcis.org.uk/pages/page_box_contents.asp?pageid=697&navcatid=11.

15. Strom JB et al. Association between operator procedure volume and patient outcomes in percutaneous coronary intervention: A systematic review and meta-analysis. *Circulation* 2014; 7(4): 560–6.

16. Levine GN et al. 2011 ACCF/AHA/SCAI guideline for percutaneous coronary intervention. A report of the American College of Cardiology Foundation/American Heart Association Task Force on Practice Guidelines and the Society for Cardiovascular Angiography and Interventions. *J Am Coll Cardiol* 2011; 58: e44–122.

17. Aversano T et al. Outcomes of PCI at hospitals with or without on-site cardiac surgery. *N Engl J Med* 2012; 366: 1792–802.

18. Jacobs AK et al. Nonemergency PCI at hospitals with or without on-site cardiac surgery. *N Engl J Med* 2013; 368: 1498–508.

19. Singh M et al. Percutaneous coronary intervention at centers with and without on-site surgery: A meta-analysis. *JAMA* 2011; 306: 2487–94.

20. Yang EH et al. Emergency coronary artery bypass surgery for percutaneous coronary intervention: Changes in the incidence, clinical characteristics, and indications from 1979 to 2003. *J Am Coll Cardiol* 2005; 46(11): 2004–9.

21. Everaert B et al. Crossover bailout revascularization after percutaneous coronary intervention and coronary artery bypass grafting. Abstracts EuroPCR 2015 Euro15A-POS209.

22. Berger PB et al. Time to reperfusion and other procedural characteristics of emergency coronary artery bypass surgery after unsuccessful coronary angioplasty. *Am J Cardiol* 1995; 76: 565–9.

23. Seshadri N et al. Emergency coronary artery bypass surgery in the contemporary percutaneous coronary intervention era. *Circulation* 2002; 106: 2346–50.

24. Zeeshan S et al. Predicting emergency coronary artery bypass graft following PCI: Application of a computational model to refer patients to hospitals with and without onsite surgical backup. *Open Heart* 2015; 2(1): e000243. Published online 2015 Dec 1.

25. Mamas M et al. Influence of arterial access site selection on outcomes in primary percutaneous coronary intervention. *J Am Coll Cardiol Intv* 2013; 6(7): 698–706.

26. Tonino P et al. Fractional flow reserve versus angiography for guiding percutaneous coronary intervention. *N Engl J Med* 2009; 360: 213–24.

27. DeBruyne B et al. Fractional flow reserve – Guided PCI versus medical therapy in stable coronary disease. *N Engl J Med* 2012; 367: 991–1001.

28. DeBruyne B et al. Fractional flow reserve-guided PCI for stable coronary artery disease. *N Engl J Med* 2014; 371: 1208–17.

29. Curzen N et al. Does routine pressure wire assessment influence management strategy at coronary angiography for diagnosis of chest pain? The RIPCORD study. *Circ Cardiovasc Interv* 2014; 7: 248–55.

30. Stone G et al. A prospective natural history study of coronary atherosclerosis. *N Engl J Med* 2011; 364: 226–35.

31. Zhang Y et al. Comparison of intravascular ultrasound versus angiography-guided drug-eluting stent implantation: A meta-analysis of one randomised trial and ten observational studies involving 19,619 patients. *EuroIntervention* 2012; 8: 855.

32. Everaert B et al. Appropriate use of bioresorbable vascular scaffolds in percutaneous coronary interventions: A recommendation from experienced users. A position statement on the use of bioresorbable vascular scaffolds in the Netherlands. *Neth Heart J* 2015; 23(3): 161–5.

33. Jiang J et al. Complex coronary lesions and rotational atherectomy: One hospitals experience. *J Zhejiang Univ Sci B* 2012; 13 (8): 645–51.

34. Tran T et al. An evidence based approach to the use of rotational and directional coronary atherectomy in the era of drug eluting stents: When does it make sense? *Catheter Cardiovasc Interv* 2008; 72(5): 650–62.

35. O'Kane P, and Redwood S. Laser. In: Redwood S et al. (editors), *Oxford Textbook of Interventional Cardiology*, 1st Edition. Kettering, Northants: Oxford University Press, 2010.

36. Banning A et al. Percutaneous coronary intervention in the UK: Recommendations for good practice 2015. *Heart* 2015; 101: 1–13.

37. Dehmer GJ et al. SCAI/ACC/AHA Expert Consensus Document: 2014 update on percutaneous coronary intervention without on site surgical backup. *J Am Coll Cardiol* 2014; 63: 2624–41.

38. Windecker S et al. 2014 ESC/EACTS Guidelines on myocardial revascularization. *Eur Heart J* 2014; 35: 2541–619.

39. Steg PG et al. ESC Guidelines for the management of acute myocardial infarction in patients presenting with ST elevation. *Eur Heart J* 2012; 33: 2569–619.

40. Dawkins KD et al. Percutaneous coronary intervention: Recommendations for good practice and training. *Heart* 2005; 91(Suppl 6): vi1–27.

41. Kumbhani DJ et al. Association of hospital primary angioplasty volume in ST elevation myocardial infarction with quality and outcomes. *JAMA* 2009; 302(20): 2207–13.

42. Academy of Medical Royal College Guidelines: Safe Sedation Practice for Healthcare Procedures: Standards and Guidelines. RCOA. October 2013. Available at https://www.rcoa.ac.uk/document-store/safe-sedation-practice-healthcare-procedures-standards-and-guidance

43. Work With Ionising Radiation. Ionising Radiations Regulations (1999) Approved Code of Practice (ACoP) and Guidance L121. Health and Safety Executive. Available at https://books.hse.gov.uk/hse/public/home.jsf (Accessed May 2016).

44. Longman K, and Curzen N. Should ischemia be the main target in selecting a percutaneous coronary intervention strategy? *Expert Rev Cardiovasc Ther* 2013; 11: 1051–9.

45. Park SJ et al. Impact of intravascular ultrasound guidance on long-term mortality in stenting for unprotected left main coronary artery stenosis. *Circ Cardiovasc Interv* 2009; 2: 167–77.

46. Souteyrand G et al. Mechanisms of stent thrombosis analysed by optical coherence tomography: Insights from the national PESTO French registry. Eur Heart J 2016; 37: 1208–16.

47. Fernandez JP et al. Beyond the balloon: Excimer coronary laser atherectomy used alone or in combination with rotational atherectomy in the treatment of chronic total occlusions, non-crossable and non-expansible coronary lesions. *EuroIntervention* 2013; 9(2): 243–50.

48. Anderson H et al. A contemporary overview of percutaneous coronary interventions: The American College of Cardiology–National Cardiovascular Data Registry (ACC–NCDR). *J Am Coll Cardiol* 2002; 39(7): 1096–103. doi:10.1016/S0735-1097(02)01733-3.

49. Kelly D et al. Percutaneous coronary angioplasty in a district general hospital: Safe and effective – the Bournemouth model September 2008. *Br J Cardiol* 2008; 15: 244–7.

50. Veasey RA et al. It's good to talk! Changes in coronary revascularisation practice in PCI centres without onsite surgical cover and the impact of an angiography video conferencing system. *Int J Clin Pract* 2011; 65(6): 658–63.

29

Interventions after coronary artery bypass surgery

DAVID R HOLMES

29.1 Introduction

Long-term follow-up of patients after coronary artery bypass graft (CABG) surgery has shown that angina may eventually recur in up to 8% of patients annually[1–3] due to graft stenoses or occlusions[4–6] or progression of disease within the native coronary arteries.[7–9] Approximately 20%, 30% and 50% of saphenous vein grafts (SVG) have significant disease or are occluded at 1, 5 and 10 years after surgery[4–6,10–15] and although 90% of internal mammary artery (IMA) grafts may be patent at 10 years, stenoses are not infrequently encountered earlier distal to the anastomosis. As the frequency of CABG surgery has increased, repeat intervention has become necessary more often (perhaps 10%–15% of post-CABG patients within 10 years)[16] and includes repeat surgery or catheter-based intervention with percutaneous coronary intervention (PCI).

The operative risks for repeat CABG are increased especially in the presence of impaired left ventricular function, left main stem and multi-vessel disease, functional class III or IV, advanced age and incomplete re-vascularisation. A 3.4%–9.2% mortality rate and up to a 15% incidence of perioperative Q-wave myocardial infarction (MI) has been reported[17–25] and the risks are even higher for a second reoperation.[21] Repeat surgery is technically more difficult

Table 29.1 Less than ideal candidates for repeat CABG

Lack of venous or arterial conduits
Advanced age
Poor LV function
Poor distal vessels
Patent grafts at risk of damage during reoperation
Previous CABG surgery, that is two previous operations
Coexisting medical problems, for example stroke,
    malignancy, renal or respiratory failure,
    immunosuppressive therapy

and also less effective in relieving symptoms. An additional issue is that whilst the vein grafts may have developed severe disease, the left internal mammary artery (LIMA) may still be patent. In this situation, reoperation may damage the LIMA. Finally if additional venous grafts are needed, they may not either be available or of as excellent quality as at the time of initial CABG; using poorer quality vein segments often results in lower graft patency rates. Adverse features for repeat CABG are shown in Table 29.1. Treatment of SVG disease carries with it increased complication rates, with increased potential for distal embolisation or no reflow as well as subsequent restenosis. Accordingly, with severely diseased or totally occluded vein grafts, percutaneous re-vascularisation should be aimed at the initial native coronary artery lesions which had been bypassed. This is particularly true in the setting of acute MI resulting from acute vein graft occlusion.

SVG percutaneous transluminal coronary angioplasty (PTCA) was first performed in 1980 with a high primary success rate. The progressive improvement in guide catheter, guidewire, balloon and stent technology has enabled more difficult cases to be performed successfully with lower complication rates,[16,26–46] but these rates are still higher than treatment of native coronary stenosis. Adjunctive therapy for treatment of vein graft disease includes the use of distal protection devices and covered stents as well as adjunctive medications such as nicardipine to treat no-reflow.

Intervention in patients with previous CABG surgery is challenging, but remains a very useful treatment for what are frequently difficult cases including patients who have undergone CABG surgery on more than one previous occasion.[47]

29.2 Indications

Patients with recurrent angina pectoris after CABG surgery may be suitable for PCI to their grafts or native coronary arteries as an alternative to medical treatment or repeat CABG surgery. The choice depends on many factors including age, coexisting medical conditions, left ventricular function, availability of conduits, the risk of damaging functioning grafts and the likelihood of a successful reoperation. The major factor which determines the suitability for PTCA or PCI is the coronary and graft anatomy defined by coronary and graft angiography.

Short, discrete stenoses in easily accessible grafts are an easier proposition than long diffuse segments of disease associated with thrombus in aged grafts which are associated with increased complications. Recently occluded grafts can be reopened although chronically blocked grafts may be impossible to recanalise and have poor prospects for long-term patency. Re-vascularisation after CABG should be considered for the following groups of stable patients:

- Significant obstruction in the proximal left anterior descending (LAD) artery and evidence of extensive anterior ischaemia on non-invasive stress testing or significant disease in other vessels. Re-vascularisation in such patients is likely to improve survival, similar to patients who have not previously undergone CABG. This would include most importantly patients without prior LIMA grafts to the LAD.
- This effect was demonstrated in an observational study of over 4600 patients with prior CABG who had a patent LIMA bypass to the LAD but had significant disease in another territory.[48] No significant difference in mortality was seen during a 20-year follow-up between those treated with PCI or CABG and those who were continued on optimal medical therapy, thus highlighting the lack of benefit of subsequent re-vascularisation if there is already a patent LIMA graft to the LAD
- Refractory angina despite optimal medical therapy. If there is a reasonable likelihood of procedural success, then re-vascularisation should be attempted.
- Stable angina with vein graft stenosis >70%. This is recommended due to the natural course of progression to total graft occlusion over time; when this occurs PCI is associated with poor outcomes.
- Patients with poor repeat CABG targets. In these patients, the suitability for PCI must be carefully considered.
- Patients with high operative risk for repeat CABG due to age or comorbid conditions. Reoperation is generally associated with less complete re-vascularisation and control of symptoms compared to the first procedure. Repeat CABG has also been shown to be associated with an increased in-hospital mortality rate compared to PCI (6%–9% vs. ≤0.5% overall and 11.2% vs. 1.6% in diabetics).[49]
- Angina or MI within 30 days after CABG is usually secondary to technical failure (e.g. kinks from redundant length of graft), a relatively small conduit size (diameter <1.5 mm or prior vein pathology), poor distal runoff or extrinsic factors. In such cases, ischaemia may persist leading to acute thrombosis complicating the stenosis. Urgent coronary angiography should be performed in this setting for diagnosis and to identify lesions that might be treated with PCI. In some of these patients, a severe graft lesion is identified which can then be treated to improve outcomes.[49]

For angina or MI after 30 days post-CABG surgery, coronary angiography should be performed immediately to rule out critical graft lesions that can be treated before irreversible loss of graft function. Such lesions can progress rapidly to a total thrombotic occlusion, if undiagnosed.[50]

29.3 Contraindications

There are few absolute contraindications to PCI in post-CABG patients. Long ectatic tortuous grafts with excessive intra-luminal material and thrombus and chronically occluded grafts are usually regarded as such. Relative contraindications include heavy calcification of the stenosis, grafts with poor distal run-off into the native coronary circulation and long diffuse lesions.

An important subset of patients in whom PCI should not be considered as first option are those in whom no arterial grafts have ever been placed such as the patients in whom only venous grafts are present. Whilst uncommon in current practice for surgeons to not use the LIMA, it should always be considered as the optimal approach to LAD re-vascularisation. Accordingly patients who present with angina post-CABG who do not have a LIMA graft implanted to the LAD should be considered for another surgical operation if feasible.

Repeat CABG should also be considered when there are large amounts of diffuse particulate debris and thrombi in patulous vein grafts that have failed trials of aspiration or rheolytic thrombectomy with the use of embolic protection devices (EPD) or would unlikely to be successful in such cases. If repeat CABG is offered, patients need to be informed of the higher mortality rates compared to first CABG. Thirty-day mortality rates of 7%–9% in stable patients and as high as 39%–50% are seen in unstable patients (hemodynamic or electrical instability).[51-55] In-hospital mortality has been reported to be 11%, 25% and 39% for first, second and third repeat CABG operations.[56] They are also associated with reduced graft patency and incomplete angina relief.

Due to the higher mortality rates, repeat CABG should only be considered if the patient cannot undergo PCI for technical reasons, or if the patient's first CABG did not include a LIMA to LAD bypass graft.

29.4 Relation of graft age to problem encountered

The effect of graft age on pathophysiology of vein graft disease and outcome after re-vascularisation has been the focus of extensive study.

29.4.1 Vein grafts

29.4.1.1 Early

SVG occlusion within 30 days after CABG is usually secondary to technical failure (e.g. kinks from redundant length of graft), a relatively small conduit size (diameter <1.5 mm or prior vein pathology), poor distal runoff or extrinsic factors.[57] In each of these cases, angina can develop leading to acute graft thrombosis.

Urgent post-operative angiography was performed in a series of such patients who had developed recurrent ischaemia immediately post-CABG. It revealed that 37%–56% of these patients had developed SVG occlusion or stenosis and 12%–29% had developed internal mammary graft occlusion or stenosis.[54,55] Out of 2052 patients in this series, 131 patients met the ischaemia criteria at 12 hours post-CABG including 23 patients who were haemodynamically unstable and required subsequent emergent surgery. Out of these 131 patients who met criteria, 108 underwent angiography which revealed the following: normal grafts in 45 patients, SVG or IMA graft occlusion in 41 patients, 29 patients with incorrect anastomosis, 12 patients with graft spasm or displacement, poor distal runoff in five patients and two patients with incomplete re-vascularisation.[54]

29.4.1.2 Early – midterm

Although graft thrombosis may still occur within 12 months after CABG, recurrent angina may be due to discrete fibroproliferative stenoses at the ostium, in the body or at the distal anastomosis of the SVG. The PREVENT IV trial of 2014 which evaluated rates and causes of vein graft failure (VGF) included 1828 patients with a total of 4343 implanted vein grafts, who underwent a 12–18-month follow-up angiography per study protocol or angiography for a clinical indication.[58] VGF which was defined as a ≥75% stenosis or occlusion was seen in 43% of patients. Of the total 4343 vein grafts that were implanted in these patients, 25% (1096 vein grafts) had VGF at this 12–18-month follow-up. Of these VGF patients only 7.1% had clinical symptoms, implying that the majority of VGFs remain clinically silent. Factors that were found to be predictive of failure included endoscopic vein harvesting, poor native artery quality and longer duration of the surgical procedure. An association between platelet $P2Y_{12}$ receptor blocker use post-operatively and VGF was also found, but was felt to be due to confounding by the authors and disregarded.

29.4.1.3 Midterm

Lipid deposition and atherosclerotic plaque may start developing in areas of intimal hyperplasia at 12–18 months causing a late occlusion.[59] Two percent of SVG's obstruct from year 1 to 6, subsequent to which rates increase at 4%–5% each passing year. Between 1 and 5 years, recurrent angina is likely to be due to atherosclerotic stenoses in the SVGs or native vessels. PTCA or PCI or other interventional techniques can be performed and an embolic protection device should always be used if possible. In the PREVENT IV trial (described in Section 29.4.1.2), long-term follow-up data were also obtained. At 4 years, the primary outcome of death, MI and repeat re-vascularisation occurred significantly more in patients who had any VGF compared to those who had none (adjusted hazard ratio, 1.68, 95% CI 1.21–2.06).[60] This was driven primarily by the higher rate of repeat re-vascularisation seen in the VGF group.

29.4.1.4 Late

Beyond 5 years, complex vein graft lesions with eccentric, ulcerated atheromatous stenoses and friable thrombotic material are more frequently encountered as well as diffuse disease and graft occlusion. Histopathological analysis of these atherosclerotic plaques document foam cells, cholesterol crystals, blood elements and necrotic debris. These lesions contain less fibrocollagenous tissue and calcification than what is seen in native coronary atherosclerosis. It is because of these factors that plaques in older SVGs are softer, larger, more friable and also more prone to thrombus formation.

Distal embolisation of material may occur during PCI in more than 20% of cases and during follow-up restenosis rates are high.[61] Nevertheless, PTCA and stenting may be worthwhile especially in patients in whom reoperation is better avoided or contraindicated.

29.4.2 Arterial grafts

Arterial grafts have superior long-term patency and survival typically greater than 90%–95% at 10 years.[62,63] LIMA to LAD graft patency rates are over 95% at 5 years and are almost comparable at 10 years.[64,65] Right internal mammary artery (RIMA) graft patency rates are also over 95% at 4 years. However, as it is typically grafted to the right coronary artery, the rate falls below 90% at 10 years (as distal anastomosis to a native vessel such as the LAD has a larger myocardial territory to supply with concomitant higher flow requirements and therefore less chances of an LAD graft becoming atretic; vis a vis the right coronary artery [RCA] which has a relatively smaller territory to perfuse).

29.4.2.1 Use of the LIMA graft

The LIMA graft has been evaluated in a study of approximately 6000 patients.[66] In this study population, the LIMA was grafted to the LAD, either alone or in combination with other SVGs and compared to patients who only had SVGs. The 10-year patient (actuarial) survival rates were superior to SVGs. LIMA alone survival rate was 93% versus 88% for SVGs. LIMA in two vessel combination with SVG was 90% versus 80% for SVGs only patients. LIMA in a three vessel combination with SVG was 83% versus 71% for SVGs only patients. The mortality benefit of arterial grafts has been shown to persist on long-term follow-up of 15 and 20 years.[67,68] These patients also have resultant fewer repeat operations and lower rates of recurrent MI and angina when compared to vein graft recipients.[68]

29.5 Strategy

The strategy for intervention should be clear to the patient and family before the procedure and the case should have been discussed with surgical colleagues and the therapeutic options agreed upon, especially when the graft supplies much of the remaining viable myocardium.[69] Multiple grafts may need to be treated and the procedure staged. If myocardium is supplied by a stenotic SVG and a stenosed native vessel, then PCI to the native vessel should be preferred because of the lower restenosis and late complication

rates.[70] Emergency surgery in patients who have previously undergone CABG surgery is difficult and the time to re-vascularisation is often prolonged.[71,72] High-risk patients including those with poor left ventricular function, last remaining graft/vessel or unstable angina associated with thrombotic occlusion of a graft should be considered for intra-aortic balloon counterpulsation, Impella or Tandem Heart placement for haemodynamic support prior to complex PCI.

29.6 Technique

29.6.1 Adjunctive pharmacology

All patients should be loaded with aspirin and clopidogrel or ticagrelor. Patients should receive 5,000–10,000 units of heparin at the start of the procedure, and heparin boluses should be given in doses of 70–100 units/kg to achieve a target Activated clotting time (ACT) between 250 and 350 seconds during the procedure. Intra-coronary vasodilators should be used as needed for the prevention and treatment of slow or no reflow.

Glycoprotein IIb/IIIa platelet receptor inhibitors have been studied for utility given the large embolic burden seen in SVG procedures. However, they were not shown to prevent periprocedural MI rates based on a pooled analysis of 3958 patients (EPIC, EPILOG, EPISTENT, IMPACT II and PURSUIT) with over 600 SVG PCI patients, which showed no benefit from these agents.[73]

In the REPLACE 1 and 2 trials, 403 SVG patients were randomised to heparin or bivalirudin.[74] No significant difference in the combined endpoint of death, MI, urgent re-vascularisation or major bleeding was found. However, bivalirudin was associated with minor bleeding. Given this, bivalirudin may theoretically increase bleeding complications and the possibility of cardiac tamponade with the higher risk of perforation seen in SVG intervention.

29.6.2 Native vessel

PTCA to suitable lesions in the native vessels should be performed with standard guide catheters, balloons and guidewires chosen according to the specific anatomical problem present. It may be useful to attempt branch vessel stenoses, for example septal, intermediate or diagonals, in order to improve the blood supply to as much myocardium as possible. It is not unusual to perform PTCA to distal native vessel stenoses through patent SVGs and IMAs and even stenoses proximal to the distal anastomosis site by retrograde passage of the guidewire and balloon catheter[75,76] Rotablator atherectomy, excimer laser coronary angioplasty (ELCA) and stenting may be appropriate depending on the coronary anatomy and/or on the presence of calcification. Intravascular ultrasound (IVUS), optical coherence tomography (OCT) or fractional flow reserve (FFR) may help in the decision-making.

29.6.3 Saphenous vein grafts

29.6.3.1 Guide catheter

The goal of a guide catheter is to ideally achieve coaxial alignment and provide adequate backup support. This is often the key to success. 7F guide catheters are ideal for most vein graft interventions as they allow optimal visualisation, and accommodate large balloons, facilitate stenting, insertion of EPD and covered stents if needed. 6F catheters with large internal lumens are also available for smaller grafts. For RCA SVGs and horizontal or inferiorly directed LAD SVGs, a right Judkins, right or left Amplatz, multipurpose or saphenous vein bypass guide catheters are helpful. For superiorly directed LAD SVGs, diagonal and LCx SVGs, a left Amplatz guide catheter may be best. However, a Hockey stick and right Judkins can also be equally effective.

29.6.3.2 Balloon catheters and guidewires

Long balloons may be necessary to prevent movement away from the lesion during inflation and balloon catheters with extended shafts may be required for long snake grafts or IMAs in very posterior locations. When encountered with SVGs that encircle around the heart or IMA grafts with far distal anastomoses, extra-long balloon catheters (e.g. shaft length 145 cm) may be needed. Tortuous IMAs and long, tortuous SVGs require flexible, steerable and low-profile devices. In some instances, shorter guide catheters can be used or the guide catheter can be shortened and a flared, short sheath (one size smaller) used to close the cut end of the catheter.

Balloon sizing is a critically important step. Although some authorities recommend slightly oversizing the balloon and stent for vein graft interventions, it may be wise to size the balloons and stents no larger than the adjacent normal reference segment. This is the result of increased risk of vein graft rupture with even modest oversizing, which has been found to be especially true in older grafts. Oversizing has been evaluated and showed no effect on target vessel re-vascularisation (TVR) (31% vs. 26%, $p = .3$) and in fact MI rates were significantly increased (29% vs. 17%, $p < .05$).[77] One study has even reported improved outcomes with under-sizing stents in SVGs with reduced post-PCI CK-MB levels.[78]

We recommend ballooning and stenting according to the normal reference vessel size.

29.6.4 Lesion site

29.6.4.1 Proximal/aorto-ostial stenosis

Proximal or aorto-ostial lesions are difficult since the guide catheter has to be backed out into the aorta and the balloon or other device balanced at the ostium. Rigid ostial stenoses often require high-pressure inflations, with relatively young (<3 years) SVGs responding best. Although technically more demanding, lesion modification with cutting balloons or atherectomy and stenting may be most appropriate for ostial lesions because of the often suboptimal acute result and high recurrence rate after PTCA.[79]

29.6.4.2 Body stenoses

Lesions in the body of SVGs are often tough and require high inflation pressures to respond to PTCA. Oversizing of the balloon and stenting can be performed for a suboptimal result but because of high restenosis rates, stenting (primary or after pre-dilatation) is probably appropriate for all such lesions.

29.6.4.3 Distal stenoses

Distal anastomotic stenoses which occur within 1 year of CABG usually respond well to low-pressure PTCA and are associated with a low complication and restenosis rate. Stenoses which occur later behave like lesions in the body of the graft and probably require stenting. Correct balloon sizing is essential to avoid rupture and dissection of the graft and distal vessel.

29.6.4.4 Acute/subacute occlusions

Acutely or subacutely thrombosed SVGs may be recanalised by PTCA, but initial and long-term success may be limited and MI due to embolisation is a real risk.[15,80–82] We initially use a 0.014 in. high-torque floppy, intermediate or standard guidewire to reach the native vessel beyond the distal anastomosis. A balloon catheter can then be passed to re-establish flow down the graft by serial inflations along its length. Thrombolytic therapy may be used in boluses but is only likely to be effective once some flow has been established[80,83] and is unfortunately associated with distal embolisation and MI.[84] Thrombolytic therapy can be infused through a Tracker™ catheter left in situ in the SVG, although several hours may be required – often an ordeal for the patient and operator, and bleeding and stroke are realistic complications,[85–88] and as such is now not a recommended strategy.

AngioJet™ thrombectomy[89–92] may be useful, but whether these techniques, Acolysis™[93] or the X-sizer™ device[94,95] are more effective in this situation than PTCA is not known.

29.6.4.5 Chronic occlusions

Chronically occluded SVGs cannot usually be entered let alone be recanalised by PTCA or PCI. It is not recommended that chronic total SVGs undergo PCI due to higher complication rates, poor long-term patency and low success rates.[81,96,97]

29.6.4.6 Restenosis lesions

PTCA for restenosis lesions in grafts is usually effective but recurrence is high. Stent implantation offers the best hope using high-pressure inflations with an appropriately sized balloon dilatation catheter.

29.6.5 Internal mammary artery grafts

8F IMA guide catheters provide the best back-up support, however they should be handled carefully to avoid dissecting the friable ostium. 6F and 7F large lumen guide catheters may be preferred if the IMA is small but visualisation of the distal vessel and the stenosis is of paramount importance during intervention. Low profile balloon catheters are essential. The left radial[98] or even brachial approach[99,100] may be useful if the femoral route fails to provide sufficient back-up support or if a proximal subclavian stenosis or occlusion interferes with access to the IMA. The RIMA is best approached from the right radial artery using an IMA guide catheter.

29.6.6 Other conduits

PTCA/PCI can be successfully performed in gastroepiploic arterial grafts and this requires cannulation of the coeliac, common hepatic, gastroduodenal and gastroepiploic arteries.[101,102] A 7F JR4 guide catheter may be used but special guide catheters (COBRA) are available to selectively engage the gastroduodenal artery. If the gastroepiploic artery originates from the superior mesenteric artery (10%–20%) the route to the graft is very tortuous and the distance to the anastomosis is longer and more challenging. Vasospasm is frequent and requires direct nitrate administration.

Large unligated side branches of IMAs may cause a coronary steal phenomenon but it may be possible to close them by coil embolisation.[103]

29.7 Results of intervention in SVGs

Despite taking on patients with more adverse characteristics for PCI, success rates are now higher than a decade ago as a result of improved technology.[104]

29.7.1 Percutaneous transluminal coronary angioplasty

PTCA in patients with previous CABG surgery generally produces high (>90%) success rates[105] and low major complication rates (Table 29.2). In a large series, Douglas et al.[106] reported a success rate of 90% with a Q-wave MI rate of 2.3%, emergency CABG rate of 3.5% and a death rate of 1.2%.

The results depend on the site of the stenosis, age of the graft, morphology of the lesion and the presence of intraluminal thrombus. Aorto-ostial lesions are fibrotic and prone to recoil and have a lower success rate with PTCA compared to lesions in the body or distal anastomosis site. Moreover, severe stenoses (>70% diameter stenosis), lesions with thrombus, complex and/or ulcerated morphology and lesions in old SVGs tend to have a lower success rate and a higher complication rate than less severe and less complex lesions. Angioscopy has shown that angiography underestimates the incidence of intra-luminal thrombus and friable plaque and this may account for the unpredictability of complications in SVG PTCA.[107]

Angiographic restenosis occurs frequently and is often more difficult to recognise clinically in patients with multivessel disease and incomplete re-vascularisation. Douglas et al.[106] reported a restenosis rate of 32% in SVGs <6 months old, 43% for SVGs 6–12 months old, 61% for SVGs 1–5 years

Table 29.2 Results of PTCA in patients after CABG surgery

Author/year	Patients	Stenoses	Success (%)	Q-wave MI (%)	Emergency CABG (%)	Death (%)	Restenosis (%)
Douglas et al. (1983)[28]	116	62	94	1.7	2.6	0	34
El Gamal et al. (1984)[29]	31	44	93	6.5	0	0	50
Dorros et al. (1984)[30]	61	33	79	4.9	1.6	3.3	46
Block et al. (1984)[31]	40	40	78	0	2.5	–	–
Corbelli et al. (1985)[32]	35	47	92	–	2	0	29
Dorros et al. (1985)[33]	–	82	90	–	–	–	20
Reeder et al. (1986)[34]	19	19	84	5.3	0	5.3	38
Ernst et al. (1987)[35]	83	33	97	2.4	0	0	31
Cote et al. (1987)[36]	82	101	85	3.6	1.2	0	23
Pinkerton et al. (1988)[37]	236	100	93	3	3	0.4	43
Cooper et al. (1989)[38]	59	24	75	5.1	0	1.7	–
Platko et al. (1989)[39]	101	107	91.8	5.9	2	2	61
Tabbalat et al. (1990)[40]	19	24	92	–	–	0	–
Webb et al. (1990)[41]	140	148	85	4	1.4	0	–
Jost et al. (1991)[42]	41	49	94	0	0	0	21
Meester et al. (1991)[43]	84	93	84	8.3	2.4	1.2	–
Plokker et al. (1991)[44]	454	–	90	2.8	1.3	0.7	–
Douglas et al. (1991)[106]	599	672	90	2.3	3.5	1.2	–
Reeves et al. (1991)[45,a]	57	64	95.3	3.5	1.8	1.8	56
Miranda et al. (1992)[26,b]	351	–	94	–	–	–	–
Morrison et al. (1994)[46]	75	89	94	3	1	3	–

[a] Reeves et al. reported a clinical success of 82.5%.
[b] Miranda et al. reported a 'major complication rate' of 5%.
Mean graft age varied from 26 to 98 months (range: 1–216 months).

old and 64% for SVGs >5 years of age. Restenosis rates average 24% for distal anastomotic lesions but 45% and 62%, respectively, for body and aorta-ostial lesions.[108] Short lesions were reported to have restenosis rates of 38% compared to virtually 100% for diffuse disease and total occlusions.[45] During clinical follow-up, Plokker et al.[44] reported that 5-year survival was 78% after successful PTCA but that event-free survival was only 26%. However, in those in whom PTCA failed, event-free survival was only 3%. Freedom from cardiac events was better in SVGs <1 year old compared to those 1–5 years and >5 years old (45% vs. 25% vs. 19%) or in those undergoing PTCA for total SVG occlusion (38%).

29.7.2 Excimer laser coronary angioplasty

Excimer laser can ablate plaque in SVGs. In 1992, a multicentre ELCA Registry reported a 91% procedural success rate (adjunctive PTCA in 80%) and 87% laser success in 514 SVG lesions in 434 patients, 80% of the SVGs were >3 years old.[109] Complications included perforation (1.1%), MI (2.3%), distal embolisation (4.1%), dissection (4.6%), acute closure (5%), death (0.9%) and emergency CABG surgery (0.7%). Restenosis occurred in 57% at 6 months. Other workers have also reported 92%–94% success rates and similar restenosis rates.[110,111] Complications are higher in lesions containing thrombus (embolisation 25% vs. 1%; MI 33% vs. 2%; abrupt closure 17% vs. 4%; restenosis 70% vs. 51%).[112,113]

Rigid, aorto-ostial lesions may be ideal for ELCA.[114] Eigler et al. reported a 90% procedural success and a 6-month restenosis rate of 47%.[115]

29.7.3 Rotablator atherectomy

Rotablator atherectomy is contraindicated in degenerated SVGs or grafts with thrombus and the technique has been used infrequently.[116–118] It may be used for rigid, balloon-resistant aorto-ostial stenosis.

When patients with SVG stenosis have lesions that are densely calcified, aorto-ostial or at the distal anastomosis they may benefit from rotational atherectomy. However, special expertise is required and these techniques albeit have unproven effect on long-term outcomes, and as such are infrequently used.[119–123]

29.7.4 Thrombolysis and thrombectomy

As lesions in SVGs have a high rate of thrombus, thrombolysis and thrombectomy techniques have been studied as adjunctive therapy for SVG stenosis or occlusion. It is not recommended to use thrombolytic therapy to treat SVG thrombus.[124] Unfortunately, intra-coronary thrombolytic therapy has been associated with thromboembolic MI, haemorrhagic complications and low long term graft patency rates. Intravenous thrombolytic therapy has similarly been found to be less effective.[125]

Catheter-based thrombectomy is an alternative to pharmacologic thrombolysis. However, none of the devices that can mechanically aspirate thrombus have been shown to improve clinically important outcomes.[122,124,126–129] These devices should rarely be used in this setting. For instance, the AngioJet device may occasionally be used in the setting of an extremely large clot burden.

29.7.5 Stenting

PTCA in SVGs >3 years old can be accompanied by a procedural complication rate of up to 15% reflecting the friable nature of late graft atherosclerosis.[36,39,45,130] Even successful PTCA often leaves a residual stenosis of almost 30% and is followed by angiographic restenosis rates of between 40% and 70% resulting in a high incidence of late cardiac events.[16,28,31,32,36,45,47,131] Endovascular stenting has therefore been proposed as an adjunctive procedure to PTCA for the management of SVG stenoses because of its ability to maximise the lumen's diameter and prevent elastic recoil after balloon dilatation,[132–134] making stents effective bail-out devices following acute failure of PTCA or atherectomy and for reducing late restenosis and reocclusion (see Figures 29.1 through 29.8).

Several studies have shown that stents can be successfully deployed (98%–100%) in SVGs with low complication rates (Table 29.3).[79,107,132,133,135–143] Preliminary data from the randomised trial of PTCA versus elective Palmaz–Schatz coronary stent placement for de novo SVG lesions (SAVED) showed stents having a higher procedural success rate (96% vs. 85%), a bigger final median lumen diameter (MLD) (2.85 mm vs. 2.12 mm), fewer clinical events (5.9% vs. 11.7%)

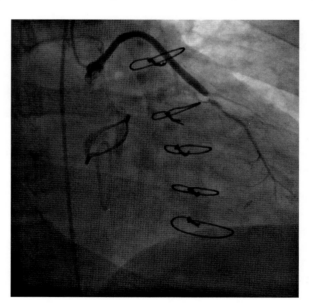

Figure 29.1 A 70-year-old male with a history of hyperlipidemia and type 2 diabetes presented with class III angina. He has a history of 3V CABG: SVG-D1, SVG-RCA, LIMA-mid LAD in 2008 following a MI. A coronary and graft angiography was performed: The SVG-first diagonal branch distal anastomotic site was found to be 90% obstructed by a single discrete lesion. The native first diagonal branch was also 100% occluded by a discrete lesion and 70% obstructed by diffuse disease.

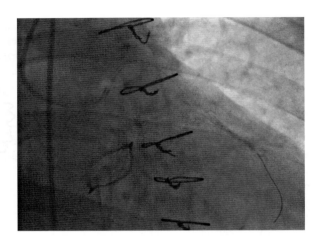

Figure 29.2 A 6 Fr LCB guiding catheter was utilised which provided reasonable fit at the vein graft origin. A balance middle weight (BMW) wire was advanced distally in the ramus and PTCA was performed initially on the native first diagonal branch with a series of dilations using a 2.0 mm × 15.0 mm Sprinter Legend Balloon. The pre-dilatation stenosis was 70%. The post-dilatation stenosis was 50%.

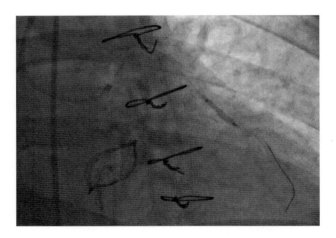

Figure 29.3 Subsequently successful PTCA of the distal anastomotic site of the SVG-first diagonal branch was performed next with a series of dilations using the same 2.0 mm × 15.0 mm Sprinter Legend Balloon. The pre-dilatation stenosis was 90%. The post-dilatation stenosis was 60%.

and a reduced need for CABG (0% vs. 6.7%), respectively.[144] Moreover unlike PTCA, the favourable early (97% vs. 97% procedural success) and 1 year clinical outcome (73% vs. 77% event free survival) after stent implantation are not diminished by advancing SVG age (<4 years vs. >4 years).[145] Early complications in the JJIS Registry included subacute thrombotic closure (1.4%), in-hospital death (1.7%), urgent CABG (2.9%) and Q-wave MI (0.3%).[136] The early regimens of aggressive anticoagulation with coumadin after stenting have been replaced by a combination of aspirin and clopidogrel, as well as high-pressure balloon inflation to ensure maximal MLDs, full stent expansion and complete wall apposition. Bleeding complications and their sequelae have diminished without any increase in acute thrombotic closures.[146]

Multi-vessel stenting has been shown to have lower overall in-hospital complications than redo CABG (death: 0% vs. 5.4%; Q-wave-MI: 1.1% vs. 2.0%; stroke 0% vs. 2.6%) and a shorter in-hospital stay (4 days vs. 9 days).[147] Although multiple SVG stenting has a similar in-hospital procedural success (97%) and major complication rate after 18 months as single SVG stenting (death/MI: 5.3%/2.9% vs. 5.6%/4.3%), periprocedural non-Q-wave-MI was higher (27.9% vs. 15.5%).[148] Stenting the native coronary vessels in post-CABG patients has a better 1 year outcome than stenting SVGs (death: 4.3% vs. 9.1%; MI: 2.3% vs. 4.5%) and a lower rate of post-procedural MI (13% vs. 18%).[70] At 30 days, an analysis of five randomised GP IIb/IIIa inhibitor trials showed that there are higher mortality rates with PCI for SVG stenosis than PCI for native disease (2.1% vs. 1.0%), with progressive increase in rates at 6 months (4.7% vs. 2.0%).[149]

A lower restenosis rate after stent implantation is almost certainly due to the greater gains in acute luminal improvement (0%–5% residual stenosis after stenting compared to 20%–30% after PTCA alone) since late intimal proliferation (late loss) after stenting may exceed that of PTCA (0.5–1.1 mm vs. 0.4–0.7 mm).[150–152] Six-month follow-up data from the SAVED trial also showed an improved clinical outcome for stenting in SVGs compared to PTCA even though restenosis rates were similar (37% vs. 46%) in the two groups.[144,153] In the JJIS Graft Registry of patients with symptomatic focal SVG stenoses, 6-month follow-up revealed an overall restenosis rate of 29.7% but lower (18.3%) in patients with de novo lesions and in patients with MLD >3 mm after final stent expansion (26%) than restenotic lesions.[139] Restenosis rates for stented SVGs were 17%–30% based on multiple observational studies[135,154,155] which are lower than the 40%–45% rate seen in previous historical controls involving PTCA and atherectomy.[16,154] The subacute thrombosis rate has been observed to be very low (approximately 1%–2%). This relatively lower rate is due to the larger luminal diameters of vein grafts in comparison to native coronary arteries.[135,155] Factors that were found to be predictive of restenosis included a restenotic lesion, stenosis at the aortic or coronary anastomosis, smaller reference vessel size, higher percent post-stent diameter stenosis and use of long or multiple stents.[155,156]

Other studies have reported low restenosis rates,[134,135] but there is significant variation relating to the site of the stenosis and the length of time to follow-up. For example, the restenosis rate after stenting non-ostial lesions (29%) has been shown to be lower than that for ostial lesions (60%–62%).[157,158]

The rate of restenosis at the distal site is lower in comparison to the aorto-ostial site or shaft portion of the vein graft, although the data is limited. In a review of PTCA versus stenting patients, a total of 182 patients were followed showing outcomes were the similar for both procedures. The success rate was 98%, with 1% having major ischaemic complications.[159] The STEMI rates were similar in both procedures (12% vs. 13% and 1% vs. 0%) after 17 months of follow-up. One major difference between the two was the higher rate of target lesion re-vascularisation (TLR) with PTCA (25% vs. 14%).

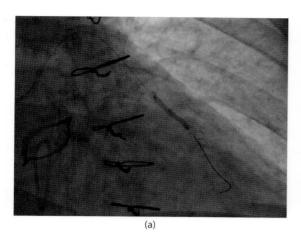
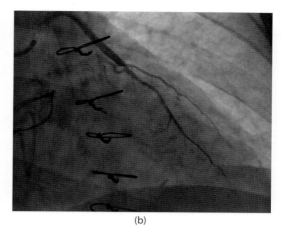

(a)   (b)

Figure 29.4 **(a)** Successful deployment of a 2.25 mm × 16 mm Taxus Liberte drug eluting stent at 14 atmospheres in the native first diagonal branch was performed. **(b)** The pre-deployment stenosis was 50%. The post-deployment stenosis was 0%.

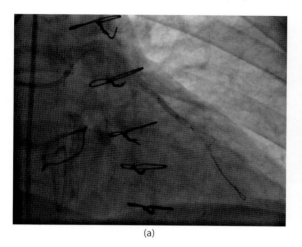
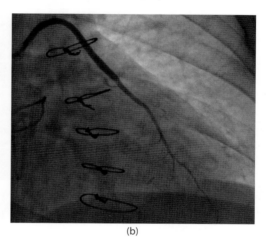

(a)   (b)

Figure 29.5 **(a)** Successful deployment of a 2.75 mm × 12.0 mm Xience drug eluting stent at 14 atmospheres in the distal anastomotic site of the SVG-first diagonal branch was performed next. **(b)** The pre-deployment stenosis was 60%. The post-deployment stenosis was 0%. The angiographic result was excellent with downstream TIMI III flow.

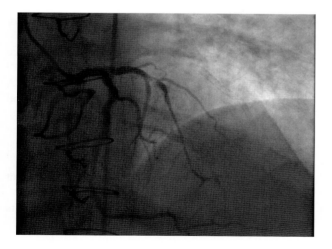

Figure 29.6 The native middle LAD artery was also found to be 90% obstructed by a calcified discrete lesion on diagnostic angiography. It partially filled antegradely from the LIMA graft. It was decided to intervene on this lesion to allow for maximal myocardial re-vascularisation.

Higher mortality rates and TLR at 1 year also occurred with SVG stenting in patients with diabetes. At 1 year, diabetic patients had a lower rate of cardiac event-free survival.[160]

Unfortunately, the longer-term results are less optimal. In the JJIS Graft Registry the 12-month event-free survival for the entire cohort was 76.3% and TVR was 13.3% (5.4% CABG and 7.9% repeat PTCA). Similarly Le May et al.[161] showed a 98% in-hospital success rate with no intraoperative deaths, but follow-up at 18 months showed a 15% death rate, 17% had MI, 20% required repeat CABG and 37% repeat PTCA. Event-free survival occurred in only 44% of cases and cumulative survival at 2.5 years was 78.7%.

Sketch et al.[162] have indicated that late (2 years) clinical outcomes after stent implantation in SVGs progressively deteriorate such that event-free survival was only 75%, 67% and 55% at 6, 12 and 24 months, respectively, and that death (5% vs. 8% vs. 14%), CABG (7% vs. 9% vs. 12%) and PTCA (6% vs. 8% vs. 12%) increased steadily. Further deterioration at the stent site (late restenosis), increasing TLR events,

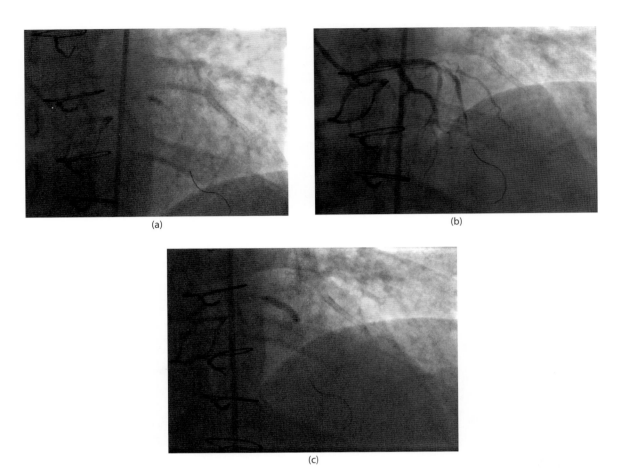

(a)

(b)

(c)

Figure 29.7 (a) Next, the operators exchanged for a 6 Fr JL-4 guide which fit reasonably well in the native left main. A BMW wire was advanced distally and was used to pre-dilate the calcified mid LAD stenosis with a 2.5 mm × 6 mm Sprinter Legend balloon, requiring up to 12 atm for lesion expansion. (b) The pre-dilation stenosis was 90%. The post-dilation stenosis was 50%. Angiography revealed some dissection at the lesion site. (c) This was covered with a 3.0 mm × 18.0 mm Xience drug-eluting stent deployed at 12 atmospheres in the native middle LAD artery.

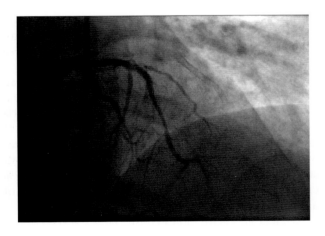

Figure 29.8 The pre-deployment stenosis was 50%. The post-deployment stenosis was 0%. The angiographic result was excellent with preserved downstream flow and competitive distal LAD filling with the LIMA graft.

less favourable baseline characteristics and progression of disease at other sites[163] are responsible.

A study of 1062 patients evaluated the in-hospital incidence and risk factors of PCI and of major cardiac events post-PCI.[164] These patients with SVG stenosis were treated with PTCA alone (42%), laser or atherectomy (16%) or stenting (42%) and followed for 3 years. The following findings were noted:

- The incidence of in-hospital major adverse cardiac events was 13%; death occurred in 8%, MI in 2% and bypass surgery was performed in 3%. Predictors of an in-hospital event were a restenotic lesion, unstable angina and heart failure.
- Late major coronary events occurred in 54% of patients and included death in 9%, MI in 9% and TVR in 36%.
- Angiographic restenosis occurred significantly less often in stented grafts (29% vs. 43% in non-stented grafts). However, there was no event-free or survival benefit with stenting, due at least in part to progressive disease at non-stented sites.

Table 29.3 Results of stent implantation for SVG disease

Author/year	Stent	Patients	Success (%)	Reference MLD mm	Stenosis MLD mm	Thrombosis (%)	Haemorrhage complications (%)	MI (%)	CABG (%)	Death (%)	Restenosis (%)	Peripheral vascular complications
Urban et al. (1989)[133]	Wallstent	13	100	–	–	0	8	0	–	0	38	–
Leon et al. (1991)[136]	P-S	192	98	–	–	–	–	1	1.6	1.6	26	–
Pomerantz et al. (1992)[132]	P-S	69	99	3.6	3.6	0	7	13	–	0	25	–
Bilodeau et al. (1992)[137]	G-R	37	100	–	–	–	21	13[c]	–	0	35	–
de Schreeder et al. (1992)[138]	Wallstent	69	100	3.3	2.7	10	33	6	–	4.3	47	–
White et al. (1993)[107]	P-S[a]	67	100	3.6	3.7	3.2	10	6.4	–	3.2	32	–
Leon et al. (1993)[139]	P-S	589	99[e]	3.2	3.4	1.4	15	0.3	2.9	1.7	30	14.3
Piana et al. (1994)[135]	P-S[b]	150	98	3.7	3.65	0.6	16	7[c]	0	0.6	17	8.5
Rechavia et al. (1995)[79,d]	P-S	29	100	3.2	3.3	0	–	7[c]	0	0	–	3
Wong et al. (1995)[141]	P-S[b]	231	99[f]	3.3	2.95	0.9	25	13[c]	0.4	1.3	–	8.4
Savage et al. (1997)[144], Wong et al. (1995)[145]	P-S	110[g]	95									

[a] Palmaz-Schatz peripheral
[b] Palmaz-Schatz coronary and biliary stents
[c] Most non-Q wave MI
[d] Aorta-ostial SVG lesions
[e] Clinical success = 97%
[f] Procedural success = 95.3%; clinical success = 93.6%
[g] Randomised SAVED Trial 110 Pts stented versus 110 Pts PTCA

Overall survival at 5 years was reported in one observational study to be 83% but event-free survival only 30%. Pooled data analysis from the literature showed similar results with 5-year survival being 26% after PTCA, 30% after stenting and 63%–76% after repeat CABG.[165] A study of SVG disease compared to native vessel disease in 175 patients at 5 years, showed poorer overall and event-free survival.[166] The increased need for repeat re-vascularisation was primarily due to progression of disease at other sites.

Most stents can be used in SVGs but because of the volume of friable atherothrombotic material often present, stents with a higher metal: artery ratio or covered stents may be most appropriate, especially since there are no side branches in SVGs. The self-expanding Wallstent® (Schneider/Boston Scientific) and the balloon-expandable Ultra™ stent (Guidant) are two stents appropriate for SVGs and are available in large diameters (2.5–6.0 mm) and a range of lengths (15–30 mm). The WINS Registry showed that the Wallstent produces good results in large (up to 5.5 mm) SVGs with 8.6% TLR and 30% angiographic restenosis rates at 6 months,[167,168] although the WINS randomised trial showed similar in-hospital and 6-month outcomes from the Wallstent and the Palmaz–Schatz® stents.[167]

For very large SVGs and those with complex disease[169,170] the Palmaz–Schatz Biliary Stent (4–9 mm) is also of use but can be a technically demanding implant procedure.[171] The greater radial strength comes from its thicker struts and is of value for treating tough aorto-ostial lesions. In the study reported by Piana et al., the lesion MLD increased from 0.98 mm to 3.7 mm, the diameter stenosis fell from 74% to 1%[135] and restenosis occurred in only 17%. Wong et al. reported a high angiographic (100% vs. 98%) and procedural success (97% vs. 96%) and a low subacute thrombosis rate (0% vs. 1.7%) in groups receiving coronary and biliary stents.[141] Major complications were infrequent – 2.9% and 1.4% for the coronary and biliary groups, respectively. Six-month event-free survival was favourable (80%) in both groups.

Now commonly procedures are combined. Severe aorto-ostial lesions or bulky eccentric stenoses in the proximal or body of SVGs can be modified and then stented to improve the acute result although the long-term result may not be any different than lesions treated by direct stenting.[121] Rigid aorto-ostial lesions may also be ablated by Rotablator atherectomy before stent implantation. Left main PCI in the setting of an occluded bypass graft to either the LAD artery or left circumflex artery should be of strong consideration, if the bypass to the opposite vessel is patent (see Figures 29.6 through 29.8).

Although restenosis is less frequent in PCI than with angioplasty alone, it still remains an important problem. Although data on native vessels predominate in trials to date, drug-eluting stents result in a lower rate of restenosis and it is expected that future outcomes data and trial results will highlight this advance.

29.7.6 Acute coronary syndrome

Urgent re-vascularisation and early angiography is recommended in an acute coronary syndrome (ACS). There are limited studies that compare this approach in patients with a prior CABG and an ACS, but in most cases PCI is preferred over CABG due to the fact of the delay in time to re-vascularisation in CABG and the higher mortality rate associated with repeat CABG.

Culprit-vessel only PCI is recommended for patients with ST elevation MI after CABG in the absence of cardiogenic shock.[172] Stabilisation in these patients is of importance. If a single culprit lesion can be identified in a patient with non-ST elevated ACS, culprit only PCI should be performed. Contrast volumes and high radiation doses can become a concern with multi-vessel PCI.

If stents are to be employed, we recommend prior administration of usual measures for the prevention of thrombosis, including loading with antiplatelet agents (e.g. aspirin and clopidogrel), and be prepared to treat bleeding complications as needed.

29.7.7 Covered stents

The Jostent® coronary stent graft is characterised by an expandable polytetrafluoroethylene (PTFE) membrane placed between two layers of stainless steel stent struts. This may prevent friable material being forced through the stent struts and into the lumen and hence reduce in-stent restenosis. Stent lengths of 9, 12, 19 and 26 mm are available and come ready mounted on a rapid-exchange balloon catheter (2.5–5.0 mm). High-pressure (>16 atm) is necessary for deployment. They can be successfully deployed and may reduce restenosis in SVGs.[173–175]. It must be remembered that re-endothelialisation, which can only start at either end of the stent due to the PTFE covering, is significantly delayed and in-stent thrombosis may be a problem unless clopidogrel is continued for 3–4 months.

29.8 Complications

The complications which occur after intervention in SVGs are shown in Table 29.4.

Table 29.4 Complications of intervention after CABG surgery

Acute occlusion
Acute dissection
Distal embolisation
Acute myocardial infarction
Perforation
Death
Restenosis

29.8.1 Acute occlusion

Abrupt closure is more common after PTCA and PCI in grafts than in the native coronary arteries (1.5% vs. 6%) and may be due to localised occlusive thrombus, dissection flaps or embolic phenomenon in older grafts. Prolonged inflation with a perfusion balloon and/or stenting may rectify the situation. Non-Q-wave and Q-wave MI (0%–8.3%) may result. CABG is necessary in 0%–3.5% and death may occur in 0%–5.3%. Emergency CABG for occlusion of SVG or native vessel has a high mortality (up to 15%) if the patient is ischaemic prior to surgery.[71,176]

29.8.2 Coronary embolism

Coronary embolism is a more common problem typically occurring during or after PCI in SVGs. It is a phenomenon involving embolisation of atherothrombotic debris downstream curing catheter intervention which can result in an elevation of cardiac enzymes, no-reflow (microvascular dysfunction), non-ST elevation MI (NSTEMI) or STEMI.[177] The theory behind this phenomenon is that the atherosclerotic plaque that develops in SVGs in particular is softer, more friable and leads to increased thrombus formation and enhanced platelet activation in comparison to atherosclerotic plaque seen in coronary arteries.[178]

Coronary embolism (3%–15%) is more common after intervention in SVGs than in native vessels due to the presence of larger volumes of friable atheromatous material and thrombus. Bulky lesions in grafts greater than 3 years old, totally occluded and diffusely diseased SVGs have a higher risk of embolism (up to 15%)[179] which may give rise to MI[180] and the 'no-reflow' phenomenon.[181] Cardiogenic shock and death may occur if important distal coronary circulation is lost or temporarily occluded by extensive embolisation. Emergency CABG is unlikely to prevent MI.[182] Major CK-MB elevations may occur after 15% of otherwise successful SVG interventions and is associated with increased late mortality.[183] Treatment includes continued heparinisation, glyceryl trinitrate infusion, intra-graft verapamil and intra-aortic balloon counterpulsation. The administration of abciximab peri-procedurally does not appear to reduce major adverse clinical events.[184] Because of the higher risk of distal embolisation during PCI of bypass grafts, PCI of the native coronary vessels is always preferred.[185] However, the development and use of novel EPD has made significant advances in lowering risk of SVG interventions and in making them safer and more effective strategies today.[73,186,187]

29.8.3 Perforation

Perforation typically occurs due to a vessel wall penetration with a stiff guidewire, balloon inflation with an oversized balloon catheter, subintimal balloon inflation or stent implantation, atherectomy device or atheroablative techniques. Pericardial and mediastinal fibrosis often protects against free rupture and cardiac tamponade, although this can occur.[202] SVGs may rupture with only slight balloon oversizing in older grafts.[203]

Prolonged inflation with a perfusion balloon, reversal of heparinisation or stenting with a covered stent may all be effective strategies to treat a perforation. In a study analysing 41 perforations, a PTFE covered stent successfully sealed the perforation completely in 92.9% cases and partially in 7.1%.[186]

29.8.4 Restenosis

Restenosis rates after intervention in SVGs are higher than in native vessels (45%–65%) and increase with age of the graft. It is also dependent on site of lesion (with ostial lesions having higher and distal lesions lower restenosis rates). Stenting has lower restenosis rates compared to other techniques (details in Section 29.7.5).

29.8.5 No–reflow

No-reflow or slow flow is multifactorial and is usually secondary to vasospasm or atheroembolisation. Vasospasm typically responds to vasodilators like calcium channel blockers (such as nicardipine), adenosine and nitroprusside.[187] Nitroglycerine has been seen to be ineffective in most cases of vasospasm in SVGs.

29.9 Use of embolic protection devices

EPD have been shown to reduce atheroembolic MI by approximately 50% across all strata of patients, which strongly support its routine use in all PCI of SVGs (especially in older grafts).[73] Unfortunately, it is used in only half of SVG PCI procedures in current interventional practice.

These devices function to trap blood and suspended debris during PCI, and enable their evacuation before normal blood flow is restored.[188] It has been revealed that during SVG PCI, large amounts of atheroembolic debris are liberated[130,188–190] including vasoactive substances that can potentially impair microvascular perfusion.[191] These substances include endothelin, serotonin and a variety of coagulation components that have been shown to be liberated during SVG PCI, removal of which is postulated to lead to improved immediate post-PCI coronary flow and microvascular perfusion.

The first EPD employed was the PercuSurge Guardwire™ (PercuSurge Inc., Sunnyvale, CA). It is an emboli-containment system which consists of a hollow 0.014 in. PTCA wire incorporating a compliant inflatable distal occlusion balloon. During occlusion of the distal graft, PTCA and stent placement can be performed after which the Export™ monorail aspiration catheter is used to remove potentially embolic debris prior to deflation of the occlusion balloon.[130,192,193]

The SAFER trial evaluated 801 patients with SVG stenosis who were assigned stent placement over the PercuSurge GuardWire or an angioplasty guidewire.[194] The use of the EPD reduced the incidence of MI (8.6% vs. 14.7%) and the no-reflow phenomenon (3% vs. 9%). Although beneficial, the PercuSurge GuardWire did not completely protect the patient from atheroembolisation and did not improve outcomes compared to PCI alone, as seen in the EMERALD study.[195]

The FilterWire EX system was later developed. Initial experience with this system showed importance of the operator learning curve as well as of device-specific and anatomic factors for achieving optimal efficacy. Operator dependent factors included inadequate filter apposition against the SVG wall, not protecting proximal native side branches and deployment in excessively distal lesions resulting in incomplete filter opening. However, with increased operator experience and attention to these details, a significant reduction in 30-day peri-procedural MI rates from 21.3% to 11.3% was seen.[196]

Subsequently, the FIRE trial was designed to compare the FilterWire EX system with the PercuSurge GuardWire. A total of 651 patients undergoing SVG PCI were included in the trial and randomised to either system. Procedural success rates were 96% for the FilterWire EX system and 97% for the PercuSurge GuardWire. The primary efficacy outcome (a composite endpoint of death, MI or TVR) at 30 days was 9.9% for the FilterWire and 11.6% for the PercuSurge.[187,197] The primary efficacy outcome remained comparable at 6 months with the two systems, but the incidence of new events increased in an additional 10% of overall patients; 19.3% in FilterWire group and 21.9% in PercuSurge group, with TVR performed in 9.1%.

Due to the slight superiority of the FilterWire over the PercuSurge and its ease of use, it has become the EPD of choice in most cardiac catheterisation laboratories across the United States.

The TriActiv system, another EPD consisting of a balloon-protection flush and extraction device, was compared to the PercuSurge GuardWire and the FilterWire EX system in the PRIDE trial. It was found to be non-inferior to the other two systems but was associated with higher bleeding complications.[198]

The AngioGuard™ device (Boston-Scientific), an EPD which employs a PVC net/filter can be deployed in the distal SVG prior to intervention to catch embolising debris and prevent it from going distally. The umbrella-shaped net behaves like a sieve with 100 μm pores which allows distal perfusion. The net can be closed once the intervention is completed and the material is then retrieved.

Distal protection devices have many limitations such as passage of the device across a stenotic lesion before distal projection is in place, debris occlusion, movement of toxic soluble mediators into the distal myocardium, and inability to use the device in distal lesions. These limitations have resulted in the development of proximal occlusion devices and plaque trapping devices.[190,199,200]

A proximal embolic protection system named the Proxis system has been developed. It consists of a proximal sealing balloon and subsequent aspiration of stagnated blood post-intervention. Its efficacy was evaluated in the PROXIMAL trial, comprising 594 patients undergoing stenting of 639 SVG lesions. These patients were randomised to proximal embolic protection (Proxis) when possible (and distal embolic protection, when proximal protection not possible) or to the established distal embolic protection when possible (and no embolic protection when not possible).[190] The primary efficacy outcome (a composite endpoint of death, MI or TVR) at 30 days was 9.2% in the Proxis group and 10.0% in the distal group. No significant difference in the primary efficacy outcome was seen between the two groups. As such, this trial has provided the interventionalist with another viable strategy in cases where distal EPDs cannot be deployed.

Patients that have in-stent restenosis in SVGs have lesions that consist primarily of neo-intimal proliferation and tend to have a lower embolic potential. The role and efficacy of an EPD in such a scenario remains equivocal. This became evident in a study of 54 patients who had PCI for in-stent restenosis in SVGs without a distal EPD.[201] No procedure related MIs and no episodes of no-reflow or slow flow occurred during the procedure. However, more robust studies are needed (due to their small sample size) to determine the validity and reliability of these findings.

Nevertheless, EPDs remain grossly underutilised in SVG interventions. This is in spite of trial data having proven their efficacy in minimising the deleterious effect of downstream debris phenomenon and as such leading to improved outcomes of PCI in SVG stenosis.[190,199]

29.10 Results of intervention in IMA grafts

IMAs seem less susceptible than SVGs to atherosclerosis, yield superior clinical results over SVGs during 20 years of follow-up[19,66,68,204,205] and 95% are patent at 10 years. However, problems do occur and up to 9% of IMAs have been reported to be stenosed or occluded within 2 years of surgery. IMA grafts most frequently develop a proliferative lesion at the distal site and less commonly at the ostium or within the shaft.[26,206–215] Occlusion of the IMA in its ostium or shaft has been typically attributed more due to trauma to the pedicle during mobilisation at the time of surgery, and may present as a late surgical complication needing interventional treatment.[216–218] IMAs are also prone to vasospasm and patients can be pretreated with nitrates and calcium channel blockers before intervention.

29.10.1 PTCA versus PCI Stenting

The ideal approach was studied in a review of 174 patients (202 lesions) where ostial lesions were treated predominantly with PCI (66% cases) and distal anastomotic lesions were treated predominantly with PTCA (71% cases).[206] Procedural success was excellent for both with 96.8% for ostial lesion PCI and 96.7% for distal anastomotic lesion PTCA. For the ostial site of the IMA graft, overall TLR was 25%; 40% for patients treated with PTCA and 18% for patients treated with PCI. For the distal anastomotic site, overall TLR was 7%; 33% for patients treated with PCI and 4.3% for patients treated with PTCA. The in-hospital mortality was 0.6%, rate of urgent CABG was 0.6%, and no cases of MI occurred. On 1 year follow-up, mortality rate was 4.4% and MI occurred in 2.9% of the patients. Thus, these results

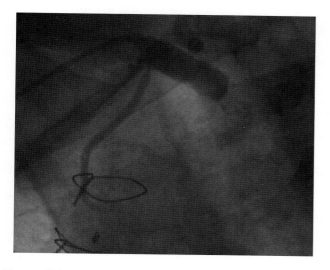

Figure 29.9 A 67-year-old male with a history of coronary artery disease, dyslipidemia, hypertension, status post–5V CABG (1987): LIMA–D1, RIMA–RCA, SVG-ramus intermedius, SVG–OM1, SVG–OM2 and re-do 3V CABG (1996): SVGs to OM1, OM2 and OM3 presented with throat tightness.

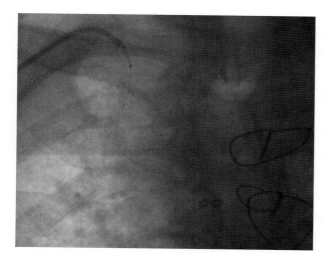

Figure 29.10 Initially, a 6-Fr JR4 guiding catheter with side holes was used to engage the ostium of the right IMA graft but this attempt was unsuccessful. A 90-cm, 6-Fr IMA guiding catheter was then utilised which provided good fit and adequate support for the entire duration of the procedure. A BMW wire was advanced through the ostial graft stenosis and then further on down the very tortuous course of the right IMA graft out into the distal RCA.

favour an approach of PCI for ostial lesions and PTCA for distal anastomotic lesions. If PTCA of a distal anastomotic lesion is suboptimal, then PCI should be considered (see Figure 29.9 through 29.15).

He underwent an adenosine sestamibi nuclear study which revealed a medium-sized area of drug-induced ischemia involving the inferior and inferolateral segments. Subsequently, a coronary and graft angiography was performed: A significant stenosis (70%) at the ostium of the RIMA graft to the distal RCA was seen.

Angiographic restenosis in LIMAs occurs in 0%–31% of successfully treated patients, although the exact incidence is unknown because follow-up angiography is infrequent in most studies.[210,211,215,219] Restenosis is especially infrequent in distal anastomotic lesions. During clinical follow-up, 73.3% had class I–III angina, after a mean of 20.5 months. Actuarial survival at 1 and 5 years was 95% and 92.3% and event-free survival was 88% and 82%, respectively.[220] Dimas et al.[221] reported similar results.

29.11 Hybrid approach

The hybrid approach is a newer re-vascularisation concept that has garnered recent attention. It involves a combination of PCI and CABG to achieve complete re-vascularisation for the patient in a staged fashion. It posits that due to the poorer long-term patency outcomes and clinical endpoints associated with SVGs, pure arterial graft re-vascularisation should be attempted during the initial CABG procedure. This has been primarily proposed to be a LIMA to the LAD graft. For re-vascularisation of the non-LAD vessels, PCI is then advocated given its relative efficacy and safety profile vis-à-vis SVGs. This would simplify the surgical procedure and reduce operation related complications and cardiopulmonary bypass time. However, randomised controlled trials are currently needed to evaluate the effectiveness of this

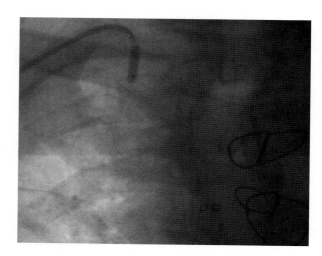

Figure 29.11 Given the non-calcified character and very discrete nature of the stenosis, it was decided on direct stenting with a 3.0 mm × 8.0 mm Xience drug eluting stent, which was deployed at 12 atm.

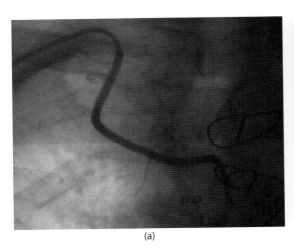
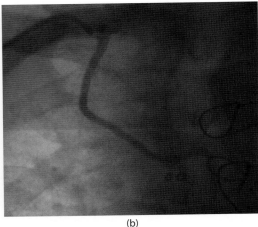

(a)   (b)

Figure 29.12 (a) Successful stent deployment in the graft origin of the RIMA to the distal right coronary artery was performed. The pre-deployment stenosis was 70%. The post-deployment stenosis was 0%. (b) Post-dilation was performed with the stent balloon to flare the ostium with two inflations up to 14 atm. The post-procedure result looked excellent with a rapid distal runoff.

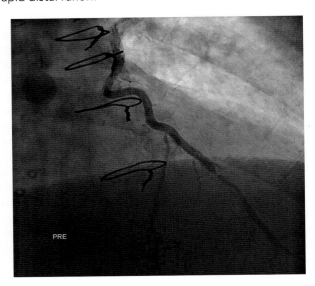

Figure 29.13 A 60-year-old male with a history of diabetes, hypertension, dyslipidemia, peripheral arterial disease and a history of 3V CABG in 2003: LIMA-mid LAD, SVG-diagonal and a radial artery graft-OM1 presents in the setting of dyspnoea and an NSTEMI. A coronary and graft angiography was performed: LIMA-mid LAD distal anastomotic site was found to be 90% obstructed by a single discrete lesion.

staged PCI-arterial CABG procedure versus a traditional CABG (arterial plus venous grafts) procedure.

29.12 Guideline recommendations

The 2011 American College of Cardiology Foundation/American Heart Association/Society for Cardiovascular Angiography and Interventions (ACC/AHA/SCAI) focused update for PCI state that in patients with early ischaemia (typically within 30 days) after CABG, PCI should be performed and is a class I indication.[97,222] When the lesion is in a SVG, the use of an embolic protection device is recommended and is a class I indication.

The ACC/AHA/SCAI guidelines recommend a class III indication for PCI in chronically occluded SVGs.

The 2011 ACC Foundation/AHA CABG guideline and the 2011 ACC Foundation/ AHA/SCAI PCI guidelines[97,222] recommend that the decision to proceed with repeat CABG rather than PCI should be undertaken only after consideration of the following factors: lesions unsuitable for PCI, chronically occluded coronary arteries, number of diseased bypass grafts, availability of the IMA for grafting and good distal targets available for bypass graft placement.

For patients with an ACS, PCI instead of CABG is recommended (*Grade 1B*). If PCI is performed, re-vascularisation of only the culprit lesion should be done at the time of the initial procedure.

For patients with a non-ACS presentation:

- Significant obstruction in the proximal LAD artery or left main artery (in unprotected and protected CABG patients) and evidence of extensive anterior ischaemia on non-invasive stress testing or significant disease in other vessels, should undergo PCI. Re-vascularisation in such patients is likely to improve survival, similar to patients with native coronary artery disease (*Grade 1B*).
- Obstructive disease but without extensive anterior ischaemia, a trial of medical therapy should be offered before attempt at re-vascularisation (*Grade 2B*).
- Refractory angina despite optimal medical therapy, PCI is recommended rather than CABG (*Grade 2B*).

29.13 Conclusions

Catheter-based intervention after CABG surgery can be an extremely useful means of alleviating angina pectoris and in

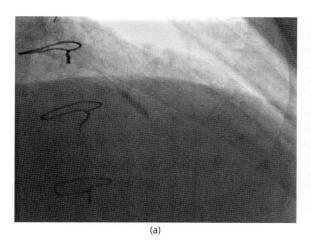
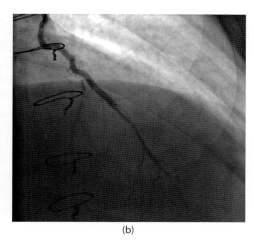

(a)　　　　　　　　　　　　　　　　　(b)

Figure 29.14 (a) A 6-Fr IMA guiding catheter was used to engage the ostium of the LIMA graft. This provided adequate support for the procedure. A Whisper wire was used to cross the 90% distal LIMA anastomotic lesion. PTCA was performed with a series of dilations using a 2.0 mm × 15.0 mm Sprinter Legend Balloon across the lesion at 12 atm for 20 seconds and repeat inflations at 12 atm for 12 seconds and 16 atm for 50 seconds. (b) The lesion was reduced to 50% post-serial dilations. Due to the suboptimal result despite serial dilations at the distal anastomotic site, it was decided to proceed with stenting.

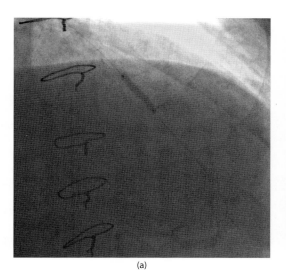
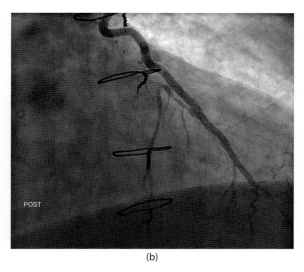

(a)　　　　　　　　　　　　　　　　　(b)

Figure 29.15 (a) Successful deployment of a 2.75 mm × 18.0 mm Driver bare-metal stent at 10 atm for 16 seconds in the distal LIMA-mid LAD anastomotic lesion was performed. (b) The pre-deployment stenosis was 50%. The post-deployment stenosis was 0%. Repeat angiogram showed an excellent result with a well-apposed stent having TIMI III flow down the distal vessel.

decreasing mortality in patients who have developed recurrent symptoms due to advancing native coronary artery disease or disease within the grafts themselves. This may delay the need for further surgical intervention or be the only alternative to medical therapy when repeat CABG is contraindicated. Wherever possible, PCI to amenable lesions in the native coronary circulation should be considered since restenosis rates are lower than in the SVGs. Maximum myocardial re-vascularisation should be sought at the least risk possible to the patient by formulating a strategy prior to the procedure after due discussion with surgical colleagues, the patient and the patient's family members. However, stent implantation is useful for improving suboptimal PTCA results and for reducing restenosis rates after balloon dilatation. Due to the lower rates of restenosis similar to what is seen in the native circulation, PCI with DES has essentially replaced balloon angioplasty as the treatment of cho ice.[16,144,154,164]. However, historically not much success has been achieved with chronically occluded SVGs or those with marked tortuosity and diffuse disease where there is a real risk of distal embolisation, MI and even death in the absence of an EPD.

It is our practice to proceed with emergent cardiac catheterisation in patients who develop acute ischaemia soon after CABG. PCI should be performed when technically feasible and especially if at least a moderate amount of myocardium is at jeopardy, and should be always preferred to repeat CABG. We recommend exercising caution and extreme care when performing interventions on fresh anastomoses. For early treatment of distal anastomoses, we recommend low-pressure balloon angioplasty, with stenting reserved only in cases of suboptimal results. The operator should be prepared and skilled to treat possible perforation amongst other complications, either with balloon angioplasty or placement of covered stents, as needed. For severely thrombotic grafts, we recommend revascularisation of the underlying native coronary system instead, due to the current reported increased risk with PCI of a totally occluded SVG.

It is important to remember that the majority of studies and centres to date have reported data and outcomes of more contemporary SVG interventions, prior to the advent of DES and EPDs and as such are likely not reflective of the true advantages of PCI in the post-CABG era. With the aging population and advancements in optimal medical therapies, the progressive development of late atherosclerosis in SVGs is inevitable and will pose an ever increasing challenge to the interventionalist.

Unfortunately, SVG PCI continues to be plagued by increased atheroembolic MI risk, subsequent in-stent restenosis and progressive vein graft disease. EPDs remain grossly underutilised today and highlight the need for more physician education to change current interventional practice and long-term outcomes. Outcome data with DES are awaited and hold promise. As such, this calls for a more aggressive and concerted effort from the interventional community, if we are to move forwards in conquering this growing and evolving complex disease process and rise to its many challenges.

References

1. Campeau L et al. Loss of the improvement of angina between 1 and 7 years after aortocoronary bypass surgery: Correlations with changes in vein grafts and in coronary arteries. *Circulation* 1979; 60(2 Pt 2): 1–5.
2. Johnson WD et al. Angina pectoris and coronary bypass surgery: Patterns of prevalence and recurrence in 3105 consecutive patients followed up to 11 years. *Am Heart J* 1984; 108(5): 1190–7.
3. Cameron A et al. Aortocoronary bypass surgery: A 7-year follow-up. *Circulation* 1979; 60(2 Pt 2): 9–13.
4. Fitzgibbon GM et al. Coronary bypass graft fate; long-term angiographic study. *J Am Coll Cardiol* 1991; 17: 1075–80.
5. Lawrie GM et al. Vein graft patency and intimal proliferation after aortocoronary bypass: Early and long-term angiopathologic correlations. *Am J Cardiol* 1976; 38(7): 856–62.
6. Bourassa MG et al. Progression of atherosclerosis in coronary arteries and bypass grafts: Ten years later. *Am J Cardiol* 1984; 53(12): 102C–7C.
7. Frick MH et al. Progression of coronary artery disease in randomized medical and surgical patients over a 5-year angiographic follow-up. *Am J Cardiol* 1983; 52(7): 681–5.
8. Hwang MH et al. Progression of native coronary artery disease at 10 years: Insights from a randomized study of medical versus surgical therapy for angina. *J Am Coll Cardiol* 1990; 16(5): 1066–70.
9. Campeau L et al. The relation of risk factors to the development of atherosclerosis in saphenous-vein bypass grafts and the progression of disease in the native circulation. A study 10 years after aortocoronary bypass surgery. *N Engl J Med* 1984; 311(21): 1329–32.
10. Bourassa MG et al. Long-term fate of bypass grafts: The Coronary Artery Surgery Study (CASS) and Montreal Heart Institute experiences. *Circulation* 1985; 72(6 Pt 2): V71–8.
11. Lytle, BW et al. Use of multiple arterial grafts and its effect on long-term outcome. *Curr Opin Cardiol* 2002; 17:594–7.
12. Campeau L et al. Atherosclerosis and late closure of aortocoronary saphenous vein grafts: Sequential angiographic studies at 2 weeks, 1 year, 5 to 7 years and 10 to 12 years after surgery. *Circulation* 1983; 68: 1–7.
13. Fitzgibbon GM et al. Coronary bypass graft fate. Angiographic grading of 1400 consecutive grafts early after operation and of 1132 after 1 year. *Circulation* 1978; 57(6): 1070–4.
14. Bourassa MG. Fate of venous grafts: The past, the present and the future. *J Am Coll Cardiol* 1991; 17(5): 1081–3.
15. Hamby RI et al. Aortocoronary saphenous vein bypass grafts. Long-term patency, morphology and blood flow in patients with patent grafts early after surgery. *Circulation* 1979; 60(4): 901–9.
16. de Feyter PJ et al. Balloon angioplasty for the treatment of lesions in saphenous vein bypass grafts. *J Am Coll Cardiol* 1993; 21(7): 1539–49.
17. Foster ED. Reoperation for recurrent coronary artery disease. *Adv Cardiol* 1988; 36: 162–4.
18. Loop FD. Repeat coronary bypass surgery: Selection of cases, surgical risks and long-term outlook. *Mod Conc Cardiovasc Dis* 1986; 55: 31–6.
19. Cameron A et al. Reoperation for coronary artery disease. 10 years of clinical follow-up. *Circulation* 1988; 78(3 Pt 2): I158–62.
20. Hall RJ et al. Reoperation for coronary artery disease. *Am J Coll Cardiol* 1986; 7: 32A.
21. Brenowitz JB et al. Coronary artery bypass grafting for the third time or more. *Circulation* 1988; 78: 166–70.
22. Jones EL et al. Percutaneous saphenous vein angioplasty to avoid reoperative bypass surgery. *Ann Thorac Surg* 1983; 36(4): 389–95.
23. Laird-Meeter K et al. Incidence, risk, and outcome of reintervention after aortocoronary bypass surgery. *Br Heart J* 1987; 57(5): 427–35.
24. Lytle BW et al. Fifteen hundred coronary reoperations. Results and determinants of early and late survival. *J Thorac Cardiovasc Surg* 1987; 93(6): 847–59.
25. Schaff HV et al. The morbidity and mortality of reoperation for coronary artery disease and analysis of late results with use of actuarial estimate of event-free interval. *J Thorac Cardiovasc Surg* 1983; 85(4): 508–15.
26. Miranda CP et al. Angioplasty of older saphenous vein grafts continues to be a sound therapeutic option. *Coll Cardiol* 1992; 19: 350A.
27. Douglas JS et al. Changing perspectives in vein graft angioplasty. *Am J Coll Cardiol* 1995; 25 A: 78–9.
28. Douglas JS., Jr et al. Percutaneous transluminal coronary angioplasty in patients with prior coronary bypass surgery. *J Am Coll Cardiol* 1983; 2(4): 745–54.

29. El Gamal M et al. Percutaneous transluminal angioplasty of stenosed aortocoronary bypass grafts. *Br Heart J* 1984; 52(6): 617–20.

30. Dorros G et al. Percutaneous transluminal coronary angioplasty in patients with prior coronary artery bypass grafting. *J Thorac Cardiovasc Surg* 1984; 87(1): 17–26.

31. Block PC et al. Percutaneous angioplasty of stenoses of bypass grafts or of bypass graft anastomotic sites. *Am J Cardiol* 1984; 53(6): 666–8.

32. Corbelli J et al. Percutaneous transluminal coronary angioplasty after previous coronary artery bypass surgery. *Am J Cardiol* 1985; 56(7): 398–403.

33. Dorros G, and Janke L.M. Complex coronary angioplasty in patients with prior coronary artery bypass surgery, in situations utilizing multiple coronary angioplasties, and in coronary occlusions. *Cardiol Clin* 1985; 3(1): 49–71.

34. Reeder GS et al. Angioplasty for aortocoronary bypass graft stenosis. *Mayo Clin Proc* 1986; 61(1): 14–9.

35. Ernst SM et al. Percutaneous transluminal coronary angioplasty in patients with prior coronary artery bypass grafting. Long-term results. *J Thorac Cardiovasc Surg* 1987; 93(2): 268–75.

36. Cote G et al. Percutaneous transluminal angioplasty of stenotic coronary artery bypass grafts: 5 years' experience. *J Am Coll Cardiol* 1987; 9(1): 8–17.

37. Pinkerton CA et al. Percutaneous transluminal angioplasty in patients with prior myocardial revascularization surgery. *Am J Cardiol* 1988; 61(14): 15G–22G.

38. Cooper I et al. Role of angioplasty in patients with previous coronary artery bypass surgery. *Cathet Cardiovasc Diagn* 1989; 16(2): 81–6.

39. Platko WP et al. Percutaneous transluminal angioplasty of saphenous vein graft stenosis: Long-term follow-up. *J Am Coll Cardiol* 1989; 14(7): 1645–50.

40. Tabbalat RA, and Haft JI. Coronary angioplasty in symptomatic patients after bypass surgery. *Am Heart J* 1990; 120(5): 1091–6.

41. Webb JG et al. Coronary angioplasty after coronary bypass surgery: Initial results and late outcome in 422 patients. *J Am Coll Cardiol* 1990; 16(4): 812–20.

42. Jost S et al. Percutaneous transluminal angioplasty of aortocoronary venous bypass grafts and effect of the caliber of the grafted coronary artery on graft stenosis. *Am J Cardiol* 1991; 68(1): 27–30.

43. Meester BJ et al. Long-term follow-up after attempted angioplasty of saphenous vein grafts: The Thoraxcenter experience 1981–1988. *Eur Heart J* 1991; 12(5): 648–53.

44. Plokker HW et al. The Dutch experience in percutaneous transluminal angioplasty of narrowed saphenous veins used for aortocoronary arterial bypass. *Am J Cardiol* 1991; 67(5): 361–6.

45. Reeves F et al. Long-term angiographic follow-up after angioplasty of venous coronary bypass grafts. *Am Heart J* 1991; 122(3 Pt 1): 620–7.

46. Morrison DA et al. Percutaneous transluminal angioplasty of saphenous vein grafts for medically refractory unstable angina. *J Am Coll Cardiol* 1994; 23(5): 1066–70.

47. Dorros G et al. Percutaneous transluminal coronary angioplasty in patients with two or more previous coronary artery bypass grafting operations. *Am J Cardiol* 1988; 61(15): 1243–7.

48. Subramanian S et al. Decision-making for patients with patent left internal thoracic artery grafts to left anterior descending. *Ann Thorac Surg* 2009; 87(5): 1392–8; discussion 1400.

49. Labinaz M et al. Outcomes of patients with acute coronary syndromes and prior coronary artery bypass grafting: Results from the platelet glycoprotein IIb/IIIa in unstable angina: Receptor suppression using integrilin therapy (PURSUIT) trial. *Circulation* 2002; 105(3): 322–7.

50. Chen L et al. Angiographic features of vein grafts versus ungrafted coronary arteries in patients with unstable angina and previous bypass surgery. *J Am Coll Cardiol* 1996; 28(6): 1493–9.

51. Fitzgibbon GM et al. Coronary bypass graft fate and patient outcome: Angiographic follow-up of 5,065 grafts related to survival and reoperation in 1,388 patients during 25 years. *J Am Coll Cardiol* 1996; 28(3): 616–26.

52. Yau TM et al. The changing pattern of reoperative coronary surgery: Trends in 1230 consecutive reoperations. *J Thorac Cardiovasc Surg* 2000; 120(1): 156–63.

53. Yap CH et al. Contemporary results show repeat coronary artery bypass grafting remains a risk factor for operative mortality. *Ann Thorac Surg* 2009; 87(5): 1386–91.

54. Fabricius AM et al. Early angiographic control of perioperative ischemia after coronary artery bypass grafting. *Eur J Cardio-Thorac Surg* 2001; 19(6): 853–8.

55. Rasmussen C et al. Significance and management of early graft failure after coronary artery bypass grafting: Feasibility and results of acute angiography and re-re-vascularization. *Eur J Cardio-Thorac Surg* 1997; 12(6): 847–52.

56. Hannan EL et al, Verbal communication.

57. Harskamp RE et al. Saphenous vein graft failure after coronary artery bypass surgery: Pathophysiology, management, and future directions. *Ann Surg* 2013; 257(5): 824–33.

58. Hess CN et al. Saphenous vein graft failure after coronary artery bypass surgery: Insights from PREVENT IV. *Circulation* 2014; 130(17): 1445–51.

59. Motwani JG, and Topol, EJ. Aortocoronary saphenous vein graft disease: Pathogenesis, predisposition, and prevention. *Circulation* 1998; 97(9): 916–31.

60. Lopes RD et al. Ferguson Project of Ex Vivo Vein Graft Engineering via (PRE-VENT IV) Investigators. Relationship between vein graft failure and subsequent clinical outcomes after coronary artery bypass surgery. *Circulation* 2012; 125: 749–56.

61. Shimshak TM, and Hartzler, GO. Percutaneous transluminal angioplasty in diffuse subtotally occluded vein grafts. *Cathet Cardiovasc Diagn* 1989; 17(2): 99–104.

62. Ferguson TB, Jr. et al. Peterson, Internal thoracic artery grafting in the elderly patient undergoing coronary artery bypass grafting: Room for process improvement? *J Thorac Cardiovasc Surg* 2002; 123(5): 869–80.

63. Leavitt BJ et al. Use of the internal mammary artery graft and in-hospital mortality and other adverse outcomes associated with coronary artery bypass surgery. *Circulation* 2001; 103(4): 507–12.

64. Tatoulis J et al. Total arterial coronary revascularization: Techniques and results in 3,220 patients. *Ann Thorac Surg* 1999; 68(6): 2093–9.

65. Sabik JF 3rd et al. Comparison of saphenous vein and internal thoracic artery graft patency by coronary system. *Ann Thorac Surg* 2005; 79(2): 544–51; discussion 544–51.

66. Loop FD et al. Influence of the internal-mammary-artery graft on 10-year survival and other cardiac events. *N Engl J Med* 1986; 314(1): 1–6.

67. Cameron A et al. Coronary bypass surgery with internal-thoracic-artery grafts – effects on survival over a 15-year period. *N Engl J Med* 1996; 334(4): 216–9.

68. Cameron AA et al. Internal thoracic artery grafts: 20-year clinical follow-up. *J Am Coll Cardiol* 1995; 25(1): 188–92.

69. Loop FD, and Whitlow PL. Coronary angioplasty in patients with previous bypass surgery. *J Am Coll Cardiol* 1990; 16(6): 1348–50.

70. Mehran R et al. Percutaneous revascularization of patients with prior coronary bypass surgery: Saphenous vein graft or native coronary stenting? *J Am Coll Cardiol* 1999; 83(Suppl A): 51A.

71. Weintraub WS et al. Results of coronary surgery after failed elective coronary angioplasty in patients with prior coronary surgery. *J Am Coll Cardiol* 1990; 16(6): 1341–7.

72. Celermajer DS et al. Emergency coronary artery bypass surgery following coronary angioplasty – favourable medium term outcome after eight years' experience. *Aust N Z J Med* 1991; 21(2): 211–6.

73. Coolong A et al. Saphenous vein graft stenting and major adverse cardiac events: A predictive model derived from a pooled analysis of 3958 patients. *Circulation* 2008; 117(6): 790–7.

74. Kao J et al. Direct thrombin inhibition appears to be a safe and effective anticoagulant for percutaneous bypass graft interventions. *Catheter Cardiovasc Interv* 2006; 68(3): 352–6.

75. Kahn JK, and Hartzler GO. Retrograde coronary angioplasty of isolated arterial segments through saphenous vein bypass grafts. *Cathet Cardiovasc Diagn* 1990; 20(2): 88–93.

76. DiSciascio G et al. Retrograde coronary angioplasty of native and branch vessels via a vein bypass graft. *J Interv Cardiol* 1989; 2: 55–8.

77. Iakovou I et al. Relation of final lumen dimensions in saphenous vein grafts after stent implantation to outcome. *Am J Cardiol* 2004; 93(8): 963–8.

78. Hong YJ et al. Outcome of undersized drug-eluting stents for percutaneous coronary intervention of saphenous vein graft lesions. *Am J Cardiol* 2010; 105(2): 179–85.

79. Rechavia E et al. Stent implantation of saphenous vein graft aorto-ostial lesions in patients with unstable ischemic syndromes: Immediate angiographic results and long-term clinical outcome. *J Am Coll Cardiol* 1995; 25(4): 866–70.

80. Halle AA 3rd et al. Angioplasty of a recently occluded coronary artery bypass graft. *Cathet Cardiovasc Diagn* 1990; 21(3): 180–4.

81. de Feyter PJ et al. Percutaneous transluminal angioplasty of a totally occluded venous bypass graft: A challenge that should be resisted. *Am J Cardiol* 1989; 64(1): 88–90.

82. Kahn JK et al. Initial and long-term outcome of 83 patients after balloon angioplasty of totally occluded bypass grafts. *J Am Coll Cardiol* 1994; 23(5): 1038–42.

83. Bell C et al. Sequential proximal and distal infusion of urokinase resulting in recanalization of acutely occluded aortocoronary bypass graft after coronary angioplasty. *Cathet Cardiovasc Diagn* 1992; 26(3): 224–8.

84. McKeever LS et al. Acute myocardial infarction complicating recanalization of aortocoronary bypass grafts with urokinase therapy. *Am J Cardiol* 1989; 64(10): 683–5.

85. Doorey AJ et al. Successful angioplasty of a chronically occluded saphenous vein graft using a prolonged urokinase infusion from the brachial route. *Cathet Cardiovasc Diagn* 1991; 23(2): 127–9.

86. Hartmann JR et al. Recanalization of chronically occluded aortocoronary saphenous vein bypass grafts by extended infusion of urokinase: Initial results and short-term clinical follow-up. *J Am Coll Cardiol* 1991; 18(6): 1517–23.

87. Hartmann JR et al. Recanalization of Chronically Occluded Aortocoronary Saphenous Vein Bypass Grafts With Long-Term, Low Dose Direct Infusion of Urokinase (ROBUST): A serial trial. *J Am Coll Cardiol* 1996; 27(1): 60–6.

88. Taylor MA et al. Intracerebral hemorrhage complicating urokinase infusion into an occluded aortocoronary bypass graft. *Cathet Cardiovasc Diagn* 1994; 31(3): 206–10.

89. Hamburger J et al. ART study: An analysis of the initial European experience with the Angiojet® rapid thrombectomy catheter. *Coll Cardiol* 1997; 29: 186A.

90. Ramee SR et al. Preliminary experience with the POSSIS coronary rheolytic thrombectomy catheter in the VEGAS I pilot study. *Coll Cardiol* 1996; 27: 69A.

91. Ramee SR et al. A randomized, prospective multicenter study comparing Intravascular uroki-nase to rheolytic thrombectomy with the Possis AngioJet® catheter for intracoronary thrombus: Final results of the VeGAS 2 trial abstract. *Circulation* 1998; 98: I–86.

92. Rodes J et al. Angioscopic evaluation of thrombus removal by the throm-bectomy catheter. *Cathet Cardiovasc Diagn* 1998; 43: 338–43.

93. Rosenschein U et al. Percutaneous transluminal therapy of occluded saphenous vein grafts: Can the challenge be met with ultrasound thrombolysis? *Circulation* 1999; 99(1): 26–9.

94. Ischinger TA et al. Thrombectomy with the X-SIZER catheter system in the coronary circulation: initial results from a multi-center study. *J Invasive Cardiol* 2001; 13:81–8.

95. Prpic R et al. Angiographic outcomes after intracoronary X-Sizer® helical atherectomy: First use in humans. *Circulation* 1999; 100(Suppl I): I–305.

96. Al-Lamee R et al. Clinical and angiographic outcomes after percutaneous recanalization of chronic total saphenous vein graft occlusion using modern techniques. *Am J Cardiol* 2010; 106(12): 1721–7.

97. Levine GN et al. 2011 ACCF/AHA/SCAI Guideline for Percutaneous Coronary Intervention: Executive summary: A report of the American College of Cardiology Foundation/American Heart Association Task Force on Practice Guidelines and the Society for Cardiovascular Angiography and Interventions. *Circulation* 2011; 124(23): 2574–609.

98. Kiemeneij F et al. Transradial artery coronary angioplasty. *Am Heart J* 1995; 129(1): 1–7.

99. Salinger M et al. Percutaneous angioplasty of internal mammary artery graft stenosis using the brachial approach: A case report. *Cathet Cardiovasc Diagn* 1986; 12(4): 261–5.

100. Dorros G, and Lewin RF. The brachial artery method to transluminal internal mammary artery angioplasty. *Cathet Cardiovasc Diagn* 1986; 12(5): 341–6.

101. Komiyama N et al. Percutaneous transluminal coronary angioplasty of gastroepiploic artery graft. *Cathet Cardiovasc Diagn* 1990; 21(3): 177–9.

102. Isshiki T et al. Percutaneous angioplasty of stenosed gastroepiploic artery grafts. *J Am Coll Cardiol* 1993; 22(3): 727–32.

103. Meier B, and Mehan, VK. Graft angioplasty. In: *Atlas of Coronary Balloon Angioplasty Dekker*. Marcel Dekker, New York, 1995, p. 123.

104. Hong MK et al. Are we making progress with percutaneous saphenous vein graft treatment? Comparison of and -98 results. *Coll Cardiol* 1999; 33 36A: 1990–4.

105. Waters D, and G. Cote. Angioplasty of bypass grafts and native arteries. *Cardiovasc Clin* 1991; 21(2): 241–56.

106. Douglas JS et al. Update of saphenous vein graft angioplasty: Restenosis and long-term outcome. *Circulation* 1991; 84(Suppl II): II–249.

107. White CJ et al. Percutaneous angioscopy of saphenous vein coronary bypass grafts. *J Am Coll Cardiol* 1993; 21(5): 1181–5.

108. Douglas J. Angioplasty of saphenous vein and internal mammary artery bypass grafts. In: Topol EJ (editor), *Textbook of Interventional Cardiology*. Philadelphia, PA: WB Saunders, 1990, p. 337.

109. Untereker WJ et al. ELCA Investigators, Excimer laser coronary angioplasty of saphenous vein grafts. *Circulation* 1992; 86(Suppl I): I–780.

110. Litvack F et al. Percutaneous excimer laser coronary angioplasty: Results in the first consecutive 3,000 patients. The ELCA Investigators. *J Am Coll Cardiol* 1994; 23(2): 323–9.

111. Bittl JA, and Sanborn TA. Excimer laser-facilitated coronary angioplasty. Relative risk analysis of acute and follow-up results in 200 patients. *Circulation* 1992; 86(1): 71–80.

112. Estella P et al. Excimer laser-assisted coronary angioplasty for lesions containing thrombus. *J Am Coll Cardiol* 1993; 21(7): 1550–6.

113. Strauss BH et al. Early and late quantitative angiographic results of vein graft lesions treated by excimer laser with adjunctive balloon angioplasty. *Circulation* 1995; 92(3): 348–56.

114. Cook SL et al. Percutaneous excimer laser coronary angioplasty of lesions not ideal for balloon angioplasty. *Circulation* 1991; 84(2): 632–43.

115. Eigler NL et al. Excimer laser coronary angioplasty of aorto-ostial stenosis: Results of the ELCA Registry. *Circulation* 1991; 84(Suppl II): II–251.

116. Ellis SG et al. Relation of clinical presentation, stenosis morphology and operator technique to the procedural result of rotational atherectomy and rotational atherectomy-facilitated angioplasty. *Circulation* 1994; 89: 882–92.

117. Borrione M et al. Treatment of simple and complex coronary stenosis using rotational ablation followed by low pressure balloon angioplasty. *Cathet Cardiovasc Diagn* 1993; 30(2): 131–7.

118. Mintz GS et al. Intravascular ultrasound evaluation of the effect of rotational atherectomy in obstructive atherosclerotic coronary artery disease. *Circulation* 1992; 86(5): 1383–93.

119. Waksman R et al. Short- and long-term outcome of narrowed saphenous vein bypass graft: A comparison of Palmaz-Schatz stent, directional coronary atherectomy, and balloon angioplasty. *Am Heart J* 1997; 134(2 Pt 1): 274–81.

120. Thomas WJ et al. Effectiveness of rotational atherectomy in aortocoronary saphenous vein grafts. *Am J Cardiol* 2000; 86(1): 88–91.

121. Ahmed JM et al. Comparison of debulking followed by stenting versus stenting alone for saphenous vein graft aortoostial lesions: Immediate and one-year clinical outcomes. *J Am Coll Cardiol* 2000; 35(6): 1560–8.

122. Stone GW et al. Prospective, randomized evaluation of thrombectomy prior to percutaneous intervention in diseased saphenous vein grafts and thrombus-containing coronary arteries. *J Am Coll Cardiol* 2003; 42(11): 2007–13.

123. Holmes DR Jr. et al. A multicenter, randomized trial of coronary angioplasty versus directional atherectomy for patients with saphenous vein bypass graft lesions. CAVEAT-II Investigators. *Circulation* 1995; 91(7): 1966–74.

124. Teirstein PS et al. Low- versus high-dose recombinant urokinase for the treatment of chronic saphenous vein occlusion. *Am J Cardiol* 1999; 83(12): 1623–8.

125. Grines CL et al. Mechanism of acute myocardial infarction in patients with prior coronary artery bypass grafting and therapeutic implications. *Am J Cardiol* 1990; 65(20): 1292–6.

126. Safian RD et al. Clinical and angiographic results of transluminal extraction coronary atherectomy in saphenous vein bypass grafts. *Circulation* 1994; 89(1): 302–12.

127. Meany TB et al. Transluminal extraction catheter for the treatment of diseased saphenous vein grafts: A multicenter experience. *Cathet Cardiovasc Diagn* 1995; 34(2): 112–20.

128. Kuntz RE et al. A trial comparing rheolytic thrombectomy with intracoronary urokinase for coronary and vein graft thrombus (the Vein Graft AngioJet Study [VeGAS 2]). *Am J Cardiol* 2002; 89(3): 326–30.

129. Cohen DJ et al. Economic assessment of rheolytic thrombectomy versus intracoronary urokinase for treatment of extensive intracoronary thrombus: Results from a randomized clinical trial. *Am Heart J* 2001; 142(4): 648–56.

130. Webb JG et al. Retrieval and analysis of particulate debris after saphenous vein graft intervention. *J Am Coll Cardiol* 1999; 34(2): 468–75.

131. Hirshfeld JW Jr. et al. Restenosis after coronary angioplasty: A multivariate statistical model to relate lesion and procedure variables to restenosis. The M-HEART Investigators. *J Am Coll Cardiol* 1991; 18(3): 647–56.

132. Pomerantz RM et al. Acute and long-term outcome of narrowed saphenous venous grafts treated by endoluminal stenting and directional atherectomy. *Am J Cardiol* 1992; 70(2): 161–7.

133. Urban P et al. Intravascular stenting for stenosis of aorto-coronary venous bypass grafts. *J Am Coll Cardiol* 1989; 13(5): 1085–91.

134. Strumpf RK et al. Palmaz-Schatz stent implantation in stenosed saphenous vein grafts: Clinical and angiographic follow-up. *Am Heart J* 1992; 123(5): 1329–36.

135. Piana RN et al. Palmaz-Schatz stenting for treatment of focal vein graft stenosis: Immediate results and long-term outcome. *J Am Coll Cardiol* 1994; 23(6): 1296–304.

136. Leon MB et al. Stents may be the preferred treatment for focal aortocoronary vein graft disease. *Circulation* 1991; 84(Suppl II): II–249.

137. Bilodeau L et al. Flexible coil stent (Cook Inc) in saphenous vein grafts: Clinical and angiographic follow-up. *J Am Coll Cardiol* 1992; 19(Suppl A): 264A.

138. de Scheerder IK et al. Stenting of venous bypass grafts: A new treatment modality for patients who are poor candidates for reintervention. *Am Heart J* 1992; 123(4 Pt 1): 1046–54.

139. Leon MB et al. Balloon expandable stent implantation in saphenous vein grafts. In: Hermann HC, Hirshfeld JW (editors), *Clinical Use of the Palmaz–Schatz Balloon Expandable Stent.* New York: Futura Publishing Company, 1993, pp. 111–21.

140. Rocha-Singh K et al. Coronary stenting for treatment of ostial stenoses of native coronary arteries or aortocoronary saphenous venous grafts. *Am J Cardiol* 1995; 75(1): 26–9.

141. Wong SC et al. Comparison of clinical and angiographic outcomes after saphenous vein graft angioplasty using coronary versus 'biliary' tubular slotted stents. *Circulation* 1995; 91(2): 339–50.

142. Diaz L et al. Stenting in old saphenous vein grafts: Early outcome and restenosis. *Circulation* 1993; 88(Suppl I): I–309.

143. Fortuna R et al. Wiktor intracoronary stent: Experience in the first 101 vein graft patients. *Circulation* 1993; 88(Suppl I): I–309.

144. Savage MP et al. Stent placement compared with balloon angioplasty for obstructed coronary bypass grafts. Saphenous Vein De Novo Trial Investigators. *N Eng J Med* 1997; 337(11): 740–7.

145. Wong SC et al. Stent placement is safe and effective in the treatment of older (>4 years) saphenous vein graft lesions. *J Am Coll Cardiol* 1995; 25(Suppl A): 79A.

146. Wong SC et al. Economic impact of reduced anticoagulation after saphenous vein graft stent placement. *J Am Coll Cardiol* 1995; 25(Suppl A): 80A.

147. Mehran R et al. Multivessel stenting reduces in-hospital complications compared with repeat aortocoronary bypass surgery. *J Am Coll Cardiol* 1999; 33(Suppl A): 51A.

148. Bhargava B et al. Procedural results and late clinical outcomes following multiple saphenous vein graft stenting. *J Am Coll Cardiol* 1999; 33(Suppl A): 50A.

149. Roffi M et al. Lack of benefit from intravenous platelet glycoprotein IIb/IIIa receptor inhibition as adjunctive treatment for percutaneous interventions of aortocoronary bypass grafts: A pooled analysis of five randomized clinical trials. *Circulation* 2002; 106(24): 3063–7.

150. Fischman DL et al. A randomized comparison of coronary-stent placement and balloon angioplasty in the treatment of coronary artery disease. Stent Restenosis Study Investigators. *N Eng J Med* 1994; 331(8): 496–501.

151. Kuntz RE et al. The importance of acute luminal diameter in determining restenosis after coronary atherectomy or stenting. *Circulation* 1992; 86(6): 1827–35.

152. Serruys PW et al. A comparison of balloon-expandable-stent implantation with balloon angioplasty in patients with coronary artery disease. Benestent Study Group. *N Eng J Med* 1994; 331(8): 489–95.

153. Douglas JS et al. Randomized trial of coronary stent placement and balloon angioplasty in the treatment of saphenous vein graft stenosis. *J Am Coll Cardiol* 1996; 27(Suppl A): 178A.

154. Brener SJ et al. Comparison of stenting and balloon angioplasty for narrowings in aortocoronary saphenous vein conduits in place for more than five years. *Am J Cardiol* 1997; 79(1): 13–8.

155. Wong SC. et al. Immediate results and late outcomes after stent implantation in saphenous vein graft lesions: The multicenter U.S. Palmaz-Schatz stent experience. The Palmaz-Schatz Stent Study Group. *J Am Coll Cardiol* 1995; 26(3): 704–12.

156. Heidland UE et al. Risk factors for the development of restenosis following stent implantation of venous bypass grafts. *Heart* 2001; 85(3): 312–7.

157. Fenton S et al. Does stent implantation in ostial saphenous vein graft lesions reduce restenosis? *J Am Coll Cardiol* 1994; 25(Suppl A): 118A.

158. Wong SC et al. Stent placement for the treatment of aorto-ostial saphenous vein graft lesions. *J Am Coll Cardiol* 1994; 25(Suppl A): 118A.

159. Gruberg L et al. In-hospital and long-term results of stent deployment compared with balloon angioplasty for treatment of narrowing at the saphenous vein graft distal anastomosis site. *Am J Cardiol* 1999; 84(12): 1381–4.

160. Ahmed JM et al. Influence of diabetes mellitus on early and late clinical outcomes in saphenous vein graft stenting. *J Am Coll Cardiol* 2000; 36(4): 1186–93.

161. Le May MR et al. Predictors of long-term outcome after stent implantation in a saphenous vein graft. *Am J Cardiol* 1999; 83(5): 681–6.

162. Sketch MH et al. 710-5 Progressive deterioration in late (2-year) clinical outcomes after stent implantation in saphenous vein grafts: The multicenter JJIS experience. *Am J Coll Cardiol* 1995; 25 A: 79–80.

163. Piana RN et al. Angiographic and clinical outcome of endoluminal stenting for stenotic saphenous vein grafts: Single center experience. *Circulation* 1993; 88: I308.

164. Keeley EC et al. Long-term clinical outcome and predictors of major adverse cardiac events after percutaneous interventions on saphenous vein grafts. *J Am Coll Cardiol* 2001; 38(3): 659–65.

165. de Jaegere PP et al. Long-term clinical outcome after stent implantation in saphenous vein grafts. *J Am Coll Cardiol* 1996; 28(1): 89–96.

166. Laham RJ et al. Long-term (4- to 6-year) outcome of Palmaz-Schatz stenting: Paucity of late clinical stent-related problems. *J Am Coll Cardiol* 1996; 28(4): 820–6.

167. Safian RD et al. Final results of the randomized Wallstent® endoprosthesis in saphenous vein graft trial (WINS). *Am J Coll Cardiol* 1999; 33: 37A.

168. Safian RD et al. Final results of the Wallstent® endoprosthesis in large saphenous vein graft. *Am J Coll Cardiol* 1999; 33: 51A.

169. Piana RN et al. Treatment of large saphenous vein graft and native coronary stenoses using the Palmaz Schatz biliary stents: Acute results. *Circulation* 1993; 88: I307.

170. Knopf WD et al. Treatment of complex saphenous vein graft disease and suboptimal native coronary angioplasty result with biliary stenting: A promising new technique. *Circulation* 1993; 88: I308.

171. Hardigan KR et al. Single-center Palmaz-Schatz experience in coronary arteries and saphenous vein grafts. *Circulation* 1993; 88: I308.

172. Blankenship JC et al. Staging of multivessel percutaneous coronary interventions: An expert consensus statement from the Society for Cardiovascular Angiography and Interventions. *Catheter Cardiovasc Interv* 2012; 79(7): 1138–52.

173. Elsner M et al. Stent-grafts containing a polytetrafluoro-ethylene membrane: Emerging indications for implantation into human coronary arteries. *J Am Coll Cardiol* 1999; 33(Suppl A): 96A.

174. Baldus S et al. Reduction of restenosis in venous bypass graft lesions after implantation of a covered graft stent. *J Am Coll Cardiol* 1999; 33(Suppl A): 37A.

175. De Gregorio J et al. Experience with the PTFE covered stent in percutaneous coronary interventional procedures: Indications and outcome. *J Am Coll Cardiol* 1999; 33(Suppl A): 96A.

176. Kahn JK et al. Early postoperative balloon coronary angioplasty for failed coronary artery bypass grafting. *Am J Cardiol* 1990; 66(12): 943–6.

177. Stone GW et al. Percutaneous recanalization of chronically occluded coronary arteries: A consensus document: Part II. *Circulation* 2005; 112(16): 2530–7.

178. Mautner SL et al. Comparison of composition of atherosclerotic plaques in saphenous veins used as aortocoronary bypass conduits with plaques in native coronary arteries in the same men. *Am J Cardiol* 1992; 70(18): 1380–7.

179. Margolis JR et al. Diffuse embolization following percutaneous transluminal coronary angioplasty of occluded vein grafts: The blush phenomenon. *Clin Cardiol* 1991; 14(6): 489–93.

180. Trono R et al. Multiple myocardial infarctions associated with atheromatous emboli after PTCA of saphenous vein grafts. A clinicopathologic correlation. *Cleve Clinic J Med* 1989; 56(6): 581–4.

181. Watson PS et al. Angiographic and clinical outcomes following acute infarct angioplasty on saphenous vein grafts. *Am J Cardiol* 1999; 83(7): 1018–21.

182. Aueron F, and Gruentzig A. Distal embolization of a coronary artery bypass graft atheroma during percutaneous transluminal coronary angioplasty. *Am J Cardiol* 1984; 53(7): 953–4.

183. Hong MK et al. Creatine kinase-MB enzyme elevation following successful saphenous vein graft intervention is associated with late mortality. *Circulation* 1999; 100(24): 2400–5.

184. Mathew V et al. The influence of abciximab use on clinical outcome after aortocoronary vein graft interventions. *J Am Coll Cardiol* 1999; 34(4): 1163–9.

185. Hoffmann R et al. Implantation of sirolimus-eluting stents in saphenous vein grafts is associated with high clinical follow-up event rates compared with treatment of native vessels. *Coro Artery Dis* 2007; 18(7): 559–64.

186. Baim DS et al. Randomized trial of a distal embolic protection device during percutaneous intervention of saphenous vein aorto-coronary bypass grafts. *Circulation* 2002; 105(11): 1285–90.

187. Stone GW et al. Randomized comparison of distal protection with a filter-based catheter and a balloon occlusion and aspiration system during percutaneous intervention of diseased saphenous vein aorto-coronary bypass grafts. *Circulation* 2003; 108(5): 548–53.

188. Grube E et al. Prevention of distal embolization during coronary angioplasty in saphenous vein grafts and native vessels using porous filter protection. *Circulation* 2001; 104(20): 2436–41.

189. Grube E et al. Evaluation of a balloon occlusion and aspiration system for protection from distal embolization during stenting in saphenous vein grafts. *Am J Cardiol* 2002; 89(8): 941–5.

190. Mauri L et al. The PROXIMAL trial: Proximal protection during saphenous vein graft intervention using the Proxis Embolic Protection System: A randomized, prospective, multicenter clinical trial. *J Am Coll Cardiol* 2007; 50(15): 1442–9.

191. Leineweber K et al. Intense vasoconstriction in response to aspirate from stented saphenous vein aortocoronary bypass grafts. *J Am Coll Cardiol* 2006; 47(5): 981–6.

192. Grube E et al. The SAFE study: Multicenter evaluation of a protection catheter system for distal embolisation in coronary venous bypass grafts SVGs. *J Am Coll Cardiol* 1999; 33: 37A.

193. Carlino M et al. Prevention of distal embolization during saphenous vein graft lesion angioplasty. Experience with a new temporary occlusion and aspiration system. *Circulation* 1999; 99(25): 3221–3.

194. Lansky AJ et al. Treatment of coronary artery perforations complicating percutaneous coronary intervention with a polytetrafluoroethylene-covered stent graft. *Am J Cardiol* 2006; 98(3): 370–4.

195. Stone GW et al. Primary angioplasty in acute myocardial infarction with distal protection of the microcirculation: Principal results from the prospective, randomized EMERALD Trial. *J Am Coll Cardiol* 2004; 43: 285A–286A.

196. Stone GW et al. Distal filter protection during saphenous vein graft stenting: Technical and clinical correlates of efficacy. *J Am Coll Cardiol* 2002; 40(10): 1882–8.

197. Halkin A et al. Six-month outcomes after percutaneous intervention for lesions in aortocoronary saphenous vein grafts using distal protection devices: Results from the FIRE trial. *Am Heart J* 2006; 151(4): 915 e1–7.

198. Carrozza JP et al. Randomized evaluation of the TriActiv balloonprotection flush and extraction system for the treatment of saphenous vein graft disease. *J Am Coll Cardiol* 2005; 46(9): 1677–83.

199. Mauri L et al. Devices for distal protection during percutaneous coronary revascularization. *Circulation* 2006; 113(22): 2651–6.

200. Gorog DA et al. Distal myocardial protection during percutaneous coronary intervention: When and where? *J Am Coll Cardiol* 2005; 46(8): 1434–45.

201. Ashby DT et al. Effect of percutaneous coronary interventions for in-stent restenosis in degenerated saphenous vein grafts without distal embolic protection. *J Am Coll Cardiol* 2003; 41(5): 749–52.

202. Teirstein PS, and Hartzler GO. Nonoperative management of aortocoronary saphenous vein graft rupture during percutaneous transluminal coronary angioplasty. *Am J Cardiol* 1987; 60(4): 377–8.

203. Drummer E et al. Rupture of a saphenous vein bypass graft during coronary angioplasty. *Br Heart J* 1987; 58(1): 78–81.

204. Singh RN et al. Green, Internal mammary artery versus saphenous vein graft. Comparative performance in patients with combined revascularisation. *Br Heart J* 1983; 50(1): 48–58.

205. Cameron A et al. Clinical implications of internal mammary artery bypass grafts: The Coronary Artery Surgery Study experience. *Circulation* 1988; 77(4): 815–9.

206. Gruberg L et al. Percutaneous revascularization of the internal mammary artery graft: Short- and long-term outcomes. *J Am Coll Cardiol* 2000; 35(4): 944–8.

207. Hosono M et al. Neointimal formation at the sites of anastomosis of the internal thoracic artery grafts after coronary artery bypass grafting in human subjects: An immunohistochemical analysis. *J Thorac Cardiovasc Surg* 2000; 120(2): 319–28.

208. Popma JJ et al. Immediate procedural and long-term clinical results of internal mammary artery angioplasty. *Am J Cardiol* 1992; 69(14): 1237–9.

209. Steffenino G et al. Percutaneous transluminal angioplasty of right and left internal mammary artery grafts. *Chest* 1986; 90(6): 849–51.

210. Shimshak TM et al. Application of percutaneous transluminal coronary angioplasty to the internal mammary artery graft. *J Am Coll Cardiol* 1988; 12(5): 1205–14.

211. Bell MR et al. Percutaneous transluminal angioplasty of left internal mammary artery grafts: Two years' experience with a femoral approach. *Br Heart J* 1989; 61(5): 417–20.

212. Zaidi AR, and Hollman JL. Percutaneous angioplasty of internal mammary artery graft stenosis: Case report and discussion. *Catheter Cardiovasc Diagn* 1985; 11(6): 603–8.

213. Kereiakes DJ et al. Percutaneous transluminal angioplasty of left internal mammary artery grafts. *Am J Cardiol* 1985; 55(9): 1215–6.

214. Crean PA et al. Transluminal angioplasty of a stenosis of an internal mammary artery graft. *Br Heart J* 1986; 56(5): 473–5.

215. Pinkerton CA et al. Percutaneous transluminal angioplasty involving internal mammary artery bypass grafts: A femoral approach. *Catheter Cardiovasc Diagn* 1987; 13(6): 414–8.

216. Tector AJ et al. The role of the sequential internal mammary artery graft in coronary surgery. *Circulation* 1984; 70(3 Pt 2): I222–5.

217. Najm HK et al. Postoperative symptomatic internal thoracic artery stenosis and successful treatment with PTCA. *Ann Thorac Surg* 1995; 59(2): 323–6; discussion 327.

218. Barner HB et al. Late patency of the internal mammary artery as a coronary bypass conduit. *Ann Thora Surg* 1982; 34(4): 408–12.

219. Dimas AP et al. Coronary artery bypass surgery vs coronary angioplasty: From antithesis to synthesis. *Eur Heart J* 1989;10 Suppl H85–91.

220. Shimshak TM et al. Percutaneous transluminal coronary angioplasty of internal mammary artery (IMA) grafts – procedural results and late follow-up. *Circulation* 1991; 84: II590.

221. Dimas AP et al. Percutaneous transluminal angioplasty involving internal mammary artery grafts. *Am Heart J* 1991; 122(2): 423–9.

222. Hillis LD et al. 2011 ACCF/AHA Guideline for Coronary Artery Bypass Graft Surgery. A report of the American College of Cardiology Foundation/American Heart Association Task Force on Practice Guidelines. Developed in collaboration with the American Association for Thoracic Surgery, Society of Cardiovascular Anesthesiologists, and Society of Thoracic Surgeons. *J Am Coll Cardiol* 2011; 58(24): e123–210.

Structural heart disease

Alcohol septal ablation in hypertrophic obstructive cardiomyopathy: Techniques and results

PAOLO ANGELINI, CARLO E URIBE, AMIR GAHREMANPOUR, ABDELKADER ALMALFI

30.1 Introduction

Hypertrophic obstructive cardiomyopathy (HOCM) is an important, progressive, lethal type of hypertrophic cardiomyopathy (HCM), which can be effectively palliated both by surgical- and catheter-based techniques: by surgical septal myomectomy (SSM) or by alcohol septal ablation (ASA).[1]

Whilst both therapeutic interventions are frequently but unevenly used at this time, ASA has shown a dramatic growth in popularity.[2]

This chapter aims primarily at summarising basic technical notions in the application of ASA.

30.2 History

Awareness of the importance, mechanisms and lethality of HOCM has become well-established during the last 40 years. The frustrating early results of medical treatment inspired medico-surgical teams to develop new interventions, such as myotomy (limited sectioning of the sub-aortic hypertrophic septum), septal myomectomy, or SSM[3] (extending the surgical approach to involve the removal of a variable amount of septal myocardium, deep in the left ventricle), or mitral valve surgery to reshape the posterior wall of the sub-aortic stenotic tract.[4]

As an alternative, ASA was developed separately, but simultaneously by Kuntz and Sigwald in Germany and Switzerland, respectively, in the mid-1990s.[2,5] Apparently, in many countries, ASA is currently de facto overcoming the early popularity of surgical myectomy (SM).[6,7] Both technique's results are quite dependent on individual operators' training and discipline.

In this chapter dedicated to ASA, we not address the genetics and the full spectrum of HCM, but only ASA for HOCM.

30.3 The mechanism of clinical manifestations and progression of HOCM

HOCM is a term used to indicate a type of HCM featuring sub-aortic obstructive outflow tract, that is the culprit of a rapid progression of this congenital condition. Longitudinal studies of HOCM showed that the appearance of a gradient clearly correlates with starting of rapid progression of the gradient and the symptoms, typically: shortness of breath, chest pain and symptoms of transient brain ischemia (dizziness, syncope). The risk of sudden cardiac death (SCD) increases greatly with the progression of the sub-aortic gradient (Figure 30.1). Onset of sub-aortic stenosis (SAS) is not usually present in the young life of genetically predisposed individuals, but it is acquired most frequently in the adult life of a carrier of HCM. HOCM should imply significant hypertrophy, meaning a wall septal thickness 'greater than 1.5 cm' in adults, or more than a standard deviation above the mean value in a large normal population: so, in children, it is necessary to depend on the analysis of such indices in a coetaneous population. Clinically, in adults, the general recommendations suggest that 'severe' HOCM should feature a thickness of the sub-aortic septum of more than 1.5–1.8 cm.[6] Only about 30% of phenotypic HCM will evolve into HOCM.[6] The essential features of HOCM are: (a) selective, asymmetric SAS (asymmetric septal hypertrophy, or ASH); (b) systolic anterior motion of the mitral valve (SAM); (c) sub-aortic dynamic (of variable degree, at different time and physiologic conditions) systolic gradient at the left ventricular (LV) outflow tract.[6]

Additionally, the following structural abnormalities may contribute to HOCM morbidity and mortality: (a) diffuse systolic coronary narrowing of intra-myocardial arterial segments in the LV territories, or myocardial bridging (MB): they are related to the presence, in HCM, of supra-systemic LV cavity and intramural pressure regimen; (b) patchy myocardial fibrosis; (c) diastolic dysfunction (mainly related to increased wall thickness); (d) mitral insufficiency (mainly due to distortion/displacement of the anterior leaflet of the mitral valve); (e) possible, late-onset systolic dysfunction, that tend to accompany diastolic dysfunction; (f) left atrial dilatation (related to the prior mechanisms), that may lead to the onset of atrial fibrillation, with significantly worsened haemodynamic compensation, whilst originating a risk for systemic embolism; (g) ventricular arrhythmias and increased risk of SCD (PVC's, ventricular tachycardia and fibrillation, that are related to both LV overload and myocardial fibrosis and ischaemia).

All these factors should be kept in mind, when managing HOCM, at any stage of the disease.

Outline of natural history of HOCM and alternative interventions

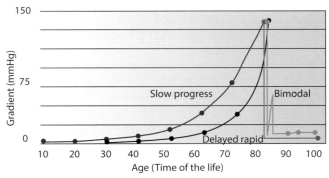

Figure 30.1 The diagrammatic illustration shows typical evolution of two patients, one with a slower and progressive (starting at 40 years of age, in green) and one with delayed and rapidly evolving hypertrophic obstructive cardiomyopathy (HOCM) form (in black): one was treated with surgical septal myomectomy (SSM) (curve in red) and one was treated with alcohol septal ablation (ASA) (in orange). Notice that ASA frequently features a transient 'rebound behaviour', after ASA, leading to long-term result only a few weeks after ASA.

30.4 The sub-aortic gradient issue

Systolic peak gradient is considered the simplest marker of severity in a given case of HOCM. This index may excessively simplify the complexity of SAS and its prognosis. In fact, SAS is greatly variable during the life of a patient in view of multiple variables. Especially, state of intravascular hydration (use of diuretics), Valsalva-like manoeuvres (like whilst lifting heavy weights), strenuous exercise, multiple drugs effects (nitroglycerin, catecholamines), or PVCs.

In clinical practice, evaluation of a given patient should involve some combination of provocation testing to evaluate the dynamic nature of the gradient (Figure 30.2).

Established guidelines suggest that a gradient of more than 30 mmHg at rest or more than 50 mmHg with provocation testing is 'significant', and condition for inclusion in ASA procedures.

In reality, the value of a gradient and its suppression with medicines or ASA comes from the fact that the gradient represents quite effectively the essence of the need and success of the procedure and the expected results on prognosis, as to the evolution of the disease. Abolishing a gradient can be safely assumed to establish stabilisation of the patient: it is more than a generic marker of haemodynamic overload.

30.5 Technique of ASA

Preoperative evaluation of a candidate for ASA should be considered one of the most critical aspects of the procedure. History and physical examination should be performed by an expert member of the ASA team on a patient (that is usually referred by another remote colleague), in order to: (a) confirm the severity of the symptoms and associated conditions (risk); (b) recognise the specific patient's risks (especially the risk of requiring a permanent pacemaker, which is highest in the presence of LBBB); (c) optimal access approach (radial arteries can be used, but they imply operational complications, in view of requiring two arterial catheters, and a venous temporary pacemaker). Similar

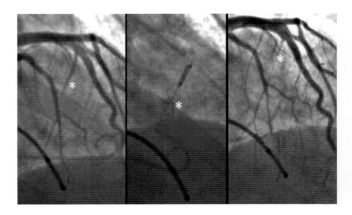

Figure 30.2 Still images of the baseline coronary angiography (left), distal balloon catheter injection and postoperative ASA. Asterisks indicate the first septal branch treated by ASA.

discussion should be entertained for SSM preoperative considerations (especially: age, gender, frail habitus, COPD, diabetes). After SSM, it is frequent to find septals left open into the left ventricle, and ASA in such context is not likely to have consistent results. A distal injection of contrast in the potential target septal (with a proximal inflated balloon) can document well such point.

Preoperative testing: (a) echocardiography is the standard for non-invasive evaluation. Data from this test should include: pulmonary peak pressure, wall thickness, severity of ASH, and SAM; LV ejection fraction; mitral insufficiency severity.

EKG: especially relevant, presence of baseline LBBB, atrioventricular (AV) block. Essential blood testing includes creatinine serum level and haemoglobin level testing. Chest x-rays: important especially for a simple postoperative follow-up (cardiomegaly).

Informed Consent: The patient and the family should be explained of the basic nature and risks of the procedure. A competent member of the team and the family should be present at this encounter. The conversation should include: the severity of the disease state and natural prognosis, expected results of the procedure, alternative treatment options, risks of complications (especially: permanent pacemaker, coronary dissection, coronary clotting, groin haematoma).

Preparation: the patient should generally withhold for 2 days any drug that may affect the gradient severity (during the procedure, one likes to monitor the worse possible gradient, not one repressed by drugs).

Sedation: ASA is a procedure that can be confidently performed with moderate sedation, whilst general anaesthesia is not generally required. The amount of pain expected from ASA is mild, especially in view of the local denervation obtained as a side effect of alcoholisation in the area.

Approach: Our group usually prefers a femoral approach, especially in view of the need for two arterial entries and a venous entry for temporary pacing. We generally use a 3.5 XB guiding catheter curve and a Run-through (Terumo) coronary guidewire.

Preoperative catheterisation laboratory evaluation and intervention: In absence of a permanent pacemaker, a temporary PM catheter is initially advanced into the right ventricular (RV) apex with mild to moderate curve to stabilise the pacing during the 2 expected days of required use. A demand mode at 50/minute rate is favoured (asynchronous pacing decreases the gradient). A 4 Fr pigtail catheter is advanced into the LV apex, trying to avoid causing ventricular premature beats, and attaining stable apical LV pressure continuous monitoring. Anticoagulation with heparin or Angiomax is established, before a coronary guidewire is advanced. A preoperative set of gradients (baseline, post-PVC, Valsalva manoeuvre, and/or after IV or IC 100 mcg nitroglycerin) are recorded for continuous monitoring during the procedure. In case of a prior, recent coronary angiography, only left coronary artery angiography is obtained in the RAO projection with a cranial tilt to optimally visualise the proximal septal

arteries. In case of unusual anatomy, it may be important to clarify it by obtaining several other projections, in order to clarify the origin, proximal course, distribution and length of the likely target branch (Figure 30.2).

The choice of the target antero-septal branch should consider the size and distribution of the vessel (it should be directed to the area of SAM contact, in a septal vessel diameter larger than 1.25 mm and longer than 3.0 cm). Neither distal vessels nor ventricles should be shown to visualise, by sub-selective angiography. We continue to hold the practice of using echocardiographic monitoring of the target region whilst using microbubbles solution to help locate the target septal (at level of SAM). The decision regarding cases with very thick interventricular septum (more than 2.5 cm) and/or many but small septals, feeding the target myocardium, follows these guidelines: 'More myocardium, more alcohol! Small septals, more septals!' (1.25 mm in balloon size, inflated at low pressure of about 6 atm, is the current smallest balloon catheter, adequate for infusion)!

30.6 ASA intervention

With a RV temporary demand mode pacemaker in place, adequate sedation, an activated clotting time of about 250 seconds, a balloon catheter of appropriate size is advanced over a coronary guidewire into the chosen septal branch, employing usual techniques of coronary angioplasty. Difficult anatomic variants could be due to proximal left coronary trunk/left anterior descending angulation, proximal left anterior descending (LAD)/septal angulation (Figure 30.3a and b), but especially the identification of the target septal branch. Periodic recording of the monitored gradients should be obtained (Figure 30.4). Then the following actions and technical rationale[8] should be taken into consideration:

1. A short (about 8 mm) balloon catheter is positioned close to the ostium (but off the LAD) with the intention of safely preventing dislodging and alcohol reflux to the rest of circulation.
2. Recording of an 'ischemic' gradient, at 2–3 minutes after balloon inflation: this sub-aortic gradient has the effective capacity of predicting adequate positioning of the balloon. A drop in gradient of more than 50% of control is clearly associated with the probability of a successful ASA. In its absence (no ischemic gradient observed), it is unlikely that ASA would be successful.
3. The ideal target area of ASA should be limited to the anterior 3 cm thickness of the upper third of the ventricular septum (the free wall thickness must be added, for a total of about 5 cm from the anterior epicardium), at SAM. ASA in areas with unwanted flow into remote regions, like the posterior descending, distal septals and diagonals should be avoided. If such objection is raised, by sub-selective injection (Figure 30.2), the required adaptation should mainly involve moving the balloon to exclude the unwanted involved branches.

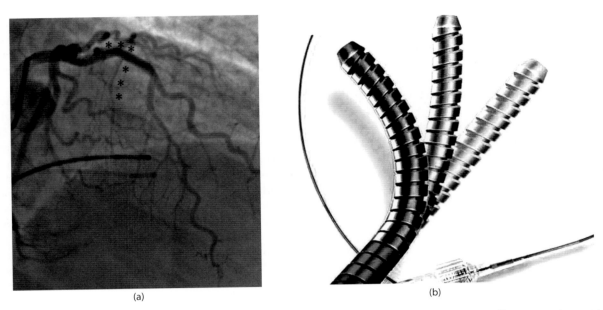

(a) (b)

Figure 30.3 **(a)** Still image of the target first septal branch (a, asterisks), in a patient with severe, rapidly progressive angina and dyspnoea. The gradients were 110 > 225 mmHg. The first septal at the level of SAM was at acute angle (about 120°) at the separation of main vessel (LAD). Initially, the coronary guidewire (run-through) could not enter distally into the distal septal, since it would prolapse into the distal LAD. A 4.1 Fr Venture catheter, Figure 2b (Vascular Solution, Minneapolis, MN) was initially located at the LAD/septal curve and the coronary guidewire could easily be advanced for 5 cm, allowing for a successful ASA. **(b)** Illustration of the mechanism of remote-control-curve **Venture catheter**. The catheter is advanced over a 0.014″ coronary guidewire, inside a 6 Fr guiding catheter, to negotiate an acute angulation. The deflectable tip outer diameter is 0.61 mm.

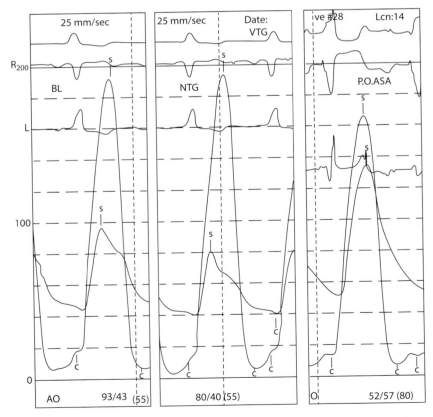

Figure 30.4 Pressure tracings during a procedure of ASA: baseline (left; gradient = 97 mmg); after nitroglycerin (middle; gradient = 120 mmHg); post-successful ASA: baseline (right; gradient = 30 mmHg). Ruling out of a residual intra-cavitary cause of residual gradient is done by careful pullback at the infundibular level.

4. Microbubbles injection also can be quite helpful to identify the ideal location of the target area for ASA, by simultaneous echocardiographic imaging in the parasternal and four chambers views.

5. ASA is generally executed by slow infusion of pure alcohol (absolute ethanol, at >96% concentration), at the continuous speed of <1 cc/ minute. Since there is very little chest pain at alcohol infusing during balloon occlusion, it is generally advisable to inject at a 2 cc/minute rate. Pressure gradient and AV block onset are to be closely monitored. In the absence of a permanent pacemaker, onset of AV advanced block (equal or > second degree) should generally advice to either stop ASA (if the results could be adequate), or change the septal and continue (if possible), or resume ASA in the same location after 2–3 minutes, at a much lower speed of infusion (1 cc /3–5 minutes).

6. After ending alcohol infusion, avoid flushing the inner lumen, because this could result in advancing distally critical amount of alcohol and increase the chance of AV block.

7. Persistent balloon inflation for a period of 5 minutes should be kept, in order to allow the alcohol in the arterial compartment to filtrate into the neighbouring tissues and for the intra-luminal blood to clot, so preventing back up into remote coronary circulation.

8. Then, the balloon catheter can be pulled out and a final coronary angiography should be done to prove the occlusion of the ASA-related branch, in absence of complications (dissection, clotting). Lack of target branch occlusion would be suspicious of technical error by superimposition of two vessels. A final sub-aortic gradient should then be recorded, to confirm success by the criterion of a less than 50%–75% of residual gradient with respect to preoperative levels (it is stated that a 50% drop is adequate, but this is not consistently correct and may be a reason for why the residual gradient is 'higher than after SSM', as commonly stated).

9. Re-evaluate the function and location of the temporary pacemaker before discharging the patient from the laboratory. In case of mental confusion from sedation side effect, a distal screw-tip pacing wire could be used, especially in cases with recurrent even though transient AV block. If the patient is totally pacemaker dependent, it is advisable to proceed to permanent AV-PM installation, if feasible, at the same session, in order to limit the danger of dislodgement (this could result in causing dramatic haemodynamic instability).

10. Usually, we pull the 6 Fr guiding catheter in the laboratory and use the Angio-Seal closure device. The 4 Fr sheath is usually left in place for 2 hours to wean the patient off anticoagulation. Rigorous bed rest in intensive care unit (ICU) is required for 2 days of observation. Such routine effectively prevents episode of serious bradycardia. The important side effect of

catheter-related (inadvertent dislodgement) ventricular tachycardia should be carefully avoided (the only cause of ventricular tachycardia in our early postoperative experience).

30.7 Additional postoperative care

Monitoring the patient in ICU implies especially documentation of any arrhythmias and PM action, whilst kept at 50/minute demand mode (in order to make a decision about the need for permanent pacing before discharge). A permanent pacemaker is indicated if the patient shows signs of advanced AV block, even though transient, before discharge (third day after ASA, as a rule).

Routine blood testing is advisable for testing the creatine kinase (CK) serum level; at *12 hours after ASA* conclusion (this time is the peak of the enzyme release curve, which correlates with infarct size). An EKG should be done at 24 hours. Echocardiography before discharge is only useful if one is studying the bimodal behaviour of the postoperative gradient, a benign and frequent, but peculiar event.[9,10] The important echocardiographic follow-up (unaffected by the presence of an early relapse at 2 days after ASA) should be at about 6 months after the procedure, when the scar has completely retracted and the residual (essentially, 'permanent') gradient can be considered the final measure of the results of ASA. Further muscle reabsorption and decrease of LV total myocardial mass will continue to occur for up to 2 years.

Medications at discharge: Beta-blockers should be generally avoided during the first month after ASA, for the residual danger of AV block, and the usual lack of their indication in case of a successful ASA. ACE inhibitors are usually indicated to enhance scar reabsorption and systemic blood pressure control (this usually increases after successful ASA). In case of inadequate early results of ASA, it is advisable to continue monitoring the patient, in hope of observing late further improvements from the results of definitive ablation, at about 6 months follow-up (initial results are only from acute infarction and a temporary flaccid myocardial state,[8] but not necessarily the definitive conclusion of the ASA process, only seen at the stage of advanced scarring). Regrowth of myocardium at the ASA site does not occur after ASA, and recurrent gradients should be generally considered the result of initially inadequate ablation, but not myocardial regrowth.

30.8 Early and late results of ASA in real-world practice

This section summarises the preliminary results of our experience, at the Texas Heart Institute, over the last 15 years. We are a single-main-operator referral centre, which includes treating HCMs, surgically and by ASA.

We are reporting a cohort of HOCM treated by ASA (continuous series of 118 patients, 133 procedures): one time in 103 cases, two times in 14 cases, and one patient treated three times. In the first 59 patients, a redo-procedure was required in 13, but only in 2 during the treatment of the last 59 patients. Our experience started with the idea of getting hands-on experience with a new, amazing technique, that dares to be a substitute for open-chest, extracorporeal-circulation, open-heart surgery (frequently successful), which at our institution was initiated several years ago by Dr. Denton Cooley.

The criterion of operative success has been the abolition of more than 50% of the baseline gradient. Further, in order to enable comparison values between patients, we proposed and used a normalised gradient, namely: the 'gradient index' in HOCM is obtained by the following formula: '(LVp – AOp)/LVp' where LVp is the LV peak pressure and AOp is the aortic peak pressure. By echo, the LVp is obtained by adding the brachial pressure to the Doppler gradient.

Early haemodynamic results: The average gradient index was found to be 0.40 at baseline and 0.04 after ASA before conclusion of the procedure (pressures obtained simultaneously, by catheter).

Hospital mortality was 1 case in 133 procedures (0.75%), or 1 in 118 patients (0.85%).

The need for insertion of *permanent pacemakers* changed during our 15 years: the incidence was 20% in the first 59 cases, but only 8.3% in the last 59 cases. This observation is only partially explained by the (mild) decrease in alcohol dose used. Most likely, the main factor associated with a decreased incidence of permanent pacing was the speed of infusion (from an average of: 1 cc/30" to 1 cc/2 minutes.

Morbidity: we saw no infections, two haematomas at the groin (one required surgery), one episode of ventricular tachycardia during the procedure, probably related to inadvertent LV irritation by the pigtail catheter. No episodes of pericardial effusion. Cerebrovascular accidents did not occur. New onset of atrial fibrillation did not occur.

At an average of 8.2-year follow-up (still incomplete!), only 2 out of 17 pacemakers inserted at time of ASA were still required (persistent dependence), whilst the other patients did not require them, any more.

Follow-up mortality: The study was complete in all 117 discharged alive patients and it resulted to be 10/117 during an average follow-up of 8.1 years. This mortality corresponds to 1.23/year, which is very close to that one expected in coetaneous persons of a general population. The causes of death in the 11 fatalities were related to pacemaker complications in two (case no. 1: a 74-year-old female with very high-risk profile, in view of the presence of systemic-level pulmonary hypertension died in the hospital at onset of advanced AV block, but malfunctioning pacemaker due to displacement; case no. 2 was due to a permanent pacemaker insertion complicated by unrecognised perforation and haemo-pericardium, after hospital discharge on warfarin for chronic atrial fibrillation). Another death was due to cocaine abuse, a few days after a repeat ASA, in a patient with an AICD (for septal thickness of >3 cm). Drug toxicity resulted in a ventricular fibrillation storm, requiring more than 200 defibrillations over 24 hours, well beyond the capacity of the AICD battery. Two cases had non-cardiac deaths, whilst no cause of death was available in the other cases. No one had signs of heart failure.

In summary, our experience is quite encouraging in term of immediate and late results. Such experience, in a continuous unselected series, may support the theory that claims that in centres adopting mature, excellent techniques, all patients with significant HOCM can be potentially treated effectively by ASA, with similar results and lower complications and inconveniencies than by SSM. Obviously, our brief review needs more extensive and prospective study, including a larger prospective multicentre study, that could objectively demonstrate that a mature ASA could be superior to SSM (contrary to the current 'imposed credo' that advises ASA only in high-risk HOCM!).

30.9 Discussion

ASA seem to have reached maturity,[11–14] 20 years after its introduction, and it appears that both peri-procedural mortality, morbidity, and especially ease of recovery could be globally assumed as attractive advantages over SSM. Additionally, if we review the results of ASA at the primary time for judgement (about 6 months after ASA, when remodelling of the septum and of the SAM mechanism are essentially complete), we could agree on the following observations:

1. Midterm success rate is quite favourable or equal to SSM, in terms of both residual sub-aortic gradient, disappearance of SAM, thinning of the upper septum, of arrhythmias (as by the important markers of mortality, SCD, aborted VF and also by pacemaker dependence, in the receivers of postoperative pacemakers). Onset of congestive heart failure is exceptional, in patients who received initial good results of ASA. Also, mitral regurgitation secondary to SAM decreases significantly and consistently.

2. On the way of maturing such experience, we learned important procedural aspects of ASA. Alcohol does not always spread uniformly all through the expected distribution area of the target vessel. Some of the alcohol must go out of the target myocardium by other routes, away from the septum (through the thebesian veins into the RV? or, through septal collaterals, to the distal septum or the papillary muscles?). Clearly, ours as well as other investigators observations (see Figure 30.5 and Veselka's Figure 1[11]) the correlation between the peak cardiac enzymes after ASA and gradient abolition is not close. Evidently, in several cases, alcohol infusion does not yield the expected results in gradient abolition as in other cases: this could be the most important limitation in using only echocardiography to identify the target area.

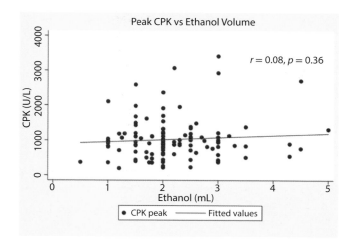

Figure 30.5 Correlation study of scar size (by peak CPK) versus administered ethanol volume. The results suggest a wide variation of the affective scar size in response to similar quantities of ethanol administration (see text).

3. It is now confirmed that slowing the speed of alcohol infusion is important both in terms of lowering the risk of AV block, need for permanent pacemaker and to expand the diffusion of alcohol laterally to the direction of the instrumented septal, leading to more efficient ablation process.

4. The original intuition by Dr. Sigwalt in proposing ASA is basically correct (myocardial alcoholisation produces shrinkage of the treated tissue) even though we must recognise the uncertainty of a general, rigid policy, which cannot be expected to be valid in all cases. The operator needs to be humble and to observe the facts, adapting to the early response of the intervention. We must realise that the operators are fortunate, since the immediate results on pressure gradient correlate with late results, even though two different mechanisms are at play: initially, an acute myocardial infarction, with a change in consistency of myocardium (flaccid state) and eventually edematous tissue, that may cause early transient recurrence of stenosis[8]) leads usually to the shrinkage of the scar, in the late results).

5. It seems possible, even though not well demonstrable as yet, that inducing necrosis of the upper septum in HOCM does more than eliminating SAS, it may also eliminate the main source of chest pain in HOCM (immediate!), whilst decreasing the substrate promoting re-entry ventricular tachycardia/fibrillation, which most frequently involve such pathway.

Finally, in a contemporary, nationwide report[16] on treatment trends and in-hospital results of SM versus ASA, in the years 2003–2011, a representative sample of 11,248 out of 71,888 patients revealed that: SM was done in 56.8% and ASA in 43.2% of cases; unadjusted incidence of use of SM decreased by 24.5% and ASA increased by 56.2%; *total hospital* mortality was 5.2% versus 0.7%; need of permanent pacemaker was 10% versus 12%; stroke was 1.8% versus 0%; important bleeding requiring transfusion was 2.2% versus 2.0%; acute renal failure was 9.7% versus 3.3%. Variance of results between hospitals was particularly important for SM (mortality varied between 15.6% and 3.8% in the lowest versus highest-volume centres).

References

1. Maron BJ et al. Prevalence of hypertrophic cardiomyopathy in a general population of young adults: Echocardiographic analysis of 4111 subjects in the CARDIA study. *Circulation* 1995; 92: 785–9.
2. Veselka J et al. Risk and causes of death in patients after alcohol septal ablation for hypertrophic obstructive cardiomyopathy. *Can J Cardiol* 2015; 31: 1245–51.
3. Kirklin JW, and Ellis FH Jr. Surgical relief of diffuse subvalvular aortic stenosis. *Circulation* 1961; 24: 739–42.
4. Krajcer Z et al. Septal myotomy-myomectomy versus mitral valve replacement in hypertrophic cardiomyopathy. Ten-year follow-up in 185 patients. *Circulation* 1989; 80(3 Pt 1): l57–64.
5. Sigwart U. Non-surgical myocardial reduction for hypertrophic obstructive cardiomyopathy. *Lancet* 1995; 346: 211–214.
6. Noble S, and Sigwart U. Therapeutic management of hypertrophic obstructive cardiomyopathy: Alcohol septal ablation or surgical myomectomy? *Expert Rev Cardiovasc Ther* 2014; 12(9): 1041–44.
7. Singh K et al. A meta-analysis of current status of alcohol septal ablation and surgical myomectomy for Obstructive hypertrophic cardiomyopathy. *Cath Cardiovasc Interv* 2015.
8. Angelini P. The "1st septal unit" in hypertrophic obstructive cardiomyopathy: A newly recognized anatomo-functional entity, identified during recent alcohol septal ablation experience. *Tex Heart Inst J* 2007; 34(3): 336–46.
9. Yorger DM et al. Time course of pressure gradient response after first alcohol septal ablation for obstructive hypertrophic cardiomyopathy. *Am J Cardiol* 97(10): 1511–14.
10. Lakkis NM et al. Echocardiography-guided ethanol septal reduction for hypertrophic obstructive cardiomyopathy. *Circulation* 1998; 97(10): 1750.
11. Veselka J et al. Early outcomes of alcohol septal ablation for hypertrophic obstructive cardiomyopathy: A European Multicenter and multinational study. *Cath Cardiovasc Interv* 2014; 84: 101–7.
12. Gersh BJ et al. 2011 ACCF/AHA guidelines for diagnosis and treatment of hypertrophic cardiomypathy. 2012; 32: 1059–1064.
13. Sorajia P et al. Survival after alcohol septal ablation for hypertrophic obstructive cardiomyopathy. *Circulation* 2012; 16: 2574–80.
14. Jensen MK et al. Alcohol septal ablation in patients with hypertrophic obstructive cardiomyopathy: Low incidence of sudden death and reduced risk profile. *Heart* 2013; 99: 1012–17.

Percutaneous transvenous mitral commissurotomy

KANJI INOUE

31.1 Introduction

In June 1982, the first clinical application of transvenous mitral commissurotomy was performed successfully by Inoue et al. by using a handmade Inoue balloon catheter. A case report of successful treatments with this balloon was published in 1984 for a total of five patients including the first one.[1] With subsequent incorporation of percutaneous procedure, the method was named as percutaneous transvenous mitral commissurotomy (PTMC), and this naming has been maintained by us until now. Extensive clinical experiences first gained in the Far East with excellent results have established the effectiveness and safety of the procedure in well-selected patients.[2–5] Consequently, PTMC has flourished beyond that region and has been widely adopted in over 90 countries in the world to date.[6,7] The American College of Cardiology and the American Heart Association

(ACC/AHA) 2014 guidelines[8] and the European Society of Cardiology (ESC) 2012 guidelines[9] recommend the PTMC as the first-line treatment for the patients with mitral stenosis having favourable valve morphology or high risk for surgery. Rheumatic heart disease, which is greatly decreased in developed countries, still remains to be a major burden in developing countries where it causes most of the cardiovascular morbidity and mortality in young people, leading to over 1 million deaths per year worldwide.[10–12] Mitral stenosis is predominant in the rheumatic heart diseases, accounting for 60%–70% of them.[13,14] Thus, the role of PTMC is being strongly anticipated as a direct means for saving many lives of patients with mitral stenosis including pregnant women together with their foetuses as well as diverse disabilities due to severe cardiac insufficiency.

As in the previous two versions,[15,16] this chapter basically aims at a concise, rather than exhaustive, introduction to PTMC enough to convey its conceptual and technical essence. At the same time, the author tries to incorporate indispensable practical know-how in performing PTMC together with updates on its recent trend and perspective towards better understanding of the technical versatility and functional potentiality of this procedure.

31.1.1 Equipment

31.1.1.1 Inoue balloon catheter

The Inoue balloon catheter (Figure 31.1) has a single balloon that is made of a double layer of latex rubber, with a synthetic micromesh inserted between the layers for reinforcement. The balloon has a low profile at the deflated state (Figure 31.1a) and can be further slenderised by inserting the metal tube to facilitate its atrial trans-septal passage (Figure 31.1b). The shape of the balloon is designed to change in four stages, depending on the extent of inflation: a small bulge (Figure 31.1c) and a larger spherical shape at the distal half with slight inflation (Figure 31.1d), an hourglass shape with moderate inflation (Figure 31.1e) and a barrel shape with full inflation (Figure 31.1f). The balloon catheter has a 12 Fr tube shaft with a coaxial double lumen. The inner lumen of the catheter permits pressure measurements, blood sampling and insertion of a metal tube, a guidewire or a stylet. The Inoue balloon catheter does not easily slip from the stenosed mitral valve orifice during its inflation. It allows for a short inflation–deflation cycle of 5–6 seconds and the diameter of the balloon can be varied. The Inoue balloon catheter has been commercialised by Toray Industry, Inc. since 1988 in Japan.

31.1.1.2 Auxiliary instruments

In addition to the Inoue balloon catheter, a number of auxiliary instruments are provided as shown in Figure 31.2:

1. Inoue balloon catheter
2. Metal tube (18 gauge, length 80 cm)
3. Dilator (14F polyethylene tube, length 70 cm)
4. Stainless steel guidewire (diameter 0.025 in., length 180 cm). Its coiled tip naturally takes a double spiral shape as shown in the inset with an arrow
5. J-tipped spring wire stylet (diameter 0.038 in., length 80 cm)
6. Syringe (30 mL) with connecting tube
7. Ruler

31.1.2 Indications/contraindications

We reported patient selection criteria for PTMC in 1990[17,18] and have since been using them without substantial changes (Table 31.1). These criteria are similar to the guidelines released in 2014 by ACC/AHA (USA) and in 2012 by ESC (Europe). However, there are important differences in a few aspects as detailed below.

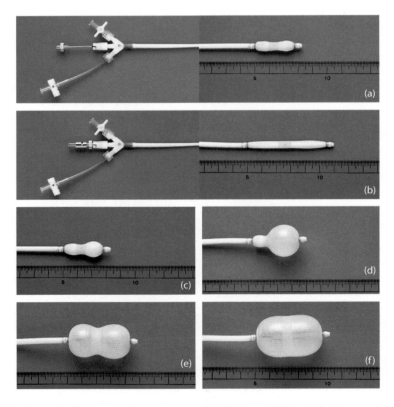

Figure 31.1 The shape of the Inoue balloon at various stages of inflation. **(a)** The default state before use. **(b)**. Stretched for crossing the atrial septum. **(c)**. Slightly inflated at the distal end. **(d)**. Moderately inflated at the distal end. **(e)**. Partially inflated in both proximal and distal ends. **(f)** Fully inflated for separating mitral commissures.

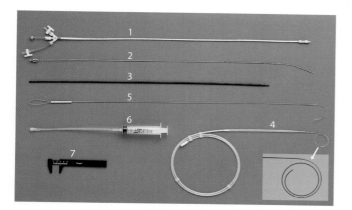

Figure 31.2 The Inoue balloon catheter and auxiliary instruments. 1, the balloon catheter; 2, metal tube; 3, dilator; 4, guidewire; 5, stylet; 6, syringe; 7, ruler.

Table 31.1 Criteria of patient selection

Criteria	Indication
1. Non-pliable valve or valve with severe sub-valvular lesions	B
2. Mitral orifice	
Very small (<0.7 cm²)	A
Relatively large (>1.5 cm²)	B
3. Left atrial thrombus[a]	B
Fresh	C
Located on the pathway of balloon catheter	C
4. Embolic history	A
5. Mitral regurgitation:	
Mild (Sellers 1+)	A
Moderate (Sellers 2+)	B
Severe (Sellers 3+)	C
6. End stage of MS	A
7. Concomitant other valvular disease (AS, AR and TSR)[a]	A
8. Associated diseases of other organs	A

A, First choice; B, conditional choice; C, contraindication; AS, aortic stenosis; AR, aortic regurgitation; TSR, tricuspid stenosis and regurgitation.
[a]Other guidelines generally indicate as C.

31.1.2.1 Valvular morphology

PTMC can be performed largely regardless of the valve orifice size or the degree of valve deformity.[19] Ideal candidates for PTMC are patients with pliable valves without severe sub-valvular lesions. Results of PTMC in these patients are comparable with those of surgical mitral commissurotomy. Although patients with rigid, calcified valves, tightly fused commissures and/or severe sub-valvular lesions may obtain sub-optimal results, PTMC is worth performing since it is very safe and the physical burden and the time required for the procedure are comparable to those for diagnostic cardiac catheterisation.

The majority of such patients show symptomatic improvements and it is rare that PTMC is completely useless.[20,21]

31.1.2.2 Left atrial thrombi

The presence of left atrial thrombus is a general contraindication for PTMC. If the thrombi are immobile, such patients should be treated with warfarin for at least 6 weeks. PTMC can then be applied safely after the thrombi have resolved.[22,23] However, if new thrombi have formed despite warfarin treatment, surgical treatment should be performed. Thrombi attached to the atrial septum, thrombi close to the mitral orifice or mobile thrombi are absolute contraindications.

Chen et al.[24] reported that in selected patients with mitral stenosis who had small and fixed left atrial appendage thrombi, PTMC could be carefully performed with acceptably low complications. From our successful experience, we also consider that thrombi confined to the left atrial appendage or outside of the balloon catheter pathway are not necessarily absolute contraindications for PTMC. PTMC can be safely performed in these patients, if the procedure is properly executed by an experienced operator under monitoring with trans-oesophageal echocardiography.

31.1.2.3 Associated mitral regurgitation

Patients with mitral regurgitation of grade 3 or above on left ventriculography in the Sellers classification are contraindicated for PTMC. In the case of grade 2 mitral regurgitation, PTMC is indicated only when the degree of mitral stenosis is severe, and clinical symptoms are mainly caused by mitral stenosis.

31.1.2.4 Other associated valvular diseases

Other valvular diseases do not hamper the procedure. In patients with aortic regurgitation, the occurrence of congestive heart failure due to acute volume loading of the left ventricle following PTMC might theoretically be a problem. However, such haemodynamic changes do not usually occur in practice because the increase in cardiac output following PTMC is mild. Patients with severe aortic regurgitation should undergo combined aortic and mitral valve replacement.

31.1.2.5 Patients at surgical high risk

PTMC can be performed safely and effectively in patients who are at unacceptably high risk for mitral valve surgery. If the clinical and haemodynamic statuses contraindicate surgical treatment, PTMC can be used as a bridge to surgical treatment.

31.1.2.6 Pregnancy

PTMC can be performed during pregnancy without significant maternal risk and foetal morbidity or mortality.[25–28] Compared with open mitral commissurotomy during pregnancy, PTMC is safe and effective and appears to be preferable for the foetus. It is recommended that PTMC is performed after 14 weeks of pregnancy, when the impact of x-ray irradiation on the foetus has decreased. However, in the presence of unstable clinical conditions, PTMC can be performed irrespective of gestational age. Of course, PTMC should be performed with total pelvic and abdominal shielding.

31.2 Selection of the balloon catheter

It is important to select the balloon catheter size properly for each individual patient. In selecting the catheter size, the patient's height is used as a first guide (Table 31.2).[4] The choice of size is then modified according to the following factors: valvular condition, age, gender, occupation and degree of surgical risk. Patients with severe valve deformity have a high risk of developing significant mitral regurgitation following the procedure. Therefore, a balloon catheter one or two sizes smaller than that dictated by the patient's height should be selected.

31.3 Preoperative and postoperative management

31.3.1 Premedication

Patients in atrial fibrillation or those with a history of paroxysmal atrial fibrillation should be anticoagulated with warfarin for at least 6 weeks.

31.3.2 Heparin during PTMC

A total dose of 100 U/kg body weight of heparin should be given to patients already receiving warfarin; 150 U/kg body weight of heparin is given to those not receiving warfarin. Half of the dose is given at the beginning of the procedure, and the rest is given after successful atrial septal puncture. In elderly patients or patients with hepatic dysfunction, the amount of warfarin should be reduced to avoid serious haemorrhagic complications.

31.3.3 Postoperative management

Patients remain at rest for 24 hours after PTMC. Doppler echocardiography is performed to confirm the absence of cardiac tamponade 4–5 hours after PTMC. When patients show an uncomplicated course after the procedure, they are

usually discharged from the hospital after 1–3 days. Patients in atrial fibrillation remain on warfarin therapy.

31.3.4 Atrial septal puncture

Trans-septal catheterisation is a prerequisite to the introduction of guidewire and balloon catheters into the left atrium. For PTMC, basically the same trans-septal technique is used and the site of puncture, *fossa ovalis*, is targeted as in ordinary diagnostic and interventional applications. However, special cautions and manoeuvres are required for PTMC, because the anatomical location and morphology of *fossa ovalis* are often deviated in patients with mitral stenosis having an enlarged left atrium, making its detection and the subsequent balloon manipulation difficult. To overcome these problems, Inoue devised the following method to determine an optimal puncture site by using well-recognisable cardiographic objects as landmarks.[17,18]

31.3.5 Landmarks for atrial septal puncture

Right atrial angiography is performed under normal respiration in the frontal view until the aorta is visualised (Figure 31.3). On the right atrial stopped-frame image at systole, the position of the upper end of the tricuspid valve is regarded as point A. On the left atrial stopped-frame image, a horizontal line is drawn from point A to the point where it intersects with the right lateral edge of the left atrium (regarded as point B). A vertical line is drawn from the midpoint of line AB, and the point where it intersects with the lower edge of the left atrium is regarded as point C. The puncture site is on the vertical line about two-thirds of the vertebral body height above point C.

Since its introduction, this method has widely been used and proved to be safe and effective. For information,

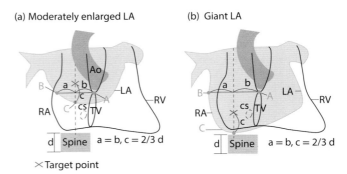

(a) Moderately enlarged LA   (b) Giant LA

✕ Target point

Figure 31.3 Schematic illustrations showing how to choose landmarks for atrial septal puncture with the guide of frontal plane right atrial angiography which is performed under normal respiration until the aorta is visualised. (a) Moderately enlarged LA. (b) Giant LA. RV, right ventricle; RA, right atrium; LA, left atrium; Ao, aorta; TV, tricuspid valve; CS, coronary sinus. (Adapted with permission from Inoue.[17])

Table 31.2 Balloon selection

Catheter grade	Diameter range (mm)	Patient height (cm)
PTMC-30	26–30	>180
PTMC-28	24–28	>160
PTMC-26	22–26	>147
PTMC-24	20–24	≤147

Figures 31.4 and 31.5 show how errors in selecting the puncture site could adversely affect the subsequent balloon catheter insertion into the mitral valve or even incur serious complications.

31.3.6 Trans-septal puncture

Trans-septal puncture is performed by the standard procedure as modified to better adapt for PTMC as previously described by Inoue and collaborators.[18,29] For technical details, operators particularly those starting to perform PTMC are recommended to study their articles.

Recently, intracardiac echocardiography is increasingly used as an aid to atrial septal puncture in developed countries. Because they can clearly show the positions of both the needle point and *fossa ovalis* on the atrial septum, it may be helpful for untrained hands to execute the procedure safely and precisely. However, serious complication including tamponade could occur even with the ultrasound guidance, so that acquisition of basic trans-septal skill together with deep understanding of the aforementioned technical requirements unique to PTMC are still essential.

31.4 PTMC procedure

31.4.1 Balloon preparation

After confirmation of the balloon diameter, the balloon is prepared for insertion. The metal tube is inserted into the inner tube of the balloon catheter and locked in place. Then, the inner tube is pushed forward until its pin is locked into the slot. In this position, the balloon is fully stretched.

31.4.2 Insertion of balloon catheter into the left atrium

After the trans-septal catheter, which was used for trans-septal puncture, is carefully pulled back 1–2 cm so that its tip does not touch the left atrial wall, the stainless steel guidewire is passed through the catheter and advanced until its coiled loop touches the roof of the left atrium. The trans-septal catheter is then removed and the 14 Fr dilator is inserted into the left atrium over the guidewire to dilate the puncture site of the femoral vein and atrial septum, and then the dilator is removed. The balloon catheter with its balloon segment stretched is passed over the guidewire across the atrial septum and advanced until its tip approaches the roof of the left atrium, with the proximal part of the balloon remaining within the right atrium (Figure 31.6a1). Pushing the balloon catheter forcefully against the roof of the atrium should be avoided, as this would bend the guidewire into an acute angle, making subsequent manipulation difficult (Figure 31.6b). After the balloon tip is advanced near the roof of the left atrium, the metal tube is released and withdrawn 2–3 cm from the inner tube (arrow), and then both the balloon catheter and metal tube are advanced (Figure 31.6a2). The balloon is inserted along the guidewire until the entire balloon is within the left atrium (Figure 31.6a3). Next, the inner tube is released and pulled back until resistance is felt, thus the stretched balloon is returned to its original length (Figure 31.6a4). Only the balloon catheter is advanced further over the coiled guidewire until the balloon tip is near the mitral valve orifice (Figure 31.6a5). Finally, both the metal tube and guidewire are removed simultaneously.

Notice: Because the tip of the balloon catheter is dull shaped so as not to injure the cardiac inner surface, it could

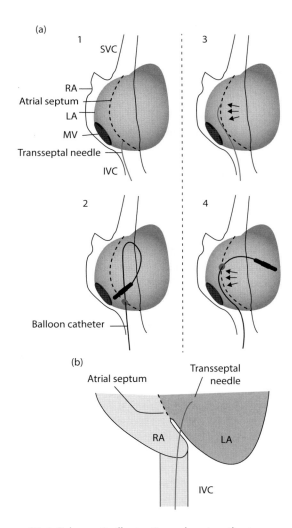

Figure 31.4 Schematic illustrations showing the transseptal puncture and balloon insertion in the case of an enlarged left atrium in the lateral view. **(a)** When puncture is properly made as in a1, the balloon can been easily directed towards the mitral valve (a2). If the puncture site is deviated upward (a3), it becomes difficult not only to make the septal puncture but also to direct the balloon towards the mitral valve (a4). **(b)** In patients with a highly enlarged left atrium, puncturing a site below the predesignated target could cause perforation through bulged walls of the left and right atriums to leading to serious cardiac tamponade. SVC, superior vena cava; IVC, inferior vena cava; RA, right atrium; LA, left atrium; MV, mitral valve.

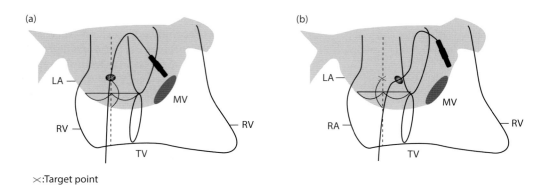

×:Target point

Figure 31.5 The effects of lateral deviation in the puncture site on the manipulation of the balloon catheter. **(a)** The balloon catheter inserted through an optimal puncture site is easily directed towards the mitral orifice. **(b)** When the septal puncture site is deviated leftward, it is difficult to direct the balloon catheter towards the mitral orifice because the catheter curves in steps at the septum. LA, left atrium; RA, right atrium; RV, right ventricle; TV, tricuspid valve; MV, mitral valve. (Adapted with permission from Inoue.[17])

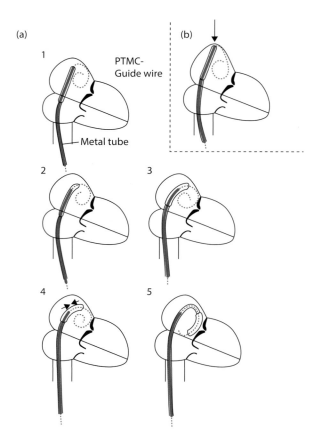

Figure 31.6 How to insert the balloon catheter into the left atrium across the atrial septum (a) Stepwise manipulations of the balloon catheter from its trans-septal passage to accession to the mitral orifice. (b) An unfavourable situation liable to occur if the balloon catheter is pushed too far into the left atrium. See section 31.4.2 in the text for details. (Adapted with permission from Inoue.[17]).

occasionally get stuck against the lid of the venous puncture site. To resolve this problem, the balloon catheter is initially pushed into the vein at a near vertical angle. Once the catheter tip enters the vein, the catheter is tilted more horizontally and is advanced along the vein. Similarly, if the balloon tip gets stuck at the atrial septum puncture site, its passage is facilitated by rotating the metal tube inside the balloon catheter about 180° and then by pushing the catheter.

31.4.3 Crossing of the mitral orifice

After the balloon catheter is inserted into the left atrium, the fluoroscopic projection is changed from frontal to 30° right anterior oblique view. The distal portion of the balloon is partially inflated to a diameter of 10–15 mm with about 1 mL of diluted contrast medium. This allows the balloon to easily pass through the mitral valve orifice into the left ventricle and ensures that the balloon will not stray among the chordal structures in the left ventricle.

There are two different methods of inserting the balloon catheter from the left atrium across the mitral valve orifice into the left ventricle (Figure 31.7a and b). In the direct method, the spring wire stylet is inserted into the balloon tip (Figure 31.7a1). The balloon catheter and the stylet are moved together while twisting the stylet counterclockwise, so that the balloon tip is directed towards the mitral valve orifice and the balloon is aligned with the long axis of the left ventricle (Figure 31.7a2). Next, with the balloon catheter held fixed in the position, the stylet is withdrawn 4–5 cm while being twisted counterclockwise by approximately 180°, or, with the stylet held fixed, the balloon catheter is advanced towards the valve orifice (Figure 31.7a3). Insertion is easier when the stylet is withdrawn 4–5 cm while being twisted counterclockwise and the balloon catheter is advanced forward 4–5 cm at the same time. In the loop method, which was developed by Hosokawa et al. in 1990,[30] the balloon catheter is inserted deeply into the left atrium and the stylet is inserted into the balloon catheter to a position 3–4 cm from the balloon base (Figure 31.7b1). By rotating the stylet clockwise by approximately 360°, a loop is formed at the catheter section in the left atrium and the balloon tip is brought towards the mitral

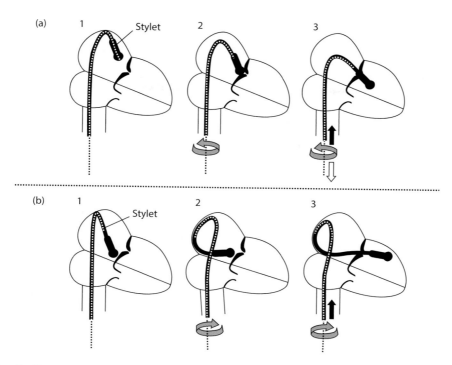

Figure 31.7 Methods of balloon insertion across the mitral orifice. **(a)** Direct method and **(b)** loop method. See section 31.4.3 in the text for details. (Adapted with permission from Inoue.[17])

valve orifice (Figure 31.7b2). While the stylet is held firm, only the balloon catheter is advanced (Figure 31.7b3). The balloon catheter can be inserted easily across the mitral valve orifice into the left ventricle. This method is available when the atrial septal puncture site is deviated upward or leftward from the target point.

If the loop becomes too large, the balloon catheter may fall short of the valve as targeted. In such a case, the loop is made smaller by appropriately pulling back the balloon catheter or the stylet, or both. Finally, the balloon catheter is advanced while the stylet is held in place.

31.4.4 Dilatation of the mitral orifice

After the balloon catheter is inserted into the left ventricle, the balloon catheter is moved back and forth two or three times inside the left ventricle to confirm that the balloon has not strayed among the chordal structures (Figure 31.8a1). If strayed among the chordae, the balloon portion tends to be curved or kinked unnaturally (Figure 31.8a2). In that case, the balloon should be pulled back into the left atrium and then reinserted across the mitral orifice.

Inflation of the balloon at the mitral orifice is performed by two individuals under fluoroscopic guidance. The operator manipulates the balloon catheter and the assistant handles the syringe. After the assistant has partially inflated the distal portion of the balloon, the operator pulls the catheter back until resistance is felt (Figure 31.8b1). Immediately after gently pressing the catheter against the valve orifice, the assistant inflates the balloon fully. As soon as the predetermined amount of diluted contrast material is rapidly injected from

the syringe, the assistant deflates the balloon quickly by pulling the syringe. The change of the balloon shape is observed on the right anterior oblique view under fluoroscopy (Figure 31.9). To be noted, a rupture of the atrial septum could occasionally happen owing to undue traction of the catheter during balloon inflation, particularly at full inflation (Figure 31.8b2). To avoid this complication, operator should release the balloon catheter from his hand immediately after the hourglass shape of balloon appears.

31.4.5 Assessment of efficacy

After each dilatation, the balloon catheter is withdrawn into the left atrium and the stylet is removed. The trans-mitral gradient, left atrial pressure and cardiac output are measured. The efficacy of valve dilatation is assessed by mean trans-mitral gradient auscultation and Doppler echocardiography examination. If necessary, left ventriculography is repeated to assess the degree of mitral regurgitation. The balloon dilatation procedure is performed using a stepwise dilatation technique described in Section 31.5. The stepwise process is repeated until the pressure gradient is reduced as much as possible without creating significant mitral regurgitation.

31.4.6 Removal of the balloon catheter

Upon withdrawal of the balloon catheter after completion of the dilatation procedure, the balloon segment is stretched to avoid injury to the atrial septum and the right femoral vein. First, the catheter is gently pulled until resistance is felt

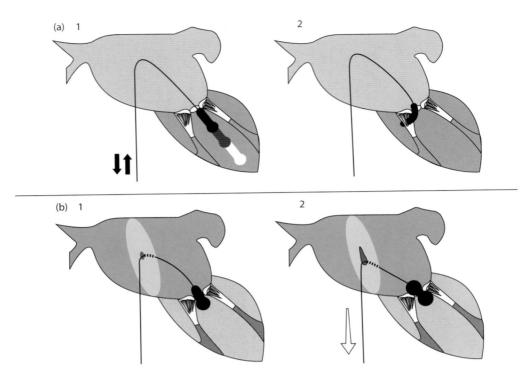

Figure 31.8 Complications due to mishandling of the balloon catheter during its insertion into the left ventricle **(a)** and its subsequent inflation **(b)**. See section 31.4.4 in the text for details. (Adapted with permission from Inoue.[17])

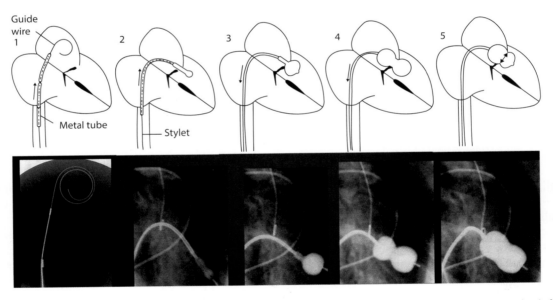

Figure 31.9 Sequential fluoroscopic images during PTMC in the right anterior oblique view (bottom row, the left four panels), and their schematic drawings (upper row). The first panel in the bottom row shows the guidewire and stretched balloon catheter as fluoroscopically imaged in vitro.

at the atrial septum puncture site. While the balloon catheter is kept fixed at this point, the metal tube with the guidewire hidden inside is inserted into the balloon catheter, and then the guidewire is advanced to make its tip coiled in the left atrium. The metal tube is advanced to the balloon tip to stretch the balloon segment. Finally, the balloon catheter is withdrawn through the atrial septum and the femoral vein.

31.5 Stepwise dilatation technique

The balloon is first inflated to a diameter of 4 mm below the maximum specified balloon diameter and the sequential inflations are repeated with stepwise increments in the balloon diameter. On each inflation, the balloon diameter is increased by 1 or 2 mm. The parameters important in deciding whether to dilate further are described below. The balloon catheter may be changed to a new one of different size grade during stepwise inflations, if necessary.

31.5.1 Commissure split

The most important factor affecting immediate results of PTMC is the separation of fused commissures. After each dilatation procedure, the degree of commissure separation is assessed by two-dimensional echocardiogram on the parasternal short-axis view. Figure 31.10 diagrammatically shows the method of stepwise dilatation.

The morphology of commissure separation is divided into three types: Type I, residual fusions left in both commissures; Type II, residual fusion left in either commissure; Type III, no separation in either commissure. Further, Type I and Type II are divided into two sub-classes depending on whether separation is effected in both commissures (B and D) or only either commissure (A and C). The need for further dilatation procedure is finally determined by assessing the degree of mitral regurgitation. For each combination of commissure splitting type and resultant mitral regurgitation, recommendable choice of incremental diameter (1 or 2 mm) or termination of dilatation is indicated in a respective rectangular box.

31.5.2 Mitral regurgitation

The degree of mitral regurgitation is assessed by left atrial pressure and Doppler echocardiography immediately after each dilatation. Left ventricular angiography should be performed if Doppler assessment is inconclusive. Colour Doppler assessment is useful to determine the severity of new or increased mitral regurgitation and to detect the site of mitral regurgitation. A regurgitation signal should be thoroughly sought using several views. When tearing of mitral leaflet is suspected, even if the development of mitral regurgitation is mild, further dilatation should be terminated. In the case of patients with pre-existing grade 2 mitral regurgitation, if any recognisable increase is detected, it is advisable to stop further dilatation. If grade 2 mitral regurgitation is newly detected following valve dilatation, further dilatation is performed only when both commissures remain fused, as in Type I. In this case, it is desirable to inflate the balloon diameter by 1 mm more than in the previous dilatation. If complete splitting is detected in only one commissure as in C and D of Type II, further dilatation may be continued to separate the remaining fused commissure only when the degree of mitral regurgitation is mild or non-existent.

Notice: Despite the above explanation, Doppler echocardiography is not always necessary, especially for young patients with favourable valve morphology as frequently encountered in developing countries. Usually, commissure adhesions in such patients are not so tough and can be separated adequately without severe regurgitation. Therefore, it is feasible to assess the degrees of both mitral stenosis and resultant regurgitation by using simpler conventional methods such as pressure measurement, left atrial pressure patterns (increase in V wave), auscultation and left ventricular angiography.

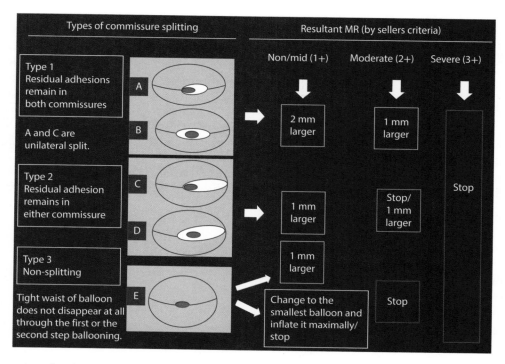

Figure 31.10 Flow chart for decision-making in the stepwise dilatation technique. See section 31.5 in the text for details.

31.5.3 Constriction of inflated balloon

A decrease or disappearance of constriction during inflation of the balloon is observed under fluoroscopy. Persistence of a marked constriction in the inflated balloon indicates either that the commissural fusions are very tight or that the internal pressure of the inflated balloon is insufficient. In either case, the balloon is inflated further by injecting a larger volume of diluted contrast medium. If this manoeuvre still fails, further dilatation using the same balloon should be stopped, because the leaflets could be ruptured before commissures are separated. To avoid this worst situation necessitating emergency surgery, the balloon catheter should be replaced with the smallest one so as to limit the degree of resultant mitral regurgitation, and then it is maximally inflated to produce a sufficient internal pressure.

31.5.4 Increase in valve area

A mitral valve area can be obtained from two-dimensional echocardiography using planimetry, the Doppler pressure half-time method or haemodynamic measurement using Gorlin's equation. However, it is cautioned that the accuracy of measurement by any method is rather limited especially in patients with unfavourable mitral valves.[31-35] Therefore, obtained values should be taken as relative measures and their comparison by face values is unadvisable, particularly when they are determined by different methods or by different centres, even if the same method is used.

31.6 Results of PTMC

During the past three decades since PTMC was first introduced, the technique has been perfected and widely confirmed to afford excellent short- and long-term results in well-selected patients. With an additional advantage of its minimally invasive nature, PTMC has been established as the first-line treatment for patient with mitral stenosis having favourable morphology or high surgical risk. Representative clinical studies supporting these contentions are reviewed below.

31.6.1 Acute outcome

Although there have been mounting reports on the results of PTMC up to the present, its excellent immediate efficacy has already been well demonstrated in large studies conducted

in late 1980s through mid-1990s. Thus, I herein pick up three such earlier series performed by the author himself and his close collaborators. Table 31.3 shows patients' baseline characteristics. Of Inoue's cases, 6.4% of patients had left atrial thrombi documented by trans-thoracic or trans-oesophageal echocardiography, or both. Patients with mitral regurgitation of three-fourth or more on left ventriculography and with fresh thrombi were contraindicated.

The immediate excellent haemodynamic effects of PTMC in these three series are summarised in Table 31.4. In Inoue's study, the mean mitral valve area measured by echocardiographic planimetry significantly increased from 1.1 ± 0.02 to 1.9 ± 0.03 cm^2. The increase in the valve area was comparable with that of surgical commissurotomy. As a result, mean mitral trans-valvular pressure gradient, left atrial pressure and mean pulmonary artery pressure were significantly reduced, and cardiac index or cardiac output was significantly increased. Hung et al. found that exercise tolerance improved after the procedure.[4] In addition, Tamai et al. documented that the mitral flow dynamics during exercise as well as the resting flow dynamics improved.[36] In more recent studies, especially those conducted in developed countries, PTMC is being increasingly performed in patients with increased age, calcified or more deformed valves and concomitant comorbidities.[37,38] Partly because of this trend, increasing procedural complication rates are noted in some recent studies.[39] Nevertheless, a systematic analysis of temporal trends over 15 years by a French group showed that the safety and efficacy of PTMC, despite increasing candidates' age and their less favourable anatomy, can be maintained at high standards by accumulating experience in improving the technique, patient selection and the timing of treatment.[37]

31.6.2 Complications

PTMC using the Inoue balloon catheter has a high technical success rate and low complication rate. Table 31.5 shows the failure and complication rates of PTMC. In Inoue's experience, there were no procedure-related deaths. The creation of (or increase in) mitral regurgitation was demonstrated in approximately 20% of patients. However, the increase was usually mild. Severe increase occurred in 1.4%–5.2%. Severe regurgitation most commonly resulted from rupture or tearing of the mitral leaflets. Embolic complications were caused by dislodging unsuspected left atrial thrombi

Table 31.3 Patient characteristics

	Inoue (n = 981)	Hung (n = 572)	Chen (n = 149)
Female (%)	74%	71%	69%
Age range (mean)	1–78 (50)	19–80 (44)	15–56 (35)
Atrial fibrillation (%)	60	67	18
Embolic history (%)	19	11	0
MR (+1 or +2) (%)	26	24	14
Previous surgical commissurotomy (%)	12	2	0
NYHA (III or IV) (%)	31		

Table 31.4 Acute haemodynamic results

	Inoue (n = 981)	Hung (n = 572)	Chen (n = 149)
LA pressure (mmHg)			
Before		24.2 ± 5.6	22.1 ± 8.2
After		15.1 ± 5.1	10.0 ± 5.7
MV gradient (mmHg)			
Before	11.7 ± 0.2	13.0 ± 5.1	17.4 ± 7.6
After	5.6 ± 0.1	5.7 ± 2.6	2.7 ± 3.1
Mean PA pressure (mmHg)			
Before		39.7 ± 13.0	34.1 ± 13.3
After		30.6 ± 10.9	22.7 ± 9.8
MV area (cm^2)			
Before	1.1 ± 0.02	1.0 ± 0.3	1.06 ± 0.21
After	1.9 ± 0.03	2.0 ± 0.7	2.04 ± 0.32
CO (L/min) or CI (L/min/m^2)			
Before	4.0 ± 0.04	4.4 ± 1.4	3.2 ± 0.7 (CI)
After	4.4 ± 0.05	4.7 ± 1.2	3.9 ± 0.5 (CI)

CI, cardiac index; CO, cardiac output; LA, left atrium; MV, mitral valve; PA, pulmonary artery.

Table 31.5 Complication rates

	Inoue (n = 981)	Hung (n = 572)	Chen (n = 149)
Mitral regurgitation (%)			
Increase	19.1	29.9	13.7
Severe	2.5	5.2	1.3
Thromboembolism (%)	0.3	2.1	1.3
Cardiac tamponade (%)	1.1	0.2	0.7
Atrial septal defect (%)	11.0	10.2	0.7
Mortality (%)	0.0	0.2	0.0

or by inadequate heparinisation in the early experience. PTMC was performed without embolic complications in patients with thrombus documented by echocardiography. Although oximetry demonstrated left-to-right shunts in approximately 10% of patients, the majority of these patients had small shunts with pulmonary-to-systemic flow ratios of 1.4 or less. Using trans-oesophageal colour Doppler echocardiography, Yoshida et al.[40] observed that the diameter of atrial septal defect decreased over time and the left-to-right shunts disappeared within 6 months after PTMC in most patients. In Inoue's case, cardiac tamponade occurred in 1.1% – as a complication of trans-septal puncture in 1.0% and of diagnostic catheterisation in 0.1%.

31.6.3 Factors affecting immediate haemodynamic results

Our analysis revealed that the immediate haemodynamic results of PTMC are influenced by the following factors: pliability of the anterior mitral leaflet, valvular calcium on fluoroscope, thickened mitral commissures, pre-existing mitral regurgitation, previous surgical commissurotomy, the presence of atrial fibrillation and patient's age. In addition, the incidence of resultant mitral regurgitation is significantly higher in patients with thickened mitral commissures and severely restricted mitral valves (mitral valve area < 1 cm^2). The importance of these factors has widely been noted in many other studies as well.

31.6.4 Late outcome

During the past decade, there begin to emerge flurry of large-scale studies reporting very long-term results of PTMC up to 15–20 years. Table 31.6 summarises the long-term outcomes presented in five such studies conducted by using Inoue balloon either exclusively[41-43] or partly with the double balloon as an alternative device.[44,45] In these studies, the rates of event-free survival in Kaplan–Meier estimate at the longest 19–20 years of follow-up performed were 30%–40%. This confirmed the excellent efficacy and durability of PTMC and lends further support to its accepted indication as the first-line treatment for mitral stenosis.[8,9] Furthermore, these studies also indicated that the long-term outcome after PTMC is mainly determined by the immediate procedural

Table 31.6 Long-term outcome after percutaneous transvenous mitral commissurotomy

Author year	No. of patients	Age at baseline (years)	Mean follow-up (years)	Balloon used	Outcomes evaluated	Event-free survival Kaplan–Meier estimate
Palacios et al. 2002	879	55 ± 15	4.2 ± 3.7	IB & DB	Death, MVR, re-PTMC	23% at 15 y
Fawzy et al. 2009	547	32 ± 11	9.52 ± 5.2	IB	Death, MVR, re-PTMC, NYHA ≥3	42% at 19 y
Kim et al. 2010	303	39.3 ± 10.8	10 ± 5	IB	Death, systemic embolism, admission for heart failure, re-PTMC, MV surgery	71% at 10 y
Bouleti et al. 2014	1024	49 ± 14	10.2	IB & DB	Death, surgery, re-PTMC, functional impairment (NYHA ≥ 3)	30.2% at 20 y
Tomai et al. 2014	441[a]	55.7 ± 11.8	11.7 ± 4.9	IB	Death, MV surgery, re-PTMC	35.9% at 20 y

DB, double balloon; IB, Inoue balloon; MV, mitral valve; MVA, mitral valve area; MVR, mitral valve replacement; NYHA, New York Heart Association functional class; PTMC, percutaneous mitral commissurotomy.
[a]A sub-cohort with procedural success and complete follow-up.

results. This prediction exactly accords with, and strongly reemphasises the importance of the goal set by the stepwise dilatation technique using the Inoue balloon, namely, a maximal possible separation of fused mitral commissures with a resultant mitral regurgitation kept at a tolerable level of grade 2 or less.

Despite the above-noted favourable results after PTMC, re-interventions were required in a substantial proportion of patients, nearly 40% in the largest study by Bouleti et al.[46] and more-or-less similar percentages in other studies as well. Among the reinterventions performed, repeat PTMC was fairly frequent (around 10%) next to mitral valve replacement (20% or more). Actually, patients with previous commissurotomy mostly surgical one were invariably included at significant rates (5%–16%) in the five studies in Table 31.6. Bouleti et al.[46] reanalysed late outcomes focusing on 163 such patients and revealed that 20% of them have good functional results at 20 years. These results are rather worse than those obtained with patients after primary PTMC, but still good enough to support the use of PTMC after previous commissurotomy, particularly in selected patients with few symptoms and favourable haemodynamic conditions.

31.7 Current status and perspective of PTMC

Rheumatic heart diseases are still imposing a huge burden on developing countries, which hold three-fourths of world's population. Among them, mitral stenosis is predominant. In general, patients with mitral stenosis in these countries are relatively young and have pliable valves without severe sub-valvular lesions and severe calcification, being suitable for PTMC. Therefore, they could largely be rescued by

PTMC from distress or death. Of such prospective candidates, an important fraction requiring special attention is occupied by female patients with pregnancy who are particularly abundant in developing countries and suffering all the more together with their foetuses from haemodynamic burdens due to mitral stenosis.

Unfortunately, the use of PTMC has been hampered in developing countries, because of economical reasons entailing lack of catheterisation laboratories, lack of equipments and devices required for PTMC including the balloon catheter and lack of doctors trained for PTMC. Thus, promoting a movement of 'Developing Countries Acceptable PTMC' is urgently anticipated. In my own clinical experiences in developing countries, I performed PTMC for up to eight cases per day by using one catheter laboratory with limited facilities. This example indicates that PTMC for favourable valves can be simplified in technique and instrumentation with concomitant shortening of the procedure time. As the PTMC inventor, I am really anxious about the enormous number of patients left untreated under the above-noted pessimistic situations.

Acknowledgments

Author deeply thanks Dr. Katsuya Shigesada for his valuable advices, Yoshimasa Nagata for his excellent assistance in drawing figures and Mitsuru Sato for his competent editorial support.

References

1. Inoue K et al. Clinical application of transvenous mitral commissurotomy by a new balloon catheter. *J Thorac Cardiovasc Surg* 1984; 87: 394–402.

2. Inoue K, and Hung JS. Percutaneous transvenous mitral commissurotomy (PTMC): The Far East experience. In: Topol EJ (editor), *Textbook of Interventional Cardiology*. Philadelphia, PA: WB Saunders, 1990, pp. 887–99.

3. Nobuyoshi M et al. Indications, complications, and short-term clinical outcome of percutaneous transvenous mitral commissurotomy. *Circulation* 1989; 80: 782–92.

4. Hung JS et al. Short- and long-term results of catheter balloon percutaneous transvenous mitral commissurotomy. *Am J Cordial* 1991; 67: 854–62.

5. Chen CR et al. Percutaneous mitral valvuloplasty with a single rubber-nylon balloon (Inoue balloon): Long-term results in 71 patients. *Am Heart J* 1990; 120: 561–8.

6. Feldman T. Hemodynamic results, clinical outcome, and complications of Inoue balloon mitral valvotomy. *Cathet Cardiovasc Diagn* 1994; 2: 2–7.

7. Vahanian A et al. Percutaneous transvenous mitral commissurotomy using the Inoue balloon: International experience. *Cathet Cardiovasc Diagn* 1994; 2: 8–15.

8. Nishimura RA et al. 2014 AHA/ACC guideline for the management of patients with valvular heart disease: Executive summary: A report of the American College of Cardiology/American Heart Association Task Force on practice guidelines. *J Am Coll Cardiol* 2014; 63(22): 2438–88.

9. Vahanian A et al. Guidelines on the management of valvular heart disease (version 2012). *Eur Heart J* 2012; 33: 2451–96.

10. Zuhlke L et al. Characteristics, complications, and gaps in evidence-based interventions in rheumatic heart disease: The global rheumatic heart disease registry (the REMEDY study). *Eur Heart J* 2015; 36: 1115–22.

11. Carapetis JR et al. The global burden of group a streptococcal diseases. *Lancet Infect Dis* 2005; 5: 685–94.

12. Remenyi B et al. Position statement of the world heart federation on the prevention and control of rheumatic heart disease. *Nat Rev Cardiol* 2013; 10: 284–92.

13. Manjunath et al. Incidence and patterns of valvular heart disease in a tertiary care high-volume cardiac center: A single center experience. *Indian Heart J* 2014; 66: 320–26.

14. Faheem M et al. Pattern of valvular lesions in rheumatic heart disease. *J Postgrad Med* 2007; 21: 99–103.

15. Inoue K, and Yoshida Y. Percutaneous transvenous mitral commissurotomy. In: Grech ED, and Ramsdale DR (editors), *Practical Interventional Cardiology*, 1st Edition. CRC Press, Boca Raton, 1996, pp. 327–341.

16. Inoue K et al. Percutaneous transvenous mitral commissurotomy. In: Grech ED, and Ramsdale DR (editors), *Practical Interventional Cardiology*, 2nd Edition. CRC Press, Boca Raton, 2001, pp. 373–387.

17. Inoue K. Technique of percutaneous transvenous mitral commissurotomy (PTMC). *Kokyu To Junkan* 1990; 38: 533–45 (Japan).

18. Inoue K. Percutaneous transvenous mitral commissurotomy using the Inoue balloon. *Eur Heart J* 1991; 12: 99–108.

19. Feldman T et al. Effect of valve deformity on results and mitral regurgitation after Inoue balloon commissurotomy. *Circulation* 1992; 85: 180–7.

20. Bouleti C et al. Relationship between valve calcification and long-term results of percutaneous mitral commissurotomy for rheumatic mitral stenosis. *Circ Cardiovasc Interv* 2014; 7: 381–9.

21. Dreyfus J et al. Feasibility of percutaneous mitral commissurotomy in patients with commissural mitral valve calcification. *Eur Heart J* 2014; 35:1617–23.

22. Hung JS et al. Successful percutaneous transvenous catheter balloon mitral commissurotomy after warfarin therapy and resolution of left atrial thrombi. *Am J Cardiol* 1989; 64: 126–8.

23. Hung JS. Mitral stenosis with left atrial thrombi: Inoue balloon catheter technique. In: Cheng TO (editor), *Percutaneous Balloon Valvuloplasty*. New York, NY: Igaku-Shoin Medical Publishers, 1992, 280–93.

24. Chen WJ et al. Safety of percutaneous transvenous balloon mitral commissurotomy in patients with mitral stenosis and thrombi in the left atrial appendage. *Am J Cardiol* 1992; 70: 117–19.

25. de Souza JAM et al. Percutaneous balloon mitral valvuloplasty in comparison with open mitral valve commissurotomy for mitral stenosis during pregnancy. *J Am Coll Cardiol* 2001; 37: 900–03.

26. Gulraze A et al. Mitral balloon valvuloplasty during pregnancy: The long term up to 17 years obstetric outcome and childhood development. *Pak J Med Sci* 2014; 30: 86–90.

27. Esteves CA et al. Immediate and long-term follow-up of percutaneous balloon mitral valvuloplasty in pregnant patients with rheumatic mitral stenosis. *Am J Cardiol* 2006; 98: 812–6.

28. Bui AH et al. Clinical problem-solving. A tight predicament. *N Engl J Med* 2014; 371: 953–9.

29. Hung JS. Atrial septal puncture technique in percutaneous transvenous mitral commissurotomy: Mitral valvuloplasty using the Inoue balloon catheter technique. *Catheter Cardiovasc Diagn* 1992; 26: 275–84.

30. Hosokawa H et al. Insertion of Inoue balloon catheter in percutaneous transvenous mitral commissurotomy. *Shin Kekkan* 1990; 5: 118–23 (Japan).

31. Thomas JD et al. Inaccuracy of mitral pressure half-time immediately after percutaneous mitral valvotomy. *Circulation* 1988; 78: 980–93.

32. Wisenbaugh T et al. Effect of mitral regurgitation and volume loading on pressure half-time before and after balloon valvotomy in mitral stenosis. *Am J Cordial* 1991; 67: 162–8.

33. Chen C et al. Reliability of the Doppler pressure half-time method for assessing effects of percutaneous mitral balloon valvuloplasty. *J Am Coll Cordial* 1989; 13: 1309–13.

34. Nakatani S et al. Acute reduction of mitral valve area after percutaneous balloon mitral valvuloplasty: Assessment with Doppler continuity equation method. *Am Heart J* 1991; 121: 770–5.

35. Chen C, and Abascal VM. Echocardiographic evaluation. In: Cheng TO (editor), *Percutaneous Balloon Valvuloplasty*. New York, NY: IgakuShoin Medical Publishers, 1992, 27–184.

36. Tamai J et al. Improvement in mitral flow dynamics during exercise after percutaneous transvenous mitral commissurotomy. Noninvasive evaluation using continuous wave Doppler technique. *Circulation* 1990; 81: 46–51.

37. Iung B et al. Temporal trends in percutaneous mitral commissurotomy over a 15-year period. *Eur Heart J* 2004; 25: 701–707.

38. Nunes MC et al. Update on percutaneous mitral commissurotomy. *Heart* 2016; 0: 1–8. doi:1136/heartjnl-2015-308091.

39. Badheka AO et al. Balloon mitral valvuloplasty in the United States: A 13-year perspective. *Am J Med* 2014; 127: 1126.e1–e2.

40. Yoshida K et al. Assessment of left-to-right atrial shunting after percutaneous mitral valvuloplasty by transesophageal color Doppler flow-mapping. *Circulation* 1989; 80: 1521–6.

41. Fawzy ME. Long-term results up to 19 years of mitral balloon valvuloplasty. *Asian Cardiovasc Thorac Ann* 2009; 17: 627–33.

42. Kim KH et al. Left atrial remodelling in patients with successful percutaneous mitral valvuloplasty: Determinants and impact on long-term clinical outcome. *Heart* 2010; 96: 1050–55.

43. Tomai F et al. Twenty year follow-up after successful percutaneous balloon mitral valvuloplasty in a large contemporary series of patients with mitral stenosis. *Int J Cardiol* 2014; 177: 881–5.

44. Palacios IF et al. Which patients benefit from percutaneous mitral balloon valvuloplasty? Prevalvuloplasty and postvalvuloplasty variables that predict long-term outcome. *Circulation* 2002; 105: 1465–71.

45. Bouleti C et al. Late results of percutaneous mitral commissurotomy up to 20 years: Development and validation of a risk score predicting late functional results from a series of 912 patients. *Circulation* 2012; 125: 2119–27.

46. Bouleti C et al. Long-term efficacy of percutaneous mitral commissurotomy for restenosis after previous mitral commissurotomy. *Heart* 2013; 99: 1336–41.

Percutaneous mitral valve repair and replacement

TED FELDMAN, MAYRA GUERRERO

Percutaneous therapy options for mitral regurgitation (MR) were the first concepts in early stages of development over a decade ago.[1] The earliest ideas were based on coronary sinus annuloplasty, since that seemed to be simple from a technical standpoint, and have the potential to mimic an established surgical procedure. In the decade that has followed, the landscape of percutaneous options for treatment of MR has evolved considerably. The entire field of percutaneous mitral repair today is synonymous with MitraClip, since this is the only repair device in wide use globally. The Cardiac Dimensions coronary sinus annuloplasty system, the Carillon, has had Conformité européenne (CE) approval, but has still relatively limited use. Several other devices have completed European approval trials, but at the time of this writing these devices are not yet available for commercial use internationally.

Percutaneous mitral valve (MV) replacement is at its beginning. Several trans-catheter mitral replacement devices have been employed in patients with technical and in some cases clinical success. The field is embryonic. Although ultimately the practice community expects mitral replacement to be similar in effectiveness to trans-catheter aortic valve replacement (TAVR), there are much greater technical challenges for developing mitral replacement devices and also the definition of clinical indications for mitral replacement.

These two frontiers of percutaneous mitral repair and trans-catheter MV replacement represent different approaches to the same clinical problem. While percutaneous repair technologies have tended to leave some residual MR, and there is an expectation that replacement devices will completely eliminate residual MR, it is increasingly clear that there is more to the clinical outcomes of these therapies than the reduction of MR. In fact, modest reductions in MR with some repair devices have led to dramatic clinical improvements and complete elimination of MR with replacement technologies has in some cases had poor clinical outcomes.

32.1 Percutaneous leaflet repair with MitraClip

MitraClip has eclipsed the field of devices in the area of catheter-based repair. Over 25,000 patients have been treated with this device, compared with the next most commonly used device having been used in about 300 patients (Table 32.1). The small number of treated patients for the remaining devices reflects their status as still under investigation. The large experience with MitraClip is well characterized by randomized trials, registry experience and a large body of accumulated analysis in single centre reports (Table 32.2 and Figure 32.1), with substantial data on the subsets of clinical populations with MR.

Table 32.1 Percutaneous mitral repair devices in clinical use

Device	Number of treated patients
(Abbott)	>25,000
CARRILON (cardiac dimensions)	300
Mitralign (Mitralign)	70
Cardioband (Valtech)	50

Table 32.2 MitraClip evidence base

Surgical candidates: 5-year Endovascular Valve Edge-to-Edge Repair Study (EVEREST II) randomised trial
- Better mitral regurgitation (MR) reduction with surgery
- Stable reductions in left ventricle (LV) chamber volumes
- Stable annular dimensions without annuloplasty

High-risk global registry experience
- Improved symptoms
- Procedural safety, short stay
- Decreased heart failure hospitalizations

High-risk degenerative MR
- US approval

High-risk Functional MR
- US Cardiovascular Outcomes Assessment of the MitraClip Percutaneous Therapy for Heart Failure Patients with Functional MR (COAPT) Trial – Randomised MitraClip vs. Guideline directed medical therapy (GDMT) ± cardiac resynchronization therapy (CRT)

Therapy for MR

	Degenerative	Functional
Low surgical risk	Surgical mitral repair	?
High surgical risk	Commercial MitraClip	Global experience COAPT

Figure 32.1 Schema for categorising therapy for function and degenerative MR in lower and higher surgical risk candidates.

32.1.1 MitraClip device and procedure

The MitraClip device is a 4-mm-wide cobalt–chromium implant with two arms that are opened and closed with the use of the delivery system. The procedure is performed under general anaesthesia with the use of fluoroscopic and trans-oesophageal echocardiographic guidance. Trans-septal puncture of the right femoral venous and left atrial access is performed. The device is navigated until it is aligned over the origin of the regurgitant jet and advanced across the mitral orifice into the left ventricle. The mitral leaflets are grasped, and the device is closed to approximate the leaflets and create a double orifice. Reduction of MR to a grade of 2+ or less is assessed in real time with the use of echocardiography. If the reduction in MR is not adequate with a single device, the device may be removed or a second device may be placed. In this trial patients with grade 3+ or 4+ MR despite device treatment were referred for elective valve surgery. Patients were treated with heparin during the procedure, with aspirin (at a dose of 325 mg daily) for 6 months and with clopidogrel (at a dose of 75 mg daily) for 30 days after the MitraClip procedure.

32.1.2 MitraClip randomized trial

The Endovascular Valve Edge-to-Edge Repair Study (EVEREST II) was a randomised comparison of percutaneous mitral repair and MV surgery to evaluate the efficacy and safety of percutaneous MV repair, as compared with conventional surgical repair or replacement.[2] This trial was a landmark investigation in several respects. It was a pivotal trial for a first in class device. It represents the only significant randomised trial in the field of MV therapy. The trial was conducted using a new device with which the investigators and little practical experience, compared with the mature field of surgical MV repair and replacement. The trial demonstrated that MV repair can be accomplished with an investigational procedure that uses the percutaneous MitraClip device, which grasps and approximates the edges of the mitral leaflets at the origin of the regurgitant jet. The trial was conducted with 279 randomly assigned patients with grade 3+ or 4+ MR, randomised in a 2:1 ratio to undergo either percutaneous repair or conventional surgery for repair or replacement of the MV. The primary composite endpoint for efficacy was freedom from death, from surgery for MV dysfunction and from grade 3+ or 4+ MR at 12 months. The primary safety endpoint was a composite of major adverse events within 30 days. After 1 year, the rates of the primary endpoint for efficacy were 55% in the percutaneous-repair group and 73% in the surgery group ($p = .007$). The respective rates of the components of the primary end point were as follows: death, 6% in each group; surgery for MV dysfunction, 20% versus 2%; and grade 3+ or 4+ MR, 21% versus 20%. Major adverse events occurred in 15% of patients in the percutaneous-repair group and 48% of patients in the surgery group at 30 days ($p < .001$). At 12 months, both groups had improved LV size, New York Heart Association (NYHA) functional class and quality-of-life measures, as compared with baseline. Although percutaneous repair was less effective at reducing MR than conventional surgery, the procedure was associated with superior safety and similar improvements in clinical outcomes. This basic conclusion that the MitraClip device is less effective at reducing MR and surgery but is safer was reached despite an early experience level with this new technology. Predictors of success analysis demonstrated that patients with poorer LV function, older age and functional MR had results most comparable with surgery. Four-year results were similar.[3] At 4 years, the rate of the composite endpoint of freedom from death, surgery or 3+ or 4+ MR in the intention-to-treat population was 39.8% versus 53.4% in the percutaneous repair group and surgical groups, respectively ($p = .070$). Rates of death were 17.4% versus 17.8% ($p = .914$), and 3+ or 4+ MR was present in 21.7% versus 24.7% ($p = .745$) at 4 years of follow-up, respectively. Surgery for MV dysfunction, however, occurred in 20.4% versus 2.2% ($p < .001$) at 1 year and 24.8% versus 5.5% ($p < .001$).

32.1.3 MitraClip in high-risk patients

During the course of the EVEREST II randomized trial it became apparent that many patients with anatomic leaflet criteria suitable for the MitraClip therapy were at high risk for surgery and could not be included in the randomised trial. This led to the development of a high-risk registry, the REALSIM High Risk Registry. This registry was a prospective study conducted in the United States and 351 patients were enrolled.[4] Inclusion criteria were 3+–4+ MR and a surgical mortality risk of ≥12% based on the Society of Thoracic Surgeons (STS) risk calculator or the estimate of a surgeon investigator using pre-specified criteria were enrolled. Patients were elderly (76 ± 11 years), with 70% having functional MR and 60% having prior cardiac surgery. MR severity was reduced to ≤2+ in 86% of patients at discharge ($p < .0001$). Major adverse events at 30 days included death in 4.8%, myocardial infarction in 1.1% and stroke in 2.6%. At 12 months, MR was ≤2+ in 84% of patients ($p < .0001$). From baseline to 12 months, LV end-diastolic volume improved from 161 ± 56 mL to 143 ± 53 mL ($p < .0001$) and LV end-systolic volume improved from 87 ± 47 mL to 79 ± 44 ml ($p < .0001$). NYHA functional class improved from 82% in Class III/IV at baseline to 83% in Class I/II at 12 months ($p < .0001$). The 36-item Short Form Health Survey physical and mental quality-of-life scores improved from baseline to 12 months ($p < .0001$). One of the most striking findings of the study was a dramatic decrease in heart failure hospitalisations. The annual hospitalisation rate for heart failure fell from 0.79% pre-procedure to 0.41% post-procedure ($p < .0001$). The Kaplan–Meier survival estimate at 12 months was 77.2%. The percutaneous MV device significantly reduced MR, improved clinical symptoms, decreased LV dimensions and dramatically reduced need for heart failure hospitalisations at 1 year in this high-surgical-risk cohort.

A prohibitive-risk degenerative MR cohort was evaluated by a multidisciplinary heart team. They evaluated high-risk degenerative MR patients enrolled in the EVEREST II studies.[5] A group 127 of these patients were retrospectively identified with prohibitive risks for surgery and also had 1-year follow-up available. These patients were elderly with a mean age of 82.4 years, severely symptomatic with 87% NYHA Class III/IV, and at prohibitive surgical risk with STS mean risk score of 13.2% ± 7.3%. MitraClip was successfully performed in 95.3%. The hospital stay was only 2.9 ± 3.1 days. Major adverse events at 30 days included death in 6.3%,

myocardial infarction in 0.8% and stroke in 2.4%. Through 1 year there were a total of 30 deaths (23.6%), with no survival difference between patients discharged with MR grade ≤1+ or MR grade 2+. At 1 year, 82.9% remained MR ≤2+ and 86.9% were in NYHA Class I or II. Left ventricular end-diastolic volume decreased, SF-36 quality-of-life scores improved and hospitalisations for heart failure were reduced in patients whose MR was reduced. This analysis led to Food and Drug Administration (FDA) approval of MitraClip in patients with degenerative MR who are at prohibitive risk for conventional surgery (Figure 32.1, lower left quadrant). A typical case example is shown in Figures 32.2 through 32.4.

32.1.4 MitraClip international experience

The MitraClip device was approved for clinical use in Europe in 2008. A large experience with many thousands of patients was accrued since then. Numerous registries have been reported. The patient populations who have been treated in clinical practice include primarily patients at high risk for conventional surgery with predominantly functional MR. One recent meta-analysis characterised the safety of MitraClip compared with surgery in high-risk patients.[6] They performed a search strategy in patients with MR and logistic EuroSCORE >18 or Society for Thoracic Surgery (STS) risk score >10% and identified 21 studies utilising MitraClip ($n = 3198$) and MV surgery ($n = 3,265$) from 2003 to 2013. Patients had a mean age of 74 ± 10 years with no differences in surgical risk, NYHA Class or MR grade comparing MitraClip and surgery patients. Technical success was achieved in 96% of patients undergoing MitraClip versus

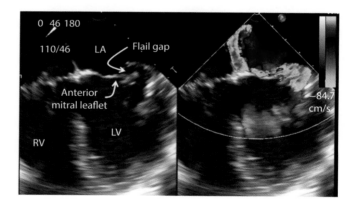

Figure 32.2 Typical case example of MitraClip in commercial Food and Drug Administration (FDA) approved use in the United Sates. The patient is an 87-year-old man with multiple hospitalisations for heart failure. His left ventricle (LV) EF is preserved at 70%. He is severely symptomatic with New York Heart Association (NYHA) Class III dyspnoea on exertion. The pulmonary artery systolic pressure is 50 mmHg. The Society for Thoracic Surgery risk score is 7.5% for repair and 11% for mitral replacement. The figure shows typical degenerative MR with a flail gap of 4–5 mm. The right-sided panel shows the severe MR colour jet. LA = left atrium, RV = right ventricle.

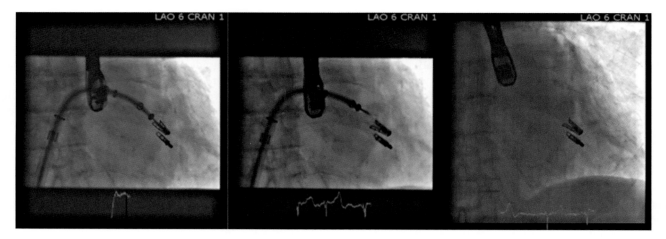

Figure 32.3 Fluoroscopic panels from a MitraClip procedure. In this case, two clips were implanted. The left panel shows the guide catheter and clipped delivery system. The first clip has been implanted and released. The second clip is manoeuvred anterior and lateral to the first clip. The right-hand panel shows both clips in their final position after complete release. The corresponding trans-oesophageal echocardiographic image is shown in Figure 32.4.

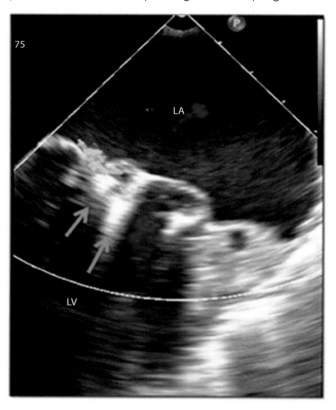

Figure 32.4 Trans-oesophageal echocardiographic imaging after implantation of two MitraClip devices. There is almost no residual mitral regurgitation (MR). The two arrows show the location to MitraClip devices. LA = left atrium, LV = left ventricle.

98% in the surgery group. The 30-day event rates for mortality were 3.3% for MitraClip versus 16.8% for surgery. The 30-day event rates for stroke were 1.1% for MitraClip versus 4.5% for surgery. Based on these studies, high-risk patients with severe MR can be safely implanted with relatively low mortality and stroke risk.

Another recent meta-analysis reviewed 12 publications[7] and reached similar conclusions. All 12 studies were prospective observational studies including a total of 878 patients. Immediate procedural success ranged from 72% to 100% and 30-day mortality ranged from 0% to 7.8%. There was a significant improvement in haemodynamic profile and functional status after MitraClip. One-year survival ranged from 75% to 90%. They concluded that MitraClip implantation is an option in managing selected high surgical risk patients with severe MR. They concluded that MitraClip can be implanted with a reproducible safety and outcome profile in this high risk group of patients and is an option in managing selected high surgical risk patients with severe MR.

32.1.5 COAPT trial

Despite the consistent findings across multiple registry trials, most prospective, and encompassing thousands of patients there remains uncertainty regarding how MitraClip might fare in comparison with best medical therapy in a randomised trial. A trial comparison in 430 patients with a 1:1 randomisation of MitraClip versus guideline-directed medical therapy has been undertaken to test this hypothesis. At the beginning of August 2015, the trial was about halfway enrolled.

32.1.6 MitraClip conclusions

Several conclusions can be drawn from the aggregate data. Based on the randomised trial data, it is clear that MitraClip is less effective at reducing MR than surgery. Despite moderate residual MR and a large proportion of patients after MitraClip, improvement in LV dimensions and symptoms is found in the majority. Among patients at high risk for traditional mitral surgery the procedure can be performed with low mortality, remarkable rate of discharge directly to home rather than a rehabilitation facility and significant improvements and quality of life. A reduced rate of hospitalisations for heart failure has also been found. Over the decade since the introduction of MitraClip into practice, the acute procedure success rate (successful implant of one or more clips and resultant MR grade ≤2+) has improved steadily, now consistently between 95% and 100% (Figure 32.5).

32.2 Indirect and direct annuloplasty

The earliest concepts for percutaneous mitral repair were based on indirect annuloplasty via the coronary sinus. The coronary sinus parallels the posterior mitral annulus. A device that would shorten or constrict the coronary sinus would thus result in diminution of the mitral circumference. Several devices were developed for this application. It seems attractive to utilise the coronary sinus for device delivery due to ease of access via the venous system and the right atrium, and a long history of coronary sinus implants for pacing without any technical difficulties. Despite these considerations, it was found that torsional motion in the coronary sinus can be a cause of device fracture. Device fracture leads to the complete failure of several devices.[8] Currently only one device in this family remains. The Cardiac Dimensions Carillon had some device fractures early during its development, but with some minor device modifications it is now a durable technology.

Direct annuloplasty has been accomplished with several devices. Two of these devices, the Mitralign system and the Valtech Cardioband, described below, have completed European approval trials. One of them is delivered using direct left atrial access and the other using retrograde trans-aortic access.

32.2.1 Indirect annuloplasty with the Carillon device

The Carillon Mitral Contour System (Cardiac Dimension Inc., Kirkland, WA) is implanted via the right internal jugular vein. The device is made of nitinol and has proximal and distal anchors connected by a wire band (Figure 32.6). The distal anchor is placed deep in the coronary sinus near the anterior commissure, and the proximal anchor near the coronary sinus ostium. Tension is placed on the delivery system to plicate the mitral annulus, thereby reducing annular circumference. The device can be recaptured if removal repositioning of the device is needed. A feasibility study, AMADEUS, was performed in a prospective, multicentre, single-arm study.[9] Of the 48 patients enrolled in the trial, 30 received the Carillon device. Eighteen patients did not receive a device because of difficult coronary sinus access, insufficient acute MR reduction or coronary artery compromise. Patients who received the device demonstrated reduction in MR and improvement in functional class and quality of life during the follow-up period through 24 months. Several patients had fractures of the nitinol wire ribbon and the device was subsequently redesigned. Wire fractures were not associated with clinical events. This led to the Trans-catheter Implantation of the Carillon Mitral Annuloplasty Device (TITAN) trial, a prospective, non-randomised study of 53 subjects with the redesigned device.[10] Inclusion criteria included functional MR, at least moderate MR (grade 2+ or greater), and LV ejection fraction (EF) <40%. Thirty-six patients underwent successful device implantation. Seventeen patients had the device removed or recaptured due to compression of the coronary artery, difficulty cannulating the coronary sinus or ineffective reduction in MR. The device was established to be safe with

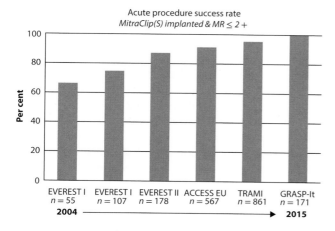

Acute procedure success rate
MitraClip(S) implanted & MR ≤ 2 +

Per cent (y-axis: 0, 20, 40, 60, 80, 100)

EVEREST I n = 55 (2004), EVEREST I n = 107, EVEREST II n = 178, ACCESS EU n = 567, TRAMI n = 861, GRASP-It n = 171 (2015)

Figure 32.5 The rate of acute procedure success (Mitraclip or Clips implanted with resultant ≤2+ MR) has improved steadily during the decade of MitraClip use. The early experience during Endovascular Valve Edge-to-Edge Repair Study (EVEREST I)[37] had an acute procedure success rate of only 66%. In more recent reports, the success rate is consistently between 95% and 100%. (From Feldman T et al., *J Am Coll Cardiol*, 46, 2134–2140, 2005).

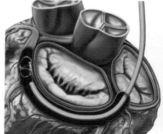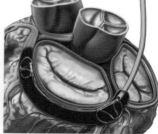

Figure 32.6 Coronary sinus annuloplasty with the Cardiac Dimensions Carillon Device. The guide catheter is introduced through jugular venous access. The device is delivered in the distal coronary sinus and the distal anchor is released (left panel), and then the guide catheter is pulled back to release the proximal anchor in the coronary sinus ostium. The right panel shows the wire form, made of nitinol wire, after release in the coronary sinus. Cinching of the mitral annulus results in compression of the septal–lateral dimension and thus the regurgitant orifice. (From Feldman T and Young A, *J Am Coll Cardiol*, 63, 2057–2068, 2014; Courtesy of Craig Skaggs.)

a low 30-day major adverse event rate (death, myocardial infarction, cardiac perforation, device embolization or surgery for device complication) of 1.9%. Cardiac perforation and device embolization did not occur. Surgery because of device failure was not observed. There was significant LV remodelling and significant reduction in quantitative measures of MR severity, LV dimensions and volume, and the septo-lateral annular dimension that were sustained at 6 and 12 months. Additionally, there was significant improvement in 6-minute walk test (MWT), functional class and quality of life sustained at 24 months. Twenty-five per cent of the patients were observed to have wire fractures on x-ray, but none were associated with adverse clinical events. Left circumflex coronary artery impingement precluded permanent placement of the device in 15% of the patients. A third generation device has not had wire fractures when tested in a model that reproduces the fractures seen in earlier versions. The Carillon device received CE mark approval in Europe in 2011.

A limitation of implantation of devices through the coronary sinus is the potential for compression of the circumflex coronary artery.[11] The circumflex artery courses between the mitral annulus and coronary sinus in between 25% and 70% of patients. While this precludes the use of the coronary sinus in some cases, experience with the Carillon has grown and this limitation has become less important.

32.2.2 Trans-catheter direct annuloplasty – Mitralign

Mitralign (Mitralign Inc., Tewksbury, MA) is a transventricular device that embeds pairs of pledgets on either side of the mitral orifice (Figure 32.7). Each pair is tensioned to reduce the mitral circumference. The procedure is done via retrograde LV catheterisation. A guiding catheter is placed into the posterior mitral annular space. Radiofrequency wires are used to traverse the annular tissue from the LV to the left atrial side of the annulus. The wires are used to pass unique pledgeted sutures through the annulus. The pledgets are introduced in pairs using a 'bident' device that spaces each pair of pledgets a predetermined distance apart. The pledgets can then be drawn together and locked into place, which reduces the distance between them and thus the circumference of the mitral annulus. Two or more pledget pairs may be used to achieve optimal reduction of the annular circumference with the goals of reversing the LV remodelling and improving symptoms. In comparison to other devices, the Mitralign platform has arguably the smallest device footprint due to the small size of the pledgets and sutures that are ultimately left behind as permanent implants.

This device has completed enrolment in a CE approval trial (ClinicalTrials.gov identifier NCT01740583).[12] The inclusion criteria include NYHA Class II–IV, structurally normal MV, at least Grade 2 LV, LV ejection fraction 20%–45% and LV end diastolic diameter 5.0–7.5 cm. The CE approval trial included 51 patients with a mean age

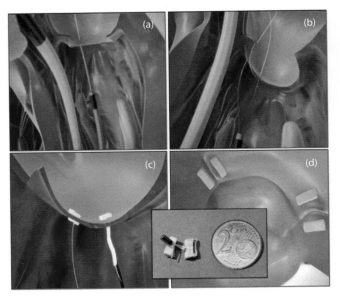

Figure 32.7 Mitralign annular plication. **(Panel a)** shows the retrograde guide catheter in the LV, with the distal catheter tip under the mitral annulus, behind the posterior leaflet. A wire has been passed from the LV through the annulus and into the LA. A second wire is introduced using a bident or two-pronged catheter **(panel b)**. Pledgets are passed over the wires, **(panel c)**. Two pairs of wires are used to place pledgets near both commissures, **(panel d)**. The pledgets are drawn together (inset) to decrease the mitral annular circumference.

of 68.5 ± 11 years, mean left ventricular ejection fraction (LVEF) 32.7% ± 8.5%, with about half NYHA Class III or IV. Thirty-day mortality was 7.8% and 30-day stroke rate 5.9%. Six-month mortality was 12.2%. After 6 months, there were significant improvements in annular dimensions, MR measures and LV remodelling. Mitral annulus anterior–posterior and septal–lateral diameters decreased by 8% and 6%, or from 3.60 ± 0.4 cm to 3.30 ± 0.3 cm and 3.56 ± 0.4 cm to 3.34 ± 0.4 cm, respectively. Effective regurgitant orifice area (EROA) decreased from 0.34 ± 0.1 cm to 0.29 ± 0.1 cm. LV end diastolic volume decreased from 186.69 ± 50.8 mL to 164.62 ± 44.2 mL ($p < .01$) and LV end systolic volume decreased from 122.21 ± 42.9 mL to 107.28 ± 33.7 mL ($p < .01$). Two pairs of pledgets could be implanted in 80% of cases and two pledget pairs were obviously more effective at reducing the mitral circumference and measures of MR than a single pair.[13] In the preliminary results from the CE study, with one pair of pledgets, 39% of patients had ≤2+ MR compared with 63% with ≤2+ MR if two pairs of pledgets were used.

Recently, the Mitralign system has been applied to the tricuspid valve in cases of severe tricuspid regurgitation. The use of pledgeted sutures to plicate the tricuspid posterior annulus is an established surgical approach.[14] Suture 'bicuspidisation' was performed by placement of a pledget-supported mattress suture from the antero-posterior to the posteroseptal commissures along the posterior annulus. Surgical bicuspidisation annuloplasty compared with ring annuloplasty in a group of 237 patients (bicuspidisation in 157 versus ring in 80) was effective at eliminating tricuspid regurgitation at 3 years post-operatively. The bicuspidisation approach utilising the Mitralign system has now been used successfully in several patients with severe tricuspid regurgitation.[15] The percutaneous approach exactly mimics the surgical procedure. The feasibility of the Mitralign system for the tricuspid application has opened the new field percutaneous treatment for tricuspid valve disease.

32.2.3 Trans-catheter direct annuloplasy – Cardioband

Among the annuloplasty devices the Cardioband (Valtech Cardio, Or Yehuda, Israel) is the one most closely resembling surgical annuloplasty rings.[16] The device is implanted into the left atrial side of the mitral annulus. The Valtech Cardioband is delivered via trans-septal atrial access. The ring is implanted directly on the atrial side of the mitral annulus (Figure 32.8). The first anchor is deployed in the lateral commissure, and then the ring is extruded from a delivery catheter in small segments, each anchored by a screw mechanism in turn, encompassing the posterior annulus, until the last anchor is implanted in the medial commissure. The band can be tensioned to reduce the annular circumference to reduce the degree of MR.

The Cardioband device has completed enrolment in a CE approval trial (ClinicalTrials.gov identifier NCT01841554). The inclusion criteria are moderate to severe functional MR, NEHA class II–IV despite optimal medical therapy, including CRT if indicated, LV ejection fraction ≥ 25%, LV end diastolic dimension ≤ 65 mm, subject is at high risk to undergo MV surgery (as assessed by a surgeon and a cardiologist, at the site) and trans-septal catheterisation and femoral vein access is feasible.

Results include patients with functional MR treated between February 2013 and July 2015. Forty-five high-risk patients with significant functional mitral regurgitation (FMR) were enrolled at six sites in Europe.[17] After a Heart Team evaluation, all patients were screened by echocardiography to assess eligibility. The mean age was 71 ± 8 years, 34 patients were male (76%). Mean Log-EuroSCORE 17% ± 12%. At baseline 87% of patients were in NYHA Class III–IV

with mean EF of 32% ± 11% (15%–59%). Device implantation was feasible in all patients (100%). MR reduction to ≤1+ was achieved in 84% of the patients (38/45) intra-procedure. After cinching the device, remodelling of the mitral annulus with an average of 20% reduction of the septo-lateral diameter was observed (from 36 ± 5 to 29 ± 6 mm; $p < .01$). No procedural mortality occurred and 30-day mortality was 4.4% (adjudicated as unrelated to the device). At 6 months follow-up, 82% of patients were in NYHA Class I–II ($N = 22, p < .05$) with significant improvement in quality of life (MLWHFQ from 38 to 18; $p < 0.05$; $N = 21$) and 86% of patients had MR ≤ 2+ ($N = 22$). At 12 months follow-up, 94% of patients had MR ≤ 2+ ($N = 17$), 68% of patients were in NYHA Class I–II ($N = 18, p < .05$) with significant improvement in quality of life (MLWHFQ from 35 to 19; $p < .05$; $N = 16$). These results suggest that trans-septal direct annuloplasty with an adjustable 'surgical-like' ring is feasible, with a good safety (safety performance similar to other trans-catheter mitral procedures). Effective reduction in MR severity is observed in most patients related to a significant septo-lateral dimension reduction. MR reduction is stable and consistent up to 12 months, with significant clinical benefit.

32.3 Trans-catheter MV replacement

The potential to replace the MV using catheter methods has been fuelled by the rapid development of TAVR. Mitral replacement is significantly more complex than TAVR due to the larger, non-circular orifice area of the MV, greater challenges for prosthesis anchoring and the potential to create LV outflow tract obstruction. Implantation of trans-catheter heart valves in native **MV**s is significantly more challenging than mitral valve-in-valve and valve-in-ring procedures due to the limitations previously mentioned. In mitral valve-in-valve, there is a scaffold the operator can use to anchor the new prosthesis and use as a landing zone. In addition, the anterior **MV** leaflet is often removed during the surgical valve replacement and therefore causing significant LV outflow tract obstruction by displacing the anterior mitral leaflet is less likely to occur than when dealing with intact native **MV**s. In addition, the association of MR with cardiomyopathy, where both valve and LV abnormalities are part of the underlying clinical syndrome further complicates the development of replacement devices. On this background, several devices are under development and have undergone some early clinical use, with a relatively small number of cases reported in total.

32.3.1 The CardiAQ valve

The CardiAQ valve (CardiAQ Valve Technologies, Inc., Irvine, CA) was the first trans-catheter valve implanted percutaneously in a native MV in humans. The first generation was made of porcine pericardium mounted on a self-expandable nitinol stent (Figure 32.9a). The first procedure was performed in Denmark in an 86-year-old male patient with severe 3–4+ MR who was not a surgical candidate.[18]

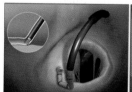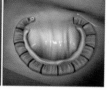

Figure 32.8 Direct mitral annuloplasty with cardioband. The left panel shows a trans-septal guide catheter delivering the annuloplasty ring in segments. Each segment is sequentially anchored into the annulus. The right panel shows the final annuloplasty ring encircling the posterior leaflet. Images used with permission from Valtech, Inc.

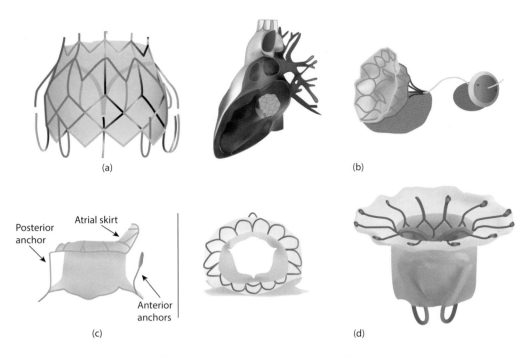

Figure 32.9 Trans-catheter mitral valves (MVs). **(a)** CardiAQ, **(b)** Tendyne, **(c)** Tiara, **(d)** Fortis.

The procedure was a technical success via trans-septal approach with circulatory support, reducing MR severity to 1+. Despite proper function of the valve, the patient expired on the third day post-procedure due to systemic inflammatory response syndrome suspected to be secondary to the use of extracorporeal assist device. There were no structural valvular abnormalities noted on autopsy. The second generation of the CardiAQ can be delivered via trans-apical or trans-femoral approach. The first three treated patients were elderly and had severe MR with Class IV heart failure symptoms.[19] Two patients had functional MR due to cardiomyopathy with ejection fraction <40% and one had chordal rupture. The procedures were successful via trans-apical approach. One patient died on post-operative day #9 due to pneumonia. The other two recovered and were discharged home. Follow-up trans esophageal echocardiography (TEE) on day 1, 30 and 60 days showed stable position of the valve, with proper function and minimal LV outflow gradient. A first case using the second generation device and an antegrade trans-septal approach was reported.[20] The antegrade path was supported by an aterio-venous loop, with the distal wire exteriorised from the femoral artery. Additional support was provided by a second trans-septal puncture, via which a snare was placed in the left atrium to hold and guide the nose cone of the valve delivery system.

32.3.2 The Tendyne valve

The Tendyne valve (Tendyne Holdings Inc., Roseville, MN) is made of porcine pericardium mounted on a nitinol frame. It is fully retrievable and is anchored with an apical tether (Figure 32.9b). The first implant was performed in February of 2013 in a 57-year-old male with severe degenerative MR

and the second in a 55-year-old female with severe MR due to combined rheumatic and degenerative aetiology. Both patients were scheduled to undergo surgical MV replacement and gave to consent to undergo trans-catheter implant of a Tendyne valve to evaluate its performance, followed by removal of the Tendyne prosthesis and traditional surgical MV replacement. The valves were deployed via a trans-apical approach. Both procedures were successful. One patient had 1+ paravalvular MR due to difficulty achieving proper position of the valve. Despite that, the haemodynamics improved. After complete evaluation of valve position and function, the patients underwent conventional MV replacement during which the Tendyne prosthesis was explanted. No damage to the MV apparatus or leaflets was noted.[21] In December of 2014, Tendyne announced the results of the first three chronic implants performed at Royal Brompton Hospital in London, England, under compassionate use.[22] The first procedure was performed in a 68-year-old female with severe functional MR who was not a surgical candidate. The subsequent patients were 75- and 87-year-old males with severe degenerative MR not candidates for conventional MV surgery. The procedures were performed using a trans-apical approach and were successful. All patients were discharged home.

32.3.3 The Tiara valve

The Tiara valve (Neovasc, Inc., Richmond, Canada) is a bovine pericardial valve mounted on a self-expandable nitinol stent. It has a 'D' shape to better adapt to the shape of the native mitral annulus and decreases the risk of LV outflow tract obstruction. It has ventricular anchoring structures that attach to the fibrous trigone and the posterior shelf of the annulus to prevent embolisation (Figure 32.9c). It is implanted via a trans-apical approach using a 32-French delivery system. The first two implants in humans were performed in early 2014.[23] The patients were 73 and 61 years old with severe functional MR and had an LV ejection fraction of 15% and 25%, respectively. They were not candidates for conventional surgery. The valves were implanted successfully via a trans-apical approach. The prosthesis had normal function with only trace paravalvular MR, the mean MV gradients were 2 and 3 mmHg, not one was noted. The patients recovered from the procedure. Echo at 4 weeks demonstrated proper function of the MV prosthesis. However, the first patient died of progressive heart failure 69 days post-procedure. The second patient improved clinically, his baseline NYHA Class IV symptoms decreased to Class II at 5 months follow-up.

32.3.4 The Fortis valve

The Fortis valve (Edwards Lifesciences, Irvine, CA) is a bovine pericardial valve mounted on a self-expandable nitinol frame covered with a fabric skirt to minimise paravalvular regurgitation and facilitate tissue ingrowth. It has two paddles attached to the central body that capture the MV leaflets to anchor the valve and prevent embolisation. It has an atrial flange made of nitinol struts covered with the same fabric as the centre body (Figure 32.9d). It is delivered via a trans-apical approach and it is only available in a 29 mm size. The first five implanted patients had severe functional MR and were not candidates for conventional MV surgery.[24] The acute procedures were successful. The first patient had an ejection fraction of 15%–20%. After a slow recovery due to persistent heart failure, the patient was discharged and then re-hospitalised on day 37 with decompensated heart failure and died on day 76. The second patient developed renal failure on day 1 followed by pulmonary oedema requiring mechanical ventilation on day 2. The echocardiogram revealed increased MR and a displaced posterior paddle with the valve partially embolised to the left atrium. The patient died on day 4. The autopsy confirmed loss of capture of the posterior leaflet and partial embolisation of the prosthesis to the left atrium. The third patient had no complications and was discharged on day 6. At 30-day follow-up, the patient had improvement in the 6-MWT (from 135 to 215 m) and adequate function of the prosthesis. The patient continues to improve slowly. The fourth patient had an uneventful procedure and was discharged on day 9 but was readmitted on day 15 with heart failure decompensation and systemic inflammatory response syndrome. Reduced leaflet mobility of the prosthesis was noted on echocardiogram with high gradients. Antibiotics and heparin were initiated but the patient deteriorated rapidly and died on day 15. The fifth patient had an uneventful procedure, was discharged on day 6 and continues to improve clinically.

Despite poor outcome on some of these patients, the two patients with good outcomes may provide proof-of-concept that trans-catheter MV replacement may be an option for non-surgical candidates. However, patient selection process is clearly important. Altisent et al. recently reported the outcome and 6-month follow-up of three patients treated with the Fortis valve.[25] The mean age was 71 ± 9 years, two were male and all had functional MR and high surgical risk with a mean STS risk score of 9.3%. The procedures were performed successfully with the standard trans-apical approach. There were no major complications. There was residual MR in two patients and no residual leak in one. The mean trans-mitral gradient post-implant was 3 mmHg. All patients were discharged between 7 and 13 days post-procedure. At 3-month follow-up, all patients showed improvement in NYHA functional class, functional status (by Duke Activity Status Index), distance walked in 6-MWT and quality of life. The functional improvement persisted at 6-month follow-up.

However, there was recently a separate report of several cases of valve thrombosis. Seventeen patients had been implanted with this device at the time. For this reason, Edwards announced in May 2015 that the Fortis valve program was going to be temporarily paused to gather additional information.

32.3.5 Calcific mitral stenosis

Recently, there has been growing interest in trans-catheter MV replacement with balloon expandable valves in patients with native mitral stenosis due to severe annular calcification who are poor candidates for standard surgery. The first successful balloon expandable trans-catheter valve implants in a native MV in a human used an Edwards Sapien XT via a surgical trans-apical approach.[26,27] Both procedures were performed in patients with severe calcific mitral stenosis and poor surgical risk. None of these early attempts have been successful, with a reported trans-catheter implantation of a Sapien XT valve in a native MV with suboptimal results.[28] After the poor initial outcome, surgical valve replacement was undertaken. Intra-operatively, the annulus was found to be extremely calcified making the surgical implantation of a bio-prosthesis impossible. A 29-mm Sapien XT was implanted under direct visualisation with good intra-operative results. An echocardiogram the following day revealed incipient valve dislocation and paravalvular leak. This was successfully treated surgically with a running 3-1 polypropylene suture to an atrial cuff. The valve function remained adequate but the patient died on post-operative day 41 from massive upper gastrointestinal bleeding.

The trans-apical approach is preferred by many operators who are familiar with this method based on their experience with TAVR. However, not all patients may be candidates for a surgical trans-apical access due their high level of risk. Therefore, an even less invasive approach may be better for some patients. A percutaneous method is preferred in these situations. However, the typical trans-venous antegrade approach may not provide adequate co-axial position and support during valve deployment, with risk of valve embolisation.[29] To improve co-axiality during trans-septal deployment, the guidewire may be externalised through the left ventricle. Guerrero et al. reported the first in human percutaneous implantation of a trans-catheter valve in a native MV.[30] A 26-mm Edwards Sapien valve was used to treat a patient with severe calcific MS who was neither a candidate for MV surgery nor a candidate for surgical trans-apical access given his extremely high surgical risk. To improve the co-axiality and support of the traditional antegrade approach, the guidewire was placed trans-septally and then exteriorised through a sheath percutaneously placed from the apex into the left ventricle (Figure 32.10). This percutaneous apical puncture approach is less invasive than the open surgical trans-apical approach and could be considered when co-axiality cannot be achieved with the antegrade trans-septal approach. The procedure was successful and the valve had adequate function with only trivial paravalvular regurgitation. However, the patient died post-operative on day 10 from non-cardiac causes including renal failure, suspected sepsis and multiorgan failure. Several cases of trans-catheter implantation of a Sapien XT valve in a native MV successfully using the trans-septal antegrade approach, which is the least invasive method, have been reported with good results.[31,32]

The combined experience of these cases suggest that trans-catheter implant of balloon expandable valves in severe calcific MV disease is feasible. However, there have been important complications including valve embolisations, LV outflow tract obstruction and catheter-induced ventricular perforation with the trans-septal approach. These complications have not all been reported in the literature. Interestingly, significant paravalvular leak has not been a frequent problem. Perhaps the native leaflets seal the gap between the round stent frame and the oval native annulus during systole, preventing significant paravalvular regurgitation.

We are currently working on a global multicentre registry to collect and report complete outcome data in a large series of cases. However, more data are needed to determine methods for annulus sizing, proper valve size selection, prevention and treatment of complications including embolisation and LV outflow tract obstruction and the best delivery method. For that reason, the MITRAL trial (Mitral Implantation of TRAnscatheter vaLves, ClinicalTrials.gov Identifier NCT02370511) was recently initiated.[33] This is a physician-sponsored FDA-approved investigational device exemption (IDE) trial aiming to evaluate the safety and feasibility of the Edwards Sapien XT in severe calcific native mitral stenosis. Enrolment started in February 2015 and is currently ongoing at six US participating sites. Details of this trial can be found at www.clinicaltrials.org.

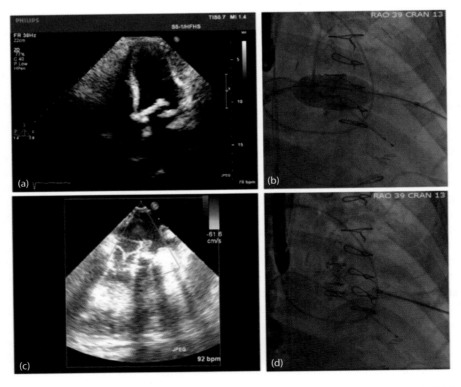

Figure 32.10 First percutaneous implant of a balloon expandable valve in a calcified native MV. (a) Echocardiogram at baseline demonstrates a severely calcified MV. (b) Fluoroscopy of a Sapien valve being implanted in a native MV via a modified antegrade approach with the guidewire externalised through a sheath percutaneously placed in the left ventricle. (c) Trans-oesophageal echocardiogram confirms a proper position of the Sapien valve in the mitral annulus with only trace to mild paravalvular regurgitation. (d) Fluoroscopy of the percutaneous ventricular access being closed with a 4-mm Amplatz VSD closure device. (From Guerrero M et al., *Cathet Cardiovasc Intervent*, 83, E287–E291, 2014; Hasan R et al., *Circulation*, 128, e74–e76, 2013.)

32.4 Conclusions

The field of percutaneous MV repair and replacement has advanced dramatically over the past decade. Two percutaneous MV repair technologies, MitraClip and Carillon, have come into international and **US**-approved clinical practice. Several other devices, including the Cardioband and Mitralign systems, have completed CE approval trials. At the same time, catheter-based MV replacement has emerged with early human implant experience. There is some discussion that replacement approaches will eclipse repair technologies completely.[34] Before the relative advantages of repair and replacement are defined, the risks and benefits, and practical limitations of each of these categories must be considered. The strength of mitral replacement is the potential to completely eliminate and a residual MR. The advantages of repair devices are their simplicity and lower risk. What remains to be defined is the degree of efficacy that can be achieved with repair relative to replacement, compared with the burden of risk associated with complete valve replacement implant devices. The acquisitions of both repair and replacement start-up companies by larger firms such as Edwards Lifesciences (acquired CardiAQ Valve Technologies trans-catheter mitral replacement), Medtronic Inc. (Twelve, Inc. trans-catheter mitral replacement), Abbott Vascular (acquired Tendyne Holdings Inc. trans-catheter mitral replacement) and Heartware International (acquired Valtech Cardio Limited trans-catheter mitral repair) highlight the level of promise of these technologies.

Historical comparisons in cardiovascular surgery of repair versus replacement have shown a paradox with the potential for better survival with repair despite a lesser reduction in the severity of MR.[35] This paradox was also shown in one of the few prospective, randomised trials ever conducted for MR, comparing the Coapsys device with standard annuloplasty.[36] In the Randomized Evaluation of a Surgical Treatment for Off-Pump Repair of the Mitral Valve (RESTOR-MV trial NCT00120276) complication-free survival (including death, stroke, myocardial infarction and valve reoperation) was significantly greater with Coapsys at 2 years compared with annuloplasty (85% vs. 71%). There was a lesser reduction of MR in the Coapsys patients, but also a lower mortality compared with annuloplasty. This analysis indicates that patients with FMR requiring revascularisation treated with ventricular reshaping rather than standard surgery can have improved survival and a significant decrease in major adverse outcomes, despite residual MR. These trial results highlight the limitations of both repair and replacement. While valve replacement may eliminate MR, it has no direct impact on the cardiomyopathy or LV dysfunction that is ultimately responsible for many of the patient's symptoms and may be the most important determinant for longer term survival. To the degree that any MR therapy can facilitate LV remodelling, there may be a greater or lesser benefit. It must also be considered that replacement can be done after repair if needed, particularly after annuloplasty. It is possible that annuloplasty will facilitate trans-septal placement of replacement devices. It is ultimately likely that there will be important roles for both percutaneous repair and replacement.

References

1. Feldman T, and Leon MB. Prospects for percutaneous valve therapies. *Circulation* 2007; 11: 2866–2877.
2. Feldman T et al. Percutaneous repair or surgery for mitral regurgitation. *New Engl J Med* 2011; 364: 1395–1406.
3. Mauri L et al. Four-year results of a randomized controlled trial of percutaneous repair versus surgery for mitral regurgitation. *J Am Coll Cardiol* 8 May 2013; 62: 317–328. doi:pii: S0735–1097(13)01791–9. 10.1016/j.jacc.2013.04.030. [Epub ahead of print]
4. Glower D et al. Percutaneous MitraClip device therapy for mitral regurgitation in 351 patients – High risk subset of the EVEREST II study. *J Am Coll Cardiol* 2014; 64: 172–181.
5. Lim DS et al. Improved functional status and quality of life in prohibitive surgical risk patients with degenerative mitral regurgitation after transcatheter mitral valve repair. *J Am Coll Cardiol* 15 July 2014; 64(2): 182–192. doi:10.1016/j.jacc.2013.10.021. Epub 2013 Oct 31.
6. Philip F et al. MitraClip for severe symptomatic mitral regurgitation in patients at high surgical risk: A comprehensive systematic review. *Catheter Cardiovasc Interv* 1 October 2014; 84(4): 581–590. doi:10.1002/ccd.25564. Epub 2014 Jul 2.
7. Munkholm-Larsen S et al. A systematic review on the safety and efficacy of percutaneous edge-to-edge mitral valve repair with the MitraClip system for high surgical risk candidates. *Heart* March 2014; 100(6): 473–478.
8. MacHaalany J et al. Fatal late migration of Viacor percutaneous transvenous mitral annuloplasty device resulting in distal coronary venous perforation. *Can J Cardiol* January 2013; 29(1): 130.e1–4. doi:10.1016/j.cjca.2012.03.014. Epub 2012 May 22.
9. Schofer J et al. Percutaneous mitral annuloplasty for functional mitral regurgitation: Results of the CARILLON Mitral Annuloplasty Device European Union Study. *Circulation* 2009; 120: 326–333.
10. Siminiak T et al. Treatment of functional mitral regurgitation by percutaneous annuloplasty: Results of the TITAN Trial. *Eur J Heart Fail* 2012; 14: 931–938.
11. Sponga S et al. Reversible circumflex coronary artery occlusion during percutaneous transvenous mitral annuloplasty with the Viacor system. *J Am Coll Cardiol* 2012; 59: 288.
12. Schueler R, Nickenig G.The Mitralign: strategies for optimal patient selection and optimised results. *EuroIntervention* 2016; Sep 18;12(Y):Y67-9
13. Schofer J. Transcatheter interventions for tricuspid regurgitation: Trialign and Mitralign. *EuroIntervention*. 2016; Sep 18;12(Y):Y119-20. doi: 10.4244/EIJV12SYA33.
14. Ghanta RK et al. Suture bicuspidization of the tricuspid valve versus ring annuloplasty for repair of functional tricuspid regurgitation: Midterm results of 237 consecutive patients. *J Thorac Cardiovasc Surg* January 2007; 133(1): 117–126.

15. Schofer J et al. First-in-human transcatheter tricuspid valve repair in a patient with severely regurgitant tricuspid valve. *J Am Coll Cardiol* 2015; 65: 1190–1195.

16. Maisano F et al. Direct access transcatheter mitral annuloplasty with a sutureless and adjustable device: Preclinical experience. *Eur J Cardiothorac Surg* September 2012; 42(3): 524–529. doi:10.1093/ejcts/ezs069.

17. Nickenig G et al. Transcatheter mitral annuloplasty in chronic functional mitral regurgitation: 6-month results with the cardioband percutaneous mitral repair system. *JACC Cardiovasc Interv.* 2016; Oct 10;9(19):2039-2047. doi: 10.1016/j.jcin.2016.07.005.

18. Sondergaard L et al. First-in-human case of transfemoral cardiac mitral valve implantation. Circulation. *Cardiovasc Intervent* 2015; 8: e002135.

19. Sondergaard L et al. Transcatheter mitral valve implantation via transapical approach: An early experience. *Eur J Cardiothorac Surg* 3 February 2015. pii: ezu546. [Epub ahead of print]

20. Ussia GP et al. Percutaneous transfemoral-transseptal implantation of a second-generation CardiAQ™ mitral valve bioprosthesis: First procedure description and 30-day follow-up. EuroIntervention, pub Sept 7, 2015, http://www .pcronline.com/eurointervention/ahead_of_print/201509-01#sthash.YVVCh9oV.dpuf

21. Lutter G et al. First-in-human off-pump transcatheter mitral valve replacement. *JACC Cardiovasc Interv* 2014; 7: 1077–1078.

22. Moat N et al. Transcatheter mitral valve replacement for the treatment of mitral regurgitation: In-hospital outcomes of an apically tethered device. *J Am Coll Cardiol* 2015; 65: 2352–2353.

23. Cheung A et al. Transcatheter mitral valve implantation with tiara bioprosthesis. *EuroIntervention* 2014; 10 Suppl U: U115–U119.

24. Bapat V et al. Transcatheter mitral valve implantation (tmvi) using the Edwards Fortis device. *EuroIntervention* 2014; 10 Suppl U: U120–U128.

25. Abdul-Jawad Altisent O et al. Initial experience of transcatheter mitral valve replacement with a novel transcatheter mitral valve: Procedural and 6-month follow-up results. *J Am Coll Cardiol* 2015; 66: 1011–1019.

26. Hasan R et al. First in human transapical implantation of an inverted transcatheter aortic valve prosthesis to treat native mitral valve stenosis. *Circulation* 2013; 128: e74–e76.

27. Sinning JM et al. Transcatheter mitral valve replacement using a balloon-expandable prosthesis in a patient with calcified native mitral valve stenosis. *Eur Heart J* September 2013; 34(33): 2609. doi:10.1093/eurheartj/eht254. Epub 2013 Jul 4.

28. Wilbring M et al. Pushing the limits-further evolutions of transcatheter valve procedures in the mitral position, including valve-in-valve, valve-in-ring, and valve-in-native-ring. *J Thorac Cardiovasc Surg* 2014; 147: 210–219.

29. Webb JG et al. Transcatheter valve-in-valve implantation for failed bioprosthetic heart valves. *Circulation* 2010; 121: 1848–1857.

30. Guerrero M et al. First in human percutaneous implantation of a balloon expandable transcatheter heart valve in a severely stenosed native mitral valve. *Cathet Cardiovasc Intervent* 15 February 2014; 83: E287–E291.

31. Fassa AA et al. Transseptal transcatheter mitral valve implantation for severely calcified mitral stenosis. *JACC Cardiovasc Intervent* 2014; 7: 696–697.

32. Himbert D et al. Transcatheter valve replacement in patients with severe mitral valve disease and annular calcification. *J Am Coll Cardiol* 2014; 64: 2557–2558.

33. www.clinicaltrials.gov/ct2/show/NCT02370511?term accessed September 6, 2015.

34. Maisano F et al. The future of transcatheter mitral valve interventions: Competitive or complementary role of repair vs replacement? *Eur Heart J* 2015; 36(26): 1651–9. doi:10.1093/eurheartj/ehv123. epub April 12, 2015.

35. Benedetto U et al. Does combined mitral valve surgery improve survival when compared to revascularization alone in patients with ischemic mitral regurgitation? A meta-analysis on 2479 patients. *J Cardiovasc Med (Hagerstown)* February 2009; 10(2): 109–114. doi:10.2459/JCM.0b013e32831c84b0.

36. Grossi EA1 et al. Outcomes of the RESTOR-MV Trial (Randomized Evaluation of a Surgical Treatment for Off-Pump Repair of the Mitral Valve). *J Am Coll Cardiol* 7 December 2010; 56(24): 1984–1993. doi:10.1016/j.jacc.2010.06.051.

37. Feldman T et al. Percutaneous mitral valve repair using the edge-to-edge technique: 6 month results of the EVEREST Phase I Clinical Trial. *J Am Coll Cardiol* 2005; 46: 2134–2140.

38. Feldman T, and Young A. Percutaneous approaches to valve repair for mitral regurgitation. *J Am Coll Cardiol* 2014; 63: 2057–2068.

Trans-catheter closure of left atrial appendage

MARIUS HORNUNG, JENNIFER FRANKE, SAMEER GAFOOR,
STEFAN BERTOG, HORST SIEVERT

33.1 Introduction

Stroke is still the leading cause of disability and the third leading cause of mortality in Western countries.[1] Approximately 80% of all strokes are ischaemic, and about one-third is caused by cardiac embolism, mostly the consequence of atrial fibrillation (AF).[2] Of note, strokes caused by AF tend to be larger, as the cardiac emboli are rather large in size and therefore occlude the cerebral arteries more proximally resulting in more severe neurological deficits. Furthermore, the resulting risk of recurrent stroke seems to be higher than that of other stroke aetiologies.[3] With AF being the most common clinically relevant arrhythmia, its estimated prevalence in the general population is about 1%–2%.[4] The average annual stroke risk in patients with non-valvular (non-rheumatic) AF is about 5% and increases with age.[5] In patients 80–89 years of age, AF causes up to 20% of all ischaemic strokes.[6] Furthermore, the annual stroke risk increases with the presence of other concomitant diseases like heart failure, hypertension, diabetes and prior thromboembolic events.[5] To assess the individual annual stroke risk, the CHADS$_2$-score took the above mentioned risk factors into account (1 point each for congestive heart failure, hypertension, age over 75 years, diabetes, and 2 points for prior stroke). Although a clear relationship

between the CHADS$_2$-score and stroke rates exists, the CHA$_2$DS$_2$-VASc-score was developed to improve risk stratification in the low-risk group. The CHA$_2$DS$_2$-VASc-score considers the presence of vascular disease and female gender as additional reasons for increasing stroke risk in patients with AF.[7] Prospective randomised trials demonstrated that oral anticoagulation with vitamin K antagonists, i.e. warfarin, significantly reduces the risk of thromboembolic events.[5,8] As warfarin reduces stroke risk by up to 84%, it is undisputed that anticoagulation therapy should be recommended to patients at increased risk. However, oral anticoagulation is still underutilised for various reasons: logistical challenges related to periodic international normalised ratio (INR) assessment with the necessity of instructions regarding dose adjustment, poor patient compliance, drug–drug and drug–diet interactions, the presence of contraindications and the risk of bleeding complications.[9–11] The narrow therapeutic window is one of the most important reasons why a significant proportion of patients, who are at high risk of stroke and would warrant anticoagulation, are not anti-coagulated.[12,13] Consequently, the development of new drugs has been advanced, which engages the coagulation cascade by direct inhibition of thrombin or inactivate factor Xa. These drugs are easier to manage as there is no need for drug monitoring, and they are less prone towards interactions with drugs and food. Nearly 90% of all thrombi in patients with AF arise in the left atrial appendage (LAA).[14] Thrombi in the LAA and a reduced peak systolic velocity are independent risk factors of thromboembolic events[15, 16] and of the recurrence of stroke in patients with AF recovering from ischaemic stroke.[17] As only about 10% of clinically relevant emboli in these patients do not originate in the LAA, the LAA became the main target for stroke prevention. Hence, its removal or occlusion may lead to a substantial reduction of stroke risk with the remaining small risk not warranting oral anticoagulation.

Various surgical and catheter-based techniques have been developed to exclude the LAA as a source for thromboembolic complications. A number of techniques have been used to seal the LAA in patients undergoing open-chest surgery for other indications (e.g. mitral valve surgery).[18] In 2001, the first percutaneous catheter-based occlusion of the LAA was reported using the Percutaneous LAA Transcatheter Occlusion system (PLAATO; Appriva Medical, Sunnyvale, California).[19] It was a self-expanding nitinol cage, which anchored in the LAA using hooks on the struts of the cage. The occluder was covered with a polytetrafluoroethylene membrane to reduce thrombogenicity (Figure 33.1). In a non-randomised trial the investigators demonstrated the feasibility of the PLAATO device to occlude the LAA in patients with AF and contraindications to oral anticoagulation. Although the observed annual ischaemic stroke risk was substantially lowered compared with predicted rates by the CHADS$_2$-Score (3.8% vs. 6.6%),[20] complications related to the procedure (e.g. cardiac tamponade after trans-septal puncture, device embolisation or severe vessel injuries at the puncture site) were reported.

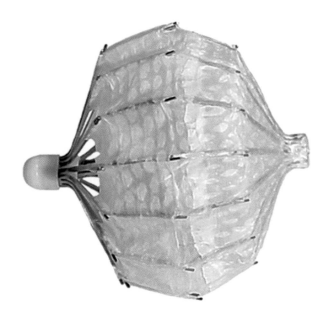

Figure 33.1 The Percutaneous LAA Transcatheter Occlusion system (PLAATO) occluder. A self-expanding nitinol cage covered with a polytetrafluoroethylene membrane.

Due to financial concerns the manufacturer discontinued the development of the device in 2006.[21] In August 2002, the first Watchman occluder (Boston Scientific Corporation, Marlborough, Massachusetts) was implanted. Today, the Watchman device is the most commonly implanted LAA occlusion system worldwide. It remains the only device comparatively studied with oral anticoagulation in randomised controlled trials (PROTECT-AF, PREVAIL).[22,23] This resulted in the US Food and Drug Administration (FDA) approval in March 2015 for the use of the Watchman device as an alternative to warfarin. The Amplatzer Cardiac Plug (St. Jude Medical, Inc., St. Paul, Minnesota) was designed specifically for percutaneous occlusion of the LAA in 2008. In December of the same year the system received the European Conformité européenne (CE) mark. In August 2013 and subsequent to the results of the WAVECREST I trial CE mark approval was granted to the Coherex WaveCrest occluder (Coherex Medical, Salt Lake City, Utah), which is the third commercially available device.

Notwithstanding these achievements, some potential problems are accompanied with the device closure of the LAA, such as the persistence of residual leaks, device-associated thrombus formation and device embolisation. In this context, minimally invasive techniques were developed to mimic surgical LAA ligation. The Lariat system (SentreHEART, Redwood City, California) combines an endocardial and epicardial approach to deliver a lasso-like suture over the LAA. Under fluoroscopic and trans-oesophageal echocardiography (TEE) guidance, the LAA can first be cinched and subsequently a suture applied.[24]

In 2012, the European Society of Cardiology included the percutaneous occlusion of the LAA as an option in the guidelines for the treatment of patients with non-valvular AF (class of recommendation II b and level of evidence B in patients with a high stroke risk and contraindications for long-term oral anticoagulation).[25]

33.2 Pre- and peri-procedural imaging

A prerequisite for the implementation of percutaneous LAA closure procedures is knowledge of the anatomy of the LAA and adjacent anatomical structures, and to recognise individual variations. The LAA is a tubular shaped, blind-ended, embryonic remnant at the lateral wall of the left atrium, localised between the pulmonary veins and the mitral valve. In the majority of patients the LAA has multiple lobes. Moreover, the presence of AF seems to influence the anatomy of the LAA and can also change it. Both the diameter of the orifice and the length of the LAA increase when comparing patients with sinus rhythm, paroxysmal and permanent AF. At the same time the eccentricity of the LAA ostium decreases with increasing duration of AF.[26, 27]

Prior to percutaneous LAA closure, all patients must undergo pre-procedural imaging to rule out thrombi in the left atrium and the LAA, and to gain familiarity with the individual cardiac anatomy. The standard imaging technique is still TEE. The presence of thrombi in the left atrium or in the LAA is a contraindication for the interventional occlusion of the LAA. Manipulation of sheaths and devices in this area significantly increases the risk of thrombus dislodgement and embolisation. In rare cases, obtaining clear images can be difficult, for example in cases with prominent pectinate muscles, which can be misinterpreted as thrombi. Although the overall incidence of thrombi in the left atrium and its appendage is rather low, it increases with higher $CHADS_2$-scores (0% for score 0, 5% for score 2 and 11% for score 4–6), TEE enables an evaluation of the LAA including its configuration, orientation, length, number of lobes, and measurements of the diameter of the ostium and the designated landing zone for an occlusion device. This information helps to choose the optimal type of occluder to implant and predicts if the procedure will be technically difficult or even impossible. With help of the x-plane function, the LAA is best viewed from a position in mid to distal oesophagus and should be displayed in at least four views (0°, 45°, 90° and 135°). Often, the presence and morphology of multiple lobes can only be detected at an angle beyond 100°. Additional imaging (computed tomography angiography or magnetic resonance imaging) may be considered in patients with complex anatomy. The length of the LAA and the maximal width of its ostial diameter are required for choosing the exact device size. At 0°, the width of the ostium is measured from the edge of the left circumflex artery (LCX) to a point at the opposite wall 1–2 cm from the left upper pulmonary vein, perpendicular to the axis of the LAA. Further measurements should be performed from mitral annulus to the opposite wall of the LAA at 45°, 90° and 135° (Figure 33.2). As the ostium is rather oval shaped, the longest value is recommended for selection of the device size (usually measured

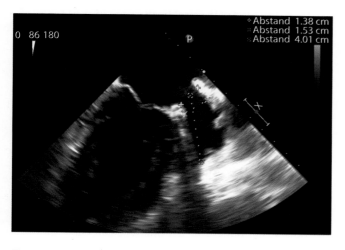

Figure 33.2 Evaluation of the LAA in trans-oesophageal echocardiography (TEE). Measurement of the device landing zone from the edge of the left circumflex artery (LCX) to a point at the opposite wall 1–2 cm from the left upper pulmonary vein, perpendicular to the axis of the LAA.

in the superior–inferior axis). The length/depth of the LAA is measured from the plane of the ostium to the apex of the LAA.

Some centres avoid using fluoroscopy only for peri-procedural imaging. The potential advantages of this approach are that the procedure may be done without any kind of sedation and may need fewer staff.[28] Nevertheless, we recommend echocardiography to enhance the safety of the operation and effectiveness of the closure device. Performing trans-septal puncture under echo-guidance facilitates accurate placement of the needle. Furthermore, TEE using 3D-imaging can provide a real-time view of the LAA for interpretation of its shape and ostium, and facilitates the evaluation of device placement success as well as the inspection for peri-device leakage. Intra-cardiac echocardiography (ICE) is an alternative to TEE although data on ICE for imaging in LAA occlusion procedures are currently limited.

33.3 Trans-septal puncture

The procedure is usually performed under local anaesthesia of the right venous femoral access site and slight sedation, if needed. The primary reason for sedation is the use of the TEE probe.

The trans-septal puncture is the first crucial step of every LAA occlusion. After insertion of a 5 Fr. sheath at the right venous femoral access site, a guidewire is advanced to the right atrium. The sheath is exchanged for a 59 cm long, 8 Fr. trans-septal sheath through which a trans-septal needle is advanced to the intra-atrial septum. The height of the puncture depends on the orientation of the LAA. Puncture should be performed under TEE guidance in the posterior and inferior segment of the fossa ovalis, which facilitates an anterior superior trajectory and optimises device delivery for most LAA configurations. Only in an anterior or rather caudal orientation of the LAA axis, the puncture should be conducted in the upper posterior part of the septum. In general the puncture site is best-seen and controlled using the bicaval (90°) and short axis (30°) view in TEE.

In 10%–38% of all humans a patent foramen ovale (PFO) persists in adulthood,[29–31] and this entity as well as an atrial septal defect (ASD) may be found incidentally. The presence of a PFO or ASD may in principle be utilised for trans-septal passage into the left atrium, thus avoiding puncture of the atrial septum. However, this depends primarily on the size and the diameter of the defect. In particular, the predetermined angles with passage of a PFO resulting in a superior and anterior path can complicate the alignment of the sheath unnecessarily and increase the risk of complications. Thus, an additional trans-septal puncture may be necessary depending on the particular anatomical circumstances.

Subsequent to trans-septal puncture and advancement of the trans-septal sheath, left atrial position can be confirmed through TEE and atrial pressure tracing. Before administering 10,000 units of heparin to achieve an activated clotting time (ACT) of at least 250 seconds, pericardial effusion should be excluded. Then, the trans-septal needle is exchanged for a 260 cm long, 0.035 inch stiff wire with a 3 cm atraumatic soft tip and a 4 Fr. angled pigtail catheter. The pigtail is placed in the distal part of the LAA under TEE and fluoroscopic guidance. It can be used for angiographic measurements of the LAA and enables an atraumatic advancement of the subsequently introduced sheaths. Next, the sheath is exchanged over the wire for the delivery sheath. To avoid air embolism, the most effective and safe method is to wait for back bleeding whilst holding the proximal end of the delivery sheath below zero. Furthermore, continuous saline infusion through the side arm of the sheath and slow removal of the dilatator are recommended to avoid air embolism caused by air suction through the valve of the sheath during removal of the sheath dilatator.

Differently shaped sheaths have been developed for each type of the available occlusion devices. Depending on the individual sheath, they have one or two curves, and some allow an additional anterior orientation. However, the anatomic variability of possible orientations of the LAA is so wide that even the available sheaths often represent only a suboptimal solution. Interventionalists have adapted the delivery sheaths individually to the anatomical conditions of their patients.[32] Following trans-septal puncture, they advanced an angled 4 Fr. pigtail catheter under fluoroscopic and TEE guidance into the distal part of the LAA. After carrying out the required measurements and deciding which occluder size to implant, the appropriate delivery sheath was chosen. The patient's chest was covered with a sterile cloth, and the delivery sheath with the dilatator inside was placed thereon. Under fluoroscopy the shape of the sheath was compared with the shape of the pigtail catheter and then gently shaped to match the configuration inside the body. Using this case-specific approach, the authors could reduce their total fluoroscopy time significantly. Furthermore, there were trends towards a decreased total procedure time as well as to a decreased number of recaptures and repositioning which may be associated with a better starting position with a shaped sheath.

33.4 Closure techniques and devices

33.4.1 Watchman (Boston Scientific Corporation)

Since the first implantation in August 2002, the device has undergone technical modifications. The Nitinol frame builds a parachute-like configuration, with 10 fixation anchors along its waist and a thin polyethylene terephthalate (PET) membrane covering the proximal part that is exposed to the left atrium after implantation. The PET membrane has a pore size of 160 μm to prevent LAA thrombus embolisation. It is designed to reduce the risk of device-associated thrombus formation and to allow rapid endothelialisation (Figure 33.3). The device is available in five different sizes ranging in 3 mm steps from 21 to 33 mm. Accordingly, the

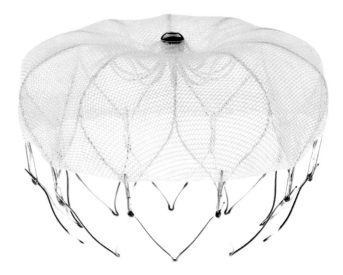

Figure 33.3 The Watchman occluder. Ten fixation barbs are placed along the waist of the parachute like configuration of the Nitinol frame. The left atrial side is covered with a polyethylene terephthalate (PET) membrane.

Watchman device can be used to occlude LAAs with landing zone diameter of up to 30 mm. Implantation in cases with ostial diameters >30 mm is not recommended, as a compression rate of at least 10% is needed to anchor the hooks within the LAA wall to prevent the risk of device embolisation.

Following trans-septal puncture a 4 Fr. pigtail catheter is placed in the LAA for angiography of the LAA in several views. In most patients, right anterior oblique (RAO 30°) caudal (20°) and cranial (20°) projections can best outline the LAA for delineation of its shape and size. Further LAA-measurements are required by TEE in at least four views (0°, 45°, 90° and 135°). When using the Watchman device, the proximal LCX is the essential landmark. To determine the landing zone for the device, the edge of the LCX to the opposite wall of the LAA about 1 cm inwards from the tip of the ridge separating the LAA from left upper pulmonary vein, perpendicular to the axis of the LAA is measured. We recommend choosing an occluder size which exceeds the largest diameter measured by 20% in order to achieve the compression rate needed to engage the fixation barbs of the device into the wall.

The Watchman system consists of three parts: the specific Watchman trans-septal access sheath that has a 14 Fr. outer diameter, the 12 Fr. delivery catheter and the preloaded Watchman occluder. To facilitate LAA access, the delivery sheath is available in three different shapes depending on the orientation of the LAA and the resulting angles caused by trans-septal puncture: The operator can chose amongst a single curved, a double curved, or an anterior curved sheath (Figure 33.4). The delivery sheath is then advanced with a dilatator into the left atrium over a 0.035 inch stiff wire. After entering the left atrium, the dilatator is removed and the pigtail catheter is then advanced into the LAA. This allows atraumatic tracking of the access sheath into

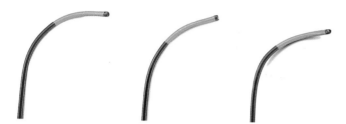

Figure 33.4 The Watchman delivery sheaths. Three available configurations of the access sheath: double-curved, single-curved access sheath, and with an anterior curve (from left to right).

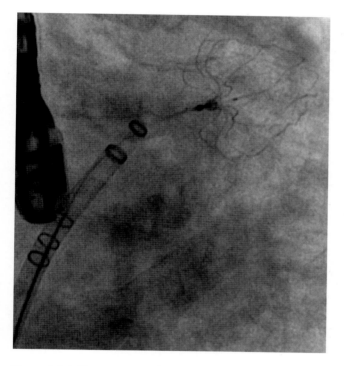

Figure 33.5 Fluoroscopy of a deployed Watchman occluder. The Watchman device is still connected to the delivery catheter. On the left side, the delivery sheath with the three radiopaque markers for optimisation of the device positioning is shown.

the LAA. The delivery sheath has four radiopaque markers. Knowledge of these specific markers is mandatory for correct and atraumatic placement of the sheath: there is one distal marker indicating the distal tip of the sheath. The three more proximal markers provide information on the position of the most proximal part of the occluder which faces the left atrium when deployed (Figure 33.5). Depending on the chosen device size, the proximal end will align with one of these three markers: the largest device size (33 mm) aligns with the most proximal placed marker, the 27 mm device aligns with the middle marker and the smallest device (21 mm) aligns with the most distal of the three markers. The 30 mm and the 24 mm devices align between the markers, respectively. The knowledge of these specifications is necessary in order to correctly position the delivery

sheath prior to release of the occluder. Depending on the selected occluder size, the appropriate marker of the sheath must align to the imaginary connecting line between the distal edge of the LCX and the opposite wall of the LAA, perpendicular to the LAA axis. This alignment allows occluder release at the level of the intended landing zone.

Whilst introducing the delivery catheter into the access sheath, the device must be flushed with heparinised saline to avoid air bubbles and air embolism. Then, the delivery catheter is advanced under fluoroscopic guidance until its distal marker aligns with the distal marker of the access sheath. Next, the access sheath must be gently pulled back to interlock the access sheath with the delivery catheter. The operator feels a click. After final fluoroscopic control of the position of the delivery system, pulling back the interlocked access and delivery sheath whilst holding the delivery cable in a stable position deploys the occluder.

Before the device is finally released, its optimal positioning has to be checked angiographically and by TEE. At this point, the occluder is still connected to the delivery core wire what allows complete retrieval of the occluder in case of unsatisfactory placement. Before final release, there are four criteria that should be evaluated to avoid device embolisation: position, anchoring, size and sealing (PASS):

1. **Position**: The maximum diameter of the device should be at or just distal to the plane of the LAA ostium, with the occluder not protruding more than 4–7 mm beyond the ostium depending on the size of the device.
2. **Anchoring**: A tug test should be performed. The delivery core wire is gently pulled with simultaneous contrast injection to see LAA movement together with the occluder.
3. **Size**: TEE measurements of the maximum diameter of the device in at least four views (0°, 45°, 90°, 135°) must confirm 10%–20% compression compared with the nominal diameter of the occluder.
4. **Sealing**: LAA occlusion is deemed sufficient when all lobes are distal to the occluder and residual peri-device leaks <3 mm in diameter. In case of gaps > 3 mm, the occluder should be repositioned.

So far, the Watchman is the only device that has been studied in randomised trials against oral anticoagulation with warfarin. In PROTECT-AF, patients with non-valvular AF and a CHADS$_2$-score of at least 1 point were randomised in a 2:1 ratio to the Watchman device ($n = 463$) or an oral anticoagulation with warfarin ($n = 244$).[22] A total of 707 patients with an average CHADS$_2$-score of 2.2 were randomised. Primary analyses proved non-inferiority of the Watchman when compared with warfarin in the prevention of the primary efficacy endpoint of stroke, systemic embolism or cardiovascular (CV) death. After 1,065 patient-years of follow-up, the primary efficacy event rate was 3.0 per 100 patient-years in the Watchman group, compared with 4.9 per 100 patient-years amongst the anti-coagulated patients. In patients with successful sealing of the LAA a

60% reduction in the composite endpoint rate of stroke, systemic embolism and CV death was achieved. A sub-study of the PROTECT-AF trial revealed that there was no clear interaction between peri-device leakage after LAA-occlusion with the Watchman device and the appearance of clinical events.[33] Depending on the size of peri-device leak-age, the hazard ratio in the presence of minor, moderate and major leaks compared with patients without peri-device flow was 0.85, 0.83 and 0.48, respectively ($p = .798$). The risk of device embolisation and peri-procedural stroke was 0.6% and 1.1%, respectively.[22] Looking specifically at indi-vidual endpoints, the absolute rate of ischaemic strokes in the Warfarin group was slightly higher, but more than com-pensated by the prevention of haemorrhagic strokes due to the lack of necessity for warfarin, resulting in an 80%–85% reduction in haemorrhagic strokes.

Despite the initially increased risk of peri-procedural complications in the interventional group, the analysis of the PROTECT-AF long-term follow-up (3.8 years) demon-strated that LAA closure with the Watchman occluder met the standards for superiority when compared with warfa-rin for the prevention of the composite primary endpoint of stroke, systemic embolism and cardiovascular or unex-plained death.[34] In total, primary endpoint events were reported in 39 patients (8.4%) treated with the Watchman versus 34 patients (13.9%) in the warfarin group. This corre-sponds to a primary event rate of 2.3 events per 100 patient-years in the interventional group versus 3.8 events in the warfarin group (relative risk [RR] = 0.6; 95% confidence interval [CI], 0.41–1.05). Therefore, the criteria for both non-inferiority and superiority were met. Furthermore, the rate of cardiovascular mortality was significantly lower in patients treated per device closure (one event per 100 patient-years vs. 2.4 events per 100 patient-years; hazards ratio [HR] = 0.4; $p = .005$). All-cause mortality was sig-nificantly lower with the Watchman (3.2 events per 100 patient-years vs. 4.8 events per 100 patient years; $p = .04$). These mortality endpoints were only secondary endpoints and it is plausible that the beneficial effect of LAA closure may further improve over time because device-related com-plications are extremely rare beyond 30 days, whereas anti-coagulants continue to cause complications over time.

For further confirmation of the PROTECT-AF results, the PREVAIL trial was initiated. The study design was almost identical to PROTECT-AF, and enrolled 407 patients who were randomly assigned in a 2:1 ratio to the Watchman device or warfarin.[23] Compared with PROTECT-AF, the implantation success rate was significantly higher in the PREVAIL trial (95% vs. 91%). At the same time, the rate of major procedural complications (composite of cardiac perforation, pericardial effusion with tamponade, stroke, device embolisation and access-related complications) was significantly lower. Surgical repair for pericardial effusion was required in only 0.4% in PREVAIL, compared with 1.6% in PROTECT-AF ($p = .027$). Pericardiocentesis was performed in 1.5% vs. 2.9% ($p = .36$). At 18 months, the Watchman failed to reach the pre-specified non-inferiority

criteria with the composite primary endpoint of stroke, systemic embolism and death of cardiovascular or unex-plained reasons with a rate of 6.4% in the Watchman group versus 6.3% in the warfarin group. The composite rate of stroke3 or systemic embolism more than 7 days after hos-pitalisation was at 18 months follow-up 2.53% in the inter-ventional group, compared with 2% in the control group. Although non-inferiority was not achieved for overall effi-cacy, event rates were low and numerically comparable in both arms.

A 2015 meta-analysis analysed the results of 2406 patients undergoing LAA-closure with the Watchman with a total follow-up of 5931 patient-years. This evaluation included the patients from PROTECT-AF and PREVAIL, and their respective registries[35] Within a mean follow-up of 2.69 years, the patients treated with the Watchman occluder had significantly fewer haemorrhagic strokes (0.15 vs. 0.96 events/100 patient-years; $p = .004$), cardiovascular and/or unexplained death (1.1 vs. 2.3 events/100 patient-years; $p = .006$) and non–procedure-related bleeding com-plications (6.0% vs. 11.3%; $p = .006$) when compared with warfarin. The all-cause stroke or systemic embolism risk was similar between both strategies (1.75 vs. 1.87 events/100 patient-years; $p = .94$). There were more ischaemic strokes in the Watchman group (1.6 vs. 0.9 events/100 patient-years; $p = .05$), but once procedure-related strokes were excluded, the rates of ischaemic stroke were no longer significantly different ($p = 0.21$). In contrast, the rate of haemorrhagic strokes occurred significantly less frequently in the inter-ventional group than with warfarin (0.15 vs. 0.96 events/100 patient-years; $p = .004$).

One potential flaw of PROTECT-AF and PREVAIL was the exclusion of patients unable to use postoperative anticoagulation, e.g. patients with a high-bleeding risk or contraindication. To evaluate the Watchman in these real-world patients, the ASAP trial studied those on anti-platelet therapy only following implantation. A total of 155 patients with a mean $CHADS_2$-scoe of 2.8 were treated with dual anti-platelet for 6 months, followed by lifelong daily aspi-rin. During the follow-up period, six patients (4%) had device-associated thrombus formation. Therefore the risk does not seem to be higher than in the PROTECT-AF study cohort. One of these thrombi caused a stroke, all the oth-ers were incidental and resolved with temporary heparin anticoagulation. The annual stroke rate was 1.7%, which is significantly lower than the calculated risk based on the $CHADS_2$-score (7.3%), and suggests that LAA closure is safe alternative, especially in patients with contraindications to oral anticoagulation.

33.4.2 Amplatzer cardiac plug/Amulet (St. Jude Medical, Inc.)

The Amplatzer cardiac plug (ACP) occluder consists of two parts: a distal cylindrical lobe with a length of 6.5 mm and a proximal disc, connected by a stretchable waist that facili-tates the positioning and conformation even to variable

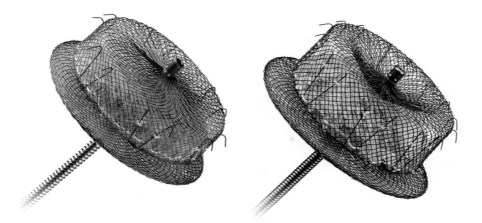

Figure 33.6 The first and second generations of the Amplatzer LAA occlusion devices – the Amplatzer Cardiac Plug (left) and the Amulet device (right).

and complex LAA shapes (Figure 33.6). It is built of a self-expanding Nitinol frame with polyester patches in both parts of the occluder to facilitate endothelialisation and decrease blood flow through the occluder. Deployed in the LAA, the distal lobe is placed in the neck of the LAA, whilst the proximal disc covers the ostium of the LAA. The system is available in 2 mm steps in sizes from 16 to 30 mm, defined by the outer diameter of the lobe. The proximal disc extends into the lobe by 4 mm for device sizes from 16 to 22 mm and by 6 mm for device sizes from 24 to 30 mm. The cylindrical lobe has six pairs of barbed stabilisation wires on its outer circumference to anchor itself in the wall of the LAA and reduce the risk of device embolisation. Selection of the correct device size should be made depending on the angiographic and echocardiographic measurements of the ostial diameter of the LAA and the landing zone for the distal lobe of the ACP. The landing zone is measured approximately 1 cm distally to the plane of the LAA. For choosing the optimal occluder size, we recommend 20% oversizing the measured diameter of the landing zone. The consecutive compression of the lobe after implantation supports the anchoring of the occluder. Due to the fact that the length of the ACP is always shorter than its diameter, implantation of the ACP can be attempted in virtually all LAAs, especially in those shorter than wide, in which the Watchman device may not be implanted. The ACP does not come preloaded and must be prepared accordingly prior to its implantation.

In January 2013, the Amulet device, the second generation of the ACP, received CE mark approval (Figure 33.6). Unlike its predecessor, the Amulet comes preloaded in the delivery sheath to ensure easier and faster use. The lobe of the Amulet is comparably longer than that of the ACP (7.5 mm in Amulet sizes 16–22 mm and 10 mm in Amulet sizes 25–34 mm compared with 6.5 mm in any size of the ACP device) has an increased number of stabilisation wires (10 pairs instead of 6 for the sizes 28–34 mm) on its outer circumference and is available in sizes reflecting the diameter of the lobe of up to 34 mm. The proximal disc extends the lobe by 6 mm in device sizes from 16 to 22 mm

and by 7 mm in sizes from 25 to 34 mm. This may be of additional advantage by sealing the ostium of complex shaped or multilobed LAAs. The occluder sizes available for the ACP and the Amulet devices fit landing zones from 11 to 31 mm.

As the size of the delivery sheath depends on the size of the occluder, we recommend placing a pigtail catheter in the LAA to ease angiographic measurements as previously described for the Watchman device. The delivery sheath itself, the Amplatzer TorqVue 45° × 45°, has two 45° bends and faces anterior at its distal end to facilitate entering of the LAA. The sheath size ranges from 9 Fr. for the 16 mm ACP, over 10 Fr. for the 18 to 22 mm ACP devices, up to 1 for all occluders with a diameter of 24 mm or larger. The Amulet requires a sheath size of 12 Fr. for occluders ranging from 16 to 25 mm and 14 Fr. for occluders with a lobe diameter of 28, 31 and 34 mm. As resistance during the introduction of the delivery sheath is often encountered at the access site in the groin and at the level of trans-septal puncture in the atrial septum, we recommend placing a 0.035-inch stiff wire in the pigtail catheter located in the LAA to advance the sheath and its dilatator into the left atrium.

By pulling back the delivery sheath whilst holding the device in position, the distal lobe of the occluder is deployed. This should be carried out carefully to ensure the entire lobe is within the neck of the LAA, and at least two-thirds of the lobe should be located distal to the left circumflex artery. When the lobe of the ACP/Amulet is positioned correctly, the proximal disc can be deployed by further pulling back of the delivery sheath.

The implantation of an ACP/Amulet device is considered successful when first, a 10%–20% compression of the distal lobe with a thereby caused slight concave configuration occurs, second, a complete separation of the lobe and the disc with correct angulation can be detected in fluoroscopy and third slightly concave shape of the proximal disc which seals the ostium of the LAA is seen (Figure 33.7).

If the position of the occluder is not satisfactory, it can be recaptured for further repositioning. However, the occluder

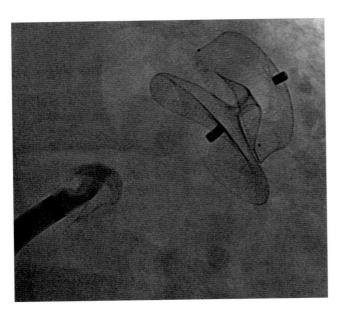

Figure 33.7 Fluoroscopy of an implanted ACP occluder. A successfully implanted ACP with a concave shaped proximal disc, a proper compression of the lobe, and a separation between the lobe and the disc.

should not be completely re-sheathed, as this may cause damage or distortion of the hooks.

Randomised trial results of the ACP device is currently ongoing (www.clinicaltrials.gov, identifier: NCT01118299) with planned enrolment of 3000 patients and 2017. Park et al. reported the results of 10 European centres. Successful device implantation was achieved in 96% (132 of 137 patients). Peri-procedural complications occurred in 10 patients (7%). Three of them experienced a peri-procedural ischaemic stroke probably because of air embolism or intra-cardiac thrombus. In 2012, data of the Amplatzer Cardiac Plug European Multicentre Prospective Observational Study were presented. Between 2009 and 2011, a total of 197 patients underwent LAA closure with the ACP device at one of 15 European centres.[36] The mean patient age was 74.2 years and the mean CHADS$_2$-score was 2.6. The majority of patients had permanent AF and 39.2% had previously suffered a stroke or transient ischaemia attack (TIA). Successful device implantation was achieved in 96.6% with an acute closure rate of 99.5%. Device- or procedure-related safety events occurred in 11 patients (5.4%). Three patients (1.5%) experienced device embolisation and all were recaptured with percutaneous methods. In three patients (1.5%), serious pericardial effusions occurred, and in five cases (2.4%) device-related thrombus formation was seen. Of note, no peri-procedural strokes occurred. The complete closure rate after 6 months was 98.9%. After 101 patient years of follow-up, the stroke rate was 1.98% compared with an expected rate of 5.6% according to the CHADS$_2$-score.

Guerios et al. performed successful occlusion using the ACP in 85 of 86 patients (99%).[37] In 2.3% of the patients, peri-procedural cerebral events occurred. Device embolisation (with successful percutaneous retrieval) and pericardial tamponade requiring percutaneous drainage were seen in

1% of the cases. Within 26 patient-years of follow-up, there appeared no thromboembolic events. Follow-up TEE confirmed the LAA completely occluded in 97%. In 6 of 69 (9%) patients who underwent TEE within follow-up, a device-associated thrombus was seen. Resolution after anticoagulation was seen in all cases. Similarly, Lopez-Minguez et al. described thrombus formation in 5 of 35 patients (14%), with resolution in all cases after temporary therapy with heparin.[38] Plicht et al. reported thrombus formation in 18% of 34 patients. They identified a high CHADS$_2$- and CHA$_2$DS$_2$-VASc-score, and low ejection fraction as risk factors for thrombus formation following LAA-closure with the ACP.[39]

In 2014, Wiebe et al. reported the results of the ACP in 60 high-risk patients with absolute contraindications to oral anticoagulation.[40] ACP-implantation was successful in 95%. Within a mean follow-up duration of 1.8 years no strokes occurred, compared with an estimated annual stroke risk of 5.8%. Major bleeding complications occurred in 1.9%. Similarly, in an analysis of Urena et al. the ACP could be successfully implanted in 98.1% of their patients with a contraindication to oral anticoagulation and a mean CHADS$_2$-score of 3.[41] At a mean time of follow-up of 20 ± 5 months, the rates of death, stroke, systemic embolism, pericardial effusion and major bleeding were 5.8%, 1.9%, 0%, 1.9% and 1.9%, respectively. After 6 months, no device-associated thrombus was detected in TEE.

The second-generation ACP, the Amulet device, carries some technical improvements. The hub has a lower profile. The distal lobe is longer with an increased number of fixation barbs to reduce the risk of embolisation, and the proximal disc is larger in diameter to minimise residual leaks. For evaluation of these improvements, Gloekler et al. compared the results of 50 ACP- and 50 Amulet-implantations.[42] The groups were similar with regard to their clinical profile and anatomical baseline criteria. Procedural success rates were similar with both devices (98% vs. 94%, $p = .61$). Severe adverse events were seen in 6% in the ACP- vs. 8% in the Amulet-group ($p = .7$), whereas the overall complication rate was insignificantly higher in the ACP-group, which was mainly driven by clinically non-relevant pericardial effusions (24% vs. 14%, $p = .31$). The rates of death (0% vs. 2%), stroke (none in both groups) or pericardial tamponade (6% in both groups) were similar between the groups. Lam et al. reported similar success rates in the use of the Amulet.[43] They implanted 17 Amulet devices successfully. Similarly, in 96% of the 25 patients (mean CHA$_2$DS$_2$-VASc-score 4.3) reported by Freixa et al. who underwent LAA occlusion with the Amulet, the device was implanted successfully without peri-procedural stroke, pericardial effusion or device embolisation.[44]

33.4.3 Coherex WaveCrest (Coherex Medical)

The Coherex WaveCrest consists of a central Nitinol structure, but due its unique design there is no exposed metal hub after implantation. The device is designed for positioning in the LAA ostium without requiring catheter

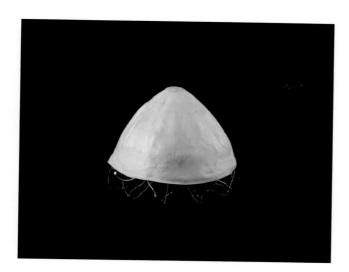

Figure 33.8 The Coherex WaveCrest occluder. An expanded polytetrafluoroethylene (ePTFE) membrane covers the part of the occluder facing the left atrium. Ten interlinked anchor struts build a total of 30 points of tissue interaction.

manipulation in the distal portion of the LAA. The part of the occluder which faces the left atrium after implantation is covered with an expanded polytetrafluoroethylene (ePTFE) membrane in order to minimise thrombogenicity and facilitate rapid endothelialisation (Figure 33.8). A rim of polyurethane located on the inner surface along the contact line between the device and the myocardium additionally stimulates tissue in-growth. Therefore, in contrast to the previously described occlusion devices, dual anti-platelet therapy with aspirin and clopidogrel is recommended for only 6 weeks after implantation of the WaveCrest occluder. Thereafter clopidogrel therapy may be stopped whilst aspirin is continued indefinitely.

The main feature of the device is that it separates positioning of the occluder and its anchoring. The positioning of the WaveCrest device proximal to all lobes guarantees best occlusion, and the risk of pericardial effusion is minimised as distal deployment may compress the device and its anchors. After placement of the device in the ostium of the LAA, 10 centrally interlinked anchor struts that build the distal part of the device are rolled out thereby allowing a very controlled release. Each of the anchor struts has a directional double microtine and a single microtine to create a total of 30 points of tissue interaction. Currently, this design specification makes the WaveCrest the occluder with the most anchoring points of all devices. Five of the ten anchors carry radiopaque tantalum markers to visualise the attachment apparatus. The device can be completely or partially recaptured for repositioning at any time of the procedure. The occluder is available in three sizes with diameters of 22, 27 and 32 mm.

The TEE measurement of the landing zone include the distance from the LCX to a point 10 mm distal to the apex of the lateral ridge in at least four projections (0°, 45°, 90° and 135°) to capture the long and the short axes of the ostium. Furthermore, measurements should include the widest part of the ostium (usually seen in 135° view), since the device will be positioned in the proximal end of the LAA mouth, allowing 5–10 mm of space for unfolding of the anchors. Regarding the selection of the device size, a mild compression of the anchors is needed for secure tissue engagement. But excessive oversizing should be avoided, as it may diminish the stability of the anchors and therefore increase the risk of delayed embolisation of the occluder. The labelled device size should be about 3 mm bigger than the average of the largest and the smallest anchor landing zone measured in TEE.

After successful trans-septal puncture and placement of a soft tipped 0.035 inch stiff wire in a pulmonary vein, the operator can choose between four different shapes of the 15 Fr. WaveCrest delivery sheath depending on the angle between the shaft and the distal tip of the sheath: 60°, 75°, 90° and 90°s (with a distal superior angle). The 75° sheath is appropriate for most LAA anatomies, whereas the 90° sheath is useful in a rather horizontal or inferior trajectory, and the 60° and 90°s sheaths are preferable in a rather superior trajectory of the LAA. After advancing the delivery sheath, the dilatator and the guidewire are removed and a pigtail catheter is placed through the delivery sheath into the LAA to enable LAA-angiography and to facilitate the placement of the delivery sheath. The sheath has an atraumatic distal tip with two radiopaque markers (5 and 15 mm from the tip) for better visualisation.

Polyurethane foam builds the leading edge of the occluder during deployment, making it soft and atraumatic. These properties allow the device to be unsheathed completely for best positioning under fluoroscopic and TEE guidance. Supplementary injection of contrast through the delivery sheath may facilitate positioning. When the system is in the desired position, the anchors can be deployed for fixation. The radiopaque anchor core is visible when the anchors are unfolded. They can be used for evaluation of the anchors' positions (Figure 33.9). As the ostium of the LAA is not planar, anchor engagement may be challenging, especially in the area of the posterior wall, which may be best controlled in TEE at 120°–135°.

Before final release of the occluder a tug-test is recommended. After pulling back the delivery sheath approximately 2 cm from the occluder, the test is carried out under simultaneous contrast injection. If the occluder fails the test, the anchors may be retracted and the device is recaptured for repositioning.

The WAVECREST I Trial included 73 patients with non-valvular AF and a $CHADS_2$ score ≥ 1. Following the implantation, patients received dual anti-platelet therapy until TEE evaluation 45 days after the implant, followed by a lifelong therapy with aspirin. The procedure was successfully conducted with implantation of an occluder in 70 patients (96%) and results of this study are awaited.

33.4.4 Lariat (SentreHEART, Red Wood City, California)

The Lariat technique mimics the surgical ligation of the LAA to achieve permanent closure without an endocardial

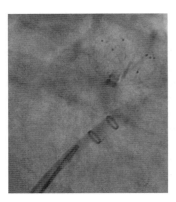

Figure 33.9 Fluoroscopy of an implanted WaveCrest occluder. The radiopaque tantalum markers incorporated into the anchor struts of the Coherex WaveCrest occluder.

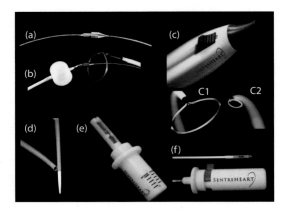

Figure 33.10 The Lariat system. The endo- and epicardial guidewires (a), the 15 mm compliant balloon catheter (b), the 12 F suture delivery device (c), the epicardial guide cannula (d), the suture tightening device (e), and the suture cutter (f).

implant. The system consists of six components: (1) a 0.025 inch endocardial and (2) a 0.035 inch epicardial guidewire (both with magnetic tips); (3) a 15 mm compliant balloon catheter (EndoCATH balloon catheter; SentreHEART); (4) a 12 Fr. suture delivery device; (5) a suture-tightening device (TenSure Suture Tightener; SentreHEART) and (6) a suture cutter (SureCut Suture Cutter; SentreHEART) (Figure 33.10).

In addition to a trans-septal approach for placing a guidewire with a magnetic tip in the most distal part of the LAA, a magnetic counterpart wire is placed epicardially using an anterior pericardial access. Then, both wires are connected by their magnetic tips and used as a rail to place the Lariat snare epicardially over the LAA. After confirmation of complete capture of the LAA by contrast injection and TEE, the snare is closed to seal the LAA.

To achieve pericardial access and to position, the snare freely over the LAA a specific pericardial space is required. Patients with a history of open chest surgery or other conditions leading to pericardial adhesions therefore have relative contraindications for this technique. Furthermore, it may

be useful to perform an additional pre-procedural imaging with computed tomography angiography to rule out the presence of LAA thrombus and to check for further anatomic exclusion criteria, which may hamper the positioning of the snare over the LAA. A width of the LAA of more than 40 mm, a superior orientation of the LAA with the apex directed behind the pulmonary trunk, the presence of a multilobed LAA in which the different lobes orient in different planes exceeding 40 mm and a posteriorly rotation of the heart are possible hindrances.

A 17-Gauge pericardial needle is used to achieve pericardial access. Fluoroscopy is used in order to align the needle towards the lateral aspect of the cardiac silhouette in an anterior–posterior view. The 90° left lateral view ensures that the puncture is on the anterior surface of the right ventricle. By injecting small amounts of contrast, tenting of the pericardium prior to puncture can be detected. Pericardial access is verified when small amount of contrast appear in the pericardial space. Next, a 0.035-inch guidewire is placed in the pericardial space, over which a 14 Fr. soft-tipped epicardial sheath is inserted. Then, the guidewire is exchanged for the 0.035 inch magnetic tipped guidewire of the Lariat system.

Using right femoral venous access, the trans-septal puncture is recommended under TEE guidance for the endocardial LAA occlusion devices. An 8.5 Fr. trans-septal delivery sheath is positioned in the atrial septum, which is used to deliver the 0.025 inch endocardial magnetic guidewire into the most distal aspect of the LAA. Over this wire the EndoCATH balloon catheter is advanced into the LAA. At its distal end a 12-mm-long balloon is mounted that has a 15 mm diameter when inflated. Next, the endocardial placed magnetic wire is connected with its epicardial counterpart (Figure 33.11a). Now, the snare can be advanced over the LAA using the connected magnetic wires as a rail. By inflation of the balloon of the EndoCATH balloon catheter proper placement of the snare at its landing zone at the LAA ostium can be facilitated (Figure 33.11b). The snare can be opened and closed multiple times to ensure proper sealing of the LAA. Once TEE and angiography confirm complete closure of the LAA, the endocardial components (EndoCATH balloon catheter and magnetic guidewire) are removed, the TenSure Suture Tightener is advanced epicardially, and the suture is cut near the ostium of the LAA (Figure 33.11c).

We recommend exchanging the magnetic guidewire placed in the epicardium for a pigtail catheter, which then can be left in the epicardial space overnight to serve as a pericardial drain. On the following day, it can be removed after echocardiographic exclusion of a relevant pericardial effusion.

As there is no foreign body left behind inside the heart, there is no need for post-interventional continuation of anticoagulation. However, the majority of the patients treated with the Lariat device so far received aspirin or clopidogrel after LAA ligation because of other concomitant diseases.

In 2013, Bartus et al. published the results of LAA ligation using the Lariat device attempted in 92 patients (mean

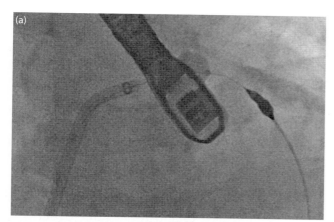

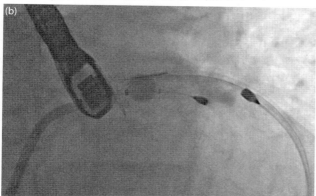

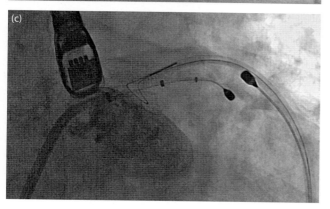

Figure 33.11 Fluoroscopy of procedural steps using the Lariat snare. The endocardial magnetic guidewire is connected with its epicardial counterpart **(a)**, and used as a rail to advance the snare over the LAA. Inflation of the EndoCATH balloon catheter facilitates placement of the snare at the LAA ostium **(b)**. Once transoesophageal echocardiography (TEE) and angiography confirm complete closure of the LAA, the endocardial components can be removed **(c)**.

$CHADS_2$-score 1.9).[45] In 85 patients (92%) the ligation was completed successfully. In four patients the procedure was aborted because of pericardial adhesions. In two patients the procedure was aborted due to complications whilst achieving pericardial access. At 1-year, complete closure was 98% (n = 77). Of note, the residual leaks in the remaining patients were less than 3 mm in size. In one patient, a

pericardial effusion was noted 2 weeks after the procedure requiring pericardial drainage. Within 12 months of follow-up no definitive thromboembolic events occurred.

Massumi et al. reported successful ligation of the LAA (defined as a residual leak of less than 5 mm) in all patients (n = 20).[46] Compared with the population of Bartus et al., these patients had an increased stroke risk with a mean $CHADS_2$-score of 3.2. The LAA remained completely sealed in 16 patients, one had a minimal residual flow. Within a mean follow-up of 352 days, no thromboembolic events occurred, and oral anticoagulation was used in only 20% of patients after the procedure. Stone et al. achieved successful LAA closure in 93% of attempted cases (n = 27, mean $CHADS_2$-score: 3.5).[47] In one patient, LAA perforation required pericardial drainage, and the LAA was closed non-emergently surgically (in conjunction with a Maze procedure). At a mean time of follow-up of 4 months, no deaths or pericardial complications were reported. One patient had a stroke that most likely was related to aortic arch atheroma at day 33 after the procedure. In TEE neither a residual leak nor thrombus formation were seen.

Patel et al. reported on their experience with complex anatomy detected by 3D cardiac computed tomography.[48] Of nine patients with complex anatomy, in seven (78%) LAA closure was achieved successfully. The two other patients had to undergo minimal invasive thoracotomy not because of major complications but for technical reasons. In one patient, pericardial adhesions precluded pericardial entry, and in the other the epicardial snare could not be released from the long C-shaped LAA. Follow-up using TEE after 3 months showed complete closure without remnant flow in all patients and there were no strokes.

In 2014, Price et al. published the results of the largest patient-group[49] A total of 154 patients were treated and procedural success was found in 86%. In nine patients, the snare could not be delivered. TEE demonstrated complete closure in 92% at the end of the procedure. A residual leak of less than 5 mm was seen in 7%. There were no in-hospital strokes or myocardial infarctions seen. A significant pericardial effusion occurred in 16 patients (10%), secondary to LAA perforation/laceration in four cases (25%), as a result of pericardial access in four cases (25%) and from unclear reasons in the remaining cases. At discharge, most patients were treated with aspirin, 19% of the patients (n = 29) received neither an anti-platelet nor oral anticoagulation and 134 patients (87%) had undergone follow-up for a median period of 112 days. The composite of out-of-hospital death, myocardial infarction or stroke occurred in four patients (2.9%). Strokes were seen in two patients, one of which was fatal.

In 2015, Chatterjee et al. published a systematic review of published reports and an analytic review of the FDA MAUDE database (Manufacturer and User Facility Device Experience) with regards to the off-label use of the Lariat device in the United States, as the device has received US FDA clearance 510(k) for soft-tissue approximation.[50] They identified five reports of Lariat device used in a total of 309 patients.

Procedural success was achieved in 90.3% (279 patients). In seven patients, urgent cardiac surgery (2.3%; $n = 7$) was needed and one patient died due to procedure-related complications (0.3%). The analysis of the FDA MAUDE database revealed 35 reports of adverse events with the use of the Lariat technique. Amongst these, five events reported about death following pericardial tamponade and additional 23 reports told about patients requiring urgent surgery for acute complications.

A multicentre prospective observational study by Pillarisetti et al. compared the LAA occlusion rates of 478 patients (219 treated with the Watchman device, 259 with the Lariat snare) up to 1 year after the procedure.[51] They found the patients treated with the Lariat system to have a higher CHADS$_2$-score and larger diameters of the left atrium and the LAA. At 1 year, 79 patients (17%) had a detectable leak. In the Watchman group, significantly more leaks were seen than in the Lariat group (21% versus 14%, $p = .019$ respectively). With regard to peri-procedural complications, three events appeared using the Watchman system: one device embolisation requiring surgery and two pericardial effusions requiring pericardiocentesis. In the Lariat group, four patients had cardiac tamponade requiring urgent surgical repair.

33.5 Other new endo- and epicardial LAA closure techniques

Whereas the above-mentioned systems have already gained access into clinical practice, the devices described below are currently in preclinical testing.

33.5.1 LAmbre (Lifetech Scientific Corp., Shenzen, China)

The LAmbre system is a self-expanding umbrella placed in the LAA for endocardial sealing. It consists of two parts connected by a short central waist: a disc covering the ostium of the LAA and a distal anchor mechanism, which has an umbrella-shaped configuration. The device is built from titanium nitride (TiN)–coated Nitinol wire mesh to reduce the risk of delayed thrombus formation and to promote faster endothelialisation. It includes two polyethylene terephthalate membranes: one inside the occlusion disc, the other covering the distal anchor-struts and thereby creating the umbrella-like shape. The distal membrane allows sealing of the LAA if that in the covering disc fails to do so. The device is available in sizes from 16 to 36 mm with the covering disc 4–6 mm larger than the diameter of the distal umbrella. Furthermore, there are special versions with sizes ranging from 16 to 26 mm with a 12–14 mm larger covering disc to facilitate occlusion of small or multilobed LAAs.

The distal umbrella includes eight anchor struts with rounded ends to lower the risk of perforation during device deployment. The delivery sheath is placed in the plane of the LAA ostium during the deployment of the occluder. This allows the rounded struts to roll into the LAA.

The anchoring of the device is achieved by a stenting-like effect of the slightly oversized umbrella with its eight individual frames trapped in the LAA tissue. Furthermore, a small hook is placed along each anchor strut to grab the LAA tissue. The struts are able to fold inwards to allow retrieval and repositioning of the device.

In the LAmbre FIM Asian registry involving six Asian centres between 2012 and 2014, 66 patients received this device.[52] Successful placement was achieved in all patients with a peri-device leakage of more than 3 mm in only one case.

33.5.2 Occlutech Occluder™ (Occlutech GmbH, Jena, Germany)

The Occlutech LAA Occluder is another system for endocardial occlusion of the LAA. It consists of a self-expanding Nitinol mesh with a tapered cylindrical shape. Its softness allows adaptation to the LAA shape with the larger diameter of the proximal part of the occluder sealing the ostium. The Nitinol wire is coated with a polycarbonate urethane layer to minimise the thromboembolic risk and improve endothelialisation of the device. Along the distal rim of the cylindrical occluder, the Nitinol wire forms loops instead of barbs to hold the device in place and reduce the risk of perforation. Furthermore, the Occlutech LAA Occluder has a special, ball-like release mechanism allowing an inclination angle of 45° between the device and the delivery cable without causing stress or tension to the implant. The occluder is available in seven sizes ranging in 3 mm steps from 15 to 33 mm, and can be delivered through a 12 Fr. sheath. The sheath itself will be available in a single- and a double-curved design.

A prospective non-randomised trial for evaluation of safety and efficacy of the device is under way and completion is estimated in 2016 (ClinicalTrials.gov Identifier: NCT02105584).

33.5.3 Cardia Ultrasept Occluder (Cardia Inc., Eagan, Minneapolis)

The Cardia Ultrasept LAA Occluder is delivered through a 12 Fr. delivery sheath which allows to collapse and reposition the occluder in case of incomplete occlusion. The device consists of two parts: a proximal sail and a distal cylindrical shaped bulb, which are connected over a 7–8 mm long waist with flexible articulation. This concept allows self-centring of the proximal disc for optimal adaption to the LAA ostium. The struts, which form the distal bulb, are composed of multiple elements forming a cable to provide the structural support for the disc, and to maintain the configuration of the occluder. In addition, the struts include lateral wall hooks. The device is available with three different sizes of the distal bulb (16, 20 or 24 mm). For all sizes of the device, the proximal disc is always 4 mm larger than the distal bulb. The device size should be 2–3 mm larger than the maximum diameter of the LAA ostium and of the landing zone measured in TEE and fluoroscopy.

33.5.4 The trans-catheter patch occlusion (Custom Medical Devices, Athens, Greece)

The trans-catheter patch occlusion technique uses an endocardial approach to implant a bioabsorbable, frameless, balloon-deliverable device that can be adjusted to the shape and size of the LAA without the risk of perforation. The patches are tailored from polyurethane foam and attached into the LAA by a two-component surgical adhesive. At the bottom of the patch, a 2 mm nylon loop is sutured, to which a nylon thread is connected for retrieval purposes. First, 1–2 ml of a polyethylene glycol–based acidic solution is applied on the distal half of the patch. The adhesive is inactive under acidic conditions. This allows advancing the patch into the LAA through a 13 Fr. trans-septal sheath and over a guidewire. Then, the supporting Latex balloon is inflated until it stretches the LAA. After confirmation of the balloon and patch position by TEE and fluoroscopy, the second component of the surgical adhesive, an alkaline solution is injected through the central lumen of the catheter. The balloon catheter can be removed 45 minutes after the activation of the surgical adhesive. The patch is then released by removal of the nylon thread. Due to subsequent water absorption the adhesive increases in volume after its placement. This allows an additional improvement in occlusion rates of the LAA within 24 hours after the implantation.

This technique was studied in 20 patients and the device was placed successful in 17 of them.[53] An injection of contrast medium for diagnostic angiography directly before the implantation was discussed a possible reason of insufficient activation of the surgical adhesive in the three remaining patients. Follow-up TEE 1 day after the implantation showed complete sealing of the LAA in 15 of the 17 successful implanted patients. TEE in the two remaining patients showed a trivial shunt in one and a partial occlusion of the LAA in the other patient.[53]

33.5.5 Sentinel (Aegis Medical, Vancouver, Canada)

Unlike the previously described systems, which are all applied endocardially, the AEGIS system represents a novel epicardial technique for LAA occlusion. It is an electrocardiogram-guided LAA capture and ligation system that requires an epicardial approach. It consists of two parts: (1) a small forceps to grasp the LAA and (2) a suture. The forceps has an articulating jaw with electrodes mounted to record the electrocardiogram and thereby help to monitor the forceps localisation and facilitate its navigation. The system is preloaded with a 0.012-inch support wire, which ensures

an anterior approach to facilitate LAA capture under fluoroscopic guidance. The LAA is grasped with the forceps and a hollow suture loop is advanced over the forceps and around the LAA to its base. In case of incomplete occlusion or unsatisfying position of the suture, further sutures can be applied more proximally.

The seven first-in-human procedures with the AEGIS system showed promising results.[54] Complete sealing of the LAA could be achieved in all seven patients. Three of the patients required more than one suture.

33.5.6 AtriClip (AtriCure, Westchester, Ohio)

Another device for epicardial occlusion of the LAA is the AtriClip system. It has been designed and is approved by the FDA for the occlusion of the LAA in patients undergoing open chest surgery for other indications. The system proved safe and atraumatic exclusion of the LAA within a multicentre trial, which analysed the results of 71 patients undergoing open cardiac surgery at seven US centers.[55] Peri-operative TEE confirmed successful occlusion of the LAA in 95.7% of the patients. In one case, the LAA was too small for clip placement. Of the 61 patients undergoing follow-up imaging (CT or TEE) 3 months after the procedure, persistent closure of the LAA was confirmed in 60 patients (98.4%). There were no TIAs or strokes seen within the time of follow-up.[55]

The main component of the device is a self-closing clip made of two parallel rigid titanium tubes with two elastic Nitinol springs. The design of the clip applies uniform pressure over the entire length of the two branches. They are covered with a polyester mesh, which serves as a matrix to improve epithelial tissue growth. The clip is available in four sizes (35, 40, 45 and 50 mm). Currently, a small thoracotomy is sufficient to position the clip around the LAA.

33.6 Procedure specific complications

As the operator is working with the catheters in the left atrium, there is the risk of embolism resulting in cerebral, peripheral and coronary air embolism. This risk can easily be reduced by correct handling of the sheaths and catheters. Generous back-bleeding of the trans-septal, the access, and the delivery sheath is recommended whilst keeping the haemostatic valve and device arm below the midline of the chest and thus allowing air to exit the sheath before any equipment or occluder is inserted. Keeping the haemostatic valve, proximal sheath end and side submerged in heparinised saline also prevents air from entering the system during back-bleeding. Furthermore, air embolism might be caused by negative pressure created during removal of the trans-septal puncture needle, dilators or catheters. This can be avoided by slow removal of devices and waiting for spontaneous blood returning into the guiding catheter. In addition, the continuous infusion of saline through the side arm of the sheath is recommended to help prevent air embolism. Accordingly, all devices and delivery catheters must be flushed generously prior to their insertion.

Trans-septal puncture is associated with the risk of falsely puncturing the aorta or perforating the atrium resulting in a pericardial effusion or even tamponade. Therefore, we recommend trans-septal puncture under fluoroscopic and echocardiographic guidance. The puncture should be performed in the posterior and inferior segment of the septum to minimise the risk to puncture the aorta, which is increased when the puncture is done in the anterior part of the septum. In general, the puncture site is best-seen and controlled using the bicaval view in TEE (90°). In addition, a lateral fluoroscopic view allows the visualisation of the needle to place it posterior and inferior the aortic valve plane. We recommend injecting small amounts of contrast before advancement of the dilatator, as cardiac tamponade may occur with advancement of dilatators and sheaths.

Perforation of the left atrium or the LAA may cause pericardial tamponade and warrants immediate pericardiocentesis with re-transfusion of the blood into a vein, or even surgical haemostasis if pericardiocentesis cannot stabilise the patient's haemodynamic. A perforation of the LAA can be caused at almost any time during the intervention and is mostly caused by traumatic manipulation within the LAA. The risk is minimised by advancing the delivery sheath over a pigtail catheter placed in the LAA. Another potential reason is suboptimal alignment of the delivery sheath with the LAA. This may be caused by insufficient shapes of the delivery sheaths as well as by using a present PFO. Therefore, we recommend a trans-septal puncture rather than using a PFO to achieve the best possible alignment of the delivery sheath, and to shape your sheath, if necessary. After successful implantation of an occluder the tug-test for checking a stable positioning should be done carefully to avoid a perforation caused by the retaining apparatus.

To decrease the risk of acute thrombotic complications the ACT should be kept at 250–300 seconds uncomplicated trans-septal puncture. Further, the device sheath time in the left atrium should be minimised, especially in a large left atrium or the pronounced smoke or sludge seen in the LAA by TEE.

Another complication is the detection of device-associated thrombus formation within the follow-up examinations. In these cases temporary oral anticoagulation is indicated. Within a few weeks, most of the thrombi dissolve completely without further complications. Acute thrombolysis is not indicated as this may lead to crumbling of the thrombus resulting in multiple emboli.

The risk of embolisation of the occluder can be reduced by careful selection and confirmation of its position at the end of the procedure. With regards to the device selection

- The implantation of a Watchman should be avoided if the LAA length is less than the device diameter and if the LAA diameter is less than 17 mm or more than 30 mm.

- The implantation of an ACP should be avoided if the landing zone is more than 29 mm (31 mm for the Amulet) and if the LAA length is less than 10 mm.
- A suture occlusion with the Lariat may be considered if the LAA is too large for either the Watchman or the ACP (but maximal diameter 40 mm for Lariat).
- A suture occlusion with the Lariat should be avoided in patients with superiorly oriented LAA or in LAAs that course behind the pulmonary artery. Furthermore, the Lariat system is contraindicated in patients with prior heart surgery (due to pericardial adhesions) and may be exceedingly difficult in patients with pectus excavatum.

The evaluation of positioning of an occluder should be performed in all standard TEE views (0°, 45°, 90° and 135°):

- Following the implantation of a Watchman device, its shoulder should not protrude beyond the LAA ostium by >20% of its diameter, and the optimal compression rate is 10%–20% (in TEE and fluoroscopy). Residual leaks of more than 3 mm should not be accepted.
- Following the implantation of an ACP device, the lobe should be slightly compressed (tyre-shaped), as a missing compression suggests too small size or too proximal positioning, whereas too much compression with alteration of the shape suggests too large size (risk of perforation) or too distal positioning. Further, the disc should be slightly concave shaped, the lobe should not protrude more than one third beyond the left circumflex artery, and the disc and the lobe should be separated slightly.

If all echocardiographic and fluoroscopic release criteria are fulfilled, embolisation of the occluder is very rare. Normally, embolisation occurs within minutes to hours after the procedure. We therefore recommend observation of the occluder a few minutes after its release before finishing the procedure. In addition, occluder position should be conformed the day after implantation using transthoracic echocardiography. Percutaneous snaring using a femoral arterial access can retrieve an embolised device and the occluder pulled out through the femoral sheath.

33.7 Medical therapy and follow-up

The anticoagulation regimen of patients referred for LAA occlusion is tailored individually, as most have either an increased bleeding risk, contraindications, or refuse oral anticoagulation. In patients with thrombi detected in pre-procedural TEE, temporary anticoagulation with short-term follow-up examination is required.

Although the femoral venous puncture does not necessitate the withdrawal of oral anticoagulation, most cardiologists mandate an INR <2.0 for the procedure and prefer the peri-procedural administration of a weight-adjusted bolus of unfractionated heparin after successful trans-septal puncture to maintain an ACT of more than 250 seconds.

Patients should receive loading doses of 500 mg aspirin and 600 mg clopidogrel prior to the procedure.

With regard to the best medical therapy following device-implantation several approaches exist that can be attributed to the different pivotal trials of the devices. The intended medication after implantation of a Watchman device consists of oral anticoagulation for at least 6 weeks after the implant, followed by dual anti-platelet therapy with aspirin and clopidogrel until 6 months of follow-up, followed by a lifelong therapy with aspirin. The oral anticoagulation is intended to reduce the risk of device-associated thrombus formation until completion of endothelialisation. This approach is based on the protocol of the PROTECT-AF trial.[22] In clinical practice, however, patients sent for LAA occlusion often already suffered severe bleeding complications for, or have contraindications to anticoagulation. Therefore, most interventional cardiologists adapt the medical therapy they use after implantation of other intra-cardiac closure devices and prescribe a dual anti-platelet therapy. When TEE 6 months after the implant shows a satisfactory result with complete sealing of the LAA, one anti-platelet agent is stopped and the other continued indefinitely. A 2014 published consensus document of the European Heart Rhythm Association (EHRA) and the European Association of Percutaneous Cardiovascular Interventions (EAPCI) recommends a differentiated approach:[57]

1. Patients with low bleeding risk who undergo implantation of a Watchman should be loaded with aspirin before the procedure and treated with 100–325 mg of aspirin indefinitely thereafter. In addition, after the implantation warfarin should be continued with INR 2–3 until TEE at day 45 or until sealing of the LAA is confirmed in a subsequent follow up TEE exam. At this point, warfarin should be switched to clopidogrel until 6 months after the implant.
2. Patients in whom implantation of an ACP, an Amulet, or a WaveCrest was implanted, or who carry an increased bleeding risk and in whom a Watchman device was implanted, should be loaded with aspirin and clopidogrel. After implantation, dual anti-platelet therapy with clopidogrel for 1–6 months (whilst ensuring adequate LAA closure) and 100–325 mg of aspirin indefinitely is recommended.

The use of TEE for follow-up can detect delayed complications at an early stage (e.g. thrombus on the device, incomplete sealing of the LAA), as these might result in relevant changes in the therapy at least for a certain period of time. The rate of thrombus-associated ischaemic strokes was 0.3 per 100 patient years in the PROTECT-AF trial. Device-associated thrombi were seen in 20 of 478 patients (4.2%), but only 3 of them caused ischaemic events.[22] The risk of thrombus formation on the occluder affects all intra-cardiac implants. Similar cases are described for the ACP, too.[58] Regardless of the implanted device, a temporary oral anticoagulation for a period of weeks to months proved effective in resolution of the thrombi, and therefore is recommended until confirmation of thrombus resolution by follow-up TEE.

Incomplete occlusion of the LAA may offset the stroke preventive effect of LAA closure necessitating continuation of oral anticoagulation, as it allows thrombus formation in the LAA with potential systemic embolisation. There is no generally accepted definition of a relevant residual leak following device implantation. In PROTECT-AF, residual shunts with a diameter of less than 5 mm were deemed not significant and that they may close over time. In TEE 45 days after Watchman implantation, a leak with a diameter of more than 5 mm was seen in 14% of the patients, and therefore warfarin was continued. The rate of relevant leaks decreased to 8% in TEE control after 6 months.[22] Although a sub-analysis of the PROTECT-AF could not show any difference in stroke rates whether oral anticoagulation was continued or not in the presence of residual leaks,[59] the persistence of leaks would require long-term anticoagulation for reduction of stroke risk. As this is complicated in this specific patient population, recurrent interventions with implantation of a second occluder may be an alternative.[60] The type and the size of the device for sealing of a residual leak should be chosen depending on the individual echocardiographic and fluoroscopic findings. A first- or second-generation ACP device might be suitable in larger leaks or cases with uncovered lobes, as its disc may provide excellent coverage. In rather small defects, or those located along another occluder, an Amplatzer Vascular Plug II or III (St. Jude Medical, Inc.) may be suitable. As these patients have an increased risk for thrombi being present in the incomplete sealed LAA, it is even more important to avoid manipulations within the appendage whenever possible. To minimise the risk of device embolization, it is necessary not to disturb the first implant during the procedure. We therefore recommend waiting 5–6 months after the original occluder implantation before proceeding with leak closure to allow endothelialisation and tissue overgrowth to provide more secure anchoring of the original device within the LAA.

References

1. Sacco RL et al. Guidelines for prevention of stroke in patients with ischemic stroke or transient ischemic attack: A statement for healthcare professionals from the American Heart Association/American Stroke Association Council on Stroke: Co-sponsored by the Council on Cardiovascular Radiology and Intervention: The American Academy of Neurology affirms the value of this guideline. *Circulation* 2006; 113(10): e409–e449.
2. Go AS et al. Executive summary: Heart disease and stroke statistics – 2014 update: A report from the American Heart Association. *Circulation* 2014; 129(3): 399–410.
3. Lin HJ et al. Stroke severity in atrial fibrillation. The Framingham Study. *Stroke* 1996; 27(10): 1760–1764.
4. Stewart S et al. Population prevalence, incidence, and predictors of atrial fibrillation in the Renfrew/Paisley study. *Heart* 2001; 86(5): 516–521.

5. Risk factors for stroke and efficacy of antithrombotic therapy in atrial fibrillation. Analysis of pooled data from five randomized controlled trials. *Arch Intern Med* 1994; 154(13): 1449–57.

6. Roger VL et al. Heart disease and stroke statistics – 2011 update: A report from the American Heart Association. *Circulation* 2011; 123(4): e18–e209.

7. Lip GY et al. Refining clinical risk stratification for predicting stroke and thromboembolism in atrial fibrillation using a novel risk factor-based approach: The euro heart survey on atrial fibrillation. *Chest* 2010; 137(2): 263–272.

8. Hart RG et al. Antithrombotic therapy to prevent stroke in patients with atrial fibrillation: A meta-analysis. *Ann Intern Med* 1999; 131(7): 492–501.

9. Bungard TJ et al. Why do patients with atrial fibrillation not receive warfarin? *Arch Intern Med* 2000; 160(1): 41–46.

10. Levine MN et al. Hemorrhagic complications of anticoagulant treatment. *Chest* 2001; 119(1 Suppl): 108S–21S.

11. Waldo AL et al. Hospitalized patients with atrial fibrillation and a high risk of stroke are not being provided with adequate anticoagulation. *J Am Coll Cardiol* 2005; 46(9): 1729–1736.

12. Hylek EM et al. An analysis of the lowest effective intensity of prophylactic anticoagulation for patients with non-rheumatic atrial fibrillation. *N Engl J Med* 1996; 335(8): 540–546.

13. Stafford RS, and Singer DE. National patterns of warfarin use in atrial fibrillation. *Arch Intern Med* 1996; 156(22): 2537–2541.

14. Blackshear JL, and Odell JA. Appendage obliteration to reduce stroke in cardiac surgical patients with atrial fibrillation. *Ann Thorac Surg* 1996; 61(2): 755–759.

15. Takada T et al. Blood flow in the left atrial appendage and embolic stroke in nonvalvular atrial fibrillation. *Eur Neurol* 2001; 46(3): 148–152.

16. Zabalgoitia M et al. Transesophageal echocardiographic correlates of clinical risk of thromboembolism in nonvalvular atrial fibrillation. Stroke Prevention in Atrial Fibrillation III Investigators. *J Am Coll Cardiol* 1998; 31(7): 1622–1626.

17. Tamura H et al. Prognostic value of low left atrial appendage wall velocity in patients with ischemic stroke and atrial fibrillation. *J Am Soc Echocardiogr* 2012; 25(5): 576–583.

18. Katz ES et al. Surgical left atrial appendage ligation is frequently incomplete: A transesophageal echocardiograhic study. *J Am Coll Cardiol* 2000; 36(2): 468–471.

19. Sievert H et al. Percutaneous left atrial appendage transcatheter occlusion to prevent stroke in high-risk patients with atrial fibrillation: Early clinical experience. *Circulation* 2002; 105(16): 1887–1889.

20. Bayard YL et al. PLAATO (Percutaneous Left Atrial Appendage Transcatheter Occlusion) for prevention of cardioembolic stroke in non-anticoagulation eligible atrial fibrillation patients: Results from the European PLAATO study. *EuroIntervention* 2010; 6(2): 220–226.

21. Park JW et al. Percutaneous left atrial appendage transcatheter occlusion (PLAATO) for stroke prevention in atrial fibrillation: 2-year outcomes. *J Invasive Cardiol* 2009; 21(9): 446–450.

22. Holmes DR et al. Percutaneous closure of the left atrial appendage versus warfarin therapy for prevention of stroke in patients with atrial fibrillation: A randomised non-inferiority trial. *Lancet* 2009; 374(9689): 534–542.

23. Holmes DR Jr et al. Prospective randomized evaluation of the Watchman Left Atrial Appendage Closure device in patients with atrial fibrillation versus long-term warfarin therapy: The PREVAIL trial. *J Am Coll Cardiol* 2014; 64(1): 1–12.

24. Bartus K et al. Feasibility of closed-chest ligation of the left atrial appendage in humans. *Heart Rhythm* 2011; 8(2): 188–193.

25. Camm AJ et al. 2012 focused update of the ESC Guidelines for the management of atrial fibrillation: An update of the 2010 ESC Guidelines for the management of atrial fibrillation. Developed with the special contribution of the European Heart Rhythm Association. *Eur Heart J* 2012; 33(21): 2719–2747.

26. Lacomis JM et al. Dynamic multidimensional imaging of the human left atrial appendage. *Europace* 2007; 9(12): 1134–1140.

27. Nucifora G et al. Evaluation of the left atrial appendage with real-time 3-dimensional transesophageal echocardiography: Implications for catheter-based left atrial appendage closure. *Circulation Cardiovasc Imaging* 2011; 4(5): 514–523.

28. Nietlispach F et al. Ad hoc percutaneous left atrial appendage closure. *J Invasive Cardiol* 2013; 25(12): 683–686.

29. Fisher DC et al. The incidence of patent foramen ovale in 1,000 consecutive patients. A contrast transesophageal echocardiography study. *Chest* 1995; 107(6): 1504–1509.

30. Hagen PT et al. Incidence and size of patent foramen ovale during the first 10 decades of life: An autopsy study of 965 normal hearts. *Mayo Clin Proc* 1984; 59(1): 17–20.

31. Konstadt SN et al. Intraoperative detection of patent foramen ovale by transesophageal echocardiography. *Anesthesiology* 1991; 74(2): 212–216.

32. Gafoor S et al. "A bend in time": Shaping the sheath facilitates left atrial appendage closure. *Catheter Cardiovasc Interv* 2015; 86(5): E224–E228.

33. Viles-Gonzalez JF et al. Incomplete occlusion of the left atrial appendage with the percutaneous left atrial appendage transcatheter occlusion device is not associated with increased risk of stroke. *J Interv Card Electrophysiol* 2012; 33(1): 69–75.

34. Reddy VY et al. Percutaneous left atrial appendage closure vs warfarin for atrial fibrillation: A randomized clinical trial. *JAMA* 2014; 312(19): 1988–1998.

35. Holmes DR Jr et al. Left Atrial Appendage Closure as an Alternative to Warfarin for Stroke Prevention in Atrial Fibrillation: A Patient-Level Meta-Analysis. *J Am Coll Cardiol* 2015; 65(24): 2614–2623.

36. Park J-W et al. TCT-86 Results of the Amplatzer Cardiac Plug European Multicenter Prospective Observational Study. *J Am Coll Cardiol* 2012; 60(17 Suppl).

37. Guerios EE et al. Left atrial appendage closure with the Amplatzer cardiac plug in patients with atrial fibrillation. *Arq Bras Cardiol* 2012; 98(6): 528–536.

38. Lopez-Minguez JR et al. Immediate and one-year results in 35 consecutive patients after closure of left atrial appendage with the Amplatzer cardiac plug. *Rev Esp Cardiol* 2013; 66(2): 90–97.

39. Plicht B et al. Risk factors for thrombus formation on the Amplatzer Cardiac Plug after left atrial appendage occlusion. *JACC Cardiovasc Interv* 2013; 6(6): 606–613.

40. Wiebe J et al. Safety of percutaneous left atrial appendage closure with the Amplatzer cardiac plug in patients with atrial fibrillation and contraindications to anticoagulation. *Catheter Cardiovasc Interv* 2014; 83(5): 796–802.

41. Urena M et al. Percutaneous left atrial appendage closure with the AMPLATZER cardiac plug device in patients with nonvalvular atrial fibrillation and contraindications to anticoagulation therapy. *J Am Coll Cardiol* 2013; 62(2): 96–102.

42. Gloekler S et al. Early results of first versus second generation Amplatzer occluders for left atrial appendage closure in patients with atrial fibrillation. *Clin Res Cardiol* 2015; 104(8): 656–665.

43. Lam SC et al. Left atrial appendage closure using the Amulet device: An initial experience with the second generation amplatzer cardiac plug. *Catheter Cardiovasc Interv* 2015; 85(2): 297–303.

44. Freixa X et al. Left atrial appendage occlusion: Initial experience with the Amplatzer Amulet. *Int J Cardiol* 2014; 174(3): 492–496.

45. Bartus K et al. Percutaneous left atrial appendage suture ligation using the LARIAT device in patients with atrial fibrillation: Initial clinical experience. *J Am Coll Cardiol* 2013; 62(2): 108–118.

46. Massumi A et al. Initial experience with a novel percutaneous left atrial appendage exclusion device in patients with atrial fibrillation, increased stroke risk, and contraindications to anticoagulation. *Am J Cardiol* 2013; 111(6): 869–873.

47. Stone D et al. Early results with the LARIAT device for left atrial appendage exclusion in patients with atrial fibrillation at high risk for stroke and anticoagulation. *Catheter Cardiovasc Interv* 2015; 86(1): 121–127.

48. Patel MB et al. Safety and effectiveness of compassionate use of LARIAT(R) device for epicardial ligation of anatomically complex left atrial appendages. *J Interv Card Electrophysiol* 2015; 42(1): 11–19.

49. Price MJ et al. Early safety and efficacy of percutaneous left atrial appendage suture ligation: Results from the U.S. transcatheter LAA ligation consortium. *J Am Coll Cardiol* 2014; 64(6): 565–572.

50. Chatterjee S et al. Safety and Procedural Success of Left Atrial Appendage Exclusion With the Lariat Device: A Systematic Review of Published Reports and Analytic Review of the FDA MAUDE Database. *JAMA Intern Med* 2015; 175(7): 1104–1109.

51. Pillarisetti J et al. Endocardial (Watchman) vs epicardial (Lariat) left atrial appendage exclusion devices: Understanding the differences in the location and type of leaks and their clinical implications. *Heart Rhythm* 2015; 12(7): 1501–1507.

52. Lam Y-Y. Sharing of LAmbre LAAO experiences. Paper presented at: 5th Asia Pacific Congenital and Structural Heart Intervention Symposium 2014. 10 October, Hong Kong, 2014.

53. Toumanides S et al. Transcatheter patch occlusion of the left atrial appendage using surgical adhesives in high-risk patients with atrial fibrillation. *J Am Coll Cardiol* 2011; 58(21): 2236–2240.

54. Bruce CJ et al. Novel percutaneous left atrial appendage closure. *Cardiovasc Revasc Med* 2013; 14(3): 164–167.

55. Ailawadi G et al. Exclusion of the left atrial appendage with a novel device: Early results of a multicenter trial. *J Thorac Cardiovasc Surg* 2011; 142(5): 1002–9, 1009 e1001.

56. Ross J Jr et al. Transseptal left heart catheterization: A new diagnostic method. *Prog Cardiovasc Dis* 1960; 2: 315–318.

57. Meier B et al. EHRA/EAPCI expert consensus statement on catheter-based left atrial appendage occlusion. *EuroIntervention* 2015; 10(9): 1109–1125.

58. Cruz-Gonzalez I et al. Thrombus formation after left atrial appendage exclusion using an Amplatzer cardiac plug device. *Catheter Cardiovasc Interv* 2011; 78(6): 970–973.

59. Viles-Gonzalez JF et al. The clinical impact of incomplete left atrial appendage closure with the Watchman Device in patients with atrial fibrillation: A PROTECT AF (Percutaneous Closure of the Left Atrial Appendage Versus Warfarin Therapy for Prevention of Stroke in Patients With Atrial Fibrillation) substudy. *J Am Coll Cardiol* 2012; 59(10): 923–929.

60. Guerios EE et al. Double device left atrial appendage closure. *EuroIntervention* 2015; 11(4): 470–476.

34

Trans-catheter aortic valve implantation

DIDIER TCHÉTCHÉ, JAVIER MOLINA MARTIN DE NICOLAS

34.1 Introduction

Aortic stenosis (AS) is the most frequent valvular heart disease in Western countries. A contemporary cohort analysis identified a prevalence constantly increasing with age and reaching up to 9.8% of the population over 80 years, the incidence rate being 4.9‰/year.[1] Due to the dismal prognosis of AS in symptomatic patients, surgery needs to be carried out in a timely manner. Surgical aortic valve replacement (SAVR) remains the gold standard in symptomatic AS patients. However, the Euro-Heart survey on valvular disease identified a need for alternative options in high or extreme-risk patients, one-third of the analysed patients not being offered SAVR because of their comorbidities.[2] Thus, trans-catheter aortic valve implantation (TAVI), first introduced in 2002, has emerged as a robust alternative to surgery in inoperable or high-risk patients.[3] To date, TAVI has been offered to more than 200,000 patients, across 65 countries worldwide and is being performed on a daily basis in numerous institutions. This field is in constant evolution in terms of indications, procedure refinements, device improvement and global comprehension of the outcomes. This chapter synthesises the key aspects of TAVI in contemporary practice.

34.2 Patient selection

In symptomatic AS patients, the final choice between SAVR and TAVI is based upon the estimated surgical risk. To make decision, a multidisciplinary 'Heart Team' including cardiologists, cardiac surgeons, anaesthesiologists and, ideally, geriatricians should be organised. Several risk scores are combined to assess the patient risk profile: The Logistic European System for Cardiac Operative Risk Evaluation (EuroSCORE), the Society of Thoracic Surgery (STS) score and the new EuroSCORE II. The European Society of Cardiology (ESC) recommends to consider TAVI when the Logistic EuroSCORE is ≥ 20% and/or the STS score is ≥ 10% (≥ 8% for ACC guidelines).[4,5] A not yet validated but realistic estimation of the patient high-risk profile is a EuroSCORE II over 7%.[6] Both the ESC and American College of Cardiology (ACC), apart from the risk profile, recommend a life expectancy greater than 1 year before considering TAVI.

Despite low surgical risk scores, several conditions, such as non-exhaustively, porcelain aorta, prior chest radiation, frailty, previous open chest surgery, right ventricle dysfunction, fixed pulmonary hypertension, chronic kidney disease, severe lung dysfunction, dementia, Alzheimer's disease, ParkinsonAlzheimerease stroke with persistent physical limitation, may favour TAVI over SAVR. The current ESC guidelines do not yet recommend TAVI for intermediate or low-risk patients but there is a worldwide trend to explore the outcome of TAVI in this population.

34.3 Access site selection

Two major TAVI techniques are regularly applied to get access to the aortic valve. The arterial retrograde approach integrates trans-femoral, subclavian/axillary, direct aortic and trans-carotid routes. The trans-apical approach is an antegrade ventricular route (Figure 34.1).

The trans-femoral approach is the most common technique in current practice, representing over 70% of the cases, trans-apical being approximately utilised in 20% of the patients whilst subclavian, direct aortic or less frequently, trans-carotid accesses represent about 10% of the procedures.[7,8] Trans-femoral is the most popular and less invasive access route, enabling fully percutaneous procedures under local anaesthesia and conscious sedation.[9] Thus, procedure time is reduced as are post-procedural pain and wound-related complications. The patients not being intubated, no intensive care unit is required after the procedure, early ambulation and shorter hospital stay are promoted. Finally, discharge from the hospital may occur earlier.[10] When trans-femoral access is not an option, because of small vessels, extreme tortuosity or calcification, an alternative access is proposed. The choice of the appropriate alternative access is based upon each individual heart team preference: apical, axillary, direct aortic or carotid access.

As coronary angiogram is routinely performed in the screening phase, the anatomy of the peripheral vasculature is usually roughly analysed at the same time (Figure 34.2). A specific and more detailed evaluation is obtained with three-dimensional contrast-enhanced multislice computed tomography (MSCT). This technique permits a better evaluation of the vessel disease (stenosis, plaque burden and distribution), vessels diameter and tortuosity as well as the amount and location of calcifications.[11] MSCT is the method of choice to assess suitability for trans-femoral TAVI. The main limitation of MSCT is the risk of contrast-induced nephropathy. Magnetic resonance imaging (MRI) is an alternative to MSCT for peripheral vasculature assessment. Its main limitation is the inability to analyse calcium burden.

MRI is also accurate in determining vessel size and tortuosity. Its only limitation is the inability to appreciate calcium burden.

34.4 Aortic root sizing

Besides confirmation of the degree of AS, trans-thoracic echocardiography (TTE) is key to assess left ventricular function and morphology, pulmonary pressures and concomitant valvular diseases. Two dimensional trans-oesophageal echocardiography (TEE) may be complementary in difficult cases but is not mandatory in contemporary practice. However, TTE or TEE is not sufficient to properly size the aortic root. These techniques tend to underestimate the true aortic annular size.

MSCT is the recommended method for sizing of the aortic root and the aortic valvular complex. The choice

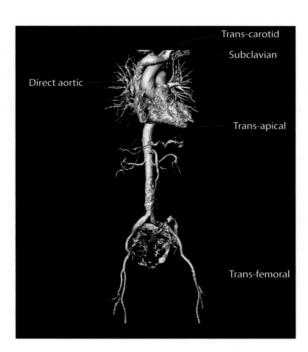

Figure 34.1 Access sites available for trans-catheter aortic valve implantation (TAVI).

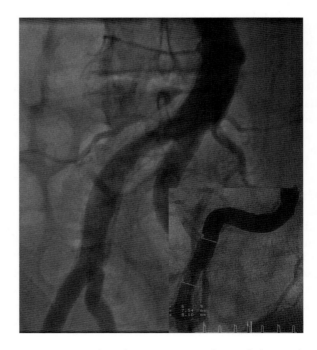

Figure 34.2 Peripheral angiogram performed during the screening for trans-femoral TAVI feasibility.

of the appropriate prosthesis type and size is based upon measurements made at the level of the aortic annulus but also the left ventricle outflow tract (typically 3–4 mm below the annulus), the sinuses of Valsalva, the sinotubular junction and the ascending aorta. The aortic root angulation (horizontal or not) combined with the degree, distribution and aspect of calcifications will be also best analysed with MSCT.

MSCT has to be electrocardiogram (ECG)-gated to dissociate systolic and diastolic phases. A multiplanar reconstruction integrating axial, sagittal and coronal planes is easily obtained with various dedicated softwares (Figure 34.3). As the annular dimension may vary between systole and diastole, sizing of the annulus is based on the maximum systolic area or perimeter. This is achieved by analysing the annulus in 5%–10% increments from 30% to 45% of the RR interval.[12] Schematically, area and perimeter-derived diameters will be identical in a circular anatomy; perimeter-derived diameter will be greater in elliptical configurations. Sizing with the area method will help in preventing annular rupture with balloon-expandable devices. For self-expanding and mechanically expanded devices, the perimeter-derived diameter will guide optimal sizing to prevent periprosthetic regurgitation.

Three-dimensional TEE is an efficient technique to determine annular dimensions. Analysis and sizing of the whole valvular complex and aortic root is, however, more precisely achieved with MSCT. All efforts should be made to obtain a good quality MSCT before TAVI, in every single patient. Proper hydration before and after dye injection is advocated to prevent contrast-induced nephropathy.

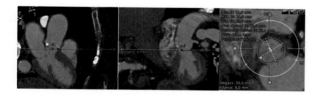

Figure 34.3 Multislice computed tomography (MSCT) multiplanar reconstruction and measurement of the aortic annulus obtained with a dedicated software.

34.5 TAVI devices

Various concepts of TAVI devices obtained Conformité européenne (CE) mark or are under investigation for CE-mark obtention (Figure 34.4). The TAVI devices most largely used across the globe are the Edwards Sapien™ (Edwards Lifesciences, Irvine, California) and the Medtronic CoreValve® (Medtronic, Minneapolis, Minnesota), latest iterations being, respectively, Sapien 3™ (S3) and Evolut R® (ER). This chapter focuses on principal second-generation TAVI devices utilised in contemporary TAVI practice.[13] The first-in-man procedure was performed with a balloon-expandable system in 2002, quickly followed by a case using a self-expanding prosthesis.[3,14]

34.5.1 Balloon-expandable technology

The Edwards Sapien family devices are the only balloon-expandable devices currently available. S3 consists of a cobalt-chromium stent mounted onto a balloon and housing a trileaflet bovine pericardial valve. It has a PTFE sleeve preventing perivalvular regurgitation. S3 is delivered via trans-femoral, trans-apical or direct aortic access routes. Trans-femoral procedures are performed with an ultra-low profile 14F to 16F expandable ESheath™.

34.5.2 Self-expanding technology

The Medtronic CoreValve and more recently ER are amongst the most popular self-expanding TAVI devices. ER consists of a nitinol stent frame, housing a supra-annular trileaflet porcine pericardial valve. It is a 14F equivalent system when delivered through trans-femoral access (In-Line Sheath™ and sheathless-like procedure) and 18F when utilised through axillary, direct aortic or trans-carotid approaches (outer sheath needed). ER is fully repositionable and retrievable up to 80% of its deployment.

The St. Jude Portico™ prosthesis (St. Jude Medical, Inc., St. Paul, Minnesota) combines a nitinol stent frame with open cell design and a trans-annular trileaflet bovine

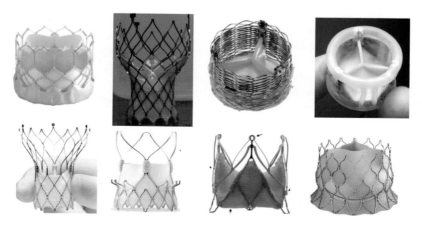

Figure 34.4 Various second generation TAVI devices with Conformité européenne (CE)-mark or under clinical investigation.

pericardial valve. It is 18F compatible, fully repositionable and retrievable up to 85% of its expansion.

The Edwards Centera™ THV (Edwards Lifesciences, Irvine, California), under clinical investigation, articulates a nitinol stent frame and a trans-annular trileaflet bovine pericardial valve. The frame has been conceived to avoid extensive protrusion within the ascending aorta. The delivery system combines a low-profile deflectable catheter and a detachable battery-powered motorised handle. It is compatible with the 14F Edwards E-Sheath™. The Centera is repositionable and recapturable up to 70% of its expansion.

The Acurate™ (Symetis SA, Ecublens, Switzerland) consists of a supra-annular trileaflet porcine tissue valve mounted within a nitinol stent frame. The upper edge of the stent frame contains three stabilisation arches to assure proper alignment with the ascending aorta. The Acurate is utilisable via trans-femoral (neo™) or trans-apical (TA™) approaches.

The JenaValve™ prosthesis (JenaValve Technology GmbH, Munich, Germany) is the only TAVI device with CE-mark for severe AS and/or regurgitation. It consists of a natural porcine aortic root fitted within an outer porcine pericardial patch and sewn onto a nitinol stent frame. Three feelers clip the prosthesis onto the native aortic valve leaflets. JenaValve is partially repositionable and retrievable. Trans-apical and trans-femoral delivery systems are available.

34.5.3 Non-balloon nor self-expanding technology

The Lotus™ valve system (Boston Scientific, Natick, Massachusetts) is made of a single nitinol wire braided and connected in the middle of the stent frame with a central radiopaque positioning marker. It is a trileaflet bovine pericardial valve and is surrounded in its inflow half by an outer polymeric sleeve, the Adaptive Seal™. The device is mechanically expanded and locked in its final configuration. It is fully repositionable and retrievable before final detachment of the coupling elements. Lotus has been used via trans-femoral and direct aortic accesses.

The Direct Flow™ Medical trans-catheter aortic valve (Direct Flow Medical, Santa Rosa, California) consists of a trileaflet bovine pericardial valve mounted over a tubular, non-metallic and inflatable structure covered with polyester fabric. An upper aortic ring is meant for positioning above the aortic leaflets and below the coronary ostia, and the lower ventricular ring below the aortic annulus. The system is fully repositionable and retrievable before final polymer exchange.

34.6 Outcomes from large registries and randomised trials

Results and outcomes may widely differ across registries and trials. Valve Academic Research Consortium (VARC) 1 and, recently updated to version 2, definitions aimed at harmonising analyses and outcomes evaluation.[15, 16]

34.6.1 Cardiovascular mortality

Mortality (all-cause and cardiovascular) is usually analysed in the peri-procedural period (within 72 hours), at 30 days and 1 year.

The randomised PARTNER trial cohort B established TAVI superiority over optimal medical management, including balloon valvuloplasty, in inoperable patients with consistency at 5 years medical follow-up.[17,18] There was an absolute 50% reduction in all-cause mortality, favouring TAVI at 1 year.

The PARTNER cohort A, randomised trial, compared TAVI, using a trans-femoral or trans-apical balloon-expandable device, to SAVR in 699 patients. Mortality rates were similar at 30 days (3.4% and 6.5%, $p = 0.07$), 1 year (24.3% and 26.8%) and up to 5 years (67.8% and 62.4%).[19]

The United States CoreValve High Risk Study randomly assigned 795 high-risk patients to TAVI using a self-expanding device or SAVR. All-cause mortality at 1 year was lower in the TAVI group: 14.2 versus 19.1%, $p = .04$ for superiority.[20] Two-year results were recently presented at 2015 ACC congress, confirming 1-year results.

The recently published TVT registry, collected contemporary data from 12,182 patients treated between November 2011 and June 2013. The 30-day mortality was 7.0%. At 1-year follow-up, overall mortality was 23.7%.[21]

34.6.2 Aortic regurgitation

Aortic regurgitation remains frequent post-TAVI, mainly due to perivalvular leakage (PVL). Intra-prosthetic central regurgitation is rarely seen in contemporary practice, particularly with second-generation TAVI devices. Moderate to severe PVL, reported on average about 10% with first generation TAVI devices, has been consistently associated with two- to threefold increase of short and long-term mortality across studies.[22,23] PVL is evaluated intra-operatively, within the first 48 hours, at 30 days and 1-year follow-up. Quantitative and semi-quantitative hemodynamic assessment of AR severity should be performed with Doppler echocardiography according to the current guidelines. PVR may originate from incomplete apposition of the prosthesis within the aortic annulus mainly due to severe calcific deposits, underestimation of the annulus diameter or a prosthesis malpositioning.

New generation TAVI devices with dedicated sealing cuffs and accurate positioning consistently decrease the rate of moderate-severe PVL below 5%.[24,25]

34.6.3 Need for a permanent pacemaker

The incidence of permanent pacemaker (PPM) implantation post-TAVI averages 17% in a recent meta-analysis.[26] Identified risk factors are male gender, baseline right bundle branch block, combination of first-degree atrioventricular block and left anterior hemiblock, the occurrence of intra-procedural atrioventricular block and deep implants. The need for PPM is higher with self-expanding devices than balloon-expandable ones.[8] Accurate positioning avoiding deep implants has been associated with a reduced need for pacemaker with a self-expanding system.[27] New generation TAVI devices, principally aiming at decreasing PVL rate, may not easily overcome the PPM issue. Improvement is needed. Need for a PPM seems associated with a decrease in left ventricle ejection fraction (LVEF) but no clear evidence of increased mortality has been reported.[28,29]

34.6.4 Vascular complications and bleeding

In the former era of large bore sheaths (18–24 Fr), major vascular complication rates ranged from 5% to 17%.[30] Vascular complications are associated with increased mortality, reduced quality of life and increased length of hospital stay. Small-vessel diameter, moderate to severe calcification and centre experience are the major risk factors for iliofemoral vascular complications. A sheath to femoral artery ratio greater than 1.05 seems associated with more frequent vascular complications.[31] Indeed, sheath size impacts the rates of vascular complications, thus several new-generation TAVI devices are available with improved 14F equivalent systems.[13,25,32]

Bleeding is classified into three categories according to its severity: minor, major and life threatening. Life-threatening and major bleedings are associated with increased overall and cardiovascular mortality rates at 30 days and 1 year.[33] The reported rates of life-threatening and major bleedings are around 13%–16% and 21%–32%, respectively. Most of bleedings originates from access site-related complications, particularly closure device failure. Two closure devices are regularly utilised to achieve haemostasis post–trans-femoral (TAVI: ProStar XL™ and Perclose ProGlide™ (Abbott Vascular, Illinois). The CONTROL multicentre study, compared vascular complications and bleeding in 944 matched patients, who underwent trans-femoral TAVI with either closure device. The primary composite primary endpoint of major vascular complications or in-hospital mortality was more frequent in the ProStar™ group (9.5% vs. 5.1%, $p = .016$), mainly driven by greater rates of major vascular complication (7.4% vs. 1.9%, $p < .001$). In-hospital mortality was equivalent in both groups (4.9% vs. 3.5%, $p = .2$).[34]

34.6.5 Stroke

The randomised PARTNER trial, cohort A, randomised trial was the first to raise concern about potential increase in stroke rates post-TAVI, as compared to SAVR. All stroke or transient ischemic attack (TIA) were 8.3% versus 4.3% at 1 year, $p = .04$. No difference was observed when only considering major stroke, without TIA (5.1% vs. 2.4%, $p = .07$).[35] Since that publication, the VARC 2 definition helped categorising cerebrovascular events by dissociating minor strokes and disabling strokes according to the modified Rankin score. The randomised US CoreValve High Risk Pivotal Study, confirmed the similarity of stroke rates between TAVI and SAVR at 1 year: 8.8% versus 10.6%, $p = .1$.[20]

A recent report from the France 2 registry, analysing 3191 patients, identified a stroke rate of 3.98% at 1 year: 55%

were major strokes, 14.5% minor strokes, and 30.5% TIA. Fifty percent of strokes were peri-procedural, occurring within 2 days and related to technical issues, for example, complex procedures with several TAVI devices needed. Moreover, patients with stroke more frequently had new-onset paroxysmal atrial fibrillation. Stroke was associated to increased 1-year mortality without any difference according to access site or device type.[36] Similarly, in the TVT registry, the incidence of stroke was 2.5% at 30 days and 4.1% at 1 year.[21] The role of cerebral embolic protection devices to peri-procedural strokes is under investigation.[37, 38] Optimal anticoagulant therapy may decrease stroke rates in the mid-term vulnerability period.

34.6.6 Acute kidney injury

According to VARC 2 definitions, three stages of acute kidney injury (AKI) are identified, according to the magnitude of increase in serum creatinine level and/or the need for renal replacement therapy. AKI may occur up to 7 days post-TAVI and affects survival. A recent series of 540 patients showed that baseline impaired renal function has a significant impact in 30 days and 1-year mortality (5.4% vs. 9%–25%; 15% vs. 32%–49%, respectively). A decrease in renal function greater than 15% was associated with increased mortality.[39] Another contemporary series of 942 patients also identified preoperative chronic kidney disease as a risk factor for 30 days and 1-year mortality post-TAVI.[40] Peri-procedural proper hydration and reduction in contrast dye volume are mandatory to prevent TAVI-related AKI.

34.6.7 Annular rupture

Annular rupture is a dreadful complication leading to death in most of the cases (Figure 34.5). It occurs in less than 1% of the procedures in contemporary practice, even with balloon-expandable devices.[24] Small and calcified annuli are more prone to rupturing. Accurate MSCT-guided sizing analysis of calcium distribution are key to avoid this complication. The emergent treatment of annular rupture is pericardial drainage

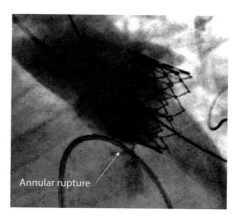

Figure 34.5 Annular rupture identified by angiography post-deployment of a balloon-expandable valve.

and open-chest surgery. Implantation of a second TAVI prosthesis has also been proposed as a bailout procedure.

34.6.8 TAVI in low- and intermediate-risk patients

Low and intermediate risks for open-chest surgery are well defined by the STS score, respectively, below 4% and between 4% and 8%, without any major organ failure or frailty item.

So far, TAVI has been proposed to high-risk or inoperable patients but data are coming about low- and intermediate-risk patients. The three centres BERMUDA registry was one the first to report a propensity matched analysis of 510 patients with STS score between 3% and 8%. There was no difference in 30-day and 1-year all-cause mortality.[41] The recently published OBSERVANT registry confirmed these findings in a larger cohort of 1300 matched patients.[42] At 1 year, all-cause death in SAVR and TAVI groups were respectively 13.6% and 13.8%, $p = .936$. Stroke rate was also equivalent in both groups.

The NOTION trial is the first trial randomising 280 patients with a mean STS score of, to TAVI or SAVR. At 1-year the composite endpoint of all-cause mortality, stroke or myocardial infarction was respectively observed in 11.3% and 15.7%, $p = .43$. Patients in the TAVI group had more pacemaker and PVL but greater effective orifice area. SAVR patients had more life-threatening bleeding, AKI II or III and new-onset atrial fibrillation.[43] More recently, two major randomized trials demonstrated the non-inferiority of TAVI, when compared to surgery, in intermediate risk patients. In the PARTNER IIA trial, at 2 years, the primary endpoint of death or disabling stroke occurred in 19.3% of the patients from the TAVI group vs. 21.1% in the surgery group (hazard ratio in the TAVI group, 0.89; 95% confidence interval [CI], 0.73 to 1.09; P = 0.25). In the transfemoral TAVI cohort, the frequency of the primary endpoint was lower than in the surgical group (hazard ratio, 0.79; 95% CI, 0.62 to 1.00; P = 0.05)[44]. The recently published SURTAVI trial confirmed TAVI non-inferiority at 2 years, when using a self-expanding platform.[45]

34.6.9 Durability of TAVI devices

Data on durability of TAVI prosthesis are scarce. Five years of analysis from the PARTNER cohort A trial, showed similar outcome between SAVR and TAVI patients. No early structural valve deterioration was observed in either group. Mean effective orifice area was larger and mean gradient was lower in the TAVI group and sustained at 5-years follow-up.[19]

34.7 Specific indications

34.7.1 Bicuspid disease

Bicuspid aortic valve (BAV) affects 0.5%–2% of the general population. Historically, it has been considered a contraindication to TAVR and an exclusion criterion in major TAVI trials, on the basis of associated risks of malpositioning, uneven and elliptical deployment or incomplete sealing,

leading to PVL and potentially accelerated leaflet degeneration.[46,47] Successful results, however, have been reported in selected patients with predominant AS.[48] Higher rates of misplacement, TAVI-in-TAVI procedures, PVL and aortic dissection are reported in recent registries.[47,49]

New generation TAVI devices, which offer better positioning and minor moderate-severe PVL could potentially achieve excellent procedural and clinical outcomes in this subset of patients.[13]

34.7.2 Pure aortic regurgitation

The main challenges of TAVI for pure aortic regurgitation are the lack of calcium to anchor the device and a more extensible aortic annulus. Thus, more oversizing of the prosthesis is advocated to allow for a stable fixation. Pure aortic regurgitation remains an off-label indication for most TAVI devices. This technique has been studied with the CoreValve™ in inoperable and high-risk patients within a multicentre registry. Procedural success rate was 74%. A second valve was required in 18.6% of the patients. Post-procedural aortic regurgitation was none-mild in 79.1% of the cases.[50]

Promising results have also been achieved with the JenaValve. It is currently the only CE-approved transcatheter device for aortic regurgitation and/or stenosis.

34.7.3 Surgical bioprosthetic valve failure

Valve-in-valve (VIV) is an alternative to redo surgery for high risk or inoperable patients experiencing failure of surgically implanted bioprostheses. The global VIV registry demonstrated the feasibility and safety of this procedure. Thirty-day mortality was 8.4%; survival at 1-year follow-up was 85.8%, without any difference between the CoreValve and the Sapien XT® valves, only CE-approved devices for VIV. This technique is challenging as it yields a higher risk of malposition and coronary obstruction in comparison with TAVI in native aortic valves. VIV in small failed bioprostheses (label size ≤21 mm) generates high residual gradients. In this scenario, the supra-annular function of the CoreValve and Evolut R family devices seems to be an asset (Figure 34.6). Stentless

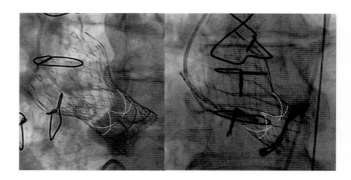

Figure 34.6 Supra-annular function of CoreValve and Evolut R prostheses in small internal diameter failed bioprostheses.

bioprostheses and those without any posts surrounding valve leaflets carry a higher risk of coronary obstruction, failed leaflets being more easily pushed towards the coronary ostiums during the procedure. A proper analysis of bioprostheses type and inner diameter, in parallel of the standard analysis of the aortic root is recommended in order to anticipate potential difficulties and appreciate the risk of coronary obstruction.

34.8 Conclusion

TAVI has demonstrated superiority over optimal medical therapy in inoperable patients and equivalence to surgery in high-risk patients. Larger studies will be necessary to confirm TAVI equivalence in low- to intermediate-risk patients. Increased operators' experience and technology refinements will help improve the outcome post-TAVI. In the future, we certainly observe more and more complex procedures, combined valvular and non-valvular transcatheter interventions in parallel of an enlargement of the indications for TAVI. The main remaining issue will certainly be the need for a permanent pacemaker. Finally, larger cohorts and longer follow-up are needed, probably in patients with greater life expectancy, to analyse prostheses' durability.

References

1. Eveborn GW et al. The evolving epidemiology of valvular aortic stenosis. The Tromso study. *Heart* 2013; 99: 396–400.
2. Iung B et al. A prospective survey of patients with valvular heart disease in Europe: The Euro Heart Survey on Valvular Heart Disease. *Eur Heart J* 2003; 24: 1231–43.
3. Cribier A et al. Percutaneous transcatheter implantation of an aortic valve prosthesis for calcific aortic stenosis: first human case description. *Circulation* 2002; 106: 3006–8.
4. Vahanian A et al. Guidelines on the management of valvular heart disease (version 2012): The Joint Task Force on the Management of Valvular Heart Disease of the European Society of Cardiology (ESC) and the European Association for Cardio-Thoracic Surgery (EACTS). *Eur J Cardiothorac Surg* 2012; 42: S1–44.
5. Nishimura RA et al. 2014 AHA/ACC guideline for the management of patients with valvular heart disease: A report of the American College of Cardiology/American Heart Association Task Force on Practice Guidelines. *J Thorac Cardiovasc Surg* 2014; 148: e1–132.
6. Arangalage et al. Agreement between the new EuroSCORE II, the Logistic EuroSCORE and the Society of Thoracic Surgeons score: Implications for transcatheter aortic valve implantation. *Arch Cardiovasc Dis* 2014; 107: 353–60.
7. Di Mario C et al. The 2011–12 pilot European Sentinel Registry of Transcatheter Aortic Valve Implantation: In-hospital results in 4,571 patients. *EuroIntervention* 2013; 8: 1362–71.
8. Gilard M et al. Registry of transcatheter aortic-valve implantation in high-risk patients. *N Engl J Med* 2012; 366: 1705–15.
9. Durand E et al. Transfemoral aortic valve replacement with the Edwards SAPIEN and Edwards SAPIEN XT prosthesis using exclusively local anesthesia and fluoroscopic guidance: Feasibility and 30-day outcomes. *JACC Cardiovasc Interv* 2012; 5: 461–7.
10. Stortecky S et al. Transcatheter aortic valve implantation: The transfemoral access route is the default access. *EuroIntervention* 2013; 9 Suppl: S14–8.
11. Toggweiler S et al. Management of vascular access in transcatheter aortic valve replacement: Part 1: basic anatomy, imaging, sheaths, wires, and access routes. *JACC Cardiovasc Interv* 2013; 6: 643–53.
12. Leipsic J et al. Multidetector computed tomography in transcatheter aortic valve implantation. *JACC Cardiovasc Imaging* 2011; 4: 416–29.
13. Tchetche D, and Van Mieghem NM. New-generation TAVI devices: Description and specifications. *EuroIntervention* 2014; 10 Suppl U: U90–100.
14. Grube E et al. First report on a human percutaneous transluminal implantation of a self-expanding valve prosthesis for interventional treatment of aortic valve stenosis. *Catheter Cardiovasc Interv* 2005; 66: 465–9.
15. Leon MB et al. Standardized endpoint definitions for transcatheter aortic valve implantation clinical trials: A consensus report from the Valve Academic Research Consortium. *Eur Heart J* 2011; 32: 205–17.
16. Kappetein AP et al. Updated standardized endpoint definitions for transcatheter aortic valve implantation: The Valve Academic Research Consortium-2 consensus document (VARC-2). *Eur J Cardiothorac Surg* 2012; 42: S45–60.
17. Leon MB et al. Transcatheter aortic-valve implantation for aortic stenosis in patients who cannot undergo surgery. *N Engl J Med* 2010; 363: 1597–607.
18. Kapadia SR et al. Long-term outcomes of inoperable patients with aortic stenosis randomly assigned to transcatheter aortic valve replacement or standard therapy. *Circulation* 2014; 130: 1483–92.
19. Mack MJ et al. 5-year outcomes of transcatheter aortic valve replacement or surgical aortic valve replacement for high surgical risk patients with aortic stenosis (PARTNER 1): A randomised controlled trial. *Lancet* 2015; 385: 2477–84.
20. Adams DH et al. Transcatheter aortic-valve replacement with a self-expanding prosthesis. *N Engl J Med* 2014; 370: 1790–8.
21. Holmes DR et al. Clinical outcomes at 1 year following transcatheter aortic valve replacement. *JAMA* 2015; 313: 1019–28.
22. Kodali S et al. Paravalvular regurgitation after transcatheter aortic valve replacement with the Edwards Sapien valve in the PARTNER trial: Characterizing patients and impact on outcomes. *Eur Heart J* 2015; 36: 449–56.
23. Athappan G et al. Incidence, predictors, and outcomes of aortic regurgitation after transcatheter aortic valve replacement: Meta-analysis and systematic review of literature. *J Am Coll Cardiol* 2013; 61: 1585–95.
24. Binder RK et al. Transcatheter aortic valve replacement with the SAPIEN 3: A new balloon-expandable transcatheter heart valve. *JACC Cardiovasc Interv* 2013; 6: 293–300.

25. Manoharan G et al. Treatment of symptomatic severe aortic stenosis with a novel resheathable supra-annular self-expanding transcatheter aortic valve system. *JACC Cardiovasc Interv* 2015; 8: 1359–67.

26. Siontis GC et al. Predictors of permanent pacemaker implantation in patients with severe aortic stenosis undergoing TAVR: A meta-analysis. *J Am Coll Cardiol* 2014; 64: 129–40.

27. Tchetche D et al. Update on the need for a permanent pacemaker after transcatheter aortic valve implantation using the CoreValve(R) Accutrak system. *EuroIntervention* 2012; 8: 556–62.

28. Urena M et al. Permanent pacemaker implantation after transcatheter aortic valve implantation: Impact on late clinical outcomes and left ventricular function. *Circulation* 2014; 129: 1233–43.

29. De Carlo M et al. Safety of a conservative strategy of permanent pacemaker implantation after transcatheter aortic CoreValve implantation. *Am Heart J* 2012; 163: 492–9.

30. Toggweiler S et al. Management of vascular access in transcatheter aortic valve replacement: Part 2: Vascular complications. *JACC Cardiovasc Interv* 2013; 6: 767–76.

31. Hayashida K et al. Transfemoral aortic valve implantation new criteria to predict vascular complications. *JACC Cardiovasc Interv* 2011; 4: 851–8.

32. Van Mieghem NM et al. Incidence, predictors, and implications of access site complications with transfemoral transcatheter aortic valve implantation. *Am J Cardiol* 2012; 110: 1361–7.

33. Tchetche D et al. Adverse impact of bleeding and transfusion on the outcome post-transcatheter aortic valve implantation: Insights from the Pooled-RotterdAm-Milano-Toulouse In Collaboration Plus (PRAGMATIC Plus) initiative. *Am Heart J* 2012; 164: 402–9.

34. Barbash IM et al. Comparison of vascular closure devices for access site closure after transfemoral aortic valve implantation. *Eur Heart J* 2015; 36: 3370–9.

35. Smith CR et al. Transcatheter versus surgical aortic-valve replacement in high-risk patients. *N Engl J Med* 2011; 364: 2187–98.

36. Tchetche D et al. Cerebrovascular events post-transcatheter aortic valve replacement in a large cohort of patients: A FRANCE-2 registry substudy. *JACC Cardiovasc Interv* 2014; 7: 1138–45.

37. Van Mieghem NM et al. Histopathology of embolic debris captured during transcatheter aortic valve replacement. *Circulation* 2013; 127: 2194–201.

38. Lansky AJ et al. A prospective randomized evaluation of the TriGuard HDH embolic DEFLECTion device during transcatheter aortic valve implantation: Results from the DEFLECT III trial. *Eur Heart J* 2015; 36: 2070–8.

39. Voigtlander L et al. Impact of kidney function on mortality after transcatheter valve implantation in patients with severe aortic valvular stenosis. *Int J Cardiol* 2015; 178: 275–81.

40. Dumonteil N et al. Impact of preoperative chronic kidney disease on short- and long-term outcomes after transcatheter aortic valve implantation: A Pooled-RotterdAm-Milano-Toulouse In Collaboration Plus (PRAGMATIC-Plus) initiative substudy. *Am Heart J* 2013; 165: 752–60.

41. Piazza N et al. A 3-center comparison of 1-year mortality outcomes between transcatheter aortic valve implantation and surgical aortic valve replacement on the basis of propensity score matching among intermediate-risk surgical patients. *JACC Cardiovasc Interv* 2013; 6: 443–51.

42. Tamburino C et al. 1-year outcomes after transfemoral transcatheter or surgical aortic valve replacement: Results from the Italian OBSERVANT study. *J Am Coll Cardiol* 2015; 66: 804–12.

43. Thyregod HG et al. Transcatheter Versus Surgical Aortic Valve Replacement in Patients With Severe Aortic Valve Stenosis: 1-Year Results From the All-Comers NOTION Randomized Clinical Trial. *J Am Coll Cardiol* 2015; 65: 2184–94.

44. Leon MB et al. Transcatheter or surgical aortic-valve replacement in intermediate-risk patients. *N Engl J Med* 2016;374: 1609–1620.

45. Reardon MJ et al. Surgical or transcatheter aortic-valve replacement in intermediate-risk patients. *N Engl J Med* 2017.

46. Rodriguez-Caulo EA et al. Transapical aortic valve implantation in bicuspid aortic valves: Must be an absolute contraindication? *Res Cardiovasc Med* 2012; 1: 37–9.

47. Mylotte D et al. Transcatheter aortic valve replacement in bicuspid aortic valve disease. *J Am Coll Cardiol* 2014; 64: 2330–9.

48. Yousef A et al. Performance of transcatheter aortic valve implantation in patients with bicuspid aortic valve: Systematic review. *Int J Cardiol* 2014; 176: 562–4.

49. Bauer T et al. Comparison of the effectiveness of transcatheter aortic valve implantation in patients with stenotic bicuspid versus tricuspid aortic valves (from the German TAVI Registry). *Am J Cardiol* 2014; 113: 518–21.

50. Roy DA et al. Transcatheter aortic valve implantation for pure severe native aortic valve regurgitation. *J Am Coll Cardiol* 2013; 61: 1577–84.

Coronary intervention in patients with aortic valve disease

ADEEL SHAHZAD, KAMRAN BAIG

35.1 Background

35.1.1 Incidence and diagnosis

The prevalence of coronary artery disease (CAD) varies between 40% and 75% in patents with aortic stenosis (AS)[1–5] and increases with age.[5,6] Patients with CAD are known to have a higher risk profile with increased frequency of diabetes, hypercholesterolemia, left ventricular (LV) dysfunction, peripheral vascular disease, ascending aorta calcification, higher Canadian Cardiovascular Society (CCS) class and longer hospital admissions.[5,7,8] Within this group, patients with significant CAD (previous percutaneous coronary intervention [PCI], previous coronary artery bypass grafting [CABG], myocardial infarction [MI] or ≥70% stenosis severity of a major epicardial coronary artery) have even higher procedural risks.[9,10]

Angina is a common indicator of CAD in the general population. In elderly patients (>70 years of age), angina is a strong determinant of CAD.[11] In AS, angina could be a manifestation of increased myocardial oxygen demand due to LV wall thickening, cavity dilatation or increased wall stress causing with sub-endocardial ischaemia. Clinically, it may be difficult to distinguish the two conditions as both may present with similar symptoms. When both conditions coexist, the clinical overlap may present a challenge in establishing the predominant condition causing the symptoms. In general, as angina is a poor marker of CAD in patients with AS, coronary angiography is recommended in symptomatic patients before intervening on the aortic valve.[12]

35.1.2 Treatment of CAD and AS

In patients with severe AS, CAD increases risks associated with surgical aortic valve replacement (SAVR).[13,14] Current guidelines recommend CABG for severe CAD.[15] aortic valve replacement (AVR) combined with concomitant CABG is associated with a higher operative mortality than AVR alone performed in patients without CAD.[14,16] The combined approach is still considered the main treatment strategy for patients with severe AS and CAD as it has shown to improve outcomes relative to AVR alone.[17,18]

35.2 Impact of CAD on trans-catheter aortic valve implantation outcomes

Significant CAD may be related to a higher risk of ischaemia associated with trans-catheter aortic valve implantation (TAVI). During TAVI, rapid pacing is performed at the time of balloon inflation and valve deployment. This may result in a significant drop in systemic blood pressure, increasing the risk of peri-procedural ischaemia and haemodynamic compromise in these patients. Other factors that could exacerbate haemodynamic compromise in this cohort are aortic regurgitation caused by attempts at valve prosthesis positioning, and mitral regurgitation induced during the procedure. The consequence of coronary occlusion or embolism during the TAVI procedure may be significantly worse, especially in patients with significant multi-vessel disease; and, other procedural complications such as cardiac rhythm disturbance and hypotension due to major bleeding may also be less well haemodynamically tolerated leading to poorer outcomes.

The influence of significant CAD on the outcomes of patients who underwent TAVI has been evaluated in several registries providing conflicting results (Table 35.1 and Figure 35.1). Currently, there are no prospective randomised studies addressing this question. The decision in all registries to date of whether to re-vascularise is commonly based on the consensus of the heart team.

35.2.1 Data showing no difference in outcomes in the presence of CAD

Recently published UK TAVI registry data with nearly 2600 patients from 31 centres examined the outcome of patients with and without CAD undergoing TAVI.[5] Overall 30 day mortality was found to be 6.3% and increased to 18.6% at 1 year and 28% at 4 years. Following multivariate analysis, the presence of CAD did not show any impact on survival at either 30 days or in the longer term.

Table 35.1 Summary of studies of coronary artery disease (CAD) around trans-catheter aortic valve implantation (TAVI) treatment.

	Presence of CAD	No. of points	EF (%)	Logistic EuroSCORE	30-day mortality (%)	1 year+ mortality (%)
Data showing no difference in outcomes in the presence of CAD						
Ussia	CAD	251	48	35	6	14
2007–2009	No CAD	408	53	22	5.9	16
					(p = .61)	(p = .33)
Masson	CAD	104	60	29	14–17	11–35
2005–2007	No CAD	32	overall	overall	6	19
					(p = .56)	(p = .63)
Gautier	CAD	83	45	31	10	24
2006–2009	No CAD	62	53	24	15	29
					(p = .37)	(p = .37)
Data showing worse outcomes in the presence of CAD						
Dewey	CAD	84	47	39	13	36
2005–2008	No CAD	87	53	29	1	18
					(p = .002)	(p = .01)
Abdel-Wahab	CAD	859	51	23	8.4	NA
2009–2010	No CAD	523	56	16	5.3	
					(p = .04)	

EF, ejection fraction; EuroSCORE, European System for Cardiac Operative Risk Evaluation; NA, not applicable.

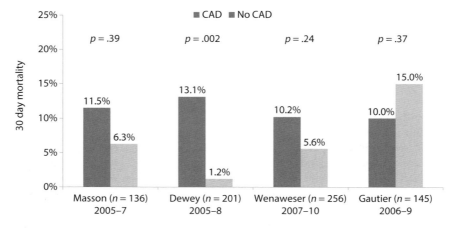

Figure 35.1 Impact of coronary disease on trans-catheter aortic valve implantation (TAVI) outcome.

Ussia et al. looked at 663 patients from 14 institutions across Italy to evaluate the clinical outcome of patients with CAD undergoing TAVI.[10] Patients with CAD had similar major adverse cardiac events (MACE) at 1 year in comparison to those who did not have CAD (15.7% vs. 18.3%; $p = .353$). The 1 year mortality was 14.5% and 15.9% in CAD group and no-CAD group, respectively ($p = .331$). Data from SOURCE registry looking at trans-apical (TA) TAVI procedures also showed no differences in 30 day mortality between patients that had CAD or not (11.8% vs. 8.3%, respectively; $p = .21$).[19]

Gautier et al. looked at 145 high-risk patients that underwent TAVI and found no significant differences in terms of 30 day mortality in patients with or without CAD (10% vs. 15%; $p = .37$) or at 1 year (23.6% vs. 29.4%; $p = .28$).[8]

35.2.2 Data showing worse outcomes in the presence of CAD

Dewey et al. studied 201 high-risk patients from two international feasibility studies and demonstrated that coexisting CAD had a negative impact on procedural outcomes and long-term survival in patients undergoing TAVI.[9] Overall mortality after TAVI was significantly higher amongst the CAD group (35.7% vs. 18.4%, $p = .01$). Abdel-Wahab et al. reviewed 1382 patients from a large German registry[20] and found that patients with CAD undergoing TAVI had significantly higher in-hospital mortality (10.0% vs. 5.5%; $p < .01$) compared with patients without CAD. The need of additional PCI was more common in patients with CAD (5.5% vs. 2.7%; $p < .05$). Incidences of MI, cerebrovascular accident (CVA), advanced conduction block and vascular complications were similar. Overall, procedural success was similar (97.1% vs. 97.7%; $p =$ not significant [ns]).

35.2.3 Using risk stratification to assess the impact of CAD

In patients undergoing TAVI, using a physiological scoring system to define the severity of CAD may be clinically useful and aid decision-making. This would define the complexity and extent of CAD and would also take into account the area of myocardium at risk. Hence in patients with CAD undergoing TAVI, Stefanini et al. used the SYNTAX score to stratify patients into low (0–22) and high (>22) SYNTAX score groups.[7] The results demonstrated that patients with high SYNTAX score had worse prognosis at 1 year follow-up compared with patients with low score. However, contrary to the above, Masson et al. used the Duke Myocardial Jeopardy Score (DMJS) to stratify the significance of CAD pre-TAVI. The presence of CAD was not associated with an increased risk of adverse events at 30 days regardless of the extent of CAD.[21] Wenaweser et al. assessed 256 patients from Bern TAVI registry for the impact of CAD on outcomes. They also used DMJS score for stratification of the myocardium at risk.[22] A stratified analysis of outcomes according to presence of CAD showed no difference during long-term follow-up (log rank $p = .16$).

The above studies highlight the variation in the results even following stratification of the extent of CAD. These discrepancies may be related to differences in patient populations, definition of CAD and presence of PCI before TAVI.

35.3 Treatment strategies for patients with severe AS and CAD

There are three principal non-conservative treatment strategies for the treatment of combined AS and CAD.

35.3.1 Conventional SAVR and CABG

Current guidelines recommend that patients undergoing SAVR should be fully re-vascularised in the presence of CAD as the outcomes are worse if this is left untreated.[12,23] However, combining CABG and SAVR is associated with higher postoperative mortality in comparison to SAVR alone.[24,25] Data from the New York Cardiac Surgery Reporting System showed that addition of CABG to SAVR increased perioperative mortality from 4.4% vs. 8.9%.[26] However, recently published data from a subgroup analysis of the PARTNER 2 trial showed that the addition of coronary re-vascularisation with CABG (performed in 14.5% of patients in the SAVR group) had no significant impact on the outcomes of mortality or CVA.[27]

35.3.2 Hybrid PCI and SAVR

Staged PCI combined with SAVR or minimally invasive valve surgery (MI-AVR) may offer an alternative to CABG with concurrent valve surgery.[28,29] In high-risk patients, combining two lower risk strategies, PCI (1% mortality in the elective settings) with either SAVR or MI-AVR approaches (0.7%–2% mortality range)[30] could reduce the overall operative risk.[31] This may potentially lower the incidence of MACE and renal injury in comparison to the conventional treatment.[28] Byrne et al. compared 26 patients who underwent PCI followed by minimally invasive or traditional SAVR. Mortality rate in the AVR group was 3.8% in comparison to the Society of Thoracic Surgeons (STS)-predicted mortality of 22%.[29] Brinster et al. studied 18 patients who underwent PCI either the same day or the evening prior to MI-AVR.[32] There was only one early post-operative death and no late mortality was observed. Santana et al. looked at 65 consecutive patients who underwent planned PCI followed by aortic or mitral valve surgery within 60 days and compared this cohort with 52 matched controls that underwent simultaneous CABG and conventional valve surgery.[28] The combined endpoint of 30 day death, renal failure or stroke occurred in 1 (1.5%) of the PCI group compared with 15 (28.8%) of the control group ($p = .001$).

The timing of PCI and the duration and risk of antiplatelet therapy remains unclear as no robust data are available in this regard. The use of dual anti-platelet therapy nevertheless increases the bleeding risk associated with SAVR and is potentially related with the timing of PCI.[28,29,32]

35.3.3 PCI and TAVI

The data regarding the management of concomitant significant CAD in patients undergoing TAVI are heterogeneous and controversial (Table 35.1). Data are available only in a high-risk population cohort and is limited to observational studies and registries. No meaningful data are available in the intermediate or low-risk cohort. However, many experienced TAVI cardiologists including ourselves favour a selective treatment strategy (Figure 35.2), treating CAD in the elderly and high-risk cohort on an either high perceived myocardial jeopardy basis (left main stem/proximal LAD lesion, critical lesion perfusing significant territory, recent acute coronary syndrome, evidence of major myocardial ischaemia, severe ischaemic LV impairment), or only on an anginal symptom led basis post TAVI. Additionally, a PCI treatment with staged procedures for those patients with complex multi-vessel CAD may reduce the procedural risks associated with TAVI and multi-vessel PCI.

35.4 Impact of PCI on TAVI outcomes

In patients with severe CAD undergoing TAVI, the optimal timing of re-vascularisation remains unclear (Table 35.2). Staged PCI before TAVI is the most frequently used strategy in current practice.

35.4.1 PCI before TAVI

Performing PCI before TAVI has the potential benefit of reduction in the risk of ischaemia or haemodynamic instability during the TAVI procedure itself. There is also less risk of contrast nephropathy as the contrast volume used is spread over two different procedural time points. However, patients undergoing staged PCI before TAVI are loaded with dual antiplatelet therapy (DAPT) that may increase the risk of bleeding complications during and after the TAVI procedure.

Most of the data in this category has shown comparable results between patients undergoing PCI before TAVI, versus TAVI alone. In the recently published UK TAVI registry data, hybrid PCI was defined as elective PCI as part of, or in the 'lead-up' to TAVI.[5] This was performed in 172 (14.7%) patients. Almost all of these (except three patients) had PCI performed before the TAVI procedure. The interval between hybrid PCI and TAVI varied widely, but in the majority of cases was performed within 3 months of valve intervention (107 patients, 62.2%). Hybrid PCI was not associated with any significant differences in in-hospital outcomes.[5]

In the PARTNER 2 trial, PCI was performed in 3.9% of patients in the TAVI group. In a subgroup analysis, no significant differences in mortality or CVA were observed between the patients that had PCI versus the rest of the cohort.[27]

Abdel-Wahab et al. studied a total of 125 patients, 55 of which received PCI before TAVI and 70 patients were treated with isolated TAVI. Thirty day all-cause mortality was 2% versus 6% for patients treated with PCI plus TAVI versus isolated TAVI, respectively ($p = .27$).[33] Van Meighem et al. looked at 263 consecutive patients that underwent TAVI. The study results showed that re-vascularisation status did not affect clinical endpoints. One year mortality for patients with and without complete re-vascularisation was 79.9% versus 77.4% ($p = .85$), respectively.[34]

Rosendael et al. assessed the timing of PCI before TAVI. The main finding of the study with 90 patients was that shortly (<30 days) or remotely (≥30 days) staged PCI before TAVI resulted in comparable TAVI outcomes with the exception of overall vascular injury (particularly minor injuries) that were more frequently observed in patients treated with staged PCI performed <30 days before TAVI.[35] The in-hospital mortality rates were comparable between the two groups (4% for <30 days and 8% for >30 days; $p = .339$).

Gasparetto et al. looked at the Padova University REVALVing Experience (PUREVALVE) Registry prospectively with

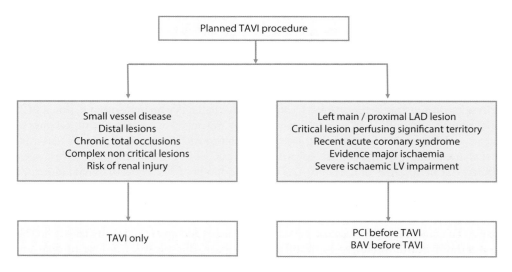

Figure 35.2 Selective coronary artery disease (CAD) treatment strategy with TAVI in high-risk patients.

Table 35.2 Summary of studies of timing of PCI treatment of CAD around TAVI treatment

	No. of pts	Reasoning for PCI	Timing (days)	DAPT	30-day mortality (%)	1 year+ mortality (%)	Conclusion
PCI prior to TAVI							
Gasparetto	CAD 113 No CAD 78	Symptom or Investigation for ischaemia	Median 27 Pre-TAVI	3 m BMS 12 m DES	4.2% No group differences	14.8% No group differences	Selective strategy safe No outcome differences
Wendt	SAVR/CABG 184 TAVI/PCI 59	MDT	82 ± 93 Pre-TAVI	NA	12.5 11.5	'Similar'	Both treatment options Similar outcomes
Abdel-Wahab	PCI + TAVI 55 Isolated TAVI 70	All significant lesions with >50% stenoses	Median 10	NA	2 6	8.1 6.1	Appears feasible and safe
PCI concomitant with TAVI							
Conradi	28 Pre-TAVI 7 with TAVI	NA	14 Zero	300 mg stat only	7.1 7.1	NA	Small numbers Feasible
Wenaweser	23 Pre-TAVI 36 with TAVI 197 no PCI	Syntax score No CTO or distal vessels	34 ± 26 Zero NA	23 16	5.6 10.2 (p = .24)	'No difference'	Feasible Similar outcomes
PCI after TAVI							
Pasic	373 TA-TAVI only 46 PCI	LMS, proximal LAD only	Immediately Post–TA-TAVI	6 m	NA 4.3	NA 13	Feasible

BMS, bare-metal stent; DES, drug-eluting stents; PCI, percutaneous coronary intervention; DAPT, dual antiplatelet therapy; CAD, coronary artery disease; CTO, chronic total occlusion; NA, not applicable.

191 consecutive patients. CAD was present in 113 (59.2%) and PCI was performed before TAVI in 39 (20.4%) patients. There was no significant difference in 30-day mortality between patients with or without CAD (5.7% vs. 2.9%, p = .32).[36] No data are available specifically looking at the cohort that underwent PCI. Wendt et al. again assessed patients that underwent PCI (n = 59) before TAVI (within 12 months) versus patients that had SAVR plus CABG (n = 184) and showed comparable results for in-hospital mortality between the two groups.[37]

Goel et al. also showed that PCI before TAVI was safe in most patients. However, patients with severe AS and reduced left ventricular ejection fraction (≤30%) or high STS score (≥10%) had a significantly increased risk of all-cause mortality 30 days after PCI.[38] Stefanini et al. reported that almost 50% of patients with significant CAD underwent PCI before TAVI. Those patients with incomplete re-vascularisation, as defined by a higher residual SYNTAX score, had significantly higher MACE (cardiovascular death, CVA or MI) rates at 1 year in comparison

to patients with low residual SYNTAX score (26.3% vs. 16.5%; p = .043).[7]

35.4.2 PCI with TAVI

A combined PCI and TAVI set of procedures may be preferred in some patients as both procedures share the same arterial access potentially reducing the risks of vascular injury and bleeding complications. Other benefits could include patient convenience and cost effectiveness.

Conradi et al. compared 21 patients who underwent staged PCI before TAVI with seven patients who underwent combined PCI and TAVI.[39] Overall in-hospital and 30-day mortality was identical between the two groups at 7.1%. Patients who underwent PCI combined with TAVI received a higher amount of contrast volume compared with those who underwent staged PCI (292.3 ± 117.5 vs. 171.9 ± 68.4 mL; p = .006). In addition, two patients of the combined PCI and TAVI group developed acute renal impairment following the procedure. Wenaweser et al. compared the outcomes of

167 patients who underwent isolated TAVI with 36 and 23 patients who were treated with staged and combined PCI, respectively.[22] No significant differences were observed in terms of 30 day all-cause mortality (5.6% vs. 11.1% and 8.7%, respectively; p = .43) or the VARC-combined safety end point (31.0% vs. 22.2% and 26.1%, respectively; p = .54). In the staged PCI cohort, the mean duration between PCI and TAVI was 34 days.

Only three patients from the UK TAVI registry data underwent PCI concomitantly with TAVI in the hybrid PCI group (n = 172)[5] highlighting the fact that this option is rarely employed in the current clinical practice in the United Kingdom.

35.4.3 PCI after TAVI

The strategy of performing PCI following valve implantation is even less established. The patients with CAD who undergo TAVI without PCI uncommonly require coronary intervention once valve implantation has been performed. This could be a reflection of symptom relief following the TAVI procedure, and the relatively reduced physical mobility of the usually elderly patient cohort that currently receive TAVI treatment. Theoretically, technical challenges associated with this approach exist, such as interference of the prosthetic valve struts with coronary cannulation or the potential dislodgement of the prosthetic valve with catheter manipulation; although in reality these are likely seldom events in experienced operators' hands.

In the UK TAVI registry data,[5] PCI after TAVI was performed only in 18 patients (1.5%). The indication for subsequent intervention was variable with six cases for stable symptoms and 11 for acute coronary syndromes. Previously, Pasic et al. studied 419 patients that underwent TA TAVI with single-stage PCI performed immediately after TAVI in 46 patients (11%).[40] Only the most significant coronary lesion or lesions were treated with achievement of 100% technical success. The 30 day mortality rate in the PCI and TAVI group was 4.3%.

35.5 Workflow and procedural efficiency

As TAVI treatments have evolved, and procedural refinements occurred, many high-volume centres look to optimise procedural workflow and efficiency. Inevitably, cost control is a pressing factor in all centres also.

There are no data that specifically address procedural or cost efficiency of either separate (but related) PCI and TAVI procedures, or where they are combined. It would appear clearly that the combined procedure would provide some economy of resource utilisation and some centres this maybe a factor in planning treatment logistics.

At the current time, it seems appropriate to continue to allow optimal clinical treatment planning to guide this decision-making although in many centres the final logistic planning will revolve around institutional and operator preferences.

35.6 Choice of valve prosthesis and coronary stent

Currently, several aortic valve design technologies are in clinical usage for TAVI treatments. No data currently exist to comprehensively guide whether any one valve prosthesis design is superior, or indeed whether any one type of coronary stent platform (principally bare-metal or drug eluting) is a more optimal choice, when considering combined therapies with TAVI and PCI.

Similarly, whether a balloon aortic valvuloplasty pre-treatment is performed prior to TAVI prosthesis deployment, particularly in the setting of impaired LV function (in the attempt to allow LV function improvement prior to PCI) remains at operator discretion, and there is currently no randomised controlled data to guide whether this treatment option has any impact on the final outcome.

35.7 Upcoming trials

The ongoing ACTIVATION (PCI prior to TAVI) trial is a randomised, controlled open-label trial of 310 patients randomised to treatment of significant CAD by PCI (test arm) or no PCI (control arm).[41] The trial is recruiting patients in the United Kingdom, France and Germany and will help define the optimum re-vascularisation strategy in this regard. The Surgical Replacement and Trans-catheter Aortic Valve Implantation (SURTAVI) trial is an ongoing large 2500 patient randomised controlled trial designed to evaluate the safety and efficacy of the Medtronic CoreValve System in the intermediate risk patients,[42] and includes patients with severe AS and significant CAD. These trials may also shed some light on the optimal antiplatelet regimen and the timing of PCI in relation to TAVI.

35.8 Conclusion

Current evidence on the impact of CAD on TAVI outcomes and for the management strategy of CAD in AS high-risk patients gives no clear guidance for optimum treatment. Data are only available in the form of registries and non-randomised studies. The lack of data and the rapidly expanding technology around TAVI has led to a large variability in clinical practice in the management of significant CAD for patients undergoing TAVI, as experienced centres and operators refine their practice and efficiency. Hence it cannot currently be said that a single optimum treatment strategy exists, and no international guidelines are currently available in this respect.

There is no compelling evidence that addition of re-vascularisation is superior to TAVI alone. Based on the evidence at hand, many operators and indeed our current practice is to employ a selective treatment strategy, which probably results in a pragmatic and the best treatment option in this setting (Figure 35.2).

When PCI is deemed necessary or appropriate, the optimal timing to proceed with coronary re-vascularisation is probably before the TAVI procedure itself. This could be a single-stage or multistage procedure depending on the operator or institutional preference and resources.

It must be recognised that these suggestions apply to the elderly cohort of high-risk patients where TAVI is currently indicated, where the limited data available do not necessarily translate into improved (CAD) survival prognosis, and hence our recommendation is that CAD treatment around TAVI treatment is symptom lead, rather than a routine re-vascularisation in all patients.

No meaningful data are available for intermediate or low-risk patients, where clearly consideration of long-term prognosis and survival from coronary disease alone becomes a more important consideration.

In the contrary, the data do, however, indicate that AS maybe safely treated with TAVI in the presence of varying degrees of CAD, and hence unlike treatment with SAVR, in the high-risk cohort complete coronary artery re-vascularisation does not appear to be mandatory at the time of TAVI; in intermediate and low-risk cohorts, this decision remains untested, and individual clinician judgement will remain although it does seem appropriate that younger patients treated with TAVI are more carefully considered for coronary re-vascularisation also.

Whether even high-risk patients with significant CAD and AS are better treated with conventional SAVR and CABG rather than TAVI and PCI, remains unknown, but this may be preferable providing they are reasonable surgical candidates.

Future studies should also address outcomes related to the use of antiplatelet therapy around the time of PCI, in relation to subsequent treatments with TAVI or SAVR.

References

1. Stewart BF et al. Clinical factors associated with calcific aortic valve disease. Cardiovascular Health Study. *J Am Coll Cardiol* 1997; 29(3): 630.
2. Moat NE et al. Long-term outcomes after transcatheter aortic valve implantation in high-risk patients with severe aortic stenosis: The UK TAVI (United Kingdom Transcatheter Aortic Valve Implantation) Registry. *J Am Coll Cardiol* 2011; 58(20): 2130–38.
3. Thomas M et al. Thirty-day results of the SAPIEN aortic Bioprosthesis European Outcome (SOURCE) Registry: A European registry of transcatheter aortic valve implantation using the Edwards SAPIEN valve. *Circulation* 2010; 122(1): 62–9.
4. Smith CR et al. Transcatheter versus Surgical Aortic-Valve Replacement in High-Risk Patients. *N Engl J Med* 2011; 364(23): 2187–98.
5. Snow TM et al. Management of concomitant coronary artery disease in patients undergoing transcatheter aortic valve implantation: The United Kingdom TAVI Registry. *Int J Cardiol* 2015; 199: 253–60.
6. Lombard JT, and Selzer A. Valvular aortic stenosis. A clinical and hemodynamic profile of patients. *Ann Intern Med* 1987; 106(2): 292–8.
7. Stefanini GG et al. Coronary artery disease severity and aortic stenosis: Clinical outcomes according to SYNTAX score in patients undergoing transcatheter aortic valve implantation. *Eur Heart J* 2014; 35(37): 2530–40.
8. Gautier M et al. Impact of coronary artery disease on indications for transcatheter aortic valve implantation and on procedural outcomes. *EuroIntervention* 2011; 7(5): 549–55.
9. Dewey TM et al. Effect of Concomitant coronary artery disease on procedural and late outcomes of transcatheter aortic valve implantation. *Ann Thor Surg* 2010; 89(3): 758–67.
10. Ussia GP et al. Impact of coronary artery disease in elderly patients undergoing transcatheter aortic valve implantation: Insight from the Italian CoreValve Registry. *Int J Cardiol* 2013; 167(3): 943–50.
11. Dangas G et al. Angina pectoris in severe aortic stenosis. *Cardiology* 1999; 92(1): 1.
12. Nishimura RA et al. 2014 AHA/ACC guideline for the management of patients with valvular heart disease. A report of the American College of Cardiology/American Heart Association Task Force on Practice Guidelines. *J Am Coll Cardiol* 2014; 63(22):e57–185.
13. Aranki SF et al. Aortic valve replacement in the elderly. Effect of gender and coronary artery disease on operative mortality. *Circulation* 1993; 88(5 Pt 2): I117.
14. Craver JM et al. Predictors of mortality, complications, and length of stay in aortic valve replacement for aortic stenosis. *Circulation* 1988; 78(3 Pt 2):185–90.
15. Bonow RO et al. ACC/AHA 2006 guidelines for the management of patients with valvular heart disease: A report of the American College of Cardiology/American Heart Association Task Force on Practice Guidelines (writing committee to revise the 1998 Guidelines for the Management of Patients With Valvular Heart Disease): Developed in collaboration with the Society of Cardiovascular Anesthesiologists: Endorsed by the Society for Cardiovascular Angiography and Interventions and the Society of Thoracic Surgeons. *Circulation* 2006; 114(5): e84.
16. Roques F et al. The logistic EuroSCORE. *Eur Heart J* 2003; 24(9): 881.
17. Lytle BW et al. Aortic valve replacement and coronary bypass grafting for patients with aortic stenosis and coronary artery disease: Early and late results. *Eur Heart J* 1988; 9(Suppl E): 143.
18. Lund O et al. The influence of coronary artery disease and bypass grafting on early and late survival after valve replacement for aortic stenosis. *J Thorac Cardiovasc Surg* 1990; 100(3): 327–37.
19. Wendler O et al. Trans-apical aortic valve implantation: Univariate and multivariate analyses of the early results from the SOURCE registry. *Eur J Cardiothorac Surg* 2010; 38(2): 119–27.
20. Abdel-Wahab M et al. Transcatheter aortic valve implantation in patients with and without concomitant coronary artery disease: Comparison of characteristics and early outcome in the German multicenter TAVI registry. *Clin Res Cardiol* 2012; 101(12): 973–81.
21. Masson Jb et al. Impact of coronary artery disease on outcomes after transcatheter aortic valve implantation. *Catheter Cardiovasc Interv* 2010; 76(2): 165–73.

22. Wenaweser P et al. Impact of coronary artery disease and percutaneous coronary intervention on outcomes in patients with severe aortic stenosis undergoing transcatheter aortic valve implantation. *EuroIntervention* 2011; 7(5): 541–8.

23. Vahanian A et al. Guidelines on the management of valvular heart disease (version 2012): The Joint Task Force on the Management of Valvular Heart Disease of the European Society of Cardiology (ESC) and the European Association for Cardio-Thoracic Surgery (EACTS). *Eur J Cardiothoracic Surg* 2012; 42(4): S1.

24. Tjang YS et al. Predictors of mortality after aortic valve replacement. *Eur J Cardiothorac Surg* 2007; 32(3): 469–74.

25. Beach JM et al. Coronary artery disease and outcomes of aortic valve replacement for severe aortic stenosis. *J Am Coll Cardiol* 2013; 61(8): 837–48.

26. Hannan EL et al. Risk index for predicting in-hospital mortality for cardiac valve surgery. *Ann Thorac Surg* 2007; 83(3): 921–9.

27. Leon MB et al. Transcatheter or surgical aortic-valve replacement in intermediate-risk patients. *N Engl J Med* 2016; 374(17): 1609–20.

28. Santana O et al. Staged percutaneous coronary intervention and minimally invasive valve surgery: Results of a hybrid approach to concomitant coronary and valvular disease. *J Thorac Cardiovasc Surg* 2012; 144(3): 634–9.

29. Byrne JG et al. Hybrid cardiovascular procedures. *JACC* 2008; 1(5): 459–68.

30. Soltesz EG, and Cohn LH. Minimally invasive valve surgery. *Cardiol Rev* 2007; 15(3): 109.

31. Byrne JG et al. Staged initial percutaneous coronary intervention followed by valve surgery ('hybrid approach') for patients with complex coronary and valve disease. *J Am Coll Cardiol* 2005; 45(1): 14–8.

32. Brinster DR et al. Effectiveness of same day percutaneous coronary intervention followed by minimally invasive aortic valve replacement for aortic stenosis and moderate coronary disease ('Hybrid Approach'). *Am J Cardiol* 2006; 98(11): 1501–3.

33. Abdel-Wahab M et al. Comparison of outcomes in patients having isolated transcatheter aortic valve implantation versus combined with preprocedural percutaneous coronary intervention. *Am J Cardiol* 2011; 109(4), 581–6.

34. Van Mieghem NM et al. Complete revascularization is not a prerequisite for success in current transcatheter aortic valve implantation practice. *JACC* 2013; 6(8): 867–75.

35. van Rosendael PJ et al. Timing of staged percutaneous coronary intervention before transcatheter aortic valve implantation. *Am J Cardiol* 2015; 115(12): 1726–32.

36. Gasparetto V et al. Safety and effectiveness of a selective strategy for coronary artery revascularization before transcatheter aortic valve implantation. *Catheter Cardiovasc Interv* 2013; 81(2): 376–83.

37. Wendt D et al. Management of high-risk patients with aortic stenosis and coronary artery disease. *Ann Thorac Surg* 2013; 95(2): 599–605.

38. Goel SS et al. Percutaneous coronary intervention in patients with severe aortic stenosis: Implications for transcatheter aortic valve replacement. *Circulation* 2012; 125(8): 1005.

39. Conradi L et al. First experience with transcatheter aortic valve implantation and concomitant percutaneous coronary intervention. *Clin Res Cardiol* 2011; 100(4): 311–16.

40. Pasic M et al. Combined elective percutaneous coronary intervention and transapical transcatheter aortic valve implantation. *Interact Cardiovasc Thorac Surg* 2012; 14(4): 463.

41. Khawaja MZ et al. The percutaneous coronary intervention prior to transcatheter aortic valve implantation (ACTIVATION) trial: Study protocol for a randomized controlled trial. *Trials* 2014; 15: 300.

42. Safety and Efficacy Study of the Medtronic CoreValve® System in the Treatment of Severe, Symptomatic Aortic Stenosis in Intermediate Risk Subjects Who Need Aortic Valve Replacement (SURTAVI). (SURTAVI). https://clinicaltrialsgov/ct2/show/NCT01586910 2016.

36

Interventional cardiac catheterisation in adults with congenital heart disease

HUSSAM S SURADI, ZIYAD M HIJAZI

36.1 Introduction

Congenital heart disease (CHD) is present in 0.7%–0.8% of live births and the vast majority of these patients are diagnosed and treated in infancy or childhood. The advances in surgical techniques for palliation of complex cardiac anomalies and the improvement in technology and post-operative care have produced survival rates for all patients with CHD in excess of 85%. The more common and less complicated diagnoses such as patent ductus arteriosus (PDA), atrial septal defect (ASD) and ventricular septal defect (VSD) have survival rates approaching 100%. The simple VSD, ASD and PDA patients can often be considered cured with elimination of their defect, and require no follow-up. The majority of the remaining patients require long-term follow-up and many have residual or recurrent structural defects that require further intervention. This has created a relatively new classification of adult cardiac disease, the adult with CHD or grown-up congenital heart disease (GUCHD).

CHD in the adult is now more prevalent than ever because of the rapid advances in surgical and medical interventions in the paediatric population. As a result, there are now an estimated one million patients included in this group in the United States.[1] The adults with CHD form two distinct groups: those with lesions that have not been previously diagnosed or not received prior intervention, and those who have had palliative procedures. There is a third group of patients, albeit rare, are those with previously diagnosed untreated lesions, that are unfortunately untreatable except with heart–lung or lung transplant. This group is not being discussed here. The first group is a rapidly diminishing group as most forms of CHD are routinely diagnosed and treated in infancy or childhood. The second group is rapidly expanding as the children with palliated CHD reach adolescence and adulthood.

Paediatric cardiologists have become increasingly experienced with trans-catheter interventional therapy for CHD. The rapid development of successful trans-catheter procedures has led to interventional procedures becoming the primary treatment for many forms of CHD. Furthermore, trans-catheter procedures have also become essential in the optimal staging of the surgical management of patients with complex anatomy. These same techniques are currently being applied to adults with CHD with excellent results. In this chapter, we focus in a defect-specific approach on the role of cardiac catheterisation and interventions for lesions encountered in adults with CHD.

36.2 Pre-procedural assessment

A thorough review of the patient's complete history and physical examination, including all previous pertinent non-invasive studies, cardiac catheterisations and reviewing operative notes from prior surgeries is essential. Patients referred for cardiac catheterisation may be severely ill or have various comorbidities and recognition of these conditions and appropriate anticipation of potential complications is vitally important. Laboratory studies should be ordered as indicated by the clinical findings and blood typing should be obtained for patients at significant complication risk and whom intervention potentially may be needed. It is also important to review all relevant imaging modalities pertinent to the procedure. Airway management and the use of conscious sedation versus general anaesthesia should be planned in advance of the catheterisation procedure. Details of the procedure and the benefits and risks of any anticipated intervention should be discussed with the patient. Alternative options including surgical treatment should be discussed and a meeting with a surgeon should be offered if patient desires.

36.3 Defect-specific conditions

36.3.1 Shunt lesions

36.3.1.1 Atrial septal defects

The ASD is the most common form of CHD to escape detection in childhood. This is due to the relatively subtle physical findings and lack of symptoms until well into the adult years. They comprise between 20% and 40% of all newly diagnosed CHD in adults. An ASD creates a source for intra-cardiac shunting at the atrial level, and if left untreated may potentially lead to chronic volume overload state with risk of late morbidity; therefore, closure of haemodynamically significant defects is recommended. There are four different types of ASDs that have different anatomical and clinical features: ostium secundum, ostium primum, coronary sinus defects and sinus venosus ASDs. Secundum ASD is the most common (75% of cases) and usually located at the level of the fossa ovalis. The primum ASD (15%–20% of cases) is located in the inferior part of the atrial septum, near the crux of the heart and is associated with atrioventricular septal defects. The sinus venosus type (5%–10% of cases) is located in the superior or inferior part of the septum, near the superior or inferior vena cavae entry to the right atrium. The superior part is usually associated with partial anomalous pulmonary venous drainage. The uncommon coronary sinus septal defect (<1%), allows shunting across the ostium of the coronary sinus.

The most common accepted indications for closure are evidence of a significant left to right shunt with Qp/Qs ratio greater than 1.5:1 or the presence of right heart enlargement (Class I recommendation). None of these defects, with the exception of secundum ASD, is amenable for device closure due to anatomical limitations.

Percutaneous closure of secundum ASD is currently the standard of care with success rate exceeding 98% of patients who have suitable margins and defect size. After an initial haemodynamic assessment is completed, the focus shifts to defining the atrial septal anatomy. Depending on the experience of the operator, the procedure may be done under conscious sedation using intra-cardiac echocardiography (ICE) or under general anaesthesia with the use of trans-oesophageal echocardiography (TEE) to define the anatomy of the defect and to guide device deployment. It is advisable to perform balloon sizing of the defect to aid in selecting the appropriate device size (Figure 36.1). The choice of device depends on its availability, the exact anatomy of the defect as well as the operator preference. In the United States, two devices are FDA approved for this indication: the Amplatzer Septal Occluder device (St. Jude Medical, Plymouth, Minnesota) and the Gore Helex Septal Occluder (Gore Medical, Flagstaff, Arizona). Both devices are variations of 'umbrella' devices that hold both sides of the atrial septum. Multiple other devices are available internationally (Figure 36.2), the most commonly used one is the Occlutech Figulla Flex II device (Occlutech GmbH, Jena, Germany), a double desk device similar in design to the Amplatzer septal occluder.

36.3.1.2 Patent foramen ovale

Patent foramen ovale (PFO) represents a congenital abnormality that is highly prevalent in the general population. Observational studies have found associations between PFO and several clinical disease states including cryptogenic stroke,[2,3] migraine headache,[4] platypnea-orthodeoxia,[5] sleep apnoea, and decompression illness.[6] The treatment of patent foramen ovale (PFO) remains controversial in the United States and marked differences exist in the treatment of this lesion across international boundaries. In the United States, two devices are predominantly used for the closure of PFOs on off-label basis using the Gore Helex Septal Occluder and the Amplatzer Cribriform Occluder with high success rates. Due to the lack of positive randomised trials, we opted not to discuss this subject here.

36.3.1.3 Ventricular septal defects

VSD comprise as many as 10% of CHD in adults. The defect may be located in the membranous or muscular portion of the ventricular septum. A thorough clinical and echocardiographic assessment is important for timely management. The common indications for closure are a significant left to right shunt greater than 1.5:1, left ventricular (LV) volume overload, or symptoms of heart failure. There are two main reasons to perform cardiac catheterisation for VSDs: (1) to define the anatomic location and level of the shunt; and (2) to exclude significant pulmonary vascular disease. Based on these data, decision for closure needs to be determined. Device closure of VSDs has become more common and can be performed safely and effectively, however, surgical closure is still reserved for inlet and supracristal defects. Since the introduction of the Amplatzer devices to close VSDs in 1998

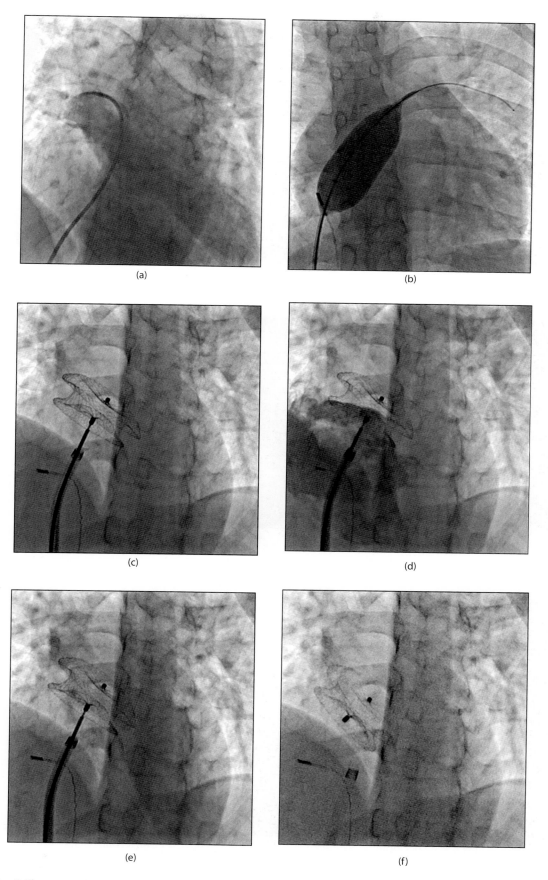

Figure 36.1 (a–f) Fluoroscopic steps in amplatzer septal occluder (ASO) device deployment and evaluation post-deployment.

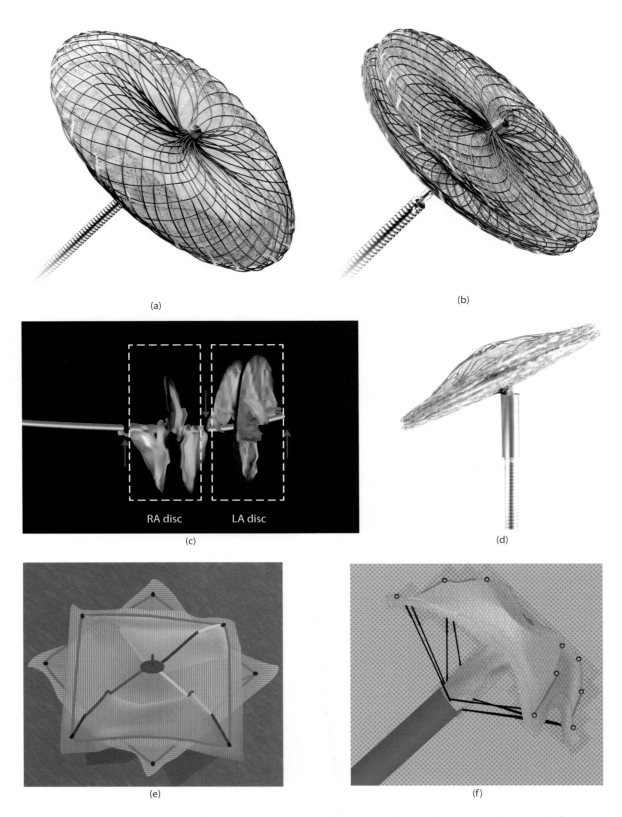

Figure 36.2 Various atrial septal defect closure devices. (a) Amplatzer septal occluder, (b) Amplatzer multifenestrated septal occluder (Cribriform) (St. Jude Medical, Plymouth, Minnesota) (c) Gore HELEX septal occluder (W.L Gore, Flagstaff, AZ) (d) Occlutech Figulla Flex II ASD occluder (Occlutech GmbH, Jena, Germany), (e) Cardioseal (f) StarFlex (NMT Medical, Boston, MA), (g) Biostar (NMT Medical, Boston, MA) , (h) Cera ASD occluder (Lifetech scientific, Shenzhen, China), (i) PFM NitOcclud ASD-R (PFM medical, Koln, Germany), (j) Transcatheter Patch device (Custom Medical Devices, Athens, Greece), (k) Solysafe Septal Occluder (Swiss Implant, Solothurn, Switzerland). (Continued)

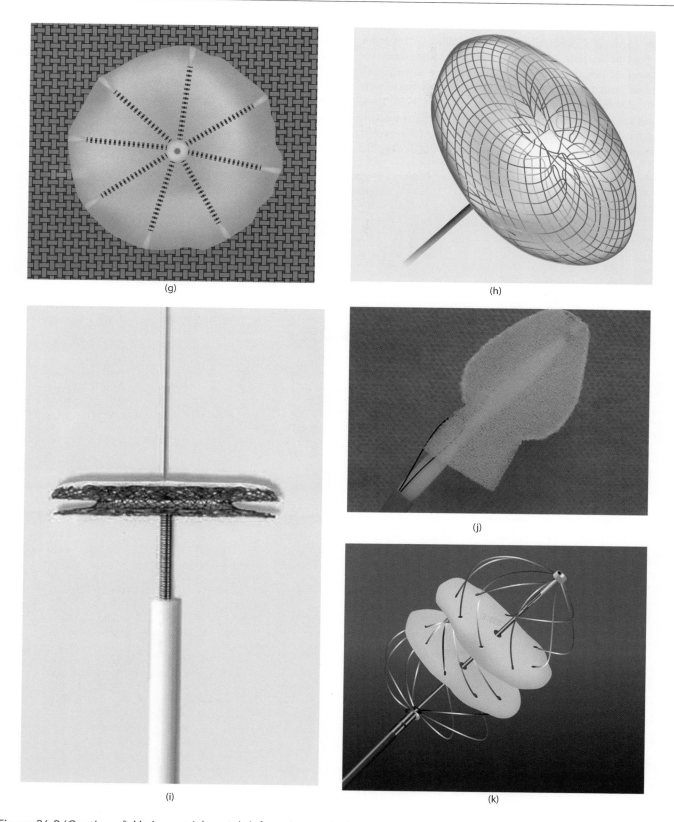

Figure 36.2 (*Continued*) Various atrial septal defect closure devices. **(a)** Amplatzer septal occluder, **(b)** Amplatzer multifenestrated septal occluder (Cribriform) (St. Jude Medical, Plymouth, Minnesota) **(c)** Gore HELEX septal occluder (W.L Gore, Flagstaff, AZ) **(d)** Occlutech Figulla Flex II ASD occluder (Occlutech GmbH, Jena, Germany), **(e)** Cardioseal **(f)** StarFlex (NMT Medical, Boston, MA), **(g)** Biostar (NMT Medical, Boston, MA) , **(h)** Cera ASD occluder (Lifetech scientific, Shenzhen, China), **(i)** PFM NitOcclud ASD-R (PFM medical, Koln, Germany), **(j)** Transcatheter Patch device (Custom Medical Devices, Athens, Greece), **(k)** Solysafe Septal Occluder (Swiss Implant, Solothurn, Switzerland).

(AGA Medical Corporation, Golden Valley, Minnesota, now part of St. Jude Medical, Plymouth, Minnesota), the outcomes of percutaneous VSD closure have significantly improved and results have been promising as these were specifically designed for closure of VSDs (Figure 36.3). These devices are self-expandable, made of nitinol wire, consisting of two flat disks that are linked via a central connecting waist, the diameter of which determines the size of the device. The wide variability in VSDs location, size and morphology led to the development of different designs of the Amplatzer VSD devices (Figure 36.4). The Amplatzer muscular VSD device has two disks that exceed the diameter of the connecting waist by 8 mm. The connecting waist itself has a length of 7 mm. The Amplatzer membranous VSD occluder is an asymmetrical device that was specifically designed for peri-membranous VSDs to account for the surrounding cardiac

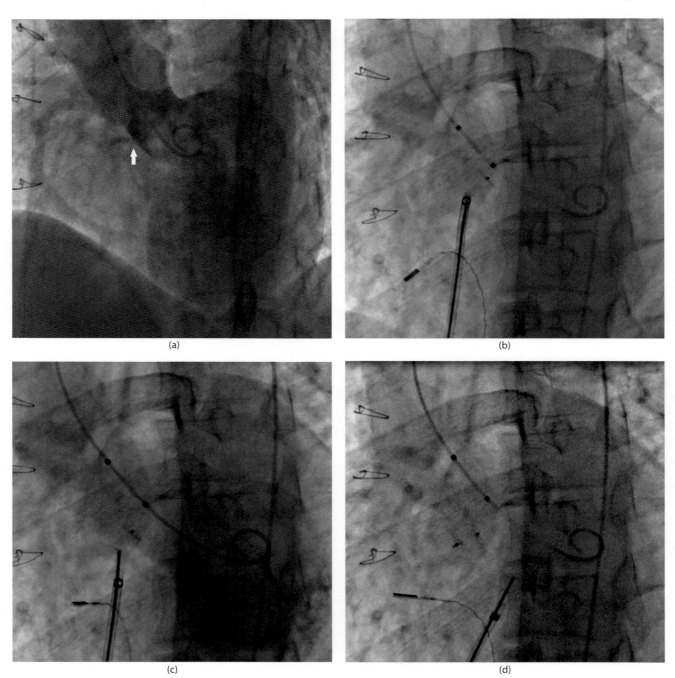

(a)

(b)

(c)

(d)

Figure 36.3 Ventricular septal defect (VSD) closure using Amplatzer muscular VSD device. (a) Left ventricular angiogram in long axial oblique (LAO 60, cranial 20) view demonstrating a membranous VSD (arrow). (b) The Left ventricular disk is deployed in the Left ventricle. (c) The right ventricular disk has been deployed and the device is still attached to the delivery cable. (d) Repeat Left ventricular angiogram after device release demonstrating good device position and no residual shunt.

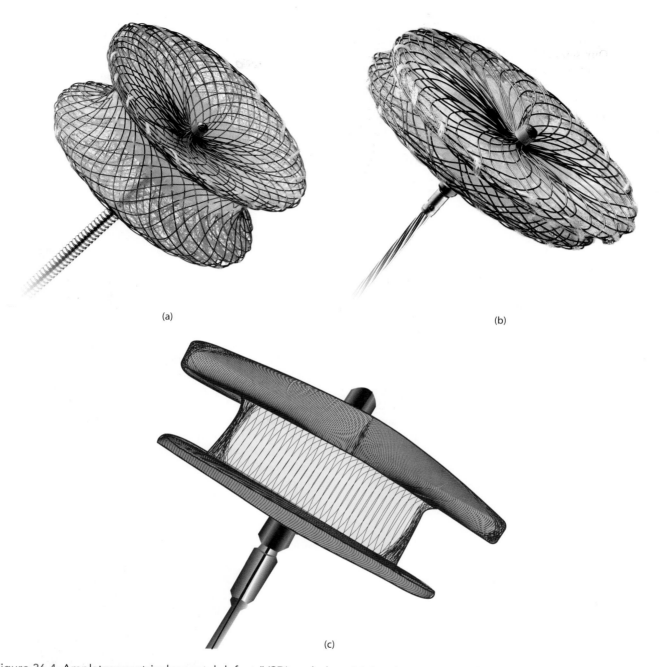

(a)

(b)

(c)

Figure 36.4 Amplatzer ventricular septal defect (VSD) occluders. **(a)** Amplatzer muscular VSD occluder, **(b)** Amplatzer membranous VSD occluder I, **(c)** Amplatzer membranous VSD occluder II. (Reprinted with permission of St. Jude Medical, St. Paul, Minnesota.)

structures. In 2002, Hijazi et al. reported the first successful attempt in humans, where six patients underwent complete VSD closure without any significant complications.[7] However, later studies raised the concern of complete heart block when using this original device due to impingement of the device on the atrioventricular node and the His-Purkinje fibres which run through that portion of the septum. The European registry reported a complete heart block rate of 5%[8]; however, some centres have cited a rate as high as 22%.[9]

This has led to the introduction of the Amplatzer membranous VSD occluder II with the hope that the new design will have a lower rate of impact on the conduction system and subsequent heart block. Initial experiences have shown to be encouraging, having no incidence of heart block reported.[10] Additionally, peri-ventricular 'hybrid' surgical approaches have been demonstrated, in which a surgical incision exposes the right ventricular free wall followed by device closure in the usual fashion.

36.3.1.4 Patent ductus arteriosus

The overwhelming majority of PDA are diagnosed and treated during childhood using a variety of catheter-based techniques. Our standard practice for PDA closure in the paediatric population is for haemodynamically significant shunt with evidence of left heart enlargement or when there is a murmur. Silent PDAs without an audible murmur is considered benign and does not warrant closure. In adults, however, PDA is a relatively uncommon finding, usually discovered incidentally whilst investigating symptoms such as dyspnoea or palpitations, evaluation of a murmur or following an episode of endarteritis. Common indications for cardiac catheterisation in the adult population are for assessment of haemodynamic data including shunt evaluation and pulmonary artery (PA) pressures and to determine the suitability for trans-catheter closure. Catheter-based closure of PDAs in adults can be more challenging and complex as compared with closure in the paediatric population as PDAs tend to be calcified and more tortuous, nevertheless, trans-catheter closure remains more desirable compared to surgery. With the availability of different devices developed specifically for PDA closure, greater than 99% of PDAs are amenable to trans-catheter closure. Devices currently available include the Amplatzer Duct Occluders (ADO 1 and 2) (St. Jude Medical, Plymouth, Minnesota) (Figure 36.5), Nit-occlud PDA Occlusion system (PFM Medical, Germany), Occlutech PDA device and detachable coils. The Amplatzer Atrial Septal and Muscular Ventricular Septal Defect Occluders have been used to close larger PDAs. The ADO comes in variety of sizes that allows it to be used effectively in PDAs up to 11 mm and it can be used in all PDA types. The trans-venous delivery route and the small 5–7 French sheath required for delivery limit the risk of vascular compromise. ADO device has a high complete closure rate and has not been noted to have recurrence of shunting (Figure 36.6).

36.3.1.5 Pulmonary arteriovenous malformations

Pulmonary arteriovenous malformations (PAVMs) are defined as defects in the terminal capillary loops which cause thin-walled vascular sacs that bypass alveolar tissue and shunt un-oxygenated blood directly into the left atrium (Figure 36.7). Most cases are isolated; however, multiple cases may be encountered (most often in Osler–Weber–Rendu syndrome). Although most cases are asymptomatic, some patients may present with unexplained hypoxia, dyspnoea or following a paradoxical embolic event. Elimination of these lesions is necessary in patients with progressive cyanosis, systemic desaturation or stroke.

Trans-catheter embolisation is the preferred therapy for elimination of a PAVM.[11] The embolisation procedure can be complicated by the presence of multiple feeding vessels requiring extensive embolisation. There are several methods of embolisation. Coil embolisation is the most commonly reported therapy. Coils are readily available and can be delivered through 4 French catheters. There is a significant rate of recanalisation of embolised PAVMs of 5%–57%.[11,12] Coils require a site of narrowing in the vessel to be occluded to prevent migration of the coil and are limited to structures less than 7–8 mm in diameter. This limitation led to the development of the Gianturco–Grifka vascular occlusion device which has been suggested as an alternative

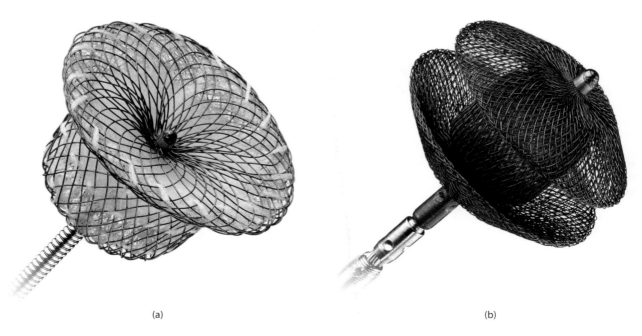

(a)   (b)

Figure 36.5 Amplatzer duct occluders (ADO) (a) I and (b) II. (Reprinted with permission of St. Jude Medical, Plymouth, Minnesota.)

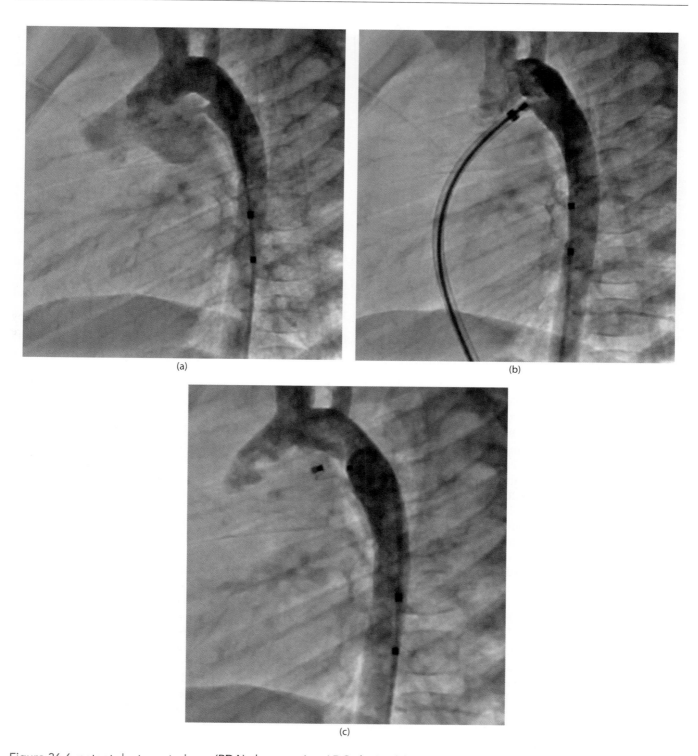

Figure 36.6 patent ductus arteriosus (PDA) closure using ADO device (a) aortic angiogram demonstrating small PDA, (b) aortic end of ADO device deployed, (c) final result after device release demonstrating good device position and no residual shunt.

therapy for PAVM occlusion. This has the advantages of increased control of delivery, limited risk of embolisation, and the ability to embolise large afferent or efferent vessels. However, this device has been discontinued.

The polyester-filled, nitinol wire frame of the Amplatzer occlusion devices and plugs produces excellent embolisation of many different vessels including PAVMs. These devices produce almost immediate complete closure and recanalisation has not been reported. Multiple devices can be delivered through a single sheath and the device can be repositioned or retrieved until the operator is sure of proper positioning.

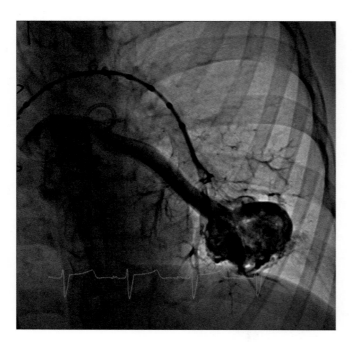

Figure 36.7 Selective injection in the left pulmonary artery demonstrating large pulmonary arteriovenous malformations (PAVM).

Trans-catheter occlusion of PAVM should be used as the primary therapeutic option for PAVM diagnosed at any age. The preservation of normal lung parenchyma and the ability to repeat the trans-catheter embolisation if recurrence is noted are important factors in its selection as primary therapy. This is very significant as 20% of patients in one series required treatment in the contralateral lung after initial therapy.[13] The use of coils and other occlusion devices has been well established; offers significantly reduced morbidity compared with surgical resection, and can be repeated as needed. Long-term follow-up is required and should include pulse oximetry, contrast echocardiograms and chest radiography.

36.3.1.6 Coronary artery fistula

Coronary artery fistulae are connections between the coronary arteries and the cardiac chambers or great vessels. Majority of fistulae originate from the right coronary artery, with the left anterior descending artery being the next most frequently involved. The major termination sites are the right cardiac chambers and pulmonary arteries. Less frequently fistulae drain into the superior vena cava, coronary sinus or left cardiac chambers. Most fistulae are small and clinically silent. However, larger fistulae can cause significant complications secondary to the magnitude of the left-to-right shunt, resulting in premature death due to myocardial ischaemia or heart failure. Selective coronary angiography is performed to delineate the origin, course, drainage point and size of the fistula.

Most coronary fistulae are amenable to percutaneous closure either via retrograde or antegrade approach, using variety of coils, plugs or duct occluders (Figure 36.8). The aim of catheter closure is to occlude the fistulous artery as distally as possible, avoiding any possibility of occluding branches to the normal myocardium. Risks of fistula closure with these devices include myocardial infarction and migration of coils or discs to extra-coronary vascular structures or within the coronary artery branches.[14]

36.4 Congenital valvular defects

36.4.1 Pulmonary valve stenosis

Valvar pulmonary stenosis is a common congenital lesion in paediatrics that may escape detection in childhood and present in adulthood with significant stenosis. It is typically caused by commissural fusion resulting in diminished valve orifice and increased right ventricular afterload. Balloon pulmonary valvuloplasty has become the procedure of choice for the treatment of pulmonary valve stenosis. Indications for intervention on isolated pulmonic stenosis include peak gradient greater than 50 mmHg or mean gradient greater than 30 mmHg in symptomatic patients. In asymptomatic patients, intervention may be considered with peak gradient greater than 60 mmHg or mean gradient greater than 40 mmHg. However, from our experience and that of others, we have found even low gradients of peak of 35 mmHg to cause symptoms. Therefore, coupled with the safety of the procedure, we have been intervening on valves with gradients as low as 35 mmHg with very good resolution of symptoms. Prior to balloon valvuloplasty, it is very important to carefully assess the pulmonary valve morphology and degree of calcification. The determinant of favourable result is the presence of commissural fusion. Dysplastic valves may be present in small percentage of patients and are characterised by thickened, nodular and redundant valve leaflets with minimal or no commissural fusion and lack of post-stenotic dilatation of the PA. Some authors consider dysplastic valves as relative contraindication for balloon dilatation; however, in our experience and that of others, balloon valvuloplasty is our initial treatment of choice. It is generally recommended that the optimal balloon size selection should not exceed 125% of pulmonary valve annulus size to achieve favourable results and to avoid the risk of significant regurgitation. Balloon pulmonary valvuloplasty has uniformly excellent results in all age groups, has low recurrence risk and can be easily repeated if necessary. The double balloon technique, which uses two smaller balloons from each femoral vein, has also been applied to pulmonary valve stenosis with equally excellent results.[15]

36.4.2 Percutaneous pulmonary valve implantation

Percutaneous pulmonary valve implantation (PPVI) is one of the most exciting recent developments in the treatment of structural heart disease and has evolved as an attractive alternative to surgery in patients with dysfunctional right ventricle-PA conduits or bioprosthetic valves. Since so many complex congenital malformations, including pulmonary valve atresia, tetralogy of Fallot, double-outlet

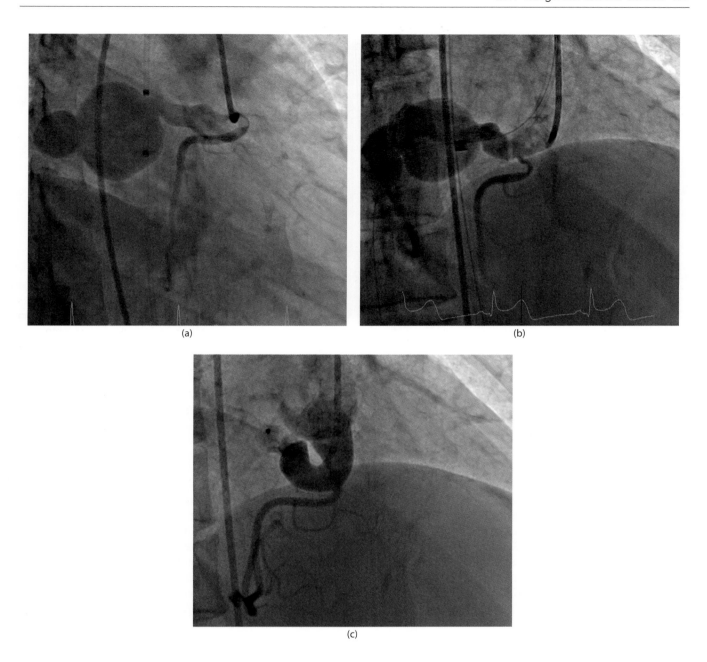

Figure 36.8 (a) Selective angiogram demonstrating a large right coronary artery fistula draining to the right atrium. (b) Wire advanced via the antegrade approach and snared out from the venous side. (c) Successful occlusion of fistula using Amplatzer muscular occluder.

right ventricle, and some of the aortic valve malformations, require intervention for, or reuse of the native pulmonary valve (Ross operation), the need for later valve replacement is growing. The advent of PPVI with Melody® (Medtronic Inc., Minneapolis, Minnesota) (Figure 36.8) and SAPIEN™ (Edwards LifeSciences, Irvine, California) (Figure 36.9) valves have dramatically altered the management of these patients (Table 36.1 outlines differences between two valves). Patients with tetralogy of Fallot who have had valved conduits or bioprosthetic valves placed, and patients who underwent the Ross procedure, where the pulmonary valve is autotransplanted to replace the diseased aortic valve

and a valved-conduit is used between the right ventricle and PA, represent the two largest patient populations who are receiving these valves. Even though PPVI is not currently a standard indication in adults with native right ventricular outflow tract (RVOT) dysfunction, many centres have performed PPVI in a select group of adults who have a native outflow tract (post-trans-annular patch repair of tetralogy of Fallot) that is of an appropriate size or one that can be altered to a suitable size by insertion of multiple stents.

To establish clinical indication criteria, all patients undergo a standardised assessment protocol to ensure appropriate patient selection. Echocardiography is usually

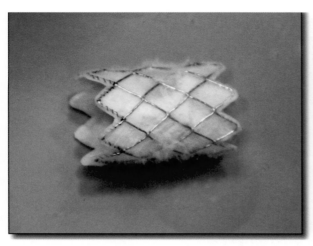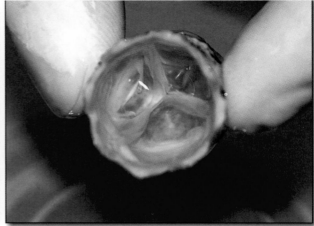

Figure 36.9 The Medtronic Melody pulmonic valve; long axis (left) and short axis views (right).

Table 36.1 Comparison of Melody and the SAPIEN valves

Characteristics	Melody valve	SAPIEN valve
Stent material	Iridium 10%, platinum 90%	Stainless steel
Valve material	Bovine jugular vein	Bovine pericardium treated with Thermafix
Available diameter (mm)	18–22	20, 23, 26, 29
Stent height (mm)	34	14.5 or 16
Delivery sheath size (Fr)	22	22 or 24 (16, 18 or 20 for XT)
Pre-stenting	Recommended	Required
Stent fracture	21%	None reported

the initial screening tool to determine the RVOT gradient and to semi-quantitatively assess the severity of pulmonary regurgitation. Recent advances in cardiac MRI imaging allow detailed quantitative assessment of the structure of the right ventricle as well as the flow dynamics in the setting of pulmonary homograft dysfunction.

Present indications for PPVI have been adapted from those accepted for surgical pulmonic valve replacement (PVR) and include:

- Presence of symptoms
- Indexed right ventricular end-diastolic volume (RVEDV) >150 mL/m^2 ± regurgitant fraction >40%
- RVOT peak instantaneous gradient >50 mmHg
- Right ventricular (RV) dysfunction (right ventricular ejection fraction [RVEF] <40%)
- Moderate-severe accompanying tricuspid regurgitation

In addition to clinical indications, several anatomical criteria need to be fulfilled to qualify for PPVI. The ideal anatomy for PPVI is a uniform diameter from RVOT to PA with adequate main PA length to avoid stenting into the PA bifurcation. With the current iterations of the Melody valve, the RVOT, pulmonary valve annulus, and proximal main PA must be 22 mm or less to prevent leaflet malcoaptation. Using the 22 mm Ensemble delivery system, the outer diameter of the Melody valve is approximately 24 mm,

and therefore any inner diameter of a conduit larger than this would be insufficient to securely anchor the valve. Nevertheless, there is limited experience with mounting the Melody valve on a 24 mm balloon delivered through a 24 French sheath.[16] On the other hand, the SAPIEN valve can be deployed in RVOT sizes up to 29 mm in diameter.

During cardiac catheterisation, routine haemodynamic data are obtained. Gradients are obtained in the RVOT/ conduit, at the level of the pulmonary valve, and the pulmonary arteries. The PA and branch morphology should be delineated by pulmonary arteriograms to define the architecture. After haemodynamic assessment, evaluation of the coronary arteries must be made with balloon inflation in the right ventricle outflow tract to assess the proximity of the coronary arteries to the outflow tract. When the conduit is placed on the anterior surface of the heart, coronary branches may pass directly beneath it, and may be potentially be compressed by placement of the stented valve and distension of the conduit.[17] If no evidence of coronary compression is noted, pre-stenting of the RVOT using bare/ covered metal stents is performed to create an appropriate landing zone for the trans-catheter valve. Pre-stenting the landing site has significantly improved the survival of the implant, minimising stent fracture which affected 23% of the initially reported cases of the Melody valve. The appropriate valve is then introduced and deployed (see Figure 36.10 for implantation steps).

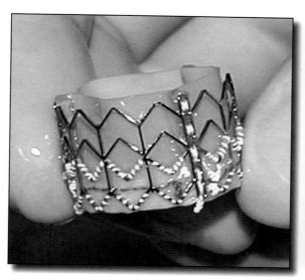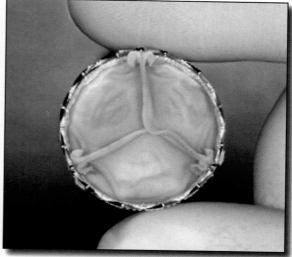

Figure 36.10 Edwards SAPIEN valve; long axis (left) and short axis views (right).

36.4.3 Aortic valve disorders

Congenital aortic stenosis is quite different from the more common calcific or senile aortic stenosis. The inherent abnormality in the valve morphology, most commonly bicuspid leaflets, can be associated with variety of sub-valvular, supravalvular, aortic root and arch abnormalities. Shone's complex comprises of defects involving the left side of the heart consisting of parachute-like mitral valve, supravalvar mitral ring, sub-aortic stenosis and coarctation of aorta. Supravalvular aortic stenosis is seen in association with William's syndrome.

Unlike senile aortic stenosis, balloon aortic valvuloplasty (BAV) remains an excellent alternative to surgical valvotomy or valve replacement in young adults with congenital valvar aortic stenosis. The pathology involved in the latter involves more commissural fusion and less leaflet rigidity compared to the calcified senile aortic valves. In the presence of heavily calcified bicuspid aortic valve, however, surgical valve replacement is the treatment of choice. Experience with trans-catheter aortic valve replacement (TAVR) in patients with bicuspid aortic valve disease remains limited with high incidence of post-implantation aortic regurgitation observed.[18] This is thought to be related to the larger annulus size, larger sinus of valsalva and ascending aortic dimension encountered with bicuspid aortic valves. Nevertheless, the enhanced paravalvular sealing effect of the third-generation SAPIEN 3 valve has shown promising results in bicuspid aortic valve stenosis.[19]

The retrograde approach is used most commonly for aortic valvuloplasty. It is important that the non-compliant balloon size do not exceed the aortic annulus size measured by aortography to prevent aortic regurgitation from occurring. In the presence of severe peripheral arterial disease, BAV via antegrade approach with trans-septal puncture can be performed.

36.4.4 Mitral valve disorders

The incidence of congenital mitral stenosis is very low and is frequently associated with other CHD. This includes cleft mitral valve seen in association with AV canal defects that may have undergone repair. Mitral stenosis may also present as a variant of 'Shone's Complex' with multiple left-sided heart abnormalities. Another uncommon presentation is 'parachute' mitral valve that involves abnormal chordal attachments. Unlike rheumatic mitral valve stenosis, congenital mitral stenosis is generally not suitable for balloon valvuloplasty.

36.5 Obstructive vascular lesions

36.5.1 Coarctation of aorta

Coarctation of the aorta (CoA) is the sixth most common congenital lesion accounting for 4%–6% of live births with CHD.[20,21] Although most patients have a discrete narrowing of the thoracic aorta at the insertion of the ductus arteriosus, the anatomical spectrum may vary from this discrete entity to tubular hypoplasia, with many variations in between these extremes. Despite these anatomical variations, the effect of the narrowing has the commonly shared features of increased afterload on the left ventricle, exposure of the upper body to hypertension, flow disturbance in the thoracic aorta, and decreased perfusion to the lower body. Depending on the balance between the degree of flow disturbance and the compensatory mechanisms available to overcome it, the clinical presentation may vary from the critically ill neonate in heart failure to the asymptomatic child or adult with hypertension. Untreated coarctation carries a poor prognosis with average survival age of 35 years of age; with 75% mortality by 46 years of age.[22] Long-term complications are the consequence of long-term hypertension including premature coronary artery disease, stroke, endocarditis, aortic dissection and heart failure.[23] Furthermore, recurrent coarctation and future aneurysm formation can occur following successful surgical and endovascular repair which mandates long-term close surveillance.

Echocardiography and MRI are the main imaging modalities used for diagnosis and evaluation of CoA. Diagnostic cardiac catheterisation may occasionally be needed for more accurate assessment of the obstruction. The main criteria for intervention include peak to peak coarctation gradient ≥20 mmHg; which is the difference in peak pressure proximal and beyond the narrowed segment. Furthermore, intervention is also recommended if the gradient is <20 mmHg in the presence of radiologic evidence of significant collateral flow. In most centres, the overwhelming majority of adult patients with CoA undergo trans-catheter repair, either using balloon angioplasty or stent implantation, with excellent results. Surgical repair is usually reserved for patients with complex arch lesions such as arch hypoplasia, long-segment coarctation, aortic aneurysms/dissection, aortic root dilatation and aortic valve stenosis/regurgitation. Surgical complications are generally more common in adults than children, and can be detrimental as surgical repair is associated with extended recovery time, potential phrenic nerve and recurrent laryngeal nerve injury, and the serious, although uncommon, lower body paralysis secondary to ischaemic spinal cord injury.

Balloon angioplasty has been an acceptable technique for three decades for the relief of coarctation.[24] It produces controlled tear of the intima and part of the media which results in an improvement of the vessel diameter. The size of the balloon selected should be no more than 1–2 mm larger in diameter than the smallest normal aortic diameter proximal to the coarctation. In cases of recurrent coarctation, the size of the balloon should not be larger than the size of the aorta at the level of the diaphragm. Due to the high incidence of future aneurysm formation (up to 9%) and re-coarctation, as well as the availability of stents in most centres, balloon angioplasty fell out of favour as first line therapy in endovascular repair.

First reported in 1995, primary stent implantation is now the procedure of choice for treatment of CoA (Figure 36.11). It reduces the complications, improves luminal diameter, results in minimal residual gradient and sustains haemodynamic benefit as compared to balloon angioplasty.[17,25,26] Data from a multicentre case series of over 500 patients demonstrated the efficacy and relative safety of stent placement for both native and recurrent coarctation with success rate exceeding 98%.[26,27]

Several different endovascular stents are commercially available, however, very few are expandable to the average diameter of a large adult aorta (21.1 ± 3.2 mm for women, 26.1 ± 4.3 mm for men). The choice of stent depends on the coarctation anatomy, size of the patient, the preference of the operator and availability. Balloon-expandable bare metal stents are the most commonly used and are made from stainless steel (Palmaz Genesis, Johnson and Johnson; Mega LD and Maxi LD series, ev3), platinum–iridium alloy (Cheatham–Platinum stent, NuMED), or chromium–cobalt alloy (AndraStent XL

and XXL, Andramed). The use of covered stents (only available under FDA's HDE use protocol in the United States) has added further safety to the short and long-term outcomes in these patients. It has been proposed that the use of covered stents reduces the risk of aneurysms, however, in a randomised trial of 120 patients with severe native coarctation, there was no difference in the rate of re-coarctation and pseudoaneurysm formation after 31 months of follow-up between patients who underwent implantation using a bare metal stent and those with a covered stent.[28] Nevertheless, covered stents offer the advantage of excluding any stretch-induced wall trauma from the endoluminal aspect of the aorta, particularly in the catastrophic event of aortic rupture.

36.5.2 Pulmonary artery stenosis

Branch PA stenosis presents in different locations and may be congenital or occur after surgical intervention. Tetralogy of Fallot repair, Blalock–Taussig shunt placement, arterial switch, or right ventricle to PA conduit placement for truncus arteriosus repair or pulmonary atresia may all lead to branch PA stenosis at suture lines. Many of these sites become technically very difficult to repair surgically and can be effectively treated in the catheterisation lab with balloon angioplasty or stent placement. All patients with a history of these types of palliative repairs should be fully evaluated for branch pulmonary stenosis, as this is a common reason for RV deterioration in previously well-palliated patients. Patients with any evidence of stenosis or increased RV pressure should receive a pulmonary perfusion scan to quantify the degree of branch PA stenosis.

Balloon angioplasty of branch PA stenosis has a variable success rate. Approximately 60% of procedures are technically successful but midterm follow-up suggests that up to two thirds have significant residual stenosis.[29] This has led interventionalists to treat branch PA stenosis with primary stent placement. The implantable stent is crimped onto a balloon catheter the size of the PA segments adjacent to the stenosis. A long sheath is passed over a wire distal to the site of stenosis and the balloon catheter is advanced over the wire to the stenotic area. The sheath is withdrawn and the balloon is inflated to dilate the stenosis. This expands the stent to the size of the balloon and the radial strength of the stent prevents elastic recoil or refolding of the stenotic site. Multiple stents can be placed sequentially in long segment stenosis. Bilateral stents can be placed at the same time using the 'kissing technique', which involves simultaneous stent implantation in the site of both proximal right and left PA stenosis. This prevents either stent from being partially collapsed or distorted by the inflation of a balloon in the contralateral PA.

Patients who require a surgical procedure and have distal pulmonary stenosis can also be treated with PA stenting in the operating room. The sites of the stenosis need to be well established prior to the surgical repair. The surgical field allows relatively easy access to the central pulmonary arteries. A stent can then be advanced into the more distal PA and expanded under direct vision and palpation. This

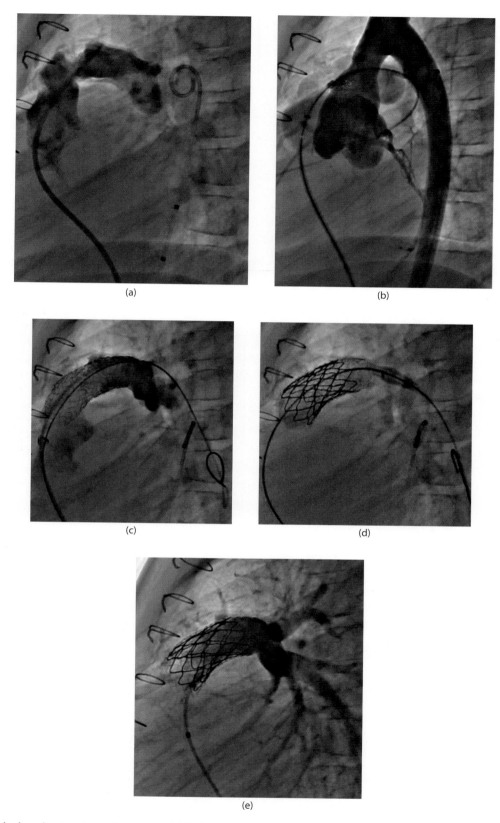

Figure 36.11 Melody valve implantation steps. **(a)** Pulmonary homograft angiography demonstrates severe pulmonic regurgitation and stenosis, **(b)** conduit balloon sizing with simultaneous aortic root angiography demonstrating left coronary artery with an acceptable distance from the conduit, **(c)** angiography post-stent deployment demonstrating no conduit stenosis with free pulmonary regurgitation, **(d)** balloon deployment of the Melody valve, **(e)** final angiography in conduit demonstrating no significant pulmonary regurgitation.

technique is useful for patients who have failed attempts at stent placement in the catheterisation lab or for patients without suitable venous access. A staged procedure with the stent placed before or after surgical repair is the more common therapy and is the preferred course.

Stents that can be expanded to accommodate branch PA size should be used (see under CoA). The results of stent placement have been impressive, with up to a 97% success rate with a 2% complication rate.[30,31] New stent technology will undoubtedly improve the results and allow smaller catheters and sheaths to be used. Future directions include self-expanding nitinol stents that can enlarge with the patient's growth and bioabsorbable stent material. Absorbable stents may remove the need for large stent placement in small children and the potential difficulties a stainless steel stent could present at the time of subsequent surgical procedures.

36.6 Complex CHD

36.6.1 D-Transposition of the great arteries

The success of the Senning and Mustard type venous switches for the treatment of the transposition of the great arteries has led to the long-term survival of many of these patients. These intra-atrial surgical baffles allow the systemic venous return to flow through the atria and cross the mitral valve to fill the left ventricle. The left ventricle then pumps the blood to the pulmonary arteries. The fully oxygenated blood returns to the left atrium and flows over the other side of the baffle to the right ventricle and out the aorta. A number of these patients have been noted to have progressive obstruction of these venous baffles. The surgical results of repair of the baffles obstruction were not favourable, therefore, trans-catheter therapy with balloon dilation

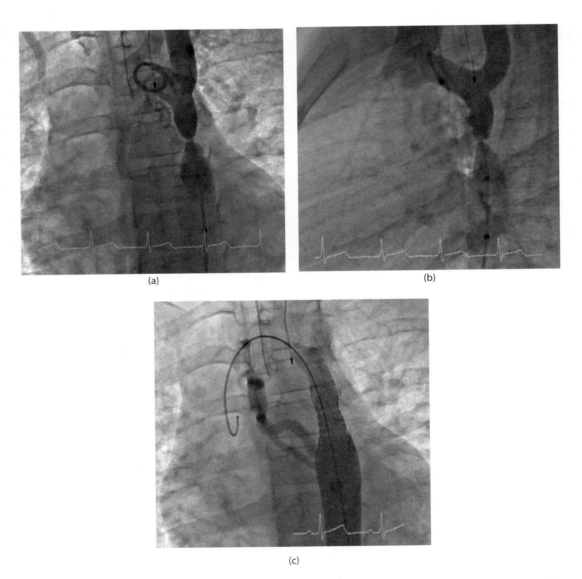

(a)

(b)

(c)

Figure 36.12 Stenting of tight native coarctation. Native coarctation with multiple collaterals in (a) LAO and (b) straight lateral views. (c) No residual stenosis following stent implantation.

and stenting emerged as the preferred therapy of choice.[32,33] Complete obstructions can be perforated and residual narrowings treated using single or multiple stents (Figure 36.12). Re-dilatation for neointimal hyperplasia induced stenosis following stent placement is also successful.[34] Furthermore, conduit leaks can be treated percutaneously via the use of covered stents or occlusion devices.

36.6.2 Post-Fontan

The growing number of patients who have palliated single ventricle physiology is a group with significant adult onset complications. These patients typically have undergone a variation of the Fontan procedure to shunt all the systemic venous blood directly into the pulmonary arteries. Common indications for catheterisation in the adults with Fontan palliation are for haemodynamic evaluation in case of clinical status change like dysrhythmia, and for preoperative assessment prior to Fontan revision or cardiac transplant. During catheterisation, it is important to record pulmonary, Fontan and aortic pressures as well as to evaluate for the presence of shunting (right-to-left or left-to-right) with oxygen saturation assessment at various levels. Angiograms should be performed to define the anatomical details of the great vessels, collateral vessels, the systemic venous drainage as well as the left ventricular

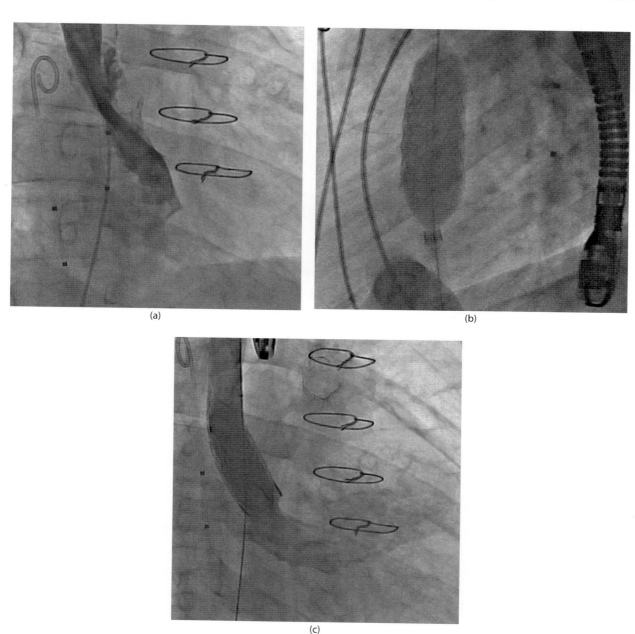

(a)

(b)

(c)

Figure 36.13 Stenting of mustard superior vena cava baffle narrowing (a) SVC baffle narrowing. (b and c) No residual narrowing following stent implantation.

volume and ejection fraction. The low, non-pulsatile flow in the systemic venous circulation and multiple suture lines can lead to significant stenosis within the Fontan circulation (see Figure 36.13). The same techniques of balloon angioplasty and stent placement are applied to relieve any anatomical obstruction in this complicated patient population. Similarly, trans-catheter closure using coils and occlusion devices are applied for abnormal vascular connections closure that may cause right-to-left (causing cyanosis and paradoxical embolism) or left-to-right shunting (causing systemic ventricular volume overload) (see Figures 36.14 and 36.15).

36.7 Summary

Paediatric cardiologists have seen vast improvements and advances in the treatment of CHD that have led to excellent long-term survival of the vast majority of the paediatric population. These patients are reaching adulthood and form a large and complicated group of patients. These patients require specialised care by physicians familiar with CHD, adult medicine, dysrhythmias and interventional procedures.

Advances in interventional cardiac catheterisation have changed the therapeutic strategy for many patients with CHD. Management of patients with CHD requires a

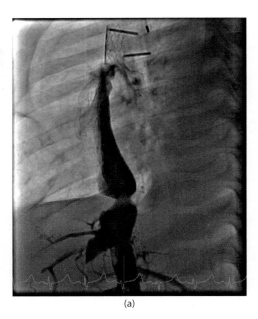
(a)

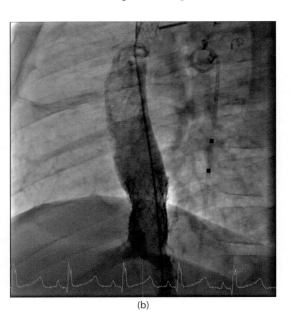
(b)

Figure 36.14 Angiogram in the Fontan conduit demonstrating (a) narrowing in its proximal portion and (b) no residual stenosis post-stent implantation.

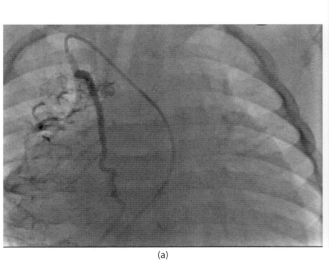
(a)

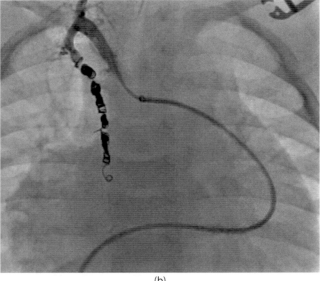
(b)

Figure 36.15 (a) Selective injection into the right internal mammary artery showing collaterals to the right lung. (b) Coil occlusion of the right internal mammary artery. (Courtesy of Dr. Damien Kenny.)

multidisciplinary approach with collaboration between adult congenital heart specialists, paediatric/adult congenital interventionalists and congenital heart surgeons. The future holds many promises with advancements in catheter-based interventions as well as hybrid surgical techniques that will improve the survival and quality of life of this complicated patient population.

References

1. Brickner ME et al. Congenital heart disease in adults. First of two parts. *N Engl J Med* 2000; 342(4): 256–63. Epub 2000/01/29.
2. Lechat P et al. Prevalence of patent foramen ovale in patients with stroke. *N Engl J Med* 1988; 318(18): 1148–52. Epub 1988/05/05.
3. Handke M et al. Patent foramen ovale and cryptogenic stroke in older patients. *N Engl J Med* 2007; 357(22): 2262–8. Epub 2007/11/30.
4. Azarbal B et al. Association of interatrial shunts and migraine headaches: Impact of transcatheter closure. *J Am Coll Cardiol* 2005; 45(4): 489–92. Epub 2005/02/15.
5. Sorrentino M, and Resnekov L. Patent foramen ovale associated with platypnea and orthodeoxia. *Chest* 1991; 100(4): 1157–8. Epub 1991/10/01.
6. Moon RE, et al. Patent foramen ovale and decompression sickness in divers. *Lancet* 1989; 1(8637): 513–4. Epub 1989/03/11.
7. Hijazi ZM et al. Catheter closure of perimembranous ventricular septal defects using the new Amplatzer membranous VSD occluder: Initial clinical experience. *Catheter Cardiovasc Interv* 2002; 56(4): 508–15. Epub 2002/07/19.
8. Carminati M et al. Transcatheter closure of congenital ventricular septal defects: Results of the European Registry. *Eur Heart J* 2007; 28(19): 2361–8. Epub 2007/08/09.
9. Predescu D et al. Complete heart block associated with device closure of perimembranous ventricular septal defects. *J Thorac Cardiovasc Surg* 2008; 136(5): 1223–8. Epub 2008/11/26.
10. Tzikas A et al. Transcatheter closure of perimembranous ventricular septal defect with the Amplatzer® membranous VSD occluder 2: Initial world experience and one-year follow-up. *Catheter Cardiovasc Interv* 2014; 83(4): 571–80. Epub 2013/05/25.
11. Haitjema TJ et al. Embolisation of pulmonary arteriovenous malformations: Results and follow up in 32 patients. *Thorax* 1995; 50(7): 719–23. Epub 1995/07/01.
12. Sagara K et al. Recanalization after coil embolotherapy of pulmonary arteriovenous malformations: Study of long-term outcome and mechanism for recanalization. *AJR Am J Roentgenol* 1998; 170(3): 727–30. Epub 1998/03/10.
13. Pick A et al. Pulmonary arteriovenous fistula: Presentation, diagnosis, and treatment. *World J Surg* 1999; 23(11): 1118–22. Epub 1999/09/29.
14. Kharouf R et al. Transcatheter closure of coronary artery fistula complicated by myocardial infarction. *J Invasive Cardiol* 2007; 19(5): E146–9. Epub 2007/05/02.
15. Mullins CE et al. Double balloon technique for dilation of valvular or vessel stenosis in congenital and acquired heart disease. *J Am Coll Cardiol* 1987; 10(1): 107–14. Epub 1987/07/01.
16. Cheatham SL et al. The Medtronic Melody(R) transcatheter pulmonary valve implanted at 24-mm diameter – it works. *Catheter Cardiovasc Interv* 2013; 82(5): 816–23. Epub 2013/01/30.
17. Chessa M et al. Results and mid-long-term follow-up of stent implantation for native and recurrent coarctation of the aorta. *Eur Heart J* 2005; 26(24): 2728–32. Epub 2005/09/28.
18. Mylotte D et al. Transcatheter aortic valve replacement in bicuspid aortic valve disease. *J Am Coll Cardiol* 2014; 64(22): 2330–9. Epub 2014/12/04.
19. Thilo C et al. Bicuspid aortic valve stenosis with successful transfemoral transcatheter aortic valve replacement (TAVI) using the Sapien 3 valve. *Eur Heart J* 2014; 35(38): 2662. Epub 2014/07/16.
20. Reller MD et al. Prevalence of congenital heart defects in metropolitan Atlanta, 1998–2005. *J Pediatr* 2008; 153(6): 807–13. Epub 2008/07/29.
21. Hoffman JI, and Kaplan S. The incidence of congenital heart disease. *J Am Coll Cardiol* 2002; 39(12): 1890–900. Epub 2002/06/27.
22. Warnes CA et al. ACC/AHA 2008 guidelines for the management of adults with congenital heart disease: A report of the American College of Cardiology/American Heart Association Task Force on Practice Guidelines (writing committee to develop guidelines on the management of adults with congenital heart disease). *Circulation* 2008; 118(23): e714–833. Epub 2008/11/11.
23. Jenkins NP, and Ward C. Coarctation of the aorta: Natural history and outcome after surgical treatment. *QJM* 1999; 92(7): 365–71. Epub 2000/01/11.
24. Singer MI et al. Transluminal aortic balloon angioplasty for coarctation of the aorta in the newborn. *Am Heart J* 1982; 103(1): 131–2. Epub 1982/01/01.
25. Hamdan MA et al. Endovascular stents for coarctation of the aorta: Initial results and intermediate-term follow-up. *J Am Coll Cardiol* 2001; 38(5): 1518–23. Epub 2001/11/03.
26. Forbes TJ et al. Intermediate follow-up following intravascular stenting for treatment of coarctation of the aorta. *Catheter Cardiovasc Interv* 2007; 70(4): 569–77. Epub 2007/09/27.
27. Forbes TJ et al. Procedural results and acute complications in stenting native and recurrent coarctation of the aorta in patients over 4 years of age: A multi-institutional study. *Catheter Cardiovasc Interv* 2007; 70(2): 276–85. Epub 2007/07/17.
28. Sohrabi B et al. Comparison between covered and bare Cheatham–Platinum stents for endovascular treatment of patients with native post-ductal aortic coarctation: Immediate and intermediate-term results. *JACC Cardiovasc Interv* 2014; 7(4): 416–23. Epub 2014/03/19.
29. Kan JS et al. Balloon angioplasty – Branch pulmonary artery stenosis: Results from the Valvuloplasty and Angioplasty of Congenital Anomalies Registry. *Am J Cardiol* 1990; 65(11): 798–801. Epub 1990/03/15.
30. O'Laughlin MP et al. Implantation and intermediate-term follow-up of stents in congenital heart disease. *Circulation* 1993; 88(2): 605–14. Epub 1993/08/01.
31. Hijazi ZM et al. Stent implantation for relief of pulmonary artery stenosis: Immediate and short-term results. *Catheter Cardiovasc Diagn* 1996; 38(1): 16–23. Epub 1996/05/01.

32. Chatelain P et al. Stenting of superior vena cava and inferior vena cava for symptomatic narrowing after repeated atrial surgery for D-transposition of the great vessels. *Br Heart J* 1991; 66(6): 466–8. Epub 1991/12/01.

33. Ward CJ et al. Use of intravascular stents in systemic venous and systemic venous baffle obstructions. Short-term follow-up results. *Circulation* 1995; 91(12): 2948–54. Epub 1995/06/15.

34. Trerotola SO et al. Palmaz stent in the treatment of central venous stenosis: Safety and efficacy of redilation. *Radiology* 1994; 190(2): 379–85. Epub 1994/02/01.

PART 3

Electrophysiology

Fundamentals of cardiac electrophysiology

SUNIL KAPUR, WILLIAM G STEVENSON, ROY M JOHN

37.1 Introduction

Clinical cardiac electrophysiology (EP) has undergone numerous technological advancements in the past 20 years, which have revolutionised the diagnosis and treatment of arrhythmias. The fundamentals have, however, remained largely unchanged, based on a thorough understanding of cardiac anatomy, cellular EP and biophysics. Navigating venous, thoracic and cardiac anatomy is essential to nearly all procedures in the EP laboratory, and numerous technologies have emerged aiming to capture cardiac anatomy with high degrees of spatial and temporal resolution. In addition, imaging techniques that combine anatomy with electrophysiological recordings allow for precise mapping and localisation of arrhythmogenic substrates. Finally, many recording/ablation techniques and pacing/defibrillation technologies require the physician to have a working knowledge of biophysics.

37.2 Cardiac anatomy relevant to EP

Right Atrium: The right atrium (RA) is bounded by the caval veins superiorly and inferiorly, the inter-atrial septum and coronary sinus medially and the crista terminalis laterally.[1] The smooth posterior wall is derived from the sinus venosum. The pectinated anterolateral portion is dominated by the right atrial appendage. The crista terminalis (terminal crest) is a well-defined fibromuscular ridge that extends from the atrial septal wall medially, courses anterior to the superior vena cava (SVC), descends inferiorly along the lateral wall and then courses anterior to the inferior vena cava (IVC) towards the septum where it meets the lateral horn of crescentic remnant of the Eustachian valve. The medial horn of the Eustachian valve joins the Thebesian valve at the orifice of the coronary sinus. The superior aspect of the crista terminalis anterior to the SVC contains the sinus node cells, but throughout its course it may contain other cells capable of automaticity giving rise to escape rhythms and ectopic atrial tachycardias. The sub-Eustachian isthmus between the opening of the IVC and the adjacent tricuspid annulus, commonly referred to as the cavo-tricuspid isthmus, is part of the re-entry path for common right atrial flutter and is targeted by ablation to treat this arrhythmia.

The atrio-ventricular node (AVN) is contained in the inter-atrial septum in the triangle of Koch that is defined anteriorly by the septal leaflet of the tricuspid valve, inferiorly by the orifice of the coronary sinus and posteriorly by the tendon of Todaro, a fibrous tendon within the atrial septal wall which extends superiorly from the fibrous Eustachian ridge to the central fibrous body. The compact AVN is located at the apex of the triangle. Many people have an extension of AV nodal tissue inferiorly along the tricuspid annulus that forms a slow AV nodal pathway that is used in atrio-ventricular nodal re-entry tachycardia (AVNRT), the most common form of paroxysmal supraventricular tachycardia encountered in adults.

Left Atrium: Unlike the right, the left atrium (LA) has a smooth-walled body except in the region of the LA appendage.[2,3] The pulmonary veins enter the posterior aspect of the LA. Extensions of the left atrial muscle into pulmonary veins are implicated in spontaneous ectopic activity that can be a trigger for atrial fibrillation. Electrical isolation of the veins by encircling ablation lesions is an essential component of interventional therapy for atrial fibrillation. The LA has a lateral ridge that is interposed between the ostia of the left pulmonary veins and the mouth of the left atrial appendage. The vein of Marshall, a remnant of the left superior vena cava, is closely related to this ridge and drains into the coronary sinus. Additionally, abundant ganglia and fibres of the autonomic nervous system are present in this ridge and can be involved in initiating atrial fibrillation.[4,5]

37.2.1 Coronary sinus

The coronary sinus extends from the inferior right atrial (RA) septum along the inferior mitral annulus. It has a muscular coat in its proximal course and transitions to the great cardiac vein that continues laterally and superiorly that is marked on the endovascular surface by the valve of Vieussen.[6] The great cardiac vein lies alongside the left circumflex artery and continues to become the anterior interventricular vein that runs parallel to the left anterior descending coronary artery. Lateral left ventricular (LV) branches join the coronary sinus at various levels and are potential targets for placement of pacing leads for LV epicardial pacing. The middle cardiac vein is a proximal branch of the coronary sinus that runs in the posterior interventricular grove, parallel to the posterior descending coronary artery. Ablation of some posterior septal accessory pathways is possible from within this branch but runs the risk of inadvertent thermal damage to adjacent branches of the right coronary artery.

37.2.2 Ventricles

The right ventricle (RV) and LV have an inlet (inflow tract), apical trabecular portion and outlet tracts. Morphologically, the RV is distinguished from the LV by having coarser trabeculae, a moderator band extending from the septum to the free wall and a lack of fibrous continuity between its inlet and outflow valves.[7] The tricuspid valve, possessing inferior, septal and antero-superior leaflets, has extensive chordal attachments to the septum and is supported by eccentric papillary muscles. The antero-lateral and postero-medial papillary muscles support the mitral valve.

The outflow segments of both ventricles are important as sources for arrhythmias in patients with and without structural heart disease.[8] The latter are referred to as idiopathic arrhythmias and are usually benign. Rarely very rapid activity from these regions causes idiopathic ventricular fibrillation. These include premature ventricular contractions (PVCs) as well as ventricular tachycardias (VTs). Some arise from muscular strands that extend superiorly along the base of the aorta where they can be ablated from within the aortic sinuses of Valsalva. The papillary muscles are also sources for idiopathic ventricular arrhythmias.

In patients with structural heart disease, regions of scar from prior myocardial infarction, cardiomyopathies or surgery are the most common causes of sustained ventricular tachycardia. In non-ischaemic cardiomyopathies, replacement fibrosis tends to involve the areas around the base of the heart along the valve structures. Distinct patterns of fibrosis have been described along the peri-mitral and lateral ventricles, infra-aortic and basal septal regions.[9]

37.3 Cardiac conduction system

The sino-atrial node (SAN) is a crescent-shaped, intramural structure with its head located subepicardially at the junction of the RA and the superior vena cava and its tail extending along the crista terminalis.[10,11] Three preferential anatomic conduction pathways from the SAN to the atrioventricular node (AVN) have been proposed (Figure 37.1), although excitation spreads from cell to cell throughout the atrial myocardium.

The AVN is a complex structure with variable extensions inferiorly and/or leftward receiving inputs from the atria. The 'compact' AVN is located at the apex of Koch's triangle where it transitions to the bundle of His.[12,13]

The specialised ventricular conduction system is comprised of Purkinje fibres that provide rapid conduction of the cardiac impulse. The His bundle courses through the central fibrous body to divide into the left and right bundle branches (RBBs) which rapidly conduct the excitation to the ventricles. The RBB divides into fibres that course through the moderator band to the free wall and papillary muscle, and spread throughout the RV. The anterior and posterior

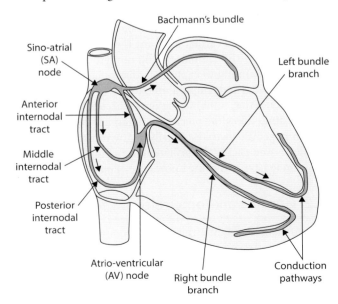

Figure 37.1 Cardiac conduction system.

fascicles of the left bundle extend to the base of each papillary muscle as well as the adjacent myocardium. There is also a LV septal fascicle. It is noteworthy that the His bundle and bundle branches are insulated along their course such that activation of the ventricular myocardium occurs at the distal arborisation of the Purkinje fibres.

37.4 Cellular EP

The cardiac action potential is a consequence of well-orchestrated ionic currents mediated by changes in membrane permeability to Na^+, K^+, Ca^{++} ions as a consequence of sequential conformational changes in ion channels (Figure 37.2). Potassium currents are outward currents that hyperpolarise the cell and are responsible for the normal resting membrane potential of ≈ -90 mV in ventricular myocardial cells. Phase 0 is the phase of rapid depolarisation mediated by the fast sodium inward current I_{Na} that occurs when the membrane potential reaches the threshold for excitation. This current is an important determinant of conduction velocity. Antiarrhythmic drugs with effects that include Na channel blockade slow conduction velocity (e.g. flecainide, propafenone, lidocaine, mexiletine, procainamide, quinidine, amiodarone). Repolarisation is primarily mediated via activation of K^+ currents. Phase 1, a phase of brief, limited rapid repolarisation due to the transient outward current, I_{to} in the ventricles, is followed by Phase 2, a plateau phase that is unique amongst excitable cells and marks the phase of calcium entry into the cell. Phase 3 is the phase of rapid repolarisation mediated by delayed rectifier potassium (I_{kr}) currents that return the membrane potential to the resting potential (Phase 4).[14,15]

Specialised 'pacemaker' cells of the sinus and AV nodal tissue are capable of spontaneous depolarisation with

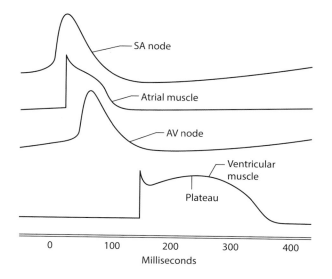

Figure 37.2 Actions potentials of the various regions in the cardiac conduction system. The sino-atrial (SA) and atrio-ventricular (AV) nodes have Ca^{++}-mediated slow action potentials whilst those in the atrial and ventricular muscle have Na^+-mediated fast action potentials.

regular periodicity.[16] Their action potential is qualitatively different from ventricular and atrial myocytes. The membrane potential at the onset of Phase 4 is less negative (−50 to −65 mV) and undergoes slow diastolic depolarisation mediated by a sodium current termed the funny current (I_f). The rate of depolarisation in Phase 0 is much slower than that in the working myocardial cells and carried primarily by the slow Ca^{++} currents that are sensitive to vagal stimulation (acetylcholine), adrenergic stimulation, adenosine and non-dihydropyridine calcium blockers. Cells in the His–Purkinje system can also show Phase 4 depolarisation.

Cell-to-cell conduction of the cardiac action potential is facilitated by gap junctions that are concentrated at the end of cells and provide low resistance channels allowing free flow of positive between cardiomyocytes. Whilst many proteins are involved, key to this are connexins, which aggregate into connexons forming pores between cells.[17]

A key feature of cardiomyocytes is the presence of a refractory period, which is the interval after depolarisation, during which the cardiac cell is resistant to re-excitation. During the absolute refractory period it cannot be re-excited. This is followed by a relative refractory period during which an early stimulus can provoke an action potential with a slower Phase 0 and hence, slowed conduction. This interaction between premature stimulation and conduction slowing is important in the genesis of re-entrant arrhythmias.

Antiarrhythmic medications are designed to target ion channels to slow conduction, prolong repolarisation or both.[18,19] Most have actions on more than one current.

Many genetic arrhythmia and sudden death syndromes occur as a consequence of abnormalities in ion channels and have provided insight into the understanding of cellular EP. Most Long QT Syndromes (LQTS) result from mutations causing loss of function of potassium channels or gain of function of sodium channels.[20,21] The common phenotype is prolongation of the QT interval with susceptibility to a characteristic type of polymorphic VT termed Torsade de Pointes VT that often leads to syncope (if self-terminating) or sudden death (if it degenerates to VF).

The Brugada syndrome is characterised by variable presence of ST elevation in the precordial leads V1 to V3 and propensity for sudden cardiac death due to polymorphic VT.[22,23] Approximately, 20%–30% of patients have mutations in a sodium channel gene (SCN5A) causing decreased sodium channel activity. In patients with latent forms of the disease, administration of a sodium channel blocker such as procainamide, flecanide or ajmaline can provoke the typical ST segment changes.[24]

37.5 Disorders of impulse formation and conduction

37.5.1 Sinus node dysfunction

Sinus node dysfunction can result from idiopathic degenerative changes, ischemia or infarction, infiltrative diseases, as well as fibrosis and degeneration with age or atrial fibrillation.[25,26] In addition, extrinsic factors such as autonomic stimulation, drugs, hypoxia and metabolic changes influence impulse generation and conduction of the impulse from sinus node cells to surrounding atrial myocytes. Bradyarrhythmias can be due to failure of impulse formation or failure of conduction from sinus node cells to atrial cells (exit block).

Similar to the atrio-ventricular node, sino-atrial exit block can display varying degrees of block that include Mobitz type I or II patterns. Overdrive suppression of the sinus node is often the mechanism of sinus pauses after periods of atrial tachy-arrhythmias.

Rarer sinus pathologies include 'atrial quiescence or standstill' in which the sinus node (as well as the rest of the atria in severe cases) has no spontaneous rhythm. Autonomic influences on the sinus node can result in sinus arrhythmia, vagally mediated sinus slowing or arrest as is commonly seen in neutrally mediated syncope.

37.5.2 Atrio-ventricular block

AV block is defined as a delay or interruption of AV conduction.[27] The conduction disturbance can be transient or permanent. Based on electrocardiogram (ECG) characteristics, AV block is classified as first, second or third degree. AV block can occur at various levels: within the AVN above the His bundle (supra-His), within the His bundle (intra-His) or below the bundle of His (infra-his). First degree and type I second degree (Wenckebach) AV block usually indicates block in the AVN. Type II second degree AV block characterised by a fixed PR interval before and after blocked beats is usually associated with widened QRS complexes and commonly indicates block within or below the His bundle. Progression to complete AV block is common. AV conduction in a 2:1 pattern can be due to block in the AVN or Purkinje system, with a wide QRS being more concerning for disease in the Purkinje system. The term 'paroxysmal high grade AV block' is used to denote two or more non-conducted sinus P waves but with resumption of conducted beats. In the setting of atrial fibrillation or flutter, a prolonged RR interval with pauses > 5 seconds, is often due to advanced second degree AV block. Third degree AV block is defined as the absence of AV conduction. When it occurs at the level of the AVN above the His, QRS complexes are usually narrow and the escape rhythm is 40–60 bpm and tends to be reliable. However, wide QRS escape rates indicate block at or below the His bundle and can be unpredictable, resulting in syncope or sudden death. In the case of atrial fibrillation, complete AV block is manifested as regularised slow ventricular rate.

Although ECG features are helpful in defining levels of AV block, they are not always reliable and occasionally an electrophysiological study is necessary. Clinical manoeuvres are sometimes helpful in determination of site of block; exercise and atropine increase AV conduction in supra-His block whilst manoeuvres that slow the atria rate such as carotid massage improve His–Purkinje conduction by allowing recovery from refractoriness.

It is important to recognise potentially reversible causes of AV block. Important examples include acute myocarditis (e.g. Lyme disease), drug toxicity, hypoxia and vagotonia. AV block related to these situations usually resolves with specific treatment of the primary condition, and although temporary pacing may be necessary, permanent cardiac pacing can often be avoided.

37.5.3 Bundle branch block

Delayed or blocked conduction in the RRBs or left bundle branches (LBBs) can manifest as widened QRS complex with typical pattern of delayed activation of the corresponding ventricle. The prevalence of bundle branch block increases with age; RBB is more common and not necessarily reflective of structural heart disease.

Beyond structural abnormalities such as degenerative disease, ischemia and iatrogenic causes, there are functional mechanisms for conduction defects in the bundle branches. These include Phase 3 aberration, Phase 4 aberration (deceleration dependent) and retrograde invasion.[28] *Phase 3 aberration* occurs when the conducted activation wave encounters a bundle branch that is refractory. It can be a physiological phenomenon when a long R–R interval prolongs the action potential duration of the bundle branch, and the next conducted excitation wavefront is sufficiently early to encounter the refractory period of the bundle branch, conducting with bundle branch block. This process referred to as the Ashman phenomenon can sometimes be observed at the initiation of paroxysmal supraventricular tachycardias or in atrial fibrillation with long and short R–R intervals. *Acceleration-dependent block* is Phase 3 block that results from R–R intervals which are short enough to encroach on the refractoriness of the bundle branch. *Phase 4 aberration* occurs after prolonged pause. During such a pause (e.g. in second degree AV block), the Purkinje fibres can slowly depolarise without generating an action potential. As they depolarise, progressively more Na channels become inactive and unavailable, resulting in conduction block.

When physiologic bundle branch block occurs, it may be maintained by concealed conduction *retrograde into the bundle branch*. This is often seen at the onset of an SVT when aberrant conduction (e.g. left bundle branch block [LBBB]) of the first beat may be due to Phase 3 block. The next beat is conducted by the non-refractory bundle (right bundle, in the example) and once the activation wave reaches the LV, it propagates into the left bundle rendering it refractory to the next antegrade impulse. This process can perpetuate until a premature ventricular beat causes a compensatory pause and 'resets' the system to normalise the QRS.

Isolated LBBB tends to be associated with structural heart disease and warrants evaluation of cardiac function and structure. In addition, LBBB can lead to worsening LV function, heart failure symptoms and mitral regurgitation caused by dysynchronous contraction of the ventricle. Bifascicular block usually refers to a combination of RBBB with block of a segment (commonly referred to as a fascicle) of the left bundle Purkinje system. This usually indicates His Purkinje system disease and a risk of AV block. In asymptomatic patients, the risk of progression is less than 1% per year whereas in patients with syncope, the annual risk is estimated to be 5%–10% and a permanent pacemaker is warranted.[29]

37.6 Mechanism of tachyarrhythmias

Tachyarrhythmias are generally produced by one of three mechanisms: enhanced automaticity, triggered activity, or re-entry.[28,30]

Enhanced automaticity refers to the accelerated generation of an action potential by either normal pacemaker tissue or by abnormal myocardium.[31] Purkinje fibres surviving myocardial infarction appear to be more sensitive to the positive chronotropic effects of catecholamines than normal Purkinje fibres, perhaps because of denervation supersensitivity. Enhanced automaticity is the likely mechanism of the accelerated idioventricular rhythms that occur during the acute phase of myocardial infarction and reperfusion.

Abnormal automaticity can arise from myocytes from hypertrophied and failing hearts have been shown to manifest spontaneous diastolic depolarisation and enhanced pacemaker currents, suggesting that abnormal automaticity may contribute to the occurrence of some arrhythmias in heart failure and LV hypertrophy. In addition, myocardial stretch increases automaticity and may promote arrhythmias in acute heart failure.

Triggered activity describes impulse initiation in cardiac fibres that is dependent on after-depolarisations that follow the upstroke of an action potential (Figure 37.3).[28] Early after depolarisations (EADs) occur during Phase 2 or 3 of repolarisation of the action potential whereas delayed (DADs) occur after completion of repolarisation. Either can potentially elicit action potentials manifest as premature beats or tachycardia.

Early after-depolarisations are the proposed mechanism for torsade de Pointes VT that is the hallmark of congenital or acquired long QT syndrome (see above). This arrhythmia is provoked by bradycardia, hypokalemia and hypomagnesemia, and drugs that affect the repolarisation currents. Delayed after-depolarisations are related to calcium overloading of cells and are the proposed mechanism of arrhythmias in digitalis toxicity, some idiopathic outflow tract VTs, and catecholaminergic polymorphic VT due to mutations that alter cellular calcium handling.

Re-entry is probably the most common and best-defined arrhythmia mechanism in the human heart, re-entrant tachycardias are due to repetitive propagation of an excitatory wave around a fixed anatomical or a functional barrier, returning to its site of origin to reactivate that site (Figure 37.4). A re-entrant circuit usually has an area of slow conduction and re-entry is initiated by a premature beat that cause unidirectional block in a part of the circuit. AVN-dependent supraventricular tachycardias such as AV nodal re-entrant tachycardia, atrio-ventricular reciprocating tachycardias due to accessory pathways are typical examples of large re-entry circuits (macro-re-entry). Other examples include common right atrial flutter that involves a circuit revolving along the tricuspid valve annulus.

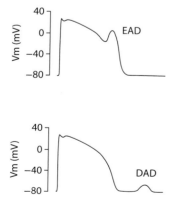

Figure 37.3 Types of after-depolarisation that lead to triggered automaticity. The top panel shows an early after depolarisation (EAD) that originates from Phase 3 of the action potential. The bottom panel shows a delayed after depolarisation (DAD) that occurs during Phase 4.

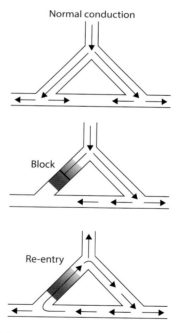

Figure 37.4 Schematic of mechanism of re-entry around an area of conduction block that may be anatomical or function (triangular dark area in centre of cartoon). In the top panel, a normally conducted beat travels bidirectionally around the area of block and collides without re-entry. The middle panel shows the formation of unidirectional block (usually due to a premature beat causing refractoriness) in one limb of the re-entrant circuit. The impulse that travels in the conducting limb can re-enter the circuit if there is sufficient conduction delay to allow recovery of conduction in the blocked limb (bottom panel).

Most infarct-related monomorphic VT result from re-entry that involves infarct scars with viable strands of muscle that may serve as slowly conducting channels. Re-entrant VT can also be due to re-entry in the Purkinje system involving the bundle branches or fascicles of the conduction system.

37.7 Common tachyarrhythmias

37.7.1 Supraventricular arrhythmias that are not AVN dependent

Atrial Flutter, atrial tachycardias and atrial fibrillation represent arrhythmias are not dependent on the AVN for their initiation or propagation. Interventions that slow conduction in the AVN reduce the ventricular rate without terminating the arrhythmia. Focal atrial tachycardias, occasionally respond to adenosine or calcium/beta-adrenergic blockade with termination of the arrhythmia.

Classical right atrial flutter (AFL) is due to re-entry revolving along the tricuspid annulus that results in continuous atrial activation seen on the surface electrocardiogram as a saw-tooth pattern with atrial rates typically between 260 and 320 beats per minute. The re-entrant wave-front can propagate in a counterclockwise (more common) or clockwise direction but both forms utilise the cavo-tricuspid isthmus (CTI) as common channel. Pacing techniques to continuously reset the arrhythmia (entrainment) can be helpful to confirm the mechanism of the tachycardia as well as help in choosing the site of ablation. Identifying the CTI-dependent nature of the flutter is important as it defines a site for ablation.[32-34]

Atrial tachycardias may be focal or re-entrant.[35] Focal tachycardias are common in patients without known atrial disease, whilst re-entrant tachycardia generally follow prior cardiac surgery, previous atrial ablation or spontaneous atrial fibrosis.

Atrial fibrillation commonly originates in the LA with passive activation of the RA, although occasionally the RA drives atrial fibrillation. Paroxysmal AF, which starts and stops spontaneously, is often mediated by focal triggers (most commonly, located around the pulmonary veins). Persistent atrial fibrillation is usually associated significant electrical and anatomic changes in the atria that provide a substrate for continued fibrillation (typically defined as lasting beyond 7 days and requiring specific interventions such as antiarrhythmic drugs or external cardioversion for conversion to sinus rhythm).[36,37]

37.7.2 AVN-dependent SVTs

The AVN forms a part of the re-entrant circuit in atrio-ventricular nodal re-entrant tachycardia (AVNRT) and atrio-ventricular reciprocating tachycardias (AVRT) mediated by accessory pathways. These AVN-dependent arrhythmias, therefore, terminate with drugs or manoeuvre that block AVN conduction.

AVNRT is the dominant cause of paroxysmal sustained regular tachycardia in adults and can vary widely in rate. The re-entrant circuit in 'typical' AVNRT involves antegrade conduction over the 'slow' pathway (inferior lobe of the AVN) and retrograde conduction from the compact node to the atrium (which comprises the 'fast' pathway). 'Atypical' forms occur where this relationship is reversed. In typical AVNRT, P waves occurs simultaneously or immediately after the QRS. When a P wave is visible, its axis is directed superiorly as the atria are activated from the region of the coronary sinus. The onset of the arrhythmia is often preceded by a premature beat and some delay in AV nodal conduction suggesting that the premature beat encountered refractoriness in the fast pathway but conducted through the slow pathway to initiate re-entry. The bundle of His and the ventricles are not an integral part of the circuit. Pacing manoeuvres from the ventricle exploit this relationship to distinguish this arrhythmia from those due to SVTs mediated by accessory pathways. Catheter ablation targeting the slow pathway of the AVN is usually curative.

Atrio-ventricular reciprocating tachycardias are mediated by atrio-ventricular accessory pathways (AP). The most common forms are comprised of strands of muscle fibres that course across the AV groove connecting atrium and ventricles. They may conduct in only one direction, or in both directions. APs that conduct from atrium to ventricle often produce ventricular pre-excitation denoted by a short PR interval and delta wave on the surface ECG. The extent of pre-excitation and hence the ECG features, vary depending on the relative fusion between conduction through the AVN and the pathway. Maximal pre-excitation is evident during AV block. Many accessory pathways conduct only in the retrograde direction (from ventricle to atrium). An AP that can only conduct from ventricle to atrium is labelled as 'concealed' because its presence is not apparent in sinus rhythm (i.e. no delta wave).

The term Wolf Parkinson White syndrome applies to manifest pre-excitation in patients with SVT. Apart from their role in SVTs, manifest accessory pathways are important for a small but finite risk of triggering sudden death due to rapid conduction of atrial fibrillation to the ventricles. This risk is higher in patients with frank symptoms of SVT or syncope. In the asymptomatic patient, the estimated risk is <0.1%.[38] The refractory period of the accessory pathway (<250 ms) and shortest RR interval during atrial fibrillation (<230 ms) are associated with increased risk.[39]

The most common arrhythmia associated with accessory pathways is a narrow complex SVT designated orthodromic re-entry in which the circulating wavefront activates the ventricles utilising the normal AVN-His Purkinje system and conducts back to the atrium over the AP to complete the circuit. P waves are present following the QRS complexes. The ventricles are integral to the circuit, a fact that is exploited in the EP laboratory with diagnostic ventricular pacing manoeuvres to distinguish it from AVNRT. Ventricular stimulation timed during refractoriness of the His bundle is capable of resetting atrial activation.

A less common arrhythmia in patients with manifest pre-excitation is anti-dromic AVRT. In this arrhythmia, antegrade activation of the ventricles occurs via the accessory pathway and retrograde activation of the atria is via the AVN. The QRS is wide and cannot be distinguished from ventricular tachycardia. Other forms of pre-excited tachycardias include those produced by any atrial arrhythmia that conducts to the ventricle predominantly via the AP.

There are a variety of other, rare types of accessory pathways that may connect specialised conduction tissue to other regions of the conduction system or myocardium.[40] A Mahaim fibre refers to an atrio-fascicular fibre between the RA and right bundle that usually causes anti-dromic tachycardia with an LBBB pattern. Fasciculo-ventricular pathways produce ventricular pre-excitation on ECG but do not cause arrhythmias.

37.7.3 Ventricular arrhythmias

Ventricular arrhythmias arise below the His bundle and typically demonstrate a wide QRS with a QRS duration in excess of 120 ms. The ECG offers clues to its mechanism. *Monomorphic VT* has the same QRS morphology from beat to beat and suggests that the ventricles are activated in a similar sequence with each tachycardia beat. These arrhythmias arise from a focal area or a stable re-entrant circuit. In patients with known structural heart disease, the source for monomorphic VT is often scar from prior infarction, surgery or replacement fibrosis related to non-ischemic cardiomyopathies. A minority of monomorphic VTs (8%–10%) in patients with structural heart disease may involve the Purkinje fibres or the bundle branches. Bundle branch re-entry involving antegrade conduction down one (usually the RBB) and retrograde through the other (usually the LBB) typically occur in patients with structural heard disease and delayed interventricular conduction.[41,42]

Polymorphic VT has a continuously changing QRS morphology and does not require a stable arrhythmia substrate. It often degenerates to ventricular fibrillation and usually results in syncope or sudden death. In patients with structural heart disease, polymorphic VT is commonly provoked by acute ischemia or infarction, electrolyte disturbances or drug toxicity. When no structural heart disease is identified, genetic arrhythmia syndromes such as the Long QT syndrome or Brugada syndrome should be considered.

Most sustained ventricular arrhythmias are associated with a risk of sudden cardiac death and warrants consideration of an implantable defibrillator. In contrast, monomorphic VT that occur in the absence of structural heart disease, termed 'idiopathic VT' is rarely life threatening. The diagnosis of idiopathic VT is one of exclusion, and it is important to exclude early cardiomyopathies such as arrhythmogenic RV cardiomyopathy. The presence of baseline abnormalities on the ECG is often a clue to underlying heart disease, and any suspicion should prompt the use of additional imaging studies such as magnetic resonance imaging of the heart with gadolinium contrast to exclude scar or inflammation.

Most idiopathic ventricular arrhythmias present as monomorphic PVCs with intermittent bursts of repetitive VT with a QRS morphology similar to the PVCs. The RV outflow tract is the most common source and show typical morphological features of LBBB with inferiorly directed QRS axis. Less commonly, the LV outflow tract musculature that extends into the aortic root in close proximity to the aortic valve cusps may generate idiopathic VT. The papillary muscles of the left and less frequently, RV are the next most common sites. A specific VT that originates from re-entry in or near the fascicles of the left bundle is termed Belhassen's VT. It most commonly has a RBBB superior axis QRS morphology. This VT is unusual in that it can be terminated by intravenous verapamil.[43]

37.8 Intracardiac electrophysiological study (EP study)

EP studies aim to determine the presence and specific type of cardiac arrhythmia. Tachyarrhythmias are induced and terminated by programmed electrical stimulation, occasionally with the need for cardioversion or defibrillation. The AV conduction system and sinus node can also be assessed. An EP study is frequently combined with interventional procedures such as ablation or implantation of a defibrillator or pacemaker, and its format is thus, tailored to the clinical indication. The role of an EP study as a purely diagnostic test is limited to patients with syncope of unknown origin, wide complex tachycardias when the diagnosis remains uncertain and for risk stratification for sudden death in the presence of mild LV dysfunction (LVEF > 35%).

Nearly every cardiac structure can be a source of arrhythmia, and therefore all four cardiac chambers may require access. Recording from multi-electrode catheters in the RA, RV, at the His bundle region and in the coronary sinus is commonly employed and provides clear evidence of the sequence and timing of atrial and ventricular activation during induced arrhythmias. For ablation, access to the LA or LV can be achieved via a trans-septal approach or retrograde to the aortic root and LV. In some patients, arrhythmia foci reside closer to the epicardial surface. Percutaneous access to the pericardial surface is possible in the majority of patients in the absence of previous cardiac surgery of pericardial inflammation.[44]

37.8.1 Signal acquisition

Intra-cardiac recordings require stable connections that are shielded against electrical noise, and patient-isolated signal amplifiers with band pass filtering to improve signal-to-noise ratio. In unipolar recordings, one pole is in contact with the tissue whose electrical activity is being recorded and the second is a distant indifferent electrode. This distant electrode may be an electrode in the IVC, a surface electrode or Wilson's central terminal (the sum of the extremity electrodes). Conversely, bipolar recordings have both electrode poles in contact with the tissue and adjacent to each other separated by a few millimetres. Unipolar recordings more accurately represent the timing of local activation but are fraught with the detection of far-field signals. Since extracellular potential decreases inversely with the square of the distance from a point source, far-field events generate relatively low amplitude signals compared to electrogram components generated by near-field sources in unipolar recordings.

Bipolar recording reduce far-field signals, and hence, are more widely employed in mapping. Given the differences in recording techniques, different patterns are expected from bipolar and unipolar recordings of the same physiologic signal.

37.8.2 Baseline intervals

In sinus rhythm, conduction intervals are helpful to determine atrio-ventricular conduction, site of conduction block if present and whether ventricular pre-excitation is present (Figures 37.5 and 37.6).

Atrio-His (AH) interval: This interval is measured on from the catheter at the His bundle region at the anterior tricuspid annulus and is the interval from the earliest rapid deflection of the atrial recording (activation of the lowest part of the RA) to the earliest onset of the His bundle deflection. This interval reflects the time for conduction through the AVN and normally ranges from 50 to 120 ms. Short AH intervals may be seen in increased sympathetic tone. Long AH intervals are most commonly due to slow AVN conduction from medications, increased vagal tone, or intrinsic disease of the atrio-ventricular node (Figure 37.5).

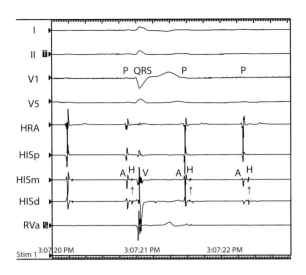

Figure 37.6 Intra-cardiac recording during spontaneous atrio-ventricular (AV) block showing block below the bundle of His. Tracing from top to bottom show surface electrocardiograms (ECGs) leads I, II, V1 and V5; bipolar recordings of high right atrium (HRA), His proximal, mid and distal; and right ventricular apex (RVa). The PR interval during the conducted beat is normal. There is abrupt loss of AV conduction for the subsequent two atrial beats (A) due to block below the His (H).

His bundle electrogram duration: This duration reflects conduction through the short length of compact His bundle that penetrates the fibrous septum. This interval is normally short (15–25 ms). His bundle disease manifests as fractionation, prolongation or splitting of the His bundle potential.

HV interval: This interval is measured from the earliest onset of the His bundle deflection to the earliest registered surface or intra-cardiac ventricular activation and reflects conduction time through the His–Purkinje system. Unlike the AVN, the His–Purkinje system is far less influenced by the autonomic nervous system, and the range in normal subjects is narrow (35–55 ms). A prolonged HV interval is consistent with diseased Purkinje system with slowed conduction. In the setting of LBBB with normal right bundle conduction the HV interval may be up to 65 ms. Longer HV intervals may reflect a risk of high grade AV block and warrants pacemaker therapy if symptoms of bradyarrhythmia are present. A short HV interval suggests one of two situations: ventricular pre-excitation via an AV bypass tract or a late premature ventricular beat. A spurious short HV interval is due to the recording of a RBB potential rather than a His potential.

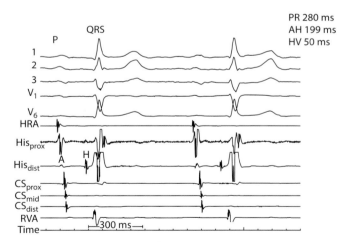

Figure 37.5 Intra-cardiac recordings during electrophysiology (EP) study. Tracings from top to bottom show surface electrocardiogram (ECG) leads I, II, III, V1 and V6; bipolar recordings from the high right atrium (HRA), His proximal and distal, coronary sinus (CS) proximal, mid and distal and right ventricular apex (RVa). There is first degree atrio-ventricular (AV) block with a PR interval of 280 ms due to prolongation of the AH interval to 199 ms with normal HV interval of 50 ms.

37.8.3 Induction of arrhythmias

In the absence of an ongoing arrhythmia, it is important to induce the suspected arrhythmia under controlled conditions to study its mechanism and origin. Programmed stimulation is useful for induction and termination of re-entrant arrhythmias, for studying atrio-ventricular conduction patterns and for diagnosis of specific arrhythmias.

For induction of arrhythmias, the chamber of interest is paced at a steady rate to stabilise its refractoriness and premature impulse are inserted at progressively shorter intervals so as to induce unidirectional block and re-entry. Often, adrenergic stimulation may be required to induce and maintain an arrhythmia for further evaluation. Once an arrhythmia is induced, routes of atrio- ventricular activation, dependence on His–Purkinje activation and responses to atrial and ventricular extra-stimulation help to differentiate the various arrhythmia mechanisms. In re-entrant arrhythmias, pacing from within a re-entrant circuit provides valuable clue as to potential targets for ablation to prevent re-entry.

Automatic arrhythmias are often induced by adrenergic stimulation using isoproterenol or epinephrine. Occasional pacing at a faster rate for brief periods of time (burst pacing) can induce these arrhythmias.

37.8.4 Mapping of arrhythmias

Once an arrhythmia is induced, its activation pattern can be discerned by simultaneous recording from multipolar catheters placed in the cardiac chambers or coronary sinus. A number of computerised mapping systems that incorporate electrical information on anatomy are available. These electro-anatomic mapping systems allow for three-dimensional reconstruction of heart chambers that incorporate voltage and activation-time criteria as well as non-fluoroscopic localisation of electrophysiological catheters within the heart. Newer multi-pronged, multi-polar catheters with smaller inter-electrode spacing have greater signal resolution and hence, are more sensitive for the identification of abnormal electrograms compared to standard ablation catheters. Automated multi-point acquisition with these catheters permit fast, high-resolution mapping to identify abnormal tissue that typically demonstrate low voltages, fractionation and late potentials. The judicious use of unipolar and bipolar voltage maps enable the identification of border zones and channels within scars.[45]

Electro-anatomic mapping systems also allow for integration of real-time intra-cardiac ultrasound images, fluoroscopy and previously acquired magnetic resonance imaging (MRI) or computer tomography (CT). Contrast enhanced MRI may be used to identify VT substrate and areas that are likely to contain critical isthmus sites prior to extensive mapping.

37.9 Catheter ablation

Once an arrhythmia is identified, controlled destruction of myocardial tissue from which it arises can prevent recurrence. Radiofrequency (RF) current remains the most convenient form of energy to effect localised tissue necrosis.[46,47] RF generators in use in the EP labs produce alternating-current energy between 300 and 750 kHz delivered in a unipolar fashion through the tip electrode of the mapping catheter positioned at the target site with the circuit completed by an indifferent cutaneous electrode patch. This high frequency current results in both resistive heating of the area of myocardium directly in contact as well as conductive heating of adjacent areas. Tissue necrosis occurs at temperatures that exceed 50°. Unfortunately, development of high temperatures at the electrode-tissue interface can lead to coagulum of denatured tissue proteins on the catheter tip that increase resistance and limit delivery of RF delivery to deeper tissue. This can be overcome by cooling the tip of the catheter with flow of saline. Such irrigated tip catheters often allow myocardial lesions 3–8 mm in depth depending on the energy, contact force and duration of delivery.

Cryothermal energy is another convenient form of energy source for ablation and has the advantage of reversibility of lesions if delivery is terminated early in the course of the application. There is higher rate of recovery of tissue viability compared to RF energy leading to arrhythmia recurrence. However, in ablation where the risk of AV block is high and in special populations such as in children, cryoablation is preferred to RF energy.

The efficacy and risks of ablation vary with the underlying heart disease, and type and location of arrhythmia. Efficacy is >90% for treatment of common paroxysmal supraventricular tachycardias. Lower for ventricular arrhythmias and atrial fibrillation. Risks include those of heart catheterisation related to vascular access, trans-septal puncture, left heart catheterisation, including perforation with tamponade and thromboembolism. Of 1676 procedures at our centre over a 2-year period, rates of major complications differed between procedure types, ranging from 0.8% for supraventricular tachycardia, 3.4% for idiopathic VT, 5.2% for AF and 6.0% for VT associated with structural heart disease.[48]

37.10 Summary

Clinical cardiac EP merges a detailed knowledge of cardiac anatomy, basic EP and pathophysiology. In addition, a working knowledge of electronics, signal processing and biophysics of energy sources is essential. Rapid advances in the field have made it possible for most arrhythmias to be effectively treated with ablation techniques or implantable devices.

References

1. Asirvatham SJ. Correlative anatomy and electrophysiology for the interventional electrophysiologist: Right atrial flutter. *J Cardiovasc Electrophysiol* 2009; 20(1): 113–22.
2. Macedo PG et al. Correlative anatomy for the electrophysiologist: Ablation for atrial fibrillation. Part I: Pulmonary vein ostia, superior vena cava, vein of Marshall. *J Cardiovasc Electrophysiol* 2010; 21(6): 721–30.
3. Macedo PG et al. Correlative anatomy for the electrophysiologist: Ablation for atrial fibrillation. Part II: Regional anatomy of the atria and relevance to damage

of adjacent structures during AF ablation. *J Cardiovasc Electrophysiol* 2010; 21(7): 829–36.

4. Hwang C et al. Vein of Marshall cannulation for the analysis of electrical activity in patients with focal atrial fibrillation. *Circulation* 2000; 101(13): 1503–05.

5. Kim DT et al. The ligament of Marshall: A structural analysis in human hearts with implications for atrial arrhythmias. *J Am Coll Cardiol* 2000; 36(4): 1324–27.

6. Habib A et al. The anatomy of the coronary sinus venous system for the cardiac electrophysiologist. *Europace* 2009; (11 Suppl 5): v15–21.

7. Haddad F et al. Right ventricular function in cardiovascular disease, part I: Anatomy, physiology, aging, and functional assessment of the right ventricle. *Circulation* 2008; 117(11): 1436–48.

8. Asirvatham SJ. Correlative anatomy for the invasive electrophysiologist: Outflow tract and supravalvar arrhythmia. *J Cardiovasc Electrophysiol* 2009; 20(8): 955–68.

9. Piers SR et al. CMR-based identification of critical isthmus sites of ischemic and nonischemic ventricular tachycardia. *JACC Cardiovasc Imaging* 2014; 7(8): 774–84.

10. Monfredi O et al. The anatomy and physiology of the sinoatrial node – A contemporary review. *Pacing Clin Electrophysiol* 2010; 33(11): 1392–406.

11. Park DS, and Fishman GI. The cardiac conduction system. *Circulation* 2011; 123(8): 904–15.

12. Wellens HJJ et al. *The Conduction System of the Heart: Structure, Function, and Clinical Implications*. Philadelphia: Lea & Febiger, 1976, p. xii, 708.

13. Tawara S et al. *Conduction System of the Mammalian Heart: An Anatomico-Histological Study of the Atrioventricular Bundle and the Purkinje Fibers*. London, Hackensack: Imperial College Press, World Scientific Publishing Company, 2000, p. 256. Online resource.

14. Grant AO. Cardiac ion channels. *Circ Arrhythm Electrophysiol* 2009; 2(2): 185–94.

15. Whalley DW et al. Basic concepts in cellular cardiac electrophysiology: Part I: Ion channels, membrane currents, and the action potential. *Pacing Clin Electrophysiol* 1995; 18(8): 1556–74.

16. Huizinga JD. *Pacemaker Activity and Intercellular Communication*. Boca Raton: CRC Press, 1995, p. 345.

17. Saffitz JE et al. Connexin expression and turnover: Implications for cardiac excitability. *Circ Res* 2000; 86(7): 723–28.

18. Singla S et al. Review of contemporary antiarrhythmic drug therapy for maintenance of sinus rhythm in atrial fibrillation. *J Cardiovasc Pharmacol Ther* 2012; 17(1): 12–20.

19. Kowey PR. Pharmacological effects of antiarrhythmic drugs. Review and update. *Arch Intern Med* 1998; 158(4): 325–32.

20. Goldenberg I, and Moss AJ. Long QT syndrome. *J Am Coll Cardiol* 2008; 51(24): 2291–300.

21. Abrams DJ, and Macrae CA. Long QT syndrome. *Circulation* 2014; 129(14): 1524–29.

22. Sheikh AS, and Ranjan K. Brugada syndrome: A review of the literature. *Clin Med* 2014; 14(5): 482–89.

23. Postema PG et al. Drugs and Brugada syndrome patients: Review of the literature, recommendations, and an up-to-date website (http://www.brugadadrugs.org). *Heart Rhythm* 2009; 6(9): 1335–41.

24. Chung EH et al. Brugada-type patterns are easily observed in high precordial lead ECGs in collegiate athletes. *J Electrocardiol* 2014; 47(1): 1–6.

25. Nof E et al. Genetics and sinus node dysfunction. *J Atr Fibrillation* 2009; 1(6): 328–36.

26. Yeh YH et al. Funny current downregulation and sinus node dysfunction associated with atrial tachyarrhythmia: A molecular basis for tachycardia-bradycardia syndrome. *Circulation* 2009; 119(12): 1576–85.

27. Epstein AE et al. 2012 ACCF/AHA/HRS focused update incorporated into the ACCF/AHA/HRS 2008 guidelines for device-based therapy of cardiac rhythm abnormalities: A report of the American College of Cardiology Foundation/American Heart Association Task Force on Practice Guidelines and the Heart Rhythm Society. *J Am Coll Cardiol* 2013; 61(3): e6–75.

28. Issa ZF et al. *Clinical Arrhythmology and Electrophysiology a Companion to Braunwald's Heart Disease*, 2nd Edition. Philadelphia, PA: Elsevier/Saunders, 2012, p. xiii, 726.

29. McAnulty JH et al. Natural history of "high-risk" bundle-branch block: Final report of a prospective study. *N Engl J Med* 1982; 307(3): 137–43.

30. Zipes DP, and Jalife J. *Cardiac Electrophysiology and Arrhythmias*. New York: Grune & Stratton, 1985, p. xxxiii, 567.

31. Rubenstein DS, and Lipsius SL. Mechanisms of automaticity in subsidiary pacemakers from cat right atrium. *Circ Res* 1989; 64(4): 648–57.

32. Bencsik G. Novel strategies in the ablation of typical atrial flutter: Role of intracardiac echocardiography. *Curr Cardiol Rev* 2015; 11(2): 127–33.

33. Tai CT, and Chen SA. Cavotricuspid isthmus: Anatomy, electrophysiology, and long-term outcome of radiofrequency ablation. *Pacing Clin Electrophysiol* 2009; 32(12): 1591–95.

34. Sawhney NS et al. Diagnosis and management of typical atrial flutter. *Cardiol Clin* 2009; 27(1): 55–67, viii.

35. Waldo AL. Mechanisms of atrial fibrillation, atrial flutter, and ectopic atrial tachycardia--a brief review. *Circulation* 1987; 75(4 Pt 2): III37–III40.

36. Andrade JG et al. Efficacy and safety of cryoballoon ablation for atrial fibrillation: A systematic review of published studies. *Heart Rhythm* 2011; 8(9): 1444–51.

37. Calkins H et al. 2012 HRS/EHRA/ECAS expert consensus statement on catheter and surgical ablation of atrial fibrillation: recommendations for patient selection, procedural techniques, patient management and follow-up, definitions, endpoints, and research trial design: A report of the Heart Rhythm Society (HRS) Task Force on Catheter and Surgical Ablation of Atrial Fibrillation. Developed in partnership with the European Heart Rhythm Association (EHRA), a registered branch of the European Society of Cardiology (ESC) and the European Cardiac Arrhythmia Society (ECAS); and in collaboration with the American College of Cardiology (ACC), American Heart Association (AHA), the Asia Pacific Heart Rhythm Society (APHRS), and the Society of Thoracic Surgeons (STS). Endorsed by the governing bodies of the American College of Cardiology Foundation, the American Heart Association, the European Cardiac Arrhythmia Society, the European Heart Rhythm Association, the Society of

Thoracic Surgeons, the Asia Pacific Heart Rhythm Society, and the Heart Rhythm Society. *Heart Rhythm* 2012; 9(4): 632–696 e21.

38. Pediatric et al. PACES/HRS expert consensus statement on the management of the asymptomatic young patient with a Wolff-Parkinson-White (WPW, ventricular preexcitation) electrocardiographic pattern: Developed in partnership between the Pediatric and Congenital Electrophysiology Society (PACES) and the Heart Rhythm Society (HRS). Endorsed by the governing bodies of PACES, HRS, the American College of Cardiology Foundation (ACCF), the American Heart Association (AHA), the American Academy of Pediatrics (AAP), and the Canadian Heart Rhythm Society (CHRS). *Heart Rhythm* 2012; 9(6): 1006–24.

39. Santinelli V et al. Asymptomatic ventricular preexcitation: A long-term prospective follow-up study of 293 adult patients. *Circ Arrhythm Electrophysiol* 2009; 2(2): 102–07.

40. Tchou P et al. Atriofascicular connection or a nodoventricular Mahaim fiber? Electrophysiologic elucidation of the pathway and associated reentrant circuit. *Circulation* 1988; 77(4): 837–48.

41. Blanck Z et al. Bundle branch reentrant ventricular tachycardia: Cumulative experience in 48 patients. *J Cardiovasc Electrophysiol* 1993; 4(3): 253–62.

42. Machino T et al. Three-dimensional visualization of the entire reentrant circuit of bundle branch reentrant tachycardia. *Heart Rhythm* 2013; 10(3): 459–60.

43. Francis J et al. Idiopathic fascicular ventricular tachycardia. *Indian Pacing Electrophysiol J* 2004; 4(3): 98–103.

44. Kumar S et al. "Needle-in-needle" epicardial access: Preliminary observations with a modified technique for facilitating epicardial interventional procedures. *Heart Rhythm* 2015; 12(7): 1691–97.

45. Chopra N et al. Relation of the unipolar low-voltage penumbra surrounding the endocardial low-voltage scar to ventricular tachycardia circuit sites and ablation outcomes in ischemic cardiomyopathy. *J Cardiovasc Electrophysiol* 2014; 25(6): 602–08.

46. Haines DE et al. Electrode radius predicts lesion radius during radiofrequency energy heating. Validation of a proposed thermodynamic model. *Circ Res* 1990; 67(1): 124–29.

47. Haines DE, and Verow AF. Observations on electrode-tissue interface temperature and effect on electrical impedance during radiofrequency ablation of ventricular myocardium. *Circulation* 1990; 82(3): 1034–38.

48. Bohnen M et al. Incidence and predictors of major complications from contemporary catheter ablation to treat cardiac arrhythmias. *Heart Rhythm* 2011; 8(11): 1661–66.

Investigations for abnormal cardiac electrophysiology

JUSTIN LEE, JONATHAN KALMAN

38.1 Introduction

Abnormalities of cardiac electrophysiology (EP) can result in brady- or tachy-arrhythmias. Bradycardia and pacemakers are discussed in a subsequent chapter. In practice, most tachycardias arise through either a focal or re-entrant mechanisms. Focal tachycardias result from abnormal cardiac activation driven from a region of the heart not involved in generation of sinus rhythm. At the cellular level, the abnormal activation may be due to increased automaticity or early or delayed after depolarisations, though in clinical practice this may be difficult to distinguish and probably does not affect the ablation strategy. Re-entry probably accounts for the majority of clinical arrhythmias and arises due to areas of slowed conduction, or barriers to conduction, allowing an electrical wavefront to continuously propagate. The clinical presentation of arrhythmias can range from chest pain, heart failure, palpitations, (pre)-syncope to rarely sudden death. There is not always a strong relationship between severity of symptoms and risk. A condition may pose risk despite the patient remaining asymptomatic, whilst more benign conditions can cause considerable symptoms. This underlies the importance of establishing a clear electrophysiological diagnosis.

38.2 Investigations

38.2.1 Initial approach

The patient history should be the starting point. Sustained episodes of palpitation should be differentiated from brief intermittent symptoms due to ectopic beats. Sudden onset and offset of episodes are typical for supraventricular tachycardia (SVT). Previous attendances to the emergency room for adenosine treatment, or the ability to terminate episodes with vagal manoeuvres is helpful information. Age of symptom onset in childhood would be more consistent with the presence of an accessory pathway. A 'red flag' symptom is syncope or pre-syncope, which may indicate significant haemodynamic compromise from arrhythmia. If one suspects ventricular arrhythmia, awareness of the presence of structural heart disease, or cardiomyopathy is important.

The 12-lead electrocardiogram (ECG) is usually the initial investigation, although it only provides a short snap shot of cardiac rhythm. Even if it has not captured an arrhythmia the 12-lead ECG can still provide significant clues to the diagnosis; e.g. the presence of conduction tissue disease or pre-excitation. However, in order to reach a diagnosis it is usually necessary to capture an episode on ECG to allow symptom rhythm correlation. This can be obtained with non-invasive continuous Holter monitoring or patient-activated ECG recordings, though in the case of infrequent but potentially serious symptoms, a subcutaneous implantable loop recorder can be considered, e.g. 'Reveal' device (Medtronic).

Non-invasive investigations may yield either a narrow complex tachycardia (usually SVT, atrial fibrillation or flutter) or a broad complex tachycardia (ventricular tachycardia [VT] or an SVT with aberrant conduction or pre-excitation). The differential diagnosis of a SVT comprises atrio-ventricular nodal re-entrant tachycardia (AVNRT), atrio-ventricular re-entrant tachycardia (AVRT) and atrial tachycardia (AT) (see Figure 38.1a through c). In some cases, the electrophysiological mechanism of arrhythmia may be apparent from the non-invasive investigations alone. The key observation in this regard is the presence of visible atrial activity (P waves) and its relationship to ventricular activity (QRS complexes). The relative timing of P and R waves can suggest whether the SVT mechanism is AVNRT (near simultaneous P and R), AVRT (short RP interval usually) or AT (long or short or variable RP interval). In a broad complex tachycardia, independent atrial activity (ventriculo-atrial dissociation, or the presence of capture or fusion beats) are diagnostic of VT. ECG algorithms based on ventriculo-atrial dissociation and morphology of the QRS complex have been reported to diagnose VT with greater than 95% sensitivity and specificity.[1,2]

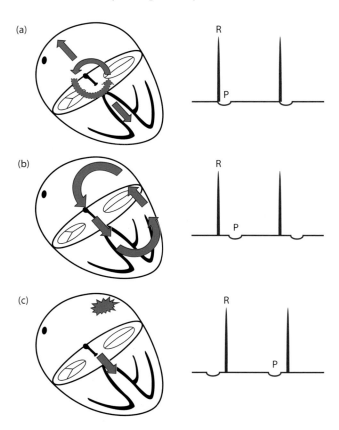

Figure 38.1 (a–c) The three-way differential diagnosis of a regular SVT is atrio-ventricular nodal re-entrant tachycardia (AVNRT), atrio-ventricular re-entrant tachycardia (AVRT) and atrial tachycardia (AT). AVNRT involves re-entry in the region around the AV node. AVRT usually utilises a circuit down the AV node and His–Purkinje system antegradely and back up an accessory pathway retrogradely (orthodromic AVRT), though more rarely the reverse situation – an anti-dromic circuit can exist with antegrade limb via accessory pathway and retrograde limb via atrioventricular (AV) node. However, this by definition is pre-excited and will not cause a narrow complex tachycardia. Focal atrial tachycardia involves ectopic atrial activation from a region other than the sinus node.

In the case of accessory pathways, the approximate location can be determined by analysis of the QRS complex,[3] provided that sufficient pre-excitation is visible. Similarly in the case of ATs, which tend to arise from specific anatomic locations, the origin of the focus can be determined from the P wave morphology on the 12-lead ECG.[4] VT origin can also be determined based on ECG morphology – on a simple level, left bundle branch morphology indicates a right ventricular origin and right bundle branch morphology indicates a left ventricular origin. The mean frontal axis and transition across the praecordial leads can help locate the origin further.

Assessment of cardiac structure and function by echocardiography or other imaging modalities, e.g.f computed tomography (CT) or magnetic resonance imaging (MRI), to determine the presence of ventricular scarring may be required to determine the aetiology of arrhythmia. Depending on symptoms, further investigations to exclude cardiac ischaemia may also be required.

38.2.2 EP studies and ablation

Once an arrhythmia has been documented, further invasive investigation with EP studies can be performed. This is often combined with therapy, e.g. radiofrequency (RF) ablation for convenience. Anti-arrhythmic drugs have an important role in the management of heart rhythm disorders, but ablation offers the potential for cure without need to take medications long-term that may impact quality of life. Prior to the development of minimally invasive catheter ablation techniques, open heart surgery was the only curative option for the treatment of selected arrhythmias.[5] This was effective but carried the potential risks associated with cardiac surgery. It is over 30 years since the original description of RF catheter ablation for atrio-ventricular (AV) node ablation to create heart block.[6] In that time, there have been significant developments in the range of arrhythmias that can now be treated using catheter ablation. RF energy is delivered through a deflectable ablation catheter with a 4–8 mm size tip, in order to heat the tissue and produce a discrete location of irreversible tissue damage and electrical inexcitability. Solid tip or irrigated catheters may be used; the latter have continuous flow of saline around the tip to cool it, allowing delivery of higher RF power without overheating the tissue to create deeper lesions.[7] RF is the mainstay of ablation treatment, but freezing therapy is also used, more frequently now in cryoballoon treatment of atrial fibrillation.

38.2.3 Technical considerations

EP studies are performed in a cardiac catheter laboratory with good quality fluoroscopic imaging and further specialised equipment including a computer-based multichannel recording system and programmable stimulator, and a RF generator for ablation. Cardiac resuscitation equipment must be available, including an external defibrillator. In addition, most laboratories will have equipment for electroanatomic mapping, intra-cardiac echocardiography and cryoablation.

Patients are prepared for elective EP studies by cessation of anti-arrhythmic drugs at least five half-lives prior to the procedure to reduce the chance of pharmacologic suppression of arrhythmia induction. Fasting is often necessary as sedation may be required, e.g. with midazolam and/or fentanyl. General anaesthesia can be used for EP studies and increases patient tolerability for long procedures but can also affect the inducibility of arrhythmias. Warfarin anticoagulation is often continued peri-procedure, particularly for atrial fibrillation (AF) ablation to reduce peri-procedural stroke risk, though international normalised ratio (INR) should be below 3.5 to reduce the risk of bleeding complications. Experience of performing EP studies and ablation on patients taking novel oral anticoagulants is limited. Many laboratories will omit these 24–48 hours prior to cardiac procedures, but early experience suggests that it may be safe to continue these during AF ablation.[8]

Central venous access is used, usually femoral but occasionally jugular, to introduce multipolar pacing and recording electrodes, typically 5–7 Fr. diameter, into key locations within the heart (see Figure 38.2). Catheter positioning is usually performed under fluoroscopic guidance, but precautions should be employed to minimize x-ray exposure to the patient and laboratory staff.[9] At a minimum, diagnostic catheters can be placed into the right ventricle and right atrium, but often catheters are positioned in the coronary sinus (for left atrial signals) and at the tricuspid annulus near the location of the His bundle.

In order to access the endocardial surface of the left side of the heart, the options lie between atrial trans-septal puncture or retrograde access across the aortic valve via the femoral artery. Trans-septal catheterisation with a specifically shaped long sheath, e.g. SL1 (St. Jude Medical, Little Canada, Minnesota) and Brockenborough needle, can be achieved using a pull down technique from the superior vena cava (SVC) into the right heart under fluoroscopic guidance to observe the catheter dropping into the fossa ovalis. The intra-cardiac catheters can be used to judge positioning of the sheath and needle, which in a right anterior oblique view should lie behind the His bundle which is adjacent to the aortic root. The angle of entry into the left

atrium should be approximately parallel to the coronary sinus catheter when viewed in the left anterior oblique view. For confirmation of needle entry into the left atrium the pressure waveform or contrast injection can be used. For greater certainty over atrial septal positioning, many centres use trans-oesophageal or intra-cardiac echo guidance (see Figure 38.3). The main complications that can arise are from inadvertent puncture of surrounding structures, e.g. the pericardial space if directed too posteriorly or the aortic root if too anterior. However, trans-septal access can now be performed routinely and safely in EP laboratories with greater than 99% success and <1% risk of complications.[10] Mapping and ablation in the left heart requires administration of intravenous heparin (e.g. 80–100 units/kg bolus with further doses titrated to activated clotting time [ACT]) to reduce the risk of thromboembolic complications.

More recently, a percutaneous approach to access the epicardial surface of the heart has been reported, initially described for the treatment of arrhythmia due to Chagas parasite infection.[11] There is increasing recognition that mapping and ablation epicardially can improve the success of treating certain arrhythmias, e.g. VT in the setting of an idiopathic dilated cardiomyopathy or an arrhythmogenic right ventricular cardiomyopathy (ARVC).[12,13] The risks of this approach relate to needle laceration of the cardiac wall or vessels, or abdominal structures including the liver. Coronary angiography is also necessary to ensure that potential sites of ablation are not adjacent to major epicardial vessels.

38.2.4 The basic EP study and common findings

Twelve-lead surface ECG and intra-cardiac electrogram data are recorded continuously onto the computer system, which also facilitates rapid review and accurate measurement of cardiac intervals using digital calipers. During EP studies, intra-cardiac electrograms are viewed at faster sweep speed than traditional surface ECG (e.g. 100–200 mm/s rather

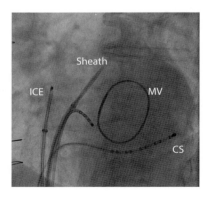

Figure 38.3 Fluoroscopic left antero-oblique view showing trans-septal access directed by intra-cardiac echo (ICE) in a patient with annuloplasty ring that marks position of the mitral valve (MV). The coronary sinus catheter (CS) is also used as landmark.

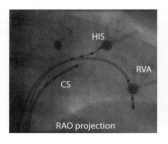 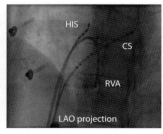

Figure 38.2 Catheter positioning. Fixed shape quadripolar catheters have been placed in the RV apex (RVA) and His bundle positions. A deflectable decapolar catheter is in the coronary sinus (CS).

25 mm/s) to allow better appreciation of the relative timing of signals and sequence of activation.

Initial cardiac intervals are recorded in order to assess the cardiac conduction system at baseline. A minimum data set consists of measurement of surface ECG PR, QRS, QT, followed by intra-cardiac Atrium-His (AH) and His-Ventricle (HV) intervals (see Figure 38.4). The AH interval is measured from septal right atrial activation to the His bundle electrogram, whilst the HV interval is measured from the His bundle electrogram to the earliest ventricular activation. The AH interval represents conduction over the AV node, whilst the HV interval represents conduction over the His bundle, left and right bundle branches and distal conduction system. Normal values for the AH interval range from 55 to 120 ms, but this is strongly influenced by autonomic tone. The HV interval is normally 35–55 ms and shows less variation. Minor prolongation of the HV interval can be seen commonly, but a HV interval of greater 100 ms indicates significant infra-nodal conduction tissue disease

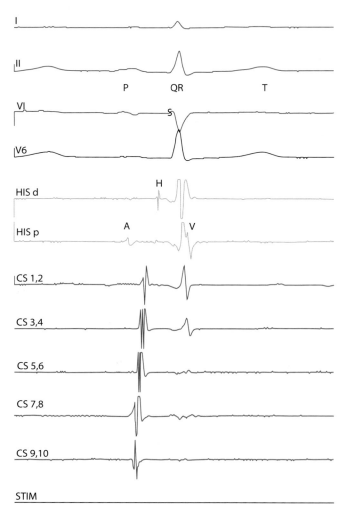

Figure 38.4 Basic intervals in sinus rhythm and relationship of these to the surface electrocardiogram (ECG). Normal AH interval = 55–125 ms and normal HV interval = 35–55 ms.

with risk of syncope. It is important to recognise that this situation can be present with a normal PR interval.

Pacing maneouvres are then performed to 'stress' the conducting system in an attempt to induce arrhythmia. The 'Retrograde curve' and 'Antegrade curve' consist of a fixed train of eight paced impulses followed a further incrementally earlier paced stimulus assessing conduction from ventricle to atrium or vice versa. In each case, this is performed until the effective refractory period of either the AV node or the chamber being paced is reached, that is, there is failure of AV conduction or failure to capture the paced chamber. Alternatively, incrementally faster pacing can be performed from atrium or ventricle until the Wenkebach point is reached when there is no longer 1:1 conduction. Due to the reliance on calcium channels rather than sodium channels for depolarization, the normal response of the AV node in the face of such stimulation is 'decremental' conduction, meaning that conduction slows down as the input stimulus gets faster. When pacing the ventricle, conduction to the atrium may be absent at baseline (ventriculo-atrial [VA] block). This is a normal finding and conduction will often return if isoprenaline is administered. When conduction from ventricle to atrium occurs normally via the AV node, atrial activation will be observed to spread from the septum laterally and as the extra-stimulus in the retrograde curve gets earlier atrial activation will delay. When conduction from ventricle to atrium occurs via an accessory pathway, atrial activation is often abnormal or 'eccentric' due to the location of the accessory pathway away from the septum and does not usually delay (non-decremental behaviour) with progressively faster pacing.

Pacing the atrium incrementally faster will cause delay in conduction via the AV node and decrement in the AH interval. A common response during gradually faster antegrade pacing is a 'jump' in the AH interval (defined as an increase in the AH interval of greater than 50 ms for a decrease in the atrial stimulus of 10 ms). This is termed dual AV nodal physiology and is accounted for by change of conduction from the 'fast pathway' to the 'slow pathway'. Dual AV nodal physiology is common, and although it is the substrate for AVNRT, not all individuals with dual nodal physiology are capable of sustained AVNRT.[14] The other key observation during antegrade studies is the presence of pre-excitation indicated by surface ECG delta waves and a short, or even negative HV interval. In the presence of an antegradely conducting accessory pathway, ventricular activation is a result of fused activation over the accessory pathway and the AV node. As the AV node conduction decrements with more rapid pacing, the degree of pre-excitation will progressively increase. When the antegrade refractory period of the pathway is reached, antegrade conduction will occur via the AV node exclusively or AV block will occur if the node is also refractory at this point. The refractory period of an accessory pathway is prognostically important as it determines whether there is a risk of future sudden death, usually due to pre-excited atrial fibrillation degenerating into ventricular fibrillation.[15]

Once tachycardia is induced the pattern of electrical activation on the catheters and response to pacing manoeuvres are used to confirm the mechanism. A brief description follows but consideration of all possible manoeuvres is beyond the scope of this chapter. However, the reader is directed to a recent comprehensive review.[16,17]

38.2.5 Entrainment

Entrainment is an important electrophysiologic principle that can also give considerable information about a tachycardia mechanism. Pacing slightly faster than the tachycardia cycle length to capture the circuit can be used to confirm that a tachycardia is re-entrant in mechanism, resulting in fixed fusion on surface ECG between the tachycardia and paced morphology. The response to entrainment then provides further information about tachycardia mechanism. In the common situation in the EP lab of a narrow complex tachycardia, entrainment from the right ventricle can be usefully employed – see Figure 38.6 for illustrative images. Recall that there is generally a three-way differential diagnosis of AVNRT, AVRT and AT. Entrainment from the right ventricle will usually accelerate the atrium to the same rate. This can occur with all three mechanisms, but if it does not occur because the ventricle becomes dissociated from the ventricle, then the mechanism cannot be AVRT because both atrium and ventricle are obligate participants in the re-entry circuit. Once the atrium has been accelerated to the pacing cycle length, pacing is discontinued and provided the tachycardia is not terminated, there are two possible responses – a VAV (ventricle, atrium, ventricle) and VAAV.[18] The VAAV response is consistent with an AT, because the AV node is the only route from ventricle to atrium and remains refractory from the last ventricular paced beat, so two atrial events occur before conduction to the ventricle. In a VAV response, which is consistent with AVRT or AVNRT, there are two limbs of the tachycardia circuit – antegrade and retrograde. In this situation, the post-pacing interval – the time from the last paced beat to the next ventricular electrogram – can be compared with the tachycardia cycle length.[19] In AVNRT, the re-entry circuit is small confined to the vicinity of the AV node, hence the last paced stimulus that captures the circuit has to travel from the RV to the AV node, around the circuit and back to the RV, and therefore the post-pacing interval is much longer than the tachycardia cycle length. However, in AVRT, the circuit is large, spanning atrium and ventricle, and the pacing site is within the circuit, so the post-pacing interval and tachycardia cycle length are similar. Entrainment can be employed whenever there is a re-entry circuit, e.g. in atypical atrial flutters or VT to determine whether the pacing location is within the arrhythmia circuit. Other common manoeuvres in the EP lab, such as critically timed (His synchronous) ventricular or atrial extra-stimuli in order to perturb the tachycardia circuit are based upon the principle of entrainment, that is, fusion and reset of the tachycardia circuit.

38.2.6 Investigation of VT

Programmed stimulation can also be performed for induction of VT. A well-known stimulation protocol has been described by Wellens et al.[20] In summary, an increasing number of extra-stimuli are applied at progressively shorter coupling intervals. As the protocol becomes more aggressive, the likelihood for VT/VF induction increases but prognostic significance decreases.[21] VT stimulation is used in studies where ablation is to be performed but less frequently employed as a stand-alone diagnostic study. Historically it was used to determine effectiveness of anti-arrhythmic drug therapy in suppressing ventricular arrhythmia. It was also used in the selection of patients for implantation of defibrillators for primary prevention of sudden cardiac death following myocardial infarction.[22] However, current international guidelines indicate that this decision should be made based on other risk factors including cardiac ejection fraction. Ventricular stimulation was previously thought to have a role in guiding implantable defibrillator programming, but increasingly this is being performed using empiric settings with longer detection to minimise shock therapy.[23]

38.2.7 Pharmacologic provocation

Tachycardia is often inducible by a particular sequence of pacing manoeuvres but may require adjunctive pharmacologic stimulation. Typically isoprenaline is given to increase sympathetic tone, either as small bolus or infusion (1–4 µg/min). Adrenaline infusion can also be used. Atropine can be used to reduce parasympathetic tone (0.5–1 mg bolus). If there is uncertainty about the presence of an accessory pathway, adenosine can be used to block the AV node temporarily, doses of up to 30 mg can be safely given provided a catheter is in place for temporary pacing if required.

Drugs can also be used to assess for underlying electrical abnormalities or 'channelopathies'. Sodium channel blockers such as flecainide or ajmaline can provoke the coved ST segment changes diagnostic of Brugada syndrome. A suggested regime for ajmaline provocation is a total of 1 mg/kg (up to maximum of 80 mg) administered in 10 mg doses over a minute every 2 minutes. No further ajmaline is given if diagnostic ECG changes are seen or ventricular arrhythmia is observed. Adrenaline can be used to assess for long QT syndrome, where failure of the QT interval to shorten or paradoxical prolongation of absolute QT interval can be observed. A common infusion regime used is 0.025 µg/kg/min for 10 minutes, followed by 5 minutes at 0.05 µg/kg/min, 5 minutes at 0.1 and 0.2 µg/kg/min. Adrenaline should be discontinued if ventricular arrhythmia or angina or heart failure occur.

38.3 Mapping of arrhythmias

38.3.1 Approaches to mapping

Once the tachycardia mechanism has been identified, some arrhythmias can be targeted for ablation at a typical anatomic location. Examples of this would include slow pathway ablation for AVNRT and cavo-tricuspid isthmus ablation for atrial flutter.[24] Where the location of the anatomic substrate is variable, e.g. an accessory pathway or a focal atrial or VT, the ideal situation is for tachycardia to be easily inducible, sustained and haemodynamically tolerated by the patient. This allows detailed activation mapping to locate the point of earliest activation. In a re-entry circuit if one can locate the isthmus of slow conduction, pacing at just faster than the tachycardia cycle length to entrain the tachycardia may result in concealed fusion, i.e. acceleration of the tachycardia to the pacing cycle length without significant change in 12-lead ECG morphology. This often indicates a likely successful location for ablation.[25] In some situations, tachycardia is difficult to induce and non-sustained and in this setting electroanatomic mapping can be useful. Pace mapping is an alternative strategy that can be employed in order to locate the origin of a tachycardia focus, by comparing the arrhythmia ECG with the paced ECG from different locations. The match of the two morphologies is conventionally described as 12/12 if all 12 surface leads appear a good match. Whilst this can serve as a rough guide, it is limited in spatial accuracy. 12/12 pace maps for ventricular arrhythmias can be obtained over a 1 cm area or larger,[26] whilst for atrial arrhythmias the spatial resolution is even worse, probably several centimetres at best.[27] Furthermore in scarred tissue, the pattern of cardiac activation during pacing may not accurately reflect that during tachycardia, due to preferential conduction via normal tissue and the absence of areas of functional block.

38.3.2 Electroanatomic mapping

Three systems are currently available commercially CARTO (Biosense Webster), NavX (St Jude Medical) and Rhythmia (Boston Scientific). The CARTO system uses low strength magnetic fields (up to 5×10^{-5} Tesla) delivered from three separate magnetic coils in a locator pad beneath the patient. The magnetic field from each coil is detected by a sensor at the tip of a specialised mapping catheter. The strength of the magnetic field measured is inversely proportional to the distance from each magnet, allowing the catheter tip location to be triangulated in space. The NavX system uses a low-level 5.6 kHz current through three pairs of orthogonally located skin patches. The voltage and impedance can be measured from multiple catheters which allows their distance from each skin patch, and therefore their location in space, to be triangulated with the help of a reference electrode. Both technologies have different strengths and weaknesses in terms of catheter location accuracy and stability of maps, and this is illustrated by the fact that Rhythmia as well as the latest versions of CARTO and NavX use a combination of magnetic and impedance-based location technology.

By collecting multiple location points, these systems allow a three-dimensional (3D) representation or 'geometry' of the cardiac chamber of interest to be created, along with real-time display of catheter positions within the map. Potentially the operator can sample several hundred locations throughout the heart. At each location, information can be collected to examine the timing of cardiac activation and also the myocardial voltage. Based on the amplitude of intra-cardiac signals recorded, scarred and fibrotic regions can be defined. In activation mapping, the relative timing of intra-cardiac signals are compared with a stable reference signal. Centrifugal activation from a single location during tachycardia indicates a focal or micro–re-entrant tachycardia. In a macro–re-entrant circuit it is possible to obtain points of cardiac activation that span the whole tachycardia cycle length. The system can also be used to document the specific points of interest, e.g. critical signals, anatomic landmarks and the locations where ablation has been performed. Mapping systems allow procedures to be performed with reduced fluoroscopy and improve the speed and success of complex ablations.[28,29]

Information is collected from catheters, which are moved around within the heart to collect information on a 'point-by-point' basis. The ability to collect several points simultaneously from multipolar catheters has been a significant advance in allowing rapid generation of detailed electro-anatomic maps. In a non-sustained, difficult to induce tachycardia it can be challenging to collect sufficient point data to accurately determine the origin and mechanism. In this situation, cardiac activation can be assessed by a non-contact device – Ensite Array (St. Jude Medical), a 64-electrode mesh mounted on a balloon placed within the chamber of interest. It detects unipolar signals within 4 cm of the surface of the array. Using complex mathematical processing it can generate over 3000 virtual electrograms and in theory collect the entire arrhythmia circuit in a single heartbeat.[30,31] A more recent development is the multielectrode ECG vest – ECVUE (Cardioinsight) with over 250 surface electrodes. This has been used in several applications including demonstration non-invasively of the origin of outflow tract VTs.[32]

38.4 Specific situations

38.4.1 Supraventricular tachycardia

Most SVTs can be investigated and treated using a simple approach of intra-cardiac catheters and fluoroscopic guidance only. The success rates are greater than 90%, whilst complication rates are low in the region of 1%. Example clinical cases are given in Figures 38.5 through 38.7 for common SVT cases. However, mapping systems can reduce fluoroscopy exposure, and may be useful in complex cases. Examples of this include (non-sustained) ATs, or septal accessory pathways, which may pass close to the AV node and where ablation carries a risk of inadvertent injury and heart block. The ability to mark and return to exact previous locations of ablation is also useful when there is recurrence of arrhythmia during the EP study.

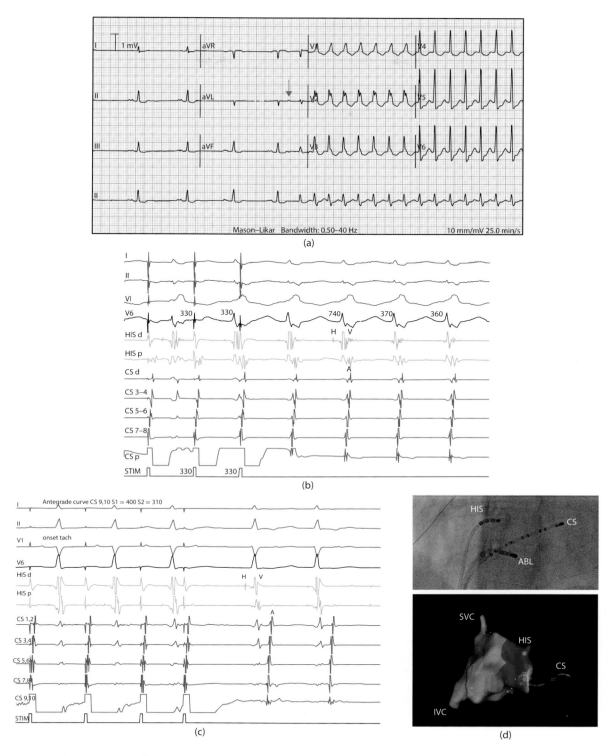

Figure 38.5 (a) This appears at first glance to show the onset of a broad complex right bundle branch block (RBBB) tachy-cardia. However, closer inspection reveals an atrial extra-systole (arrow) with prolongation of the PR interval and that the first beat of tachycardia is narrow. This strongly suggests that this in fact is an SVT with abberrant conduction, most likely atrio-ventricular nodal re-entrant tachycardia (AVNRT) and highlights the importance of careful inspection of the 12-lead electrocardiogram (ECG). (b) Atrial pacing has induced typical AVNRT utilising the slow pathway antegradely and the fast pathway retrogradely. Ventricle-atrium (VA) interval is 15 ms. (c) Atrial pacing has induced atypical AVNRT using a slow pathway antegradely and a separate slow pathway retrogradely. The VA interval is longer compared to (b). (d) Fluoroscopy and electroanatomic mapping from a case of atypical AVNRT. On the fluoroscopic image, the ablation catheter is at the slow pathway region. Note that on the activation map, earliest atrial activation (white region) is from the slow pathway near the coronary sinus (CS) or mouth rather than the fast pathway which is located near the His bundle.

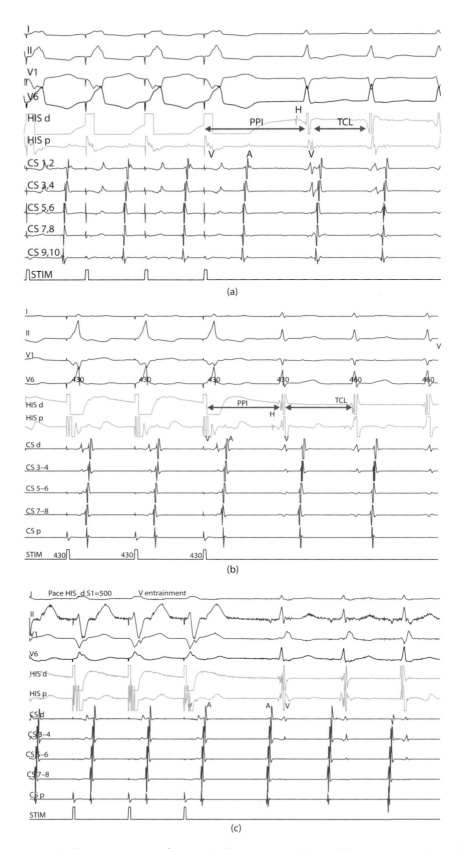

Figure 38.6 **(a)** Following ventricular entrainment of an atypical atrio-ventricular nodal re-entrant tachycardia (AVNRT), the post-pacing interval (PPI) is much longer than the tachycardia cycle length (TCL). **(b)** In atrio-ventricular re-entrant tachycardia (AVRT) via a septal accessory pathway, tachycardia appears similar to atypical AVNRT. However following entrainment the PPI and tachycardia cycle length (TCL) are similar. **(c)** In atrial tachycardia, following ventricular entrainment there is a VAAV response.

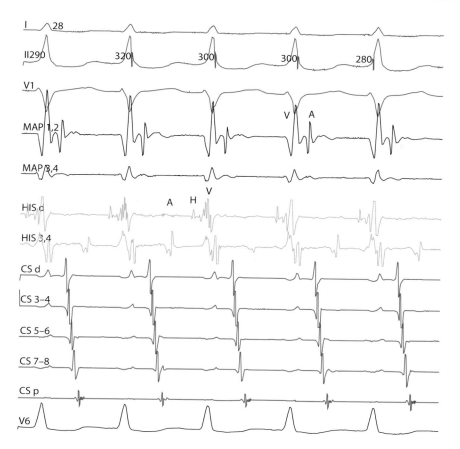

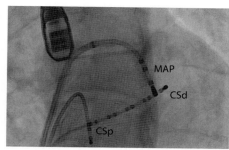

Figure 38.7 Left-sided accessory pathway causing orthodromic atrio-ventricular re-entrant tachycardia (AVRT). Note the eccentric coronary sinus activation with distal electrode first. Mapping the accessory pathway using fluoroscopic guidance and timing of intra-cardiac electrograms. On the mapping catheter the local atrial signal is earlier than any other atrial signals.

38.4.2 Atrial fibrillation and flutter

AF is the commonest sustained cardiac arrhythmia, characterised by rapid and chaotic atrial electrical activity without significant mechanical contraction. The prevalence is rising, with an ageing population and as metabolic health declines. In the young patient presenting with AF it is wise to check for an unusual trigger such as an SVT that degenerates to AF, as this may be more easily addressed.[33] However, following the initial description of pulmonary vein triggers for initiation of atrial fibrillation,[34] AF ablation (pulmonary vein isolation) has become the commonest indication for invasive EP studies. Following recognition of the risk of pulmonary vein stenosis due to ablation distally within the vein, ablation is now performed more proximally in the atrial body guided by a mapping system (see Figure 38.8). If desired the map can be fused with a CT or MRI of the heart for greater anatomic detail.[35] Complete electrical disconnection or 'isolation' of the pulmonary veins is achieved by delivering a continuous series of ablation points around each vein or left or right-sided pair of veins using a steerable

ablation catheter. Alternatives to point-by-point ablation have been developed to try and speed up the procedure of pulmonary vein isolation, including cryoballoon (Medtronic) (see Figure 38.9), and multipolar ablation catheter technologies, e.g. nMARQ (Biosense Webster) and PVAC (Medtronic). Catheter ablation is superior to anti-arrhythmic drugs in maintaining sinus rhythm and is indicated in current guidelines to treat symptoms refractory to medication.[36] Clinical success is dependent on the category of disease. Paroxysmal AF has a high success rate from a single procedure in the order of 70%, rising to 80%–90% after multiple procedures. Persistent AF presents more of a challenge with lower first procedure success around 30%–50%.[37] Multiple procedures and further ablation of atrial substrate may improve outcomes. Mapping systems allow the operator to locate and ablate complex fractionated signals (CFAE) within the atria,[38] or perform linear ablation to compartmentalise the atrium in similar fashion to a surgical 'maze' procedure.[39,40] These approaches can be combined to perform 'stepwise' ablation with the goal of ablating until sinus rhythm is restored.[41] Another approach is to target the autonomic

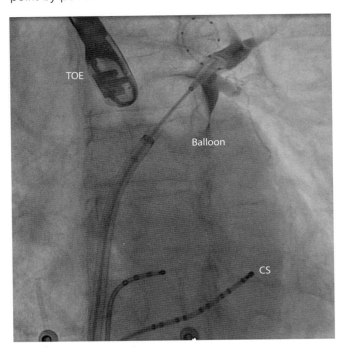

Figure 38.8 Electroanatomic maps of the left atrium. The four pulmonary veins, left superior (LSPV), left inferior (LIPV), right superior (RSPV), right inferior (RIPV) and left atrial appendage (LAA) are marked. Red dots represent point-by-point antral ablation lesions.

Figure 38.9 Trans-septal access has been achieved with trans-oesophageal echocardiography (TOE) guidance and coronary sinus (CS) as landmark. Cryoballoon ablation of left upper pulmonary vein is being performed. Contrast is injected distal to the balloon to ensure a good seal against the vein ostium. Liquid nitrous oxide is delivered into the balloon, which converts to gas and cools the balloon down to −70°. The balloon is mounted on a hybrid guide wire/circular catheter that can be used to check pulmonary vein isolation.

ganglia innervating the atrium.[42] Recently an approach of focal ablation guided by high-density multipolar basket catheter and proprietary software to map 'rotors' during atrial fibrillation has been described.[43] If the results can be

replicated, this may significantly improve outcomes. The variation in approach to ablation of persistent AF means that the optimum strategy is not yet known.[44]

Mapping systems are often combined with contact force sensing technology to feedback in real time the pressure exerted by the ablation catheter tip. The success of RF ablation is dependent on good catheter contact with the myocardium in order to produce a permanent lesion. Acute tissue injury and oedema can result from poor contact ablation and give the impression of success, but when tissue recovers arrhythmia will recur. This is a particular issue with atrial fibrillation where reconnection of pulmonary veins is a common finding at repeat ablation. Considerable variation in the contact force can be observed during cardiac and respiratory motion and also in different regions of the heart.[45] Adequate tissue contact, without excessive force, improves the success of AF ablation and may avoid complications such as cardiac perforation and tamponade.[46,47]

Atrial flutter is a classic example of a macro–re-entrant circuit which in typical or common right atrial flutter involves activation rotating counter-clockwise around the right atrium (see Figure 38.10).[48] It is ablated in a linear fashion at the cavo-tricuspid isthmus, between the tricuspid annulus and the inferior vena cava. Mapping systems are particularly useful for 'atypical' flutters due to atrial scarring that can occur spontaneously or following cardiac surgery or catheter ablation. These situations can be very complicated with 'figure of eight' or multiple circuits around the atria.[49]

38.4.3 Ventricular tachycardia

VT in structurally normal hearts usually originates from the outflow tract, more commonly from the right ventricle.[50] Rarely VT can arise from alternative sites including the His–Purkinje system or papillary muscles.[51,52] Arrhythmia is usually non-sustained, or may take the form of frequent ectopic beats. If the burden of ectopy is high, LV function can become impaired due to dys-synchrony. Electroanatomic mapping is used to locate the abnormal focus and ablation can reverse LV dysfunction.[53,54] In cases

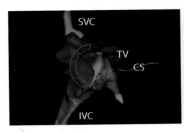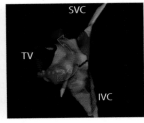

Figure 38.10 Typical atrial flutter with counter-clockwise wavefront around the right atrium displayed on a mapping system (activation timing represented on a 'rainbow' scale red to purple). Catheter ablation (red markers) has been performed at the isthmus between the tricuspid annulus (TV) and the inferior vena cava (IVC).

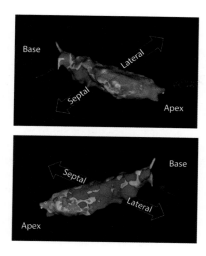

Figure 38.11 Voltage maps of a left ventricle showing previous antero-septal infarction. Dense scar areas are marked grey, normal myocardium is purple, whilst abnormal tissue is red–green. Red markers indicate where ablation has been performed.

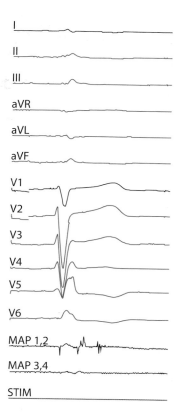

Figure 38.12 Damaged myocardium shows slowed conduction with local late activation (late potentials), here observed beyond the QRS in sinus rhythm. If haemo-dynamically tolerated activation mapping of VT can be performed. During VT mid-diastolic potentials are seen on the MAP (roving mapping) catheter.

with infrequent ectopic beats, pharmacologic provocation or the Ensite non-contact array can be employed.

More often VT occurs in the setting of structural heart disease, with impaired ventricular function and scarring. Following myocardial infarction surviving cells near the infarct zone conduct more slowly allowing a re-entry circuit to be sustained.[55] There are often multiple regions of the scar that can give rise to VT and multiple ECG morphologies of VT can be seen in a single patient. Several approaches to investigation and ablation of VT have been described. General anaesthetic may be preferable for VT ablation. Use of an electroanatomic mapping system (see Figure 38.11) is vital to determine the presence and extent of scarred regions. Voltage criteria for damaged ventricle have been established as <1.5 V, with <0.5 V representing dense scar on the endocardial surface.[56] Use of mechanical support with intra-aortic balloon pump or catheter based axial flow pump, e.g. Impella (Abiomed) has been described and may be helpful in haemodynamically unstable cases.[57] If tachycardia occurs spontaneously or is inducible and haemodynamically tolerated, activation mapping of the circuit can be performed[58] (see Figure 38.12). Critical isthmuses can be identified by diastolic signals at sites during VT that show concealed entrainment (paced morphology and VT morphology are identical) and also good pace maps during sinus rhythm.[59] An approach gaining popularity is to ablate the VT substrate by targeting all abnormal electrical signals including 'late potentials' within scarred regions of the ventricle.[60] This substrate-based approach involves more extensive ablation but is likely to get rid of more potential VT circuits. Success rates of VT ablation in ischaemic cardiomyopathy are reported from experienced centres in the region of 50%–80%.[61,62]

38.5 Conclusions

The investigation of abnormal EP starts with simple investigations such as the 12-lead ECG and Holter monitoring to obtain symptom rhythm correlation. The surface ECG often holds clues to the diagnosis. Invasive studies can then be performed and combined with curative treatment. This chapter describes the principles of conducting a basic invasive EP study using fluoroscopic guidance and analysis of intra-cardiac electrograms, as typically applied to cases of SVT. Sound knowledge of the basic principles is required to perform more advanced EP studies such as those using electroanatomic mapping to treat complex atrial and ventricular arrhythmias. More detailed information on ablation of specific arrhythmias is found in subsequent chapters.

References

1. Brugada P et al. A new approach to the differential diagnosis of a regular tachycardia with a wide qrs complex. *Circulation* 1991; 83: 1649–59.
2. Vereckei A et al. Application of a new algorithm in the differential diagnosis of wide qrs complex tachycardia. *Eur Heart J* 2007; 28: 589–600.

3. Fitzpatrick AP et al. New algorithm for the localization of accessory atrioventricular connections using a baseline electrocardiogram. *J Am Coll Cardiol* 1994; 23: 107–16.

4. Kistler PM et al. P-wave morphology in focal atrial tachycardia: Development of an algorithm to predict the anatomic site of origin. *J Am Coll Cardiol* 2006; 48: 1010–17.

5. Guiraudon GM et al. Surgical treatment of supraventricular tachycardia: A five-year experience. *Pacing Clin Electrophysiol* 1986; 9: 1376–80.

6. Scheinman MM et al. Catheter-induced ablation of the atrioventricular junction to control refractory supraventricular arrhythmias. *Jama* 1982; 248: 851–55.

7. Calkins H et al. Catheter ablation of ventricular tachycardia in patients with structural heart disease using cooled radiofrequency energy: Results of a prospective multicenter study. Cooled rf multi center investigators group. *J Am Coll Cardiol* 2000; 35: 1905–14.

8. Potpara TS et al. Oral anticoagulant therapy for stroke prevention in patients with atrial fibrillation undergoing ablation: Results from the first European snapshot survey on procedural routines for atrial fibrillation ablation (ess-prafa). *Europace* 2015; 17: 986–93.

9. Walters TE et al. Impact of collimation on radiation exposure during interventional electrophysiology. *Europace* 2012; 14: 1670–73.

10. De Ponti R et al. Trans-septal catheterization in the electrophysiology laboratory: Data from a multicenter survey spanning 12 years. *J Am Coll Cardiol* 2006; 47: 1037–42.

11. Sosa E et al. A new technique to perform epicardial mapping in the electrophysiology laboratory. *J Cardiovasc Electrophysiol* 1996; 7: 531–36.

12. Bai R et al. Ablation of ventricular arrhythmias in arrhythmogenic right ventricular dysplasia/cardiomyopathy: Arrhythmia-free survival after endo-epicardial substrate based mapping and ablation. *Circ Arrhythm Electrophysiol* 2011; 4: 478–85.

13. Della Bella P et al. Epicardial ablation for ventricular tachycardia: A european multicenter study. *Circ Arrhythm Electrophysiol* 2011; 4: 653–59.

14. Denes P et al. Demonstration of dual a-v nodal pathways in patients with paroxysmal supraventricular tachycardia. *Circulation* 1973; 48: 549–55.

15. Klein GJ et al. Ventricular fibrillation in the Wolff-Parkinson-White syndrome. *N Engl J Med* 1979; 301: 1080–85.

16. Veenhuyzen GD et al. Diagnostic pacing maneuvers for supraventricular tachycardia: Part 1. *Pacing Clin Electrophysiol* 2011; 34: 767–82.

17. Veenhuyzen GD et al. Diagnostic pacing maneuvers for supraventricular tachycardias: Part 2. *Pacing Clin Electrophysiol* 2012; 35: 757–69.

18. Knight BP et al. A technique for the rapid diagnosis of atrial tachycardia in the electrophysiology laboratory. *J Am Coll Cardiol* 1999; 33: 775–81.

19. Michaud GF et al. Differentiation of atypical atrioventricular node re-entrant tachycardia from orthodromic reciprocating tachycardia using a septal accessory pathway by the response to ventricular pacing. *J Am Coll Cardiol* 2001; 38: 1163–67.

20. Wellens HJ et al. Programmed electrical stimulation of the heart in patients with life-threatening ventricular arrhythmias: What is the significance of induced arrhythmias and what is the correct stimulation protocol? *Circulation* 1985; 72: 1–7.

21. Brugada P et al. Significance of ventricular arrhythmias initiated by programmed ventricular stimulation: The importance of the type of ventricular arrhythmia induced and the number of premature stimuli required. *Circulation* 1984; 69: 87–92.

22. Moss AJ et al. Improved survival with an implanted defibrillator in patients with coronary disease at high risk for ventricular arrhythmia. Multicenter automatic defibrillator implantation trial investigators. *N Engl J Med* 1996; 335: 1933–40.

23. Moss AJ et al. Reduction in inappropriate therapy and mortality through icd programming. *N Engl J Med* 2012; 367(24): 2275–83.

24. Jackman WM et al. Treatment of supraventricular tachycardia due to atrioventricular nodal reentry, by radiofrequency catheter ablation of slow-pathway conduction. *N Engl J Med* 1992; 327: 313–18.

25. Morady F et al. Concealed entrainment as a guide for catheter ablation of ventricular tachycardia in patients with prior myocardial infarction. *J Am Coll Cardiol* 1991; 17: 678–89.

26. Kadish AH et al. Differences in qrs configuration during unipolar pacing from adjacent sites: Implications for the spatial resolution of pace-mapping. *J Am Coll Cardiol* 1991; 17: 143–51.

27. Man KC et al. Spatial resolution of atrial pace mapping as determined by unipolar atrial pacing at adjacent sites. *Circulation* 1996; 94: 1357–63.

28. Earley MJ et al. Radiofrequency ablation of arrhythmias guided by non-fluoroscopic catheter location: A prospective randomized trial. *Eur Heart J* 2006; 27: 1223–29.

29. Rotter M et al. Reduction of fluoroscopy exposure and procedure duration during ablation of atrial fibrillation using a novel anatomical navigation system. *Eur Heart J* 2005; 26: 1415–21.

30. Higa S et al. Focal atrial tachycardia: New insight from non-contact mapping and catheter ablation. *Circulation* 2004; 109: 84–91.

31. Schilling RJ et al. Feasibility of a noncontact catheter for endocardial mapping of human ventricular tachycardia. *Circulation* 1999; 99: 2543–52.

32. Jamil-Copley S et al. Noninvasive electrocardiographic mapping to guide ablation of outflow tract ventricular arrhythmias. *Heart Rhythm* 2014; 11: 587–94.

33. Sauer WH et al. Atrioventricular nodal reentrant tachycardia in patients referred for atrial fibrillation ablation: Response to ablation that incorporates slow-pathway modification. *Circulation* 2006; 114: 191–95.

34. Haissaguerre M et al. Spontaneous initiation of atrial fibrillation by ectopic beats originating in the pulmonary veins. *N Engl J Med* 1998; 339: 659–66.

35. Kistler PM et al. Validation of three-dimensional cardiac image integration: Use of integrated ct image into electroanatomic mapping system to perform catheter ablation of atrial fibrillation. *J Cardiovasc Electrophysiol* 2006; 17: 341–48.

36. Calkins H et al. 2012 HRS/EHRA/ECAS Expert Consensus Statement on catheter and surgical ablation of atrial fibrillation: Recommendations for patient selection, procedural techniques, patient management and follow-up, definitions, endpoints, and research trial design: A report of

the heart rhythm society (hrs) task force on catheter and surgical ablation of atrial fibrillation. Developed in partnership with the european heart rhythm association (ehra), a registered branch of the european society of cardiology (esc) and the european cardiac arrhythmia society (ecas); and in collaboration with the american college of cardiology (acc), american heart association (aha), the asia pacific heart rhythm society (aphrs), and the society of thoracic surgeons (sts). Endorsed by the governing bodies of the american college of cardiology foundation, the american heart association, the european cardiac arrhythmia society, the european heart rhythm association, the society of thoracic surgeons, the asia pacific heart rhythm society, and the heart rhythm society. *Heart Rhythm* 2012; 9(4): 632–96.

37. Rostock T et al. Long-term single- and multiple-procedure outcome and predictors of success after catheter ablation for persistent atrial fibrillation. *Heart Rhythm* 2011; 8: 1391–97.

38. Nademanee K et al. A new approach for catheter ablation of atrial fibrillation: Mapping of the electrophysiologic substrate. *J Am Coll Cardiol* 2004; 43: 2044–53.

39. Knecht S et al. Left atrial linear lesions are required for successful treatment of persistent atrial fibrillation. *Eur Heart J* 2008; 29: 2359–66.

40. Sanders P et al. Complete isolation of the pulmonary veins and posterior left atrium in chronic atrial fibrillation. Long-term clinical outcome. *Eur Heart J* 2007; 28: 1862–71.

41. O'Neill MD et al. Long-term follow-up of persistent atrial fibrillation ablation using termination as a procedural endpoint. *Eur Heart J* 2009; 30: 1105–12.

42. Nakagawa H et al. Pathophysiologic basis of autonomic ganglionated plexus ablation in patients with atrial fibrillation. *Heart Rhythm* 2009; 6: S26–S34.

43. Narayan SM et al. Treatment of atrial fibrillation by the ablation of localized sources: Confirm (conventional ablation for atrial fibrillation with or without focal impulse and rotor modulation) trial. *J Am Coll Cardiol* 2012; 60: 628–36.

44. Verma A et al. Approaches to catheter ablation for persistent atrial fibrillation. *N Engl J Med* 2015; 372: 1812–22.

45. Kumar S et al. Prospective characterization of catheter-tissue contact force at different anatomical sites during antral pulmonary vein isolation. *Circ Arrhythm Electrophysiol* 2012; 5(6): 1124–29.

46. Kuck KH et al. A novel radiofrequency ablation catheter using contact force sensing: Toccata study. *Heart Rhythm* 2012; 9: 18–23.

47. Reddy VY et al. Randomized, controlled trial of the safety and effectiveness of a contact force-sensing irrigated catheter for ablation of paroxysmal atrial fibrillation: Results of the tacticath contact force ablation catheter study for atrial fibrillation (toccastar) study. *Circulation* 2015; 132: 907–15.

48. Kalman JM et al. Activation and entrainment mapping defines the tricuspid annulus as the anterior barrier in typical atrial flutter. *Circulation* 1996; 94: 398–406.

49. Saoudi N et al. A classification of atrial flutter and regular atrial tachycardia according to electrophysiological mechanisms and anatomical bases; A statement from a joint expert group from the working group of arrhythmias of the european society of cardiology and the north american society of pacing and electrophysiology. *Eur Heart J* 2001; 22: 1162–82.

50. Buxton AE et al. Repetitive, monomorphic ventricular tachycardia: Clinical and electrophysiologic characteristics in patients with and patients without organic heart disease. *Am J Cardiol* 1984; 54: 997–1002.

51. Lin D et al. Idiopathic fascicular left ventricular tachycardia: Linear ablation lesion strategy for noninducible or nonsustained tachycardia. *Heart Rhythm* 2005; 2: 934–39.

52. Yamada T et al. Idiopathic ventricular arrhythmias originating from the papillary muscles in the left ventricle: Prevalence, electrocardiographic and electrophysiological characteristics, and results of the radiofrequency catheter ablation. *J Cardiovasc Electrophysiol* 2010; 21: 62–69.

53. Bogun F et al. Radiofrequency ablation of frequent, idiopathic premature ventricular complexes: Comparison with a control group without intervention. *Heart Rhythm* 2007; 4: 863–67.

54. Yarlagadda RK et al. Reversal of cardiomyopathy in patients with repetitive monomorphic ventricular ectopy originating from the right ventricular outflow tract. *Circulation* 2005; 112: 1092–97.

55. Arenal A et al. Tachycardia-related channel in the scar tissue in patients with sustained monomorphic ventricular tachycardias: Influence of the voltage scar definition. *Circulation* 2004; 110: 2568–74.

56. Marchlinski FE et al. Linear ablation lesions for control of unmappable ventricular tachycardia in patients with ischemic and nonischemic cardiomyopathy. *Circulation* 2000; 101: 1288–96.

57. Miller MA et al. Percutaneous hemodynamic support with impella 2.5 during scar-related ventricular tachycardia ablation (permit 1). *Circ Arrhythm Electrophysiol.* 2013; 6: 151–59.

58. Stevenson WG et al. Identification of reentry circuit sites during catheter mapping and radiofrequency ablation of ventricular tachycardia late after myocardial infarction. *Circulation* 1993; 88: 1647–70.

59. Bogun F et al. Isolated potentials during sinus rhythm and pace-mapping within scars as guides for ablation of postinfarction ventricular tachycardia. *J Am Coll Cardiol* 2006; 47: 2013–19.

60. Jais P et al. Elimination of local abnormal ventricular activities: A new end point for substrate modification in patients with scar-related ventricular tachycardia. *Circulation* 2012; 125(18): 2184–96.

61. Vergara P et al. Late potentials abolition as an additional technique for reduction of arrhythmia recurrence in scar related ventricular tachycardia ablation. *J Cardiovasc Electrophysiol* 2012; 23(6): 621–27.

62. Tanner H et al. Catheter abla00tion of recurrent scar-related ventricular tachycardia using electroanatomical mapping and irrigated ablation technology: Results of the prospective multicenter Euro-VT-study. *J Cardiovasc Electrophysiol* 2010; 21: 47–53.

Catheter ablation of supraventricular tachycardia

CHRISTOPHER MADIAS, MARK S LINK

39.1 Introduction

Supraventricular tachycardia (SVT) is not a universally agreed upon term. Some define it as any non-ventricular rhythm with a heart rate >100 bpm.[1,2] In this definition, sinus tachycardia (ST), atrial fibrillation (AF) and atrial flutters (AFLs) are designated SVTs. Some exclude only ST, while others use a much more restricted definition that only includes atrioventricular nodal re-entrant tachycardia (AVNRT), atrio-ventricular reciprocating tachycardia (AVRT) and atrial tachycardia (AT); sometimes with a qualifier of paroxysmal, so that these three may be described as paroxysmal supraventricular tachycardias (PSVTs). For interpretation of surface electrocardiograms (ECGs), an expanded definition is favoured that incorporates ST in the differential diagnosis;[1] however, for the ablationist the more restricted definition is preferred.

39.2 Presentation

Patients with SVT can exhibit a variety of symptoms. The majority present with acute onset and termination of palpitations often described as a sensation of both fast and strong heartbeats. Associated symptoms might include light-headedness, dyspnoea on exertion and chest pain. In general, the more rapid the SVT, the more likely these associated symptoms occur. The description of palpitations is rarely helpful in the differential diagnosis of SVTs, with the possible exception of an irregular pattern more often being reported by patients with AF. Patients can also have asymptomatic SVTs, particularly if the heart rate is relatively slow. Notably, not all patients presenting with palpitations will have a clinically significant arrhythmia. Palpitations are not specific for SVTs and are also observed in patients with appropriate and inappropriate ST, anxiety, panic attacks, hyperthyroidism, pheochromocytoma and various other conditions.

SVT can affect individuals of all ages; however, the differential diagnosis is shaped by the age at presentation. Children and adolescents are more likely to have Wolff–Parkinson–White (WPW) syndrome, while AT is more likely to present later in life.[3,4] AVNRT can present at all ages. AF and AFL are rare in the young. Patients with AVRT are slightly more likely to be male (54%), while patients with AVNRT and AT are more likely to be female (70% and 62%, respectively).[5]

39.3 Diagnostic workup

In general, it is important to obtain an ECG recording at the time of symptoms. Although these tracings might not be diagnostic, they document the presence of SVT and can provide important clues as to the underlying cause of the arrhythmia. A 12-lead ECG is preferable to a rhythm strip but can only be obtained if the arrhythmia persists for an extended time. For those patients with shorter episodes, ambulatory monitoring is often necessary. For those with daily episodes, a 24- or 48-hour Holter is useful. For those with more sporadic events, a 30-day event ('loop') monitor might be required to capture an arrhythmic episode. Over the last few years, mobile devices have been developed that can record rhythm strips onto a cell phone. While these are not likely to capture onset of a tachycardia, they can be very useful and avoid inconveniences associated with extended ambulatory monitors.

If SVT is diagnosed and an ablation is contemplated, assessment for structural heart disease is useful. If the patient has risk factors for coronary disease, exercise or pharmacologic, stress testing might also be warranted. Thyroid function assessment is often useful, particularly if the SVT is AF.

39.4 Differential diagnosis

VTs can be first categorised as irregular or regular (Figure 39.1 and Table 39.1).[1] Irregular SVTs include AF, multifocal atrial tachycardia (MAT) and AFL and AT with variable atrioventricular (AV) conduction. Regular tachycardias include ST, AVNRT, AVRT, AT, AFL and junctional tachycardia (JT). With acquisition of ECG

tracings, particularly if they include onset or termination, one can often narrow the differential. AVNRT often starts with a premature atrial beat and consequent PR interval prolongation from slow pathway conduction in the beat that initiates SVT. During a regular, narrow complex SVT, the absence of P waves or a very short RP interval (<70 ms) can be suggestive of AVNRT (Figure 39.2). An asymptomatic, baseline 12-lead ECG might also be useful by revealing the presence of delta waves. If delta waves are noted, AVRT is likely. Right or left atrial enlargement on ECG or documented by an echocardiogram increases the likelihood of AF or AT. The response to adenosine is also helpful. Adenosine will terminate AVNRT and AVRT and can also terminate many ATs. In patients with rapid AF and AFL, adenosine will slow AV conduction, often revealing fibrillatory or flutter waves.[6] Arrhythmia circuits that are dependent on AV nodal conduction will often terminate with an atrial beat, such as AVNRT and AVRT. Thus, the last beat of the tachycardia on a surface ECG will be a P wave (Figure 39.2). AT does not depend on the AV node and thus, termination is usually with a QRS complex.

(a)

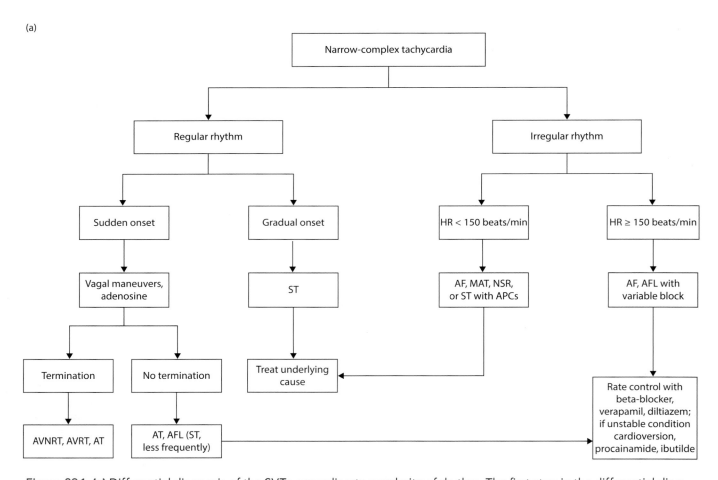

Figure 39.1 **(a)** Differential diagnosis of the SVTs, according to regularity of rhythm. The first step in the differential diagnosis of narrow-complex tachycardias is to determine whether the rhythm is regular or irregular. Further delineation of SVTs can be established according to onset (sudden or gradual), heart rate and response to vagal manoeuvres or administration of adenosine.

(Continued)

(b)

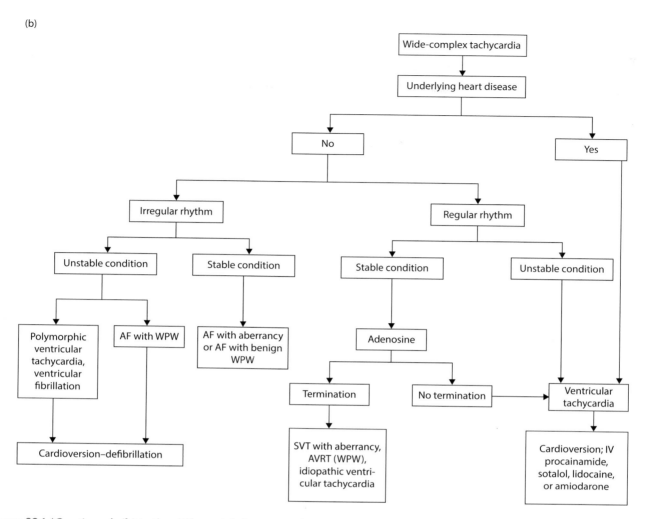

Figure 39.1 (*Continued*) **(b)** In the differential diagnosis of wide-complex tachycardias, the initial step is to determine whether there is underlying heart disease. If the patient has known or suspected cardiac disease, the tachycardia is probably a ventricular tachycardia, and treatment for that condition should be initiated. If heart disease is not thought to be present, the strategy is to separate the ventricular response into regular and irregular rhythms. If a patient with a regular wide-complex tachycardia is in stable condition, administration of adenosine is reasonable, since this will terminate many of the SVTs. If the patient's condition is unstable or if the tachycardia does not terminate with adenosine, treatment for presumptive ventricular tachycardia (i.e. cardioversion) should be given. Irregular wide-complex tachycardias are always worrisome, since they are frequently unstable. Patients with unstable irregular wide-complex tachycardias should undergo cardioversion; if the tachycardias are stable, monitoring and cardiac consultation are appropriate. AF, atrial fibrillation; AFL, atrial flutter; APC, atrial premature contraction; AT, atrial tachycardia; AVNRT, atrioventricular nodal re-entrant tachycardia; AVRT, atrioventricular reciprocating tachycardia; HR, heart rate; MAT, multifocal atrial tachycardia; NSR, normal sinus rhythm and ST, sinus tachycardia; IV, intravenous; SVT, supraventricular tachycardia and WPW, Wolff–Parkinson–White syndrome. (Reproduced from Link MS, *N Engl J Med*, 367, 1438–1448, 2012. With permission.)

39.5 Treatment decisions

Once SVT has been documented, decisions regarding management with medications or catheter ablation can be discussed. Medical management might include AV nodal agents, such as beta blockers, calcium channel blockers and digoxin. These medications are effective in AVNRT, AVRT and some ATs. They also slow the ventricular response of AF and AFL. Antiarrhythmic drugs can prevent and terminate many SVTs including AF, AFL, AVNRT, AVRT and AT; however, these medications possess toxicities and

risks that need to be considered prior to administration. Ablation has high success rates for re-entrant arrhythmias, such as AFL, AVNRT and AVRT. Ablation of automatic rhythms, such as AT, can be performed with high success as well; however, induction and maintenance of AT can be affected by sympathetic tone, sometimes limiting success of mapping and ablation at the time of electrophysiology (EP) study. Ablation for AF has a variable success depending on patient characteristics such as underlying valvular heart disease, left atrial size, heart failure and the duration of AF.

Table 39.1 The differential diagnosis of the supraventricular tachycardias (SVTs) arranged by regularity

SVT	Underlying conditions	Regularity	Rate (in bpm)	Onset	P-QRS ratio	Adenosine response	Electrocardiogram
Atrial fibrillation (AF)	Cardiac disease, pulmonary disease, pulmonary embolism, hyperthyroidism, post-operative	Irregular	100–220	Acute gradual (if in chronic AF)	None	Transient slowing of ventricular rate	
Multifocal atrial tachycardia (MAT)	Pulmonary disease, theophylline	Irregular	100–150	Gradual	Changing P morphology prior to QRS	None	
Frequent atrial premature contractions (APCs)	Caffeine stimulants	Irregular	100–150	Gradual	P prior to QRS	None	
Sinus tachycardia (ST)	Sepsis, hypovolaemia, anaemia, pulmonary embolism, pain, fear, fright, exertion, myocardial ischaemia, hyperthyroidism, heart failure	Regular	220-age	Gradual	P prior to QRS	Transient slowing	
Atrial flutter (AFL)	Cardiac disease	Regular (occasionally irregular if variable AV conduction)	150	Acute	Flutter waves	Transient slowing of ventricular rate	
Atrioventricular (AV) nodal re-entrant tachycardia (AVNRT)	None	Regular	150–250	Acute	No apparent atrial activity or R' at termination of QRS	Terminate	
AV re-entrant tachycardia (AVRT)	Rarely Epstein's anomaly	Regular	150–250	Acute	In narrow complex-P following QRS In wide complex-P rarely observed In irregular (AFib) no apparent P waves	Terminate	Orthodromic AVRT / Antidromic AVRT / AFib with Wolff–Parkinson (WPW)
Atrial tachycardia (AT)	Cardiac disease, pulmonary disease	Regular	150–250	Acute	P prior to QRS	Terminates 60%–80%	

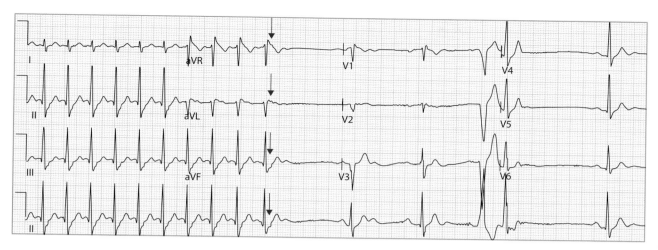

Figure 39.2 A 12-lead electrocardiogram (ECG) demonstrating termination of atrioventricular nodal re-entrant tachycardia (AVNRT). Note the retrogradely conducted P waves located at the terminal portion of the QRS complexes, appearing as slightly positive deflections in V1 (pseudo R' wave) and negative deflections in lead II (pseudo S wave). Also, the last beat of the tachycardia is a retrogradely conducting P wave, which can be seen just at the terminal portion of the QRS complex (blue arrow). Termination of SVT with an atrial beat would be expected with AVNRT and atrioventricular reciprocating tachycardia (AVRT). These two arrhythmias are re-entrant and both dependent on AV nodal conduction to maintain the tachycardia circuit. Any interruption of AV nodal conduction, such as would be provoked with vagal manoeuvres or with administration of adenosine will normally terminate these tachycardias. The mechanism of atrial tachycardia (AT) is not dependent on the AV node and thus, AT almost always terminates with a ventricular complex.

Management of SVT, including the use of catheter ablation, should be tailored to each specific patient, taking into account several factors including symptom severity and frequency, tolerance of medical therapy, age and underlying comorbidities. Patients and physicians should have a clear understanding of goals of care, individual procedural risk and realistic expectations of ablation outcomes, especially in regard to AF ablation. For some patients, medical therapy is quite viable; however, younger patients tend to have poor compliance and intolerance to medications. Ablation is more often pursued in younger patients or for those in whom atrioventricular (AV) nodal agents or antiarrhythmic medications fail. In addition, if a patient has associated symptoms of chest pain, lightheadedness or dyspnoea, they might be more likely to be offered ablation.

39.6 EP studies

Patient preparation includes withdrawal of AV nodal agents or antiarrhythmic medications for up to six doses and fasting after midnight. AF ablation is often performed with general anaesthesia, while most other SVT ablations can be safely performed with conscious sedation. Automatic rhythms such as AT can be suppressed by any sedation, and thus sedation should be minimised during the diagnostic portion of EP study. Venous access is obtained via the right and left femoral veins and traditionally catheters are placed in the high right atrium, the bundle of His, at the right ventricular (RV) apex and in the coronary sinus (CS). Some laboratories access the CS from the subclavian or internal jugular veins.

After catheters are placed, an evaluation of the underlying electrical substrate is undertaken. AVNRT requires dual AV nodal physiology with the presence of a slow pathway revealed with pacing manoeuvres. AVRT requires the presence of a bypass tract that is often observed early in the EP study. Bypass tracts might be concealed on a surface ECG (lack of a delta wave) because they only conduct in a retrograde fashion or because of rapid AV nodal conduction – in which case AV nodal conduction precedes conduction via the bypass tract.[7] The pattern of retrograde conduction and pacing to AV and ventriculoatrial (VA) Wenckebach and 2-1 heart block will generally rapidly uncover bypass tracts. By pacing in the ventricle, retrograde conduction and activation of the atrial tissue as observed on the CS, His bundle and right atrial catheters can be concentric or eccentric. A concentric pattern refers to midline VA conduction through or near the AV node. Eccentric conduction suggests initial activation of the atria is via a discrete bypass tract apart from the AV node (Figure 39.3). Concentric VA conduction can also be present with septal bypass tracts, but these can be differentiated from AV nodal conduction, as they usually do not show decremental properties. Para-Hisian pacing is another helpful manoeuvre to uncover septal bypass tracts (Figure 39.4).[8] Para-Hisian pacing is performed by pacing from the distal pole of the His catheter and measuring VA conduction times. In addition to capturing local ventricular myocardium, by pacing at maximal energy outputs, the insulation surrounding the His–Purkinje fibres can be penetrated and ventricular activation proceeds via the specialised conduction system, resulting in a narrow QRS. With decreased pacing outputs, the His–Purkinje system will no longer be captured and the QRS will widen. In the absence

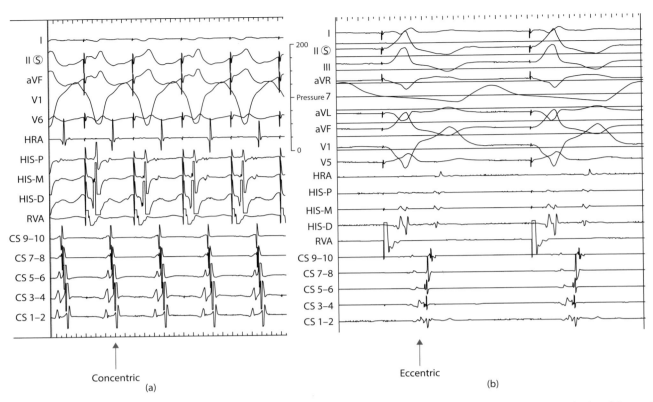

Figure 39.3 Concentric and eccentric retrograde atrial activation. **(a)** Concentric activation. During a ventricular drive train the atria are activated retrogradely via the His–Purkinje system and the AV node. The earliest atrial signal is via the His catheter and activation of the coronary sinus (CS) follows a proximal (CS 9,10) to distal activation pattern. **(b)** Eccentric activation in a patient with a left free wall accessory pathway. Ventricular pacing results with eccentric atrial activation with the earliest atrial signal noted on the distal CS catheter (CS 1,2).

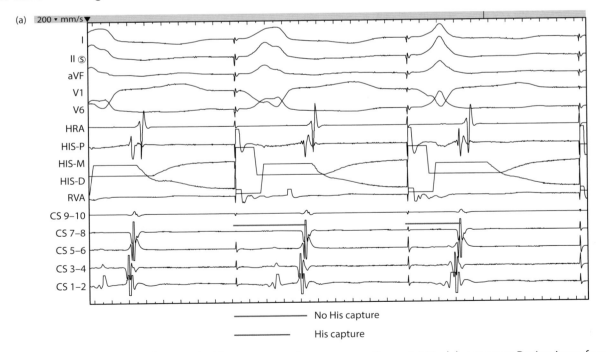

Figure 39.4 Para-Hisian pacing without and with a para-septal accessory pathway. **(a)** Nodal response: Pacing is performed from the His catheter. When pacing does not penetrate the His, the QRS is wide and the stim to A time is longer (red line), as the activation wavefront must reach the distal right bundle branch and traverse the entire length of the right bundle before reaching the His, atrioventricular node (AVN) and atria. When high output pacing results in direct capture of the His bundle and the local myocardium the stim to A time is comparably short (blue line) and the QRS is narrow. *(Continued)*

(b)

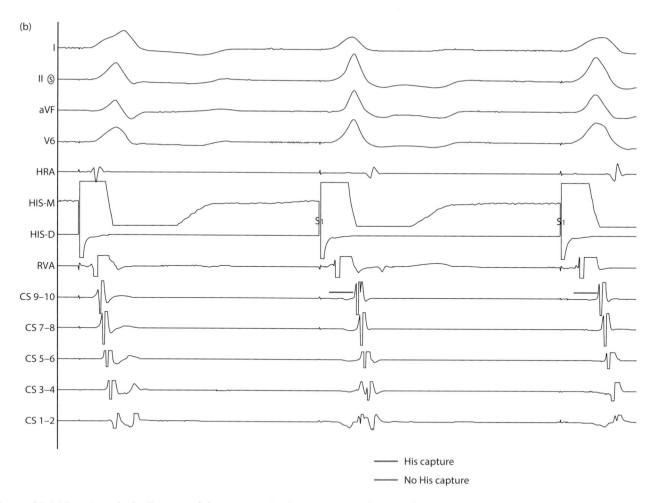

——— His capture

——— No His capture

Figure 39.4 (*Continued*) **(b)** Extra-nodal response: In the presence of a septal accessory pathway, VA conduction is not dependent on capture of the His bundle. The stim to A time is identical due to retrograde conduction solely across the bypass tract, regardless of His capture.

of a septal bypass tract, retrograde activation of the atrium travels through the His–Purkinje system and the AV node. If there is capture of the His then retrograde conduction occurs rapidly and the VA time is short; however, when the His is no longer captured, the impulse must travel down to the apex of the RV and then retrogradely through the His–Purkinje system, thereby lengthening the VA time. In the presence of a septal bypass tract, VA conduction time and activation sequence will be similar whether or not the His–Purkinje network is captured.

Anterograde curves are performed with pacing from the right atrium. The atrium is paced at a fixed cycle length (CL) (often at 600 ms) for 8–10 beats with single extra-stimuli given at decreasing CLs (often starting at 580 ms). This manoeuvre is sequentially repeated with a decrease of 10–20 ms in the CL of the extra-stimuli. With each pacing sequence, measurements are made of the atrial to His (AH) and AV conduction times. Decremental conduction in the AV node should result in a steady increase in AH conduction times as the CL of the extra-stimuli decrease. As decremental conduction is noted through the AV node, curves can also uncover bypass tracts or specialised bypass tracts

known as Mahaim fibres. If dual AV nodal physiology is present – the substrate for AVNRT – the refractory period of the fast AV nodal pathway will eventually be reached and AV conduction will switch to the slow pathway. This will manifest as a sudden increase in atrial to His bundle conduction (i.e. an AH 'jump') (Figure 39.5). Retrograde curves are performed in a similar manner by pacing in the RV and measuring the VA conduction time.

Most patients with AVNRT and AVRT will have the underlying electrophysiologic substrate uncovered by the above pacing manoeuvres; however, induction of the clinical arrhythmia is important, not only to verify the diagnosis, but also to establish an endpoint for assessment of the efficacy of ablation. Induction is performed with burst atrial pacing at decreasing CLs or by introducing single or double atrial extra-stimuli. Some patients will have easily inducible arrhythmias, while others will require more aggressive stimulation. Some patients will also require the concomitant administration of adrenergic agonists such as isoproterenol or less commonly, epinephrine. Arrhythmias such as AF and AFL will often require induction with rapid atrial pacing.

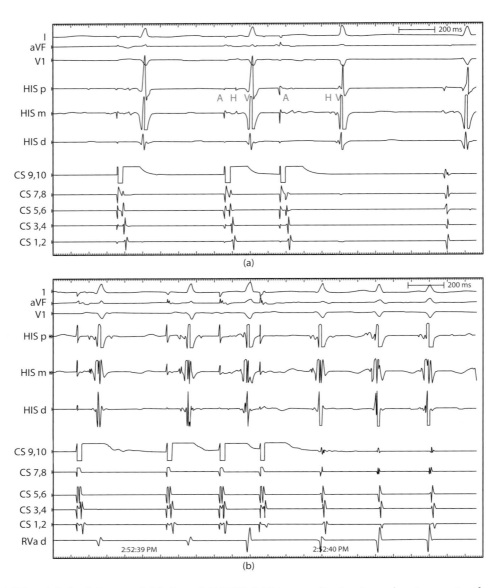

Figure 39.5 Dual AV nodal physiology an initiation of AVNRT. **(a)** Intra-cardiac tracings showing pacing from the proximal CS (CS 9,10). The first beat of the tracing represents that last beat of a drive train followed by two early extra-stimuli. With the second extra-stimulus (the last paced beat), conduction via the fast pathway is refractory and AV conduction switches to the slow pathway. This is manifest as a sudden increase in atrial to His bundle conduction (i.e. an AH 'jump'). **(b)** After initiation of isoproterenol, appropriately timed extra-stimuli initiate AVNRT after an AH jump. Note the very short VA time in during AVNRT with atrial electrograms virtually simultaneous with ventricular electrograms.

With induction of SVT, a diagnosis can be established by assessing the timing and relationship of atrial and ventricular depolarization, by evaluating activation patterns on the CS catheter and by examining the response to various pacing manoeuvres. In general, with intra-cardiac catheters in place, AF and AFL are relatively easy to discern. Distinguishing between the three primary regular SVTs – AVNRT, AVRT and AT – often requires more thorough appraisal. If the septal VA time at the His catheter is 70 ms or less, the diagnosis of AVNRT is most likely. The ventricle is a mandatory component of the circuit in AVRT, and thus, a one to one AV relationship is obligatory to sustain AVRT. During tachycardia, if there is noted to be two to one AV or

VA conduction, AVRT is ruled out (Figure 39.6). Two to one AV conduction can be seen in AVNRT (rarely) or AT. If the tachycardia terminates in the atrium (last beat is an atrial beat) or with AV block, the mechanism is unlikely to be AT. If the tachycardia terminates with V pacing without atrial activation, it is not likely to be AT. Variability in the CL of the SVT can also be revealing. If changes in individual A–A CLs precede H–H alterations, then the SVT is likely to be AT; whereas, if fluctuations in H–H intervals drive A–A intervals, then AVNRT or AVRT are more likely.

Entrainment of the tachycardia from the RV apex can also be used to differentiate AVNRT from AVRT and AT. A V–A–V response is typical of AVNRT and AVRT, whereas

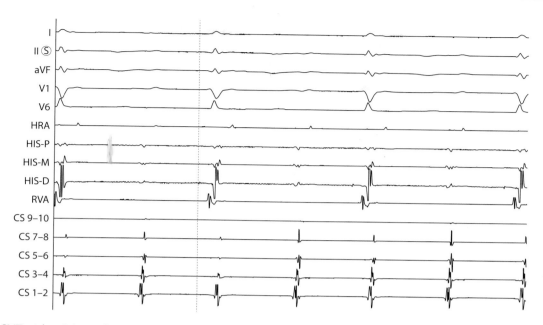

Figure 39.6 SVT with a 2:1 atrial to ventricular ratio. The ventricle is a mandatory component of the circuit in AV reciprocating tachycardia (AVRT), and thus, a one-to-one AV relationship during tachycardia is obligatory. Two to one AV conduction, as is demonstrated in the figure rules out AVRT as the mechanism. A two to one atrial to ventricular ratio can be seen in AT and more rarely in AVNRT. The eccentric atrial activation pattern points to an AT as the mechanism of this tachycardia.

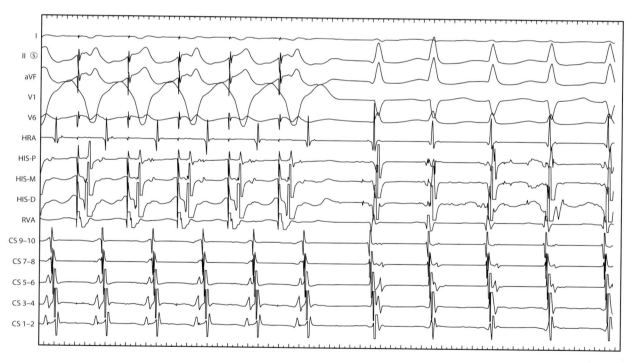

Figure 39.7 Ventricular entrainment during SVT. Ventricular pacing is performed at a CL of 20–30 ms shorter than the tachycardia. The presence of 1:1 VA conduction and acceleration of the atrial rate to the pacing CL is confirmed. Following cessation of pacing, the tachycardia continues. The retrograde atrial activation sequence during ventricular pacing matches that of the tachycardia, showing a concentric activation pattern. Following cessation of ventricular pacing, a VAV response is noted, ruling out AT as a mechanism, and suggesting AVNRT.

AT will show a V–A–A–V response (Figure 39.7). The post-pacing interval of the RV catheter is also diagnostic. With AVNRT, the RV is not part of the re-entrant circuit and thus, the post-pacing interval is longer than that of AVRT.[9] If the V post-pacing interval is ≥115 ms, the tachycardia is likely to be AVNRT.

39.7 Specific arrhythmias

39.7.1 AV nodal re-entrant tachycardia

AVNRT is the most common mechanism of regular SVT.[5] In typical (slow-fast) AVNRT, the re-entrant circuit consists of anterograde conduction down the slow AV nodal pathway and retrograde conduction up the fast pathway. Due to near simultaneous atrial and ventricular activation, the P wave in typical AVNRT is often buried in the QRS complex or is visible just at the tail end of the QRS (Figure 39.2).[1] Other variants of AVNRT are less common, including reverse typical (fast-slow) AVNRT, in which re-entry proceeds anterogradely down the fast pathway and retrogradely up the slow. In slow–slow AVNRT, re-entry proceeds anterogradely down a slow pathway and uses a second slow pathway for the retrograde limb. In atypical forms of AVNRT, the P wave is visible and can result in long RP tachycardia with the P-wave morphology being negative in the inferior leads, consistent with retrograde atrial activation (Figure 39.8).

The target of AVNRT ablation is the slow pathway. The catheter is guided to the posteroinferior base of the triangle of Koch, which is defined by the ostium (os) of the CS posteriorly, the tricuspid annulus inferiorly, and the tendon of Todaro anteriorly and superiorly. A small atrial electrogram and larger ventricular electrogram should be notable on the distal electrode of the ablation catheter and the catheter is carefully manipulated to identify slow pathway potentials (Figure 39.9). During radiofrequency (RF) ablation at effective sites, accelerated junctional beats are noted. The absence of junctional beats during RF ablation usually signifies an unsuccessful lesion and the catheter should be repositioned. During ablation, intra-cardiac and surface electrograms are carefully monitored for PR prolongation or AV block during sinus rhythm and for VA block during junctional beats. Rapid junctional tachycardia (CL > 350 ms) during ablation can signify thermal injury of the His bundle and the RF application should be immediately terminated.

Acute success rates for AVNRT ablation are quite high, ranging up to 98%.[10] Although the ultimate outcome of AVNRT ablation is non-inducibility with complete elimination of the slow pathway, studies suggest that slow pathway modification with a residual AH jump or a single echo beat can result in durable success with a low recurrence rate (<5%).[11] The risk of serious complications from AVNRT ablation is quite low, with AV block requiring permanent pacemaker implant being the most common serious complication.[10]

39.7.2 Focal AT

Focal AT is characterised as a SVT with centrifugal conduction that originates from a discrete location in either the left or right atrium. ATs are usually paroxysmal but can be incessant and in some patients can result in tachycardia

mediated cardiomyopathy. The mechanism for focal AT can be abnormal automaticity, triggered activity or micro-re-entry. As opposed to triggered and automatic ATs, micro-re-entrant AT is less likely to terminate with adenosine.[12] Distinguishing the underlying mechanism is not essential, as the mapping and ablation strategy will not be altered. ATs often originate from characteristic anatomic sites and more commonly from the right than the left atrium.[13] The P-wave morphology on a 12-lead ECG can be useful in predicting the anatomic site of origin and can aid in preparing a mapping and ablation strategy.[14]

39.7.3 AV re-entrant tachycardia

Normally, the atria and ventricles are electrically isolated from each other, except for conduction via the AV node. Bypass tracts are additional, congenital electrical connections. Although most commonly occurring in patients with normal cardiac anatomy, bypass tracts can be associated with structural congenital heart disease, most notably Ebstein's anomaly. Bypass tracts can conduct in anterograde direction only, in retrograde direction only or in both directions. Early, partial activation of the ventricular tissue via the bypass tract (bypassing conduction via the AV node/His–Purkinje system) is manifest on a surface ECG as a delta wave and is termed pre-excitation (Figure 39.9). Pre-excitation is absent in patients where there is no or slow anterograde conduction and in some patients where the bypass tract is distant from the AV node, such as on the left free wall. Patients who have manifest pre-excitation and have clinical SVT are characterised with WPW syndrome.[1]

Four potential arrhythmias can be seen with bypass tracts: (1) a regular narrow QRS tachycardia, with anterograde conduction down the normal AV node/His–Purkinje system and retrograde conduction up the bypass tract (orthodromic AVRT); (2) a regular wide QRS tachycardia, with anterograde conduction down the bypass tract and retrograde conduction up the AV node (antidromic AVRT); (3) a regular wide QRS tachycardia due to AT or AVNRT with ventricular pre-excitation via a 'bystander' bypass tract and (4) wide irregular tachycardia due to AF with atrioventricular conduction through the bypass tract (Figure 39.10). Orthodromic AVRT is the most common arrhythmia associated with bypass tracts.

Both spontaneous and inducible AF can be quite commonly associated with WPW. Rapid anterograde conduction over a bypass tract during AF can potentially result in precipitation of ventricular arrhythmias and sudden death. Risk stratification for sudden death in WPW can be necessary. Risk factors include younger age (<30 years old), male gender, prior history of AF, prior syncope, congenital heart disease and familial WPW.[15,16] Non-invasive risk stratification can include ECG or ambulatory monitoring, as well as an exercise stress test. Intermittent loss of pre-excitation during ECG or ambulatory monitor suggests a low risk pathway. Complete loss of pre-excitation with elevated heart rates during a treadmill test also suggests a lower risk pathway.

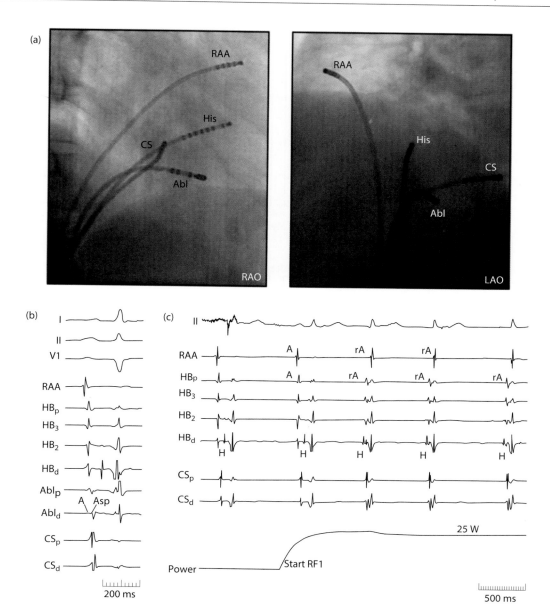

Figure 39.8 Ablation of the slow pathway for AVNRT. **(a)** Catheter positions during ablation of AVNRT. Radiographs taken in the right and left anterior oblique views are shown (RAO and LAO). An octopolar His bundle catheter (His) is noted. A catheter in the proximal CS helps to delineate the triangle of Koch. The ablation catheter (Ab1) is positioned in the right posteroseptal (inferoseptal) area, between the ostium of the CS and the tricuspid annulus. A fourth catheter, positioned in the right atrial appendage is used during atrial programmed stimulation. **(b)** Electrograms recorded from the catheters as shown in (a). The electrogram at the distal bipole of the ablation catheter (Ab1) shows a large and sharp 'slow pathway potential (Asp)', preceded by a small 'atrial deflection (a)', and followed by a large ventricular deflection. Note that the Asp is recorded after atrial activation in the proximal CS. RAA, right atrial appendage; HB, His bundle, proximal to distal. **(c)** Radiofrequency (RF) energy delivered at this site immediately resulted in the induction of an accelerated junctional rhythm. Note the retrograde atrial activation over the fast pathway (rA) during each consecutive junctional beat, ensuring integrity of the physiological AV nodal conduction axis. Later during RF delivery, the junctional rhythm slowed down and gave way to sinus rhythm. After this single application (60 seconds), one-to-one antegrade slow pathway conduction was eliminated, and AVNRT was no longer inducible. (Modified from Heidbüchel H, *Europace*, 2, 15–19, 2000. With permission.)

Measurement of the shortest pre-excited R–R interval on an ECG during AF with pre-excitation can be used as a non-invasive surrogate to assess accessory pathway properties. A rapid shortest pre-excited R–R interval (SPERRI) during pre-excited AF can be associated with a higher risk pathway (<250 ms). During invasive EP study, a SPERRI of <220–250 ms is used to stratify patients as having high-risk pathways.[15] The accessory pathway effective refractory period (APERP) can also be directly measured, though overall it is felt to be a less predictive variable than the SPERRI.[15,17,18]

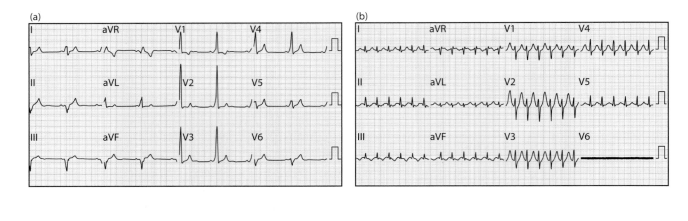

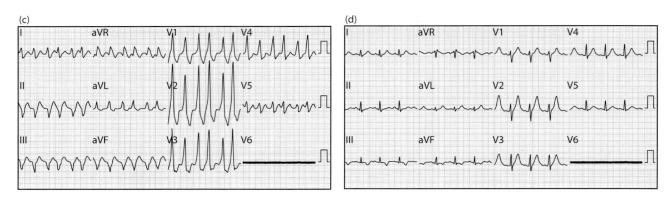

Figure 39.9 Twelve-lead ECGs in a patient with WPW syndrome an AV re-entrant tachycardia from a left free wall bypass tract. **(a)** Twelve-lead ECG in sinus rhythm showing ventricular pre-excitation manifest as a delta wave. **(b)** A regular narrow complex tachycardia consistent with orthodromic AVRT. **(c)** A wide irregular tachycardia due to atrial fibrillation with pre-excitation and AV conduction via the bypass tract. **(d)** Twelve-lead ECG in sinus rhythm post-ablation showing absence of the delta wave. Note lead V6 is disconnected in some of the tracings.

Catheter ablation of bypass tracts can offer definitive management for those with symptomatic SVT or for those with high-risk pathways. There are several types of bypass tracts and their location can be distributed throughout the AV annuli; however, certain locations tend to be more common than others.[15] The vector of the delta wave on the surface ECG can be helpful in localizing the anatomic location of the bypass tract, which can aid pre-procedure planning and patient counselling prior to ablation.[19] The target of ablation is the bypass tract, which is most commonly mapped on the atrial side of the annulus. Left-sided bypass tracts are usually approached with a trans-septal technique, though some will approach them from a retrograde ventricular approach. If there is pre-excitation, mapping can be performed in sinus rhythm or during atrial pacing. Successful ablation sites should have short AV intervals with continuous electrical activity or pathway/bypass tract potentials noted between the atrial and ventricular signals. The ventricular electrogram on the distal pole of the ablation catheter should precede the onset of the delta wave. If a bypass tract is concealed, retrograde activation mapping can be performed during SVT or with ventricular pacing. Successful ablation sites should have short VA intervals,

with continuous electrical activity and pathway/bypass tract potentials often noted at successful sites (Figure 39.11). Successful ablation should result in non-inducibility of SVT, complete loss of pre-excitation on the surface ECG and elimination of bidirectional (anterograde and retrograde) conduction across the bypass tract. Adenosine is often given post-ablation to confirm pathway elimination and complete absence of conduction during AV nodal block.

39.7.4 Atrial flutter

In AFL or macro-re-entrant AT, the re-entrant circuit encompasses a large area of the left or right atrium. The most common form of AFL is termed *typical* AFL, in which the circuit propagates around the tricuspid valve annulus in a counter-clockwise pattern. Typical AFL is generally characterised by an atrial rate of 280–300 beats/min with 2:1 conduction in the AV node resulting in a ventricular rate of 140–150 beats/min.[1] In patients with AV nodal disease or in those who have received rate slowing medications, the characteristic 'saw-tooth' appearing flutter waves can be clearly visualised on the surface ECG. An area of slowed conduction between the tricuspid valve and the inferior vena cava – the cavotricuspid

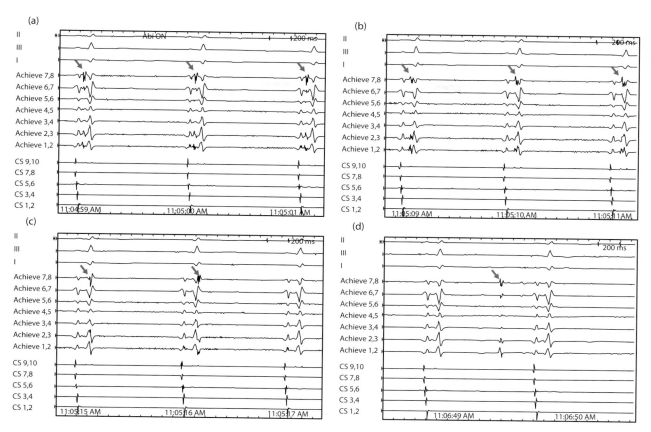

Figure 39.10 Pulmonary vein isolation with cryoballoon. (a) The cryoballoon catheter is positioned in the left superior pulmonary vein with the balloon inflated. Atrial and ventricular electrograms are recorded with distinct pulmonary vein potentials noted after the initial atrial signals (arrows). (b) Initiation of cryoablation results in delay of the pulmonary vein potentials (arrows). (c) During continuation of the ablation lesion, the pulmonary vein potentials are shown to further delay, until the vein is isolated (third beat). (d) Later on during the lesion, an isolated pulmonary vein potential is noted to fire in between two beats of sinus rhythm.

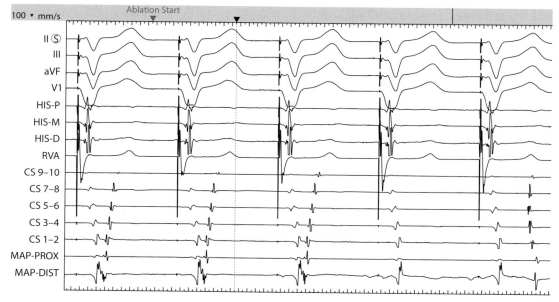

Figure 39.11 Ablation of left free wall bypass tract. Successful ablation site of a left free wall bypass tract during ventricular pacing. Note the earliest atrial signal is on the ablation catheter with continuous electrical activity noted between the VA signals. Retrograde conduction via the bypass tract is eliminated within seconds of ablation. Of note, post-ablation there is no VA conduction via the AV node. The last atrial beat on the tracing is a dissociated sinus beat.

isthmus – is critical for the perpetuation of the arrhythmia and is the target for ablation in typical AFL. Successful ablation results in termination of the tachycardia and creation of bidirectional electrical block across the isthmus (medial to lateral and vice versa). Bidirectional block is often confirmed by placing a multi-electrode catheter along the lateral tricuspid annulus and performing differential pacing manoeuvres from this catheter and from a catheter in the CS. Although typical AFL ablation is normally uncomplicated, anatomic variation including sub-Eustachian pouches or large pectinate muscles encroaching on the isthmus can result in challenging ablation.[20]

39.7.5 Atypical atrial flutter

Atypical AFLs can occur in either the left or right atria and sometimes are found in normal hearts; however, more commonly, atypical AFL is associated with atrial enlargement as a result of structural heart disease, including heart failure and mitral regurgitation. Atypical AFL can also occur around areas of scar created by prior surgeries or as a result of AF ablation. When associated with prior AF ablation, AFL can typically be mapped around the pulmonary veins or to gaps in prior ablation lines, such as roof lines or mitral isthmus lines.

39.7.6 Atrial fibrillation

The recognition that triggers of AF could be focal targets for ablative therapy led to the concept of pulmonary vein isolation as a predominant strategy for AF ablation.[21] In pulmonary vein isolation, lesions are created around the antrum of the pulmonary veins resulting in non-conducting scar. Traditionally, this is performed with catheters using RF energy to deliver connecting, point-by-point, circumferential lesions around each vein.[22] Balloon-based catheters using cryoablation or laser energy have also been created with the objective of generating uninterrupted, contiguous lesions around the pulmonary veins (Figure 39.10).[23,24]

Catheter ablation of AF with pulmonary vein isolation as the predominant approach has become safer and more effective for patients with paroxysmal AF. The success rates of pulmonary vein isolation in patients with persistent or long-standing persistent AF remain comparatively poor.[25] Patients with persistent or long-standing persistent AF often need additional ablation in the left (and sometimes the right) atrium to target the substrate of AF. The optimal targets for substrate modification in more advanced AF remain unclear, resulting in the examination of a number of different approaches. One such strategy attempts to replicate surgical 'debulking' of the left atrium with connecting point-by-point RF lesions in a pattern of lines across the left atrium. The most common lines include a roof line connecting the left and right superior pulmonary veins and a mitral line connecting the left inferior vein to the mitral annulus.[26,27] In addition, complex fractionated atrial electrograms have been mapped and targeted as areas theorised to

represent slowed conduction or pivot points of wavelets that might be essential to the maintenance of AF.[28] Adoption of these techniques has shown mixed success in clinical trials and over time.[29]

More recent strategies have shifted the focus in an attempt to identify patient specific AF substrates. These approaches are influenced by mechanistic insights that focal impulses and organised sources of functional re-entry, termed *rotors*, might play key roles in the perpetuation of AF. Focal impulse and rotor modulation (FIRM) ablation employs a 64-pole basket catheter placed in the left and right atria, and a computational mapping approach to identify areas of localised rotors and focal impulses that are then targeted for ablation.[30,31] Another approach uses non-invasive electrical data obtained from a 252 electrode body vest combined with individual atrial anatomic geometry obtained from a cardiac computed tomography (CT) scan to create a non-invasive map of AF drivers.[32,33] These data are then used to guide electrical substrate ablation. Randomised trials assessing the short- and long-term success of these approaches are ongoing.

A combined surgical and percutaneous approach has also been developed and termed *hybrid ablation* or the *convergent procedure*.[34] In hybrid ablation, a surgeon uses a closed-chest, minimally invasive strategy to deliver transmural, linear ablation lesions guided by direct visualization of the epicardial surface of the atrium. A percutaneous endocardial ablation is then performed by an electrophysiologist, either immediately after the surgical ablation or in a staged approach. Further research is necessary to determine optimal patient selection for this modality; however, hybrid ablation might provide an effective approach in patients with substantial structural heart disease.

39.8 Mapping systems

Three-dimensional electroanatomic mapping has evolved into a very accurate method of visualizing the cardiac anatomy and physiology. Multiple systems exist and are now widely utilised for AF ablation as well as in mapping and ablation of atypical AFL, AT and other SVTs. These systems share similar abilities to create three-dimensional maps of cardiac structures and incorporate electrophysiologic information, including tachycardia activation patterns and local voltage. Multipole catheters of different shapes have been developed, allowing for more efficient and accurate mapping of cardiac anatomy and arrhythmic activation.

39.9 Energy sources

Energy sources for ablation include cryoenergy and RF. The most commonly used energy source for SVT ablation is RF, especially in adults. RF has been used for over 25 years and has a long record of safety and efficacy.[35,36] Cryoablation catheters are more recently utilised. They do not possess the flexibility of RF catheters but they do have the advantage of reversibility of the lesion if unintended injury of the native conduction system is noted during ablation. Thus, cryoablation can be used to target bypass tracts that have been localised near the His–Purkinje system and it is more frequently employed for SVT ablation in young children. Notably, recurrence rates are generally higher with cryoablation compared to RF. Novel ablation energy sources continue to be developed, including laser energy for the ablation of AF.[24]

39.10 Success rates

The success rates of ablation depend on the type of SVT. For typical AFL, AVNRT and AVRT success rates are generally greater than 95%. For AT, the success rate is lower for the prime reason that if the patient is non-inducible at the time of EP study, one might not be able to map the AT. Success rates for atypical AFL are also lower than typical AFL. Finally, success rates are lower and recurrence rates are higher for AF than for any other SVT. Success rates for AF range from 50% to 80% and importantly depend on whether the AF is paroxysmal or persistent and whether there is underlying structural heart disease.

39.11 Complications

The more common complications of SVT ablations are local haematomas at the groin access site. Vascular damage such as AV fistulas and aneurysms are less common. Cardiac inflammation may cause mild chest pain and atrial premature beats. The more serious but less common complications include pericardial effusion from a cardiac tear or perforation, heart block from collateral damage with ablation near the His–Purkinje system and systemic thromboembolism when ablation is performed in the left atrium. Ablations that require longer procedure times and more extensive ablation, such as AF ablation, are associated with higher risk.

References

1. Link MS. Clinical practice. Evaluation and initial treatment of supraventricular tachycardia. *N Engl J Med* 2012; 367: 1438–48.
2. Page RL et al. 2015 ACC/AHA/HRS guideline for the management of adult patients with supraventricular tachycardia: A report of the American College of Cardiology/American Heart Association task force on clinical practice guidelines and the heart rhythm society. *Circulation* 2016; 133: e506–74.
3. Rodriguez LM et al. Age at onset and gender of patients with different types of supraventricular tachycardias. *Am J Cardiol* 1992; 70: 1213–15.
4. Goyal R et al. Comparison of the ages of tachycardia onset in patients with atrioventricular nodal reentrant tachycardia and accessory pathway-mediated tachycardia. *Am Heart J* 1996; 132: 765–7.
5. Porter MJ et al. Influence of age and gender on the mechanism of supraventricular tachycardia. *Heart Rhythm* 2004; 1: 393–6.
6. Yamabe H et al. Analysis of the anatomical tachycardia circuit in verapamil-sensitive atrial tachycardia originating from the vicinity of the atrioventricular node. *Circ Arrhythm Electrophysiol* 2010; 3: 54–62.
7. Katritsis DG, and Camm AJ. Atrioventricular nodal reentrant tachycardia. *Circulation* 2010; 122: 831–40.
8. Hirao K et al. A new method for differentiating retrograde conduction over an accessory AV pathway from conduction over the AV node. *Circulation* 1996; 94: 1027–35.
9. Michaud GF et al. Differentiation of atypical atrioventricular node re-entrant tachycardia from orthodromic reciprocating tachycardia using a septal accessory pathway by the response to ventricular pacing. *J Am Coll Cardiol* 2001; 38: 1163–7.
10. Feldman A et al. Predictors of acute and long-term success of slow pathway ablation for atrioventricular nodal reentrant tachycardia: A single center series of 1,419 consecutive patients. *Pacing Clin Electrophysiol* 2011; 34: 927–33.
11. Stern JD et al. Meta-analysis to assess the appropriate endpoint for slow pathway ablation of atrioventricular nodal reentrant tachycardia. *Pacing Clin Electrophysiol* 2011; 34: 269–77.
12. Markowitz SM et al. Adenosine-insensitive focal atrial tachycardia: Evidence for de novo micro-re-entry in the human atrium. *J Am Coll Cardiol* 2007; 49: 1324–33.
13. Hoffmann E et al. Clinical experience with electroanatomic mapping of ectopic atrial tachycardia. *Pacing Clin Electrophysiol* 2002; 25: 49–56.
14. Kistler PM et al. P-wave morphology in focal atrial tachycardia: Development of an algorithm to predict the anatomic site of origin. *J Am Coll Cardiol* 2006; 48: 1010–17.
15. Cohen MI et al. Paces/hrs expert consensus statement on the management of the asymptomatic young patient with a Wolff-Parkinson-White (WPW, ventricular pre-excitation) electrocardiographic pattern: Developed in partnership between the pediatric and congenital electrophysiology society (paces) and the Heart Rhythm Society (HRS). Endorsed by the governing bodies of paces, HRS, the American College Of Cardiology Foundation (ACCF), the American Heart Association (AHA), the American Academy of Pediatrics (AAP), and the Canadian Heart Rhythm Society (CHRS). *Heart Rhythm* 2012; 9: 1006–24.
16. Al-Khatib SM et al. Risk stratification for arrhythmic events in patients with asymptomatic pre-excitation: A systematic review for the 2015 ACC/AHA/HRS guideline for the management of adult patients with supraventricular tachycardia: A report of the American College of Cardiology/American Heart Association task force on clinical practice guidelines and the heart rhythm society. *Circulation* 2016; 133: e575–86.
17. Santinelli V et al. Asymptomatic ventricular preexcitation: A long-term prospective follow-up study of 293 adult patients. *Circ Arrhythm Electrophysiol* 2009; 2: 102–107.
18. Santinelli V et al. The natural history of asymptomatic ventricular pre-excitation a long-term prospective follow-up study of 184 asymptomatic children. *J Am Coll Cardiol* 2009; 53: 275–80.

19. Arruda MS et al. Development and validation of an ECG algorithm for identifying accessory pathway ablation site in Wolff-Parkinson-White syndrome. *J Cardiovasc Electrophysiol* 1998; 9: 2–12.

20. Asirvatham SJ. Correlative anatomy and electrophysiology for the interventional electrophysiologist: Right atrial flutter. *J Cardiovasc Electrophysiol* 2009; 20: 113–22.

21. Haissaguerre M et al. Spontaneous initiation of atrial fibrillation by ectopic beats originating in the pulmonary veins. *N Engl J Med* 1998; 339: 659–66.

22. Calkins H et al. 2012 HRS/EHRA/ECAS expert consensus statement on catheter and surgical ablation of atrial fibrillation: Recommendations for patient selection, procedural techniques, patient management and follow-up, definitions, endpoints, and research trial design: A report of the heart rhythm society (hrs) task force on catheter and surgical ablation of atrial fibrillation. Developed in partnership with the European Heart Rhythm Association (EHRA), a registered branch of the European Society Of Cardiology (ESC) and the European Cardiac Arrhythmia Society (ECAS); and in collaboration with the American College of Cardiology (ACC), American Heart Association (AHA), the Asia Pacific Heart Rhythm Society (APHRS), and the Society of Thoracic Surgeons (STS). Endorsed by the governing bodies of the American College of Cardiology Foundation, the American Heart Association, the European Cardiac Arrhythmia Society, the European Heart Rhythm Association, the Society of Thoracic Surgeons, the Asia Pacific Heart Rhythm Society, and the Heart Rhythm Society. *Heart Rhythm* 2012; 9: 632–96 e621.

23. Packer DL et al. Cryoballoon ablation of pulmonary veins for paroxysmal atrial fibrillation: First results of the north American Arctic Front (stop AF) pivotal trial. *J Am Coll Cardiol* 2013; 61: 1713–23.

24. Dukkipati SR et al. Pulmonary vein isolation using a visually guided laser balloon catheter: The first 200-patient multicenter clinical experience. *Circulation Arrhythmia Electrophysiol* 2013; 6: 467–72.

25. Weerasooriya R et al. Catheter ablation for atrial fibrillation: Are results maintained at 5 years of follow-up? *J Am Coll Cardiol* 2011; 57: 160–66.

26. Jais P et al. Technique and results of linear ablation at the mitral isthmus. *Circulation* 2004; 110: 2996–3002.

27. Hocini M et al. Techniques, evaluation, and consequences of linear block at the left atrial roof in paroxysmal atrial fibrillation: A prospective randomized study. *Circulation* 2005; 112: 3688–96.

28. Nademanee K et al. A new approach for catheter ablation of atrial fibrillation: Mapping of the electrophysiologic substrate. *J Am Coll Cardiol* 2004; 43: 2044–53.

29. Verma A et al. Catheter ablation for persistent atrial fibrillation. *N Engl J Med* 2015; 373: 878–79.

30. Narayan SM et al. Treatment of atrial fibrillation by the ablation of localized sources: Confirm (conventional ablation for atrial fibrillation with or without focal impulse and rotor modulation) trial. *J Am Coll Cardiol* 2012; 60: 628–36.

31. Miller JM et al. Initial independent outcomes from focal impulse and rotor modulation ablation for atrial fibrillation: Multicenter firm registry. *J Cardiovasc Electrophysiol* 2014; 25: 921–9.

32. Dubois R et al. Non-invasive cardiac mapping in clinical practice: Application to the ablation of cardiac arrhythmias. *J Electrocardiol* 2015; 48: 966–74.

33. Lim HS et al. Noninvasive mapping to guide atrial fibrillation ablation. *Card Electrophysiol Clin* 2015; 7: 89–98.

34. Kumar P et al. Hybrid treatment of atrial fibrillation. *Prog Cardiovasc Dis* 2015; 58: 213–20.

35. Jackman WM et al. Catheter ablation of accessory atrioventricular pathways (Wolff-Parkinson-White syndrome) by radiofrequency current. *N Engl J Med* 1991; 324: 1605–11.

36. Jackman WM et al. Treatment of supraventricular tachycardia due to atrioventricular nodal reentry, by radiofrequency catheter ablation of slow-pathway conduction. *N Engl J Med* 1992; 327: 313–18.

40

Ablation of ventricular arrhythmias

ERIK WISSNER, WILLIAM H SPEAR

40.1 Introduction

Catheter ablation has become an important treatment modality for patients suffering from ventricular arrhythmias (VAs). The advent of implantable cardioverter defibrillators (ICDs) has resulted in greater survival of patients at risk for or survivors of sudden arrhythmic death.[1,2] Whilst ICDs successfully abort VAs, their use has no meaningful impact on prevention of VAs since the arrhythmogenic substrate remains unaltered or may progress over time. Recurrent ICD shocks can be harmful and negatively affect the quality of life.[3–5] Anti-arrhythmic drugs reduce the incidence of new or recurrent VAs, but may not be tolerated long-term resulting in drug discontinuation in nearly 25% of patients.[6] Hence, definitive therapy targeting the pathologic substrate is desirable. Catheter ablation reduces the incidence of recurrent VAs through modification of the arrhythmogenic substrate. This chapter focuses on the use of catheter ablation in patients suffering from scar-related VAs and discusses its role in patients without structural heart disease.

40.2 General principles of catheter ablation of VAs

Since VAs in patients with underlying cardiac disease often arise from abnormal substrate in the form of scar, differentiating normal from abnormal ventricular myocardium is

of paramount importance. Regions of scar form the most common substrate for VAs in patients with ischaemic cardiomyopathy (ICM), dilated cardiomyopathy (DCM), cardiac sarcoidosis and arrhythmogenic right ventricular dysplasia (ARVD). Surviving myocyte bundles within the scar promote slow conduction resulting in anatomical or functional conduction block and macro–re-entry.[7] The critical isthmus is defined as the region within the re-entry circuit that displays slowed conduction. Catheter ablation commonly targets the exit site of the critical isthmus where depolarisation away from scar gives rise to the QRS complex.

40.2.1 Mapping techniques

Different mapping techniques are available and often used in conjunction when treating a patient with VA. Utilising a three-dimensional electroanatomical mapping system, mapping during ongoing VA (activation and entrainment mapping) can define the macro–re-entrant circuit but will require haemodynamic stability to complete. The local electrogram is annotated to a stable reference, for example, the surface QRS complex, until the full cycle length of the tachycardia is covered. If the activation map covers less than 70% of the tachycardia cycle length, a focal rather than a macro–re-entrant tachycardia may be present. In the presence of a macro–re-entrant tachycardia, entrainment mapping is performed by placing the catheter at an anatomic site in the ventricle and pacing at slightly faster rate (usually 20 ms faster than the VA cycle length) during VA. This accelerates the VA to the paced cycle length and allows the operator to determine if that anatomic site is within the VA circuit. Entrainment mapping can delineate if the pacing site is in a critical isthmus, in an isolated scar or remote from the VA circuit. Characteristics such as whether the entrainment is manifest or concealed and the post-pacing intervals help to identify whether the pacing site is located in a critical isthmus and these would then serve as a reasonable ablation target.

If the VA is haemodynamically unstable, haemodynamic compromise is anticipated, or if VA is non-inducible, mapping can be performed in sinus rhythm utilising a three-dimensional electroanatomical mapping system to complete an anatomical map. Many commercially available mapping systems exist to create three-dimensional maps of the ventricle. These include the CARTO 3 system by Biosense Webster, the Ensite Velocity system by St. Jude Medical and the Rhythmia mapping system by Boston Scientific. During substrate mapping in sinus rhythm, point-by-point acquisition of bipolar voltage signals allows differentiation between normal ($\geq$1.5 mV) and scarred (<1.5 mV) ventricular myocardium. The amplitude of bipolar voltage is markedly diminished in areas of dense scar (<0.5 mV).[8] Varying degrees of bipolar voltage can be colour-coded on the three-dimensional electroanatomical map (Figure 40.1).

Scars typically display fractionated, low-amplitude electrograms. Sometimes, electrograms are separated by an isoelectric interval and the late components are defined as late potentials. Late potentials during sinus rhythm are a marker of slowed conduction at the site of the critical isthmus during VT.[9] Targeting late potentials during ablation in patients with ischaemic VT was associated with good outcome.[10] During substrate mapping, local abnormal ventricular activities (LAVAs) may be seen in patients with ischaemic VT.[11] Ventricular pacing or a spontaneous premature ventricular contraction (PVC) may facilitate identification of LAVA. The resultant alteration in the direction of local activation may cause slowing of conduction in areas of the scar and fractionation of local electrograms. Elimination of LAVA in patients with ischaemic VT lowered the rate of VT recurrence during a median follow-up of 22 months.[11] In recent years, substrate mapping has increased in acceptance and is the preferred strategy in patients in whom haemodynamic compromise is anticipated. Many centres may utilise substrate mapping as the sole strategy in any patient presenting with scar-related VA.

Pace mapping can facilitate identification of the site of VA origin. Pace mapping typically requires a 12-lead electrocardiogram (ECG) documentation of the clinical VA. Alternatively, stored ICD electrograms may serve as surrogate if clinical documentation of the VT is unavailable.[12] Once the mapping catheter is positioned at the site of VA origin, pacing at the cycle length of the clinical tachycardia

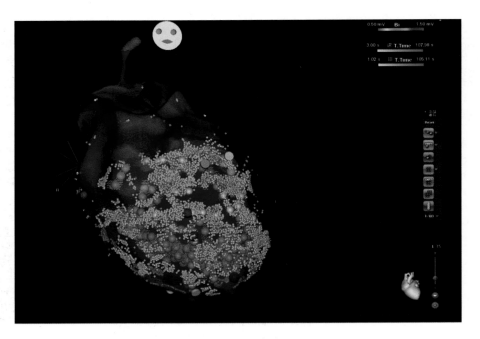

Figure 40.1 A patient with a large scar burden due to previous myocardial infarction resulting in recurrent ventricular tachycardia (VT) and ICD shocks. Shown is a three-dimensional electroanatomical CARTO 3 (Biosense Webster) bipolar voltage map of the left ventricle (LV) (apical projection). Normal voltage is coloured in purple ($\geq$1.5 mV), dense scar in red (<0.5 mV) and the scar border zone in blue, green and yellow. Extensive ablation was performed. Ablation lesions (light red dots) are automatically annotated by the CARTO 3 system if they meet preset criteria for stability over time (Visitag feature). The small white dots highlight the position of the ablation catheter during energy delivery where the preset criteria for an ablation lesion were not met. Blue dots are sites demonstrating late potentials.

at twice the diastolic threshold will result in identical QRS morphology between the pace map and clinical VA (Figure 40.2).

In patients with focal VA from the right ventricular outflow tract (RVOT), pace mapping is limited by its low resolution (1.8 cm²), but may identify the region of interest that needs further exploration using high-density mapping.[13]

During ischaemic injury, the wavefront of necrosis traverses from endo- to epicardium. Hence, mapping and ablation of ischaemic VT targets endocardial scar and rarely necessitates an epicardial approach.[14] Epicardial mapping and ablation is indicated in patients with ARVD. In these patients, scar formation initiates from the epicardium and advances towards the endocardium. Epicardial access is obtained first in patients with a high likelihood for an epicardial substrate, since endocardial mapping will require heparinisation to prevent intra-cardiac thrombus formation. In DCM, an endocardial approach as the initial step may be preferred. Only if the clinical VT demonstrates typical morphology of an epicardial origin, should a combined epi- and endocardial approach serve as the initial step.[15] Endocardial bipolar voltage signals provide accurate detail of tissue composition within the immediate vicinity (near field) of the distal electrode pair of the ablation catheter. Extending the range of view, endocardial unipolar voltage recorded between the distal tip of the ablation catheter and Wilson's central terminal may identify epicardial scar in patients with ARVD or non-ICM supporting the need for additional epicardial mapping and ablation.[16,17]

40.2.2 Ablation technology and techniques

Catheter ablation most commonly utilises radiofrequency energy delivered to the distal tip of the ablation catheter resulting in resistive heating of tissue in immediate contact with the catheter tip. Energy transfer to deeper tissue layers is mediated through conductive heating, which is counterbalanced by convective cooling from nearby blood flow. Lesion size is determined by the amount of energy delivered, the temperature setting during ablation, convective cooling and the duration of energy delivery. Insufficient energy delivery may result from sudden rise in temperature in areas of low blood flow (e.g. in trabeculated portions of the ventricle). For sufficient lesion penetration, customarily an open-irrigated tip ablation catheter is utilised that provides constant irrigation irrespective of tissue characteristics. The addition of contact force sensing to current catheter designs has resulted in further improvement of energy delivery and lesion formation.

Once an adequate ablation target is identified, unipolar radiofrequency energy is delivered typically via an open-irrigated tip catheter. Utilisation of an open-irrigation system allows for adequate cooling of the tip, which avoids overheating and char formation at the proximal ring location. This is thought to reduce the incidence of stroke related to embolisation during the procedure. Typically, power delivered can range between 30 and 50 W. The addition of contact force sensors to contemporary catheters allows for added feedback to titrate energy levels. Typical force settings would range between 10 and 50 g. Force levels which exceed 40 g are more likely to result in a steam pop. Force levels less than 10 g are likely to result in ineffective lesion formation. With open-irrigated catheters, temperature control of the ablation lesion is typically less reliable because of uniform cooling by heparinised saline. In an open-irrigated system, temperature at the catheter tip should rarely exceed 40°C–42°C. The duration of an effective lesion is dependent on the amount of power delivered, the amount of force at the catheter tip/tissue interface and the coupling of the catheter to the tissue. Effective ablation lesions in the ventricle typically last between 60 and 90 seconds. An ablation lesion located in a critical isthmus on the endocardium may have effect within 2 seconds, although most operators would stay on to complete the full 60–90-second lesion.

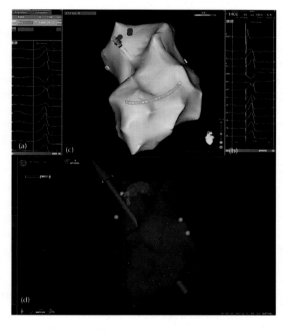

Figure 40.2 Premature ventricular contractions (PVCs) emanating from the LV summit. **(a)** 12-lead surface ECG of the spontaneous clinical PVC demonstrating right bundle branch block (RBBB) morphology and inferior axis. **(b)** Perfect pace map from the LV summit with 12/12 match between spontaneous PVC and paced QRS morphology. **(c)** Anatomical three-dimensional electroanatomical CARTO 3 (Biosense Webster) map of the LV (apical projection). Yellow dot annotates the His-bundle potential. The coronary sinus catheter is visualised in the background. The tip of the ablation catheter is positioned at the site where a perfect pace map was recorded (green dot). Successful ablation is performed and individual ablation lesions are annotated in red. **(d)** Identical three-dimensional map using the magnetic navigation system Stereotaxis. The summation of radiofrequency energy (ablation history) delivered at the LV summit is depicted as a red cloud.

An anterograde trans-septal or retrograde aortic access may be utilised for mapping and ablation within the left ventricle. A combined approach may be the preferred strategy as access to the basal-anterior, mid-anterior and mid-lateral left ventricular wall is facilitated by an anterograde trans-septal access. By contrast, septal and inferior sites are better targeted using a retrograde aortic approach.[18]

Percutaneous left ventricular assist devices may facilitate activation mapping and catheter ablation in patients presenting with haemodynamically unstable VA.[19,20] However, a pure substrate-based approach often precludes the need for haemodynamic support.

Several studies could demonstrate that the rate of recurrence is lower if VT is non-inducible following catheter ablation.[21,22] Hence, the preferred acute procedural endpoint should be non-inducibility of any VT. Induction of VA during programmed stimulation is dependent on several factors including the aggressiveness of the stimulation protocol, the level of sedation and the use of sympathetic drugs. If a lengthy stimulation protocol is unfeasible at the end of the procedure, abolition of all late potentials and/or LAVA should be sought. Alternatively, an abbreviated programmed stimulation protocol may be used that begins with a maximum number of extra stimuli.

Despite these advances in the ablative armamentarium, in patients with sustained VT fulfilling ICD eligibility, catheter ablation is yet to be shown to be an alternative to ICD implantation.

Complications of catheter ablation of VAs include damage to valves, cardiac perforation resulting in pericardial effusion and tamponade, complications related to vascular access, complete AV block, myocardial infarction and stroke. Procedural mortality ranges from 0% to 3%.[23] Acute haemodynamic decompensation may occur in 11% of the patients.[24] Close attention should be paid to the volume of saline delivered by the open-irrigated catheter as many patients have congestive heart failure. Diuretics are useful both during and after the procedure to balance the fluid administration from the catheters and infusions. Using an epicardial approach, additional complications may include damage to the coronary vasculature, left phrenic nerve palsy or accidental puncture of nearby non-cardiac structures during epicardial access.

40.3 Catheter ablation in patients with structural heart disease

40.3.1 Patients with VT due to ischaemic scar-related heart disease

The greatest evidence for superiority of catheter ablation for the prevention of recurrent VT has been collected in patients with ICM. Two prospective, randomised, multicentre trials provide the highest evidence that catheter ablation should be first-line treatment in patients with ICM presenting with VT.[25,26] The Substrate Mapping and Ablation in Sinus Rhythm to Halt Ventricular Tachycardia

(SMASH VT) study demonstrated that a substrate-based mapping approach in patients presenting with unstable VT lowered the incidence of recurrent VT compared to anti-arrhythmic therapy only.[25] All patients received an ICD for secondary prevention of sudden arrhythmic death. SMASH VT was not powered to assess mortality, although there was a trend to lower mortality in those patients undergoing catheter ablation. The Ventricular Tachycardia Ablation in Coronary Heart Disease (VTACH) study demonstrated the superiority of an ablative approach followed by ICD implantation in patients with ICM presenting with a first episode of VT compared with anti-arrhythmic therapy and ICD implantation only.[26] The VTACH trial more closely resembled the 'real-world' scenario as a higher number of centres participated in the study, and the incidence of recurrent VT was higher in both the treatment and control arm. Targeting conductive channels within the scar may limit the need for extensive ablation and has demonstrated good outcome during 2-year follow-up.[27] A recent randomised multicentre study in patients with ischaemic VT compared limited ablation of clinical and mappable VTs with extensive scar homogenisation.[28] VT recurrence was significantly lower in patients undergoing extensive substrate-based scar ablation (Figure 40.1).

Further evidence for the superiority of a catheter-based approach in patients with ischaemic VT comes from several observational studies.[7] In patients presenting with electrical storm (≥3 VT episodes during a 24-hour period), anti-arrhythmic therapy often is insufficient in controlling repetitive ICD shocks, and catheter ablation of VT should strongly be considered if performed in an experienced centre.[29]

Occasionally, an electrical storm may arise in the setting of acute myocardial infarction. PVC originating from the Purkinje network may trigger polymorphic VT, ventricular fibrillation (VF) and electrical storm, and catheter ablation targeting the PVC trigger has demonstrated encouraging results.[30,31]

40.3.2 Patients with VT due to non-ischaemic scar-related heart disease

Patients with non-ICM exhibit scar at distinct regions that may serve as a substrate for macro–re-entrant VT. In DCM, the scar is commonly found along the basal lateral mitral annulus and epicardial involvement is common.[32] Magnetic resonance imaging (MRI) can be particularly helpful in delineating the extent of endo- and epicardial scar and aid in selecting the proper ablation strategy.[33] In patients with cardiac sarcoidosis, scar is often confined to the basal right ventricular region.[34] Epicardial scar is virtually always present in patients presenting with VA due to ARVD and often extends to the endocardial layer. A combined epi- and endocardial ablation strategy was superior to endocardial ablation alone in patients with ARVD.[35] In addition, an ablative strategy targeting conducting channels (dechannelling) within epi- and endocardial scar has demonstrated encouraging outcome in this patient population.[36]

To date, prospective randomised trials are lacking for evaluating the role of catheter ablation of VT in patients with non-ICM. Observational and retrospective studies suggest that catheter ablation is superior to anti-arrhythmic therapy for the prevention of recurrent VT.[7] Overall, the reported success rates following catheter ablation are less favourable in patients with VA in the setting of non-ICM. This may be due to a more complex substrate with a higher incidence of intra-mural and epicardial scar.

40.4 Catheter ablation in patients without overt structural heart disease

In patients without overt structural heart disease, idiopathic VAs most commonly originate from the outflow tracts. The region surrounding the outflow tracts is complex and comprises the RVOT, the pulmonary artery, the left ventricular outflow tract (LVOT) and the aortic cusps. The RVOT is positioned leftward and anterior to the aortic valve, whilst the right and left coronary cusps oppose the septal RVOT.

40.4.1 Mapping strategies

A stepwise mapping approach assures that catheter ablation will result in a successful outcome.[37] Initial mapping should focus on the RVOT as the most common site of focal origin and proceed to alternative sites as needed. The use of a three-dimensional electroanatomical mapping system greatly facilitates mapping and ablation. Activation mapping is performed if PVCs are frequent. At the successful site of ablation, the local ventricular electrogram will precede the onset of the earliest QRS on the surface ECG by 10–60 ms. Pace mapping is used if infrequent PVCs preclude completion of an activation map. Angiography of the aortic root or selective angiography to delineate the course of the coronary arteries may facilitate mapping within the aortic cusps. Intra-cardiac echocardiography can be helpful to define anatomy and assure proper catheter tip-to-tissue contact during mapping and ablation.

40.4.2 VAs emanating from the RVOT

In patients without overt structural heart disease, focal VAs most commonly emanate from the RVOT. The underlying pathophysiologic mechanism for PVC or VT is a calcium-dependent triggered activity due to delayed after-depolarisations.[23] Sympathomimetic drugs such as isoproterenol can facilitate induction of VA due to triggered activity. The anteroseptal RVOT is the most common site of origin and clinical PVCs will demonstrate a narrow QRS complex. Notching of the QRS complex implies delayed ventricular activation from sites emanating from the RVOT free wall.[38] A positive QRS complex in lead I indicates a posterior site of origin within the RVOT.[38] Successful ablation

targets an area 1–2 cm inferior to the pulmonic valve, although in rare cases the clinical VA may originate within the pulmonary artery.[39] The clinical VA should terminate within 10 seconds of energy delivery; otherwise, an alternative site is sought. Mapping and ablation of RVOT VA is often curative,[23] however, the presence of undiagnosed ARVD needs to be excluded, if multiple PVC or VT morphologies are identified from the RV or RVOT.

40.4.3 Ventricular arrhythmia origin from the aortic cusps and the LVOT

If the RVOT has been excluded as the focal site of VA origin, mapping should expand to the aortic root. The left coronary cusp is the most common site of origin within the aortic root. Characteristic 12-lead ECG criteria include an R wave to QRS duration ratio ≥50% and an R/S amplitude ratio ≥30% in surface leads V1 and V2.[40] Activation mapping is typically required to confirm the coronary cusps as the site of focal origin, since pace mapping often fails to reproduce the clinical PVC morphology. An aortic root angiogram facilitates proper localisation and safe catheter ablation targeting the individual coronary cusps. Intra-cardiac echocardiography may be used in conjunction or as an alternative to angiography. Furthermore, a three-dimensional electroanatomical mapping system will aid in accurate identification of the earliest site of origin and delineation of complex anatomy. Successful ablation targets the nadir of the left coronary cusp ≥6–7 mm inferior to the left coronary ostium. A low-amplitude presystolic or late diastolic potential precedes the local ventricular signal during the clinical VA, and this activation sequence reverses in sinus rhythm.[40]

The right coronary cusp is a less frequent site of origin and mapping is performed in a similar manner to that for the left coronary cusp. Due to their close proximity, 12-lead ECG criteria may not reliably differentiate between a focal site originating from the right coronary cusp and the RVOT. Earliest local ventricular activity recorded on the His catheter rather than within the RVOT may indicate a focal origin from the right coronary cusp.[41]

VAs from the LVOT may originate from above or below the aortic sinus of Valsalva. The LV summit, a region immediately below the aortic valve, is confined laterally by the anterior interventricular vein, posteriorly by the left circumflex artery and medially by the left anterior descending artery.[42] A retrograde trans-septal approach using a reverse S-curve configuration on the ablation catheter in right anterior oblique (RAO) projection is required to complete successful manual ablation of VA from the LV summit.

Potential complications during catheter ablation of outflow tract VAs include cardiac perforation, damage to the left main coronary artery that traverses immediately posterior of the RVOT, complete AV block if ablation is performed below the aortic valve, air embolism or stroke.[43]

40.4.4 VAs originating from other sites within the ventricles

The aortomitral continuity may give rise to VAs. The aortomitral continuity is made of fibrous tissue, but may contain muscle bundles that promote VAs. A characteristic ECG pattern, a qR complex or monomorphic R wave in lead V1, suggests an origin from the aortomitral continuity and catheter ablation targets the earliest site during activation mapping.[44]

VAs may arise from the papillary muscles.[45] The clinical PVC may demonstrate varying QRS morphologies implying a deeper intra-mural origin with multiple breakthrough exit sites.[46] Catheter stability may be suboptimal requiring ablation at the base of the papillary muscle from multiple angles. Using a three-dimensional electroanatomical mapping system, separate maps of the left ventricle and the papillary muscle should be created. Intra-cardiac echocardiography is helpful in guiding mapping and ablation.[45]

Papillary muscle VAs need to be differentiated from fascicular VT that exhibits a narrower QRS complex. Fascicular VT has also been termed Belhassen VT, verapamil-sensitive VT or idiopathic left VT (ILVT). Most ILVT involve the posterior fascicle. Ablation targets presystolic Purkinje potentials preceding the local ventricular electrogram during ongoing VT.[45] A three-dimensional electroanatomical mapping system facilitates mapping and ablation. Catheter manipulation within the LV can result in premature mechanical termination of ILVT, rendering the patient non-inducible for the remainder of the procedure. Iatrogenic induction of complete or partial left posterior fascicular block by linear lesion deployment has been proposed as an acceptable procedural endpoint.[47] Since most affected patients are of young age, partial or complete conduction block of the left posterior fascicle may not be desirable. A previous study demonstrated that only in patients with a history of ILVT involving the posterior fascicle, sharp low-amplitude retrograde Purkinje potentials (retro-PP) are recorded that follow the local ventricular electrogram, during sinus rhythm.[48] Retro-PPs are confined to a small region along the posterior mid-septal LV. Targeting the earliest retro-PP during sinus rhythm resulted in long-term freedom from recurrent ILVT without development of left posterior fascicular block.[49]

40.4.5 Idiopathic ventricular fibrillation and VAs due to underlying genetic disease

A monomorphic short-coupled PVC emanating from the Purkinje network that is identical in morphology to the first beat of ventricular fibrillation may trigger idiopathic ventricular fibrillation. Targeting the PVC trigger during catheter ablation has resulted in successful prevention of ventricular fibrillation with a low rate of recurrence during long-term follow-up.[50]

Similarly, in patients with long QT syndrome, PVCs originating from the Purkinje network may trigger ventricular fibrillation.[51] Targeting the initiating PVC has shown to prevent recurrent episodes of ventricular fibrillation.

The risk for ventricular fibrillation resulting in sudden cardiac death (SCD) is increased in patients with Brugada syndrome.[23] In some patients, episodes of ventricular fibrillation are initiated by monomorphic PVCs from the Purkinje network and targeting the PVC trigger during ablation results in reduction of arrhythmia recurrence.[51,52] Recently, an anatomical correlate to the genetic abnormality in patients suffering from Brugada syndrome presenting with ventricular fibrillation was described.[53] The pathognomonic changes found in patients presenting with type 1 Brugada ECG pattern were associated with abnormal, low voltage, fractionated electrograms located exclusively along the anterior epicardial RVOT. Catheter ablation targeting the abnormal epicardial substrate rendered ventricular fibrillation non-inducible and resulted in disappearance of the characteristic surface ECG pattern in the majority of patients. Additional studies are needed to support these interesting findings.

40.5 Future outlook

A mortality benefit for patients undergoing catheter ablation of ischaemic VT has yet to be demonstrated and future prospective, randomised trials are needed. In addition, there is paucity of data from randomised trials comparing the appropriate timing of catheter ablation in patients with ischaemic VT, although an early ablative strategy appears beneficial.[54,55] Two randomised multicentre trials are currently enrolling patients to assess proper timing of catheter ablation. (1) The PARTITA trial compares early catheter ablation after an appropriate ICD shock, with a delayed ablative strategy after an episode of electrical storm[56] and (2) the BERLIN study will randomise patients with documented VT to immediate ICD implantation and catheter ablation versus delayed ablation after the third appropriate ICD shock.[57]

Non-invasive imaging can guide the mapping and ablation procedure. MRI has been utilised to delineate the endo- and epicardial substrate.[58,59] A non-invasive epicardial and endocardial electrophysiology system accurately localised the site of PVC origin, guiding the operator to the region of interest during invasive mapping[60] (Figure 40.3).

For patients with an intra-mural VT substrate who have failed conventional ablative efforts, an extendable/retractable irrigated needle catheter may provide sufficient depth to target the arrhythmogenic focus.[61] Remote magnetic navigation may offer certain advantages in patients presenting with ischaemic VT including enhanced manoeuvrability of the mapping and ablation catheter and increased catheter stability. The Magnetic-VT study, a prospective, randomised, multicentre trial is currently enrolling patients with ischaemic VT for treatment between conventional catheter ablation and ablation using the magnetic navigation system.[62]

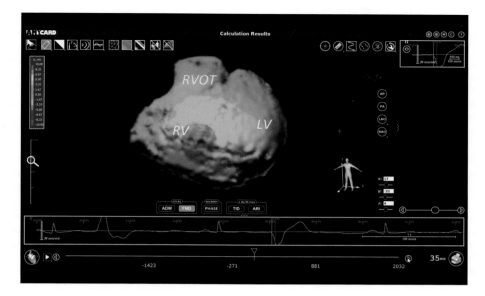

Figure 40.3 Earliest epicardial activation (dark blue circle) of a PVC visualised on an isopotential map using a novel non-invasive epicardial and endocardial electrophysiology system (Amycard, EP Solutions, apical projection). Surface ECG lead II demonstrates two different PVC. The second premature contraction is mapped by the non-invasive system. Note that the earliest epicardial activation depicted by the red line is later in time than the onset of the QRS complex (orange line). This implies an endocardial site of origin and can be visualised by a separate non-invasive endocardial map.

40.6 Conclusions

As more patients undergo implantation of an ICD for primary and secondary prevention of SCD, a subset of patients will present with recurrent VAs and ICD shocks that increase mortality and reduce quality of life. Since anti-arrhythmic drugs demonstrate disappointing results in suppressing VA recurrence, catheter ablation is increasingly used in experienced centres. A substrate-based ablation approach minimises intra-procedural haemodynamic compromise and decreases the rate of VA recurrence during follow-up. In patients with scar-related VA, an early ablative strategy appears beneficial but requires further research. In patients without overt structural heart disease, catheter ablation is usually curative.

References

1. Bardy GH et al. Amiodarone or an implantable cardioverter-defibrillator for congestive heart failure. N Engl J Med 2005; 352(3): 225–37.
2. Connolly SJ et al. Meta-analysis of the implantable cardioverter defibrillator secondary prevention trials. AVID, CASH and CIDS studies. Antiarrhythmics vs Implantable Defibrillator study. Cardiac Arrest Study Hamburg. Canadian Implantable Defibrillator Study. Eur Heart J 2000; 21(24): 2071–8.
3. Poole JE et al. Prognostic importance of defibrillator shocks in patients with heart failure. N Engl J Med 2008; 359(10): 1009–17.
4. Powell BD et al. Survival after shock therapy in implantable cardioverter-defibrillator and cardiac resynchronization therapy-defibrillator recipients according to rhythm shocked. The ALTITUDE survival by rhythm study. J Am Coll Cardiol 2013; 62(18): 1674–9.
5. Kamphuis HC et al. Implantable cardioverter defibrillator recipients: Quality of life in recipients with and without ICD shock delivery: A prospective study. Europace 2003; 5(4): 381–9.
6. Hohnloser SH et al. Effect of amiodarone and sotalol on ventricular defibrillation threshold: The optimal pharmacological therapy in cardioverter defibrillator patients (OPTIC) trial. Circulation 2006; 114(2): 104–9.
7. Wissner E et al. Catheter ablation of ventricular tachycardia in ischaemic and non-ischaemic cardiomyopathy: Where are we today? A clinical review. Eur Heart J 2012; 33(12): 1440–50.
8. Marchlinski FE et al. Linear ablation lesions for control of unmappable ventricular tachycardia in patients with ischemic and nonischemic cardiomyopathy. Circulation 2000; 101(11): 1288–96.
9. Arenal A et al. Ablation of electrograms with an isolated, delayed component as treatment of unmappable monomorphic ventricular tachycardias in patients with structural heart disease. J Am Coll Cardiol 2003; 41(1): 81–92.
10. Bogun F et al. Isolated potentials during sinus rhythm and pace-mapping within scars as guides for ablation of post-infarction ventricular tachycardia. J Am Coll Cardiol 2006; 47(10): 2013–9.
11. Jais P et al. Elimination of local abnormal ventricular activities: A new end point for substrate modification in patients with scar-related ventricular tachycardia. Circulation 2012; 125(18): 2184–96.
12. Yoshida K et al. The value of defibrillator electrograms for recognition of clinical ventricular tachycardias and for pace mapping of post-infarction ventricular tachycardia. J Am Coll Cardiol 2010; 56(12): 969–79.
13. Bogun F et al. Spatial resolution of pace mapping of idiopathic ventricular tachycardia/ectopy originating in the right ventricular outflow tract. Heart Rhythm 2008; 5(3): 339–44.

14. Yoshiga Y et al. Correlation between substrate location and ablation strategy in patients with ventricular tachycardia late after myocardial infarction. *Heart Rhythm* 2012; 9(8): 1192–9.

15. Valles E et al. ECG criteria to identify epicardial ventricular tachycardia in nonischemic cardiomyopathy. *Circ Arrhythm Electrophysiol* 2010; 3(1): 63–71.

16. Polin GM et al. Endocardial unipolar voltage mapping to identify epicardial substrate in arrhythmogenic right ventricular cardiomyopathy/dysplasia. *Heart Rhythm* 2011; 8(1): 76–83.

17. Hutchinson MD et al. Endocardial unipolar voltage mapping to detect epicardial ventricular tachycardia substrate in patients with nonischemic left ventricular cardiomyopathy. *Circ Arrhythm Electrophysiol* 2011; 4(1): 49–55.

18. Tilz RR et al. In vivo left-ventricular contact force analysis: Comparison of antegrade transseptal with retrograde transaortic mapping strategies and correlation of impedance and electrical amplitude with contact force. *Europace* 2014; 16(9): 1387–95.

19. Reddy YM et al. Percutaneous left ventricular assist devices in ventricular tachycardia ablation: Multicenter experience. *Circ Arrhythm Electrophysiol* 2014; 7(2): 244–50.

20. Miller MA et al. Percutaneous hemodynamic support with Impella 2.5 during scar-related ventricular tachycardia ablation (PERMIT 1). *Circ Arrhythm Electrophysiol* 2013; 6(1): 151–9.

21. Yokokawa M et al. Predictive value of programmed ventricular stimulation after catheter ablation of post-infarction ventricular tachycardia. *J Am Coll Cardiol* 2015; 65(18): 1954–9.

22. Ghanbari H et al. Noninducibility in postinfarction ventricular tachycardia as an end point for ventricular tachycardia ablation and its effects on outcomes: A meta-analysis. *Circ Arrhythm Electrophysiol* 2014; 7(4): 677–83.

23. Priori SG et al. 2015 ESC Guidelines for the management of patients with ventricular arrhythmias and the prevention of sudden cardiac death: The Task Force for the Management of Patients with Ventricular Arrhythmias and the Prevention of Sudden Cardiac Death of the European Society of Cardiology (ESC)Endorsed by: Association for European Paediatric and Congenital Cardiology (AEPC). *Eur Heart J* 2015; 36(41): 2793–867.

24. Santangeli P et al. Acute hemodynamic decompensation during catheter ablation of scar-related ventricular tachycardia: Incidence, predictors, and impact on mortality. *Circ Arrhythm Electrophysiol* 2015; 8(1): 68–75.

25. Reddy VY et al. Prophylactic catheter ablation for the prevention of defibrillator therapy. *N Engl J Med* 2007; 357(26): 2657–65.

26. Kuck KH et al. Catheter ablation of stable ventricular tachycardia before defibrillator implantation in patients with coronary heart disease (VTACH): a multicentre randomised controlled trial. *Lancet* 2010; 375(9708): 31–40.

27. Berruezo A et al. Scar dechanneling: New method for scar-related left ventricular tachycardia substrate ablation. *Circ Arrhythm Electrophysiol* 2015; 8(2): 326–36.

28. Di Biase L et al. Ablation of Stable VTs versus Substrate Ablation in Ischemic Cardiomyopathy: The VISTA Randomized Multicenter Trial. *J Am Coll Cardiol* 2015; 66(25): 2872–82.

29. Carbucicchio C et al. Catheter ablation for the treatment of electrical storm in patients with implantable cardioverter-defibrillators: Short- and long-term outcomes in a prospective single-center study. *Circulation* 2008; 117(4): 462–9.

30. Bansch D et al. Successful catheter ablation of electrical storm after myocardial infarction. *Circulation* 2003; 108(24): 3011–6.

31. Marrouche NF et al. Mode of initiation and ablation of ventricular fibrillation storms in patients with ischemic cardiomyopathy. *J Am Coll Cardiol* 2004; 43(9): 1715–20.

32. Cano O et al. Electroanatomic substrate and ablation outcome for suspected epicardial ventricular tachycardia in left ventricular nonischemic cardiomyopathy. *J Am Coll Cardiol* 2009; 54(9): 799–808.

33. Bogun FM et al. Delayed-enhanced magnetic resonance imaging in nonischemic cardiomyopathy: Utility for identifying the ventricular arrhythmia substrate. *J Am Coll Cardiol* 2009; 53(13): 1138–45.

34. Jefic D et al. Role of radiofrequency catheter ablation of ventricular tachycardia in cardiac sarcoidosis: Report from a multicenter registry. *Heart Rhythm* 2009; 6(2): 189–95.

35. Bai R et al. Ablation of ventricular arrhythmias in arrhythmogenic right ventricular dysplasia/cardiomyopathy: Arrhythmia-free survival after endo-epicardial substrate based mapping and ablation. *Circ Arrhythm Electrophysiol* 2011; 4(4): 478–85.

36. Berruezo A et al. Combined endocardial and epicardial catheter ablation in arrhythmogenic right ventricular dysplasia incorporating scar dechanneling technique. *Circ Arrhythm Electrophysiol* 2012; 5(1): 111–21.

37. Tanner H et al. Outflow tract tachycardia with R/S transition in lead V3: Six different anatomic approaches for successful ablation. *J Am Coll Cardiol* 2005; 45(3): 418–23.

38. Dixit S et al. Electrocardiographic patterns of superior right ventricular outflow tract tachycardias: Distinguishing septal and free-wall sites of origin. *J Cardiovasc Electrophysiol* 2003; 14(1): 1–7.

39. Sekiguchi Y et al. Electrocardiographic and electrophysiologic characteristics of ventricular tachycardia originating within the pulmonary artery. *J Am Coll Cardiol* 2005; 45(6): 887–95.

40. Ouyang F et al. Repetitive monomorphic ventricular tachycardia originating from the aortic sinus cusp: Electrocardiographic characterization for guiding catheter ablation. *J Am Coll Cardiol* 2002; 39(3): 500–8.

41. Yamada T et al. Idiopathic ventricular arrhythmias originating from the aortic root prevalence, electrocardiographic and electrophysiologic characteristics, and results of radiofrequency catheter ablation. *J Am Coll Cardiol* 2008; 52(2): 139–47.

42. Ouyang F et al. Ventricular arrhythmias arising from the left ventricular outflow tract below the aortic sinus cusps: Mapping and catheter ablation via transseptal approach and electrocardiographic characteristics. *Circ Arrhythm Electrophysiol* 2014; 7(3): 445–55.

43. Suleiman M, and Asirvatham SJ. Ablation above the semilunar valves: When, why, and how? Part I. *Heart Rhythm* 2008; 5(10): 1485–92.

44. Lin D et al. Twelve-lead electrocardiographic characteristics of the aortic cusp region guided by intracardiac echocardiography and electroanatomic mapping. *Heart Rhythm* 2008; 5(5): 663–9.

45. Good E et al. Ventricular arrhythmias originating from a papillary muscle in patients without prior infarction: A comparison with fascicular arrhythmias. *Heart Rhythm* 2008; 5(11): 1530–7.

46. Yamada T et al. Electrocardiographic and electrophysiological characteristics in idiopathic ventricular arrhythmias originating from the papillary muscles in the left ventricle: Relevance for catheter ablation. *Circ Arrhythm Electrophysiol* 2010; 3(4): 324–31.

47. Fishberger SB et al. Creation of partial fascicular block: An approach to ablation of idiopathic left ventricular tachycardia in the pediatric population. *Pacing Clin Electrophysiol* 2015; 38(2): 209–15.

48. Ouyang F et al. Electroanatomic substrate of idiopathic left ventricular tachycardia: Unidirectional block and macro–reentry within the Purkinje network. *Circulation* 2002; 105(4): 462–9.

49. Wissner E et al. Long-term outcome after catheter ablation for left posterior fascicular ventricular tachycardia without development of left posterior fascicular block. *J Cardiovasc Electrophysiol* 2012; 23(11): 1179–84.

50. Knecht S et al. Long-term follow-up of idiopathic ventricular fibrillation ablation: A multicenter study. *J Am Coll Cardiol* 2009; 54(6): 522–8.

51. Haissaguerre M et al. Mapping and ablation of ventricular fibrillation associated with long-QT and Brugada syndromes. *Circulation* 2003; 108(8): 925–8.

52. Priori SG et al. Executive summary: HRS/EHRA/APHRS expert consensus statement on the diagnosis and management of patients with inherited primary arrhythmia syndromes. *Europace* 2013; 15(10): 1389–406.

53. Nademanee K et al. Prevention of ventricular fibrillation episodes in Brugada syndrome by catheter ablation over the anterior right ventricular outflow tract epicardium. *Circulation* 2011; 123(12): 1270–9.

54. Tanner H et al. Catheter ablation of recurrent scar-related ventricular tachycardia using electroanatomical mapping and irrigated ablation technology: results of the prospective multicenter Euro-VT-study. *J Cardiovasc Electrophysiol* 2010; 21(1): 47–53.

55. Dinov B et al. Early referral for ablation of scar-related ventricular tachycardia is associated with improved acute and long-term outcomes: Results from the Heart Center of Leipzig ventricular tachycardia registry. *Circ Arrhythm Electrophysiol* 2014; 7(6): 1144–51.

56. Does Timing of VT Ablation Affect Prognosis in Patients with an Implantable Cardioverter-defibrillator? (PARTITA). Available at: https://clinicaltrials.gov/ct2/show/NCT01547208 (Accessed 14 February 2017).

57. Preventive aBlation of vEntricular tachycaRdia in Patients With myocardiaL INfarction (BERLIN VT). Available at: https://clinicaltrials.gov/ct2/show/NCT02501005?term=NCT02501005&rank=1 (Accessed 14 February 2017).

58. Arenal A et al. Noninvasive identification of epicardial ventricular tachycardia substrate by magnetic resonance-based signal intensity mapping. *Heart Rhythm* 2014; 11(8): 1456–64.

59. Dickfeld T et al. MRI-guided ventricular tachycardia ablation: Integration of late gadolinium-enhanced 3D scar in patients with implantable cardioverter-defibrillators. *Circ Arrhythm Electrophysiol* 2011; 4(2): 172–84.

60. Wissner E et al. Noninvasive epicardial and endocardial mapping of premature ventricular contractions. *Europace* 2016; pii: euw103. [Epub ahead of print]

61. Sapp JL et al. Initial human feasibility of infusion needle catheter ablation for refractory ventricular tachycardia. *Circulation* 2013; 128(21): 2289–95.

62. Di Biase L et al. MAGNETIC VT study: A prospective, multicenter, post-market randomized controlled trial comparing VT ablation outcomes using remote magnetic navigation-guided substrate mapping and ablation versus manual approach in a low LVEF population. *J Interv Card Electrophysiol* 2017. doi:10.1007/s10840-016-0217-3.

41

Pacemakers for the treatment of bradyarrhythmias

GERRY KAYE

Pacemaker support for bradycardia has been a reality since the first human implant in 1958. Although syncope and bradycardia had been noted for hundreds of years, it wasn't until Stokes together with Adams, made the link between a slow pulse and syncope. They originally described "a very remarkable pulsation in the right jugular vein more than double the number of the manifest ventricular contractions" which was confirmed to be due to heart block with the advent of the electrocardiogram.[1] Over the past 60 years advances in electronics and battery technology has revolutionised the clinical application of cardiac implantable electronic devices such that pacemakers are the mainstay of management for bradycardias. Increasing device complexity has widened their applicability such that they now form a ubiquitous part of cardiology management, considered by some to have become a specialty of their own.

41.1 Natural history of bradycardias

There have been no large randomised trials of the effect of pacemakers on mortality associated with bradycardias and heart block. Much of our knowledge arises from observational studies and the mortality benefit of pacing is more inferred than proven by trials. In the main, death from untreated atrioventricular block (AVB) occurs due to prolonged asystole, bradycardia-related ventricular arrhythmias or heart failure. It is generally accepted, mainly from observational studies, that pacing prevents syncope and improves survival. For sinus node disease, however, mortality and sudden death are similar to the general population and there is little evidence to support a survival benefit from pacing. Whatever the underlying conduction pathology at presentation, pacing, for the most part, confers a morbidity benefit and although a mortality benefit may accrue, it is unproven.[2–5]

41.2 Bradycardia

The exclusion of a reversible cause is paramount as long-term pacing is not indicated. In a study of patients presenting acutely to an emergency department with symptomatic bradycardia, 21% were drug-related, 14% associated with myocardial infarction, 6% with intoxication and 4% with a reversible electrolyte disturbance.[6] Thyroid disease also needs to be excluded. Temporary pacing may be required in cases with a reversible cause and the decision will depend upon the severity of symptoms and how quickly the primary cause can be reversed.

Symptoms due to bradycardias are related to a decrease in cardiac output, although in some patients compensation in stroke volume may allow the patient to remain asymptomatic. For others, syncope, presyncope, breathlessness, fatigue and lack of exercise tolerance are common presenting symptoms.[6]

41.2.1 Indications for pacing

Recommended European guidelines for pacing are shown in Figure 41.1.[6] The US guidelines are similar.

The diagnosis of bradycardia, which may be persistent or intermittent, is confirmed by electrocardiogram (ECG). In order to diagnose the latter, a prolonged period of monitoring, either ambulatory or by implanted loop recorder, may be required.

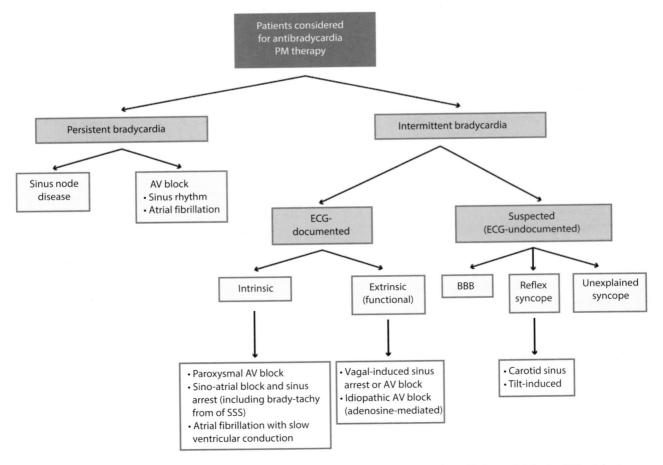

Figure 41.1 Classification of bradycardias based upon clinical presentation. BBB, bundle branch block; SSS, sick sinus syndrome. (From Brignole M et al., *Eur Heart J*, 34, 2013.)

Pacemaker support for bradycardia is generally indicated in

- Symptomatic sinus node disease (sick sinus syndrome)
- Heart blocks
- Atrial fibrillation (AF) with a slow ventricular response (the tachy-brady syndrome)

41.2.2 Persistent bradycardias

41.2.2.1 Sinus node disease

- Sinus bradycardia: When symptoms can be clearly related to the degree of bradycardia (sometime difficult to prove) pacing may be indicated. Symptoms may be present at rest but more often with exercise, manifesting as a lack of exercise capacity. Failure of an adequate increase in heart rate on exercise associated with symptoms (chronotropic incompetence) may help to determine the requirement for pacing. In a randomised study of 107 patients with symptomatic sinus node disease, paced patients had less syncope or heart failure compared with both those on drug therapy and controls.[7] As pacing for sinus bradycardia has not been shown to prolong survival, it should only be offered where there is a direct correlation between symptoms and heart rate. If this causal relationship cannot be established, then pacing should be avoided. However, there is no generally accepted definition for chronotropic incompetence, as the range of heart rate with exercise is wide, and an individualised approach needs to be taken. For example, a resting heart rate of 40–45 bpm may be acceptable in trained athletes with good exercise reserves but perhaps not to the same degree at the age of 70 years, particularly if associated with symptoms.
- Sinus node disease and brady-tachy syndrome: This is often manifest by prolonged sinus pauses (i.e. >3 seconds), slow persistent sinus rate 40–50 bpm and prolonged pauses at the termination of a tachyarrhythmia. Paroxysmal AF is common (less so paroxysms of atrial flutter) and has been shown to occur in 30%–55% of patients.[7,8] Pacing is indicated with syncope or presyncope. When symptoms cannot be definitively correlated with a bradycardia, but documented pauses or persistent bradycardia (with the exception of trained athletes or during sleep) is/are present, cardiac pacing also may be a very reasonable approach. In addition, anti-arrhythmia medication for AF or flutter, where definitive treatment such as ablation is not indicated, may exacerbate any tendency to bradycardia. A pacemaker is therefore a reasonable treatment strategy.
- AVB or heart block is categorised as first-, second- or third-degree (complete). Heart block in one of these forms accounts for about 40%–60% of patients who have pacemakers implanted. Acquired AVB may be intermittent or persistent and requires pacing, provided reversible causes are excluded. The concern is that

during block the rhythm may be dependent upon subsidiary pacemaker sites which are often unreliable.

- First-degree heart block (Figure 41.2) defined as a PR interval of greater than 200 ms and does not usually require pacing unless the AV delay is such that there are either symptoms and/or haemodynamic impairment.
- Second-degree heart block: Mobitz type I block (also known as the Wenckebach phenomenon) in which there is a gradual prolongation of the PR interval in sinus rhythm, culminating in a dropped beat (Figure 41.2), pacing is controversial unless symptoms are correlated or there is evidence of infra-His block. However, symptom correlation can sometimes be difficult to determine as they may be subtle or non-specific. The presence of a wide QRS may augur progression to complete heart block.
- Mobitz type II block in which there is no lengthening of the PR interval in sinus rhythm but a sudden dropped atrial beat, that is no conducted QRS complex (Figure 41.2), pacing is mandatory due to the unpredictable risk of sudden ventricular standstill.
- Third-degree or complete heart block is characterised by a slow regular ventricular response usually 40 bpm and the sinus beats are not conducted to the ventricles (Figure 41.3). Complete heart block may be congenital or acquired. Acquired irreversible heart block requires pacing.
- Trifascicular block is defined as either left bundle branch block and first-degree block or a combination of left anterior or posterior hemiblock, complete right bundle branch block and first-degree block. In left anterior hemiblock, the QRS axis is markedly leftwards and in left posterior hemiblock it is markedly rightwards.

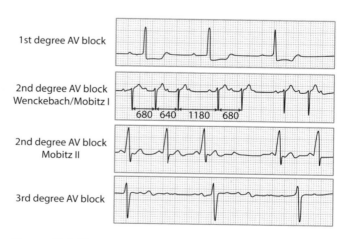

Figure 41.2 The top electrocardiogram (ECG) shows first degree heart block with a prolonged PR interval at 240 ms. Below is an example of Mobitz type 1 or Wenckebach block. There is progressive lengthening of the PR interval culminating in a loss of conduction to the ventricles. The third example is Mobitz type II block where the PR interval remains constant with sudden loss of conduction to the ventricles. The final ECG shows a slow regular ventricular rhythm with independent P-wave activity.

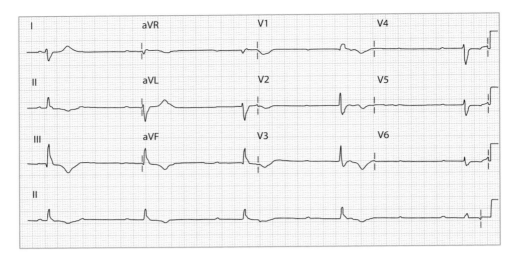

Figure 41.3 Complete heart block showing a slow regular ventricular rate at 40 bpm and independent P-wave activity. There is complete right bundle branch block and right anterior hemiblock compatible with advanced conduction disease.

Prophylactic pacing may be recommended but is not mandatory. These patients usually have heart disease, other co-morbidities and the conduction disease may progress to heart block.

- Atrial fibrillation: Some patients with AF have an intermittently slow ventricular rate, associated with symptoms of presyncope or syncope. Patients with pauses of 5 seconds or greater, even if asymptomatic, should receive a pacemaker. Even if there are pauses of more than 3 seconds with symptoms of presyncope or syncope, a pacemaker should be considered. Frequently, drug treatment is also given to slow the ventricular rate during AF and this will often exacerbate any bradycardia requiring pacemaker support.

- Congenital AV block: The incidence of congenital AV block (CAVB) ranges between 1:15 and 20,000 births.[9] Pacing is indicated in the following circumstances:
  - Syncope: There is a consensus that patients presenting with syncope should be paced urgently
  - Congestive heart failure
  - Chronotropic incompetence with limitation of physical activity
  - Prolonged pauses (>3 seconds)
  - Long QT interval: There is some evidence of an increased risk of sudden cardiac death in this sub-group

A more difficult decision is where patients are genuinely asymptomatic. The issue is not *if* pacing is required but *when*, particularly when the patients present with the symptoms in adulthood. Observational data suggest that where there is left ventricular (LV) dilatation or systolic impairment then pacing reverses these changes and current international guidelines recommend pacing in this setting. The heart rate threshold for pacing is controversial but many centres suggest rates persistently less than 50 bpm and/or pauses of >3 seconds irrespective of whether in the day or night should be paced. Although data are not clear, it is also generally accepted that where the QRS duration is ≥120 ms, pacing is advisable.[9]

- Reflex syncope and carotid hypersensitivity: This is a complex area and is not covered in detail in this section. However, the syndrome is defined as the reproduction of symptoms of syncope with carotid sinus massage yielding either a pause of >3 seconds or a fall in blood pressure of >50 mmHg or often both. This condition is benign, and therefore pacing should be made with careful consideration of symptomatology and the long-term benefits and complications of pacing. Overall, it is felt that pacing will reduce syncopal events in the majority of patients but in up to 20% syncope may recur. Careful selection of patients is therefore required.[6,10]

- Unexplained syncope and conduction disease (bundle branch block [BBB]): Although the presence of BBB may suggest the cause of syncope is cardiac, less than half of patients with BBB and syncope have a cardiac cause proven.[11,12] Management is mainly related to LV function at presentation. Where function is significantly impaired with a LV ejection fraction of <35% then consideration should be given to a prophylactic defibrillator. Where LV function is preserved and no other clear cause is found, electrophysiological (EP) studies can be helpful. The demonstration of infra-His block with prolongation of the HV interval predicts an increased risk of AVB.[13] Where the HV interval is greater than 70 ms the risk of AVB increases, particularly so when the HV is >100 ms, and pacing is recommended. If the EP is negative, an implanted loop recorder is suggested to better correlate the rhythm with any future syncope/symptoms. Reassuringly, mortality in these patients appears to be relatively low while they are being investigated.[12] However, pacing is recommended where there is alternating left and right BBB, even in the absence of symptoms. There is a general consensus that such patients progress to complete AVB.[6]

41.3 Pacemaker nomenclature

Pacemaker mode and function are described in shorthand using a four-letter coding. The first two letters refer to the chamber which is paced and sensed. The third refers to the mode setting for the device: D for a dual chamber device where there is pacing and sensing in both chambers; I for inhibited (either in a single or dual chamber device), or T for triggered, which is rarely used nowadays. The fourth letter refers to whether the rate sensor programme is present, whereupon an R is added. For example, a VVI system is a single-lead system which paces and senses in the right ventricle. VVI pacemakers are almost obsolete now as all have rate sensors and thus are referred to as VVIR system. A rate sensing dual chamber pacemaker which senses and paces in the atrium and ventricle is a DDDR system. A single-lead system which is able to sense in the atrium and pace and sense in the ventricle is a VDD system. This type of pacemaker tracks the sinus rate but cannot pace in the atrium and thus should only be used if the sinus node is functional. If it is ever decided to turn off pacing function in a DDD system, for whatever reason, then this is an ODO system.

- **Mode of pacing – I for inhibited:** All modern pacing systems are programmed to inhibited mode. A pacing impulse is not delivered when there is an adequate underlying rhythm. This allows the heart's intrinsic rhythm to come through, but when there is failure of the cardiac impulse, the pacemaker will then deliver a pacing output.
- **T for triggered:** Triggered mode is a pacemaker safety back up function and is very rarely used nowadays. This can be employed where patients who require extensive periods of ventricular pacing and where there is a sensing problem of the underlying R wave, the device can be programmed to deliver a pacing output upon each sensed R wave. Should there be a failure of the intrinsic underlying rhythm, the device will continue to pace, overcoming any problems with sensing. The down side of this approach is that the pacemaker paces continuously and the battery will be depleted prematurely.
- **Noise reversion mode:** All pacemakers are heavily shielded against external electrical noise. This prevents the pacemaker from misinterpreting noise as an underlying R wave and inappropriately inhibiting a potentially serious problem in patients who are pacing dependent (Figure 41.4). No pacemaker is completely immune from noise and eventually the sensing circuits will be

overcome. In order to avoid complete pacemaker inhibition, the pacemaker will switch to a non-sensing mode forcing it to pace continuously until the external interference is removed. This is known as the noise reversion mode. Situations where this may occur are, for example, during arc welding or faulty electrical equipment where a sufficient corporeal current can be induced in the body which is sensed by the device. Electrocautery/diathermy during surgery (see Section 14.14.1 – General Surgery) or a transcutaneous electrical nerve stimulation (TENS) machine applied in close proximity to the pacing generator, which may alter pacing function. If it is known that the pacemaker might be exposed to such external interference, then a strong magnet can be placed directly over the generator. The magnet temporarily alters pacemaker function and will revert to its pre-programmed state once the magnet is removed.

The other circumstance where external interference may alter and possibly damage the generator is magnetic resonance imaging (MRI) scanning. Recent changes in pacemaker design now allow MRI scanning under most circumstances (see Section 41.14 – MRI Scanning).

41.4 Choice of pacing mode: Single or dual chamber

Originally, all pacemakers used a single pacing lead placed in the right ventricle. This type of pacemaker ignored any contribution of the atria and dual chamber pacemakers (DDD) were developed to mimic the normal conduction of the heart. Although it was felt that more complex pacing systems would carry a significant benefit, randomised studies have not shown a mortality advantage from dual chamber over ventricular pacing. However, atrial-based pacing systems (DDD) do confer a morbidity benefit as manifest by less AF, stroke, pacemaker syndrome (see Section 41.11 – complications) and increased exercise capacity. This has to be weighed against an increased complication rate from dual chamber pacing such as atrial lead displacement.[14,15]

41.4.1 Specific pacing modes[6]

41.4.1.1 Sinus node disease

- Where there is chronotropic incompetence or exercise-related symptoms then dual chamber rate responsive

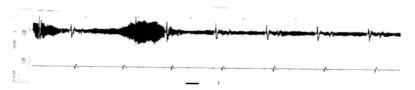

Figure 41.4 An example of noise reversion mode. The upper ECG shows baseline noise and the marker channels on the lower recording show a regular pacing rhythm at the programmed lower rate.

pacing (DDDR) is the first choice, promoting atrial pacing and minimising ventricular pacing
- Where the atrial rate with exercise is adequate, then DDD pacing with minimisation of ventricular pacing is the choice

Previous studies have suggested that for sinus node disease with intact AV nodal function, AAI or AAIR is an alternative pacing mode; but recent trials have shown an increase in paroxysmal AF and an annual incidence of AVB between 0.6% and 1.9% (Figure 41.5). This supports the routine use of DDD(R) pacing rather than AAIR in sinus node disease.[3,16]

41.4.1.2 Atrioventricular block

- In persistent block without concomitant sinus node disease (an adequate atrial response to exercise), then DDD pacing is indicated. VDD can be used in selected cases, where there is only one lead capable of sensing the atrial rate and pacing in the ventricle. VDD leads are a single lead, which in addition to a bipolar tip to pace in the ventricle also have an electrode within the body of the right atrium but within the same lead. This electrode senses the atrial signal but is unable to pace the atria as the electrode is not in direct contact with atrial myocardium. This may suffice where there is no sino-atrial disease.
- In AVB with sinus node disease, a DDDR system is indicated.
- In some circumstances, a VVIR pacemaker may be appropriate, particularly when life expectancy is short or the patient is very infirm.

41.4.1.3 Permanent AF

- With complete AVB or symptomatic bradycardias, a VVIR system is indicated.

41.4.1.4 Reflex syncope

- A dual chamber system is indicated where clinically relevant.

41.5 Specific issues related to DDD pacing

41.5.1 Upper rate behaviour

DDD pacing is effectively a truly 'physiological' pacing system as it senses the atrium and in the presence of atrioventricular nodal disease will pace in the ventricle as required. However if the atrial rate should increase significantly, such as atrial fibrillation, the device has a software algorithm which prevents the ventricular rate from becoming too rapid. There are a number of ways the pacemaker can deal with the increased atrial rate – one is called upper rate behavior and the other is mode switching. In upper rate behavior the device allows the ventricle to track the increase in atrial rate but once the atrial rate becomes too rapid the device allows the paced AV interval to increase producing initially Wenckebach block and, if the atrial rate continues to increase, intermittent AV block. There are advantages and disadvantages. In the elderly, inappropriately high rates of pacing in the ventricle can be avoided. In younger patients however, during vigorous exercise where a rapid heart rate is required it may become a serious problem as during exercise the ventricular rate can suddenly drop (Figure 41.6). Algorithms have been developed to avoid this and may involve individualised programming to allow rapid ventricular paced rates to occur where appropriate. Early

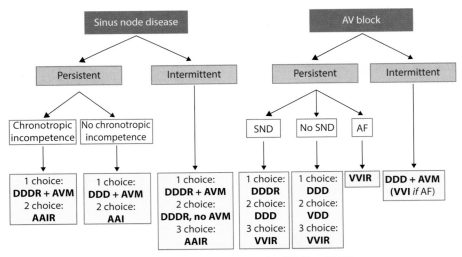

Figure 41.5 Suggested optimal pacing mode for patients with sinus node disease and for atrioventricular block. AF, atrial fibrillation; AV, atrioventricular; AVM, AV delay management for minimise ventricular pacing if possible. DDD, dual chamber pacing; DDDR, rate responsive dual chamber pacing; SND, sinus node disease; VVIR, rate responsive ventricular pacing. (From Brignole M et al., *Eur Heart J*, 34, 2013.)

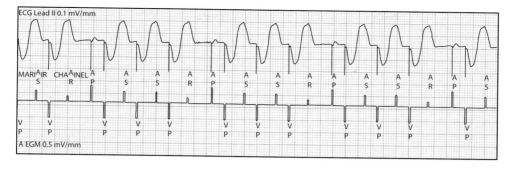

Figure 41.6 An irregular pacing rate in a dual chamber pacemaker showing what looks initially like dropped pacing beats. The atrial rate has increased producing a Wenckebach phenomenon where the ventricular paced rate appears to intermittently fail. The key to interpreting the ECG is shown by the ECG markers on the lower line which shows the high atrial rate. This is normal upper rate pacemaker behaviour and can produce symptoms during exercise.

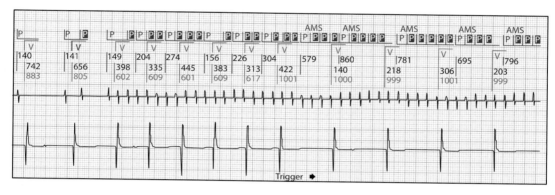

Figure 41.7 An example of mode switching. The upper blue ECG recording shows that atrial intra-cardiac electrogram (IEGM) and the red ECG the ventricular IEGM. The first two atrial beats are sinus followed by two atrial ectopics which initiate atrial fibrillation. At the onset of fibrillation, the ventricular response is irregular as the pacemaker tracks the increased atrial rate. To avoid a persistent increase in ventricular rate, the device switches automatically to a non-atrial sensing mode, thus pacing regularly in the ventricle. Automatic mode switch (AMS) in blue at the top of the recording confirms the devices has correctly switched.

systems employed a ventricular rate smoothing algorithm, sometime referred to as 'fly wheeling' but modern devices have programmes which essentially avoid sudden changes in the ventricular pacing rate. However to the uninitiated it can appear as though the device is malfunctioning.

41.5.2 Atrial arrhythmias and mode switching

When DDD pacing was first established it became clear that during atrial arrhythmias, the most common being AF, the device sensed the increase in the atrial rate and attempted to track this at the ventricular level. This resulted in both a rapid and irregular ventricular pacing response often felt by the patient. To overcome this problem, modern devices have a software algorithm known as 'mode switching' where the sudden change in atrial rate automatically alters the pacing function to inhibit tracking of atrial events and pace only in the ventricle at the programmed base or sensor rate. Each pacing company has developed a slightly different response but all switch temporarily to a non-tracking state known as either DDI or DDIR pacing. Figure 41.7 shows an example

where as soon as AF has developed, the device switches to pace and senses only in the ventricle. The atrial channel still senses but does not allow tracking of the atrial rate. When the rhythm reverts to sinus, the device automatically switches back to its dual chamber function.

41.5.3 Pacemaker-mediated tachycardia

This is only seen with DDD pacing and is a rapid and inappropriate ventricular paced rhythm due to retrograde sensing of an atrial signal in patients with dual chamber pacemakers. If a paced ventricular beat conducts retrogradely to the atria, then that atrial signal can be mis-interpreted as a sinus beat. In turn, the pacemaker paces the ventricle with a programmed AV delay and sets up a re-entrant loop which results in the pacemaker rate suddenly increasing. Such pacemaker mediated tachycardias (PMTs) can also be initiated by a ventricular ectopic with retrograde conduction to the atria. Software algorithms were developed to prevent this by avoiding either sensing the retrograde atrial signal or by terminating the PMT shortly after its onset. They have proven very effective and PMT is now rare.[17]

41.6 Minimising right ventricular pacing

Although right ventricular (RV) pacing, particularly at the apex, has been the traditional site for transvenous pacing, there is concern that this may increase the risk of LV dysfunction (see Section 41.7). Many studies suggest that RV pacing should be avoided, if at all possible.[15,18] All modern pacemakers have software-based pacing algorithms capable of determining the paced AV delay and allowing intrinsic ventricular conduction to occur, if possible. Each pacemaker company has its own version and these are variably referred to as AV search hysteresis, managed ventricular pacing (MVP), AV delay management or ventricular intrinsic preference (VIP). The philosophy is to avoid ventricular pacing, if possible.

41.7 Controversies: Optimal lead position

Since the inception of transvenous pacing, the right ventricular apex (RVA) has been the traditional site of choice for chronic lead placement. Early lead design coupled with the muscular trabeculations within the RVA region and the relative ease of vascular access to the right heart provides a stable and effective means for lead placement. As a result, this has proven to be an effective technology from which millions of patients worldwide have benefitted. However, there is a body of clinical and experimental evidence which suggests that chronic RVA pacing in some patients is implicated in the deterioration of LV function over time leading to increased risk of heart failure and premature death. The exact reason for this is unknown. As a result of concerns over RVA pacing, other sites within the RV have been studied including the RV septum, outflow tract, the His-bundle and dual-site pacing (where two leads are placed within the RV, one at the apex and one at the septum). A recent large-scale randomised trial comparing apical to septal pacing did not show any difference in outcome for LV function where baseline LV systolic function is preserved.[19] Other data suggest that where LV function is impaired septal lead placement may provide a protective effect on LV function over time compared to RVA pacing.[20] His-bundle pacing has recently received renewed interest and although the implant can be a challenge, pacing the His-bundle improves cardiac haemodynamics and may prevent deterioration in LV function.[21] Cardiac re-synchronisation therapy is also being suggested as an alternative to RV pacing where patients present with high-grade AV block and require a high percentage of pacing.[22] As yet, there remains controversy about which is the optimal pacing lead position and whether further clinical trials are required. Direct LV pacing has also been studied as there are supporting data that this has haemodynamic benefit over RV pacing.[23,24]

41.8 Pacemaker implantation – Technique

Pacemakers are inserted under local anaesthesia with light sedation in a surgically sterile environment usually in a standard cardiac catheter laboratory.[25,26]

41.8.1 Antibiotic prophylaxis

Infection either early or late is the most feared complication of device implantation as it necessitates complete system removal. To minimise infection, antibiotics are mandatory prior to implant: 1 g of amoxycillin or 2 g cephazolin is given an hour prior to surgery. In penicillin-sensitive patients, vancomycin 0.15 mg/kg with or without gentamycin is given intravenously. Post-implant approaches vary. Many centres continue to use oral antibiotics in the form of amoxicillin 250 mg qds or cephalexin 500 mg qds for up to 1 week. The use of antibiotics will also depend upon the patient's perceived risk. In high-risk cases, advice from the infectious diseases department is recommended. In Methicillin-resistant *Staphylococcus aureus* (MRSA)-positive patients, aggressive skin preparation prior to implant is justified. Some centres use additional topical antibiotics to the nasal passages, a common source of MRSA. Careful patient assessment together with adequate antibiotic usage is mandatory.

41.8.2 Surgery

Patients are often given a pre-medication. By convention, the device is usually inserted under the skin in the left or right prepectoral position beneath the clavicle. The procedure takes between 30 and 60 minutes. Access to the right heart is gained either via direct subclavian or axillary vein puncture or by dissection of the cephalic vein with direct introduction of the pacing lead(s). The pacing leads are screened into position, one at the high right atrium and the other in the RV. Patients are mobilised within a few hours and allowed home the following day. Some centres implant as a day-case procedure.

41.9 Pacemaker implantation and anticoagulation

Many centres implant devices without interruption of warfarin therapy although allowing the international normalized ratio (INR) to drift to around 2.0–2.5 is preferable. Careful surgical technique reduces the risk of pocket haematoma. Dual anti-platelet therapy is of more concern and ideally anti-platelet agents such as clopidogrel or ticagrelor may need to be withheld for 3–5 days depending upon clinical circumstances. With increasing use of drug-eluting stents, there may be no alternative to continued drug use during pacemaker implantation, and although scrupulous attention to haemostasis is mandatory, uninterrupted dual anti-platelet therapy is not a contraindication to implant. Post-operative heparin should be avoided as this significantly increases the risk of haematoma.

41.9.1 Complications

Bruising around the wound is common as is some discomfort, all usually short-lived. Patients are encouraged to keep the left shoulder mobile to a degree. Fear of activity can lead to frozen shoulders.

41.9.1.1 Acute

- Pocket haematoma is common (Figure 41.8).[27] Rarely, this may be significant requiring drainage. Careful surgical technique avoids late bleeding even in anticoagulated patients. A small drain can be used, if there is a high risk of local bleeding. Most pocket haematomas can be managed conservatively and re-opening the pocket should be avoided to minimise the risk of subsequent infection. Often, simple compression and time resolve the situation.
- 1% risk of a pneumothorax.
- Haemothorax is rare, as is death.
- Cardiac perforation has been described but rarely leads to tamponade (Figure 41.9).

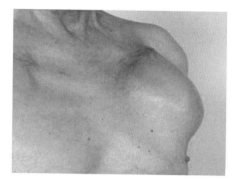

Figure 41.8 Large pacemaker haematoma. Haematomas of this size may require drainage if painful or increasing in size. (From Gul EE and Kayrak M www.intechopen.com.)

- Lead displacement: Uncommon; it is more so with atrial leads than ventricular and is often operator dependent.
- Acute infection is uncommon.

41.9.1.2 Chronic

- Late infection is a serious but uncommon complication. An infected pacemaker site mandates system removal including the generator and the leads (see Section 41.11).
- Pacemaker erosion (Figure 41.10) is also a rare complication now that generators are so small. Erosion is always associated with infection and again results in the need to remove the system completely.
- Lead fracture due to subclavian crush (Figure 41.9): Sometimes, the lead insulation is damaged, often after many years at the insertion site into the subclavian vein. Crush fractures do not occur with a cephalic approach and are rare with subclavian and axillary approaches.
- Twiddler's syndrome (Figure 41.11): This is patient-induced due to repeated rotation of the pacing generator within the pocket which results in rotation and possible displacement of the pacing leads often resulting in failure of pacing. The treatment is to revise the leads and system either to suture the generator to the pectoralis muscle or in extreme cases to place the device in a special pouch within the pocket which causes fibrosis around the generator thereby limiting the ability to rotate the device.

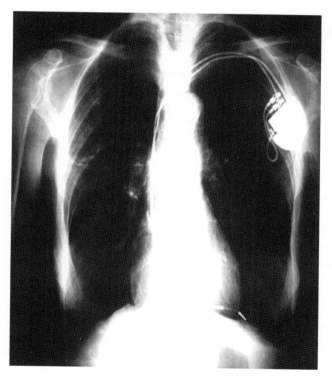

Figure 41.9 Showing the tip of the ventricular lead outside the cardiac silhouette.

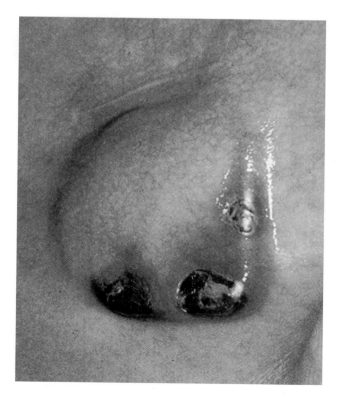

Figure 41.10 Device erosion showing parts of the pacing generator exposed.

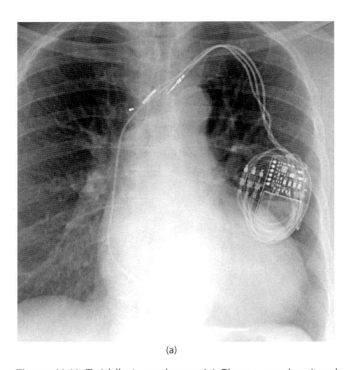
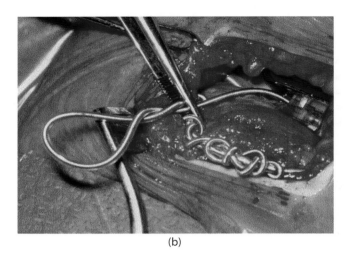

(a)

(b)

Figure 41.11 Twiddler's syndrome: **(a)** Chest x-ray showing the leads twisted around each other in the pocket resulting in two leads being pulled out of the heart. **(b)** During the pacemaker revision the leads are clearly seen wrapped around each other.

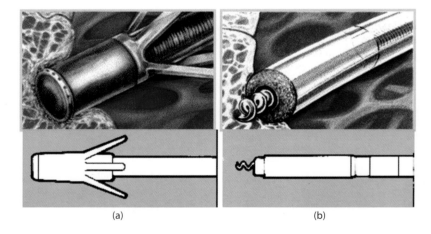

(a)

(b)

Figure 41.12 An example of a passive tip lead **(a)** which has tines which lock into the ventricular myocardium and an active tip lead **(b)** which has a screw mechanism which anchors directly to the cardiac muscle.

41.9.1.3 Pacemaker syndrome

This is rare with modern pacing systems. It occurs most commonly with single-lead ventricular pacing and can occur both early after implantation and late. There is loss of synchronised physiological timing of atrial and ventricular contractions which occurs when there is retrograde ventriculo-atrial conduction during ventricular pacing. Symptoms may be varied and include dizziness, near syncope, symptomatic hypotension as well as dyspnoea. The treatment is to either re-programme the device if possible or upgrade to a dual chamber system to re-synchronises atrial and ventricular contraction.[15,28,29]

41.10 Transvenous pacing leads

Leads consist of an inner metallic core insulated from blood and body fluids by an external synthetic coat nowadays usually made from polyurethane, although newer compounds have been developed. Pacing leads are either active or passive (Figure 41.12). The latter utilise a series of tines, similar to an arrowhead, which simply anchor the lead tip between the muscle bundles of the RV and atrial endocardium. Active leads have a mechanism which extends a screw from the tip into the myocardium. Passive leads are designed primarily to pace from the RVA or high right atrium/appendage, whereas screw-in leads can be placed almost anywhere in the right heart. All leads eventually become fibrosed to the myocardium making late displacement impossible. The lead body is highly resilient, flexing and twisting to accommodate daily cardiac contractions. Lead failure is rare (<0.05% fracture/year) and longevity is around 10–15 years. Fractures do occur either within the inner conducting core or the outer insulation. Commonly, insulation failure occurs at the insertion of the lead to the subclavian vein. Lead integrity can be assessed non-invasively via the pacemaker generator, and modern devices now have the capability of self-checking lead function on a daily basis and allow automatic reprogramming to maintain patient safety. A broken lead needs replacement or, uncommonly, removal.

41.10.1 Unipolar versus bipolar pacing

All modern leads are bipolar having both pacing electrodes at the tip of the lead. Early lead design was unipolar where there was a single pacing electrode at the tip and the generator can act as the second electrode. Although unipolar leads are less complex to manufacture than bipolar and have very good longevity, the major disadvantage is that they are more sensitive to external interference causing inappropriate pacemaker inhibition. Modern systems use bipolar leads exclusively.

41.10.2 Pacemakers implant rates

Results of a worldwide survey show a steady increase, year on year, in the rate of pacemaker implants with over a million implants. The implant rate per country varies widely, for example in 2011, there were 518 implants per million in the United Kingdom, 767 in the United States, 927 in Germany and 565 per million population in Australia.[30] Developing countries lag behind but rates are steadily increasing.[30]

41.10.3 Living with a pacemaker

41.10.3.1 Quality of life

41.10.3.1.1 Driving

Patients who have had blackouts and an identifiable cause treated by a pacemaker are able to drive 1 week after the procedure. Strenuous exertion (e.g. swimming) is best avoided for 1 month. Heavy goods (HGV) and passenger (PSA) vehicle license holders also need to be assessed.

41.10.3.1.2 Flying

Pacemaker implantation precludes the flying of a commercial airplane. Non-commercial pilots need to have their license assessed by the National Aviation Authority.

41.10.3.1.3 Pregnancy

Pacemakers in women of child-bearing age are rare. There is no contraindication to pregnancy and the only limitation will relate to the underlying cardiac disorder.

41.10.3.1.4 General surgery

The major risk during surgery, although small, pertains to the use of diathermy. Diathermy should be kept at least 10 cm away from the pacing generator and an ECG recording throughout. If close diathermy cannot be avoided, the pacemaker can be protected by placing a strong magnet over the generator. As soon as the magnet is withdrawn, the pacemaker reverts to normal function.

41.10.3.1.5 MRI scanning

Devices have been developed which are MRI-conditional allowing certain MRI scans to be performed, in some cases even a cardiac MRI. Patients should be informed that they can have an MRI scan with this pacemaker. The device often requires re-programming to MRI mode prior to the scan, although newer devices can detect MRI scan and automatically re-programme themselves to a protected mode during the procedure.

41.10.3.1.6 TENS machines

It is not advised to use a TENS machine close to a pacing generator due to potential pacemaker inhibition.

41.10.3.1.7 Daily activities

There are very few restrictions on daily activity. Normal sexual function and exercise are allowed and purely depend on the underlying cardiac abnormality. The use of microwave ovens is permitted providing the wearer does not stand very close to the machine.

41.10.3.1.8 Mobile/cellular phones

These can interfere with pacemaker function and it is recommended that the phone be used at the ear opposite to the pacemaker and stored away from breast pockets.

41.10.3.1.9 External interference

All modern pacemakers are well shielded and considerable interference is required to alter or damage a pacemaker. Under normal daily living, exposure to high-level electromagnetic fields is unlikely. Any machine capable of generating a high-density current, like an arc-welding unit, may be capable of disturbing pacing function. Airport and department store security systems are safe. If a pacemaker is overwhelmed by external interference, it has an additional safety feature where sensing circuits are temporarily switched off and the device paces continuously until the interference is resolved. Nowadays, it is rare for a device to sense extrinsic noise and interpret it as an underlying QRS complex.

41.10.3.1.10 After death

If patients are to be cremated, the pacemaker *must* be removed beforehand as incineration can cause an explosion.

41.11 Pacemaker removal and lead extraction

The presence of infection mandates removal of all parts of the system, leads and generator. Lead extraction carries a small but significant risk. Once leads are implanted for more than 6–12 months, it is unlikely they will be removed easily with simple traction. Currently, leads are removed percutaneously either with a laser or less commonly using radiofrequency ablation around the lead. There are also mechanical cutters able to break through the fibrosis around the leads. The common areas where the leads become densely fibrosed are the RV myocardial/lead interface, at the superior vena cava and at the insertion to the subclavian veins. Percutaneous lead extraction has an overall mortality of 1%–3% and should be performed in specialised centres only. Tearing of the major intra-thoracic venous structures or the RV is a particular hazard and many centres now perform lead extraction with the capability of performing emergency open heart surgery (so-called hybrid catheter laboratories). Lead extraction should be the last resort and patients must be counselled accordingly. Although leads are remarkably resilient, they are the Achilles' heel of pacing, as removal is often difficult and potentially hazardous. As a result, technology is being developed to make implantation of transvenous leads redundant (see below).

41.12 Pacemaker technology

41.12.1 Batteries

Device longevity is an important issue for implanters. Currently, batteries are lithium-based (lithium-iodine over the last few decades, but recently, lithium carbon monofluoride/silver vanadium oxide hybrid batteries are being used). Most dual chamber systems will endure usually 8–10 years. Battery depletion is gradual and current devices can estimate longevity (often a warning of battery depletion of at least 1 year is given). Battery replacement involves day-case surgery.

41.12.2 Data storage

Large amounts of data over long periods of time can now be stored on a device. Information about lead integrity (impedance), pacing threshold, arrhythmias either atrial or ventricular, or from the sensor (see below) can be stored for up to 1 year continuously. Thus, trends in how the device, and to a degree the patient, is behaving can be seen. Figure 41.13 demonstrates a years' worth of information showing how frequently AF was detected and the amount of atrial and ventricular pacing, sensor data which indirectly give a

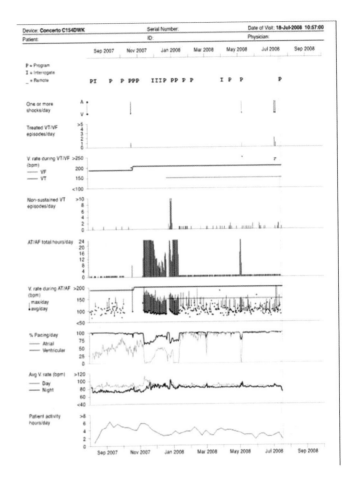

Figure 41.13 Data storage – this figure shows a number of parameters monitored simultaneously and stored within the device. This example shows a period of 10 months. Data concerning the detection of atrial arrhythmias (fibrillation), percentage of ventricular pacing, the ventricular rate, and patient activity trend derived from the sensor are shown allowing earlier detection of problems and also providing a picture of how the patient is progressing during this 10-month period.

picture of how active the patient was. In some cases, this allows pre-emptive treatment to be given before a patient decompensates clinically. For example, if sustained AF occurs, rather than wait until the patient presents with symptoms, a possible stroke or heart failure, this information can be made available earlier allowing the physician to intervene, if appropriate.

41.12.3 Cardiac sensors

All pacemakers have a sensor capable of reacting to the demands of exercise known as rate-responsive pacing (referred to with an 'R' in pacemaker nomenclature). There are two main types: activity and metabolic sensors. One type of activity sensor relies upon changes in the signal emitted from an accelerometer. During body movement, the signal from the accelerometer is amplified and variations in frequency are used to increase the heart rate, usually commensurate with the patient's exercise demand. Such sensors have proven highly effective and software programming allows significant individualisation. Another type of activity sensor involves a piezo-electric crystal within the pacing generator. Metabolic sensors measure changes in the paced QT interval, the respiratory rate or cardiac contractility and again are effective at responding to both exercise and other stimuli such as mental stress. Devices with two sensors, activity and metabolic, overcome the limitations of each separate sensor but increase device complexity and battery drain.

Sensors have also been used in different ways, for example, changes in the respiratory rate facilitate the diagnosis of obstructive sleep apnoea. Newer algorithms are also under investigation, which are capable of determining changes in ST segments possibly predicting ischaemic events or myocardial infarction. Clinical studies are underway.

41.12.4 Remote monitoring

For the past 10 years, devices have been capable of transmitting data from the pacemaker over either a mobile or land telephone line, allowing real-time monitoring. All the information described above, such as lead integrity, battery longevity and arrhythmias can be determined remotely, from the patients' home. Any sudden changes such as a lead failure or the development of new arrhythmias can be detected promptly. Recent studies have confirmed a mortality benefit with remote monitoring. Although a number of studies have suggested a mortality benefit, a recent randomised trial in over 750 patients demonstrated a clear clinical benefit, and in particular, reduced mortality in patients in the remote monitoring arm.[31] Remote monitoring is now standard of care for follow-up of paced patients. A detailed picture of changes within individual patients can be determined. This may be particularly useful for patients with heart failure

where alterations in certain parameters may predict early cardiac decompensation allowing intervention before the patient requires acute admission (Figure 41.13).

41.13 Basic troubleshooting

An understanding of basic pacing malfunction is useful. Serious complications are uncommon with modern systems and troubleshooting of more complex devices is beyond the scope of this chapter.

41.13.1 Failure of pacing

Acutely, this might be due to a lead displacement occurring immediately or shortly after implantation. Following implantation of a new lead, there is usually an acute tissue reaction around the tip which produces an increase in the pacing threshold over time. The threshold nearly always stabilises at the 6–8-week point (Figure 41.14) after which it usually remains stable for years. Sometimes, the threshold increases dramatically due to the intensity of the lead/myocardial interface or occasionally a micro-displacement of the tip occurs and may result in loss of capture (Figure 41.15). Modern pacemakers are able to continually test capture threshold, known as capture control, where the device will retest the threshold, usually on a daily basis, and automatically increase output to ensure safe capture at all times. Failure to capture may also signify a lead fracture.

41.13.2 Failure of sensing

All pacemakers sense the underlying rhythm and inhibit pacing output accordingly. Undersensing occurs when the pacemaker fails to adequately sense the native cardiac signal. Causes include increased stimulation threshold at

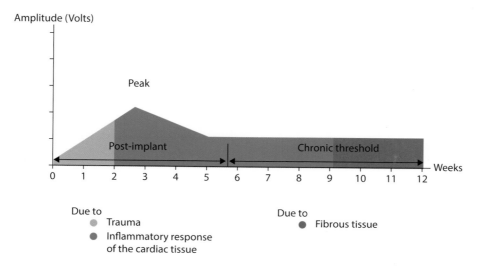

Figure 41.14 Changes in pacing threshold over time. There is an acute rise within 2–3 weeks due to a combination of initial lead tip-induced trauma and an inflammatory tissue response which gradually falls to a stable chronic threshold which often holds steady for years. (Courtesy of St. Jude Medical.)

electrode site (exit block), poor lead contact, new BBB or programming problems. Undersensing is manifest on the surface ECG when pacing spikes occur during QRS complex or P waves (Figure 41.16). Oversensing occurs when extrinsic electrical signals are inappropriately recognised as native cardiac activity and pacing is inhibited. This may be due to large far-field signals such as P waves or inappropriate sensing of T waves (Figure 41.17). Signals such as skeletal muscle contractions (usually pectoral) or external interference may be the source. Sometimes, this may not be evident from the surface ECG but interrogation of the internal electrograms may give a clue. Figure 41.4 shows 50-Hz interference detected from external electrical equipment. This sort of signal can also be seen with lead

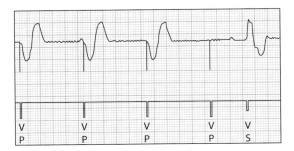

Figure 41.15 Loss of capture: The first three paced beats result in a ventricular complex but the fourth spike does not indicating loss of capture of the ventricle.

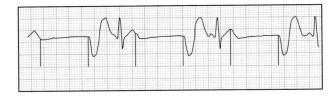

Figure 41.16 Loss of sensing: pacing spikes are seen during T waves. This may be due to a loss of adequate sensing or similar changes can be seen as a result of noise reversion mode where sensing is temporarily turned off to avoid inappropriate inhibition of pacing. This usually occurs where external noise is sensed.

insulation fractures, sometimes before electrical breakdown of the lead is obvious. Figure 41.17 shows pacemaker inhibition due to oversensing during contraction of the pectoralis muscle.

41.13.3 Lead failure

There are two main types of lead failure: external insulation failure or a fracture of the internal metallic core. In insulation failure, the lead impedance falls and in a conductor fracture, it rises.

41.13.4 Pacemaker-related tachycardias

41.13.4.1 Pacemaker-mediated tachycardia (PMT)

This only occurs with DDD systems. It has been referred in the past as endless-loop tachycardia or pacemaker circus movement tachycardia. PMT is usually initiated by a ventricular ectopic which has retrograde conduction to the atria (Figure 41.18). The retrograde P wave is sensed as a sinus P wave and initiates ventricular pacing. The pacemaker forms the antegrade part of a re-entry loop with the retrograde part being conduction through the AV node. Ventricular pacing results in further retrograde conduction with retrograde P-wave generation thus forming a continuous cycle resulting in a paced tachycardia with the maximum rate limited by the pacemaker programmed upper rate. All DDD pacemakers have automatic programmed algorithms capable of recognising and terminating PMT soon after initiation. PMT is now a rare complication of DDD pacemakers.

41.13.4.2 Sensor driven tachycardia

Rarely, sensors may misinterpret stimuli such as external vibrations, fever or, rarely, electrocautery (e.g. during surgery) and pace at an inappropriately fast rate. Interrogation of the device will usually provide the answer and if in doubt rapid pacing can be terminated with application of a magnet externally.

41.13.4.3 Runaway pacemaker

This is a rare malfunction of older pacing systems implanted

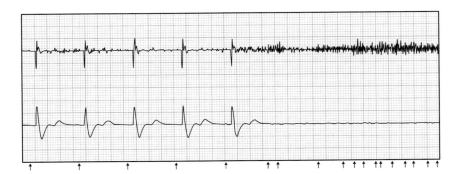

Figure 41.17 An example of myopotential oversensing: A patient complaining of intermittent presyncope was asked to contract the pectoralis muscle in the clinic resulting in oversensing of the myopotentials resulting in inhibition of pacing output.

over the last 15 years or more. It is potentially life threatening and occurs due to low battery voltage (e.g. overdue pacemaker replacement). The pacemaker delivers either paroxysms of rapid pacing spikes or paces at a continuously rapid rate. Immediate pacemaker replacement is required.

41.13.4.4 Hysteresis

This is a normal pacemaker function but is often mis-interpreted as a pacing malfunction. Hysteresis is a programmable function which allows the underlying cardiac

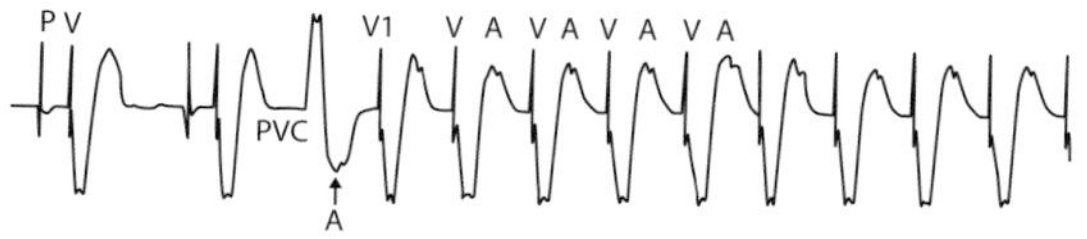

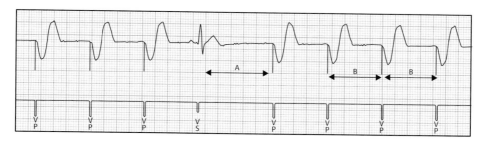

Figure 41.18 An example of the initiation of a pacemaker mediated tachycardia (PMT): The first two beats represent normal dual chamber pacing with an atrial paced beat (P) and a ventricular paced beat (V). There is a ventricular ectopic (PVC) with retrograde conduction to the atrium (arrow) which is sensed by the device as a sinus beat and this initiates a paced AV delay. The first paced ventricular beat (V1) is also conducted retrogradely to the atrium (A) and this establishes a re-entrant loop between the retrograde P wave (A) and ventricular pacing (V) giving rise to a tachycardia.

rhythm time to occur and thus minimises the amount of pacing. An example is shown in Figure 41.19. As the heart rate slows, the device is programmed to wait until the heart rate drops to a very low level giving the heart as much time as possible to generate an underlying rhythm. The device then paces at a much faster base rate to maintain an adequate cardiac output.

41.14 External cardioversion in pacemaker patients

If external cardioversion is required, either emergent or elective, the paddles or patches should be placed at a distance, at least 10 cm from the pacing generator. The paddles can be placed in the usual position over the cardiac apex and to the right of the sternum. Patches can also be placed in the anteroposterior position. The device should be interrogated after external shock delivery.

41.14.1 Radiotherapy

Radiotherapy produces ionising radiation which can damage the electronic circuitry within the generator. The dose is cumulative. The generator should be shielded if possible. Ionising radiation damage to the lead is rare. If the cumulative dose is high (>1 gray) and the generator cannot be

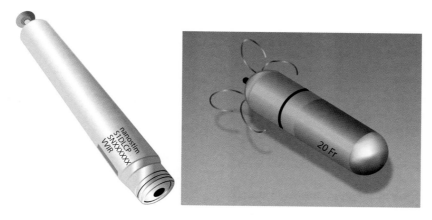

Figure 41.19 An example of pacing hysteresis: The first three beats are ventricular pacing. The fourth beat is an intrinsic beat which inhibits pacing output. The next paced beat is delayed (interval A) to allow time for an intrinsic beat to occur but the subsequent pacing rate (B) is faster to provide adequate cardiac output. Hysteresis should not be used where there is marked variation in the underlying heart rate such as in atrial fibrillation or sinus rhythm with frequent ectopy.

Figure 41.20 Current examples of two leadless pacemakers. The device on the right has a screw mechanism at one end designed to fix to the endocardium and the other has tines which anchor to the muscle bundles within the right ventricle.

adequately shielded or there is concern that the generator will be exposed to high dose backscatter, then consideration should be given to moving the generator outside the field of radiation, particularly in pacing dependency. Radiation treatment may also result in temporary pacing at the upper sensor rate.

41.14.2 The near future: Leadless pacing

The long-term downside of pacing relates to the intra-cardiac lead. Lead extraction for whatever reason still carries a small mortality risk and thus avoiding intra-cardiac leads would negate this requirement. Clinical trials are currently underway to determine the safety of implanting miniaturised pacing generators directly into the RV myocardium.[32,33] Two such devices are currently available. They are delivered to the endocardium via the femoral vein using a specially designed catheter. One such device is screwed directly into the myocardium and the other has tines which expand to lock into the RV muscular trabeculations (Figure 41.20). At present, they are only single chamber (although dual chamber devices are in development). Leadless devices are proving effective and safe. Their size is approximately 80% less than a standard pacing generator and battery life is expected to exceed 10 years. Once depleted, it is planned that another device would be placed alongside without the need to remove the first device. The effect on the mechanical function of the RV with more than one device is unknown.

Miniaturised generators have also been developed which can be implanted directly into the left ventricle. A recent proof of concept clinical study in man has proven effective and more data are required to determine long-term safety.

41.14.3 The far future: Genetic engineering

Over the past 10 years, significant progress has been made in identifying the molecular components of the mammalian conduction system. Advances in stem cell therapy and genetic manipulation may also offer the possibility of repairing the hearts' intrinsic conduction system. As yet, these possibilities are far off but some progress has been made and the scenario that an implantable device may not be required is a real one. A recent proof of concept publication provided an insight into the possibility of re-engineering the mammalian conduction system in complete heart block to electrically reconnect the atria and ventricles.[34] Undoubtedly, more work is required but the concept of re-establishing the hearts' own pacemaker may be genuine.

41.15 Conclusions

Developments in pacemaker technology have revolutionised the management of bradycardia. Advances in miniaturisation, lead and battery technology and, in particular, data acquisition and storage have extended the reach of these devices from being simply a means of preventing slow heart rates to providing detailed and continuous information about previously undiagnosed arrhythmias. Remote monitoring has provided the ability to determine changes in the heart rhythm as well to determine any problems with the pacemaker itself increasing the benefit and safety to patients. Whereas traditionally patients were reviewed annually, data about their heart now can be accessed daily and thus provide an almost immediate diagnosis of new events. The wealth of data in combination with new sensing technology allows the possibility of pre-emptive intervention before patients decompensate clinically and is an area of great interest particularly in the management of heart failure. Although controversies remain about the optimal pacing site, the RV still remains the chamber of choice for chronic pacing in many patients. However, cardiac re-synchronisation or His-bundle pacing may be increasingly used in future for patients requiring a high burden of ventricular pacing. Although pacing technology has proven remarkably safe, the Achilles' heel remains transvenous leads, hence the development of leadless pacemakers implanted directly into the heart. Current clinical studies in single chamber ventricular leadless pacing show promise and future developments into dual chamber leadless systems are awaited. In the interim, research on genetic manipulation of cardiac cells may ultimately make an implanted system redundant but such developments are many years away and until then we remain dependent on sophisticated electronics surrounded by a metallic can.

References

1. Ovsyshcher IE, Ed. Cardiac Arrhythmias and Device Therapy. New York, NY: Futura Publishing Company, 2000.
2. Sasaki Y et al. Long-term follow-up of patients with sick sinus syndrome: A comparison of clinical aspects among unpaced, ventricular inhibited paced and physiological paced groups. Pacing Clin Electrophysiol 1988; 11: 1575–83.
3. Andersen HR et al. Prospective randomized trial of atrial versus ventricular pacing in sick-sinus syndrome. Lancet 1994; 334: 1523–28.
4. Adan V and Crown LA. Diagnosis and treatment of sick sinus syndrome. Am Fam Physician 2003; 67: 1725–32.
5. Benditt DG et al. Sinus node dysfunction: Pathophysiology, clinical features, evaluation, and treatment. In: Zipes DP, Jalife J, (editors), Cardiac Electrophysiology: From Cell to Bedside, 2nd Edition. Philadelphia, PA: WB Saunders Company, 1995, pp. 1215–47.
6. Brignole M et al. 2013 Guidelines on cardiac pacing and cardiac resynchronization therapy. Eur Heart J 2013; 34: 2281–329.
7. Alboni P et al. Effects of permanent pacemaker and oral theophylline in sick sinus syndrome: The THEOPACE study. Circulation 1997; 96: 260–67.
8. Lamas GA et al. Ventricular pacing or dual chamber pacing for sinus-node dysfunction. N Eng J Med 2002; 346: 1854–62.

9. Bordachar P et al. Pathophysiology, clinical course, and management of congenital atrioventricular block. *Heart Rhythm* 2013; 10: 760–66.

10. Brignole M et al. Pacemaker therapy in patients with neutrally mediated syncope and documented asystole: Third International Study on Syncope of Uncertain Etiology (ISSUE-3): A randomized study. *Circulation* 2012; 125: 2566–71.

11. Sud S. Implications of mechanism of bradycardia in response to pacing in patients with unexplained syncope. *Europace* 2007; 9: 312–18.

12. Moya A et al. Diagnosis, management, and outcomes of patients with syncope and bundle branch block. *Eur Heart J* 2011; 32: 1535–41.

13. Scheinman MM et al. Value of the H-Q interval in patients with bundle branch block and the role of prophylactic permanent pacing. *Am J Cardiol* 1982; 50: 1316–22.

14. Nielsen JC et al. A comparison of single-lead atrial pacing with dual chamber pacing in sick sinus syndrome. *Eur Heart J* 2011; 32: 686–96.

15. Sweeney MO et al. Minimizing ventricular pacing to reduce atrial fibrillation in sinus-node disease. *N Eng J Med* 2007; 357: 1000–8.

16. Castelnuovo E et al. The effectiveness and cost-effectiveness of dual chamber pacemakers compared with single chamber pacemakers for bradycardia due to atrioventricular block or sick sinus syndrome: A systematic review and economic evaluation. *Health Technol Assess* 2005; 9: iii, xi–xiii:1–24617.

17. Richter S et al. Ventriculoatrial conduction and related pacemaker-mediated arrhythmias in patients implanted for atrioventricular block: An old problem revisited. *Int J Cardiol.* 2013 Oct 9; 168(4): 3300–8.

18. Wilkoff BL et al Dual chamber pacing or ventricular back-up pacing in patients with an implantable defibrillator: The dual chamber and VVI implantable defibrillator (DAVID) Trial. *JAMA* 2002; 288: 3115–23.

19. Kaye GC et al. Effect of right ventricular pacing lead site on left ventricular function in patients with high-grade atrioventricular block: Results of the Protect-Pace study. *Eur Heart J* 2015; 36(14): 856–62.

20. Hussain MA et al. The effect of right ventricular apical and non-apical pacing on the short- and long-term changes in left ventricular ejection fraction: A systematic review and meta-analysis of randomized-controlled trials. *Pacing Clin Electrophysiol* 2015; 38(9): 1121–36.

21. Lustgarten D et al. His-bundle versus biventricular pacing in cardiac resynchronization therapy patients: A cross over design. *Heart Rhythm* 2015; 12: 1548–57.

22. Barold SS. Editorial: Biventricular pacing for bradycardia: Are we there yet? *J Electrocardiol* 2015; 48: 236–40.

23. Rademakers LM et al. Mid-term follow-up of Thromboembolic complications in left ventricular endocardial cardiac resynchronization therapy. *Heart Rhythm* 2014; 11(4): 609–13.

24. Shetty AK et al. A comparison of left ventricular endocardial, multisite, and multipolar epicardial cardiac resynchronization: An acute haemodynamic and electroanatomical study. *Europace* 2014; 16(6): 873–9.

25. Rajappan K. Permanent pacemaker implantation technique: Part I. *Heart* 2009; 95: 259–64.

26. Rajappan K. Permanent pacemaker implantation technique: Part II. *Heart* 2009; 95: 334–42.

27. Furman S. Pacemaker syndrome. *Pacing Clin Electrophysiol.* 1994 Jan; 17(1): 1–5.

28. Gul EE and Kayrak M www.intechopen.com.

29. Epstein AE et al. ACC/AHA/HRS 2008 Guidelines for Device-Based Therapy of Cardiac Rhythm Abnormalities: A report of the American College of Cardiology/American Heart Association Task Force on Practice Guidelines (Writing Committee to Revise the ACC/AHA/NASPE 2002 Guideline Update for Implantation of Cardiac Pacemakers and Antiarrhythmia Devices) *J Am Coll Cardiol.* 2008 May 27; 51(21): e1–62.

30. Mond HG, and Crozier I. The Australian and New Zealand cardiac pacemaker and implantable cardioverter-defibrillator survey: Calendar year 2013. *Heart Lung Circ* 2015; 24: 291–97.

31. Hindricks G et al. Implant-based multiparameter tele-monitoring of patients with heart failure: A randomised controlled trial. *Lancet* 2014; 384: 583–90.

32. Reddy VY et al. Permanent leadless cardiac pacing: Results of the LEADLESS trial. *Circulation* 2014; 129(14): 1466–71.

33. Seriwala HM et al. Leadless pacemakers: A new era in cardiac pacing. *Cardiology* 2015 Oct 9; pii: S0914–087(15): 00293–2. doi: 10.1016/j.jjcc.2015.09.006

34. Cingolani E et al. Engineered electrical conduction tract restores conduction in complete heart block. *J Am Cardiol* 2014; 64(2): 2575–85.

Other resources

Fast Facts: *Management of Cardiac Arrhythmias.* Authors: Gerry Kaye, Stephen Furniss, and Robert Lemery Editors: Healthpress@UK

Useful websites: www.arrhythmiaalliance.org www.hrsonline.or

Cardiac resynchronisation therapy (CRT)

DOMINIC ROGERS, ABDALLAH AL-MOHAMMAD

42.1 Introduction

Heart failure (HF) is a syndrome that occurs in 2% of young adults and in 10%–20% of the older adult population.[1] The incidence of HF may well be constant, but its prevalence is increasing. HF is associated with a high morbidity burden characterised by an increased need for hospitalisation and with an increased risk of mortality that varies according to the severity of the HF symptoms.[2] Irrespective of the aetiology and severity of the HF, it is recognised that up to 50% of the patients die suddenly, presumably due to arrhythmias, usually ventricular tachycardia and ventricular fibrillation. Ischaemic heart disease and systemic hypertension are the most common causes of HF. Other causes include diabetes mellitus, primary myocardial diseases (cardiomyopathies including dilated, hypertrophic, restrictive and arrhythmogenic ventricular cardiomyopathy), secondary myocardial diseases (which could be caused by infective factors such viruses and trypanosome; chemical factors such as alcohol or chemotherapeutic agents such as doxorubicin and Herceptin; physical

factors such as radiotherapy). Rarely the syndrome of HF is caused by constrictive pericarditis.

42.1.1 Medical treatment of HF

Since 1986, the treatment options in HF associated with reduced left ventricular ejection fraction (HFREF, and previously labelled as HF due to left ventricular systolic dysfunction [LVSD]), have improved with the introduction of hydralazine and nitrate[3] as the first treatment for HF (beyond heart transplantation) to have a positive impact on the prognosis of patients with HF. This was followed by a string of landmark studies investigating agents that altered the profile and outcomes of patients with HFREF, including angiotensin converting enzyme inhibitor (ACEi),[4–6] angiotensin receptor blockers (ARB),[7,8] beta-blockers (BB),[9–11] aldosterone antagonists (AA),[12,13] the addition of combined hydralazine and nitrates to the classic therapy in black patients with HFREF[14] and ivabradine.[15] More recently the combined agent LCZ696 (valsartan and Neprilysin Inhibitor, or ARNI) was shown to be superior to the ACEi enalapril in reducing the morbidity and mortality of patients with HFREF.[16] These interventions dramatically altered the poor prognosis of patients with HFREF.

In contrast, much more recently it has been recognised that almost 45% of the patients with symptoms of HF present with the syndrome in the absence of significant left ventricular (LV) systolic impairment, but with varying degrees of diastolic impairment, and were grouped, in the absence of primary valvular disease, as patients with 'heart failure and preserved left ventricular ejection fraction' (HFPEF). Although not mandatory for the definition of this group, these patients are frequently affected by systemic hypertension, LV hypertrophy, have diabetes mellitus, underlying ischaemic heart disease or suffer from being overweight. Not infrequently, these patients tend to be older than those presenting with HFREF and, probably due to the epidemiology of the older population, HFPEF tends to affect more women than men. Attempts at testing the same agents that proved to be effective in treating HFREF have thus far yielded either negative outcome such as the trials of ARB[17] or were rather inconclusive such as those with ACEi,[18] or BB.[19] More recently, in the TOPCAT trial, spironolactone at a low dose of 15 mg per day was used in patients with HFPEF; this demonstrated no survival benefit, but perhaps a trend towards reducing the risk of HF hospitalisation.[20] There is currently an ongoing trial of the ARNI LCZ696 in patients with HFPEF (the PARAGON trial).

42.2 The development of pacing in HF

42.2.1 Atrio-ventricular conduction delay

Patients with significant atrio-ventricular (AV) nodal conduction delay lose the coordinated timing of atrial filling, reducing diastolic filling time and cardiac output. Several studies suggested improvement of heart failure in such patients using dual chamber pacing programmed with short AV delay. Historically, the right ventricular (RV) pacing lead was normally positioned in the RV apex as this is easy to identify during implantation and usually results in a stable lead position, a factor that was particularly important before active fixation leads were available. However, pacing from the RV apex can significantly delay LV activation, impairing both systolic function and ventricular filling and resulting in the neurohormonal imbalances and remodelling seen in chronic HF.[21] Prolonged RV pacing can induce HF symptoms and worsening cardiac function even in patients without a previous history of HF[22] and in those with impaired ventricles, higher ventricular pacing burden correlates with death and HF hospitalisation rates.[23]

Given these detrimental effects many operators attempt to pace the right ventricle in a way which more closely involves or mimics the intrinsic conduction system of the heart. This 'selective site pacing' has produced inconsistent

evidence in favour of any particular pacing site,[24-26] probably explained in part by the greatly varying electrical effect of pacing from even relatively close sites around the RV septum,[27] such that it is the effect on ventricular depolarisation (as measured by QRS duration) rather than the anatomic pacing site *per se* that is important for LV function (Figure 42.1).

42.2.2 Intraventricular conduction delay

Disruption of the normal, rapid intraventricular activation occurs commonly in HF; most common is left bundle branch block (LBBB) which is associated with increased rates of sudden death and total mortality in HF patients, with an inverse relationship between the duration of the QRS complex and life expectancy in HFREF.[28] The consequences of LBBB include decreased mechanical efficiency, impaired LV filling and exacerbation of mitral regurgitation.[29] To overcome these factors, the concept of biventricular (BiV) pacing – simultaneous stimulation of both the LV free wall and the septum – led to trials of this therapy in Small cohorts of patients. LV pacing was initially achieved using surgical application of an epicardial pacing wire but with the development of an entirely transvenous approach and a demonstrated haemodynamic benefit of BiV pacing, larger series were undertaken to confirm the feasibility and safety of this technique.

42.2.3 Evidence for the benefit of cardiac resynchronisation therapy

A number of prospective randomised trials assessed the longer term effects of what became known as cardiac resynchronisation therapy (CRT). These have shown improvements in clinical measures of HF such as New York Heart Association (NYHA) class, 6-minute walk distance (6MW), quality of life scores and oxygen transport[30-33] and in echocardiographic parameters such as LV volumes and mitral regurgitation.[34-36] Unlike inotropic agents, BiV pacing can improve systolic function without increasing myocardial energy demands[37] leading to improvements in autonomic function and possibly a reduction in arrhythmias.[38,39] Given these effects, it might be expected that CRT alone (without implantable cardioverter defibrillator [ICD] functionality) could reduce deaths in patients with HF.

In the COMPANION trial of approximately 1500 patients with HF and prolonged QRS duration, a significant reduction in the primary end point (time to death or hospitalisation from any cause) was seen for BiV pacing both with (CRT-D) and without (CRT-P) ICD capability.[32] However, although the secondary end point of all-cause mortality was reduced by CRT-D, the reduction failed to reach significance in the CRT-P arm. In 2005, the landmark CARE-HF study was published and for the first time demonstrated that CRT-P alone could improve mortality

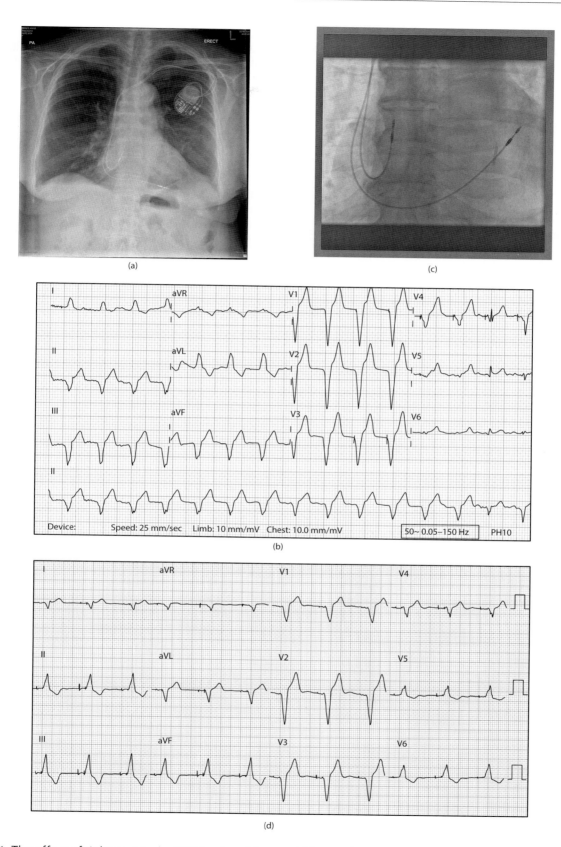

Figure 42.1 The effect of right ventricular (RV) lead position on QRS complexes. (a) Chest x-ray showing a dual chamber pacemaker with the RV lead positioned in the apex. (b) An electrocardiogram (ECG) showing paced complexes from the apex. (c) Fluoroscopic image of a dual chamber pacemaker with the RV lead attached to the high septum. (d) An ECG showing the corresponding paced complexes.

including a reduction in the risk of sudden cardiac death. After a mean follow up of 29 months, the mortality rates were 20% in the CRT-P group compared to 30% in the medical therapy group.[33]

42.2.4 CRT in patients with milder symptoms of HF

The majority of patient recruited into the early trials of CRT were classified as NYHA Class III or IV patients. Given the adverse prognostic implications of LBBB, whether induced by RV pacing or intrinsic conduction abnormalities, it has been suggested that BiV pacing may slow the progression of HF, even in less symptomatic stages. The MADIT-CRT trial recruited over 1800 patients in NYHA Class I or II (85% in the latter class) and randomised them to either ICD alone or CRT-D. The CRT group had a significant reduction in the primary end point of death or a major HF event, driven by the reduction in HF events.[40] Similarly, the RAFT trial compared ICD to CRT-D in almost 1800 patients with NYHA II or III followed up for over 3 years and demonstrated a reduction in death or hospitalisation for HF with CRT-D, implying that even in clinically milder forms of HF, earlier intervention with CRT appears to be of benefit.[41]

42.2.5 BiV pacing in atrial fibrillation

Early trials of CRT principally recruited patients in sinus rhythm; however, numerous trials have shown acute haemodynamic, symptomatic and remodelling benefits in patients with atrial fibrillation (AF) receiving CRT and a meta-analysis suggested that CRT is a beneficial therapy in this population.[42] The remodelling produced by CRT, including reductions in mitral regurgitation and left atrial dimensions may lead to a lower burden of arrhythmia in patients with paroxysmal AF or allow restoration

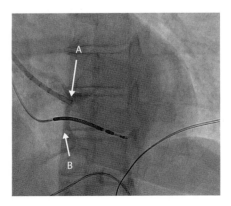

Figure 42.2 **(A)** Contrast injected through a coronary sinus (CS) guide catheter, positioned in the RA, aids location of the os of the CS. **(B)** An implantable cardioverter defibrillator (ICD) lead has already been implanted, showing approximate location of the tricuspid valve.

or maintenance of sinus rhythm.[43,44] The benefit of BiV pacing relies on a very high level of BiV pacing and some authors have advocated that AV nodal ablation should be mandatory.[45]

42.3 Implantation of a BiV pacing system

42.3.1 Pre-procedure

Preparation of the patient should include formal assessment of HF symptoms, analysis of an ECG and measurement of LV function. Assessment of other parameters, such as measures of dyssynchrony, including echocardiographic tissue Doppler imaging or strain, or CT or magnetic resonance imaging (MRI) for scar are of less certain relevance, as discussed below. Patients must of course be consented in the full knowledge of potential complications of device implantation. An example of the scope of potential complications of cardiac re-synchronisation comes from a recent publication describing experience from the Danish National registry.[46] These authors described real life experience in almost 6000 consecutive patients who underwent device implantation between May 2010 and April 2011. The findings demonstrated an incidence of complications ranging from 15% for new dual chamber ICD implantation through 16% for a new CRT-D implant and rising to 23% for a procedure involving an upgrade to a CRT-D device (Table 42.1).

42.3.2 Procedure

Sterile preparation of the patient in the catheter lab or operating theatre has been covered in Chapter 41 on pacing along with approaches to venous access. Given that patients in sinus rhythm will require three leads, it is uncommon for implantation to be achieved with cephalic venous access alone and expertise in multiple venous puncture, preferably extra-thoracic, is advantageous.

42.3.3 Which order for the leads?

In many centres it is customary to implant the RV lead first, although historically some operators have argued that in a patient with no indication for a device other than CRT (no bradycardic indication, nor a need for an ICD), that the LV lead should be attempted first. The reasoning was that in the case of failure of LV lead implantation, the procedure would be abandoned without having implanted, and therefore having to remove, redundant leads. With the advancement of implant techniques and equipment, failure of LV lead implantation is now relatively unusual via the transvenous route and, where this occurs, there is the possibility of implanting a LV lead using minimal access surgery.[47] One advantage of implanting the RV lead first is that, given most

Table 42.1 Overall complication rates

	All (5918)	New implant (4355)	Generator replacement (1136)	Upgrade/Lead revision (427)
Any complication	9.5%	9.9%	5.9%	14.8%
Any major complication	5.6%	5.8%	3.5%	8.4%
Any minor complication	4.2%	4.3%	2.6%	7.3%
Minor Complications				
Haematoma	2.3%	2.4%	1.8%	3.3%
Wound infection treated with antibiotics	1.2%	1.1%	1%	2.3%
Pneumothorax treated conservatively	0.7%	0.7%	0	1.6%
Lead dislodgement without re-intervention	0.2%	0.2%	0	0.2%
Major Complications of Pacing				
Lead related re-intervention	2.4%	2.8%	0.9%	3%
Infection	0.8%	0.6%	1.5%	1.9%
Local infection	0.4%	0.2%	0.7%	1%
Systemic infection/endocarditis	0.5%	0.3%	0.8%	0.9%
Pneumothorax requiring drainage	0.9%	1%	0	1.4%
Cardiac perforation	0.6%	0.8%	0	0.7%
No intervention	0.4%	0.4%	0	0.7%
Intervention	0.3%	0.4%	0	0
Pocket revision because of pain	0.4%	0.2%	0.8%	1.4%
Generator-lead interface problem with re-intervention	0.1%	0.1%	0.4%	0
Haematoma requiring re-intervention	0.2%	0.2%	0.1%	0
Other	0.3%	0.4%	0	0

Source: From Kirkfeldt RE et al., *Eur Heart J,* 35, 1186–1194, 2014.

patients have pre-existing conduction disease in the form of LBBB, if temporary stunning of the right bundle occurs during manipulation of the leads or guide catheters, urgent temporary pacing can easily be provided via the RV lead to overcome the resulting complete heart block.

Many operators move next to the implantation of the atrial lead (where indicated); however, implanting the LV lead as the second lead keeps a 'spare' route of access available for those cases where an intervention is required to achieve LV lead implantation or stability (see below), with the right atrial lead being implanted last.

42.3.4 LV lead implantation

In early studies of BiV pacing, LV free wall pacing was achieved through surgical attachment of an epicardial pacing lead. However, the coronary sinus (CS) tracks round the area of the mitral valve annulus and tributaries of the coronary venous system usually track to an appropriate location for LV pacing, thus providing a route from the right atrium (RA) to the epicardial surface of the lateral wall of the LV, via a completely transvenous route. Electrophysiology

studies usually involve cannulation of the CS and this has been performed for many decades – however, this is usually achieved from a femoral approach. In order to achieve CS access from a superior approach (left or right subclavian vein) LV lead delivery systems have evolved with differing shapes to allow for the anatomical variety.

To access the CS, the guide catheter is introduced into the RA and steered towards the tricuspid valve. It is often advantageous at this point to screen in left anterior oblique angulation to better align with the plane of the coronary venous system. Using a guidewire (e.g., a 0.035″ standard or hydrophilic wire) to probe from this point it may be possible to identify the CS. Where this is difficult, contrast injection in the RA can aid identification (Figure 42.2). To further aid location, the CS os is posterior to the tricuspid valve and passage of the guide catheter or guidewire through the valve will often cause ventricular ectopics. A slight withdrawal of the catheter or wire back into the RA, and a small amount of anticlockwise rotation will move it towards the CS os. Approaching from a posterior or inferior position may be more difficult due to the presence of the Eustachian ridge and variations in the size, fenestration and location of the

Thebesian valve can also impede access and advancement of catheters (Figure 42.3).[48] The range of CS guide catheters allows for the variation in right atrial size, position of the CS os and the angulation of the proximal coronary vein. Steerable LV catheters can be actively angulated to help cannulation. The use of inner catheters, or diagnostic coronary catheters as well as guidewires advance the sheath up the body of the CS (Figure 42.4).

It is helpful, where a patient who is likely to receive a CRT system is undergoing coronary angiography, for images to be acquired in the venous phase after contrast injection to highlight the location and anatomy of the CS (Figure 42.5). This should be obtained with the image intensifier at the same angulation used for CS intubation. In exceptionally difficult cases, coronary artery injection can be performed *during* the implantation procedure to allow CS access. In

patients with persistent left-sided superior vena cava (SVC) this is often found to drain into the CS – this is correspondingly often very dilated. Despite the easy access into the CS it can be very difficult to cannulate a side branch; achieving a position for the RV lead (pacing or ICD lead) may require individualised approaches between patients including guide catheters, shaped stylets and extra-long leads.[49]

Following cannulation of the CS, contrast injection is used to delineate the anatomy and identify potential target vessels for LV lead placement. It is recommended that an occlusive balloon is used due to the variable presence of valves in the coronary veins – given the retrograde flow of blood with respect to contrast injection, there may be coronary venous branches that are not visible on the initial injection (Figure 42.6). Additionally, in cases where lead displacement, intractable phrenic nerve stimulation (PNS) or non-response subsequently occur, the venogram images are invaluable in planning further intervention options.

Once the coronary venous anatomy is known, a target for LV lead placement can be chosen. As discussed below, a lateral or posterolateral position is generally preferred. A number of sub-selecting catheters now exist to allow direct intubation of smaller sub branches providing greater support for lead placement. Leads can be steered using stylets or angioplasty wires and the 'buddy wire' technique can help navigate or straighten tortuous vessels. In some cases, where it proves impossible to advance a lead sufficiently far down the vein, it is possible to steer a guidewire through small coronary venous branches and back into the main body of the CS allowing this to be snared retrogradely and secured to support lead advancement.[50] Where vessel calibre prevents LV lead placement, balloon venoplasty can be used to dilate veins and achieve lead positioning (Figure 42.7).

42.3.5 Choice of LV leads

Factors to consider when selecting an LV lead include its calibre, shape and the number and position of electrodes. Smaller

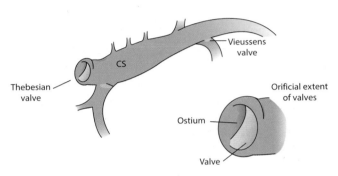

Valves in ventricular veins

Figure 42.3 Valves in the coronary venous system may impede left ventricular (LV) lead placement. (From Habib A. et al., *Europace*, 11, v15–v21, 2009.)

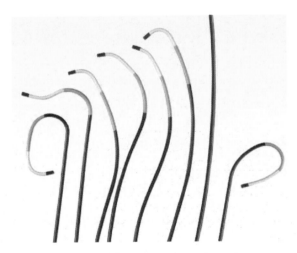

Figure 42.4 A range of CS guide catheters and inner (sub-selecting) catheters are now available to aid cannulation of the CS and delivery of pacing leads into sub-branches. (From http://www.medtronic.com/for-healthcare-professionals/products-therapies/cardiac-rhythm/cardiac-resynchronization-therapy-devices/fully-integrated-crt-implant-system/delivery-systems/#tab2.)

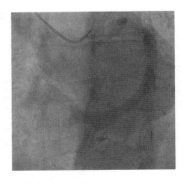

Figure 42.5 Venous phase picture from coronary angiogram. During injection of the left coronary arteries, a late acquisition has been obtained to show drainage of contrast through the coronary veins. This image was obtained in LAO 30°, to aid intubation of the CS performed in the same projection during cardiac resynchronisation therapy (CRT) implantation.

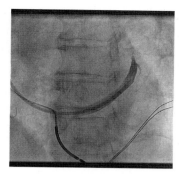

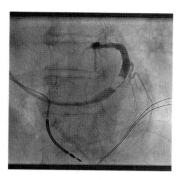

Figure 42.6 (Top) Contrast injection through the CS guide catheter alone reveals no obvious target for LV lead placement. (Bottom) An occlusive balloon has been used, revealing a lateral coronary vein which was used for LV lead placement.

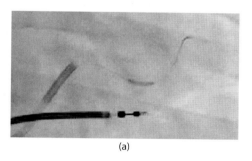

(a)

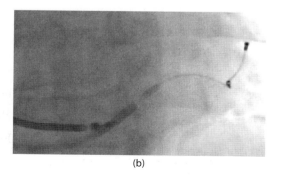

(b)

Figure 42.7 (a) Angioplasty balloon inflated within a narrowed part of a lateral coronary vein, through which it had not been possible to advance a pacing lead. (b) Following inflation, the LV lead is passed to a lateral position.

calibre leads are clearly required when the target vein is of small diameter but may be less stable. Stability is achieved by either 'wedging' the lead into the distal vessel, often aided by tines on the distal electrode, or by 'S' shaped, canted or coiled leads, designed to use the in-built lead shape to maintain position. Active fixation leads or the use of coronary artery stents to 'jail' the lead can also be used but may result in difficulties if the need for extraction arises at a later date.

In a parallel way to the development of simple pacing, the leads available for CRT have evolved to provide more variety in shape, smaller calibre delivery systems and increasing numbers of electrodes. Unipolar leads are now rarely used due to the limited options for programming; bipolar leads can be programmed with a variety of vectors including those involving the RV lead electrodes or RV coil in the case of an ICD lead. This development allowed a number of options with a single LV lead position – potentially improving response or overcoming PNS. The now widely available quadripolar leads give further options in programming and have been shown to reduce the incidence of PNS requiring an intervention.[51]

42.4 Alternative approaches to achieve CRT

42.4.1 Trans-septal approaches

Despite advances in LV lead systems and delivery systems, it may not be possible to achieve a satisfactory position for an LV lead in an area appropriate to provide CRT which is stable and does not cause PNS. Pacing from the endocardial surface allows more freedom of choice of position for the LV lead (unconstrained by coronary venous anatomy) and more closely mimics intrinsic LV myocardial activation (from the endocardial surface outwards). A number of methods have evolved to deliver endocardial pacing, most using an atrial trans-septal puncture to obtain access to the left heart from the RA and this approach appears to be feasible and increases clinical response.[52] The disadvantages of this approach include the increased complexity of the implant procedure, the need for lifelong anticoagulation, given the presence of lead in the systemic circulation and the as yet unknown chronic effects of a pacemaker lead crossing the mitral valve. This last issue is avoided in the alternative approach involving a ventricular trans-septal lead which has proved successful in a small series of patients[53] (Figure 42.8).

42.4.2 Epicardial leads

In cases where a transvenous approach does not result in an effective LV pacing site – whether due to venous access difficulties, poor thresholds or intractable PNS, a lack of a suitable coronary vein for an LV lead or indeed a lack of response after technically successful placement of a lead, surgical implantation of an epicardial lead, via mini-thoracotomy, remains an option. It is unclear whether this approach is associated with a tendency to more unpredictable lead

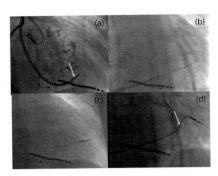

Figure 42.8 Fluoroscopic images from a trans-septal LV lead implantation. **(a)** Sheath opposed to interventricular septum. **(b)** Wire advanced into LV. Final position of LV lead in **(c)** right anterior oblique and **(d)** antero-posterior views. (From Betts T et al., *Circ Arrhythm Electrophysiol*, 7, 17–22, 2014.)

parameters, in particular rising thresholds, but small studies have suggested this is a successful approach and that this may be achieved using robotic assisted surgery.[54]

42.4.3 Dual RV pacing

Pacing simultaneously at two disparate sites within the RV might be expected to produce some improvement in depolarisation compared to single site pacing. In an acute study, dual site RV pacing improved both ejection fraction and measures of dys-synchrony, but was inferior to conventional BiV pacing.[55] Two randomised crossover studies of this technique produced conflicting results so this approach may be considered a possible alternative to conventional BiV pacing where anatomical or technical factors preclude this and surgical epicardial or trans-septal approaches are not felt to be viable.

42.4.4 'LV only' pacing

In LBBB, septal depolarisation may occur through intrinsic AV nodal conduction and therefore stimulation of the LV free wall alone, timed to coincide with intrinsic depolarisation through the AV node, can produce electrical synchronisation. Given that, in general, the implantation of fewer leads is associated with reduced procedure time, reduced complications and less infection risk , a number of studies investigated the potential for 'LV only' pacing with medium-term results suggesting significant improvement in symptoms, exercise capacity and echocardiographic remodelling similar to BiV pacing.[56,57] The DECREASE-HF trial compared simultaneous BiV pacing, sequential BiV (with V-V delays optimised acutely) and LV only pacing and showed significant reductions in LV dimensions for all groups, with no difference between the groups except for LV end-systolic diameter (LVESD), where simultaneous BiV was best.[35]

Whether chronic 'LV only' pacing is superior to standard BiV pacing may never be elucidated. The prospective randomised BELIEVE study showed a (non-inferior) response rate of 75% of patients in the LV group compared to 70% in the BiV group[58] but the wide 95% confidence intervals of the difference between these proportions mean that a sample size of 1100 patients would be needed in a theoretical trial to demonstrate an *advantage* of LV only pacing over BiV.

42.5 Non-responders

Whilst the advent of BiV pacing was a major advance in the treatment of patients with HFREF and intraventricular conduction abnormalities, it became increasingly clear that not all such patients benefit from CRT. This remains a major hurdle presently facing practitioners of CRT. The proportion of patients reported as 'non-responders' varies widely, due largely to a lack of consensus for the definition of response. Most early studies used either symptomatic or exercise improvement to assess response. With emerging evidence that CRT can result in significant ventricular remodelling and that this may herald improved prognosis, other authors have used echocardiographically defined end points to define response to therapy. On the whole, the latter, more stringent, definitions result in lower response rate.[59]

42.5.1 Improving response – LV pacing site

One factor determining response to CRT may be the site of LV pacing. In general it is agreed that a lateral position is preferable for the LV lead but the optimal position varies between patients.[60] Figure 42.9 shows how the anatomical location of coronary venous branches is normally described. Retrospective analyses of several large trials have shown that anatomy alone cannot be used to determine a specific area to target; however, apical positions seem to offer no advantage and may even be harmful.[61,62] The separation distance between the RV and LV leads may be another important factor.[63]

The properties of the tissue underlying the LV lead are also likely to be relevant: electrophysiological mapping studies have shown that the response to BiV pacing is adversely affected when the pacing lead is positioned in an area of slow myocardial conduction and that pacing away from these areas significantly increases haemodynamic response.[64] The presence of scar tissue at the area of LV pacing in CRT recipients, detected on MRI scanning, profoundly reduced their response rate[65] (Figure 42.10). Thus, the presence of viable myocardium in the left ventricle may also determine response.[66]

Several series have shown that the best response to CRT occurs in those in whom the LV pacing lead is situated over the site of latest mechanical contraction determined by, for example, Tissue Doppler Imaging or circumferential strain.[67] The randomised controlled TARGET study used echocardiographic speckle-tracking strain imaging to determine areas of the LV which were both free of scar and late contracting and demonstrated a significant increase in the proportion of patients responding to CRT.[68]

42.5.2 Improving response – Optimisation

The relative timing of atrial contraction within the ventricular cycle affects diastolic filling and therefore cardiac output.

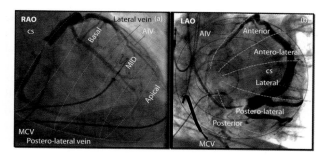

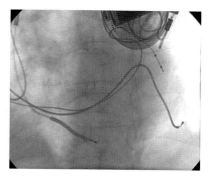

Figure 42.9 These fluoroscopic images show an occlusive venogram of the CS in (a) right anterior oblique (RAO) and (b) left anterior oblique (LAO). LV lead position is normally classified using the areas defined on these images. (From Singh JP et al., *Circulation*, 123, 1159–1166, 2011.)

Figure 42.11 Triventricular pacing. A fluoroscopic image of a triventricular system implant. Two pacing leads are seen in lateral branches of the coronary venous system.

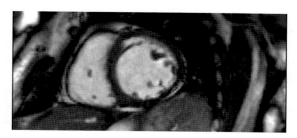

Figure 42.10 Posterolateral scar seen in cardiac magnetic resonance short-axis views of the left and right ventricles.

A wealth of studies have explored how AV timing affects the efficacy of BiV pacing and many suggested that AV optimisation can improve clinical outcomes in CRT.[69,70] However, these have tended to be small studies with relatively short follow-up; a larger prospective trial demonstrated no benefits for either remodelling or symptomatic measures.[71] Minimising intra-ventricular dyssynchrony may require an offset interval between the pacing stimuli from LV and RV leads (V-V interval) and there have been many studies examining the effects of V-V optimisation. Encouraging results from acute or small studies have again not been borne out in larger or longer term series.[72,73]

The findings of these trials should not perhaps be surprising when traditionally, and due to the obvious limitations in programming devices and performing echocardiography on moving patients, most optimisations are performed at rest. However, optimal settings may differ at rest versus during exercise[74] and, in a remodelling heart, they may evolve with time.[75] Devices with automatic algorithms to repeatedly assess and alter AV and V-V lead timings provide an attractive solution to this situation and will hopefully produce data to support the benefit of this function on mortality and HF hospitalisation.[76,77]

42.5.3 Improving response – Multisite and multipoint pacing

BiV pacing is limited by the variable position of scar and electrical properties of the myocardium, so it follows that stimulation at additional sites might further improve

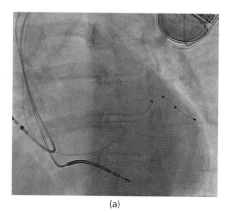

(a)

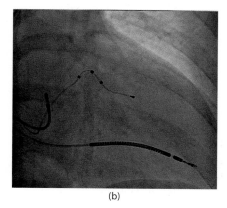

(b)

Figure 42.12 Final position of pacing leads in CRT-D implant: (a) LAO and (b) RAO projections.

response. Case series suggested that the addition of a third lead in either the RV or the LV could help patients who had deteriorated despite BiV pacing. Other reports confirmed the feasibility of triple-site ventricular pacing with both dual-RV and dual-LV configurations[78,79] but prospective studies have had variable outcomes (Figure 42.11).[80,81] Multipoint pacing – using multiple electrodes within the same pacing lead – is increasingly available due to the widespread use of quadripolar leads and may have benefits in both acute haemodynamic improvement and longer term outcomes (Figure 42.12).[82]

42.6 Predicting response

The early major trials of CRT recruited almost exclusively patients with prolonged QRS duration and, usually, LBBB and it was suggested that prolonged QRS duration may be necessary for improvement with CRT and that the degree of reduction in QRS width or baseline LBBB (as opposed to other patterns of conduction delay) might determine response.[83,84] However, even with similar surface ECGs, intraventricular conduction and depolarisation can be markedly varied. The interval known as QLV represents the time delay from the onset of the QRS complex on a surface ECG to the LV electrogram obtained from an LV lead within the coronary venous system (Figure 42.13).[85] This is easily obtained during device implantation and BiV pacing using an LV lead in a position with relatively long QLV has been proposed as a predictor of acute response to CRT, reverse remodelling[86] and of longer term outcome.[87]

42.6.1 Electrical delay or mechanical dyssynchrony?

As acquisition and processing of imaging techniques developed, the concept of mechanical dyssynchrony was introduced as a superior parameter to be addressed by resynchronisation. A number of studies looked at a vast array of echocardiographic parameters in this context, including

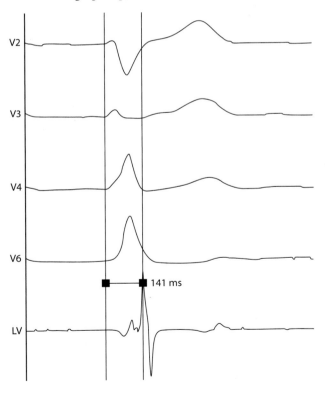

Figure 42.13 Measurement of Q-LV interval during CRT implantation. QLV is calculated by measuring the time from the onset of the QRS complex on a surface ECG to the peak deflection in the LV electrogram. (From Zanon F et al., *Circ Arrhythm Electrophysiol*, 7, 377–383, 2014.)

AV, inter-ventricular and intra-ventricular dyssynchrony and combinations of two or all three of these. AV dyssynchrony is most commonly assessed using trans-mitral pulsed-wave Doppler measurements in the four chamber apical view. The total duration of filling time can be expressed as a ratio of the corresponding cycle length (R-R interval) and AV dyssynchrony is defined to be present if ratio is <40%.[88]

Inter-ventricular dyssynchrony is said to be present when there is a delay of over 40 ms between the aortic and the pulmonary pre-ejection times. The latter are measured by comparing the delay between the onset of the QRS complex on the ECG and the onset of Doppler flow waves through the aortic and the pulmonary valves, respectively.[89] An alternative method relies on tissue Doppler imaging and compares the delay to peak S waves in the lateral wall of the right ventricle to that of the left ventricle.

Intra-ventricular dyssynchrony has attracted the largest variety of methods of assessment, with different groups using M mode, pulsed wave tissue Doppler or colour tissue Doppler imaging parameters to measure mechanical dyssynchrony and successfully correlate this with clinical response. Tissue Doppler imaging approaches have used 2, 4 or even 12 sampling points within the ventricles to create cut-off points or indices thought to represent significant dyssynchrony (Figure 42.14).[90,91] Using these parameters as the new 'gold standard' of dyssynchrony, there was found to be poor correlation between electrical (prolonged QRS duration) and mechanical dyssynchrony. For example, it was suggested that up to 30% of patients with widened QRS on an ECG did not have dyssynchrony and that 25%–30% of individuals with normal QRS width on ECG may have a form of concealed dyssynchrony.[92]

Based on largely retrospective studies, the PROSPECT trial was designed to assess the expected potential of a large variety of echocardiographic measures of dyssynchrony to predict clinical response to CRT implant.[93] Despite recruiting 498 patients in 53 centres, there was poor sensitivity and specificity of these methods for assessing dyssynchrony with respect to predicting clinical outcomes; this was partly due to a wide variation in the number of required measurements supplied by different centres and in their approaches to analysing the imaging data. Other potential approaches to assessing dys-synchrony include assessment during exercise, real-time 3D echocardiography and cardiac MRI. These techniques, along with further developments in echocardiographic imaging and processing require further prospective study to demonstrate their clinical benefit.

42.6.2 Patients with 'narrow' QRS complexes

Several small series suggested that CRT could be effective in patients without overt electrical delay – for example in right bundle branch block or narrow (normal) QRS complexes. However, more recently, attempts to extend the indication

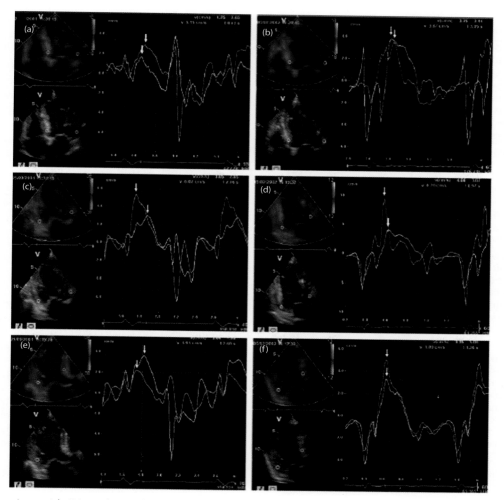

Figure 42.14 A patient with LV mechanical dyssynchrony in multiple segments before (a, c, e) and after (b, d, f) CRT. Before CRT, the apical four chamber view **(a)** shows only mild delay of basal lateral segment over the basal septal segment of 30 ms. In the apical two-chamber view **(c)**, there was severe delay in the basal inferior wall over the basal anterior wall of 130 ms which was significantly improved after CRT **(d)**. In the apical long-axis view **(e)**, the basal posterior wall was delayed over the basal anteroseptal wall of 90 ms which was totally abolished after CRT **(f)** The peak systolic velocity during the ejection phase in each view are shown by the arrows. (From Yu CM et al., *Heart*, 90, vi17–vi22, 2004.)

for CRT into those patients who may have demonstrable mechanical dyssynchrony with relatively narrow QRS complexes have suggested no benefit in the ReThinQ trial,[94] and even excess harm in the ECHO-CRT trial.[95]

42.7 Patient selection – current best practice

Before considering CRT in patients with HFREF, they should be optimally treated pharmacologically. The minimum requirement for the patient with HFREF is to be on an ACEi, a BB effective in HFREF and an aldosterone antagonist. The latter three agents should be given at either the maximum doses tried in randomised controlled trials or at the maximum doses tolerated by the individual patient. Patients who are in sinus rhythm and whose heart rate remains above 70–75 bpm despite beta-blockade (or in those who are genuinely intolerant of BB) should be considered for ivabradine to be added to their therapy. LCZ696 is expected to become an integral part of optimal therapy particularly those patients with severe left ventricular systolic impairment (left ventricular ejection fraction <35%). Such patients who remain symptomatic, and have evidence of severe LV systolic impairment, and electromechanical dyssynchrony – currently considered to be evidenced by a QRS complex of any morphology with a duration of at least 150 ms, or between 120 and 149 ms with LBBB – should be considered for CRT (although more recent evidence restricts the range to those with QRS duration >130 m sec). These criteria are reflected in current guidelines from the American Heart Association/American College of Cardiology, the European Society of Cardiology and the UK advisory body NICE (Figure 42.15).[96]

Accepting that the quality of the myocardium to be paced is an important consideration prior to implantation,

Recommendations	Class[a]	Level[b]
1) LBBS with QRS duration >150 ms. CRT is recommended in chronic HF patients and LYEF ≤35% who remain in NYHA functional class II, III and ambulatory IV despite adequate medical treatment[d]	I	A
2) LBBB with QRS duration 120–150 ms. CRT is recommended in chronic HF patients and LVEF ≤35% who remain in NYHA functional class II, III and ambulatory IV despite adequate medical treatment[d]	I	B
3) Non-LBBB with QRS duration >150 ms. CRT should be considered in chronic HF patients and LYEF ≤35% who remain in NYHA functional class II, III and ambulatory IV despite adequate medical treatment[d]	IIa	B
4) Non-LBBB with QRS duration 120–150 ms. CRT may be considered in chronic HF patients and LVEF ≤35% who remain in NYHA functional class II, III and ambulatory IV despite adequate medical treatment[d]	IIb	B
5) CRT in patients with chronic HF with QRS duration <120 ms is not recommended.	III	B

Figure 42.15 2013 European Society of Cardiology Guidelines on cardiac pacing and cardiac resynchronisation therapy. (From Brignole M et al., *Eur Heart J*, 34, 2281–2329, 2013).

if one knows that there is extensive LV scarring particularly of the lateral wall, then the plan for CRT may need to be altered, or even reconsidered. However, there is no mandate based on evidence to demand formal assessment of myocardial scarring (whether by MRI or echocardiography) prior to CRT implantation.

42.7.1 Who should not receive CRT?

Many patients with symptomatic HFREF have multiple comorbidities and many are older adults; it is good practice to carefully consider the potential adverse impact some of those comorbidities have on any patient's ability to derive meaningful benefit from CRT. The most important desired effects of CRT are the reduction of the patient's symptom burden, the reduction of the risk of HF hospitalisation, the improvement of the patient's functional class and also improvement of the patient's survival rate. Therefore, comorbidities that are too severe to permit the patient to become less breathless (such as end-stage

chronic obstructive pulmonary disease – COPD), or to become more mobile (such as disabling arthritis) or to be able to enjoy the survival benefit (e.g., life-limiting illnesses suh as cancers with poor prognosis or advanced CKD IV-V with no prospect of renal replacement therapy) should be carefully considered before offering a CRT device and raising the patient's hopes unrealistically. Patients with evident signs of end-stage HF such as cardiac cachexia, severe pulmonary hypertension or severe end-stage disease of other organs such as those with severe COPD, should normally not be subjected to these devices as their likelihood of deriving significant symptomatic improvement is low and their poor outlook could be worsened by the high incidence of potentially significant complications associated with the implantation of these devices.

References

1. Davies M et al. Prevalence of left-ventricular systolic dysfunction and heart failure in the Echocardiographic Heart of England Screening study: A population based study. *Lancet* 2001; 358(9280): 439–44.
2. Mehta PA et al. Improving survival in the 6 months after diagnosis of heart failure in the past decade: Population-based data from the UK. *Heart* 2009; 95(22): 1851–6.
3. Cohn JN et al. Effect of vasodilator therapy on mortality in chronic congestive heart failure. Results of a Veterans Administration Cooperative Study. *N Engl J Med* 1986; 314(24): 1547–52.
4. Effects of enalapril on mortality in severe congestive heart failure. Results of the Cooperative North Scandinavian Enalapril Survival Study (CONSENSUS). The CONSENSUS Trial Study Group. *N Engl J Med* 1987; 316(23): 1429–35.
5. Effect of captopril on mortality and morbidity in patients with left ventricular dysfunction after myocardial infarction. Results of the survival and ventricular enlargement trial. The SAVE Investigators. *N Engl J Med* 1992; 327(10): 669–77.
6. Effect of ramipril on mortality and morbidity of survivors of acute myocardial infarction with clinical evidence of heart failure. The Acute Infarction Ramipril Efficacy (AIRE) Study Investigators. *Lancet* 1993; 342(8875): 821–8.
7. Pfeffer MA et al. Effects of candesartan on mortality and morbidity in patients with chronic heart failure: The CHARM-Overall programme. *Lancet* 2003; 362(9386): 759–66.
8. Cohn JN, and Tognoni G. A randomized trial of the angiotensin-receptor blocker valsartan in chronic heart failure. *N Engl J Med* 2001; 345(23): 1667–75.
9. The Cardiac Insufficiency Bisoprolol Study II (CIBIS-II): A randomised trial. CIBIS II Study Group. *Lancet* 1999; 353(9146): 9–13.
10. Effect of metoprolol CR/XL in chronic heart failure: Metoprolol CR/XL Randomised Intervention Trial in Congestive Heart Failure (MERIT-HF). MERIT-HF Study Group. *Lancet* 1999; 353(9169): 2001–7.
11. Dargie HJ. Effect of carvedilol on outcome after myocardial infarction in patients with left-ventricular dysfunction: The CAPRICORN randomised trial. *Lancet* 2001; 357(9266): 1385–90.

12. Pitt B et al. The effect of spironolactone on morbidity and mortality in patients with severe heart failure. Randomized Aldactone Evaluation Study Investigators. *N Engl J Med* 1999; 341(10): 709–17.

13. Pitt B et al. Eplerenone, a selective aldosterone blocker, in patients with left ventricular dysfunction after myocardial infarction. *N Engl J Med* 2003; 348(14): 1309–21.

14. Taylor AL et al. Combination of isosorbide dinitrate and hydralazine in blacks with heart failure. *N Engl J Med* 2004; 351(20): 2049–57.

15. Swedberg K et al. Ivabradine and outcomes in chronic heart failure (SHIFT): A randomised placebo-controlled study. *Lancet* 2010; 376(9744): 875–85.

16. McMurray JJ et al. Angiotensin-neprilysin inhibition versus enalapril in heart failure. *N Engl J Med* 2014; 371(11): 993–1004.

17. Yusuf S et al. Effects of candesartan in patients with chronic heart failure and preserved left-ventricular ejection fraction: The CHARM-Preserved Trial. *Lancet* 2003; 362(9386): 777–81.

18. Cleland JG et al. The perindopril in elderly people with chronic heart failure (PEP-CHF) study. *Eur Heart J* 2006; 27(19): 2338–45.

19. Flather MD et al. Randomized trial to determine the effect of nebivolol on mortality and cardiovascular hospital admission in elderly patients with heart failure (SENIORS). *Eur Heart J* 2005; 26(3): 215–25.

20. Pitt B et al. Spironolactone for heart failure with preserved ejection fraction. *N Engl J Med* 2014; 370(15): 1383–92.

21. Moe GW, and Armstrong P. Pacing-induced heart failure: A model to study the mechanism of disease progression and novel therapy in heart failure. *Cardiovasc Res* 1999; 42(3): 591–9.

22. Lamas GA et al. Ventricular pacing or dual-chamber pacing for sinus-node dysfunction. *N Engl J Med* 2002; 346(24): 1854–62.

23. Wilkoff BL et al. Dual-chamber pacing or ventricular backup pacing in patients with an implantable defibrillator: The Dual Chamber and VVI Implantable Defibrillator (DAVID) Trial. *JAMA* 2002; 288(24): 3115–23.

24. Victor F et al. Optimal right ventricular pacing site in chronically implanted patients: A prospective randomized crossover comparison of apical and outflow tract pacing. *J Am Coll Cardiol* 1999; 33(2): 311–6.

25. Gold MR et al. The acute hemodynamic effects of right ventricular septal pacing in patients with congestive heart failure secondary to ischemic or idiopathic dilated cardiomyopathy. *Am J Cardiol* 1997; 79(5): 679–81.

26. Giudici MC et al. Comparison of right ventricular outflow tract and apical lead permanent pacing on cardiac output. *Am J Cardiol* 1997; 79(2): 209–12.

27. Schwaab B et al. Influence of right ventricular stimulation site on left ventricular function in atrial synchronous ventricular pacing. *J Am Coll Cardiol* 1999; 33(2): 317–23.

28. Gottipaty VK et al. The resting electrocardiogram provides a sensitive and inexpensive marker of prognosis in patients with chronic congestive heart failure. *J Am Coll Cardiol* 1999; 33(2): 145A.

29. Grines CL et al. Functional abnormalities in isolated left bundle branch block. The effect of interventricular asynchrony. *Circulation* 1989; 79(4): 845–53.

30. Cazeau S et al. Effects of multisite biventricular pacing in patients with heart failure and intraventricular conduction delay. *N Engl J Med* 2001; 344(12): 873–80.

31. Abraham WT et al. Cardiac resynchronization in chronic heart failure. *N Engl J Med* 2002; 346(24): 1845–53.

32. Bristow MR et al. Cardiac-resynchronization therapy with or without an implantable defibrillator in advanced chronic heart failure. *N Engl J Med* 2004; 350(21): 2140–50.

33. Cleland JG et al. The effect of cardiac resynchronization on morbidity and mortality in heart failure. *N Engl J Med* 2005; 352(15): 1539–49.

34. Saxon LA et al. Effects of long-term biventricular stimulation for resynchronization on echocardiographic measures of remodeling. *Circulation* 2002; 105(11): 1304–10.

35. Rao RK et al. Reduced ventricular volumes and improved systolic function with cardiac resynchronization therapy: A randomized trial comparing simultaneous biventricular pacing, sequential biventricular pacing, and left ventricular pacing. *Circulation* 2007; 115(16): 2136–44.

36. Yu CM et al. Left ventricular reverse remodeling but not clinical improvement predicts long-term survival after cardiac resynchronization therapy. *Circulation* 2005; 112(11): 1580–6.

37. Nelson GS et al. Left ventricular or biventricular pacing improves cardiac function at diminished energy cost in patients with dilated cardiomyopathy and left bundle-branch block. *Circulation* 2000; 102(25): 3053–9.

38. Hamdan MH et al. Biventricular pacing decreases sympathetic activity compared with right ventricular pacing in patients with depressed ejection fraction. *Circulation* 2000; 102(9): 1027–32.

39. Arya A et al. Effect of cardiac resynchronization therapy on the incidence of ventricular arrhythmias in patients with an implantable cardioverter-defibrillator. *Heart Rhythm* 2005; 2(10): 1094–8.

40. Moss AJ et al. Cardiac-resynchronization therapy for the prevention of heart-failure events. *N Engl J Med* 2009; 361(14): 1329–38.

41. Tang AS et al. Cardiac-resynchronization therapy for mild-to-moderate heart failure. *N Engl J Med* 2010; 363(25): 2385–95.

42. Upadhyay GA et al. Cardiac resynchronization in patients with atrial fibrillation: a meta-analysis of prospective cohort studies. *J Am Coll Cardiol* 2008; 52(15): 1239–46.

43. Kies P et al. Cardiac resynchronisation therapy in chronic atrial fibrillation: Impact on left atrial size and reversal to sinus rhythm. *Heart* 2006; 92(4): 490–4.

44. Gasparini M et al. Resumption of sinus rhythm in patients with heart failure and permanent atrial fibrillation undergoing cardiac resynchronization therapy: A longitudinal observational study. *Eur Heart J* 2010; 31(8): 976–83.

45. Gasparini M et al. Four-year efficacy of cardiac resynchronization therapy on exercise tolerance and disease progression: The importance of performing atrioventricular junction ablation in patients with atrial fibrillation. *J Am Coll Cardiol* 2006; 48(4): 734–43.

46. Kirkfeldt RE et al. Complications after cardiac implantable electronic device implantations: An analysis of a complete, nationwide cohort in Denmark. *Eur Heart J* 2014; 35(18): 1186–94.

47. Mair H et al. Surgical epicardial left ventricular lead versus coronary sinus lead placement in biventricular pacing. *Eur J Cardiothorac Surg* 2005; 27(2): 235–42.

48. Habib Aet al., The anatomy of the coronary sinus venous system for the cardiac electrophysiologist. *Europace* 2009; 11: v15–21.

49. Polewczyk A et al. Complications of permanent cardiac pacing in patients with persistent left superior vena cava. *Cardiol J* 2014; 21(2): 128–37.

50. Worley SJ et al. Goose neck snare for LV lead placement in difficult venous anatomy. *Pacing Clin Electrophysiol* 2009; 32(12): 1577–81.

51. Behar JM et al. Cardiac Resynchronization Therapy Delivered Via a Multipolar Left Ventricular Lead is Associated with Reduced Mortality and Elimination of Phrenic Nerve Stimulation: Long-Term Follow-Up from a Multicenter Registry. *J Cardiovasc Electrophysiol* 2015; 26(5): 540–6.

52. Morgan JM et al. ALternate Site Cardiac ResYNChronization (ALSYNC): A prospective and multicentre study of left ventricular endocardial pacing for cardiac resynchronization therapy. *Eur Heart J* 2016; 37(27): 2118–27.

53. Betts TR et al. Development of a technique for left ventricular endocardial pacing via puncture of the interventricular septum. *Circ Arrhythm Electrophysiol* 2014; 7(1): 17–22.

54. Garikipati NV et al. Comparison of endovascular versus epicardial lead placement for resynchronization therapy. *Am J Cardiol* 2014; 113(5): 840–4.

55. Lane RE et al. Comparison of temporary bifocal right ventricular pacing and biventricular pacing for heart failure: Evaluation by tissue Doppler imaging. *Heart* 2008; 94(1): 53–8.

56. Blanc JJ et al. Midterm benefits of left univentricular pacing in patients with congestive heart failure. *Circulation* 2004; 109(14): 1741–4.

57. Boriani G et al. A randomized double-blind comparison of biventricular versus left ventricular stimulation for cardiac resynchronization therapy: The Biventricular versus Left Univentricular Pacing with ICD Back-up in Heart Failure Patients (B-LEFT HF) trial. *Am Heart J* 2010; 159(6): 1052–8.

58. Gasparini M et al. Comparison of 1-year effects of left ventricular and biventricular pacing in patients with heart failure who have ventricular arrhythmias and left bundle-branch block: The Bi vs Left Ventricular Pacing: An International Pilot Evaluation on Heart Failure Patients with Ventricular Arrhythmias (BELIEVE) multicenter prospective randomized pilot study. *Am Heart J* 2006; 152(1): 155–7.

59. Birnie DH, and Tang AS. The problem of non-response to cardiac resynchronization therapy. *Curr Opin Cardiol* 2006; 21(1): 20–6.

60. Rossillo A et al. Impact of coronary sinus lead position on biventricular pacing: Mortality and echocardiographic evaluation during long-term follow-up. *J Cardiovasc Electrophysiol* 2004; 15(10): 1120–5.

61. Singh JP et al. Left ventricular lead position and clinical outcome in the multicenter automatic defibrillator implantation trial-cardiac resynchronization therapy (MADIT-CRT) trial. *Circulation* 2011; 123(11): 1159–66.

62. Thebault C et al. Sites of left and right ventricular lead implantation and response to cardiac resynchronization therapy observations from the REVERSE trial. *Eur Heart J* 2012; 33(21): 2662–71.

63. Heist EK et al. Radiographic left ventricular-right ventricular interlead distance predicts the acute hemodynamic response to cardiac resynchronization therapy. *Am J Cardiol* 2005; 96(5): 685–90.

64. Lambiase PD et al. Non-contact left ventricular endocardial mapping in cardiac resynchronisation therapy. *Heart* 2004; 90(1): 44–51.

65. Bleeker GB et al. Effect of posterolateral scar tissue on clinical and echocardiographic improvement after cardiac resynchronization therapy. *Circulation* 2006; 113(7): 969–76.

66. Ypenburg C et al. Impact of viability and scar tissue on response to cardiac resynchronization therapy in ischaemic heart failure patients. *Eur Heart J* 2007; 28(1): 33–41.

67. Becker M et al. Impact of left ventricular lead position on the efficacy of cardiac resynchronisation therapy: A two-dimensional strain echocardiography study. *Heart* 2007; 93(10): 1197–203.

68. Khan FZ et al. Targeted left ventricular lead placement to guide cardiac resynchronization therapy: The TARGET study: A randomized, controlled trial. *J Am Coll Cardiol* 2012; 59(17): 1509–18.

69. Meluzin J et al. A fast and simple echocardiographic method of determination of the optimal atrioventricular delay in patients after biventricular stimulation. *Pacing Clin Electrophysiol* 2004; 27(1): 58–64.

70. Sawhney NS et al. Randomized prospective trial of atrioventricular delay programming for cardiac resynchronization therapy. *Heart Rhythm* 2004; 1(5): 562–7.

71. Ellenbogen KA et al. Primary results from the SmartDelay determined AV optimization: A comparison to other AV delay methods used in cardiac resynchronization therapy (SMART-AV) trial: A randomized trial comparing empirical, echocardiography-guided, and algorithmic atrioventricular delay programming in cardiac resynchronization therapy. *Circulation* 2010; 122(25): 2660–8.

72. Perego GB et al. Simultaneous vs. sequential biventricular pacing in dilated cardiomyopathy: An acute hemodynamic study. *Eur J Heart Fail* 2003; 5(3): 305–13.

73. Boriani G et al. Randomized comparison of simultaneous biventricular stimulation versus optimized interventricular delay in cardiac resynchronization therapy. The Resynchronization for the HemodYnamic Treatment for Heart Failure Management II implantable cardioverter defibrillator (RHYTHM II ICD) study. *Am Heart J* 2006; 151(5): 1050–8.

74. Bordachar P et al. Echocardiographic assessment during exercise of heart failure patients with cardiac resynchronization therapy. *Am J Cardiol* 2006; 97(11): 16202–5.

75. O'Donnell D et al. Long-term variations in optimal programming of cardiac resynchronization therapy devices. *Pacing Clin Electrophysiol* 2005; 28(Suppl 1): S24–6.

76. Abraham WT et al. Rationale and design of a randomized clinical trial to assess the safety and efficacy of frequent optimization of cardiac resynchronization therapy: The Frequent Optimization Study Using the QuickOpt Method (FREEDOM) trial. *Am Heart J* 2010; 159(6): 944–8.

77. Brugada J et al. Automatic optimization of cardiac resynchronization therapy using SonR-rationale and design of the clinical trial of the SonRtip lead and automatic AV-VV optimization algorithm in the paradym RF SonR CRT-D (RESPOND CRT) trial. *Am Heart J* 2014; 167(4): 429–36.

78. Lenarczyk R et al. Triple-site biventricular pacing in patients undergoing cardiac resynchronization therapy: A feasibility study. *Europace* 2007; 9(9): 762–7.

79. Yoshida K et al. Effect of triangle ventricular pacing on haemodynamics and dyssynchrony in patients with advanced heart failure: A comparison study with conventional bi-ventricular pacing therapy. *Eur Heart J* 2007; 28(21): 2610–9.

80. Leclercq C et al. A randomized comparison of triple-site versus dual-site ventricular stimulation in patients with congestive heart failure. *J Am Coll Cardiol* 2008; 51(15): 1455–62.

81. Rogers DP et al. A randomized double-blind crossover trial of triventricular versus biventricular pacing in heart failure. *Eur J Heart Fail* 2012; 14(5): 495–505.

82. Pappone C et al. Improving cardiac resynchronization therapy response with multipoint left ventricular pacing: Twelve-month follow-up study. *Heart Rhythm* 2015; 12(6): 1250–8.

83. Auricchio A et al. Clinical efficacy of cardiac resynchronization therapy using left ventricular pacing in heart failure patients stratified by severity of ventricular conduction delay. *J Am Coll Cardiol* 2003; 42(12): 2109–16.

84. Zareba W et al. Effectiveness of Cardiac Resynchronization Therapy by QRS Morphology in the Multicenter Automatic Defibrillator Implantation Trial-Cardiac Resynchronization Therapy (MADIT-CRT). *Circulation* 2011; 123(10): 1061–72.

85. Zanon F et al. Determination of the longest intrapatient left ventricular electrical delay may predict acute hemodynamic improvement in patients after cardiac resynchronization therapy. Circ Arrhythm Electrophysiol 2014; 7: 377–83.

86. Gold MR et al. The relationship between ventricular electrical delay and left ventricular remodelling with cardiac resynchronization therapy. *Eur Heart J* 2011; 32(20): 2516–24.

87. Roubicek T et al. Left Ventricular Lead Electrical Delay Is a Predictor of Mortality in Patients With Cardiac Resynchronization Therapy. *Circ Arrhythm Electrophysiol* 2015; 8(5): 1113–21.

88. Cazeau S et al. Echocardiographic modeling of cardiac dyssynchrony before and during multisite stimulation: A prospective study. *Pacing Clin Electrophysiol* 2003; 26(1 Pt 2): 137–43.

89. Bax JJ et al. Echocardiographic evaluation of cardiac resynchronization therapy: Ready for routine clinical use? A critical appraisal. *J Am Coll Cardiol* 2004; 44(1): 1–9.

90. Serri K et al. Echocardiographic evaluation of cardiac dyssynchrony. *Can J Cardiol* 2007; 23(4): 303–10.

91. Yu CM et al. Echocardiographic evaluation of cardiac dyssynchrony for predicting a favourable response to cardiac resynchronisation therapy. *Heart* 2004; 90(Suppl VI): vi17–22.

92. Ghio S et al. Interventricular and intraventricular dyssynchrony are common in heart failure patients, regardless of QRS duration. *Eur Heart J* 2004; 25(7): 571–8.

93. Gold MR et al. Comparison of stimulation sites within left ventricular veins on the acute hemodynamic effects of cardiac resynchronization therapy. *Heart Rhythm* 2005; 2(4): 376–81.

94. Beshai JF et al. Cardiac-resynchronization therapy in heart failure with narrow QRS complexes. *N Engl J Med* 2007; 357(24): 2461–71.

95. Ruschitzka F et al. Cardiac-resynchronization therapy in heart failure with a narrow QRS complex. *N Engl J Med* 2013; 369(15): 1395–405.

96. Brignole M et al. 2013 ESC Guidelines on cardiac pacing and cardiac resynchronization therapy: The Task Force on cardiac pacing and resynchronization therapy of the European Society of Cardiology (ESC). Developed in collaboration with the European Heart Rhythm Association (EHRA). *Eur Heart J* 2013; 34: 2281–329.

43

Implantable cardioverter defibrillators

DOMINIC ROGERS, ABDALLAH AL-MOHAMMAD

43.1 Introduction

Sudden cardiac death (SCD) – a death occurring within a short period after the onset of symptoms and from a cardiac cause – is a major mode of mortality worldwide. It is the outcome in a not insignificant proportion of patients with the syndrome of heart failure (HF), especially those with heart failure with reduced left ventricular (LV) ejection fraction (HFREF).[1] SCD also occurs in patients with acute coronary syndrome,[2] the cardiomyopathies (hypertrophic cardiomyopathy [HCM], arrhythmogenic cardiomyopathy, dilated cardiomyopathy [DCM]), or channelopathies. In many cases, it occurs through the development of ventricular tachyarrhythmias (VA) including ventricular tachycardia (VT), ventricular flutter and ventricular fibrillation (VF). In these circumstances, early defibrillation (within minutes) can avert the death; however, the chance of surviving an out-of-hospital cardiac arrest is low (8%).[3] In 1998, cardiac arrest was reported in 450,000 cases in the United States.[4] The European annual incidence of reported out-of-hospital cardiac arrest varies between countries and ranges from 50 to 123 cases per 100,000 population.

43.2 The development of ICDs

Early attempts to abort VAs occurred in hospitals using externally applied defibrillators, first in the coronary care units and then in other hospital settings. This was principally utilised in the course of treating patients with acute ST elevation myocardial infarction (MI). A major advance in the field following the development of the external defibrillators was the first implantable cardioverter-defibrillator (ICD) by Mirowski et al. in 1980.[5] The first implant was bulky, implanted in the abdomen and required thoracic surgery to position a pericardial patch and the leads. Since then several developments have occurred including miniaturisation of the device, allowing implantation of the device in the subcutaneous tissue of the thoracic wall, the development of leads which can be implanted transvenously and increasingly sophisticated algorithms within the ICD including anti-tachycardia pacing (ATP) programmes that can terminate VAs without the need to deliver shocks (Figure 43.1).[6] Recently, subcutaneous ICD devices with no intravenous component were developed as an option for patients who have no pacing indications to reduce the risk from intravascular complications.

First device 1980
289 g, 150 cc, 22 mm

2010 device
72 g, 30.5 cc, 9.9 mm

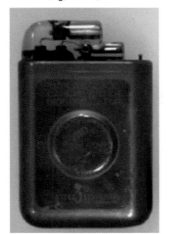
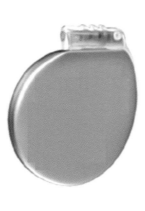

Figure 43.1 The evolution of ICDs: since the first implant, ICDs have become smaller, with longer battery life and greatly increased functionality. (From Gasparini M, Nisam S, *Europace*, 14, 8, 1087–93, 2012.)

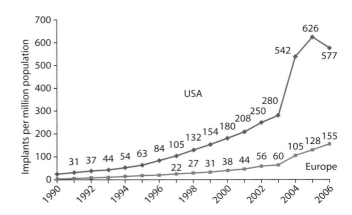

Figure 43.2 Graph showing annual ICD implant rates per million population since 1990 in the United States (blue line) and Europe (red line). (From John CA, Nisam S, *Europace*, 12, 1063–9, 2010.)

ICD implant rates vary from country to country. In 2006, Germany was ahead of the rest of Europe in the annual rate of ICD implantation per million population at 226 p/m, whilst the United Kingdom lagged behind at 69 p/m. The corresponding rate in the United States was 557 p/m. By 2008, the UK rate showed a minor improvement to 74 p/m; Germany's rate went up to 262 p/m becoming surpassed by the Italian rate at 310 p/m[7,8] (Figure 43.2).

43.3 Aetiologies associated with ICD implantation

There are a number of aetiologies associated with a risk of VA and therefore the potential for SCD; thus, the following conditions might provide an indication for ICD.

43.3.1 Heart failure (ischaemic and non-ischaemic cardiomyopathy)

Patients with severe LV systolic impairment have a markedly increased risk of SCD. The major causes of HF remain ischaemic heart disease (IHD) and systemic hypertension. Dilated or non-ischaemic cardiomyopathy (DCM) refers to patients with LV dilatation and systolic impairment not caused by IHD or valvular heart disease. It has many types and causes including genetically determined abnormalities of the myocardium. Reduced LV ejection fraction (LVEF) and widening of the QRS complexes in patients with HF are major defining factors of risk of death. The risk is modified by treatment for HFREF with angiotensin converting enzyme inhibitor (ACEI), beta blockers and aldosterone antagonists. Many of the major trials examining the role of ICDs in primary prevention included patients with HF; the sudden

cardiac death in heart failure trial (SCD-HeFT), for example, required patients to have either New York Heart Association (NYHA) Class II or III symptoms and showed a 23% relative risk reduction in death with an ICD.[9]

43.3.2 Hypertrophic cardiomyopathy

HCM is characterised by increased thickness of the myocardial wall without dilatation of the LV cavity in the absence of any trigger for the increased LV thickness. The prevalence is 0.2%, which is much higher than is seen in clinical practice. Whilst some patients with HCM are at an increased risk of arrhythmias and SCD, not everyone with the disease is at that risk, but SCD could be in those the first manifestation of the disease. SCD in patients with HCM may occur at any age, but in particular it occurs in adolescents and young adults before the age of 35 years. In addition to secondary prevention in patients who survived a cardiac arrest, primary prevention is determined in those with risk factors such as family medical history of SCD related to HCM, recurrent non-sustained VT on 24-hour electrocardiogram (ECG), hypotension or attenuated blood pressure response to exercise, those with unexplained recent syncope, massive LV hypertrophy (wall thickness $\geq$ 30 mm) or those with extensive or diffuse late gadolinium enhancement on contrast cardiac magnetic resonance (MR) imaging.[10] ICDs in these patients are effective in preventing SCD whether used for secondary prevention (where appropriate therapies occur at approximately 11%/year) or for primary prevention (4%/year).[11]

43.3.3 Arrhythmogenic cardiomyopathy

Arrhythmogenic cardiomyopathy (formerly known as ARVC) is a genetically determined disorder characterised by replacement of the myocardial cells by fibro-fatty tissue, which is rather patchy and leads to the formation of small aneurysmal dilatations that were initially thought to exclusively affect the right ventricle (RV), hence the acronym ARVC. However, it became recently evident that the left ventricle is affected in up to 50% of the cases. This disease can result in HF, thromboembolism and life-threatening VAs. ICDs are recommended in these patients following an aborted sudden death, syncope or decreased LV function.

43.3.4 Infiltrative/restrictive cardiomyopathies

Of the restrictive cardiomyopathies, amyloidosis is one of the more common and potentially devastating ones. Even though syncope and SCD are common eventual outcomes, the role of ICD in these is less clear than in dilated and HCM. This is because in patients with amyloidosis who have received an ICD have yet died suddenly, interrogation of their devices often shows electromechanical dissociation due to the infiltrative cardiomyopathy. It is, therefore, uncommon to recommend an ICD for patients with amyloidosis unless a syncopal attack could be clearly linked to a documented sustained ventricular arrhythmia.

Cardiac sarcoidosis is another type of infiltrative cardiomyopathy that could lead to reduced LV contraction, brady-arrhythmias and tachy-arrhythmias. Patients with cardiac sarcoidosis and high-grade atrioventricular conduction defects who require pacing may be recommended to have an ICD. Some recommend prophylactic ICD if the LVEF is significantly reduced. As a marker of the appropriateness of this recommendation in these patients, Schuller et al. have shown that over a 31-month follow up of their series of 83 patients with cardiac sarcoidosis who received an ICD as a primary prevention, 28% of them had an appropriate ICD therapy delivered.[12] However, it remains unclear as to whether an ICD is appropriate in patients with cardiac sarcoidosis in the absence of atrio-ventricular conduction problems and in whom the LVEF is either normal or mildly reduced. In those with mildly reduced LVEF, an ICD may be justified if VT is inducible on electrophysiological testing.

The treatment with ICD for patients with Fabry's disease falls within the indications used for patients with HCM. The latter is the usual phenotypical presentation of cardiac Fabry's disease. This disease was found in 0.5% of the screened European men and women with presumed HCM above the ages of 35 and 40 years, respectively.

43.3.5 Channelopathies

This is a group of inheritable electrical abnormalities that could lead to potentially lethal arrhythmias that occur in otherwise structurally normal hearts. They are labelled as cardiac channelopathies and include the congenital long QT syndromes, Brugada syndrome and catecholaminergic polymorphic VT (CPVT) and related disorders. These are thought to be responsible for a third of the cases of negative autopsy sudden unexplained deaths in the young.[13]

43.3.5.1 Long QT syndrome

Prolonged repolarisation of the heart makes the heart vulnerable to potentially serious ventricular arrhythmias usually triggered by a premature ventricular contraction falling within the extended period of vulnerability manifested by a prolonged corrected QT interval (typically > 480 ms) on the ECG. More than 10 genes have been identified as responsible for the non-syndromic long QT disorders. Three disorders are complex, as they involve problems beyond just those associated with a long QT interval. These have previously been labelled as Long QT4 (Ankyrin-B syndrome), Long QT7 (Anderson-Tawil syndrome) and Long QT8 (Timothy syndrome). The incidence of long QT syndrome probably exceeds 1 in 2500 persons. The arrhythmia caused is classically Torsades-de-Pointes and may be self-terminating, or present with syncope. The triggers include exertion (such as swimming), emotion and auditory stimuli. Occasionally, the arrhythmia can occur in the post-partum period. Up to 5% of the patients with this abnormality may develop fatal arrhythmia. Congenital long QT syndromes are responsible for 20% of the autopsy-negative cases of unexplained sudden death in the young and for 10% of the sudden infant death syndrome.[13,14]

43.3.5.2 Brugada syndrome

This is another channelopathy involving the sodium channel, resulting in a heritable arrhythmia that frequently occurs during sleep resulting in sudden death and more commonly in males. It is particularly prevalent in Southeast Asia and can be triggered by fever or a variety of medications. The abnormality on the ECG is coved ST segment elevation (>2 mm) followed by a negative T wave in the right chest leads (V_1–V_3) (Type 1 Brugada ECG). The genetics are complex and not as well characterised as those of the congenital long QT syndrome. The arrhythmia induced is normally polymorphic VT.[15]

43.3.5.3 CPVT

CPVT is a heritable arrhythmia triggered classically by heavy exertion such as swimming in a patient with QT interval <460 ms and presenting with syncope. The diagnosis should be particularly suspected in the presence of ectopy induced by exercise in someone whose resting ECG may not show more than sinus bradycardia. It should not be confused with the similar Long QT_1.

43.4 The evidence base for the use of ICDs

ICDs are indicated for both secondary prevention (i.e. in patients who have survived a resuscitated ventricular arrhythmia), or for primary prevention of SCD in patients without previous arrhythmic syncope or arrest who are judged to be at high risk of ventricular arrhythmia.

43.4.1 Secondary prevention

The strong consensus on the use of ICDs for secondary prevention is based on multiple randomised controlled trials (RCTs) that compared antiarrhythmic drugs with ICDs and in particular three important studies in the 1990s.[16–18] The Antiarrhythmics Versus Implantable Defibrillators (AVID) trial enrolled patients who had survived a cardiac arrest or with documented sustained ventricular arrhythmias, and they were randomised to receive amiodarone therapy or an ICD. The primary endpoint was all-cause mortality. There was a 28% reduction in all-cause mortality in the ICD group. Using a similar design, the Canadian Implantable Defibrillator Study (CIDS) trial showed a 20% reduction in mortality in the ICD group, compared with amiodarone treatment. The Cardiac Arrest Study Hamburg (CASH) trial randomised patients who survived an episode of cardiac arrest to either ICD or antiarrhythmic drug therapy, and showed a 23% mortality reduction in the ICD group.

Five points need to be made about these trials of secondary prevention. The first is that the reduction in mortality with ICD reached statistical significance only in the AVID trial. Second, this significance may be overestimated due to the threefold higher use of β-blockers in the ICD arm.[19] The third point is that whilst the reduction in the mortality in the ICD arm in both CIDS and CASH trials did not reach statistical significance, it pointed in the same direction as that of AVID, and was of a similar degree. The justification for lack of statistical significance in the CIDS trial was its early termination when AVID was published, and thus an insufficient number of patients was recruited. Similarly, the CASH study is of a small size which may explain the non-significance of the reduction in the mortality by ICD in this study. The fourth point is that a meta-analysis of these three trials by Connolly et al. demonstrated a statistically significant 28% reduction of all-cause mortality in patients randomised to ICD.[20] Finally, the combination of the results of AVID, the meta-analysis of the three trials and the trend demonstrated in the CIDS trial led to establishing ICDs place in the secondary prevention of SCD.

43.4.2 Primary prevention

More than 80% of ICDs are implanted for primary prevention. Amongst patients with reduced LVEF, those with high risk are identified by their HF functional class and an LVEF at or lower than 35%. This is based on a number of trials.

The Multicenter Automatic Defibrillator Implantation Trial (MADIT), enrolled patients with a prior MI, LVEF < 35%, non-sustained VT and inducible, non-suppressible VT on electrophysiological study (EPS). MADIT randomised the patients to amiodarone therapy or ICD and showed a 54% reduction in mortality in the ICD group.[21] There were some methodical issues with the trial, and some questioned its validity. However, publication of the Multicenter Unsustained Tachycardia Trial (MUSTT), which enrolled patients with coronary artery disease, LVEF < 40%, nonsustained VT and

inducible, nonsuppressible VT on EPS showed a survival benefit from ICD comparable with MADIT.[22]

Following on from those studies, the MADIT II trial randomised patients with a history of MI and an LVEF < 30% to either ICD therapy or no ICD; in this study, no EPS was needed. This showed a 31% reduction for mortality in patients treated with an ICD.[23] Both the MADIT II and the subsequent SCD-HeFT trials are randomised controlled trials which demonstrated absolute mortality reductions of 5%–7% over a period of 2–4 years in high-risk patients with ischaemic or non-ischaemic cardiomyopathy.[9] Further confirmation of benefit from primary prevention by ICD in patients with LV reduced contraction came from a meta-analysis published in 2004 showing a significant 25% reduction in all-cause mortality in the ICD-treated patients.[24]

Additional markers, although admittedly based on a more limited evidence-base, are used to identify subgroups of high-risk patients with less common diseases, including HCM and ion channelopathies.

In clinical practice, patients who receive ICDs are older and have more serious comorbid conditions than did the patients who were enrolled in the RCTs. There are retrospective analyses indicating that ICDs (excluding CRT-D) do not prolong life in identifiable subgroups of primary-prevention patients with extensive comorbidity. In addition, approximately 15–20 primary-prevention ICDs must be implanted in asymptomatic patients to save one life. Not surprisingly, patients vary in their willingness to accept implantation of ICDs to treat statistical risk. The NICE guidelines are summarised in Table 43.1.

43.5 ICDs in combination with CRT

The indications for an ICD significantly overlap those for biventricular pacing (cardiac resynchronisation therapy [CRT]). In the context of HF symptoms despite medical therapy, reduced LV ejection fraction and intraventricular conduction abnormalities (particularly left bundle branch block) are qualifying criteria for CRT. Both therapies are combined in a biventricular ICD (CRT-D). A meta-analysis of randomised controlled trials suggested that when compared to ICD alone, CRT-D improved rates of hospitalisation, and clinical outcomes including survival; this was though at a cost of higher procedural complications.[25] The addition of CRT to ICD function may also reduce the rates of both arrhythmias and inappropriate shocks, particularly if there is a clinical response to CRT.[26] Patients meeting the criteria for ICD who have heart failure with reduced left ventricular ejection fraction, who are likely to require at least a moderate percentage of pacing, will benefit from biventricular pacing and again should be offered CRT-D[27] – see Chapter 42.

43.6 Implantation
43.6.1 Pre-procedure

Preparation of the patient should include a full history to assess symptoms, analysis of an ECG and measurement of

Table 43.1 NICE guidelines (June 2014)

ICDs are recommended as options for:
A. Treating people with previous serious VAs, that is, people who, without a treatable cause:
  1. Have survived a cardiac arrest caused by either VT or VF or
  2. Have spontaneous sustained VT causing syncope or significant haemodynamic compromise or
  3. Have sustained VT without syncope or cardiac arrest, and also have an associated LVEF of 35% or less but their symptoms are no worse than NYHA class III.
B. Treating people who:
  1. Have a familial cardiac condition with a high risk of sudden death, such as long QT syndrome, hypertrophic cardiomyopathy, Brugada syndrome or arrhythmogenic cardiomyopathy or
  2. Have undergone surgical repair of congenital heart disease.

ICDs, CRT-D or CRT-P are recommended as treatment options for people with heart failure who have left ventricular dysfunction with an LVEF of 35% or less as specified as follows:

HFREF, LVEF ≤ 35%	NYHA I	NYHA II	NYHA III	NYHA IV
QRS < 120 ms	ICD	ICD	ICD	No device
QRS 120–149 ms no LBBB	ICD	ICD	ICD	CRT-P
QRS 120–149 ms + LBBB	ICD	CRT-P	CRT-P/CRT-D	CRT-P
QRS ≥ 150 ms no LBBB	CRT-D	CRT-D	CRT-P/CRT-D	CRT-P
QRS ≥ 150 ms + LBBB	CRT-D	CRT-D	CRT-P/CRT-D	CRT-P

Note: There is no indication for primary prevention using ICD in patients with IHD, outside the concomitant presence of significant left ventricular systolic impairment. In addition, it is advised that an ICD implantation is postponed for 40 days after the incidence of myocardial infarction (MI). Secondary prevention with ICD in patients with IHD is only indicated following MI if the VA occurred more than 48 hours after the onset of the MI and was not caused by a transient and correctable cause. Other international guidelines exist and vary somewhat from the stance proposed by NICE (which is informed by both clinical evidence appraisal and cost-effective analysis); most notably the ACC/AHA guidelines published in 2013. HFREF, heart failure with reduced ejection fraction; ICDs, implantable cardioverter-defibrillators; LVEF, left ventricular ejection fraction; NYHA, New York Heart Association.

LVEF. Assessment for CRT should be considered as discussed earlier and in Chapter 42. Where possible, patients should be counselled regarding ICD implantation at a date before the implantation. Psychological support can be of value before and after ICD implantation.[28] It is good practice to discuss the potential for deactivation of therapies, if a future situation rendered this appropriate. It is also useful to outline the role of remote patient monitoring at this stage and to discuss the implications for driving. In the United Kingdom, the current guidance for driving with an ICD is available through the Driver and Vehicle Licensing Agency (DVLA) website: www.gov.uk/guidance/cardiovascular-disorders-assessing-fitness-to-drive. The patient must provide informed consent following discussion of the potential complications, including infection, surgical issues such as bruising and bleeding, pneumothorax, cardiac perforation and tamponade as well as delayed complications such as lead displacement and inappropriate shocks.

43.6.2 Procedure

ICD implantation normally takes place in a catheter lab or operating theatre. The patient must be monitored and have external pads applied in case of the need for defibrillation or cardioversion during the procedure. Pre-procedural antibiotics are given, ideally within an hour before the start of the procedure. Strict aseptic technique is mandatory. Venous access for lead(s) – (the ICD lead ± other leads as necessary) can be via cephalic, axillary or subclavian veins and is covered in Chapter 41.

43.6.2.1 Choice of leads (dual vs. single coil)

Contemporary ICD leads are implanted transvenously and consist of pacing and sensing electrodes at their distal tip along with either one or two coils along their length, through which the defibrillation energy is delivered. In some systems, the ring electrode (the proximal pace/sense electrode) is integrated into the RV coil. This 'integrated bipole' reduces the risk of T-wave over-sensing but is more susceptible to external electromagnetic interference, and R-wave double counting.[29]

In early systems, the generator was not part of the shocking circuit and two coils were needed. Initial implants required epicardial placement of at least one part of this combination along with a separate coil positioned in the superior vena cava (SVC). The next iteration of ICD technology included two shock coils within a single lead, between which the electrical energy was delivered. Later, the generator became part of the circuit ('active can'), enabling a defibrillation vector between three points (the ICD generator body, a coil in the RV and a coil within the SVC). However, as extraction of ICD leads became increasingly necessary, whether for infection or lead malfunction, it became apparent that adhesions of the proximal coil to the SVC significantly increased the risks of vascular damage during extraction. Specialised coatings or 'backfilling' of the coils are designed to reduce ingrowth of tissue into the coils and may aid extraction,[30,31] but it is preferable to consider leads with a single coil. As energy outputs from ICDs have increased, the use of single-coil leads has substantially increased in the last decade and their use does not appear to be associated with more frequent failure of defibrillation or with increased mortality or worsening outcomes.[32]

The position of the distal part of the ICD lead (containing the anode and cathode electrodes – 'pace/sense' portion) needs to be stable with good parameters for both sensing and pacing threshold – however, compared to bradycardia pacing devices the former may be considered to be the more critical, particularly if the amount of expected pacing is minimal. Indeed, given that a significant proportion of patients receiving ICDs will have reduced LVEF, and therefore a high likelihood of HF symptoms, if a significant proportion of pacing is expected to take place, the patient should be considered for CRT-D (see Chapter 42). Similarly, if CRT is not required but some pacing is expected, positioning the lead at a septal site might reduce the potentially detrimental effects.[33] The position of the ICD shock coil(s) is also important – contact between the distal (RV) coil and myocardium is critical to deliver sufficient energy. This contact is normally reflected in the 'shock impedance' registered through the device.

43.6.2.2 Positioning the generator

The majority of operators favour the left-sided approach and therefore a device positioned in the left sub-clavicular area. However, where there is strong patient preference, where there has been previous device extraction (e.g. for infection) on the left-hand side or where left-sided approach may not be feasible due to venous access obstruction or extensive surgery or use of lines for renal replacement therapy or chemotherapeutic agents, a right-sided approach can be used. Defibrillation energy thresholds are likely to be higher in a right-sided device but with contemporary devices, providing higher energy outputs, this does not seem to be associated with higher mortality.[34]

In most cases, the generator is positioned subcutaneously but on top of the pectoral muscles. As an alternative, subpectoral pockets provide extra tissue coverage of the device – this can be very important in very thin patients, where erosion of the device presents a real risk. It is also preferred by some patients for cosmetic reasons. Where the cosmetic issue is greater, particularly in younger female patients, a sub-mammary position for the generator, or a sub-mammary or axillary approach with the sub-muscular position for the generator, have been used.[35]

43.6.2.3 MR compatibility

It has been conventionally held that patients with implantable devices cannot enter an MR scanner. However, an increasing proportion of the ICDs currently available have either been developed for use in, or retrospectively approved for, MR scanning. Most will have an 'MRI safe' or 'MRI conditional' mode to be programmed on for the duration of the scan. Consideration for MR scanning of a patient with an ICD depends on a number of factors including the device type, the number of leads, the presence of redundant leads and patient factors such as pacing dependence. Manufacturer-specific advice should be sought before scanning.[36]

43.6.2.4 Defibrillation testing

The implantation of an ICD was previously not considered complete until a threshold for defibrillation (the lowest amount of energy required to terminate VF) was determined. Thus, defibrillation threshold testing (DFT) was a routine part of an implant procedure. To avoid repeated inductions, it became more common to perform one or two VF inductions with attempted defibrillation at a specified energy (10 J or 15 J) below the maximum output of the implanted device; successful defibrillation demonstrated at these outputs suggested an adequate safety margin of defibrillation energy. Thus, rather than defining a defibrillation threshold, this is an assessment of the efficacy of defibrillation, termed defibrillation testing (DT). With a reduction in the amount of energy required to defibrillate, and the increased energy available from contemporary devices, it has been questioned how necessary the DT is as part of a procedure, particularly as the circumstances of a planned defibrillation in the cath lab (a supine, unmoving, often sedated patient with an electrically induced ventricular arrhythmia) differ so much from a 'real-life' spontaneous VF in the context of ischaemia, hypoperfusion and acidosis.

There are potential risks from DT, from both the arrhythmia induced and the shock applied; these include failure to defibrillate, prolonged hypotension, embolic events, myocardial injury and the risks associated with anaesthetic or deep sedation. These events are relatively rare but several studies have assessed the risks to patients in whom DT during routine ICD implant is not performed. The SIMPLE trial of 2500 patients, randomised to DT or not and followed up for a mean of 3.1 years showed no advantage for DT in terms of shock efficacy or arrhythmic death.[37] The NORDIC-ICD prospective randomised multicentre trial, assessed the average first shock efficacy for all VT and VF episodes occurring in over 1000 patients during a median follow-up of just under 2 years and showed that first shock efficacy was non-inferior in the patients undergoing ICD implantation without DT.[38] In summary, in standard, left-sided ICD implants with lead parameters within normal range, routine DT is not indicated. It should be noted that for right-sided implants (where the defibrillation vector is very different), it remains standard practice in most centres to perform a DT.

43.7 Programming

The programming of an ICD has several aims in addition to the obvious one of avoiding death from cardiac tachyarrhythmia. The ideal device will monitor and record VT episodes, delay therapies to the point of haemodynamic compromise, accurately discriminate SVTs and other non-lethal causes of tachyarrhythmias and have a variety of options to treat ventricular arrhythmias. ICD therapies consist of ATP (overdrive) and defibrillation shocks (Figure 43.3). There is a wealth of evidence that early delivery of defibrillation energy saves lives in cardiac arrest; however, the delivery of therapies in the absence of life-threatening rhythms, termed inappropriate shocks, increases morbidity including psychological stress and has been demonstrated to occur at very high rates in the past. In both MADIT II and the SCD-Heft trials, inappropriate shocks were associated with a more than doubling in the risk of death.

The programming of high-energy devices (ICDs including biventricular ICDs) has evolved significantly in the last decade due to emergence of trial data exploring outcomes following what might have been considered extreme programming values. The PAINFREE studies showed that ATP can be used to reduce the frequency of shocks in rapid VT with an associated improved quality of life and without an increase in mortality.[39] The PREPARE cohort study showed that employing a strategic programming, including longer detection periods before therapies are given can reduce shocks and other morbidities without an increase in adverse effects.[40] The prospective RELEVANT trial (in patients with a non-ischaemic aetiology undergoing an implant for primary prevention) showed that longer detection times reduced both appropriate and inappropriate shocks and reduced HF hospitalisation, again without increasing mortality.[41]

The important MADIT-RIT study prospectively enrolled 1500 patients with a primary-prevention indication who were then randomised to one of three programming configurations. These compared 'standard' programming to 'high-rate therapy' (treating only heart rates ≥200 beats per minute) or 'delayed therapy' (programmed with unusually long delays before therapies – 60-second delay before therapies for rates of 170–199 beats per minute and a 12-second delay at 200–249 beats per minute). During an average follow-up of 1.4 years, both high-rate therapy and delayed ICD therapy strategies were associated with reductions in a

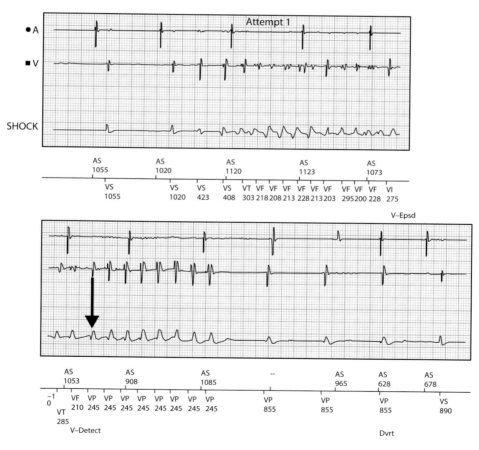

Figure 43.3 Printout from a dual chamber ICD showing successful termination of ventricular fibrillation (VF) using ATP. The three signal traces show the atrial (A), ventricular (V) and far-field (shock) electrograms, with the device markers below. In the top printout, onset of arrhythmia is seen following two ventricular ectopics. The atrial rate is unchanged but the ventricular cycle length is close to 200 ms (300 bpm). This rate, and the morphology on the shock electrogram suggests this is VF. In the bottom printout, the device delivers eight-paced beats at a faster rate (arrow), terminating the tachycardia which reverts to sinus rhythm, without the need for a shock.

first occurrence of inappropriate therapy and reductions in all-cause mortality. There were no significant differences in procedure-related adverse events amongst the three treatment groups (Figure 43.4).[42] Recently released guidance incorporates the findings from these recent trials of programming and provides manufacturer-specific programming advice.[43]

43.8 Home monitoring

The vast majority of ICD implanted have the facility for data to be transmitted from the device to a clinician via a monitor within the patient's home – usually this can be achieved wirelessly. This is often performed automatically with scheduled transmissions of information relayed at intervals via a secure server. Most systems will also use remote monitoring to advise clinicians of a potentially serious issue within the ICD systems such as suspected lead failure or battery depletion. Many series and trials have looked at the benefits of remote monitoring and have shown a reduction in inappropriate shocks and in some cases a reduction in mortality.[44]

43.9 Complications

Complications relating to ICD procedures include pocket haematoma, bleeding, lead displacement, pneumothorax, infection, tamponade and death. The first five of these constitute the majority of complications; in-hospital mortality is very low.[45] Published series of complication rates have varied, largely because there is no agreed definition of what constitutes a complication – important factors include whether or not a further intervention is required and how long surveillance follow-up for potential complications is continued.[46,47] Rates may well exceed 10% per year, but are greater for CRT devices than non-CRT ICDs and greater in dual-chamber than single-chamber systems.[48] Generator

replacement procedures carry a relatively high risk of complications, particularly if a further lead intervention is required.[49]

Implanted materials will always carry a risk of malfunction or damage, due to the stresses imposed within their operating environment. Although the absolute risk is low – a study of over 2000 leads followed for 3 years suggested an overall incidence for clinical lead failure of 1.3 per 100 lead-years – the implications for system failure with an ICD are obviously potentially serious.[50] Important ICD advisories involving both pulse generators and leads have occurred in recent years (Figure 43.5).[51,52] The Sprint Fidelis lead (Medtronic) is associated with a high rate of lead fracture which might involve both the pace-sense and high-voltage components – this defect resulted in inappropriate shocks and failure to deliver therapies. Distribution of the lead was stopped in 2007. The Riata lead (St. Jude Medical, St. Paul, MN) has a high incidence of externalisation of the components of the lead, particularly in the distal portion. Although the structural abnormalities have been associated with a loss of function, the incidence of externalisation, normally detected on fluoroscopy or incidental x-ray, is much higher than that of lead malfunction. Riata leads were recalled in 2011 but a high number of these leads remain implanted. The radiographic appearances do not reliably predict either current or future performance of the lead – therefore replacing or removing the lead remains a decision on a case by case basis.[53] Home monitoring has greatly helped manage patients with components under advisories such as these.

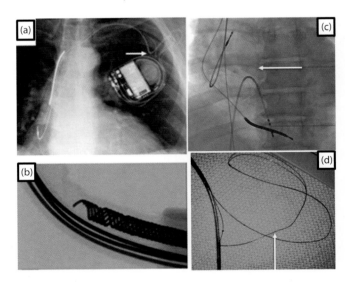

Figure 43.5 Left: Radiographs of Medtronic Sprint Fidelis lead showing **(a)** sharp angulation of lead associated with fracture of pace-sense coil to helix (arrow) and **(b)** coil fracture. Right: St. Jude Medical Riata lead with extensive externalisation of conduction cables (arrows) **(c)** image from fluoroscopic screening and **(d)** following extraction of the lead. (Adapted from Swerdlow C, Ellenbogen K, *Circulation*, 128, 2062–71, 2013 and Wazni O, Wilkoff B, *Nat Rev Cardiol*, 13, 221–9,2016.)

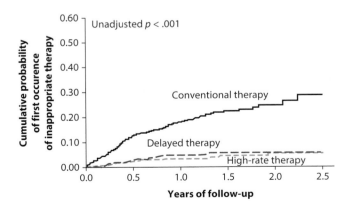

Figure 43.4 This Kaplan–Meier graph demonstrates the primary endpoint of the MADIT-RIT trial. Both the 'delayed' and 'high-rate' programming strategies resulted in a reduction in the occurrence of inappropriate ICD therapies. (From Moss AJ et al., *N Engl J Med*, 367, 2275—83, 2012.)

43.10 Extraction

Extraction of a device and the leads may be indicated to provide venous access (particularly in a patient undergoing upgrade of function of an implanted device – e.g. permanent pacemaker [PPM] to ICD), very rarely for venous obstructive symptoms or a lead defect that requires its removal, but most commonly for infection. Occasionally, an infective process may be limited to the skin and very superficial tissue – in those circumstances this can be treated with antibiotics. However, if there is any extension of infection into the generator pocket or around the leads, full extraction of the entire system is required. Extraction should take place at a specialist centre with cardiothoracic surgical back up; if possible these cases should be performed in a hybrid catheter lab or operating theatre.

A number of factors should be taken into account when assessing the complexity and risk of an extraction (and therefore when consenting the patient) – whether the system includes ICD leads and how many coils the lead(s) have; the total number of leads and dates of implant and whether the patient requires continuous pacing. Explanting the generator is normally straightforward. However, lead extraction is much more complex and a number of techniques and adjunctive tools have been developed for lead extraction (Figure 43.6).[54] This may be achieved by simple traction using a locking stylet, using sheaths with an active cutting tip or with a laser. Occasionally, an additional approach from the femoral vein is required to achieve complete extraction.

In patients with no or limited underlying rhythm (where the device was providing regular pacing), there is the adequate complexity as the patient will require a means of pacing during and after the extraction. If the indication was infection, it is probably undesirable to reimplant a permanent device at the same sitting. In this situation, a temporary/permanent, or externalised, pacing system can be employed. Similarly, where pacing is not required, but it is considered high risk to discharge leave a patient without an ICD, there is the option of a covering a period out of hospital using a wearable defibrillator.[55]

43.11 Subcutaneous ICDs

The subcutaneous ICD system consists of a pulse generator and lead, both positioned subcutaneously. This provides

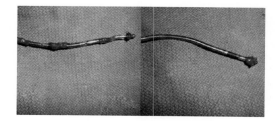

Figure 43.6 Extracted ICDs with adherent tissue to the distal coil (left) and distal pacing electrode (right). (From O to A et al., *Europace*, 13, 543–7, 2011.)

an entirely extravascular system and therefore reduces the infection and of other vascular complications such as venous occlusion. The use of this system is steadily increasing and where it was initially targeted at younger patients with rare causes of arrhythmia, such as the channelopathies, it is increasingly used in patients requiring primary prevention of SCD, including those with HF symptoms (Figure 43.7).[56] However, it does not provide pacing, so cannot protect against bradycardia, nor provide pacing as part of CRT.

The defibrillation energy required for therapies is higher than an intravascular system and the generator can is larger than contemporary ICDs. The lack of an endocardial contact electrode does not appear to be associated with decreased detection of ventricular arrhythmias but problems such as 'T wave oversensing' can lead to inappropriate therapies. Patients therefore undergo screening using specific ECG vectors obtained with the patient both supine and standing to assess the potential for inadequate sensing.

The implantation procedure requires different techniques to those used in conventional intravascular implants, and is generally performed under general anaesthetic although increasingly operators are using conscious sedation. Before preparing the skin and draping the patient, a mock generator and lead are often used, with fluoroscopic screening, to mark the positions for the pocket and lead incisions. The generator should be positioned within a pocket in a lateral, mid-axillary line, either subcutaneously or under the latissimus dorsi. A second incision is made in the xiphisternal area and the lead tunnelled subcutaneously from there to the pocket. The distal end of the lead is then tunnelled parallel to the sternum, normally to its left-hand side, either using a third incision, allowing pull-through of the lead or using an introducer sheath which is then removed by splitting ('two incision technique') (Figure 43.8). It is still standard practice to perform a defibrillation test as part of the implantation of a subcutaneous device.

43.12 Deactivation

There are two important issues here: the first is deactivation of the ICD device in patients whose comorbidities make further resuscitation from ventricular arrhythmia in-appropriate; and the second one is what to do when the lifetime of the device comes to an end in an elderly patient?

The advancing age of the patient is an issue because, in addition to the development of comorbidities (such as atrial fibrillation, congestive HF, chronic lung disease, cerebrovascular disease, diabetes and renal dysfunction) which may render the benefit of resuscitation by an ICD less desirable, those comorbidities along with older age predict worse survival in patients with these devices. Deactivation should be considered after careful consideration of the status of the patient at the time and after considering the opinion of the patient. The basis of deactivation has to be futility of further resuscitation attempts, or a decision that resuscitation is not wanted.

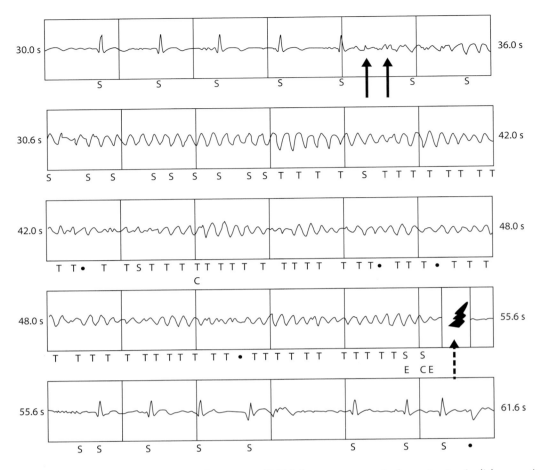

Figure 43.7 Printout from a subcutaneous ICD. The onset of VF follows two ventricular ectopics (solid arrows). The device charges and delivers a shock (dotted arrow) restoring normal rhythm.

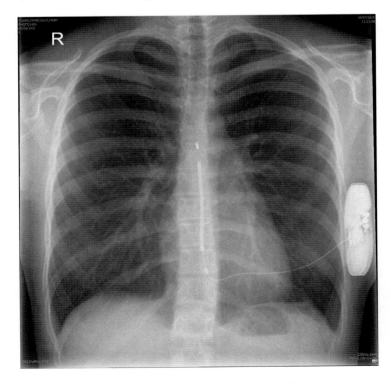

Figure 43.8 X-ray of a patient following implantation of a subcutaneous ICD. The generator is seen end-on.

The second problem is a significant one as many ICD implant procedures are device generator replacements. In some of these patients, it may no longer be appropriate for the patient to be provided with an ICD, either because their LV impairment has improved or because they had developed a contraindication to the procedure. Of course, if there had been evidence of ATP or shocks, it would be unethical to not provide them with a new device unless a total contraindication to the device had occurred. In these patients, replacing the generator by a pacing generator might be appropriate. A study by Kini et al. found that 26% of those coming to have the ICD generator replaced no longer fulfil the indication for an ICD. The latter were found to have significantly lower chance of receiving ICD therapies than the remaining patients.[57]

Goonewardene et al. reported their 20-year experience with ICDs implanted in octogenarians for planned end of generator replacement and found the median additional years of life after that to be 1.2; 50% of deceased patients died within the first year. Importantly, ICD therapies were not delivered in patients who had not had ICD interventions prior to the replacement.[58] On the other hand, however, there is evidence that 21.4% of the patients with ICD who had no prior appropriate therapy may still receive appropriate ICD intervention within the 3 years following generator replacement.[59]

43.13 Who should not get a device?

One has to remain sensible when selecting patients for this intervention and consider the rate of considerably serious complications of the implantation and the cost implications of the implantation and the follow up. National and international guidelines agree on the basic principles but may differ in the level of recommendation for certain groups.

It is universally accepted that in patients with severe symptoms of HF (NYHA Class IV), ICD therapy is not appropriate as it offers no improvement in quality of life in this group who have the highest chance of death from pump failure (rather than arrhythmia). Similarly, it would normally not be appropriate to implant ICDs in patients with evident signs of end-stage HF such as cardiac cachexia, patients with severe end-stage disease of other organs such as those with severe COPD, advanced chronic kidney disease (CKD) IV–V with no prospect of renal replacement therapy or patients with advanced or incurable malignant disease.

The patient's age should also be taken into account: a meta-analysis by Santangeli et al. had reported on pooled data of the DEFINITE, SCD-HeFT and MADIT trials, but was unable to demonstrate significant survival benefit of the ICD in the elderly.[60] A different meta-analysis pooled individual patient data from all three secondary prevention trials comparing ICD to amiodarone (AVID, CIDS and CASH) and concluded that ICD therapy did not seem to offer a survival benefit in secondary prevention patients ≥75 years of age.[61]

References

1. Uretsky BF, and Sheahan RG. Primary prevention of sudden cardiac death in heart failure: Will the solution be shocking? *J Am Coll Cardiol* 1997; 30(7): 1589–97.
2. Myerburg RJ, and Junttila MJ. Sudden cardiac death caused by coronary heart disease. *Circulation* 2012; 125(8): 1043–52.
3. de Vreede-Swagemakers JJ et al. Out-of-hospital cardiac arrest in the 1990's: A population-based study in the Maastricht area on incidence, characteristics and survival. *J Am Coll Cardiol* 1997; 30(6): 1500–5.
4. Lloyd-Jones D et al. Heart disease and stroke statistics – 2010 update: A report from the American Heart Association. *Circulation* 2010; 121(7): e46–215.
5. Mirowski M et al. Termination of malignant ventricular arrhythmias with an implanted automatic defibrillator in human beings. *N Engl J Med* 1980; 303(6): 322–4.
6. Gasparini M, and Nisam S. Implantable cardioverter defibrillator harm? *Europace* 2012; 14(8): 1087–93.
7. Lubinski A et al. Determinants of geographic variations in implantation of cardiac defibrillators in the European Society of Cardiology member countries – data from the European Heart Rhythm Association White Book. *Europace* 2011; 13(5): 654–62.
8. John Camm A, and Nisam S. European utilization of the implantable defibrillator: Has 10 years changed the 'enigma'? *Europace* 2010; 12: 1063–9.
9. Bardy GH et al. Amiodarone or an implantable cardioverter-defibrillator for congestive heart failure. *N Engl J Med* 2005; 352(3): 225–37.
10. Chan RH et al. Prognostic value of quantitative contrast-enhanced cardiovascular magnetic resonance for the evaluation of sudden death risk in patients with hypertrophic cardiomyopathy. *Circulation* 2014; 130(6): 484–95.
11. Maron BJ. Contemporary insights and strategies for risk stratification and prevention of sudden death in hypertrophic cardiomyopathy. *Circulation* 2010; 121(3): 445–56.
12. Schuller JL et al. Implantable cardioverter defibrillator therapy in patients with cardiac sarcoidosis. *J Cardiovasc Electrophysiol* 2012; 23(9): 925–9.
13. Tester DJ et al. Cardiac channel molecular autopsy: Insights from 173 consecutive cases of autopsy-negative sudden unexplained death referred for postmortem genetic testing. *Mayo Clin Proc* 2012; 87(6): 524–39.
14. Arnestad M et al. Prevalence of long-QT syndrome gene variants in sudden infant death syndrome. *Circulation* 2007; 115(3): 361–7.
15. Ruan Y et al. Sodium channel mutations and arrhythmias. *Nat Rev Cardiol* 2009; 6(5): 337–48.
16. A comparison of antiarrhythmic-drug therapy with implantable defibrillators in patients resuscitated from near-fatal ventricular arrhythmias. The Antiarrhythmics versus Implantable Defibrillators (AVID) Investigators. *N Engl J Med* 1997; 337(22): 1576–83.
17. Connolly SJ et al. Canadian implantable defibrillator study (CIDS): A randomized trial of the implantable cardioverter defibrillator against amiodarone. *Circulation* 2000; 101(11): 1297–302.
18. Kuck KH et al. Randomized comparison of antiarrhythmic drug therapy with implantable defibrillators in patients

resuscitated from cardiac arrest: The Cardiac Arrest Study Hamburg (CASH). *Circulation* 2000; 102(7): 748–54.

19. Tung R et al. A critical appraisal of implantable cardioverter-defibrillator therapy for the prevention of sudden cardiac death. *J Am Coll Cardiol* 2008; 52(14): 1111–21.

20. Connolly SJ et al. Meta-analysis of the implantable cardioverter defibrillator secondary prevention trials. AVID, CASH and CIDS studies. Antiarrhythmics vs Implantable Defibrillator study. Cardiac Arrest Study Hamburg. Canadian Implantable Defibrillator Study. *Eur Heart J* 2000; 21(24): 2071–8.

21. Moss AJ et al. Improved survival with an implanted defibrillator in patients with coronary disease at high risk for ventricular arrhythmia. Multicenter Automatic Defibrillator Implantation Trial Investigators. *N Engl J Med* 1996; 335(26): 1933–40.

22. Buxton AE et al. A randomized study of the prevention of sudden death in patients with coronary artery disease. Multicenter Unsustained Tachycardia Trial Investigators. *N Engl J Med* 1999; 341(25): 1882–90.

23. Moss AJ et al. Prophylactic implantation of a defibrillator in patients with myocardial infarction and reduced ejection fraction. *N Engl J Med* 2002; 346(12): 877–83.

24. Nanthakumar K et al. Prophylactic implantable cardioverter-defibrillator therapy in patients with left ventricular systolic dysfunction: A pooled analysis of 10 primary prevention trials. *J Am Coll Cardiol* 2004; 44(11): 2166–72.

25. Chen S et al. The efficacy and safety of cardiac resynchronization therapy combined with implantable cardioverter defibrillator for heart failure: A meta-analysis of 5674 patients. *Europace* 2013; 15(7): 992–1001.

26. Thijssen J et al. Implantable cardioverter-defibrillator patients who are upgraded and respond to cardiac resynchronization therapy have less ventricular arrhythmias compared with nonresponders. *J Am Coll Cardiol* 2011; 58(22): 2282–9.

27. Curtis AB et al. Biventricular pacing for atrioventricular block and systolic dysfunction. *N Engl J Med* 2013; 368(17): 1585–93.

28. Dunbar SB et al. Effect of a psychoeducational intervention on depression, anxiety, and health resource use in implantable cardioverter defibrillator patients. *Pacing Clin Electrophysiol* 2009; 32(10): 1259–71.

29. Powell BD et al. Noise, artifact, and oversensing related inappropriate ICD shock evaluation: ALTITUDE noise study. *Pacing Clin Electrophysiol* 2012; 35(7): 863–9.

30. Hackler JW et al. Effectiveness of implantable cardioverter-defibrillator lead coil treatments in facilitating ease of extraction. *Heart Rhythm* 2010; 7(7): 890–7.

31. Kohut AR et al. Percutaneous extraction of ePTFE-coated ICD leads: A single center comparative experience. *Pacing Clin Electrophysiol* 2013; 36(4): 444–50.

32. Aoukar PS et al. No benefit of a dual coil over a single coil ICD lead: Evidence from the Sudden Cardiac Death in Heart Failure Trial. *Heart Rhythm* 2013; 10(7): 970–6.

33. Mond HG, and Gammage MD. Selective site pacing: The future of cardiac pacing? *Pacing Clin Electrophysiol* 2004; 27(6 Pt 2): 835–6.

34. Gold MR et al. Comparison of defibrillation efficacy and survival associated with right versus left pectoral placement for implantable defibrillators. *Am J Cardiol* 2007; 100(2): 243–6.

35. Obeyesekere MN et al. Long-term performance of submammary defibrillator system. *Europace* 2010; 12(9): 1239–44.

36. van der Graaf AW et al. MRI and cardiac implantable electronic devices; current status and required safety conditions. *Neth Heart J* 2014; 22(6): 269–76.

37. Healey JS et al. Cardioverter defibrillator implantation without induction of ventricular fibrillation: A single-blind, non-inferiority, randomised controlled trial (SIMPLE). *Lancet* 2015; 385(9970): 785–91.

38. Bansch D et al. Intra-operative defibrillation testing and clinical shock efficacy in patients with implantable cardioverter-defibrillators: The NORDIC ICD randomized clinical trial. *Eur Heart J* 2015; 36(37): 2500–7.

39. Wathen MS et al. Prospective randomized multicenter trial of empirical antitachycardia pacing versus shocks for spontaneous rapid ventricular tachycardia in patients with implantable cardioverter-defibrillators: Pacing Fast Ventricular Tachycardia Reduces Shock Therapies (PainFREE Rx II) trial results. *Circulation* 2004;110(17): 2591–6.

40. Wilkoff BL et al. Strategic programming of detection and therapy parameters in implantable cardioverter-defibrillators reduces shocks in primary prevention patients: Results from the PREPARE (Primary Prevention Parameters Evaluation) study. *J Am Coll Cardiol* 2008; 52(7): 541–50.

41. Gasparini M et al. A simplified biventricular defibrillator with fixed long detection intervals reduces implantable cardioverter defibrillator (ICD) interventions and heart failure hospitalizations in patients with non-ischaemic cardiomyopathy implanted for primary prevention: The RELEVANT [Role of long dEtection window programming in patients with LEft VentriculAr dysfunction, Non-ischemic eTiology in primary prevention treated with a biventricular ICD] study. *Eur Heart J* 2009; 30(22): 2758–67.

42. Moss AJ et al. Reduction in inappropriate therapy and mortality through ICD programming. *N Engl J Med* 2012; 367(24): 2275–83.

43. Wilkoff BL et al. 2015 HRS/EHRA/APHRS/SOLAECE expert consensus statement on optimal implantable cardioverter-defibrillator programming and testing. *Heart Rhythm* 2016; 13(2): e50–86.

44. Parthiban N et al. Remote monitoring of implantable cardioverter-defibrillators: A systematic review and meta-analysis of clinical outcomes. *J Am Coll Cardiol* 2015; 65(24): 2591–600.

45. van Rees JB et al. Implantation-related complications of implantable cardioverter-defibrillators and cardiac resynchronization therapy devices: A systematic review of randomized clinical trials. *J Am Coll Cardiol* 2011; 58(10): 995–1000.

46. Pakarinen S et al. Short-term implantation-related complications of cardiac rhythm management device therapy: A retrospective single-centre 1-year survey. *Europace* 2010; 12(1): 103–8.

47. Duray GZ et al. Complications leading to surgical revision in implantable cardioverter defibrillator patients: Comparison of patients with single-chamber, dual-chamber, and biventricular devices. *Europace* 2009; 11(3): 297–302.

48. Kirkfeldt RE et al. Complications after cardiac implantable electronic device implantations: An analysis of a complete, nationwide cohort in Denmark. *Eur Heart J* 2014; 35(18): 1186–94.

49. Poole JE et al. Complication rates associated with pacemaker or implantable cardioverter-defibrillator generator replacements and upgrade procedures: Results from the REPLACE registry. *Circulation* 2010; 122(16): 1553–61.

50. Borleffs CJ et al. Risk of failure of transvenous implantable cardioverter-defibrillator leads. *Circ Arrhythm Electrophysiol* 2009; 2(4): 411–6.

51. Swerdlow C, and Ellenbogen K. Implantable cardioverter-defibrillator leads: Design, diagnostics, and management. *Circulation* 2013; 128: 2062–71.

52. Wazni O, and Wilkoff B. Considerations for cardiac device lead extraction. *Nat Rev Cardiol* 2016; 13: 221–9.

53. Kubala M et al. Progressive decrease in amplitude of intracardiac ventricular electrogram and higher left ventricular ejection fraction are associated with conductors' externalization in Riata leads. *Europace* 2013; 15(8): 1198–204.

54. O to A et al. Percutaneous extraction of cardiac pacemaker and implantable cardioverter defibrillator leads with evolution mechanical dilator sheath: A single-centre experience. *Europace* 2011; 13: 543–7.

55. Healy CA, and Carrillo RG. Wearable cardioverter-defibrillator for prevention of sudden cardiac death after infected implantable cardioverter-defibrillator removal: A cost-effectiveness evaluation. *Heart Rhythm* 2015; 12(7): 1565–73.

56. Lambiase PD et al. Worldwide experience with a totally subcutaneous implantable defibrillator: Early results from the EFFORTLESS S-ICD Registry. *Eur Heart J* 2014; 35(25): 1657–65.

57. Kini V et al. Appropriateness of primary prevention implantable cardioverter-defibrillators at the time of generator replacement: Are indications still met? *J Am Coll Cardiol* 2014; 63(22): 2388–94.

58. Goonewardene M et al. Cardioverter-defibrillator implantation and generator replacement in the octogenarian. *Europace* 2015; 17(3): 409–16.

59. Inada K et al. Mortality and safety of catheter ablation for antiarrhythmic drug-refractory ventricular tachycardia in elderly patients with coronary artery disease. *Heart Rhythm* 2010; 7(6): 740–4.

60. Santangeli P et al. Meta-analysis: Age and effectiveness of prophylactic implantable cardioverter-defibrillators. *Ann Intern Med* 2010; 153(9): 592–9.

61. Healey JS et al. Role of the implantable defibrillator among elderly patients with a history of life-threatening ventricular arrhythmias. *Eur Heart J* 2007; 28(14): 1746–9.

Miscellany

The role of the interventionalist in peripheral vascular interventions

ALFRED HURLEY, JAYANT KHITHA, TANVIR BAJWA

44.1 Introduction

Over time, many advances have been made in the management of peripheral artery disease (PAD), a disorder of the non-cardiac vasculature. Increasingly, interventional cardiologists are able to manage many of these disorders using a percutaneous approach. In many practices, >40% of pathology can include PAD management. This chapter discusses the various options for management, including the research data that help guide clinical decision-making.

44.2 Epidemiology, pathophysiology and diagnosis

The prevalence of PAD is 5.9% in people >40 years of age, according to National Health and Nutrition Examination Survey data. PAD has shown increased all-cause mortality compared to patients with matched Framingham risk scores. This is most likely due to undertreated co-morbidities. Unfortunately, only 33% of PAD patients are treated, despite 50%–60% having concomitant cerebrovascular or coronary disease.[1,2]

PAD can be categorised as an atherosclerotic occlusive disease (about 90% of cases), non-atherosclerotic occlusive disease (i.e. fibromuscular dysplasia, vasculitis, trauma, embolism) or aneurysmal. Amongst the risk factors, a relationship has been observed between the development of PAD and both diabetes and pack-year of smoking.[3]

PAD has a wide range of clinical presentations, including intermittent claudication,[3] critical limb ischaemia (CLI) (rest pain, non-healing ulcer, and dry gangrene), acute limb ischaemia, vague leg discomfort or most commonly, no symptoms at all. Treatment is often directed by the Rutherford classification system (Table 44.1).

A detailed clinical history in patients with atypical symptoms can differentiate it from non-vascular etiology and determine the degree and progression of symptoms. The clinician also should assess for symptoms of cardiovascular and neurovascular disease, in addition to taking a complete family history and conducting a vascular examination.

Ankle-brachial index (ABI) is recommended to detect angiographically significant PAD. If there is high suspicion in a patient with a normal at-rest ABI, they should undergo an exercise ABI. Arterial duplex ultrasound is the

Table 44.1 Rutherford classification of peripheral artery disease

Grade	Category	Clinical presentation
0	0	Asymptomatic
I	1	Mild claudication
I	2	Moderate claudication
I	3	Severe claudication
II	4	Ischemic rest pain
II	5	Minor tissue loss
III	6	Major tissue loss

Source: (Adapted from J Vasc Surg, 45, Norgren L et al., Inter-Society Consensus for the Management of Peripheral Arterial Disease (TASC II), S5–67, Copyright (2007), with permission from Elsevier.)

preferred imaging modality in patients with an abnormal ABI, and if they are candidates for re-vascularisation, they should undergo computed tomography angiography (CTA), magnetic resonance angiography (MRA) or invasive angiography for definitive assessment.

44.3 Treatment

Patients with PAD should be encouraged to modify behaviours (quit smoking and control low-density lipoprotein levels, blood pressure and blood sugar levels) leading to higher risk or severity of co-morbidities. Further, PAD management includes anti-platelet therapy (aspirin, clopidogrel as alternative)[4–7] and treatment of claudication symptoms (exercise therapy/supervised walking program, cilostazol, pentoxifylline and statins).

Re-vascularisation is indicated for patients with CLI requiring limb salvage, acute limb ischaemia and claudication that is refractory to medical therapy, supervised walking program and management of risk factors. Re-vascularisation can take place endovascularly or surgically. Percutaneous re-vascularisation techniques include angioplasty, stent, stent graft, plaque debulking, thrombolysis and percutaneous thrombectomy. Synthetic bypass, autogenous bypass and endarterectomy are the mainstays of surgical re-vascularisation.

Recently, there is an increased preference for endovascular re-vascularisation over surgical. The choice of percutaneous approach is driven by the anatomic complexity (based on TransAtlantic Inter-Society Consensus [TASC] II classification) of aortoiliac (Figure 44.1)[8] and femoropopliteal lesions (Figure 44.2). Sustained patency is based on anatomic factors. Success rate and duration of patency worsens with increased length and the number of stenotic lesions treated. Also, patency rate is negatively affected when there is more severe disease in the distal run-off arteries. Severity of ischaemia decreases patency rates and can be evaluated by measuring the gradient across the stenotic lesion.

44.3.1 Suprainguinal (aortoiliac) re-vascularisation

Patients with aortoiliac occlusive disease benefit the most from a percutaneous approach (Figure 44.3), with endovascular re-vascularisation having lower mortality and morbidity rates.[9] Clinical presentation consists of buttock, thigh or hip claudication; CLI; or Leriche's syndrome (impotence and absent femoral pulses). Lesion morphology (Types A-D according to TASC II) dictates re-vascularisation choice. Surgical re-vascularisation for aortoiliac disease has been reserved for patients with diffuse disease that is not amenable to the percutaneous approach (Type D). However, newer technologies like re-entry devices, drug-coated balloons and covered stent grafts make catheter-based intervention in diffuse disease an option. This is determined case by case. In the iliac artery territory, primary stent placement is a Class I indication due to the success rate and patency duration without the 8.3% morbidity and 3.3% mortality rates associated with surgery; it is preferred over percutaneous transluminal angioplasty (PTA) alone (Table 44.2).[10]

44.3.2 Infrainguinal re-vascularisation

Anatomically, because the common femoral artery lies over the hip joint, stent placement has been associated with stent thrombosis and restenosis (Figure 44.4). In this region, iliofemoral bypass or endarterectomy with patch angioplasty has been the best treatment. Percutaneous atherectomy, cutting balloon PTA or a drug-coated balloon can be second-line therapy for patients who are poor surgical candidates. Likewise, the deep femoral artery (which serves as collateral blood supply with superficial femoral artery [SFA] disease) is typically treated surgically and only approached percutaneously in poor surgical candidates with limb-threatening ischaemia.

In femoropopliteal disease (superficial femoral and popliteal arteries), the extent of the disease dictates treatment choice. If symptoms persist after medical management and an exercise program, TASC types A and B are primarily approached percutaneously, whereas types C and D are usually managed surgically with venous conduit.[4] Long-term stent durability is affected by lesion characteristics and distal runoffs as well as mechanical forces on the artery that can cause stent fracture and restenosis.[11] In general, the increased number and length of stents (including overlapping stents) negatively affect patency rates. Based on this, lesions in this segment are only stented if angioplasty yields suboptimal results (>50% residual stenosis, flow-limiting dissection, persistent gradient >10 mmHg) (Figures 44.5 and 44.6).[12]

Invasive treatment also can be beneficial in infrapopliteal disease for both limb salvage and severe claudication (Figure 44.7). Percutaneous re-vascularisation with low-profile balloons has shown >90% technical success. Unfortunately, the restenosis rate has remained high at 1 year. Stent use has been provisional with suboptimal outcomes in this region; however, studies have demonstrated improved outcomes with each generation of devices. The

Type A lesions
- Unilateral or bilateral stenoses of CIA
- Unilateral or bilateral single short (≤3 cm) stenosis of EIA

Type B lesions
- Short (≤3 cm) stenosis of infrarenal aorta
- Unilateral CIA occlusion
- Single or multiple stenosis totalling 3–10 cm involving the EIA not extending into the CFA
- Unilateral EIA occlusion not involving the origins of internal iliac or CFA

Type C lesions
- Bilateral CIA occlusions
- Bilateral EIA stenoses 3–10 cm long not extending into the CFA
- Unilateral EIA stenoses extending into the CFA
- Unilateral EIA occlusion that involves the origins of internal iliac and/or CFA
- Heavily calcified unilateral EIA occlusion with or without involvement of origins of internal iliac and/or CFA

Type D lesions
- Infrarenal aortoiliac occlusion
- Diffuse disease involving the aorta and both iliac arteries requiring treatment
- Diffuse multiple stenoses involving the unilateral CIA, EIA and CFA
- Unilateral occlusions of both CIA and EIA
- Bilateral occlusions of EIA
- Iliac stenoses in patients with AAA requiring treatment and not amenable to endograft placement or other lesions requiring open aortic or iliac surgery

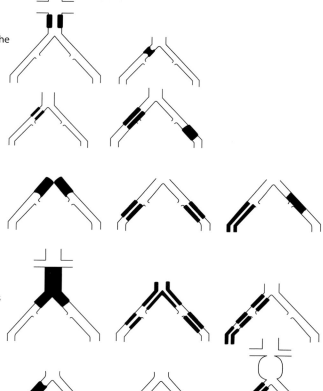

Figure 44.1 Trans-Atlantic Inter-Society Consensus (TASC) II classification of aortoiliac lesions. AAA, abdominal aortic aneurysm; CIA, common iliac artery; CFA, common femoral artery; EIA, external iliac artery. (Adapted from *J Vasc Surg*, 45, Norgren L et al., Inter-Society Consensus for the Management of Peripheral Arterial Disease (TASC II), S5–67, Copyright (2007), with permission from Elsevier.)

ACHILLES trial showed improved 12-month restenosis rates in sirolimus drug-eluting stent (DES) versus standard balloon angioplasty (22.4% vs. 41.9%, respectively).[13] The Drug Eluting Stents in the Critically Ischemic Lower Leg (DESTINY) trial compared Xience V everolimus DES with bare-metal stents (BMS) in Rutherford class 4 to 5 disease and showed improved patency (85% vs. 54%, respectively) at 12 months and freedom from target lesion re-vascularisation (TLR) (91% vs. 66%, respectively).

In addition to stenting, drug-coated balloons have shown promise in recent trials. The randomised Drug Eluting Balloon in PeripherAl InTErvention for Below The Knee Angioplasty Evaluation (DEBATE-BTK) trial showed improved 12-month restenosis (27% vs. 63%) and reocclusion (29% vs. 44%) outcomes over uncoated balloons.[14] In patients with both SFA and infrapopliteal disease, the Drug-Eluting Balloon Evaluation for Lower Limb Multilevel Treatment (DEBELLUM) trial showed improved 6-month restenosis (9.1% vs. 28.9%) and TLR rates (6.1% vs. 23.6%)

as well as improvements in ABI and clinical outcomes over standard balloon angioplasty.[15]

Surgical intervention for infrainguinal disease has demonstrated only marginal benefits in the younger population as more aggressive atherosclerotic disease has neutralised the symptomatic relief. Autologous vein bypass has shown superior patency at 5 years over synthetic grafts to the popliteal segment (74% vs. 39%). Axillofemoral–femoral bypass is currently not recommended, whereas femoral–tibial bypass with the autogenous vein is recommended in patients with claudication who have been refractory to pharmacotherapy and an exercise program.

44.3.3 Types of stents and outcomes

BMS have shown improved patency rates over balloon angioplasty, as shown in Figure 44.8.[16] Covered stents, which are used most commonly in vessel perforation and aneurysms, have not demonstrated improved outcomes over

Type A lesions

- Single stenosis ≤10 cm in length
- Single occlusion ≤5 cm in length

Type B lesions

- Multiple lesions (stenoses or occlusions), each ≤5 cm
- Single stenoses or occlusion ≤15 cm not involving the infrageniculate popliteal artery
- Single or multiple lesions in the absense of continuous tibial vessels to improve inflow for a diatal bypass
- Heavily calcified occlusion ≤5 cm in length
- Single popliteal stenosis

Type C lesions

- Multiple stenoses or occlusions totalling >15 cm with or without heavy calcification
- Recurrent stenoses or occulsions that need treatment after two endovascular interventions

Type D lessions

- Chronic total occlusions of CFA or SFA (>20 cm, involving the popliteal artery)
- Chronic total occlusion of popliteal artery and proximal trifurcation vessels

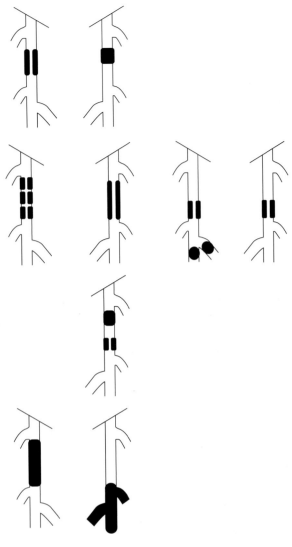

Figure 44.2 Trans-Atlantic Inter-Society Consensus (TASC) II classification of femoropopliteal lesions. CFA, common femoral artery; SFA, superficial femoral artery. (Adapted from *J Vasc Surg*, 45, Norgren L et al., Inter-Society Consensus for the Management of Peripheral Arterial Disease (TASC II), S5–67, Copyright (2007), with permission from Elsevier.)

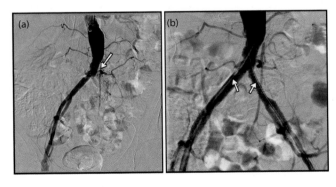

Figure 44.3 A 65-year-old female presented with an occluded femoral–femoral bypass and recurrent claudication. The left common iliac artery was totally occluded (**arrow, Panel a**) and treated with bilateral self-expanding common iliac stents via kissing technique (**arrows, Panel b**).

non-covered stents in the most recent study (VIBRANT Trial). Rather, increased edge restenosis and re-thrombosis rates were observed.[17]

DES in femoropopliteal disease have demonstrated increased benefits over balloon angioplasty, but have failed to show better long-term results compared to BMS. In a population of femoropopliteal disease patients, the Zilver PTX trial exhibited better long-term results with primary use of DES over balloon angioplasty with provisional stenting. Of 238 patients in the angioplasty group, 120 had unsuccessful angioplasty and were subsequently randomised to provisional paclitaxel DES or BMS. Event-free survival (90.4% vs. 82.6%, $p = .004$) and primary patency (83.1% vs. 32.8%, $p < .001$) were both in favour of primary DES use (Figure 44.8).

High rates of stent fractures and restenosis led to the advent of drug-coated balloons for femoropopliteal disease.

Table 44.2 PTA versus PTA plus stenting in iliac occlusive disease: Results of meta-analysis of 14 studies

	PTA		PTA + STENT	
	Stenosis (%)	Occlusion (%)	Stenosis (%)	Occlusion (%)
Immediate technical success	96	80	100	80
Primary patency[a]	65	54	77	61
Secondary patency	80	–	80	–
Major complications	4.3	–	5.2	–

Source: From Khitha et al., *Cardiology: An Illustrated Textbook*, Jaypee Brothers Medical Publishers, New Delhi, India. 2017. With permission.
PTA: *percutaneous transluminal angioplasty.*
[a] Four-year patency rate.

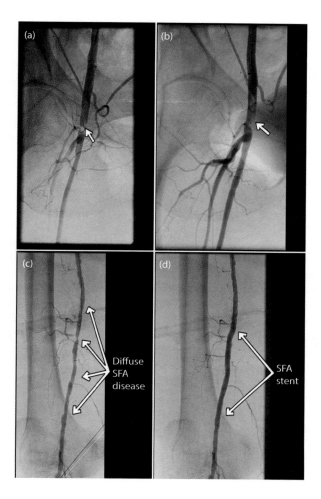

Figure 44.4 Panels **(a)** and **(b)**: A 64-year-old female with recent coronary angiogram status post-closure of right common femoral arteriotomy site with Perclose closure device complained of right lower extremity pain, numbness and pallor for 1 week. She was found to have severe 90% right common femerol artery stenosis (arrow, Panel a) with thrombus formation and treated with balloon angioplasty (arrow, Panel b). An 81-year-old female with diabetes mellitus presented with non-healing ulcers of the right lower extremity. Angiogram showed multiple sequential severe stenotic lesions **(arrows, Panel c)** in the distal SFA which was treated with drug eluting stent **(arrows, Panel d)**.

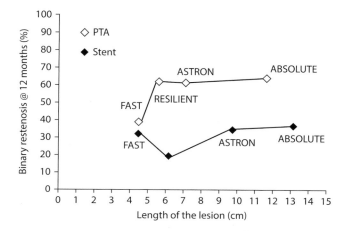

Figure 44.5 Studies reporting 12-month primary patency rates of different stent types in the SFA according to mean lesion length. Trend line shows decrease in patency rates with increasing lesion length. PTA, percutaneous transluminal angiography. (From Schillinger M, and Minar E, *Circulation*, 1263, 2433–40, 2012. With permission from Wolters Kluwer Health.)

A recent meta-analysis of four randomised controlled trials included the Lutonix Paclitaxel-Coated Balloon for the Prevention of Femoropopliteal Restenosis (LEVANT I) trial. The LEVANT I trial showed significantly reduced TLR in paclitaxel-coated balloon versus standard balloon angioplasty (12.2% vs. 27.7%, odds ratio (OR): 0.23; 95% confidence interval (CI): 0.13–0.40).[18]

Similarly, the recently published LEVANT II trial randomised 476 patients with claudication or ischaemic rest pain in a 2:1 ratio to drug-eluting balloon versus standard angioplasty and showed primary 12-month patency superiority in the drug-eluting balloon group (65.2% vs. 52.6%, $p = .02$).[19]

The IN.PACT SFA trial randomised 331 patients with symptomatic SFA and/or popliteal artery disease in a 2:1 ratio to treatment with paclitaxel-coated balloon or PTA. At 12 months, the paclitaxel-coated balloon demonstrated higher rates of primary patency (82.2% vs. 52.4%; $p < .001$), clinically driven TLR (2.4% vs. 20.6%, $p < .001$) and a low

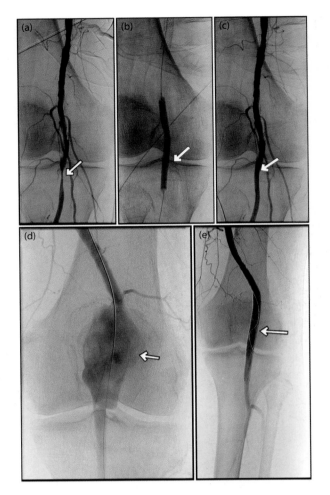

Figure 44.6 A 69-year-old female (Panels a–c) with history of coronary artery bypass graft and previous peripheral stents presented with right lower extremity critical limb ischemia (right ankle-brachial index [ABI] 0.48 and unable to obtain toe pressures). Severe stenosis was seen in the right popliteal artery behind the knee (arrow, Panel a), and was managed with atherectomy and subsequent balloon angioplasty (arrow, Panel b). Postre-vascularisation images show restoration of flow (Panel c). An 81-year-old male (Panels d and e) with left lower extremity pain and ulcers. Angiogram noted left popliteal aneurysm (arrow, Panel d) which was treated with 2 Viabahn stents, restoring flow (Panel e).

rate of vessel thrombosis (1.4% vs. 3.7%). These results persisted with more complex anatomy. The IN.PACT global study followed 655 patients with longer, more calcified lesions and chronic total occlusions and showed a TLR rate of 8.7% at 12 months. Because previous studies with stents showed increased rates of restenosis in long lesions, there is hope drug-coated balloons may one day be used with only provisional stenting in areas with suboptimal results.

Bioabsorbable stents are the newest frontier in stent development, and both organic polymer-based and metal-based bioabsorbable DES are in the early stages of evaluation.[20] Biodegradable stents showed a 30% 6-month restenosis rate in the TAXUS Element Paclitaxel-Eluting Coronary

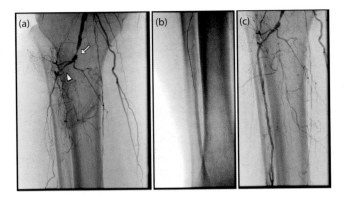

Figure 44.7 A 69-year-old male with a history of previous SFA stenting presented with non-healing ulcer of the right lower extremity. Angiogram showed a severe distal popliteal region, subtotal occlusion of the proximal anterior tibial artery (arrow, Panel a) and a totally occluded tibioperoneal trunk. A wire was passed through the anterior tibial occlusion (arrow, Panel b) with subsequent angioplasty. In Panel (c), distal flow is improved despite there still being diffuse disease.

Stent System (PERSEUS) study.[21] Study and development of newer technologies are ongoing.

44.3.4 Challenges to the endovascular approach

Chronic total occlusion remains a challenging area despite advances in endovascular techniques and devices. Specialised re-entry devices such as the Outback (Cordis, Fremont, California) and Pioneer (Volcano Corp., San Diego, California) catheters have shown procedural success rates of 70%–90%. In addition, the Frontrunner catheter (LuMend, Inc., Redwood City, California) offers a different technique, creating a channel through the plaque in order to subsequently perform angioplasty or stenting.

Calcified lesions add to the difficulty of endovascular intervention, often being difficult to dilate even with a high-pressure balloon. Atherectomy and use of an excimer laser have increased procedural success. Unfortunately, long-term patency rates have not improved, and these devices continue to be used solely as salvage therapy (Figure 44.9).[22–24]

Therapeutic angiogenesis is a type of gene therapy aimed at creating new mature collateral vessels to better perfuse an ischaemic limb. Early trials have been encouraging; however, only a modest benefit has been observed. Studies are ongoing as long-term effects are not yet known.[25]

44.4 Limb ischaemia

Acute limb ischaemia usually occurs due to embolisation or sudden thrombus formation in a diseased artery and results in rapidly declining limb perfusion. Intravenous heparin, the preferred anticoagulation method as it minimises the interference with urgent re-vascularisation, should be immediately administered. Imaging is then necessary to identify

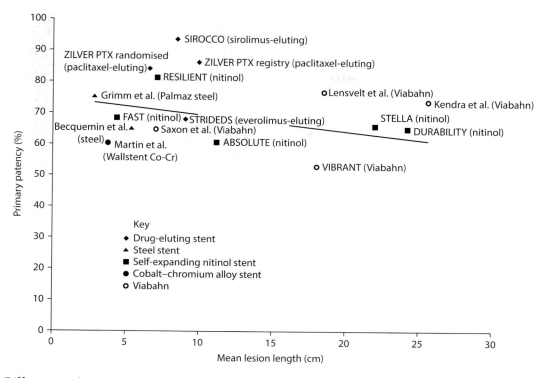

Figure 44.8 Different studies reporting 12-month primary patency rates of different stent types in the SFA according to mean lesion length. Trend line shows decrease in patency rates with increasing lesion length. (From Nfor T et al., *Advances in Cardiology*, Jaypee Brothers Medical Publishing, New Delhi, India, 2014. With permission.)

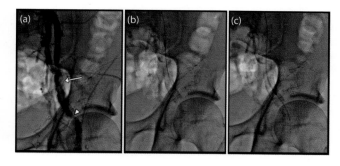

Figure 44.9. An angiogram demonstrates severe in-stent calcified lesions in the external iliac artery **(arrow, Panel a)** and a severe stenosis in the common femoral artery **(arrowhead, Panel a).** An orbital atherectomy catheter can be seen preparing the vessel prior to angioplasty **(Panels b and c).**

the region of occlusion and extent of disease in order to plan the best-suited method of re-vascularisation. Intra-arterial thrombolysis is a Class I recommendation if at a capable endovascular centre (especially if <14 days since onset).[4] Alternatively, mechanical thrombectomy is an option for debulking a clot. However, if there are concerns the limb may be close to being unsalvageable (i.e. paralysis), then surgery may be the best method to immediately obtain perfusion.

CLI is characterised by >2 weeks of ischaemic rest pain or ulcers/gangrene attributed to known PAD. The Rutherford classification grades severity (Table 44.1), and typically classes 4–6 are representative of CLI in which permanent

loss of limb, life or functional status may be imminent. The mechanism of treatment is based solely on feasibility and patient characteristics, including co-morbidities. Endovascular and surgical re-vascularisation are options, and the decision is made according to a modality's ability to provide improved inflow and then outflow perfusion. Inflow, in general, takes priority and should be addressed before the outflow lesion (Class 1 recommendation). However, if there is extensive necrosis or increased risk of mortality, then primary amputation may be the best treatment.

The Bypass versus Angioplasty in Severe Ischaemia of the Leg (BASIL) trial randomised 452 patients with infrainguinal CLI to surgical bypass versus balloon angioplasty. Overall, there was no significant difference in survival free of amputation between the groups at 1 or 3 years (68% vs. 71%, 57% vs. 52%) with an overall hazard ratio of 0.89 (95% CI: 0.68–1.17).[26] Quality-of-life measures also were similar. The major separation was the increased hospital costs at 1 year in the surgical group over angioplasty. Currently, endovascular re-vascularisation is preferred, but surgery remains an option if the anatomy is poorly suited for a percutaneous approach (long calcified lesions, poor distal runoff).

In addition to re-vascularisation, patients with non-healing ulcers from CLI can benefit from a comprehensive wound care program. In diabetic patients and those with low transcutaneous oximetry, hyperbaric oxygen therapy has shown evidence of efficacy. Also, these programs have access to specialised dressings and debridement that can improve outcomes.[27–29]

44.5 Subclavian artery disease

Subclavian artery stenosis has an incidence of ≈4% and has multiple etiologies including atherosclerotic disease (most common), arteritis, radiation exposure, compression syndrome and fibromuscular dysplasia. Half of these patients may also have underlying coronary artery disease. Treatment is indicated if there is evidence of upper-extremity ischaemia (claudication), lower-extremity ischaemia (related to axillofemoral bypass), preservation of flow for a dialysis arteriovenous fistula or subclavian steal syndrome/subclavian coronary steal syndrome.

Re-vascularisation with subclavian artery stenosis is indicated when medical therapy does not resolve symptoms. There are no randomised trials comparing invasive procedures. However, in trials, axillary–axillary bypass and carotid–subclavian bypass have shown >80% 10-year patency rates with a stroke rate of ≈2%–3%.[30] Endovascularly, BMS and nitinol stents that are typically used for iliac artery disease have a demonstrated primary success rate of 98% with a peri-procedural stroke rate of only 0.6% according to a published series of 170 patients.[31,32] At the 5-year follow-up, these stents also displayed impressive outcomes with 83% primary patency, 96% secondary patency and overall 89% of patients remaining asymptomatic (Figure 44.10).

44.6 Cerebrovascular disease

Atherosclerotic disease is the most common cause of stroke (88% manifesting as ischaemic). Incidence of stroke increases with age, and 20% of survivors become significantly disabled.

During the Framingham Heart Study, 10% of patients >65 years had asymptomatic >50% carotid stenosis and <1% of patients had >80% stenosis (annual stroke risk 1%–4.3%). Any patient who has focal stroke-like symptoms should initially be evaluated with carotid ultrasound and likely CTA or MRA to define vasculature. Aspirin (first-line), clopidogrel and aspirin plus extended-release dipyridamole are Class I recommendations for ischaemic stroke.[33] The only indication for screening imaging is for patients undergoing coronary artery bypass graft.

44.6.1 Re-vascularisation for extracranial carotid disease

The benefit of carotid endarterectomy (CEA) over medical therapy alone was initially demonstrated in the North American Symptomatic Carotid Endarterectomy Trial (NASCET),[34–36] with 22% of patients with moderate stenosis and 26% of patients with severe stenosis experiencing stroke. However, as current medical therapy is more aggressive, there may be less relative benefit from CEA. CEA carries a 7.1% rate of 30-day stroke incidence and death as seen in a meta-analysis of randomised studies.[36] Additional

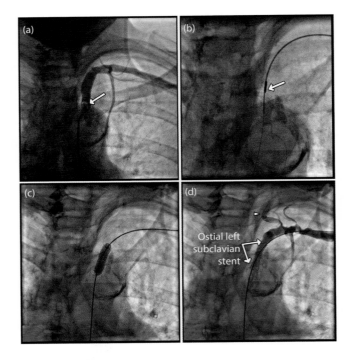

Figure 44.10 A 72-year-old female with a history of tobacco use and hypertension (HTN) presented as an outpatient complaining of left-hand paresthesias. Carotid ultrasound was performed that showed reversal of flow in the left vertebral artery, indicating severe proximal subclavian stenosis (subclavian steal syndrome). Initial angiogram showed a severe ostial calcified lesion (**arrow, Panel a**) with failed attempt at balloon angioplasty. A subsequent procedure was performed from the brachial artery and orbital atherectomy was performed (**arrow, Panel b**). A stent was then deployed (**Panel c**) in the ostial left subclavian artery. A final image (**Panel d**) was taken to confirm adequate flow into the distal subclavian artery and anterograde flow into the vertebral artery (arrowhead).

complications include cranial nerve palsy, peri-operative myocardial infarction and wound infection or haematoma.

More recently, carotid artery stenting (CAS) has been introduced with promising outcomes (Figures 44.11 and 44.12; Table 44.3).

A recent meta-analysis involving 5,796 symptomatic patients demonstrated a 7.2% 30-day incidence of stroke and death in the CAS group versus 3.9% in the CEA group.[37] Outcomes in asymptomatic patients were expectedly lower (2.3% vs. 1.3%). Myocardial infarction rates at 30-day and 1-year follow-up were significantly lower amongst patients receiving CAS than patients receiving CEA.

The Carotid Revascularization versus Endarterectomy Trial (CREST) contributed to the meta-analysis and randomised 2,502 patients with severe carotid stenosis.[38] There was no significant difference in the 4-year composite endpoint (peri-procedural stroke, myocardial infarction, death or post-procedure ipsilateral stroke, 7.2% CAS vs. 6.8% CEA), peri-procedural death (0.7% vs. 0.3%) or 30-day ipsilateral stroke (2.0% vs. 2.4%). However, CAS had higher rates

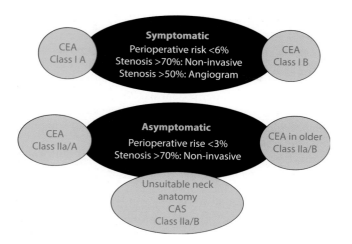

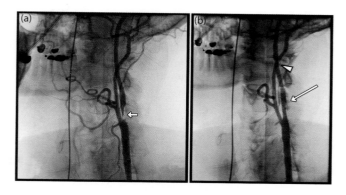

Figure 44.11 American College of Cardiology/American Heart Association 2011 guidelines on methods of re-vascularisation for extracranial carotid stenosis. CAS, carotid artery stenting; CEA, carotid endarterectomy. (From Nfor T et al., *Advances in Cardiology*, Jaypee Brothers Medical Publishing, New Delhi, India, 2014. With permissions.)

Figure 44.12 A 58-year-old male with a history of HTN and peripheral artery disease developed acute left-sided weakness and slurred speech. He was diagnosed with right middle cerebral artery stroke and on ultrasound was found to have a totally occluded right internal carotid artery and an 85% stenotic left internal carotid artery **(Panel a, arrow)**. He was deemed high risk for CEA and was subsequently re-vascularised with a left internal carotid artery stent **(Panel b, arrow)** under the protection of a distal embolisation device (arrowhead) to prevent debris migration.

of peri-procedural stroke (0.1% vs. 2.3%, $p = .01$) and myocardial infarction (1.1% vs. 2.3%, $p = .03$). Complications as a whole were more common in patients age >75 years and lower in patients <69 years.

Factors such as operator experience, anatomical feasibility and surgical risk are the main determinants in the choice between CAS and CEA. At select higher-volume centres, lower peri-procedural stroke rates have been observed, likely due to patient selection and providers' technical experience. Currently, CAS is the preferred treatment for patients with difficult neck anatomy or high surgical/anaesthesia risk. CREST 2 (*clinicaltrials.gov* identifier: NCT02089217), involving patients with 70% stenosis, is ongoing. One arm

randomises to CEA + optimal medical therapy (OMT) versus OMT alone and a second arm randomises to CAS + OMT versus OMT alone.

44.6.2 Vertebral artery disease

Vertebrobasilar system disease comprises 20% of all ischaemic strokes and at 1 year symptomatic patients have a 6%–11% risk of stroke or death. Up to 40% of patients with vertebrobasilar disease have vertebral artery stenosis. Symptoms typical of brainstem ischaemia, including dizziness, ataxia and visual or sensory/motor deficit, usually

Table 44.3 Clinical and anatomic features associated with increased procedural risks after carotid stenting and CEA

	Carotid stenting	Carotid endarterectomy
Clinical	Age ≥80 years	Age ≥80 years
	Recent stroke	Recent stroke
	Multiple lacunar infarcts	Severe heart disease
	Intracranial microangiopathy	Severe pulmonary disease
		Concomitant cardiac surgery
		Renal insufficiency or failure
Anatomic	Ulcerated plaque/thrombus	Ulcerated plaque/thrombus
	Long subtotal ICA lesion (string sign)	Long subtotal ICA lesion (string sign)
	Excessive tortuosity	Prior CEA
	Calcification	Prior neck radiation/surgery
	Multiple lesions	Contralateral ICA occlusion
	Contralateral carotid occlusion	High ICA lesion
		Low CCA lesion

Source: From Khitha et al., *Cardiology: An Illustrated Textbook*, Jaypee Brothers Medical Publishers, New Delhi, India, 2017. With permission.
CCA, common carotid artery; CEA, carotid endarterectomy; ICA, internal carotid artery.

require concomitant carotid artery or contralateral vertebral artery obstruction to be present. In these circumstances, CTA or MRA are the best choice for diagnosis.

Initial management with anti-platelet or anti-thrombotic therapy is indicated when symptomatic, but if patients are refractory, surgical or endovascular re-vascularisation is the next step.

Surgical re-vascularisation has demonstrated 5-year patency rates of 80%. Typically when lesions are distal, bypass is performed, and when proximal, transposition is the most common technique.[39]

Currently, there are no large, randomised trials for endovascular management, but Carotid and Vertebral Artery Transluminal Angioplasty Study (CAVATAS) randomised 16 patients to vertebral artery stenting and medical therapy. At 4.7 years, however, there were no vertebral strokes.

The technical success rate of vertebral artery stenting was 98% in a systematic review of more than 600 cases of vertebral artery stenting.[40] Anatomically, procedural mortality was 0.3% proximally and 3.2% distally. Neurological complications were 5.5% proximally and 17.3% distally.

44.7 Renal arterial disease

Renal artery disease is largely due to atherosclerosis (95%), but also can be related to fibromuscular dysplasia (5%). Prevalence is 10%–20%, but significant stenosis was seen on ultrasound in 6.8% of patients >65 years.[41]

When symptomatic, patients usually present with resistant/malignant hypertension (HTN), renal failure or congestive heart failure (CHF) with acute pulmonary edema. If duplex ultrasound is not sufficient, CTA and MRA are alternatives. If there is high suspicion or all noninvasive evaluations are inconclusive, invasive angiography can be performed.

Medical management consists of atherosclerotic disease secondary prevention and optimisation of antihypertensives.

Percutaneous re-vascularisation in renal artery stenosis (RAS) is preferred over surgical reconstruction. Current American College of Cardiology (ACC)/American Heart Association (AHA) guidelines for RAS re-vascularisations:

- Class I recommendation – Haemodynamically significant RAS, unexplained CHF or acute pulmonary edema
- Class 2a recommendation – Accelerated, resistant or malignant HTN; progressive renal insufficiency or unstable angina

Atherosclerotic disease typically causes ostial stenosis and usually is treated with a stent. In contrast, fibromuscular dysplasia (diffuse or midsegment stenosis) is primarily treated with balloon angioplasty and only stented if there is a suboptimal result.

44.7.1 Renal artery stenting

As a whole, renal artery stenting (Figure 44.13) has shown overall better outcomes compared to balloon angioplasty. A meta-analysis of 24 studies showed higher technical success (98% vs. 77%), lower restenosis (17% vs. 26%) and more improvement in HTN with renal artery stenting. Renal function did favour balloon angioplasty. Overall complication rates were the same in both groups.[42]

However, a recent meta-analysis which included studies such as The Angioplasty and Stent for Renal Artery Lesions (ASTRAL) study[43] and Cardiovascular Outcomes in Renal Atherosclerotic Lesions (CORAL) study,[44] showed no benefit of stenting over OMT, thereby causing scepticism about its efficacy. Regardless, OMT remains the first-line of treatment. There have been studies indicating that elevated brain natriuretic peptide and fractional flow reserve <0.8 during peak hyperaemia may predict improvement in HTN after renal artery stenting.[45,46] Further randomised trials are needed.

44.7.2 Renal denervation therapy

Percutaneous ablation of the renal sympathetic nerves (renal denervation) is meant to reduce sympathetic activity from the afferent network and thereby prevent resistant HTN. It is contraindicated with multiple renal arteries, main renal artery diameter <4 mm, short main renal artery <20 mm, previous renal stenting, severe RAS and glomerular filtration rate <45 mL/min/1.73 m^2.

In the Symplicity HTN-1 trial, 153 patients with resistant HTN were treated with denervation.[47] At follow-up, the change from baseline blood pressure (176/98 ± 17/15 mmHg) was 20/10 mmHg at 1 month, 2/11 mmHg at 12 months and 32/14 mmHg at 24 months. There were three groin pseudoaneurysms and only one renal artery dissection. The Symplicity HTN-2 trial randomised 106 patients to renal denervation plus medical treatment versus medical treatment alone.[48] At 6 months, the baseline blood pressure

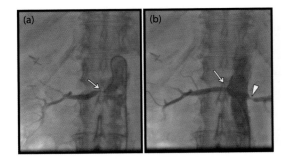

Figure 44.13 An 82-year-old female with a history of poorly controlled HTN and Stage III chronic kidney disease had a renal ultrasound that showed bilateral renal artery stenosis. Selective angiogram showed a severe left ostial stenosis (arrow, Panel a) that was treated with a renal express stent (arrow, Panel b). The left renal artery stenosis (arrowhead) was subsequently treated endovascularly

of 178/96 mmHg improved by 32/12 ± 23/11 mmHg compared to 1/0 ± 21/10 mmHg in the control group (p <.0001). Symplicity HTN-3 randomised 535 patients to renal denervation or a sham procedure at a 2:1 ratio.[49] At 6 months, both groups showed a similar significant difference from baseline at (−14.13 ± 23.93 mmHg vs. −11.74 ± 25.94 mmHg; p < .001). The 24-hour ambulatory systolic blood pressure also showed no difference (−6.75 ± 15.11 mmHg vs. −4.79 ± 17.25 mmHg, denervation vs. sham, for a difference of −1.96 mmHg). Despite the results, the study was deemed underpowered, and there was concern adequate denervation was not achieved.

44.8 Mesenteric ischaemia

44.8.1 Chronic mesenteric ischaemia

Chronic mesenteric ischaemia (Figure 44.14) has multiple etiologies, including atherosclerosis (most common), arteritis, fibromuscular dysplasia or iatrogenic causes. The superior mesenteric artery is most commonly affected, but because of additional blood supply from the celiac and inferior mesenteric artery, patients often are not symptomatic. However, when patients do present, they often complain of postprandial pain, bloating and weight loss. The preferred diagnostic imaging modalities are CTA, MRA and, when the first two are inadequate, invasive angiography. Ultrasound can be technically difficult in this region and is not widely used.

Re-vascularisation options include endarterectomy, bypass grafting (preferred surgical route) and angioplasty with stenting (Class Ib recommendation). Even though there are no randomised comparisons between endovascular and surgical strategies, stenting has shown promising outcomes in symptom relief (89.8%) and sustained longevity, with 61% of patients showing no recurrence of symptoms at 36 months.[50] Additionally, treatment of two vessels during the index intervention has protected against symptomatic recurrence and repeat re-vascularisation. In contrast, surgery is associated with higher complication rates (36% vs. 18%, p <.001) and longer hospital stays (12 ± 8 vs. 3 ± 5 days, p <.001).[51] Despite this, surgery has shown 5-year results with lower rates of restenosis (12% vs. 59%) and symptomatic recurrence (11% vs. 49%). Overall, endovascular re-vascularisation has been the preferred initial choice in treatment.

44.8.2 Acute mesenteric ischaemia

Acute mesenteric ischaemia can be due to the progression of chronic mesenteric ischaemia or thromboembolism.[52] Additionally, patients with poor perfusion from shock can develop non-occlusive acute mesenteric ischaemia. It should be suspected in any patient with cardiovascular disease or atrial fibrillation with an acute presentation of severe abdominal pain out of proportion to the physical exam. Multi-detector computed tomography using a biphasic mesenteric angiography protocol has sensitivity of 93% and specificity of 100% and is key to early diagnosis and treatment.[53] After the initiation of aspirin, heparin and volume resuscitation, more invasive angiography is performed with the possibility of endovascular treatment with catheter-directed thrombolysis, balloon angioplasty and stenting (Class 2b recommendation). Alternatively, in the setting of 'non-occlusive' acute mesenteric ischaemia, transcatheter vasodilator therapy can be administered at the time of diagnosis (Class 2a recommendation).

A combined endovascular and surgical approach has yielded the best outcomes. Endovascular re-vascularisation, surgical exploration with resection of necrotic bowel and even a 'second look' surgical exploration at 24–48 hours (Class I recommendation) have demonstrated lower morbidity and mortality compared with a singular total surgical approach (surgical re-vascularisation and laparotomy). This has been supported by previously reported peri-operative mortality rates of 36% with primary endovascular treatment and 50% with primary surgical treatment, p < .05.[54]

44.9 Aortic aneurysm and dissection

44.9.1 Abdominal aortic aneurysm

Abdominal aortic aneurysm (AAA) is widely described as a maximal diameter of ≥3 cm measured coaxial to the vessel, however dilatation >1.5 times the expected normal diameter better compensates for ranges across body surface area and sex.

The overall prevalence of AAA is about 1.3%, but risk increases with age (0.1% in age 45–55 to 12.5% in men and 5.2% in women >75 years). Therefore, ultrasound screening is indicated for men >60 years of age who have a first-degree relative with AAA and men ages 65–75 with tobacco history (both Class 1).

The major consequences of untreated AAA are rupture and distal embolisation. Unfortunately, 64% of patients with ruptured AAA die before arriving at the hospital and peri-operative mortality with repair is >50%; therefore, the focal

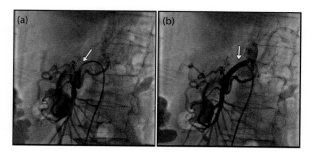

Figure 44.14 An 82-year-old female with a history of chronic lymphocytic leukaemia, HTN and hyperlipidemia was hospitalised after 1-day history of severe abdominal pain and diarrhea. Computed tomography of the abdomen and pelvis showed colitis in the ascending colon. Subsequent angiography showed a severe ostial stenosis of the superior mesenteric artery (arrow, Panel a) that was treated with balloon angioplasty and stenting (arrow, Panel b).

point of management is to repair high-risk patients prior to rupture[55] (Figure 44.15). Because aneurysm size correlates with risk of rupture, current ACC/AHA indications for repair are AAA ≥5.5 cm (Class I), 5–5.4 cm (females – 4.6–5.0 cm) (Class IIa) or rapid expansion (0.7–1.0 cm/year). Smaller aneurysms (4.0–5.0/5.4 cm) should undergo ultrasound or CTA surveillance every 6–12 months.

Unfortunately, size is not a perfect predictor; ongoing research with MRA has detected cellular inflammation that may correlate with risk of expansion. In a study of 29 patients with stable AAA, distinct uptake of ultrasmall superparamagnetic particles of iron oxide (USPIO) indicated an increased risk of expansion (0.66 cm/year vs. 0.22 cm/year, $p = .02$).[56]

Imaging at 1 month, 6 months and yearly after repair is necessary to monitor the size of the residual aneurysm, as well as assess for graft migration and endoleak.

44.9.2 Endovascular versus open surgical repair

Both endovascular aneurysm repair (EVAR) and open surgical repair (OSR) carry a Class I indication, according to the 2011 ACC/AHA guidelines, and the decision is typically made based on surgical risk, anatomic factors, provider experience, patient preference and the ability to continue follow-up.

There have been several randomised trials comparing EVAR and OSR. The UK Endovascular Aneurysm Repair 1 (EVAR 1) trial randomised 1,252 patients with AAA ≥5.5 cm to EVAR or OSR and showed 30-day mortality of 1.8% and 4.3%, respectively.[57] Despite this early mortality benefit, after 6 months there was no difference in deaths or even aneurysm-related deaths. EVAR cost more due to the increased complication rate (12.6% EVAR vs. 2.5% OSR) and need for re-intervention (5.1% vs. 1.7%).

The Dutch Randomised Endovascular Aneurysm Repair (DREAM) trial showed similar results with a lower in-hospital mortality rate in EVAR (1.2% vs. 4.6%, $p = .06$) and no difference long-term (31.1% vs. 30.1%, $p = .97$ at median

6.4 years).[58] Again, EVAR had higher rates of re-intervention (29.6% vs. 18.1%, $p = .03$).

Finally, the Open Versus Endovascular Repair (OVER) trial randomised 881 patients, but also included AAA of 4.5 cm with either rapid expansion or an associated iliac aneurysm ≥3 cm.[59] The short-term mortality benefits of EVAR (0.5% vs. 3%, $p = .004$) persisted up to 3 years before equilibrating. The rates of repeat procedures, hospitalisation related to aneurysm and all-cause hospitalisation were similar amongst groups.

In a cost analysis, although initial hospital cost was lower in EVAR, there was no significant difference after 2 years in total healthcare cost.[60] The differences in cost results between trials may be related to timing (increases in inpatient costs over time) and differences between inpatient costs in the United Kingdom versus United States with similar costs of the actual graft.

Patients with pararenal AAA can benefit from fenestrated stent grafts (Figure 44.16), which are custom-made composite grafts with predetermined openings for the renal arteries and celiac trunk that are connected to the main graft body. Alternatively, the chimney technique (Figure 44.17) is used when there is a short infrarenal neck. A covered stent is deployed in each renal artery to maintain patent flow prior to the deployment of the aortic endograft. The renal artery stent and the aortic endograft are simultaneously dilated with balloons.

44.9.3 Descending thoracic and thoracoabdominal aortic aneurysms

Thoracic aortic aneurysms (TAA) and thoracoabdominal aortic aneurysms (TAAA) (defined as diameter ≥2 standard deviations above the mean), when symptomatic, typically present as life-threatening emergent dissection or rupture. However, the majority are asymptomatic and incidentally found. Current recommendations are for annual surveillance with CTA or MRA for a TAA <4 cm or 6-month surveillance for ≥4 cm. According to the University Health System Consortium, of all the hospitalisations involving

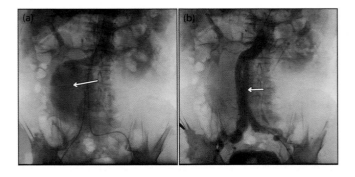

Figure 44.15 A 79-year-old asymptomatic male was seen as an outpatient and on exam a large pulsatile abdominal mass was appreciated. Computed tomography showed a large 10 cm × 10 cm infrarenal AAA (**arrow, Panel a**), which was repaired with an endovascular graft (**arrow, Panel b**).

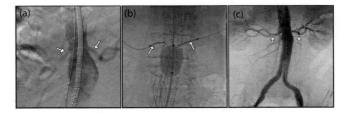

Figure 44.16 A 68-year-old male with an AAA (**Panel a**) had endovascular aneurysm repair performed with a fenestrated graft due to the short distance between the renal arteries (arrow) and the superior portion of the aneurysm. The pre-formed renal arterial fenestrations (**arrows, Panel b**) can be seen during expansion of the graft. The final image demonstrates patent flow without endovascular leak and preserved perfusion of bilateral renal arteries (**arrows, Panel c**).

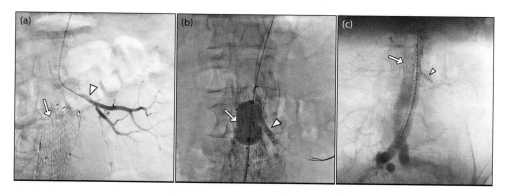

Figure 44.17 A 79-year-old male with an AAA underwent endovascular aortic repair **(Panel a)**. Due to the short infrarenal neck, patency of the renal artery was maintained with simultaneous expansion of the graft **(arrow, Panels b and c)** and a covered stent (arrowhead) via the chimney technique.

aortic disease, AAA accounted for 62.7%, TAA 25.9% and TAAA 8.3%. TAA and TAAA have a more aggressive natural history; of the dissection or rupture admissions, 8.4% had AAA and 30%–37% had TAA or TAAA.[61]

Sixty percent of aneurysms involve the root and arch, 40% the descending aorta, 10% the arch alone and 10% the thoracoabdominal aorta. The normal range of size is based on body surface area and age. This is particularly important for identifying younger patients (<40 years old) who may have a genetic predisposition for aneurysm (e.g. Marfan syndrome 5 cm, Loeys-Dietz syndrome 4.4–4.6 cm); genetic sequencing is recommended for first-degree relatives.[61]

Initial medical management consists of beta-blockers, angiotensin-converting enzyme inhibitors, angiotensin II receptor blockers, statins and smoking cessation.[62–66] Repair is currently indicated when the diameter is ≥ 5.5 cm, growth rate is >0.5 cm/year, symptoms related to TAA occur (chest pain, back pain, aortic insufficiency with CHF) or the diameter is >4.5 cm in patients who need valve surgery or coronary bypass.

Repair can be performed endovascularly or with open surgery. Because OSR carries increased risk of paralysis from ischaemic spinal cord injury and acute renal failure, thoracic EVAR (TEVAR) was introduced in the late 1990s; TEVAR was noted to have lower procedure times and complication rates. To date, there has been no randomised trial comparing TEVAR to OSR; however, there was a meta-analysis with 5,888 patients that showed lower peri-operative mortality with TEVAR (5.8% vs. 13%, $p < .0001$).[67] This persisted up to 1 year, but no mortality difference was seen at 2–3 years (23% vs. 24.8%). There also was no significant difference in myocardial infarction, repeat aortic procedures, stroke or limb or mesenteric ischaemia. There was a notable decrease in risk of paraplegia and paraparesis with TEVAR (3.4% vs. 8.2%; $p < .0001$). In contrast to this meta-analysis, another study showed 5-year outcomes with persistently reduced aneurysm-related mortality in TEVAR (2.8% vs. 11.7%; $p = .008$) despite all-cause mortality remaining similar (68%

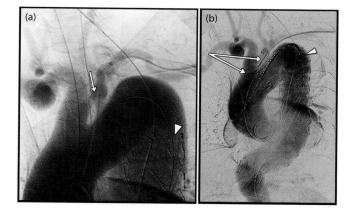

Figure 44.18 An 83-year-old female with a thoracic aortic aneurysm underwent an endovascular thoracic aortic repair with two overlapping stent grafts. Due to extension of the aneurysm to the left subclavian artery **(arrow, Panel a)**, perfusion was preserved with a covered stent via the chimney technique **(arrow, Panel b)**.

vs. 67%).[68] Additionally, major adverse events also were lower with TEVAR (57.9% vs. 78.7%, $p = .0001$).

Based on these studies, endovascular repair is the treatment of choice for descending TAA; surgery is recommended for aneurysms located in the ascending aorta or the aortic arch. Other technical factors include a 20-mm proximal landing zone, distal landing zones of normal size and a straight aorta that adequately seals and fixates the graft. However, there is a hybrid 'elephant trunk' procedure that uses a Dacron graft to surgically reconstruct the ascending aorta and arch, allowing the distal graft to provide a landing zone for the endovascular stent graft.[69]

In circumstances in which the proximal landing zone is inadequate, proximal extension may be achieved via a left common carotid to subclavian bypass. This minimises ischaemic complications involving the arm, spinal cord, vertebrobasilar circulation and stroke, which is seen in 4%–8% of patients.[70] Alternatively, the chimney graft technique (Figure 44.18) can be used to cannulate the branching left subclavian or left common carotid artery by pre-wiring and deploying a covered stent. With the covered stent protruding into the aortic arch, simultaneous inflation with a balloon assures an adequate seal whilst maintaining patency of the branching vessels.[71] This technique also is used for the abdominal viscera in the presence of a TAAA.

Fenestrated stent grafts for TAA are still undergoing trials.

44.9.4 Aortic dissection

There are approximately 7000 cases of aortic dissection each year, carrying a mortality rate of 25% in the first 24 hours after presentation. Dissection is more likely in aneurysmal areas and therefore prevention is most important with long-term survival. Diagnosis and Sanford classification (ascending type A, arch and descending type B) can be achieved with CTA, MRA and transoesophageal echocardiography. Type A dissections usually require resection and urgent surgical repair with or without aortic valve replacement (in the setting of aortic regurgitation). Type B dissections can initially be managed medically when haemodynamically stable. Intravenous beta-blockers can be administered with a goal blood pressure of <120 mmHg and a heart rate <60 bpm. In-hospital mortality is significantly higher in unstable (pain, rupture, organ dysfunction, aneurysm expansion, dissection extension, uncontrolled HTN) dissections compared to a stable patient's (35.7% vs. 1.5%).[61] There are recent data that stable type B dissections also may benefit from repair. The Investigation of Stent Grafts in Aortic Dissection (INSTEAD) trial randomised 140 patients with stable type B thoracic dissections; it showed an absolute risk reduction of 12.4% in TEVAR compared to OMT.[72] Disease progression was reduced (46.1% vs. 27%), likely due to remodelling of the aorta.

44.10 Conclusion

PAD carries a significant morbidity and mortality due to its associated co-morbidities and is still largely undertreated. With advances in technology, endovascular re-vascularisation is becoming the intervention of choice. Whilst stenting in aortoiliac disease is well established, long-term patency and durability in femoropopliteal disease has not been as promising. Drug-eluting balloons and bioabsorbable stents currently are being studied with hopes of improving outcomes. Additional technologies, such as debulking and re-entry devices, have not shown significant improvement in limb salvage or stent patency, but still are used as tools for addressing calcified chronic lesions. Renal artery stenting has not demonstrated the expected benefits, and renal denervation for resistant HTN is still being investigated due to questionable outcomes on most recent studies. Carotid stenting has replaced CEA when anatomically and clinically favourable. Endovascular repair of TAA and AAA is rapidly becoming the preferred therapy, and as devices continue to develop, complicated anatomy will be less of a limitation. In time, we foresee continued improvements in outcomes for endovascular treatment of PAD.

References

1. Baumgartner I et al. Cardiovascular risk profile and outcome of patients with abdominal aortic aneurysm in outpatients with atherothrombosis: Data from the Reduction of Atherothrombosis for Continued Health (REACH) Registry. *J Vasc Surg* 2008; 48: 808–14.
2. Fowkes FG et al. Ankle-brachial index and extent of atherothrombosis in 8891 patients with or at risk of vascular disease: Results of the international AGATHA study. *Eur Heart J* 2006; 27: 1861–7.
3. McDermott MM et al. Prevalence and significance of unrecognized lower extremity peripheral arterial disease in general medicine practice. *J Gen Intern Med* 2001; 16: 384–90.
4. Hirsch AT et al. ACC/AHA 2005 guidelines for the management of patients with peripheral arterial disease (lower extremity, renal, mesenteric and abdominal aortic): Executive summary a collaborative report from the American Association for Vascular Surgery/Society for Vascular Surgery, Society for Cardiovascular Angiography and Interventions, Society for Vascular Medicine and Biology, Society of Interventional Radiology and the ACC/AHA Task Force on Practice Guidelines (Writing Committee to Develop Guidelines for the Management of Patients with Peripheral Arterial Disease) endorsed by the American Association of Cardiovascular and Pulmonary Rehabilitation; National Heart, Lung and Blood Institute; Society for Vascular Nursing; TransAtlantic Inter-Society Consensus; and Vascular Disease Foundation. *J Am Coll Cardiol* 2006; 47: 1239–312.
5. Sobel M et al. Antithrombotic therapy for peripheral artery occlusive disease: American College of Chest Physicians Evidence-Based Clinical Practice Guidelines (8th Edition). *Chest* 2008; 133: 815S–43S.
6. CAPRIE Steering Committee. A randomised, blinded, trial of clopidogrel versus aspirin in patients at risk of ischaemic events (CAPRIE). CAPRIE Steering Committee. *Lancet* 1996; 348: 1329–39.
7. Bhatt DL et al. Clopidogrel and aspirin versus aspirin alone for the prevention of atherothrombotic events. *N Engl J Med* 2006; 354: 1706–17.
8. Norgren L et al. Inter-Society Consensus for the Management of Peripheral Arterial Disease (TASC II). *J Vasc Surg* 2007; 45: S5–67.
9. Zafar AM et al. Lower-extremity endovascular interventions for Medicare beneficiaries: Comparative effectiveness as a function of provider specialty. *J Vasc Interv Radiol* 2012; 23: 3–9.e14.
10. Khitha J et al. Peripheral artery disease. In: London B (editor), *Cardiology: An Illustrated Textbook*. New Delhi, India: Jaypee Brothers Medical Publishers, 2017.
11. Early M. Stresses in peripheral arteries following stent placement: A finite element analysis. *Comput Methods Biomech Biomed Engin* 2009; 12: 25–33.
12. Schillinger M, and Minar E. Percutaneous treatment of peripheral artery disease: Novel techniques. *Circulation* 2012; 1263: 2433–40.

13. Scheinert D et al. A prospective randomized multicenter comparison of balloon angioplasty and infrapopliteal stenting with the sirolimus-eluting stent in patients with ischemic peripheral arterial disease: 1-year results from the ACHILLES trial. *J Am Coll Cardiol* 2012; 60: 2290–5.

14. Liistro F et al. Drug-eluting balloon in peripheral intervention for below the knee angioplasty evaluation (DEBATE-BTK): A randomized trial in diabetic patients with critical limb ischemia. *Circulation* 2013; 128: 615–21.

15. Fanelli F et al. Lower limb multilevel treatment with drug-eluting balloons: 6-month results from the DEBELLUM randomized trial. *J Endovasc Ther* 2012; 19: 571–80.

16. Nfor T et al. Advances in peripheral arterial and aortic diseases. In: Chatterjee K, Horwitz PA (editors), *Advances in Cardiology*, Chap. 4, New Delhi, India: Jaypee Brothers Medical Publishing, 2014.

17. Geraghty PJ et al. Three-year results of the VIBRANT trial of VIABAHN endoprosthesis versus bare nitinol stent implantation for complex superficial femoral artery occlusive disease. *J Vasc Surg* 2013; 58: 386–95.e4.

18. Mohler ER 3rd et al. Cholesterol reduction with atorvastatin improves walking distance in patients with peripheral arterial disease. *Circulation* 2003; 108: 1481–6.

19. Cassese S et al. Paclitaxel-coated versus uncoated balloon angioplasty reduces target lesion revascularization in patients with femoropopliteal arterial disease: A meta-analysis of randomized trials. *Circ Cardiovasc Interv* 2012; 5: 582–9.

20. Peeters P et al. Are bio-absorbable stents the future of SFA treatment? *J Cardiovasc Surg (Torino)* 2010; 51: 121–4.

21. Biamino G et al. Treatment of SFA lesions with PLLA biodegradable stents: Results of the PERSEUS study (abstract). *J Endovasc Ther* 2005; 12: 1–5.

22. Safian RD et al. Orbital atherectomy for infrapopliteal disease: Device concept and outcome data for the OASIS trial. *Catheter Cardiovasc Interv* 2009; 73: 406–12.

23. Ramaiah V et al. Midterm outcomes from the TALON Registry: Treating peripherals with SilverHawk: Outcomes collection. *J Endovasc Ther* 2006; 13: 592–602.

24. Shammas NW et al. Safety and One-Year revascularization outcome of excimer laser ablation therapy in treating in-stent restenosis of femoropopliteal arteries: A retrospective review from a single center. *Cardiovasc Revasc Med* 2012; 13: 341–4.

25. Lederman RJ et al. Therapeutic angiogenesis with recombinant fibroblast growth factor-2 for intermittent claudication (the TRAFFIC study): A randomised trial. *Lancet* 2002; 359: 2053–8.

26. Adam DJ et al. Bypass versus angioplasty in severe ischaemia of the leg (BASIL): Multicentre, randomised controlled trial. *Lancet* 2005; 366: 1925–34.

27. Hopf HW et al. Guidelines for the treatment of arterial insufficiency ulcers. *Wound Repair Regen* 2006; 14: 693–710.

28. Hinchliffe RJ et al. A systematic review of the effectiveness of revascularization of the ulcerated foot in patients with diabetes and peripheral arterial disease. *Diabetes Metab Res Rev* 2012; 28(Suppl 1): 179–217. Erratum in: *Diabetes Metab Res Rev* 2012; 28: 376. Fiedrichs, S [corrected to Friederichs, S].

29. Kranke P et al. Hyperbaric oxygen therapy for chronic wounds. *Cochrane Database Syst Rev* 2012; 4: CD004123.

30. Kretschmer G et al. Obliterations of the proximal subclavian artery: To bypass or to anastomose? *J Cardiovasc Surg (Torino)* 1991; 32: 334–9.

31. Ochoa VM, and Yeghiazarians Y. Subclavian artery stenosis: A review for the vascular medicine practitioner. *Vasc Med* 2011; 16: 29–34.

32. Patel SN et al. Catheter-based treatment of the subclavian and innominate arteries. *Catheter Cardiovasc Interv* 2008; 71: 963–8.

33. Brott TG et al. 2011 ASA/ACCF/AHA/AANN/AANS/ACR/ ASNR/CNS/SAIP/SCAI/SIR/SNIS/SVM/SVS guideline on the management of patients with extracranial carotid and vertebral artery disease: A report of the American College of Cardiology Foundation/American Heart Association Task Force on Practice Guidelines, and the American Stroke Association, American Association of Neuroscience Nurses, American Association of Neurological Surgeons, American College of Radiology, American Society of Neuroradiology, Congress of Neurological Surgeons, Society of Atherosclerosis Imaging and Prevention, Society for Cardiovascular Angiography and Interventions, Society of Interventional Radiology, Society of NeuroInterventional Surgery, Society for Vascular Medicine, and Society for Vascular Surgery. *J Am Coll Cardiol* 2011; 57: e16–94. Erratum in: *J Am Coll Cardiol* 2012; 60: 566.

34. North American Symptomatic Carotid Endarterectomy Trial Collaborators. Beneficial effect of carotid endarterectomy in symptomatic patients with high-grade carotid stenosis. *N Engl J Med* 1991; 325: 445–53.

35. Barnett HJ et al. Benefit of carotid endarterectomy in patients with symptomatic moderate or severe stenosis. North American Symptomatic Carotid Endarterectomy Trial Collaborators. *N Engl J Med* 1998; 339: 1415–25.

36. Rothwell PM et al. Reanalysis of the final results of the European Carotid Surgery Trial. *Stroke* 2003; 34: 514–23.

37. Liu ZJ et al. Updated systematic review and meta-analysis of randomized clinical trials comparing carotid artery stenting and carotid endarterectomy in the treatment of carotid stenosis. *Ann Vasc Surg* 2012; 26: 576–90.

38. Brott TG et al. Stenting versus endarterectomy for treatment of carotid-artery stenosis. *N Engl J Med* 2010; 363: 11–23. Erratum in: *N Engl J Med* 2010; 363: 198; *N Engl J Med* 2010; 363: 498.

39. Berguer R et al. Surgical reconstruction of the extracranial vertebral artery: Management and outcome. *J Vasc Surg* 2000; 31: 9–18.

40. Eberhardt O et al. Stenting of vertebrobasilar arteries in symptomatic atherosclerotic disease and acute occlusion: Case series and review of the literature. *J Vasc Surg* 2006; 43: 1145–54.

41. Hansen KJ et al. Prevalence of renovascular disease in the elderly: A population-based study. *J Vasc Surg* 2002; 36: 443–51.

42. Leertouwer TC et al. Stent placement for renal arterial stenosis: Where do we stand? A meta-analysis. *Radiology* 2000; 216: 78–85.

43. ASTRAL Investigators et al. Revascularization versus medical therapy for renal-artery stenosis. *N Engl J Med* 2009; 361: 1953–62.

44. Cooper CJ et al. Stenting and medical therapy for atherosclerotic renal-artery stenosis. *N Engl J Med* 2014; 370: 13–22.

45. Silva JA et al. Elevated brain natriuretic peptide predicts blood pressure response after stent revascularization in patients with renal artery stenosis. *Circulation* 2005; 111: 328–33.

46. Mitchell JA et al. Predicting blood pressure improvement in hypertensive patients after renal artery stent placement: Renal fractional flow reserve. *Catheter Cardiovasc Interv* 2007; 69: 685–9.

47. Symplicity HTN-1 Investigators. Catheter-based renal sympathetic denervation for resistant hypertension: Durability of blood pressure reduction out to 24 months. *Hypertension* 2011; 57: 911–7.

48. Symplicity HTN-2 Investigators et al. Renal sympathetic denervation in patients with treatment-resistant hypertension (The Symplicity HTN-2 Trial): A randomised controlled trial. *Lancet* 2010; 376: 1903–9.

49. Bhatt DL et al. A controlled trial of renal denervation for resistant hypertension. *N Engl J Med* 2014; 370: 1393–401.

50. Peck MA et al. Intermediate-term outcomes of endovascular treatment for symptomatic chronic mesenteric ischemia. *J Vasc Surg* 2010; 51: 140–7.e1–2.

51. Oderich GS et al. Open versus endovascular revascularization for chronic mesenteric ischemia: Risk-stratified outcomes. *J Vasc Surg* 2009; 49: 1472–9.e3.

52. Herbert GS, and Steele SR. Acute and chronic mesenteric ischemia. *Surg Clin North Am* 2007; 87: 1115–34, ix.

53. Aschoff AJ et al. Evaluation of acute mesenteric ischemia: Accuracy of biphasic mesenteric multi-detector CT angiography. *Abdom Imaging* 2009; 34: 345–57.

54. Arthurs ZM et al. A comparison of endovascular revascularization with traditional therapy for the treatment of acute mesenteric ischemia. *J Vasc Surg* 2011; 53: 698–704; discussion 704–5.

55. Mealy K and Salman A. The true incidence of ruptured abdominal aortic aneurysms. *Eur J Vasc Surg* 1988; 2: 405–8.

56. Richards JM et al. Abdominal aortic aneurysm growth predicted by uptake of ultrasmall superparamagnetic particles of iron oxide: A pilot study. *Circ Cardiovasc Imaging* 2011; 4: 274–81.

57. United Kingdom EVAR Trial Investigators et al. Endovascular versus open repair of abdominal aortic aneurysm. *N Engl J Med* 2010; 362: 1863–71.

58. De Bruin JL et al. Long-term outcome of open or endovascular repair of abdominal aortic aneurysm. *N Engl J Med* 2010; 362: 1881–9.

59. Lederle FA et al. Long-term comparison of endovascular and open repair of abdominal aortic aneurysm. *N Engl J Med* 2012; 367: 1988–97.

60. Stroupe KT et al. Cost-effectiveness of open versus endovascular repair of abdominal aortic aneurysm in the OVER trial. *J Vasc Surg* 2012; 56: 901–10.

61. Hiratzka LF et al. 2010 ACCF/AHA/AATS/ACR/ASA/SCA/SCAI/SIR/STS/SVM Guidelines for the diagnosis and management of patients with thoracic aortic disease. A Report of the American College of Cardiology Foundation/American Heart Association Task Force on Practice Guidelines, American Association for Thoracic Surgery, American College of Radiology, American Stroke Association, Society of Cardiovascular Anesthesiologists, Society for Cardiovascular Angiography and Interventions, Society of Interventional Radiology, Society of Thoracic Surgeons, and Society for Vascular Medicine. *J Am Coll Cardiol* 2010; 55: e27–e129. Erratum in: *J Am Coll Cardiol* 2013; 62: 1039–40.

62. Genoni M et al. Chronic beta-blocker therapy improves outcome and reduces treatment costs in chronic type B aortic dissection. *Eur J Cardiothorac Surg* 2001; 19: 606–10.

63. Shores J et al. Progression of aortic dilatation and the benefit of long-term beta-adrenergic blockade in Marfan's syndrome. *N Engl J Med* 1994; 330: 1335–41.

64. Ahimastos AA et al. Effect of perindopril on large artery stiffness and aortic root diameter in patients with Marfan syndrome: A randomized controlled trial. *JAMA* 2007; 298: 1539–47.

65. Brooke BS et al. Angiotensin II blockade and aortic-root dilation in Marfan's syndrome. *N Engl J Med* 2008; 358: 2787–95.

66. Diehm N et al. Statins are associated with decreased mortality in abdominal, but not in thoracic aortic aneurysm patients undergoing endovascular repair: Propensity score-adjusted analysis. *Vasa* 2008; 37: 241–9.

67. Cheng D et al. Endovascular aortic repair versus open surgical repair for descending thoracic aortic disease a systematic review and meta-analysis of comparative studies. *J Am Coll Cardiol* 2010; 55: 986–1001.

68. Makaroun MS et al. Five-year results of endovascular treatment with the Gore TAG device compared with open repair of thoracic aortic aneurysms. *J Vasc Surg* 2008; 47: 912–8.

69. Azizzadeh A et al. The hybrid elephant trunk procedure: A single-stage repair of an ascending, arch, and descending thoracic aortic aneurysm. *J Vasc Surg* 2006; 44: 404–7.

70. Brozzi NA, and Roselli EE. Endovascular therapy for thoracic aortic aneurysms: State of the art in 2012. *Curr Treat Options Cardiovasc Med* 2012; 14: 149–63.

71. Kolvenbach RR et al. Urgent endovascular treatment of thoraco-abdominal aneurysms using a sandwich technique and chimney grafts – A technical description. *Eur J Vasc Endovasc Surg* 2011; 41: 54–60.

72. Nienaber CA et al. Endovascular repair of type B aortic dissection: Long-term results of the randomized investigation of stent grafts in aortic dissection trial. *Circ Cardiovasc Interv* 2013; 6: 407–16.

Training programs and certification in interventional cardiology in European countries

LINO GONÇALVES, CARLO DI MARIO

45.1 Introduction

Cardiovascular disease (CVD) remains the leading cause of death around the world. The Global Burden of Disease study estimated that 30% of all deaths worldwide were caused by CVD in 2010, which represents twice the number of deaths caused by cancers.[1] Despite the observed recent decreases in mortality rates in many European countries, CVD is still the leading cause of death, and being responsible for over four million deaths per year, which represents about half of all deaths in Europe.[2]

In the last four decades, major achievements in the treatment of CVD were achieved. Invasive cardiology, and particularly interventional cardiology, is amongst those areas that experienced the most important developments and constitutes nowadays one of the cornerstones for the treatment of many CVD, even replacing the surgical approach in many areas.

Interventional cardiology is a rapidly evolving field of cardiology, bringing a continuous flow of new information that improves the diagnosis and treatment of several CVD. As a consequence, interventional cardiology training needs to be updated and modified on a continuous basis in order to keep pace with all these new developments. The training of interventional cardiology is, however, highly heterogeneous across the different European countries.

Harmonisation of training in interventional cardiology and training credentialing in Europe became more important as the field expanded tremendously with the development of several novel diagnostic and therapeutic techniques. Moreover, major differences in the curricula for the field of cardiovascular interventions and non-coronary peripheral endovascular therapy are currently seen in Europe. Therefore, harmonisation of the training and education as well as certification is of utmost importance to guarantee high-quality treatment standards and patient safety across the different European countries.

45.2 Historical background

One of the main challenges that we currently face in Europe is the lack of harmonisation of interventional cardiology training across the different countries. Indeed, interventional cardiology training is largely heterogeneous as training programs are devised and run at a National level, with significant differences amongst them. This lack of harmonisation results from the subsidiary principle, the EU rule assigning to each member country the right to organise all aspects of high education and certifying effective completion of the study program. In 2005, a European directive, the 'Luxembourg Declaration on Patient Safety', was published. This document presents the importance of the standardisation of training in optimising patient safety.[3] Still specific regulations have not been passed in this field.

In order to address this lack of training harmonisation at the European level, European scientific medical societies, such as the European Society of Cardiology (including the European Association for Percutaneous Cardiovascular Intervention [EAPCI]), have an important role to lead the process.

The first step in the direction of the harmonisation of the cardiology training and education in Europe was taken when the document 'Recommendations of the European Board for the Specialty Cardiology (EBSC) for education and training in basic cardiology in Europe' was published in 1996.[4] This document presents the recommendations for education and training in General Cardiology in Europe. The most important relevant EBSC document 'The Core Curriculum for the General Cardiologist', was published in 2006,[5] and updated in 2008[6] and 2013.[7] All together, these documents provide a potential framework for the education, training and certification of general cardiologists across Europe, by defining teaching, learning and assessment methods as well. The 2013 version of the General Cardiology Core Curriculum outlined the knowledge, the skills, and professionalism needed for the European general cardiologist, rather than those required for the sub-specialties. The Core curriculum can also be used for the continuing medical education of qualified European General Cardiologists. Beyond General Cardiology, other sub-specialties inside the EBSC (including percutaneous interventional cardiology) have also developed and defined their own core curricula.[8–11] Furthermore, EBSC Nurses and Allied Professionals also published recently their own core curriculum.[12] EAPCI Nurses and Allied Professionals are also preparing their own core curriculum.

Thus, the standards are already available and published. We now need to move forward and implement them in a uniform way across all European countries.

A formal interventional cardiology training program is in place in only a few countries in Europe and is not supported by binding legislation in the majority of cases. The practical consequences of this situation is that all cardiologists (and other doctors as well) are legally entitled to perform percutaneous interventions after finishing their specialty.

45.3 Interventional cardiology training in Europe: Current situation

A number of surveys on training and education in Europe, performed along the years showed very disappointing results:

- The assessment of trainees at the end of the training is largely heterogeneous throughout Europe, ranging from multiple choice questions (MCQs), to interview, oral examination and/or log book assessment.
- Training is not always organised in accordance with the recommendations of the European core curriculum.

- Duration of interventional cardiology training is highly variable throughout Europe (from 6 months to more than 3 years).
- The number of procedures required to be performed during training and the duration of the different parts of training is not clearly established and harmonised.
- Implementation, endorsement and the impact over the years of the core curriculum at a national level is highly variable in all the European countries.

A number of reasons were identified in some of these surveys that potentially explain the lack of implementation of the core curriculum at a national level:

- It is being implemented or it is a work in progress.
- Technically not achievable.
- Could be implemented at regional level, but difficult at national level.
- The certification process is under the responsibility of Government/Ministry of Health/Regional Health Authorities and National Cardiac Societies have no authority or are not involved.

Therefore, it is quite obvious that the harmonisation of interventional cardiology training in Europe is a top priority and many efforts should be developed to achieve this goal in the years to come.

It is therefore essential to establish the minimum standards for a training of excellence in interventional cardiology in all European countries. This proposal of a minimum standard of training and education for interventional cardiologists would provide a significantly improvement to the standard of care for cardiovascular patients in Europe, and it would facilitate the free movement of interventional cardiologists and patients across borders.

This harmonisation should be able to fit the national reality and deal with the specific requirements, health strategies, legislation and regulations that govern safe medical practice at the national level.

45.4 Interventional cardiology training in Europe: The standards

The 2013' ESC Core Curriculum establishes during the General Cardiology training no specific numbers needed to be achieved by the trainees. However, it states that the trainees are expected to obtain a Level III competence for coronary and LV angiography, and a Level I competence for percutaneous interventions.[7]

According to this document,[7] Level I means experience of selecting the appropriate diagnostic or therapeutic modality and interpreting results or choosing an appropriate treatment for which the patient should be referred. This level of competency does not include performing a technique, but participation in procedures during training may be valuable. In Level III, the trainee must be able independently to recognise the indication, perform the technique or procedure, interpret the data and manage the complications.

The recommended duration of postgraduate education and training for the Subspecialty of Interventional Cardiology has been defined in a document published in 2006 after extensive discussion within EAPCI and the national working groups of interventional cardiology. It defined a minimum duration of 2 years, divided into four semesters with a stepwise approach.[8]

At the beginning, the trainee is expected to start dealing with the preparation of the patient for the diagnosis and/or intervention and assist the supervisor or other experienced operator performing the interventional procedure. It is recommended that the trainee starts to act as primary operator in simple interventions under close supervision and assists in the most complex percutaneous procedures till they reach a level of competence to allow them to act as a primary independent operator. Therefore, apprenticeship is key for the training process in interventional cardiology. Since the beginning, the trainees must be involved in assessment of indications and contraindications, patient risk based on their clinical and angiographic characteristics, and in the procedure planning. The trainee must attend at least 240 hours of training sessions (study and postgraduate courses) during the 2 years of the training in order to allow the trainee to master the different topics included in the EAPCI syllabus.

The minimum requirements for interventional training according to the EAPCI curriculum are presented in Table 45.1.

The interventional cardiologist may decide, after completion of general training, to develop additional knowledge and skills in specific areas such as peripheral or valve interventions. However, beyond specific interventional cardiology experience in these specific areas must also be part of the general training in order to have a basic high standard knowledge of these areas.[8]

Assessment of skills is an essential aspect of the training period, without which it is impossible to evaluate the excellence of a training program. Implementation of a regular, structured and formally documented assessment is crucial for the successful application of the core curriculum and evaluation of the excellence of training.

This should include assessments of knowledge (formative and summative), directly observed procedures and practical skills (online) logbooks. Where available, the appropriate use of simulation (applicable both to training and assessment) is also recommended. A dedicated website has been developed to assist interventional trainees and trainers to acquire and certify their knowledge, using on-line resources or entering certificates of attendance and their procedures, confirmed by their supervisor. The ESCeL/EAPCI platform can provide all these features and harmonise training across the different European countries and beyond.

45.5 The harmonisation of interventional cardiology training in Europe: The ESCeL/EAPCI platform role

The EAPCI education committee has worked to develop an e-learning electronic tool intended to support the harmonisation of education and training, as well as the assessments necessary to make sure that the different objectives of training are fulfilled by the trainees. One example of these electronic tools is the ESCeL platform (Figure 45.1) which can deliver the EAPCI Core Curriculum standards worldwide (http://learn.escardio.org/percutaneous-interventions/homepage.aspx). ESCeL/EAPCI provides up-to-date knowledge to the trainee, allows formative assessment, verifies the implementation of the training curriculum and allows practical skills assessment through a patient logbook, a patient safety logbook, a procedure logbook and a direct observation of practical skills (DOPS). Moreover, it allows (on a voluntary basis) assessment of the professional development of the trainee during the training period. In the absence of European or national defined standards a tool like the ESCeL/EAPCI platform is highly recommended as

Table 45.1 Minimum requirements for interventional training according to the EAPCI curriculum

Duration	
Number of PCIs as first operator	200
Number of primary PCIs as first operator	50
Preparation of the patient and follow-up after the procedure	mandatory
Formal training	30 full days
Peripheral interventions	optional
Structural interventions	optional
MSCT analysis and interpretation	optional

Source: Carlo di Mario Gilard M et al., *The PCR-EAPCI Textbook*, 2012.

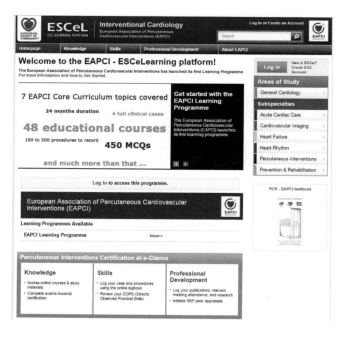

Figure 45.1 The ESCeL/EAPCI platform.

a guarantee of the excellence in education and training in interventional cardiology.

To support this harmonisation of standards, after successfully finishing the training program contained as outlined within ESCeL, the trainee should undertake a summative MCQ exam. This must be a standardised examination, developed at European level, and based upon the EAPCI Core Curriculum and EAPCI/EuroPCR textbook. These MCQs must be produced by a specialised committee and be audited by an independent committee. It is clear, however, that the focus must be centred on the need to pass a summative exam in order to receive the final diploma, certifying that the trainee went through an excellent training program and acquired the required level of knowledge.

45.6 Interventional cardiology training in Europe: The level of excellence

In order to become an independent operator, the trainee should be involved in the management of an appropriate number of patients with a various mix of indications, taking into consideration several well-defined requirements.[8]

45.7 Requirements for the training institutions and local trainers

45.7.1 Requirements for training institutions

To reach excellence the training institution alone or as part of a structured and organised collaboration should have the necessary facilities to ensure that trainees can fulfil all the aspects of the EAPCI Core Curriculum together with the regulatory requirements for cardiology and postgraduate training at national level and ensure that they will be exposed to a sufficient number of patients and procedures in order to develop the required skills and experience.[8]

45.7.2 Requirements for local trainers

The trainers should be recognised by the National Training Authority, they should be training experts and they should fulfil specific criteria.[8]

45.8 The future training of interventional cardiology training in Europe

With the help of education experts, it will be possible in the near future to include within the ESCeL/EAPCI project totally new concepts such as evidence-based education and training and objective clinical performance evaluation. With the continuous use of ESCeL we will be able to analyse an extraordinary amount of valuable data (evidence). Moreover, randomised clinical trials on education and training will generate additional, high-quality evidence in this much-neglected area. All this information will allow us to identify gaps (needs assessment) and to design better education and training for the future.

Thus far, clinical performance evaluation has been limited to demonstrating the number of procedures the trainee needs to achieve in a specific period of time, together with a subjective evaluation of the trainee's technical and cognitive skills by the mentor. There are, however, better ways of evaluating clinical performance by using innovative techniques within the ESCeL platform. One of these techniques is certainly biomedical simulation.[13–15] Biomedical simulation allows the objective evaluation of performance by measuring the number of errors, the quality of the decisions that are taken, the time needed to achieve the goal and if the goal is achieved. However, simulation is not widely available, and this lack of availability is expected to continue for the near future. One good alternative is the development of 'micro clinical cases' that are created with the purpose of measuring the trainees' performance in the presence of their mentor. By using these 'micro clinical cases' the mentors will be able to evaluate in an objective way several clinical performance parameters and to measure trainees' progression.

These concepts are the new frontiers of the medical education and training in cardiology and are expected to be available within the ESCeL/EAPCI project in the near future.

The final goal of all these projects is to improve and harmonise education and training across Europe. In this harmonisation process national intervention cardiovascular societies play a key role. The role of the EAPCI in this process is to propose a consensus framework and provide tools for its implementation (methodology, technology, products). Using this combined strategy at the European level and at the national level harmonisation is likely to occur.

45.9 Conclusion

There is a large heterogeneity of interventional cardiology training and education in European countries. Taking into consideration the reality of the free movement of doctors and patients across borders, the cardiology community feels a strong need for the harmonisation of training and education of European health care professionals. The EAPCI already produced and published the standards, and recently developed the tool to deliver these standards: the ESCeL/EAPCI platform. A challenge for the future is the diffusion of the platform to include thousands, and not hundreds, of trainees from all European countries. Although this project meets many challenges it also opens a universe of new possibilities for the future of our profession and particularly for the delivery of a high standard of interventional treatment to our cardiovascular patients.

References

1. Lozano R et al. Global and regional mortality from 235 causes of death for 20 age groups in 1990 and 2010: A systematic analysis for the Global Burden of Disease Study 2010. *Lancet* 2012; 380: 2095–128.

2. Townsend N et al. Cardiovascular disease in Europe—Epidemiological update 2015. *Eur Heart J* October 21, 2015; 36(40): 2696–705. doi:10.1093/eurheartj/ehv428. Epub 2015 Aug 25.

3. European Commission DG Health and Consumer Protection & Présidence Luxembourgeoise du Conseil de l'Union européenne.The Luxembourg Declaration on Patient Safety. Available at http://ec.europa.eu/health/ph_overview/Documents/ev_20050405_rd01_en.pdf

4. The Executive Committee of the European Board for the Specialty of Cardiology. Recommendations of the European Board for the Specialty Cardiology (EBSC) for education and training in basis cardiology in Europe. *Eur Heart J* 1996; 17: 996–1000.

5. Core Curriculum for the General Cardiologist. The ESC Education Committee. 2006. Booklet published by the European Society of Cardiology.

6. Core Curriculum for the General Cardiologist. The ESC Education Committee. 2008. Booklet published by the European Society of Cardiology.

7. Gillebert TC et al. ESC core curriculum for the general cardiologist. *Eur Heart J* August 2013; 34(30): 2381–411.

8. Di Mario C et al. Curriculum and syllabus for interventional cardiology subspeciality training in Europe. *Eurointervention* 2006; 2: 31–36.

9. Acute Cardiovascular Care Association Core Curriculum. Available at http://www.escardio.org/static_file/Escardio/Subspecialty/ACCA/core-curriculum-ACCA-2014-FINAL.pdf

10. European Association of Cardiovascular Imaging Core Syllabus. Available at http://www.escardio.org/Sub-specialty-communities/European-Association-of-Cardiovascular-Imaging-(EACVI)/Education/Core-Syllabus

11. Merino JL et al. Core curriculum for the heart rhythm specialist: Executive summary. *Europace* 2009; 11: 1381–6. doi:10.1093/europace/eup214 1381–1386.

12. Astin F et al. A core curriculum for the continuing professional development of nurses: Developed by the Education Committee on behalf of the Council on Cardiovascular Nursing and Allied Professions of the ESC. *Eur J Cardiovasc Nurs* 2015; 14(Suppl 2): S1–S17.

13. Carlo di Mario Gilard M et al. Percutaneous interventional cardiovascular medicine. In: *The PCR-EAPCI Textbook*, Europa edition, Vol. IV, Chap. 10, pp. 107–16, 2012.

14. Gosai J et al. Simulation in cardiology: State of the art. *Eur Heart J* April 1, 2015; 36(13): 777–83.

15. McGaghie WC et al. A critical review of simulation-based medical education research: 2003–2009. *Med Educ* 2010; 44: 50–63.

Training in interventional cardiology in the United States: Program accreditation and physician certification

SASAN RAEISSI, TAREK HELMY

46.1 Introduction

Physician competence is an essential component in the provision of optimal healthcare. Physicians must have the appropriate training, fund of knowledge, clinical decision-making and technical skills to deliver their services in a competent, caring manner and to attain optimal patient outcomes. Optimal outcome is most likely when operators select clinically appropriate patients for interventional procedures and perform these procedures at a requisite level of proficiency and competency. The United States has been at the forefront in training clinicians and setting quality standards in medical training, including the field of interventional cardiology.

The field has rapidly expanded since the early days of Andreas Gruentzig pioneering the first coronary balloon angioplasty in 1977, and has now evolved into a sub-specialty treating a wide range of both stable and acutely ill patients. Interventional cardiologists manage a broad spectrum of not only increasingly complex coronary artery diseases, but also other cardiovascular conditions like peripheral vascular and structural heart disease. This has been accompanied by rapid proliferation of scientific information facilitating the practice of evidence-based clinical medicine. However, these advances have led us to another challenge in the optimal training of fellows and physicians to assure achievement and maintenance of competence in this rapidly changing environment. This overview provides a perspective on the certification process of sub-specialty training in interventional cardiology in the United States. Since there can be variations amongst operators in cognitive knowledge and skill amongst procedures in technical difficulty, there is a potential for substantial variation in procedure safety and efficacy. Credentialing physicians in the United States to perform certain procedures is the responsibility of the governance of the local healthcare facility, as the healthcare systems and payers expect optimal care delivered in an efficient and cost-sensitive manner. The Joint Commission on the Accreditation of Healthcare Organizations (JCAHO) requires that medical staff privileges be granted to applicants by the Medical Executive Committee (MEC) and the Credentialing Committee in each hospital, based on their training, experience and skill set. Physicians are charged with the responsibility to establish the criteria that constitute professional competence and to evaluate their peers on the basis of such criteria. Obtaining a medical license in the respective state is usually one of the requirements for practice in a medical facility in the state. The US healthcare system relies, in part, on this process of granting and renewing clinical privileges to maintain quality.

The achievement and maintenance of standards for 'physician proficiency' in interventional cardiology is done through the American Board of Internal Medicine (ABIM) and the American Board of Medical Specialties (ABMS). Board certification is achieved after completing an American Council on Graduate Medical Education (ACGME) accredited training program and passing a standardized test administered through the ABMS. Interventional cardiology has recently been granted a sub-specialty designation, rather than the previous status as a sub-discipline of cardiovascular disease. The ACGME is the organization responsible for evaluating the standards that 'training programs' have to meet to receive accreditation. The initial guidelines for training in adult cardiovascular medicine were published in 1995 as a consensus statement from the American College of Cardiology (ACC); COre CArdiology Training Symposium (COCATS) held in Bethesda, Maryland. Subsequent updates were published as Core Cardiovascular Training Statement 2 (COCATS 2) in 2002, including additional task force reports to address training in vascular medicine, peripheral catheter-based interventions and cardiovascular magnetic resonance. Further revisions published in COCATS 3 in 2008 not only included how fellows-in-training (FITs) could develop expertise as comprehensive, multimodal cardiovascular imaging specialists, but also underscored the importance of the six core competencies formulated by the Accreditation Council for Graduate Medical Education (ACGME) in 1999:

1. Medical knowledge
2. Patient care
3. Interpersonal and communication skills
4. Professionalism
5. Practice-based learning and improvement
6. Systems-based practice

The latest iteration of COCATS 4 has the potential to transform cardiovascular fellowship training, making perhaps its most important advancement in 20 years. COCATS 4

is also corresponding to the development of the ACGME's Next Accreditation System (NAS). The NAS addresses public expectations for physician training. It stems from the philosophy that the twenty-first century physician should participate in a team-based healthcare system, use information technology, practice cost-effective medicine and function as a healthcare leader. With NAS, the ACGME sought to accomplish three missions:

1. Prepare physicians for team-based, cost-effective twenty-first century practice
2. Accelerate the ACGME's movement towards outcome-based rather than time-based accreditation
3. Mitigate the burden of the structure and process-based approach to facilitate innovative learning paradigms.

Most notably, COCATS 4 transitions to a competency-based curriculum with specific 'milestones'. Milestones are defined as the knowledge, skills, attitudes and other attributes for each of the ACGME competencies that describe the competence of a trainee from the beginning of training up to and beyond the level expected for unsupervised practice. The current competency-based curriculum in COCATS 4 not only represents a shift in focus from minimal case volume and exposure time requirements, but also underscores the emphasis on outcome-based evaluations, specific learner objectives and bidirectional evaluations. COCATS 4 allows programs and trainees more flexibility in structuring the fellowship training.

46.2 ACGME core competency components and curricular milestones for interventional cardiology fellowship training

Admission to an interventional cardiology training fellowship program requires completing an accredited fellowship in general cardiology, including all the core competencies associated with such training. Interventional cardiology training follows the same overall outline and requirements as relate to core competency components and curricular milestones for training.

46.2.1 Medical Knowledge for invasive diagnostic cardiology includes but is not limited to the following

1. Locate, appraise and assimilate information from scientific studies, guidelines and registries in order to identify knowledge and performance gaps, including indications/contraindications and potential complications of cardiac catheterisation for assessment of coronary, valvular, myocardial and basic adult congenital heart diseases.
2. Principles of radiation safety, and use and complications of contrast media and the role of renal protection measures.

3. Indications for, and clinical pharmacology of, anti-platelet and anticoagulant drugs and vasopressor and vasodilator agents used in the cardiac catheterization laboratory.
4. Normal cardiovascular haemodynamics of valvular, pericardial, pulmonary, and myocardial diseases
5. Methods to detect and estimate the magnitude of intra-cardiac and extra-cardiac shunts.
6. Vascular anatomy and physiology of the coronary and peripheral vasculature, and the indications and contraindications for, and complications of diagnostic procedures.
7. Indications and contraindications for, and the complications of, endomyocardial biopsy and pericardiocentesis.
8. Indications for, and the mechanisms of action of, mechanical circulatory support devices.
9. Indications for, and complications of, vascular access and closure strategies and devices.

46.2.2 Medical Knowledge for interventional cardiology includes but is not limited to the following

- Basic pathophysiology of development of atherosclerosis and coronary and peripheral vascular disease
- Advanced knowledge of performance and interpretation of invasive procedures including coronary and peripheral angiography, as well as hemodynamics of valvular and pericardial disease.
- Knowledge of interventional equipment including catheters, wires, and specialized devices used in the catheterization laboratory
- Knowledge of various types of balloons, stents, scaffolds, thrombectomy and atherectomy devices, and appropriate indications for use.
- Potential complications and how to manage them.
- Adjunctive pharmacologic therapy pre, intra, and post procedure.
- Different strategies for management of acute ST elevation myocardial infarction.
- Knowledge and management of cardiogenic shock, and mechanical circulatory support devices

46.2.3 Patient care and procedural skills

1. Skill to perform pre-procedural evaluation, assess appropriateness, obtain informed consent and plan procedure strategy.
2. Skill to perform venous and arterial access and obtain haemostasis.
3. Skill to perform right and left heart catheterization, including coronary and peripheral angiography
4. Skill to analyse haemodynamic, ventriculographic and angiographic data and to integrate with clinical findings for patient management.
5. Skill to manage post-procedural patients, including

complications andcoordination of care.
6. Skill to perform pericardiocentesis, and endomyocardial biopsy.
7. Skill to perform percutaneous coronary interventions.
8. Skill to perform peripheral, carotid, valvular and structural heartinterventions.
9. Skill to insert and manage percutaneous left ventricular support devices.

46.2.4 Systems-based practice

1. Coordinate care in an interdisciplinary approach for patient management, including transition of care.
2. Utilise cost-awareness and risk/benefit analysis in patient care.
3. Recognizes system deficiencies and strives for improvements.

46.2.5 Practice-based learning and improvement

1. Obtain knowledge and information from scientific studies, guidelines and registries in order to identify knowledge and performance gaps within the practice.
2. Review the practice with the objective to identify deficiencies, and improve on them.
3. Be receptive to audits and feedback, and initiate quality improvement efforts accordingly.

46.2.6 Professionalism

1. Practice within the scope of expertise and technical skills.
2. Know and promote adherence to guidelines and Appropriate Use Criteria.
3. Interact respectfully with patients, families and all members of the healthcare team, including ancillary and support staff.
4. Exhibits ethical behavior and integrity in the practice.
5. Accepts responsibility for actions and mistakes and learns from them.

46.2.7 Interpersonal and communication skills

1. Communicate with and educate patients and families across a broad range of socioeconomic, ethnic and cultural backgrounds, including obtaining informed consent.

2. Communicate and work effectively with physicians and other professionals on the healthcare team regarding procedure findings, treatment plans and follow-up care coordination.
3. Complete procedure records and communicate testing results to physicians and patients in an effective and timely manner.

46.3 ACGME requirements for interventional cardiology training programs

46.3.1 Duration and qualifications

Interventional cardiology is a sub-specialty training program, allowing candidates who complete the program to achieve level 3 certification and to qualify for the interventional cardiology board examination sponsored by the ABIM/ABMS. The duration of the interventional fellowship is at least 12 dedicated months, although some programs offer longer training fellowships to include research time or further sub-specialty training in peripheral or structural heart disease. Candidates must complete an ACGME-accredited general cardiology fellowship prior to starting interventional training

46.3.2 Faculty

According to the ACGME requirements, there must be a sufficient number of 'key' clinical faculty with documented qualifications to supervise the interventional cardiology fellows. A specific ratio of the number of key faculty to the number of fellows (1: 1.5 respectively) in the program must be observed Key clinical faculty must maintain current certification in interventional cardiology by the ABIM. They also must foster an environment of learning, scholarship, and research. They must regularly participate in clinical, rounds, journal clubs and conferences. Faculty are encouraged to participate in publication in peer-reviewed journals or chapters in textbooks; publish or present case reports or clinical series at local, regional or national professional and scientific meetings; participate in national committees or educational organisations. The program should provide the faculty with resources for faculty development to ensure the progression of both faculty members and the program

46.3.2.1 Training program director

There must be a single program director to be available at the primary clinical site with the responsibility for the operation of all aspects of the program; clinical, educational and research, as well as compliance with ACGME requirements. The program director should have protected and dedicated percentage of time and effort to the fellowship, including time for administration of the program. The program director must board certified in the field of cardiology and interventional cardiology and have at least 5 years of experience as an active faculty member in an ACGME-accredited cardiovascular disease fellowship or interventional cardiology fellowship.

46.3.3 Resources

Inpatient and outpatient systems should be available to facilitate both patient care and the educational experience of the fellows.

46.3.3.1 Equipment

Cardiac catheterisation laboratories, each equipped with high-quality x-ray digital imaging, and hemodynamic recording devices, a wide spectrum of interventional devices and resuscitative equipment. The primary site catheterization laboratory must perform a minimum of 400 interventional procedures per year, and each secondary training site must perform a minimum of 200 interventional procedures per year. The laboratory must have access to the support personnel to ensure radiation exposure to patients and staff is both monitored and minimised. The presence of equipment for assessing both coronary physiology, such as fractional flow reserve, and coronary and structural heart anatomy, such as intravascular or intra-cardiac ultrasound, is strongly recommended. Programs must have onsite access to all core cardiovascular services, including a cardiac critical care facility, cardiac surgery, anaesthesia, echocardiography and stress testing. Furthermore, the fellows must maintain a continuity out-patient clinic supervised by a core clinical faculty for patient evaluation, as well as post procedure follow-up.

46.3.4 Training components: curriculum, clinical experience and scholarly activities

46.3.4.1 Didactic elements

The core curriculum includes a didactic program based upon the core knowledge content. In addition to becoming familiar with the many manifestations of coronary artery disease, trainees must also gain experience evaluation and management of patients with valvular, myocardial, peripheral vascular and congenital heart disease. The program must afford each fellow the resources to achieve these educational goals. The curriculum should coincide with the ACGME and COCATS outlines for medical knowledge required for interventional cardiology trainees. Several documents from the ACC and SCAI, as well as online resources (fellow in Training FIT program from SCAI as one example) have also attempted to provide a platform for the interventional cardiology didactic curriculum. Beyond the didactic component, other forms of educational activities are encouraged, which may include all or some of the following:

- Case discussion conferences, which may be a combined medical/surgical conference. in context with history, physical examination and non-invasive findings – indications, complications and management strategies
- Journal clubs and research conferences
- Patient safety or quality improvement conferences
- Peer-review conferences

46.3.4.2 Clinical and procedural experience

Variation in case exposure for the trainees is strongly recommended. The nature of a trainee's participation in a given procedure varies depending on the procedure's complexity and the trainee's experience level. Faculty members must teach and supervise the fellows in the performance and interpretation of procedures, which must be documented in each fellow's record. Procedural components include the following: Pre-procedural evaluation is performed to assess appropriateness and plan procedure strategy. This should include a history and physical examination, an informed consent and a pre-procedural note that includes indications for the procedure as per Appropriate Use Criteria (AUC), risks of the procedure, alternatives to the procedure and understanding by the patient. Performance of the procedure by the trainee is allowed at a level appropriate to their experience, always under the direct supervision of a faculty member. Trainees are expected to progress in procedural exposure and skills throughout their training. Trainees should participate in the interpretation of the haemodynamic and angiographic data obtained during the procedure, and the preparation of the procedure report as well as formulation of treatment plans. Fellows should have active involvement in pre- and post-procedural management inside and outside of the catheterisation laboratory, including management of any complications, patient education and arranging follow-up. The interventional fellow must maintain a continuity outpatient clinic supervised by an attending interventional cardiologist.

46.3.4.3 Fellows' scholarly activities

Each program must provide an opportunity for fellows to participate in research or other scholarly activities, including

1. A research project (with faculty mentorship)
2. Participation with the faculty in the initiation and conduct of clinical trials within the department
3. Participation in quality assurance/quality improvement or process improvement projects
4. Fellows are strongly encouraged to submit cases for peer-reviewed publication, or presentation in conferences.

46.3.5 Evaluation of competency

Fellow evaluation is ultimately the responsibility of the program director.

The program director appoints the Clinical Competency Committee, which is composed of at least three members of the program faculty. The committee reviews all fellow evaluations semi-annually and assures the reporting of milestones evaluations of each fellow to ACGME as well as providing each fellow with documented semi-annual evaluation of performance with feedback. The committee also advises the program director regarding fellow progress, including promotion, remediation and dismissal. The faculty must discuss evaluations with each fellow at least every 3 months.

46.3.5.1 The program provides objective assessments of the fellows' competencies on

1. Patient care
2. Procedural skills
3. Medical knowledge
4. Practice-based learning and improvement
5. Interpersonal and communication skills
6. Professionalism
7. Systems-based practice

The evaluation tools include Chart-stimulated recall, conference presentation, direct observation, multi-source evaluation, reflection and self-assessment, logbook and simulation. Evaluations of the fellows are also provided by technical staff, nurses, and other members of the multidisciplinary team.

Trainees should maintain records of participation and advancement in the form of a Health Insurance Portability and Accountability Act (HIPAA)-compliant electronic database or logbook that meets ACGME/ABIM reporting standards and summarises pertinent clinical information (e.g. number of cases, diversity of referral sources, diagnoses, disease severity, outcomes and disposition).

46.3.5.2 Milestones

The progress of the fellows in all aspects of training is monitored and evaluated based on the "milestones" system proposed in the "New Accreditation System" (NAS). Specific competencies are evaluated in a gradated manner based on the level of training of the fellows. The evaluation has different levels ranging from "unsatisfactory" where specific deficiencies are identified, up to the level of "competent to practice independently". There is also an aspirational designation for fellows who exceed expectations in certain aspects of their training. The overall performance of each fellow in training is then reported to the local institution Graduate Medical Education (GME) and periodically reported to the ACGME.

46.3.6 Fatigue management/mitigation

Programs must educate all faculty members and fellows to recognise the signs of illness, fatigue and sleep deprivation. Fellows who suffer from fatigue must inform faculty and are encouraged to refrain from patient care until fatigue is managed and resolved. Strategic napping, especially after 16 hours of continuous duty is strongly suggested.

46.3.7 Fellows duty hours (daytime and night float)

Duty periods of fellows may be scheduled to a maximum of 24 hours of continuous duty in the hospital. Duty hours must be limited to 80 hours/week, averaged over a 4-week period, inclusive of all in-house call activities and all moonlighting. Fellows must be scheduled for a minimum of 1 day free of duty every week, averaged over 4 weeks. Fellows must not be assigned additional clinical responsibilities after 24 hours of continuous in-house duty. Fellows must not be scheduled for more than six consecutive nights of night float. Moonlighting is voluntary, compensated, medically related work not related with training requirements. This activity is allowed by most training programs as long as it does not interfere with the ability of the fellow to achieve the goals and objectives of the educational program. The time spent by fellows in moonlighting must be counted towards the 80-hour maximum weekly hour limit.

The principles and practice of audit in coronary intervention

PETER F LUDMAN

47.1 Introduction to clinical audit

For patients to benefit from our increasingly comprehensive understanding of the pathophysiology of disease and its treatment, we need to be able to apply correct therapies to appropriate patients in a timely fashion guided by the results of clinical trials and observational studies.

Clinical audit is the process by which we can assess whether or not we are applying this knowledge to treat patients in the best possible way and as such underpins the delivery of high-quality care. An accepted definition has been provided by the National Institute for Health and Clinical Excellence (NICE) in their 'Principles for Best Practice in Clinical Audit':[1]

a quality improvement process that seeks to improve patient care and outcomes through systematic review of care against explicit criteria and the implementation of change. Aspects of the structure, processes and outcomes of care are selected and systematically evaluated against explicit criteria. Where indicated, changes are implemented at an individual, team or service level and further monitoring is used to confirm improvement in healthcare delivery.

Thus actual care provided is measured and compared with what would be considered optimal care, and a process is incorporated that seeks to improve care if found to fall short of expectations. Clinical audit is therefore founded on evidence from research, addresses the practicalities of providing routine care to patients, highlights both good practice and deficiencies and provides a framework to enable improvements to be made.

To place clinical audit in perspective, it is helpful to look at other ways in which clinical practice can be assessed. 'Peer review' is an important example, where clinicians have their practice assessed by others in their profession. The aim is to provide feedback and thereby support reflection on practice. The intent is that this will lead to improvements in the quality of care. Often, individual patient cases are discussed with peers to determine, with the benefit of hindsight, whether the best care was given. Peer review might look at the entire case load or focus on cases with specific characteristics (unusual cases, cases where a specific issue needs to be addressed such as appropriateness of care or cases deemed potentially problematic for other reasons). 'Morbidity and Mortality' meetings should be a routine part of clinical practice and describe peer review when the focus is on cases where outcomes have been poor, to see if lessons can be learnt.

Peer review may take place within a hospital or be organised between care settings. Some of the professional societies organise national peer review schemes as part of their ongoing commitment to professional development.[2]

47.2 Clinical governance

A disparate group of service improvement processes and concepts were brought together in a framework called 'Clinical Governance' in the United Kingdom in a 1997

White Paper entitled 'The New NHS: Modern, Dependable'. A coherent structure was thus formally established and set clinical audit in a wider context. 'Clinical Governance', was defined as the systematic approach to maintaining and improving the quality of patient care in a health system. It is a framework that embodies three key attributes: recognisably high standards of care; transparent responsibility and accountability for those standards and a constant dynamic of improvement.

Clinical governance is composed of six service improvement processes that work together to improve patient care. These include

1. Clinical audit.
2. Education and training: A recognition of a continually evolving scientific evidence base, such that much of what was learned during training becomes outdated. Continued professional development is required to ensure physicians are aware of current medical literature and thus able to provide best care for their patients.
3. Clinical effectiveness: Efficacy of therapies should not be considered in isolation. Decisions regarding optimal practice include an understanding of appropriateness, comparative cost-effectiveness and safety of different therapies.
4. Research and development: The application of new research findings into clinical practice and guideline development is pivotal to improving patient care and underpins the mechanism of clinical audit. The professional societies in both Europe (European Society of Cardiology) and the United States (American College of Cardiology and American Heart Association) have formed comprehensive and carefully structured guideline groups whose remit is to provide a synthesis of current evidence resulting in up-to-date recommendations for best practice across all the sub-specialty areas of cardiology and cardiothoracic surgery.
5. Openness: Poor practice can thrive if it occurs in isolation, out of the scrutiny of peers. Openness for both the profession and the public increasingly dominates an era where information via the Internet is ubiquitous. Whilst a careful balance must be struck to respect appropriate individual patient and practitioner confidentiality, it is clear that in the past, the traditional paternalistic approach to medicine biased this balance far too much towards professional secrecy. This has not been an acceptable position for many years and has been slow to change. The concept of openness was part of the specific recommendations of the 2013 Berwick report into patient safety after poor standards of care were identified in a hospital in England (Mid Staffordshire NHS Trust)[3], 'transparency should be complete, timely and unequivocal. All data on quality and safety, whether assembled by government, organisations, or professional societies, should be shared in a timely fashion with all parties who want it, including, in accessible form, with the public.'

6. Risk management: Addressing and minimising risks to patients, physicians and organisations.

47.3 Domains of clinical audit

Clinical audit can be divided into four domains, addressing different aspects of patient care:

1. Structure: This defines the environment in which treatment is being delivered. This includes issues such as the number of percutaneous coronary intervention (PCI) labs for a given population, the equipment available, the staffing of such labs, the level of services available and the volume of activity undertaken.
2. Appropriateness: An assessment of whether or not an intervention was indicated given the clinical setting and patient's presenting features and co-morbidities. Included would be appropriate use of PCI (rather than alternative therapies), the use of correct adjunctive therapies and so on.
3. Process: The mechanisms by which care was delivered, for example, the speed of delivery of primary PCI, length of stay, completeness of re-vascularisation and timing of staged procedures.
4. Outcome: Whilst a focus on major adverse cardiac and cerebrovascular events is appropriate in higher risk PCI, these events are extremely rare in PCI for stable angina, and other measures dominate in providing a picture of the quality of care such as improvement in symptoms and quality of life, and other patient reported outcomes.

47.4 Mechanisms of clinical audit

47.4.1 The classical audit cycle

The process of clinical audit has been described as a loop or spiral. An area of interest is selected and standards that define optimal care are identified from the literature. Clinical practice is then measured against these standards using either prospectively or retrospectively collected data. If there are areas where practice falls short of these standards, then a strategy to improve care is defined and implemented. Closing the 'loop' involves a repeat audit to assess, if the suggested changes to practice have occurred and standards have improved. Continued loops are needed to monitor practice. The first part of this process involves a 'Quality Assurance' process – a way in which care provision can be measured, and if satisfactory provides assurance that all is well. The second part of the process places emphasis on implementing change and using repeat assessment to aim for sustained improvement. This has been described as a 'Quality Improvement' process.

It is in the first part of this cycle that key aspects of the national audits dominate. Here, the use of observational data for benchmarking and risk adjustment have a pivotal role, and so are more focused on the quality assurance aspect of a clinical audit. Benchmarking facilitates the full classical audit cycle, that underpins a subsequent focused assessment of specific aspects of care and also the ongoing monitoring of standards.

47.4.2 Registry data for audit – 'Benchmarking'

The literature of randomised clinical trials (RCT) cannot provide us with a measure of what might be achievable in the treatment of patients presenting in a variety of different healthcare settings. The national assessment of a primary PCI program requires us to compare the rapidity with which each centre treats patients presenting with stent thrombosis (ST) elevation myocardial infarction. These comparisons will highlight centres performing well and also by comparison those centres where improvements are required. These comparative data can stimulate a more focused assessment using classical audit cycles to address specific issues, and lessons can be learnt from the better performing units. Thus 'benchmarking' has an important role in the audit process. The comparison of centres, even for a statistic as simple as the number of cases treated within a certain time window, is not completely without difficulty. The data need to be presented in a way that helps to provide an intuitive understanding of issues that relate to statistical variation. As an example, Figure 47.1 shows the way data regarding delays to primary PCI are presented in the British Cardiovascular Intervention Society's audit of PCI in the United Kingdom.

Centres treating fewer cases towards the left of the plot may have a larger range of time delays by random statistical variation than those treating large numbers. This is why the confidence limits are funnel-shaped and using these limits

helps us understand which centres fall outside the variation that might be expected by chance. In this figure, there is unlikely to be a statistically significant difference in the performance between centres A and B even though there are large differences in the actual percentage of patients being treated within 90 minutes. Centre C appears to be doing well, but a focus on the delays in centre D is warranted, though centre A has even poorer results. This is because the larger number of cases performed by D increases the confidence with which they can be identified as performing poorly, and they lie below the red line that represents the 3 standard deviation (SD) boundary, whilst centre A is actually above the green 2 SD boundary. As with all analyses of data, this sort of display can only serve as a guide because of methodological issues that include the problems of multiple statistical comparisons and of over dispersion (some of which are discussed below).

The audit process is dependent on the standards selected to define optimal care, and yet, these 'standards' may be elusive. The difficulty lies with the application of RCT data to the treatment of unselected populations. Whilst RCTs provide a very high level of scientific rigor when assessing therapeutic effects of different treatments in a clinical arena, there are important limitations to RCTs that limit the validity of their application to treat patients. The process of randomisation is an excellent way to ensure that the characteristics of patients in each of the arms of a trial are similar, leaving the only difference being the therapy under investigation. Nevertheless, patients recruited into such trials usually have characteristics quite different from the features of the overall population being treated. The problem is that because of the logistics of being involved in a trial, the requirement for informed consent, the ability for patients to understand the principles of trial recruitment and a long list of exclusion

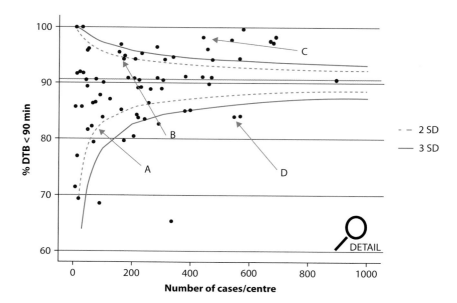

Figure 47.1 Treatment of patients with ST elevation myocardial infarction by primary PCI. Each dot represents a PCI centre and shows the percentage of cases that centre treated within 90 minutes of the patient's arrival time. The green and red lines show the 2 and 3 SD confidence limits respectively. (DTB, door-to-balloon time; SD, standard deviation.)

criteria for most trials patients who end up being recruited are often markedly different from the general population of patients in the 'real world' with the condition being treated. They are usually fitter, of a higher socio-economic group and with less co-morbid conditions than patients treated in every day practice. These features and the study protocols also mean they are more likely to have higher levels of compliance with medication during follow-up. This limits the ability for RCTs to assess treatment effects and safety in high-risk populations and limits the applicability of trial results, because many of the patients being treated would have been excluded from the trials on which we base the evidence of benefit from a particular treatment. High cost also limits the number of patients who can be recruited and the length of time they can be followed after intervention.

An illustration of these issues was provided by Hordijk-Trion[4] who looked at the characteristics of the participants of 14 major RCTs that had compared coronary artery bypass surgery and percutaneous intervention and set these against the 4713 patients enrolled into the 'all comer' registry of the Euro Heart Survey on Coronary Revascularisation. As few as about 11% in the survey would have been eligible for inclusion in the RCTs, and even using only the major exclusion criteria, only 36% would have been trial eligible. In an analysis of the ACC/AHA clinical practice guidelines, Tricoci showed that only 11% of the recommendations were based on level A evidence (i.e. from multiple RCT).[5]

If we look at some recent trials, the randomised trial of preventive angioplasty in myocardial infarction (PRAMI) screened 2428 patients for randomisation, but less than 20% (465) were actually randomised, leaving less than 10% in each of the arms of the trial.[6] In an open label 'all comers' trial COMPARE II, only 26% of screen patients were enrolled.[7]

These limitations highlight the role for registry data and observational research to help inform us about the outcomes of interventions in 'all comer' populations, many of whom would never have been randomised into the trial that supports the treatment they are being offered. National audit involves the collection of data on entire populations being treated, and provides not only data that can be analysed for benchmarking, but also that can be fed into observational research.

47.5 Risk adjustment

The limitations in RCTs mean that we need to use registry data to provide benchmarks in clinical audits where we are assessing the quality of treatment provided to unselected patients, including those at high risk and with extensive co-morbidities. Whilst a benchmark for simple parameters is not problematic, if we are to try to audit outcomes from interventions, we need to develop tools to adjust for the disparate risk of patients being treated.

If we consider mortality after PCI, a patient's presenting syndrome and co-morbidity dominates the likely outcome, irrespective of quality of care. A patient presenting to a hospital in cardiogenic shock has a probability of dying

that approaches 50% in spite of high quality treatment, and conversely even with unimpressive attention to detail, a stable patient being treated by PCI will have a mortality of less than 1%. This is because the possible influence of the quality of PCI on outcomes is relatively limited. A study into cause of death provides some insight. Of those patients who died within 30 days of a PCI, 42% died of a non-cardiac cause (mainly sepsis, neurological or pulmonary causes) and of the remainder, 16% died from a cardiac cause unrelated to PCI (for example pump failure), leaving 42% of deaths potentially related to the PCI procedure itself.[8]

To attempt to dissect out the quality of care provided from the background risk requires the development of methods that can be used to compare expected outcomes with those observed, and the use of statistical tools to decide whether any differences measured are likely to be due to the play of chance or genuinely poor or excellent performance.

47.6 Models

The first stage in the development of a risk adjustment model is to identify a large dataset that includes all the types of patients being treated in a contemporary era. That dataset needs to have a high degree of data completeness and accuracy and include all the factors which are likely to have an impact on the outcome being measured. Finding such datasets is difficult. In PCI, many models have been developed using the data collected as part of national audit programs and attempts have also been made to use administrative datasets – which are large and comprehensive but may lack sufficient clinical detail.[9–11]

The dataset is then analysed using logistic regression to find independent risk factors that are associated with the outcome of interest and mathematical techniques are used to create a model that takes into account the fact that these factors may have differing 'influences' on outcome. A factor such as the presence of pre-procedural cardiogenic shock is more strongly associated with adverse outcome than, for example, being a diabetic. The model takes the form of a formula that when provided with the specific characteristics of a patient being treated, gives a prediction of expected outcome (for example a 5% risk of mortality at 30 days). Most models are then analysed to see how well they work. This is done by assessing their calibration and discrimination. Calibration assesses the agreement between observed and predicted outcomes. It can be assessed by looking at the 'goodness of fit' using the Hosmer–Lemeshow statistic. Discrimination measures how well the model correctly separates those that go on to have the outcome from those who do not. The c-statistic is usually used, though it has limitations.[12] It corresponds to the area under the receiver operating characteristic curve (AUC). The higher the value the better the model discriminates between true positive predictions and true negative predictions. An AUC of 0.5 is no better than a random coin toss (i.e. it has no ability to discriminate at all). AUCs of over 0.75 are generally considered to have clinical utility. A model is usually developed in a training dataset and then applied to data collected over a different time period for validation.

There are several potential problems to be considered. If a data item is not part of the dataset, then it cannot be used in the model. An example is 'frailty'. This may be an important determinant of outcome but if not in the dataset its role remains undefined. All data items should be capable of objective measurement. Age is usually easy to define, as for example is serum creatinine. However, some of the most important features are more difficult to define objectively, such as cardiogenic shock. Data such as cardiac output and left atrial pressure are usually not available at the time of emergency PCI and so the diagnosis often remains a subjective clinical one, with the possibility of disparate identification by different operators. It must be remembered that a procedural dataset will only include those patients who actually received treatment. In addition, as treatment techniques, equipment and adjunctive pharmacology change, a model will become out of date, and calibration and discrimination may drift.

47.7 Definition of outliers

Once a model has been developed, it can be used to assess outcomes from centres or individual operators by taking into account differences in case mix. The observed outcomes are compared with those predicted from the model, and statistical tools are used to decide if the differences are statistically significant or not.

Though this process is at the heart of clinical audit and the concept is clear, the statistical methodology is fraught with complexity. There is no single 'correct' way to make these assessments and getting the balance right can be difficult. Considering only extreme outlying performance to define an outlier risks inadequately protecting patients, yet, taking lower cut points risks incorrectly criticising perfectly acceptable performance. Understanding the potential limitations of the methods used helps guide an appropriate balance and gives perspective in the overall assessment of an individual's or a centre's performance.

47.7.1 Public reporting

In embracing openness, there has been a move towards the public reporting of individual operator outcomes which has increased the focus on the methods used to try to identify poor and excellent practice.

In New York State, public reports of cardiothoracic surgical outcomes started in the mid-1990s. In the United Kingdom, outcomes from cardiothoracic surgery have been reported for several years and for PCI since 2012. Whilst this is an important step that embraces a much needed increase in transparency and openness, there is the potential for unintended consequences that may reduce the very quality of care that is intended to be enhanced. The concern is that of causing risk-averse behaviour. This term is used to describe a situation where an operator might be reluctant

to treat patients at high risk because if they do badly, that operator will appear to have poor performance. Yet, it is just those patients with the most co-morbidity and at highest risk of dying, who often have the most to gain from intervention. A risk adjustment model should be able to adjust for these factors, but anxiety that the model may fail to adequately adjust might be enough to alter behaviour. Studies of human behaviour strongly support the concept that negative emotions carry more weight than positive ones.[13]

Observational evidence for risk-averse behaviour is persuasive, with good studies both in cardiothoracic surgery and PCI.[14-19]

One way to try and limit this potential problem is to exclude certain clinical scenarios from risk-adjusted outcomes reporting. A good example is patients who present with out-of-hospital cardiac arrest. It is acknowledged that no model has yet been validated to adjust for risk of PCI performed in this setting.[20] It is likely that there are even more factors than usual that are unrelated to PCI quality than those that might influence patient survival. Examples include the location of cardiac arrest, the quality of CRP, the presenting rhythm and timing of defibrillation. A high quality or timely PCI cannot help a patient who has irreversible neurological injury and neurological status cannot be assessed until after emergency PCI has been performed.

47.7.2 Statistical considerations

All risk-adjusted methods are dependent on the appropriate calibration and sensitivity of the risk adjustment model, and the accuracy of the data recorded for the cases being analysed. In addition, the mathematics behind the application of models to the assessment of outlier status is complex, and several different statistical methods can be used. Each method has benefits and limitations, and different methods can lead to identification of different outliers. The issues include problems such as over dispersion and adjustments that might need to be made when multiple statistical comparisons are made. This can result in some unintuitive conclusions. Commonly cut points are used to define outliers if they fall outside either 2 or 3 SDs from the mean, and these cut offs have been labelled 'alert' (2 SD) and 'alarm' (3 SD). If we use the example of 3 SDs, and we assume that all operators are performing to a satisfactory level (i.e. there are no actual poor performers in the cohort being assessed) then 99.8% should be within the limits, and we find 0.2% outside the limits purely by random chance. This means, 0.1% will be above expected and 0.1% below and inadvertently identified as an outlier, a 'false alarm'.

If we consider 100 hospitals, this means that each year the chance of incorrectly identifying as outlier is 0.1% of 100 = 0.1, so that this will occur every 10 years (reciprocal of 0.1). However, as the number of comparators rise so does the chance of a false alarm. If we assess 600 PCI operators, a false alarm would occur every 2 years.

But the full interpretation is more complex. The statistical certainty that an outlier is correctly identified is not 99.9%, rather it is dependent on the total number of operators being assessed and the total that appear to be outliers. The concept of a 'false discovery rate' was first proposed in the mid-1990s[21] and has since been used to deal with the statistical problems that arise from multiple comparisons.[22] The calculation for the 'false discovery rate' is given in the equation

$$p = 1 - \left(\frac{E}{K} \right)$$

where p is the probability that someone identified as an outlier is actually an outlier, E is the expected number of false alarms (at the 3 SD level that is number of individuals being assessed × 0.001) and K is the number of outliers actually observed.

So if there were 1000 cardiologists being assessed, we would expect one false alarm (1 × 0.001). If five were found to be outliers, then the chances they are correctly identified as truly performing below an expected level is 80%. Thus there is a 20% chance the observation is incorrect and that satisfactory practice is being incorrectly labelled as sub-standard.

The examples above underscore the point that we need to look at more than a single metric in trying to correctly identify poor performance. In addition it is self evident that although the outcomes discussed above are dichotomised (i.e. a binary decision is made – they fall 'within' or 'outside' a cut off), there is in fact a graded relationship. Of two outliers, the one further from the cut point is more likely to be a genuine outlier than the one who is closer. Other factors need to be taken into account to give face validity to the assessment such as the actual and predicted rates of adverse outcomes. A sensitivity analysis can be performed to see how the assessment changes with a single extra case with good or poor outcome and longitudinal measures to see if outlying performance is isolated or repeated over several time periods. These methods, therefore, can only be used as a guide to finding potentially poor practice. In the end, it is important to try to make a balanced judgment that seeks to protect the rights of both the operators and patients. An alert or alarm, however defined should trigger appropriate individual and organisational scrutiny to try to identify potential issues and try to improve the quality of care provided.

47.8 Data presentation

There are a variety of ways in which the results of the national audit of PCI can be presented. The data can be made available for benchmarking and be used to support local audit cycles if areas of concern are identified. Regular feedback to centres with reports of activity and outcomes promote better engagement with the process and this in itself encourages more complete and timely data collection by centres.

Data can be presented at fixed time points, as in the display of 'Door-to-Balloon' times for primary PCI (Figure 47.1), but the application of statistical process control charts first developed in industry[23] is valuable in tracking progressive changes in performance and activity. These tools can serve to provide an early warning of unexpected changes in and help to increase the timeliness with which potential problems can be identified and corrected. In the United Kingdom, cumulative funnel plots developed by Kunadian[24] have been used to help centres keep track of contemporaneous outcomes and are e-mailed to key contacts in all centres every quarter. An example is provided in Figure 47.2. The occurrence of major adverse cardiac or cerebrovascular events (MACCE) after PCI is recorded for every procedure. This is then plotted as a cumulative mean, represented by the pale blue line. Using a risk model, the predicted MACCE for each case is calculated and this is then plotted also as a cumulative mean (dark blue line). In this case, the North West Quality Improvement Programme (NWQIP) model was used,[25] but any model could be applied. The 95% and 99.8% confidence intervals (approximating to the 2 and 3 SD limits) are shown in green and red. Providing the 'observed MACCE' line remains within the two sigma lines, the observed outcomes are not statistically different from those that would be predicted by the risk model used. If the observed line rises above the predicted, and then crosses one of the boundaries, this would be a signal of performance that is statistically less good than the model would predict and should trigger further exploration of the practice of PCI at that site.

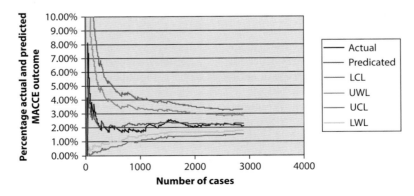

Figure 47.2 Cumulative funnel plot. Cumulative mean of actual outcomes (dark blue) and predicted outcomes (light blue) with confidence limits (3 standard deviations control limits, and 2 standard deviations warning limits). LCL, lower confidence limit; LWL, lower warning limit; MACCE, major adverse cardiovascular and cerebrovascular event; UCL, upper control limit; UWL, upper warning limit.

47.9 Conclusions

The practicalities of healthcare delivery are challenging and can impede optimal patient care. Clinical audit is therefore fundamental to our attempts to optimise patients care so that they can benefit from enormous advances in the treatment of cardiological conditions. It is not enough to know a therapy that will save lives; we need to check that the treatment is actually being provided for patients to benefit.

There are many hurdles to performing a good clinical audit. Having defined an area of interest, it starts with accurate and complete data collection which in itself can be problematic and requires resource. The process of comparing observed practice with benchmarks, clinical guidelines and risk-adjusted outcomes can also be complex. The identification of unsatisfactory performance must lead to reflection and an investigation into the causes. In turn, this should lead to changes in practice and re-evaluation to confirm improvement and monitor ongoing standards of care.

Clinical audit must occur in an open and transparent way, and we must guard against the possibility of risk-averse behaviour. Patients expect that the medical profession places their optimal care at the very centre of all its endeavours, and we should be able to reassure them that the quality of their care is being monitored in a fair, open, honest, robust and responsive way.

References

1. Scrivener R et al.. *Principles for Best Practice in Clinical Audit. National Institute for Clinical Excellence.* Oxford: Radcliffe Medical Press, 2002, p. 206.

2. Blows LHJ et al. Prospective peer review of regional percutaneous interventional procedures : A tool for quality control and revalidation. *EuroIntervention* 2012; 8(8): 939–44.

3. Berwick D. A Promise to Learn – A Commitment to Act Improving the Safety of Patients in England. 2013. Available at https://www.gov.uk/government/publications/berwick-review-into-patient-safety. London: Department of Health.

4. Hordijk-Trion M et al. Patients enrolled in coronary intervention trials are not representative of patients in clinical practice: Results from the Euro Heart Survey on Coronary Revascularization. *Eur Heart J* 2006; 27(6): 671–8.

5. Tricoci P et al. Scientific evidence underlying the ACC/AHA. *J Am Med Assoc* 2009; 301(8): 831–41.

6. Wald DS et al. Randomized trial of preventive angioplasty in myocardial infarction. *N Engl J Med* 2013; 369(12): 1115–23. Available from http://www.ncbi.nlm.nih.gov/pubmed/23991625

7. Smits PC et al. Abluminal biodegradable polymer biolimus-eluting stent versus durable polymer everolimus-eluting stent (COMPARE II): A randomised, controlled, non-inferiority trial. *Lancet* 2013; 381(9867): 651–60. Available from http://linkinghub.elsevier.com/retrieve/pii/S0140673612618522

8. Aggarwal B et al. Cause of death within 30 days of percutaneous coronary intervention in an era of mandatory outcome reporting. *J Am Coll Cardiol* 2013; 62(5): 409–15. Available from http://www.ncbi.nlm.nih.gov/pubmed/23665371

9. Hannan EL et al. The New York state risk score for predicting in-hospital/30-day mortality following percutaneous coronary intervention. *JACC Cardiovasc Interv* 2013; 6(6): 614–22.

10. Petersen ED et al. Contemporary mortality risk prediction for percutaneous coronary intervention: Results from 588, 398 procedures in the national cardiovascular data registry. *Rev Port Cardiol* 2010; 29(11): 1767–70.

11. Chowdhary S et al. The Toronto score for in-hospital mortality after percutaneous coronary interventions. *Am Heart J* 2009; 157(1): 156–63.

12. Steyerberg EW and Vergouwe Y. Towards better clinical prediction models: Seven steps for development and an ABCD for validation. *Eur Heart J* 2014; 35: 1925–31. Available from http://www.ncbi.nlm.nih.gov/pubmed/24898551

13. Baumeister RF et al. Bad is stronger than good. *Rev Gen Psychol* 2001; 5(4): 323–70. doi: 10.1037/1089-2680.5.4.323

14. Resnic FS and Welt FGP. The public health hazards of risk avoidance associated with public reporting of risk-adjusted outcomes in coronary intervention. *J Am Coll Cardiol* 2009; 53(10): 825–30. Available from http://content.onlinejacc.org/cgi/content/abstract/53/10/825

15. Moscucci M et al. Public reporting and case selection for percutaneous coronary interventions an analysis from two large multicenter. *J Am Coll Cardiol* 2005; 45(11): 1759–65.

16. Joynt KE et al. Association of public reporting for percutaneous coronary intervention with utilization with acute myocardial infarction. *JAMA* 2012; 308(14): 1460–8.

17. Apolito RA et al. Impact of the New York State Cardiac Surgery and Percutaneous Coronary Intervention Reporting System on the management of patients with acute myocardial infarction complicated by cardiogenic shock. *Am Heart J* 2008; 155(2): 267–73. Available from http://www.ncbi.nlm. nih.gov/pubmed/18215596

18. Waldo SW et al. Association between public reporting of outcomes with procedural management and mortality for patients with acute myocardial infarction. *J Am Coll Cardiol* 2015; 65(11): 1119–26.

19. McCabe JM et al. Impact of public reporting and outlier status identification on percutaneous coronary intervention case selection in Massachusetts. *JACC Cardiovasc Interv* 2013; 6(6): 625–30. Available from http://www.ncbi.nlm.nih.gov/pubmed/23787236

20. Peberdy MA et al. Impact of percutaneous coronary intervention performance reporting on cardiac resuscitation centers: A scientific statement from the American Heart Association. *Circulation* 2013; 128(7): 762–73. Available from http://www.ncbi.nlm.nih.gov/pubmed/23857321

21. Benjamini Y and Hochberg Y. Controlling the false discovery rate: A practical and powerful approach to multiple testing. *J R Stat Soc Ser B* 1995; 57(1): 289–300. Available from http://www.jstor.org/stable/2346101

22. Jones HE et al. Use of the false discovery rate when comparing multiple health care providers. *J Clin Epidemiol* 2008; 61(3): 232–40.

23. Shewhart WA. The application of statistics as an aid in maintaining quality of a manufactured product. *J Am Stat Assoc* 1925; 20(152): 546–8.

24. Kunadian B et al. Cumulative funnel plots for the early detection of interoperator variation. *BMJ* 2008; 336(7650): 931–4.

25. Grayson AD et al. Multivariate prediction of major adverse cardiac events after 9914 percutaneous coronary interventions in the north west of England. *Heart* 2006; 92(5): 658–63.

48

What's on the horizon?

STEVEN L GOLDBERG

The editor of this textbook made the observation to me that the authors of this chapter in the previous edition, published 10 years ago, had no discussion of structural heart disease. This seems remarkable given the dominance of structural heart disease in interventional cardiology today. Therefore, the prediction most likely to come true is that something revolutionary will occur that I do not mention in this chapter. This is actually something very exciting – the field of interventional cardiology moves so rapidly that disruptive technologies become established extraordinarily quickly – something we have seen since the dawn of interventional cardiology with balloon angioplasty. Since then we have experienced stent mania – now the standard of care. We have witnessed the ridiculing (or ignoring) of early structural interventional cardiologists (and surgeons) that the placement of prosthetic valves was an unnecessary and even silly proposition, only to now be rivalling traditional surgical valve replacement. It is humbling when trying to predict the future when the pace of change is so rapid. However, there are some areas that are almost certainly going to take hold, because the seeds are implanted even today. This chapter touches upon a few of those areas, and something fascinating to consider is the convergence of multiple areas of innovation which may well provide even greater value to patients.

48.1 Information technology

It is obvious to all of us that we are in the midst of a revolution with regards to information technology, and it seems to be an easy prediction that this is going to lead to many important developments in identifying patient characteristics of disease processes. The use of cell phones (as well as smartwatches, wrist bands, etc.) is ubiquitous, and they are almost certainly going to be taken advantage of to provide health information beyond simply how many steps a person takes in a day.[1] To be sure that in of itself may represent an important advancement in cardiovascular health, given the crucial role of exercise and activity in reducing the risk of heart disease, and an important therapy in patients with a variety of cardiovascular disorders. More sophisticated sensory modalities may be imbedded in the skin to provide information that may communicate to an individual that there are subclinical changes occurring which may preface clinical events.[2] To some extent, this type of approach is already available (although to a less sophisticated degree) in the form of the CardioMEMS device (Figure 48.1).[3,4] This device is placed by a cardiologist into the pulmonary artery and can provide daily feedback on pulmonary artery pressures in patients with congestive heart failure. When pressures are seen to rise (which occurs before a patient develops increase in symptoms or even an increase in weight), increase in diuretics may be prescribed. This approach has been shown to reduce heart failure hospitalisations and improve patient well-being. It is likely that technologies in the future will be able to communicate directly to the patient via a smartphone and prescribe changes in medical therapy based upon a predefined algorithm, simplifying the demands on the healthcare system (something of a current limitation with today's CardioMEMS). Tattoo technology with built-in electrocardiograms, or troponin sensors, may perhaps identify when a patient is having ischaemia and alert them to seek medical attention before the symptoms of a myocardial infarction even develop. Imagine how useful that might be after stenting, perhaps allowing for targeted use of anti-platelet therapy. Even more lifesaving, perhaps future technology will be able to detect patients at risk for sudden cardiac death from arrhythmias before they present with their first episode of cardiac arrest.

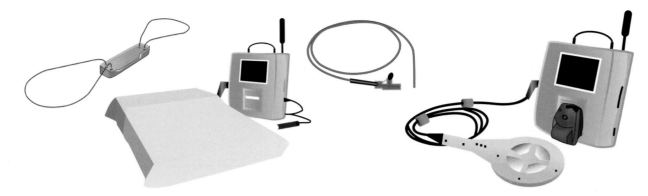

Figure 48.1 CarioMems device and equipment. Seen here is the CardioMEMS sensor, with nitinol loops to fix the device in a pulmonary artery branch. Next to it is a transmitting pillow with a recording device. The patient lies on the pillow every day for a few moments to transmit pulmonary artery pressures to the receiver. Next to this is the delivery catheter and finally is a transmitting wand, which can be placed on the patient's chest to record the pulmonary artery pressure (as an alternative to the pillow). From www.sjm.com.

48.2 Reducing recurrent disease events and quality control

As mentioned, the CardioMEMS device has evidence that the use of this diagnostic technology can reduce recurrent hospitalisations. Several regulatory bodies have begun addressing the need to standardise the quality of patient care, with recurrent hospitalisations as one key component. This has become an interest based upon controlling costs of medicine as well as in ensuring quality of patient care, and is likely to become ever increasingly present in the field of interventional cardiologist. This is already seen in the requirement to contribute patient data into registries in order to be paid for Medicare patients (such as the trans-catheter valve therapy [TVT] registry for valve procedures). This is also seen in the increasing role of appropriateness criteria and clinical guidelines being used for reimbursement as well as in establishing quality assessments of different hospital environments. We have seen that these tools have been combined with diagnostic tools more sophisticated than simple angiography alone to refine who should or should not receive a percutaneous coronary intervention (PCI). Thus, fractional flow reserve has become a standard practice in the United States, along with intra-vascular ultrasound, to provide greater sophistication and justification in proceeding with an interventional procedure, versus turning to greater rigor in medical management.[5,6] There are two components in this paradigm, both of which are likely to progress in the next several years. First is the role of external controls, guidelines, quality-based reimbursement models and reporting requirements. Greater refinements, modifications and requirements are going to lead to increasing demands on interventional cardiologists in documentation and ensuring that specific criteria are being met.

48.3 Improved diagnostic capabilities

The second component to the paradigm hopefully will be increasingly sophisticated diagnostic technologies allowing interventional cardiologists to refine the role of invasive

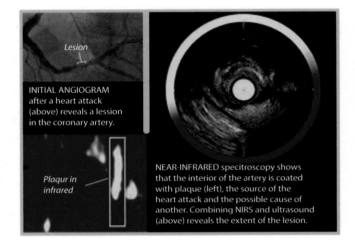

Figure 48.2 Coronary angiogram, intra-vascular ultrasound and near-infrared spectroscopy imaging demonstrating characteristics of plaque composition. From www.infraredx.com.

coronary artery management. It is likely that a greater role of non-invasive technologies will become established, cardiac computed tomography (CT) imaging and physiological testing on the precipice of redefining who needs an invasive cardiac catheterisation.[7] More importantly, the holy grail of identification of the high-risk or vulnerable plaque has been sought after for the past 25 years, and continues to be of great interest today.[8] Although several innovative approaches have not yet proven to be clinically meaningful, a modality able to identify a plaque at a high risk of rupture would certainly be a disruptive technology (pun intended). At the present time, near-infrared spectroscopy, in combination with intra-vascular ultrasound, has been shown to increase the identification of potentially high-risk lesions (Figure 48.2).[9] Perhaps, within the next 10 years, we will have a study showing that prophylactic revascularisation of high-risk lesions may reduce the risk of the development of unstable ischaemic syndromes, including myocardial infarction and cardiac death.

48.4 Bioabsorbable scaffolds

Bio-absorbable stents or scaffolds are present today but the clinical utility remains to be proven.[10,11] There certainly is an attractiveness to leaving no scaffold behind, potentially allowing resumption of normal endovascular function and allowing for later surgical graft implantation, as well as protection of side branches, but the clinical significance of these possibilities remains unclear at the present time. In the next 10 years, we may see trials demonstrating a clear clinical benefit over metal stents, which has the potential to change how we approach PCI.

48.5 The impact of the chronic total occlusion revolution

It is possible we are in the initial stages of a revolution in coronary revascularisation given the dramatic recent advances in opening chronic total occlusions (CTOs), relying to a large degree on in situ bypasses.[12] These dissection re-entry techniques use the adventitial space to effectively bypass the hard obstructive segments and re-enter the vasculature beyond the obstructions, either from an anterograde or a retrograde approach (Figure 48.3). This has not only revolutionised the approach to CTOs, but also has allowed progress in more traditional approaches going directly through the occluded segment, encouraging the development of newer technologies, and giving greater

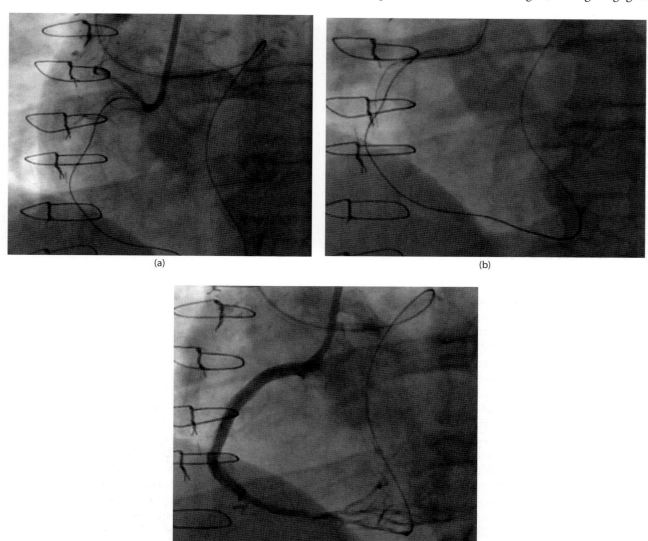

(a)

(b)

(c)

Figure 48.3 Opening a CTO with retrograde re-entry. (a) Coronary angiography of a CTO of an ostial right coronary artery (RCA). On the left is the injection of the RCA, with a retrograde wire from the left coronary artery. Note the loop in the artery at the ostium of the RCA – this loop is inside a dissection plane. (b) In the middle panel, a balloon is inflated in the dissection plane – from the anterograde direction. A wire is then passed from the retrograde direction into the dissection plane created by the balloon, into the guiding catheter and snared. (c) On the right is the final result after stenting.

confidence to the experienced CTO operator that if one approach does not work than other options are available. Currently, these more advanced techniques are primarily limited to a small group of enthusiasts, who have worked to hone their techniques in addressing complex CTOs.[13] However, if these techniques become more widespread and accepted, it is possible that the approach to revascularisation of coronary artery disease may be significantly altered. Amongst the most common reasons, a patient is referred for a coronary artery bypass graft surgery is the presence of a CTO. Although surgery may be a suitable alternative, the durability of vein grafts remains a problem. If CTO revascularisation becomes more standardised across the discipline, a complete re-evaluation of the relative role of bypass surgery versus percutaneous approaches may be worth re-evaluating with randomised trials. The value of an internal mammary artery for a conduit may well remain established, but the role of stenting versus vein graft revascularisation may be better studied with the confounding role of CTOs a lesser issue. A better understanding of what occurs with failure and/or complications in attempting to open a CTO will need to be evaluated closely, especially as these techniques become more widespread. To be truly disruptive, the opening of CTOs will need to become part of the arsenal of the standard interventional cardiologist or at least available within the interventional cardiology group.[13]

48.6 Invasive stem cell therapy

Even with the ability to create an in situ bypass around an occluded vessel, there are many patients with vessels that are too small, or too diffusely diseased to revascularise, whether by surgery or percutaneous techniques. Although many mechanical approaches have been attempted to provide greater vascularity to such patients, the results have been mixed. Some disappointing approaches have included percutaneous direct myocardial revascularisation as well as direct injections of multiple compounds, such as protein and gene angiogenic agents. However, several small studies have been done in a variety of clinical scenarios, using injectable compounds. These have included patients with angina and no revascularization options, as wells as patients post large myocardial infarctions. Both ischemic and non-ischemic cardiomyopathy patients have been studied. There have been some successful preliminary studies with a variety of different types of selective stem cells, such as autologous stimulated CD34 bone marrow-derived stem cells, and larger studies have been initiated.[14–18] These are administered using direct myocardial injections, taking advantage of intra-myocardial mapping techniques, reminiscent of the tools used by electrophysiologists. Thus, this type of therapy would require the development of a new skill set for interventional cardiologist, and has the possibility to impact 6%–29% of patients who are unable to have optimal revascularisation, due to anatomical considerations, even allowing for newer CTO techniques.

48.7 Structural heart disease

As mentioned at the onset of this chapter, the explosion and rapid acceptance of percutaneous management of structural heart disease has been the most dramatic development in interventional cardiology in the last decade, and it is clear that rapid advancements are likely to continue. Other chapters in this textbook are addressing the future of trans-catheter aortic valve replacement (TAVR), and there is a chapter devoted to the currently less well-established role of percutaneous mitral valve repair and replacement. It is anticipated that the role of percutaneous treatment of mitral regurgitation will dwarf that of TAVR, given the larger patient population.[19] This is driven by the relatively unrecognised prevalence of functional mitral regurgitation, which is seen in around half or more of patients with congestive heart failure.[20,21] Although there is currently no Food and Drug Administration (FDA)-approved device available in the United States to treat functional mitral regurgitation, there are ongoing studies of various devices. If any of these devices show convincing clinical data that such treatment can improve the quality of life of a patient with congestive heart failure and functional magnetic resonance (MR), such procedures could become quite common for interventional cardiologists. Combinations of such therapies may also be useful, adding to the role of the interventional cardiologist in the management of the heart failure patient. Percutaneous placement of mitral valves is well on its way to demonstrating clinical efficacy, however, there are likely to be many challenges to overcome, and it is possible even when successful there may be a risk of complications such that there may be a role for attempting a repair procedure first. It remains to be seen if they will be used strategically, after a repair technology has first been attempted, provided that repair does not preclude a valve replacement.

The next valve likely to benefit from trans-catheter therapy is the 'forgotten valve' – the tricuspid valve. Treatments for tricuspid regurgitation, using percutaneous techniques, are just now being explored.[22–24] Valve implantation into failed bio-prosthetic valves has been performed to a limited degree and long-term outcomes are not yet available in large series, but as more experience is gained the pitfalls and limitations will be identified. It is likely that this will become the preferred treatment for a failed surgically placed valve. It is less clear what the role might be in surgically repaired valves, but there is some experience of success in this condition as well. Of more interest is the possibility of treating native valve tricuspid regurgitation with percutaneous techniques. Although limited to only a few patients worldwide, there have been some successful percutaneous treatments of patients with native tricuspid valve regurgitation. One approach has used a trans-catheter valve in the inferior vena cava. Another approach has imitated the surgical Kay technique to bicuspidise the valve, using a variation of the Mitralign technology (Figure 48.4).[25] Another approach, the TriCinch system has been to place a corkscrew in the anteroposterior commissure of the tricuspid valve, which

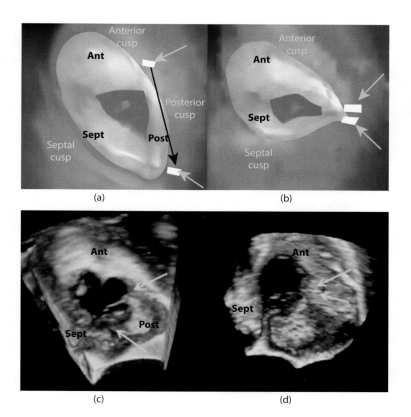

(a) (b)

(c) (d)

Figure 48.4 A dedicated plication lock device was used to bring two percutaneously placed pledgeted sutures, plicating the annulus and effectively bicuspidising the tricuspid valve. (a) Illustration of the sutures placed in the posterior-anterior commissure and the septo-posterior commissure (yellow arrows). (b) Illustration of the two sutures after plication. Patient's three-dimensional trans-oesophageal echocardiographic images are shown (c) before plication and (d) after plication. Ant = anterior leaflet, Post = posterior leaflet, Sept = septal leaflet. (Reproduced from *J Am Coll Cardiol*, 65, Schofer J et al., First-in-human transcatheter tricuspid valve repair in a patient with severely regurgitant tricuspid valve, 1190–95, Copyright (2015), with permission from Elsevier.)

is then connected to a self-expanding stent in the inferior vena cava. The tension created effectively bicuspidises the tricuspid valve. Each of these approaches has successfully reduced, or even resolved, tricuspid regurgitation acutely, although only in a very small number of patients. However, because severe tricuspid regurgitation carries such a poor prognosis, and confounds other cardiac pathology, the ability to reduce pathologic tricuspid regurgitation may be of great utility.

Several lessons have been learned from the TAVR experience. One of these has been the value of advanced imaging and it is likely that further advancements in imaging will enhance structural interventions. For example, three-dimensional printing of echo or CT or MR scans allow for guidance of individualised valve or structural elements to be prepared and tested ex vivo, prior to the performance of a procedure, to tailor the device specifications to that person's precise anatomy.[26–29] Initial work on this has been done in congenital heart disease (Figure 48.5) as well as in vascular endograft repair.[26,30,31] In vascular endograft repair, precise identification of important side branches can allow for a customised stent graft, which allows for access to those side branches, allowing a glove-like fit for the endograft repair. Other diagnostic imaging enhancements will likely include

further development of co-registration techniques, allowing for superimposition of one modality of imaging (such as CT imaging) on fluoroscopic imaging, or of combining fluoroscopic and intra-vascular imaging, to allow a greater appreciation as to where the precise location of intra-vascular ultrasound images are in the coronary angiogram. These technologies are already available and in use in selected centres, but are likely to be developed further to allow them to be more user-friendly and mainstream.

Another peripheral lesson from the TAVR experience is the power of combining disciplines as the interventional cardiologists and cardiac surgeons forged relationships which became ever more symbiotic. Not only these two disciplines, but also greater partnership with imaging specialists has grown out of this experience as well. These types of partnerships create possibilities with education across disciplines which can be very useful. For example, electrophysiologists may adopt techniques of interventional cardiologists in the placement of coronary sinus leads (Figure 48.6), which can be facilitated by having the interventional cardiologists and electrophysiologists working together.[32] Combining forces even outside of cardiology may have meaningful benefits to patients. Involving specifically trained interventional cardiologists in acute stroke teams may allow for greater

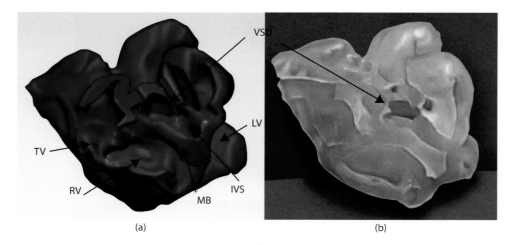

(a)   (b)

Figure 48.5 3D imaging of a patient with a ventricular septal defect. Comparison of the digital (left) and printed (right) 3D models. The 3D echocardiographic data are segmented to create a digital 3D model of the heart (a). The digital model is then printed to create a realistic, tangible 3D model of the heart (b), which has been derived from the original 3D echocardiographic images. 3D, three dimensional; IVS, intra-ventricular septum; LV, left ventricle; MB, moderator band; RV, right ventricle; TV, tricuspid valve; VSD, ventricular septal defect. (Reprinted from Olivieri et al., *J Am Soc Echocardiogr*, 28, 392–7, 2015. With permission.)

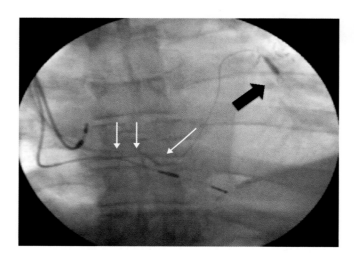

Figure 48.6 Fluoroscopic image of a challenging coronary sinus access for placement of a CRT lead. A multipurpose catheter is seen (white arrows) not readily entering into the proximal coronary sinus, due to tortuosity. A coronary guide wire has been placed from the coronary sinus/great cardiac vein into the anterior interventricular vein (AIV). A balloon is inflated in the AIV to provide support for the catheter in negotiating the proximal tortuosity. This demonstrates the possibility of a partnership between electrophysiologists and interventional cardiologists. (From Seth Worley, Lancaster (Pennsylvania) Hospital.)

availability of acute stroke interventions than what might be possible given current work force in neurointerventional radiology.[33] Interventional pulmonology has adapted several techniques from interventional cardiology, such as stenting, and opening occluded structures.[34] Joining forces with those involved in that fledgling discipline may allow them to benefit from the experience interventional cardiologists have in problem-solving, both in achieving a desired result, as well as in recovering from complications occurring during the attempts.

Many of the operators performing peripheral interventions are experienced interventional cardiologists, so many already have expertise in trans-radial approaches. As longer equipment becomes available, a trans-radial approach to renovascular and lower extremity work is likely to become increasingly common, not only due to the lower vascular complication risk but also to take advantage of the more physiologically stable approach by reducing curvature into the system.[35] Trans-radial approach to coronary intervention appears to be on the rise and this is likely to continue as fellows coming out of training are adopting this approach more rapidly than more experienced operators. The use of trans-radial access for structural heart disease is likely to become ever more common as well.[36] Although it may seem preposterous to propose that a TAVR could be performed trans-radially, perhaps that is not as farfetched as it sounds. Consider that in just a few years, sheath sizes for TAVR have decreased from 26 to 14 Fr. It is certainly possible to place an 8- or even a 9-Fr sheath into many radial arteries, so to go from 14 to 8 Fr is not so unreasonable (since going from 26 to 14 Fr has happened so quickly). Balloon aortic valvuloplasty has been successfully done via the radial artery using 8- and 9-Fr sheaths, so technically the performance of a TAVR should not be much different. The two challenging considerations are miniaturisation and vascular protection, which are preserving vascular patency when stretched. Whether technologies will be developed to allow this, or greater reliance on vascular imaging for vascular access becomes commonplace, it is likely that increased interest in relying upon the safer route of radial access for a large number of interventional cardiology procedures is likely to be seen.

Finally, a therapy which has been around for years may or may not turn out to be a procedure commonly done by interventional cardiologists in the near future – the closure of patent foramen ovales (PFOs). In 2016, the Amplatzer PFO occlude device is anticipated to be presented to the FDA for approval. Given the prevalence of PFOs (occurring in ~25% of hearts), and the ease of the procedure, the availability of an FDA-approved device would potentially allow this to become one of the most common procedures for interventional cardiologists to be asked to perform. There are a variety of conditions wherein a PFO closure may be a reasonable consideration, including stroke (and other paradoxical embolisation) prevention, migraines, obstructive sleep apnoea, decompression illness, platypnoea-orthodeoxia and so on.[37–42] Studies in cryptogenic stroke and migraine patients have strongly suggested benefit, even if the statistics are confounded by relatively small numbers studied, as well as the use of challenging endpoints, which may have diminished the true benefit of the therapy. Should it be the case that one or more PFO occluder devices become available, the interventional cardiology community should be mindful of the harm to indiscriminate application of this procedure/technology. It would be very important to ensure that interventional cardiologists are good stewards and be wary of overuse of PFO closure, given the widespread prevalence of these anatomical variations. We have seen a backlash with somewhat indiscriminate use of PCI in the past and would be well served to learn from those mistakes.

References

1. Topol E. TED Talks. 2010. Podcast. Available from https://www.ted.com/talks/eric_topol_the_wireless_future_of_medicine
2. Fittzgerald P. *New Technology & Innovation in Medicine from Dotter to Discovery.* Stanford, CA: Stanford University School of Medicine. Presented by IGI50. VuMedi, 2015.
3. Abraham WT et al. Wireless pulmonary artery haemodynamic monitoring in chronic heart failure: A randomised controlled trial. *Lancet* 2011; 377(9766): 658–66.
4. Adamson PB et al. Wireless pulmonary artery pressure monitoring guides management to reduce decompensation in heart failure with preserved ejection fraction. *Circ Heart Fail* 2014; 7(6): 935–44.
5. Levine GN et al. 2011 ACCF/AHA/SCAI Guideline for Percutaneous Coronary Intervention. A report of the American College of Cardiology Foundation/American Heart Association Task Force on Practice Guidelines and the Society for Cardiovascular Angiography and Interventions. *J Am Coll Cardiol* 2011; 58(24): e44–122.
6. Task Force on Myocardial Revascularization of the European Society of Cardiology et al. Guidelines on myocardial revascularization. *Eur Heart J* 2010; 31(20): 2501–55.
7. Min JK et al. Noninvasive fractional flow reserve derived from coronary CT angiography: Clinical data and scientific principles. *JACC Cardiovasc Imaging* 2015; 8(10): 1209–22.
8. Libby P, and Pasterkamp G. Requiem for the 'vulnerable plaque'. *Eur Heart J* 2015; 36(43): 2984–7.
9. Puri R et al. Near-infrared spectroscopy enhances intravascular ultrasound assessment of vulnerable coronary plaque: A combined pathological and in vivo study. *Arterioscler Thromb Vasc Biol* 2015; 35(11): 2423–31.
10. CADTH Rapid Response Reports. *Bioabsorbable Stents for Adults with Coronary Artery Disease: A Review of the Clinical Effectiveness, Cost-Effectiveness, and Guidelines.* Ottawa, ON: Canadian Agency for Drugs and Technologies in Health, 2013.
11. Patel N, and Banning AP. Bioabsorbable scaffolds for the treatment of obstructive coronary artery disease: The next revolution in coronary intervention? *Heart* 2013; 99(17): 1236–43.
12. Brilakis ES et al. A percutaneous treatment algorithm for crossing coronary chronic total occlusions. *JACC Cardiovasc Interv* 2012; 5(4): 367–79.
13. Carlino M et al. Treatment of the chronic total occlusion: A call to action for the interventional community. *Catheter Cardiovasc Interv* 2015; 85(5): 771–8.
14. Fisher SA et al. Bone marrow stem cell treatment for ischemic heart disease in patients with no option of revascularization: A systematic review and meta-analysis. *PLoS One* 2013; 8(6): e64669.
15. Kandala J et al. Meta-analysis of stem cell therapy in chronic ischemic cardiomyopathy. *Am J Cardiol* 2013; 112(2): 217–25.
16. Losordo DW et al. Intramyocardial, autologous CD34+ cell therapy for refractory angina. *Circ Res* 2011; 109(4): 428–36.
17. Losordo DW et al. Intramyocardial transplantation of autologous CD34+ stem cells for intractable angina: A phase I/IIa double-blind, randomized controlled trial. *Circulation* 2007; 115(25): 3165–72.
18. Povsic TJ et al. A phase 3, randomized, double-blinded, active-controlled, unblinded standard of care study assessing the efficacy and safety of intramyocardial autologous CD34+ cell administration in patients with refractory angina: Design of the RENEW study. *Am Heart J* 2013; 165(6): 854–61.e2.
19. Asgar AW et al. Secondary mitral regurgitation in heart failure: Pathophysiology, prognosis, and therapeutic considerations. *J Am Coll Cardiol* 2015; 65(12): 1231–48.
20. Koelling TM et al. Prognostic significance of mitral regurgitation and tricuspid regurgitation in patients with left ventricular systolic dysfunction. *Am Heart J* 2002; 144(3): 524–9.
21. Trichon BH et al. Relation of frequency and severity of mitral regurgitation to survival among patients with left ventricular systolic dysfunction and heart failure. *Am J Cardiol* 2003; 91(5): 538–43.
22. Bouleti C et al. Tricuspid valve and percutaneous approach: No longer the forgotten valve! *Arch Cardiovasc Dis* 2016; 109(1): 55–66.
23. Lancellotti P et al. Targeting the tricuspid valve: A new therapeutic challenge. *Arch Cardiovasc Dis* 2016; 109(1): 1–3.
24. Rogers JH. Functional tricuspid regurgitation: Percutaneous therapies needed. *JACC Cardiovasc Interv* 2015; 8(3): 492–4.
25. Schofer J et al. First-in-human transcatheter tricuspid valve repair in a patient with severely regurgitant tricuspid valve. *J Am Coll Cardiol* 2015; 65: 1190–5.

26. Leotta DF, and Starnes BW. Custom fenestration templates for endovascular repair of juxtarenal aortic aneurysms. *J Vasc Surg* 2015; 61(6): 1637–41.

27. O'Neill B et al. Transcatheter caval valve implantation using multimodality imaging: roles of TEE, CT, and 3D printing. *JACC Cardiovasc Imaging* 2015; 8(2): 221–5.

28. Schmauss D et al. Three-dimensional printing in cardiac surgery and interventional cardiology: A single-centre experience. *Eur J Cardiothorac Surg* 2015; 47(6): 1044–52.

29. Samuel BP et al. Ultrasound-derived three-dimensional printing in congenital heart disease. *J Digit Imaging* 2015; 28(4): 459–61.

30. Olivieri et al. Three-dimensional printing of intracardiac defects from three-dimensional echocardiographic images: Feasibility and relative accuracy. *J Am Soc Echocardiogr* 2015; 28: 392–7.

31. Poterucha JT et al. Percutaneous pulmonary valve implantation in a native outflow tract: 3-dimensional DynaCT rotational angiographic reconstruction and 3-dimensional printed model. *JACC Cardiovasc Interv* 2014; 7(10): e151–2.

32. Worley SJ. How to use balloons as anchors to facilitate cannulation of the coronary sinus left ventricular lead placement and to regain lost coronary sinus or target vein access. *Heart Rhythm* 2009; 6(8): 1242–6.

33. Widimsky P, and Hopkins LN. Catheter-based interventions for acute ischaemic stroke. *Eur Heart J* 2016 Oct 21; 37(40): 3081–89.

34. Beaudoin EL et al. Interventional pulmonology: An update for internal medicine physicians. *Minerva Med* 2014; 105(3): 197–209.

35. Posham R et al. Transradial approach for noncoronary interventions: A single-center review of safety and feasibility in the first 1,500 cases. *J Vasc Interv Radiol* 2016; 27(2):159–66.

36. Allende R et al. The transradial approach during transcatheter structural heart disease interventions: A review. *Eur J Clin Invest* 2015; 45(2): 215–25.

37. Carroll JD et al. Closure of patent foramen ovale versus medical therapy after cryptogenic stroke. *N Engl J Med* 2013; 368(12): 1092–100.

38. Carroll J. Patent Foramen Ovale (PFO): Implicated as Major Cause of Cryptogenic Strokes Especially in People < 60 Years Old. Available from RESPECT Trial Extended Follow-up. TCT2015. TCTMD.com

39. Tobis JCA et al. Results of the PREMIUM trial: Patent Foramen Ovale Closure with the Amplatzer PFO Occluder for the Prevention of Migraine. Available from TCT2015. TCTMD.com.

40. Smart D et al. Joint position statement on persistent foramen ovale (PFO) and diving. South Pacific Underwater Medicine Society (SPUMS) and the United Kingdom Sports Diving Medical Committee (UKSDMC). *Diving Hyperb Med* 2015; 45(2): 129–31.

41. Mojadidi MK et al. The effect of patent foramen ovale closure in patients with platypnea-orthodeoxia syndrome. *Catheter Cardiovasc Interv* 2015; 86(4): 701–7.

42. Meier B. Closure of the patent foramen ovale, perhaps the best thing interventional cardiology has to offer. *Catheter Cardiovasc Interv* 2015; 86(6): 1085–6.

Index